Essential Orthopaedics

Essential Orthopaedics

Mark D. Miller, MD
S. Ward Casscells Professor of Orthopaedic Surgery
Head, Division of Sports Medicine, University of Virginia
Charlottesville, Virginia
Adjunctive Clinical Professor and Team Physician
James Madison University
Harrisonburg, Virginia

Jennifer A. Hart, MPAS, PA-C
Physician Assistant
University of Virginia
Charlottesville, Virginia

John M. MacKnight, MD
Associate Professor
Clinical Internal Medicine and Orthopaedic Surgery
Co-Medical Director for Sports Medicine
Primary Care Team Physician
University of Virginia
Charlottesville, Virginia

SAUNDERS

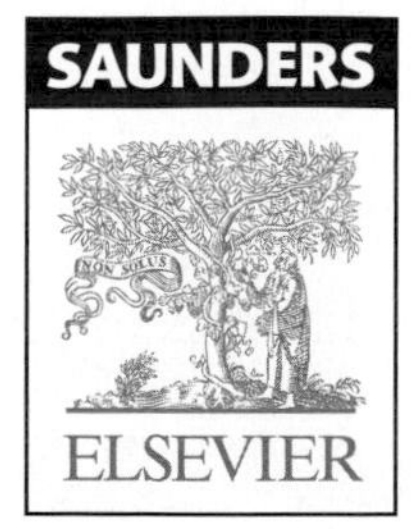

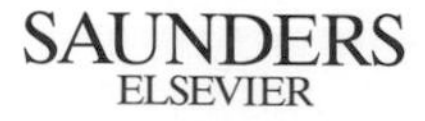

1600 John F. Kennedy Blvd.
Ste 1800
Philadelphia, PA 19103-2899

ESSENTIAL ORTHOPAEDICS ISBN: 978-1-4160-5473-3

Notice

Knowledge and best practice in this field are constantly changing. As new research and experience broaden our knowledge, changes in practice, treatment, and drug therapy may become necessary or appropriate. Readers are advised to check the most current information provided (i) on procedures featured or (ii) by the manufacturer of each product to be administered, to verify the recommended dose or formula, the method and duration of administration, and contraindications. It is the responsibility of the practitioner, relying on his or her own experience and knowledge of the patient, to make diagnoses, to determine dosages and the best treatment for each individual patient, and to take all appropriate safety precautions. To the fullest extent of the law, neither the Publisher nor the Editors assume any liability for any injury and/or damage to persons or property arising out of or related to any use of the material contained in this book.

Library of Congress Cataloging-in-Publication Data
Essential orthopaedics / [edited by] Mark Miller, Jennifer Hart,
John MacKnight.—1st ed.
p. ; cm.
Includes bibliographical references.
ISBN 978-1-4160-5473-3
1. Orthopedics. I. Miller, Mark D. II. Hart, Jennifer. III. MacKnight, John.
[DNLM: 1. Orthopedics. WE 168 E775 2009]
RD731.E77 2009
616.7—dc22

2008034181

Acquisitions Editor: Druanne Martin
Developmental Editor: Julia Bartz
Editorial Assistant: John Ingram
Marketing Manager: William Veltre
Design Direction: Gene Harris
Multi-Media Producer: Bruce Robison

Printed in China
Last digit is the print number: 9 8 7 6 5 4 3 2 1

To my children, who have allowed me to work on yet another book. To the residents and fellows that I teach. To my teachers, who have taught me the importance of life-long learning. And to the Great Physician, who has given me the aptitude and ability to help others.

MDM

To my past teachers, from whom I learned what it takes to be a PA; to my current mentors, Drs. Diduch and Miller, who have taught me what I know about orthopaedics; and to all of the students that I encounter with whom I hope to share this knowledge. Also, to my husband, Joe, and my children Jordyn, Julia, and the one on the way, who have supported all of my projects and taught me what I know about life and love.

JAH

To my wife, Melissa, for her undying love and support. To my children, Abby, Hannah, Eliza, and Josh, for their sacrifice and understanding. And to my parents for the inspiration to live a life of service.

JMM

List of Contributors

R. Todd Allen, MD, PhD
Assistant Clinical Professor, University of California San Diego Medical Center; San Diego Veterans Affairs Hospital, San Diego, CA

Annunziato (Ned) Amendola, MD
Professor, Department of Orthopaedic Surgery and Rehabilitation, University of Iowa College of Medicine; Director, University of Iowa Sports Medicine Center; University of Iowa Hospitals and Clinics, Iowa City, IA

Howard S. An, MD
The Morton International Professor and Director, Division of Spine Surgery, Department of Orthopaedic Surgery, Rush University Medical Center, Chicago, IL

D. Greg Anderson, MD
Associate Professor, Department of Orthopaedics, Rothman Institute, Thomas Jefferson University, Philadelphia, PA

Mark W. Anderson, MD
Associate Professor and Chief, Musculoskeletal Imaging, Department of Radiology, University of Virginia, Charlottesville, VA

Ivan J. Antosh, MD
Division of Orthopaedics, Madigan Army Medical Center, Tacoma, WA

Adam W. Anz, MD
Resident, Department of Orthopaedic Surgery, Wake Forest University Baptist Medical Center, Winston-Salem, NC

Joseph Armen, DO
Faculty, Primary Care Sports Medicine Fellowship, East Carolina University; Team Physician, East Carolina University Student Health Services, Greenville, NC

Geoffrey S. Baer, MD, PhD
Assistant Professor, Department of Orthopaedic Surgery, Division of Sports Medicine, University of Wisconsin, Madison, WI

James Beazell, DPT
Residency Director, University of Virginia, Charlottesville, VA

Claire F. Beimesch, MD
Resident, Orthopaedic Surgery, West Virginia University, Morgantown, WV

David J. Berkoff, MD
Assistant Professor, Department of Surgery, Division of Emergency and Sports Medicine, Duke University, Durham, NC

Meenakshi Bindal, MD
Director of Pain Management, Pain and Rehabilitation Medicine, Riverside Tappahannock Hospital, Tappahannock, VA

Jason Blackham, MD
Clinical Assistant Professor, Department of Internal Medicine; Team Physician, The University of Iowa, Iowa City, IA

Gary Blum, MD
Fellow, Hand and Microvascular Surgery, The Hand Center of San Antonio, San Antonio, TX

Eric M. Bluman, MD, PhD
Assistant Professor, Uniformed Services University of the Health Sciences, Bethesda, MD; Chief, Orthopaedic Foot and Ankle Surgery, Madigan Army Medical Center, Tacoma, WA

Blake Boggess, DO
Assistant Professor, Duke University Medical Center, Durham, NC

Mark Bouchard, MD
Associate Professor, University of Vermont School of Medicine, Burlington, VT; Associate Professor, University of Southern Maine, Gorham, ME; Assistant Director, Sports Medicine Fellowship; Medical Director, Family Medicine Residency Program, Maine Medical Center, Portland, ME

César J. Bravo, MD
Assistant Professor of Clinical Orthopaedics, University of Virginia, Charlottesville, VA; Co-Director, Divisions of Hand and Upper Extremity and Microvascular Surgery, Carilion Bone and Joint Center, Carilion Clinic, Roanoke, VA

Jason Brayley, MD
Fellow, Primary Care Sports Medicine, Cleveland Clinic Foundation, Cleveland, OH

Thomas E. Brickner, MD
University of North Carolina, Chapel Hill, NC

Per Gunnar Brolinson, DO
Virginia College of Osteopathic Medicine, Virginia Tech Sports Medicine, Blacksburg, VA

Brandon D. Bushnell, MD
Steadman Hawkins Sports Fellow, Steadman Hawkins Clinic, Vail, CO

R. Bryan Butler, MD
Chief Resident, University of Maryland School of Medicine, Baltimore, MD

Jeffrey R. Bytomski, DO
Assistant Professor and Physician, Duke Sports Medicine, Duke University Medical Center, Durham, NC

James E. Carpenter, MD
Chair, Department of Orthopaedic Surgery, University of Michigan, Ann Arbor, MI

Robert C. Chadderdon, MD
Resident, Department of Orthopaedic Surgery, Virginia Commonwealth University Health System, Richmond, VA

A. Bobby Chhabra, MD
Associate Professor and Vice Chair, Department of Orthopaedic Surgery; Division Head, Hand and Upper Extremity Surgery, University of Virginia, Charlottesville, VA

Luke S. Choi, MD
Resident, Department of Orthopaedic Surgery, University of Virginia, Charlottesville, VA

Alfred Cianflocco, MD
Staff Physician, Department of Orthopaedic Surgery, Cleveland Clinic Sports Health Center, Cleveland Clinic Foundation, Cleveland, OH

Mario Ciocca, MD
Clinical Assistant Professor, Department of Medicine; Team Physician, University of North Carolina, Chapel Hill, NC

John P. Colianni, MD
Sports Medicine Fellow, Maine Medical Center, Portland, ME

M. Truitt Cooper, MD
Fellow, Idaho Foot and Ankle Fellowship, Coughlin Clinic, Boise, ID

Colin G. Crosby, MD
Resident, Department of Orthopaedic Surgery, Vanderbilt University Medical Center, Nashville, TN

Rashard Dacus, MD
Assistant Professor, University of Virginia, Charlottesville, VA

Barry C. Davis, MD
Resident, Orthopaedic Surgery, West Virginia University, Morgantown, WV

Marc De Jong, MD
Director, Southern Illinois Sports Medicine, Belleville, IL

Christopher J. DeWald, MD
Assistant Professor, Department of Orthopedic Surgery, Rush University Medical Center, Chicago, IL

Kevin deWeber, MD, FAAFP
Assistant Professor of Family Medicine; Director, Military Primary Care Sports Medicine Fellowship, Uniformed Services University of the Health Sciences, Bethesda, MD; Director, Military Primary Care Sports Medicine Fellowship, Dewitt Army Community Hospital, Ft. Belvoir, VA

William Dexter, MD, FACSM
Professor, University of Vermont College of Medicine, Burlington, VT; Adjunct Professor, University of Southern Maine, Gorham, ME; Director, Sports Medicine Program; Assistant Director, Family Medicine Residency Program, Maine Medical Center, Portland, ME

Matthew J. Dietz, MD
Resident, Orthopaedic Surgery, West Virginia University, Morgantown, WV

Robert Dimeff, MD
Medical Director of Sports Medicine, Cleveland Clinic Foundation, Cleveland, OH

George S. Edwards III, MD
Resident, Department of Orthopaedics, University of North Carolina Hospitals, Chapel Hill, NC

Josef K. Eichinger, MD
Division of Orthopaedics, Madigan Army Medical Center, Tacoma, WA

Hany El-Rashidy, MD
Resident, Rush Medical College, Chicago, IL

Norman Espinosa, MD
Head of Foot and Ankle Surgery, Department of Orthopaedic Surgery, University of Zurich, Zurich, Switzerland

Michael Feldman, MD
Department of General Surgery, Division of Plastic Surgery, Virginia Commonwealth University Health System, Richmond, VA

Marifel Mitzi F. Fernandez, MD
Sports Medicine Fellow, University of Kentucky, Lexington, KY; Associate Physician, Marshfield Clinic Cornwell Center, Cornwell, WI; Staff Physician, Saint Joseph's Hospital, Chippewa Falls, WI

Brian J. Finnegan, MD
Clinical Instructor, Duke University, Durham, NC

Daniel T. Fletcher, Jr., MD
Orthomemphis, Memphis, TN

Brett A. Freedman, MD
Chief, Spine and Neurosurgery, Landstuhl Regional Medical Center, Landstuhl, Germany

Eric J. Gardner, MD
Resident, Department of Orthopaedic Surgery, University of Wisconsin, Madison, WI

Sanjitpal S. Gill, MD
Adjunct Assistant Professor, Department of Bioengineering, Clemson University, Clemson, SC; Steadman Hawkins Clinic, Vail, CO

George S. Gluck, MD
Resident, Department of Orthopaedics, University of North Carolina School of Medicine, Chapel Hill, NC

Laura D. Goldberg, MD, FAAP
Clinical Staff, Department of Orthopedics, The Cleveland Clinic Foundation, Cleveland, OH

S. Raymond Golish, MD, PhD
Administrative Chief Resident, University of Virginia Health System, Charlottesville, VA

Thomas A. Goodwin, DO
Sports Medicine Fellow, Edward Via Virginia College of Osteopathic Medicine, Blacksburg, VA; Family Medicine, ProMed Family and Sports Medicine, Portage, MI

Chancellor F. Gray, AB
Jefferson Medical College, Thomas Jefferson University, Philadelphia, PA

Paul Gubanich, MD, MPH
Director, Primary Care Sports Medicine Research; Director, Wellness Institute, Cleveland Clinic Sports Health Center; Team Physician, Cleveland Browns, Cleveland, OH

Theresa Guise, MD
Division of Endocrinology, University of Virginia, Charlottesville, VA

Steven L. Haddad, MD
Associate Professor of Clinical Orthopaedic Surgery, Northwestern University Feinberg School of Medicine, Chicago, IL; Section Head, Foot and Ankle Surgery, North Shore University Healthcare System, Evanston, IL

Robin J. Hamill-Ruth, MD
Associate Professor, Department of Anesthesiology and Critical Care Medicine; Director, Pain Management Center, University of Virginia Health System, Charlottesville, VA

Emily Harold, MD
Staff Physician, Sports Medicine, Granger Medical Clinic, Salt Lake City, UT

Jennifer A. Hart, MPAS, PA-C
Physician Assistant, University of Virginia, Charlottesville, VA

John Hatzenbuehler, MD
Central Maine Sports Medicine, Lewiston, ME

Daniel S. Heckman, MD
Resident, Department of Orthopaedic Surgery, University of North Carolina Hospitals, Chapel Hill, NC

Duane R. Hennion, MD
Director, Primary Care Sports Medicine, Keller Army Community Hospital, West Point, NY

Steven L. Henry, MD
Faculty, Institute of Reconstructive Plastic Surgery of Central Texas, Austin, TX

Ailleen Heras-Herzig, MD
Clinical Assistant Professor of Medicine, School of Medicine and Public Health, University of Wisconsin, Madison, WI

Aaron Hoblet, MD
Division of Orthopaedics, Madigan Army Medical Center, Tacoma, WA

Michael P. Horan, MD
Resident, Orthopaedic Surgery, University of Kentucky, Lexington, KY

Robert G. Hosey, MD
Associate Professor, Primary Care Sports Medicine, University of Kentucky, Lexington, KY

Clinton W. Howard, MD
Fellow, Texas Medical Center, Houston, TX

Thomas M. Howard, MD
Assistant Professor, Department of Family Medicine, Virginia Commonwealth University School of Medicine, Richmond, VA; Program Director, Sports Medicine Fellowship, Fairfax Family Practice, Fairfax, VA

Jack Ingari, MD
Staff Attending Hand Surgeon and Associate Professor of Surgery, The Hand Center of San Antonio, University of Texas Health Science Center, San Antonio, TX; Assistant Professor of Surgery, Uniformed Services University of the Health Sciences, Bethesda, MD

Jonathan E. Isaacs, MD
Associate Professor, Department of Orthopaedic Surgery, Virginia Commonwealth University Health System, Richmond, VA

Henry J. Iwinski, Jr., MD
Associate Professor, Department of Orthopaedic Surgery, University of Kentucky; Assistant Chief of Staff, Shriners Hospital for Children, Lexington, KY

Benjamin J. Jacobs, MD
Resident, Northwestern University Feinberg School of Medicine, Chicago, IL

Joseph A. Janicki, MD
Assistant Professor of Orthopaedic Surgery, Northwestern University Feinberg School of Medicine; Attending Pediatric Orthopaedic Surgeon, Children's Memorial Hospital, Chicago, IL

Jeffrey G. Jenkins, MD
Assistant Professor and Assistant Program Director, Department of Physical Medicine and Rehabilitation, University of Virginia School of Medicine, Charlottesville, VA

Sheryl Johnson, MD
Assistant Professor, Psychiatry and Neurobehavioral Science and Anesthesia, University of Virginia, Charlottesville, VA

Peter S. Johnston, MD, MS
Resident, University of North Carolina Hospitals, Chapel Hill, NC

Anish R. Kadakia, MD
Chief, Division of Foot and Ankle Surgery; Clinical Instructor, Department of Orthopaedic Surgery, University of Michigan, Ann Arbor, MI

Jerrod Keith, MD
General Surgery Resident, University of Colorado, Denver, CO

A. Jay Khanna, MD
Assistant Professor, Department of Orthopaedic Surgery, Johns Hopkins University; Co-Director, Division of Spine Surgery, Johns Hopkins Orthopaedic Surgery at Good Samaritan Hospital, Baltimore, MD

Joseph S. Kim, MD
Spine Surgeon, West End Orthopaedic Clinic, Saint Francis Medical Center, Richmond, VA

Jeremy Kinder, MD
Resident, Northwestern Memorial Hospital, Chicago, IL

Mininder S. Kocher, MD, MPH
Associate Professor of Orthopaedic Surgery, Harvard Medical School; Associate Director, Division of Sports Medicine, Children's Hospital Boston, Boston, MA

Kevin L. Krasinski, MD
Orthopaedic Surgeon, The Bone and Joint Center, Saint Elizabeth's Medical Center, Boston, MA

Justin Kunes, MD
Resident, Department of Orthopaedic Surgery, University of Kentucky, Lexington, KY

Michael Kwon, MD
Resident, Department of Orthopaedics, University of Virginia, Charlottesville, VA

Christian Lattermann, MD
Director, Center for Cartilage Repair and Restoration; Assistant Professor, Orthopaedics and Sports Medicine, University of Kentucky, Lexington, KY

Alan C. League, MD
Assistant Clinical Professor, Department of Orthopaedics, University of Illinois Medical Center, Chicago, IL; Private Practice, Illinois Bone and Joint Institute, Morton Grove, IL

Simon Lee, MD
Assistant Professor, Department of Orthopaedic Surgery, Rush University Medical Center, Chicago, IL

Edward J. Lewis, MD
Sports Medicine Fellow, Fairfax Family Practice, Fairfax, VA

Joy L. Long, MD
Orthopedic Surgeon, Lancaster Orthopedic Group, Lancaster, PA

Daniel Luppens, MD
Division of Plastic Surgery, Department of General Surgery, Virginia Commonwealth University Health System, Richmond, VA

James MacDonald, MD
Primary Care Sports Medicine Fellow, Children's Hospital of Boston, Boston, MA

John M. MacKnight, MD
Associate Professor, Clinical Internal Medicine and Orthopaedic Surgery; Co-Medical Director for Sports Medicine; Primary Care Team Physician, University of Virginia, Charlottesville, VA

Scott D. Mair, MD
Associate Professor, Sports Medicine, University of Kentucky, Lexington, KY

Gerardo Juan Maquieira, MD
Deputy Head of Foot and Ankle Surgery, Department of Orthopaedic Surgery, University of Zurich, Zurich, Switzerland

Rex Marco, MD
Associate Professor, University of Texas Health Science Center at Houston, Houston, TX

David M. Marcu, MD
Resident, Department of Orthopaedic Surgery, University of Wisconsin, Madison, WI

Medardo R. Maroto, MD
Resident, Department of Orthopaedic Surgery, Rush University Medical Center, Chicago, IL

Sameer Mathur, MD
Assistant Professor, Department of Orthopaedic Surgery, University of North Carolina, Chapel Hill, NC

Sarah McGinley, DO
Assistant Professor, Department of Sports and Family Medicine, Edward Via Virginia College of Osteopathic Medicine; Team Physician, Virginia Tech University, Blacksburg, VA

Jasmin L. McGinty, MD
Department of Orthopaedic Surgery, University of Virginia Hospital, Charlottesville, VA

Howard McGowan, MD
Sports Medicine Physician, Eglin Air Force Base Family Medicine Residence, Eglin Air Force Base, FL

Nancy M. McLaren, MD
Medical Director, Teen Health Center; Assistant Professor, Department of Pediatrics, University of Virginia, Charlottesville, VA

Robert Meehan, MD
Clinical Orthopaedic Instructor, Department of Foot and Ankle Surgery, Detroit Medical Center/ Providence Hospital Orthopaedic Surgery Program, Detroit, MI

Cay Mierisch, MD, MS
Assistant Professor of Clinical Orthopaedics, University of Virginia, Charlottesville, VA; Co-Director, Microvascular, Hand and Upper Extremity Surgery, Carilion Bone and Joint Center, Roanoke, VA

Todd Milbrandt, MD, MS
Assistant Professor, Department of Pediatric Orthopaedic Surgery, University of Kentucky; Attending Orthopaedic Surgeon, Shriners Hospital for Children, Lexington, KY

Bruce S. Miller, MD
Assistant Professor, Department of Orthopaedic Surgery, University of Michigan, Ann Abor, MI

Mark D. Miller, MD
S. Ward Casscells Professor of Orthopaedic Surgery; Head, Division of Sports Medicine, University of Virginia, Charlottesville, VA; Adjunctive Clinical Professor and Team Physician, James Madison University, Harrisonburg, VA

Andrew Molloy, MB ChB, MRCS, FRCS Tr&Orth
Consultant Orthopaedic Surgeon, University Hospital Aintree, Liverpool, England

Andrew Moore, MD
Chief Resident, Department of Orthopaedic Surgery, University of Michigan, Ann Arbor, MI

Michael P. Mott, MD
Associate Professor and Head, Division of Musculoskeletal Oncology, Department of Orthopaedic Surgery, Henry Ford Hospital, Detroit, MI

Timothy D. Murphy, MD
Resident, Department of Orthopaedics, University of North Carolina, Chapel Hill, NC

Robert Neff, MD
Department of Orthopaedic Surgery, Virginia Commonwealth University Health System, Richmond, VA

Maria Nguyen, MD
Interventional Pain Management Physician, Kaiser Permanente, Kensington, MD

Olabode Ogunwole, AB
Research Coordinator, Department of Orthopaedic Surgery, Children's Hospital Boston, Boston, MA

Oana Panea, MD
Team Physician and Faculty, Primary Care Sports Medicine Fellowship, Department of Family and Community Medicine, Wake Forest University; Faculty, Wake Forest University Baptist Medical Center, Winston-Salem, NC

Chris Pappas, MD
Adjunct Assistant Professor, Uniformed Services University of the Health Sciences, Bethesda, MD; Director of Primary Care Sports Medicine, Family Medicine Residency Teaching Staff, Womack Army Medical Center, Fort Bragg, NC

Daniel K. Park, MD
Resident, Department of Orthopaedic Surgery, Rush University Medical Center, Chicago, IL

Richard D. Parker, MD
Chairman and Professor of Surgery, Department of Orthopaedic Surgery, Orthopaedic Rheumatology Institute, Cleveland Clinic Foundation, Cleveland, OH

Lucien Parrillo, MD
Primary Care Sports Medicine, Maine Medical Center, Portland, ME

Theodore W. Parsons III, MD, FACS
Professor and Breech Chair, Department of Orthopaedic Surgery, Henry Ford Medical Group, Detroit, MI

Jayesh Patel, MD
Resident, University of Kentucky, Lexington, KY

Khurram Pervaiz, MD
Department of Orthopaedic Surgery, Virginia Commonwealth University Health System, Richmond, VA

Frank M. Phillips, MD
Director, Minimally Invasive Spine Surgery, Rush University Medical Center, Chicago, IL

Tracy Ray, MD
Director, Primary Care Sports Medicine Fellowship, St. Vincent's East Family Medicine Sports Medicine Residency Program, American Sports Medicine Institute, Birmingham, AL

Conor Regan, MD
Orthopaedic Resident, University of North Carolina Hospitals, Chapel Hill, NC

Nathan Richardson, MD
Department of Orthopaedic Surgery, Virginia Commonwealth University Health System, Richmond, VA

Scott A. Riley, MD
Orthopaedic Surgeon, Hand and Upper Extremity Surgery, Shriners Hospital for Children, Lexington, KY

Jeffrey Roberts, MD
Primary Care Sports Medicine Fellow, Duke University, Durham, NC

Mark B. Rogers, DO, MA
Department of Family and Sports Medicine, Edward Via Virginia College of Osteopathic Medicine; Team Physician, Virginia Tech University, Blacksburg, VA

Mark Romness, MD
Assistant Professor of Orthopaedic Surgery, Division of Pediatric Orthopaedic Surgery, University of Virginia, Charlottesville, VA

Elizabeth Rothe, MD
Sports Medicine Fellow, Maine Medical Center, Portland, ME

M. Brennan Royalty, MD
Primary Care Sports Medicine Fellow, University of Kentucky, Lexington, KY

Robert N. Royalty, MD
Resident, Department of Orthopaedic Surgery, University of Kentucky, Lexington, KY

James H. Rubright, MD
Clinical Instructor, University of Vermont School of Medicine; Staff Physician, Department of Orthopaedics, Fletcher Allen Health Care, Burlington, VT

Sara D. Rynders, MPAS
Physcian Assistant, Orthopaedic Hand and Upper Extremity Surgery, University of Virginia, Charlottesville, VA

Michael J. Salata, MD
Chief Resident, Department of Orthopaedic Surgery, University of Michigan Hospitals, Ann Arbor, MI

Brian P. Scannell, MD
Resident, Carolinas Medical Center, Charlotte, NC

David Schnur, MD
Clinical Assistant Professor, University of Colorado Health Science Center, Denver, CO

Joseph J. Schumann, BS
Medical Student, Medical College of Wisconsin, Milwaukee, WI

Benson A. Scott, MD
Physician, Knoxville Orthopedic Clinic, Knoxville, TN

Nicholas R. Seibert, MD
Resident, Department of Orthopaedics, University of Michigan, Ann Arbor, MI

Jon K. Sekiya, MD
Associate Professor and Team Physician, MedSport, Department of Orthopaedic Surgery, University of Michigan, Ann Arbor, MI; Team Physician, Eastern Michigan University, Ypsilanti, MI

Franklin D. Shuler, MD, PhD
Director, Orthopaedic Research; Assistant Professor, Orthopaedic Trauma, Department of Orthopaedics, West Virginia University, Morgantown, WV

Michael Simpson, DO, MC
Major, U.S. Army, Fort Jackson, SC

Jonathan Smerek, MD, MS
Clinical Assistant Professor, Indiana University School of Medicine; Methodist Sports Medicine/The Orthopaedic Specialists; Clarian North Medical Center, Indianapolis, IN

Kyle Smoot, MD
Fellow, Primary Care Sports Medicine, University of Kentucky, Lexington, KY

Umasuthan Srikumaran, MD
Resident, Department of Orthopaedics, Johns Hopkins School of Medicine, Baltimore, MD

Harry C. Stafford, MD
Primary Care Sports Medicine, Duke University, Durham, NC

Trevor Starnes, MD, PhD
Resident, Department of Orthopaedic Surgery, University of Virginia, Charlottesville, VA

Timothy N. Taft, MD
Max Novich Distinguished Professor of Sports Medicine, Department of Orthopaedics; Adjunct Professor, Department of Exercise and Sport Science, University of North Carolina School of Medicine, Chapel Hill, NC

Vishwas Talwalkar, MD
Assistant Professor, Department of Orthopaedic Surgery, University of Kentucky; Attending Physician, Shriners Hospital for Children, Lexington, KY

Chin Khoon Tan, MB ChB, MRCS
Specialist Registrar, Department of Trauma and Orthopaedics, University of Liverpool, Liverpool, England

Tony Y. Tannoury, MD
Assistant Professor, Department of Orthopaedic Surgery, Boston University, Boston, MA

John B. Thaller, MD
Augusta Orthopaedic Associates, Augusta, ME

Jared Toman, MD
Resident, Department of Orthopaedic Surgery, Boston Medical Center, Boston, MA

Michael A. Townsend, PA-C
Steadman Hawkins Clinic of the Carolinas, Greenville, SC

List of Contributors

Scott Van Aman, MD
Orthopaedic Surgeon, Ohio Orthopedic Center of Excellence, Columbus, OH

Anand Vora, MD
Clinical Assistant Professor, University of Illinois, Illinois Bone and Joint Institute, Chicago, IL

Kelly Waicus, MD
Clinical Assistant Professor, Departments of Orthopaedics and Pediatrics, University of North Carolina School of Medicine; Team Physician, University of North Carolina Sports Medicine, Chapel Hill, NC

Jeffrey C. Wang, MD
Professor, Orthopaedic Surgery and Neurosurgery, University of California, Los Angeles School of Medicine; Chief, Orthopaedic Spine Service, University of California, Los Angeles Spine Center, Los Angeles, CA

Robert P. Waugh, MD
Chief Resident, Department of Orthopaedics, University of Maryland Medical School, Baltimore, MD

Jeffrey W. Webb, MD
Assistant Professor, Emory University, Atlanta, GA

Thomas S. Weber, MD
Medical Director, Valley Orthopedics and Sports Medicine, Rockingham Memorial Hospital, Harrisonburg, VA

Modern Weng, DO
Primary Care Physician, Department of Orthopedics, Walnut Creek Medical Center, Walnut Creek, CA

Robert P. Wilder, MD, FACSM
Associate Professor, Department of Physical Medicine and Rehabilitation, University of Virginia, Charlottesville, VA

Edward M. Wojtys, MD
Professor, Department of Orthopaedic Surgery; Chief, Sports Medicine Service; Medical Director, MedSport, University of Michigan, Ann Arbor, MI

Edward V. Wood, MB ChB, FRCS Tr&Orth
Consultant Orthopaedic Surgeon, Countess of Chester Hospital, Chester, England

Megan M. Wood, MD
Clinical Assistant Professor, Department of Orthopaedics, University of Texas Southwestern Medical School, Dallas, TX

Ramon Ylanan, MD
Assistant Professor, Family and Preventative Medicine; Team Physician, University of South Carolina, Columbia, SC

S. Tim Yoon, MD, PhD
Assistant Professor, Department of Orthopaedic Surgery, Emory University, Atlanta, GA; Chief of Orthopaedic Surgery, Atlanta VA Medical Center, Decatur, GA

Dan A. Zlotolow, MD
Assistant Professor, University of Maryland School of Medicine, Baltimore, MD

Matthew G. Zmurko, MD
Orthopaedic Spine Surgeon, Vermont Orthopaedic Clinic, Rutland Regional Medical Center, Rutland, VT

Foreword

In this era of publication overload, it is often difficult to determine which medical texts will make the best investments. *Essential Orthopaedics,* edited by Dr. Mark Miller and colleagues, is an outstanding contribution to the field. It is replete with excellent chapter selection that uses an uncomplicated approach to presenting information. The text is complemented by excellent imaging, graphics, and data tables. Its easy reading style will be a delight to orthopaedists—both junior and senior—and non-orthopaedists alike. The chapters are well referenced to highlight many expert opinions in the field.

The discussions of clinical problems are thought provoking and will serve clinicians well as they ponder the best treatment choices for their patients. This text offers keen insights provided by experienced clinicians.

It is very difficult to coalesce state-of-the-art orthopaedics into a single text because of the range and depth of topics. However, Dr. Miller and his contributors have certainly accomplished this task. My congratulations to Mark and his team for a big job well done!

Edward M. Wojtys, MD

Foreword

I am honored for the invitation to provide a foreword for *Essential Orthopaedics.* As a longtime sports medicine practitioner, educator, and fellowship director, I am often asked, "What is a good sports medicine book to use for reference?" I usually deflect the answer with a comment that the rapidly changing face of sports medicine does not permit the publication of a good, "current" sports medicine reference. Now, *Essential Orthopaedics* allows me to offer a quality answer to that very question.

The chapter authors are highly skilled and experienced clinicians who have successfully identified the most relevant details of each injury and condition and have effectively synthesized the data into an easily readable format. A brief review of each chapter reflects the thoroughness and depth of each contribution.

Essential Orthopaedics is a clear, concise, easy-to-consult volume. Excellent line drawings, photographs, and tables enhance the text and emphasize significant details. The outline format offers chapter-by-chapter consistency that simplifies and expedites use. The references at the end of each brief section permit easy access to more detailed information should the reader require a more comprehensive discussion.

Any clinician whose practice involves an active athletic population will find this a very welcome addition to his or her medical library. I congratulate the editors and authors for a most successful sports medicine reference text.

Rob Johnson, MD

Contents

Section 9
Pediatric Orthopaedics

SECTION 1

General Principles

Chapter 1 How to Use This Book

Mark D. Miller, John M. MacKnight, and Jennifer A. Hart

Welcome to what we hope will be the most comprehensive and useful textbook of orthopaedics you will ever own. Appreciating that the vast majority of orthopaedic care takes place not in the orthopaedic surgeon's office or operating room but rather in a myriad of primary care settings, this work is designed to be a user-friendly reference to assist primary care physicians, physician's assistants, nurse practitioners, physical therapists, and athletic trainers. Having a reliable, thorough resource of clinical information is essential to ensure timely and appropriate management of all orthopaedic concerns. As such, we have produced *Essential Orthopaedics* to be your go-to resource in the clinic or the training room.

As you peruse the text, you will find that the initial sections are devoted to a number of general topics important to orthopaedic care. A review of orthopaedic anatomy and terminology is followed by information on the nuances of radiologic evaluation of orthopaedic conditions. Subsequent chapters are dedicated to such vital topics as pharmacology, impairment and disability, and principles of rehabilitation. Additional chapters are dedicated to special populations and conditions such as the obese, elderly, pediatric, and female and pregnant patients, and those with multiple comorbid conditions, arthritides, and trauma.

The remainder of the text is divided into six major anatomic groups: shoulder, elbow, wrist/hand, spine, pelvis/hip, knee and lower leg, ankle and foot, and pediatrics. Each section begins with an anatomic graphic that will direct you to likely diagnoses based on the location of the patient's symptoms or findings. The following pages include a review of regional anatomy, pertinent history that is characteristic for each anatomic area, a review of specific physical examination techniques, and practical management of imaging strategies.

Within each specific topic chapter, you will find a consistent format designed to aid efficiency in finding the information that you need as quickly as possible. After alternative condition names and ICD-9 codes are provided, topic headings include Key Concepts, History, Physical Examination, Imaging, Additional Tests (if applicable), Differential Diagnosis, Treatment, Troubleshooting, Patient Instructions, Considerations in Special Populations, and Suggested Reading. We have placed great emphasis on including multiple drawings, photographs, and radiologic images to enhance the quality of each topic. In addition, we have added an accompanying DVD that covers in great detail the key orthopaedic physical examination techniques and procedures that any provider should know. We want you to feel comfortable that you have seen before what you will be presented with for care.

It is our sincere hope that you will find *Essential Orthopaedics* to be the finest orthopaedic reference for primary care providers of all types. Having a comprehensive reference designed for rapid access of information is crucial for busy practitioners. This text will help you find the right answer quickly and will help enhance your comfort with orthopaedic diagnosis, management, and appropriate referral. Musculoskeletal care accounts for a sizable percentage of medical encounters; let *Essential Orthopaedics* help enhance the care of every orthopaedic patient whom you see.

Chapter 2 Orthopaedic Terminology

Paul Gubanich

Introduction

Orthopaedic complaints account for some of the most common presentations to physicians. A thorough working knowledge of basic anatomy, function, and movement is essential for prompt diagnosis and appropriate management of these conditions. The following terms are commonly used in an orthopaedic practice. Mastery of these basic terms will allow you to better understand the material presented in the following chapters.

Anatomy

- *Allograft*: Tissue or specimen that comes from the same species but a different individual. Examples include the use of cadaver grafts in reconstruction of the anterior cruciate ligament.
- *Anterior cruciate ligament*: The primary stabilizer that prevents anterior translation of the tibia on the femur. The anterior cruciate ligament also is a primary stabilizer for rotary movement. It is one of the most commonly injured knee ligaments. It heals poorly due to its limited blood supply and often requires surgical reconstruction.
- *Articular cartilage*: Hyaline cartilage that lines the end of long bones and forms the surface of a joint
- *Autograft*: Tissue specimen that comes from the same individual but from a different anatomic site. Examples include the use of bone–patellar tendon–bone or hamstring grafts in the reconstruction of the anterior cruciate ligament in the same individual.
- *Bipartite*: Meaning two parts, it refers to the anatomic variant in which the ossification centers of a sesamoid bone fail to properly fuse. This is most commonly seen in the patella and the sesamoids of the foot.
- *Diaphysis*: The shaft of long bone. Bone elongation occurs toward the diaphysis.
- *Discoid meniscus*: Anatomic variant in which the typical C-shaped fibrocartilage meniscus assumes a flat contour
- *Epiphyseal plate (physis)*: Also called the growth plate, this hyaline cartilage structure is the site of elongation of long bones. Growth plates are inherently weak compared with the surrounding bone and are often sites of injury in children and adolescents.
- *Epiphysis*: The end of a long bone. This ultimately forms the articular cartilage–lined ends of a long bone.
- *Labrum*: A fibrocartilage ring that surrounds the articular surface of a joint. The labrum helps to deepen and stabilize the joint. Examples include the labrum of the glenoid in the shoulder and acetabulum of the hip.
- *Lateral collateral ligament*: Primary knee stabilizer to varus stress
- *Ligament*: Fibrous connective tissue that attaches one bone to another, providing structural support to the joint
- *Medial collateral ligament*: The primary knee stabilizer to valgus stress
- *Meniscus*: C-shaped fibrocartilage that helps cushion the knee and distribute load between the femur and the tibia
- *Metaphysis*: The portion of a long bone between the epiphysis and the diaphysis
- *Posterior cruciate ligament*: The primary stabilizer that prevents posterior translation of the tibia on the femur. The posterior cruciate ligament also contributes to rotary stability. In contrast to the anterior cruciate ligament, the posterior cruciate ligament has a better blood supply and less commonly requires surgical reconstruction.
- *Tendon*: Fibrous connective tissue that attaches muscle to bone
- *Triangular fibrocartilage complex*: A collection of ligaments and fibrocartilage located on the ulnar side of the wrist that stabilizes the distal radius, ulnar, and carpal bones
- *Tuberosity*: A bony prominence that serves as the site of attachment for tendons and/or ligaments

Injury

- *Apophysitis*: Repetitive stress injury with inflammation in the growth plate of a bony prominence such as the point of insertion of a tendon (tuberosity). Commonly affected sites include the knee (tibial tubercle [Osgood-

Schlatter disease], elbow [medial epicondyle], and pelvis [iliac crest]).
- *Bursitis*: Inflammation of the synovial sac (bursa) that protects the soft-tissue structures (muscles, tendons) from underlying bony prominences. Common areas of involvement include the shoulder (subacromial bursa), knee (prepatellar bursa), elbow (bursa of olecranon bursa), and hip (trochanteric bursa).
- *Dislocation*: Complete disassociation of the articular surfaces of a joint. Commonly affected sites include the patella and glenohumeral joint of the shoulder.
- *Impingement*: The process by which soft tissues (e.g., tendons, bursas) are compressed by bony structures. This often is dynamic in nature. The shoulder and ankle are two commonly affected sites.
- *Myositis ossificans*: Condition of heterotopic bone formation at the site of previous trauma and hematoma formation. The most common site of involvement is the thigh after a contusion, but this disorder does occur less frequently in other muscle groups.
- *Osteoarthritis*: Degenerative condition that causes inflammation, breakdown of synovial fluid, and destruction of the articular cartilage with resultant abnormal new bone formation
- *Osteochondritis dissecans*: Injury (often traumatic) to the joint surface of bone that involves detachment of the subchondral bone and its overlying articular cartilage. Commonly affected sites include the knee (femur), elbow (ulna), and ankle (talus).
- *Salter-Harris*: Classification system used to categorize injuries to the growth plate (physis)
    - Type I: Transverse fracture through the physis without other injury. Widening of the physis can be seen.
    - Type II: Physeal fracture that extends into the metaphysis
    - Type III: Physeal fracture that extends into the epiphysis
    - Type IV: Fracture that involves the epiphysis, metaphysis, and physis
    - Type V: Fracture that involves compression of the epiphyseal plate
- *Spondylolisthesis*: The abnormal translation of one vertebra with respect to another
- *Spondylolysis*: A fracture of the pars articularis of the vertebra. This injury is usually caused by repetitive stress and most commonly affects the lower lumbar vertebrae.
- *Sprain*: An injury to the ligaments that support a joint. Mild (first-degree) injuries involve microscopic tearing. Second-degree injuries involve a partial tear of the ligament, and third-degree injuries involve a complete disruption of the ligament.
- *Strain*: An injury to muscle or tendon around or attached to a joint. Grading scale is similar to sprains with mild (first-degree) injuries involving microscopic tearing, second-degree injuries involving a partial tear of the muscle or tendon, and third-degree injuries involving a complete disruption of muscle or tendon fibers.
- *Stress fracture*: A microscopic fracture in bone caused by repetitive loading. Bone breakdown/resorption occurs at a faster rate than bone deposition in response to overuse.
- *Subluxation*: Partial dislocation of the articular surfaces of a joint
- *Syndesmotic ankle (high ankle) sprain*: An ankle sprain that involves injury to the syndesmotic ligament that connects the tibia and fibula. These are often more severe than routine ankle sprains.
- *Tendinitis*: Acute inflammation of a tendon. Symptoms are typically present for several (1 to 3) weeks. Commonly affected sites include the shoulder (rotator cuff tendons), knee (patellar tendon), elbow (extensor tendon), and heel (Achilles tendon).
- *Tendonosis/tendonopathy*: Degenerative breakdown of the tendon and abnormal vascularization due to chronic, repetitive stress. Symptoms are often present for several weeks to months.
- *Tenosynovitis*: Inflammation of the sheath surrounding a tendon. This can occur concomitantly with tendon involvement or independently.

Movement

- *Abduction*: Movement away from the body's midline
- *Adduction*: Movement toward the body's midline
- *Eversion*: Rotation of the foot or ankle outward
- *Inversion*: Rotation of the foot or ankle inward
- *Pronation*: Rotary movement described at the wrist, where the palm of the hand rotates from a superior facing position to one facing inferiorly. Similarly, at the ankle, the plantar aspect of the foot rotates outward or laterally.
- *Supination*: Rotary movement described at the wrist, where the palm of the hand rotates from an inferior facing position to one facing superiorly. Similarly, at the ankle, the plantar aspect of the foot rotates inward or medially.
- *Valgus*: Anatomic alignment of a joint where the distal portion is angulated away from the midline, for example, knock knees

- *Varus*: Anatomic alignment of a joint where the distal portion is angulated toward the midline, for example, bowlegs

Treatment

- *Arthrocentesis*: Aspiration of synovial fluid from a joint
- *Arthroscopy*: A surgical technique that uses a small camera (endoscope) in a joint space for the diagnosis and treatment of joint-related conditions
- *Iontophoresis*: Process by which an electrical current is used to deliver a drug (often a corticosteroid) to the surrounding soft tissues or joint transdermally
- *Phonophoresis*: Process by which ultrasound is used to deliver a drug (often nonsteroidal anti-inflammatory drugs) to the surrounding soft tissues or joint transdermally
- *Physical therapy*: The branch of medicine that specializes in treatment, prevention, and functional optimization of disorders of the musculoskeletal system. It encompasses numerous treatment modalities including mobilization, strengthening, flexibility, massage, heat, and water.
- *Rehabilitation*: The process of restoring one's health functionality

Suggested Reading

- DeLee JC, Drez D (eds): Orthopaedic Sports Medicine: Principles and Practices, 2nd ed. Philadelphia: Elsevier Science, 2003.
- Griffin LY, Greene WB (eds): Essentials of Musculoskeletal Care, 3rd ed. Rosemont, IL: American Academy of Orthopaedic Surgeons, 2005.
- O'Connor FG, Sallis RE, Wilder RP, St. Pierre P: Sports Medicine: Just the Facts. Chicago: McGraw-Hill, 2005.
- Thompson JC: Netter's Concise Atlas of Orthopaedic Anatomy. Teterboro, NJ: MediMedia, 2002.

Chapter 3 Imaging of the Musculoskeletal System

Mark W. Anderson

Key Concepts

- Imaging studies should be used as an adjunct to the history and physical examination.
- Obtain the least number of imaging studies needed to arrive at a diagnosis (or reasonable differential diagnosis).
- Each imaging modality has specific strengths and weaknesses that must be taken into account when considering which test to perform.

Imaging

Radiography

- Technique: A beam of x-rays is projected through the body to a detector that constructs a two-dimensional image based on the differential attenuation of the beam by various tissues.
- The primary modality for investigating the musculoskeletal system; should be the first imaging study ordered for most indications
- Four basic tissues are recognizable on a radiograph: metals, which are the densest structures on a film (this category includes bone because of its calcium content); air, which is the most lucent (black); fat, which is dark gray; and soft tissue, which appears as intermediate gray (this category includes fluid that cannot be differentiated from muscle, etc.) (Fig. 3-1).
- At least two views are usually obtained, most often in the frontal and lateral projections (Fig. 3-2).

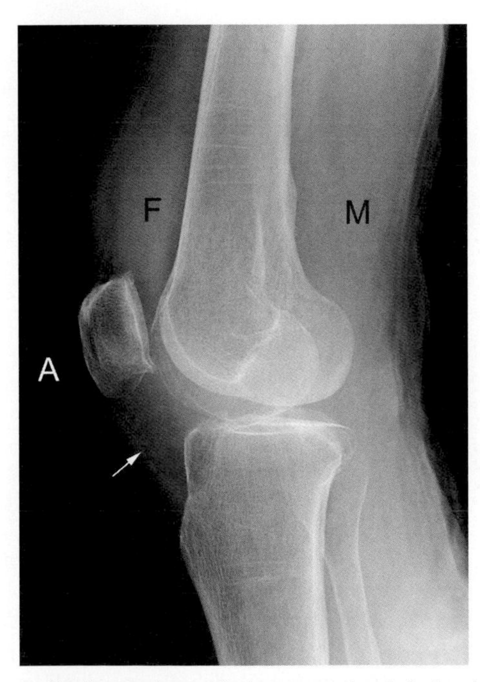

Figure 3-1 Radiography: soft-tissue contrast. Lateral radiograph of the knee demonstrates dark, lucent air (A); dark gray fat in Hoffa's fat pad (*arrow*); intermediate gray fluid in the suprapatellar bursa (F) related to a large joint effusion (note the similarity in density between the fluid and the hamstring muscles [M] posteriorly); and the relatively dense bones (related to their calcium content).

Strengths

- Relatively inexpensive
- Widely available

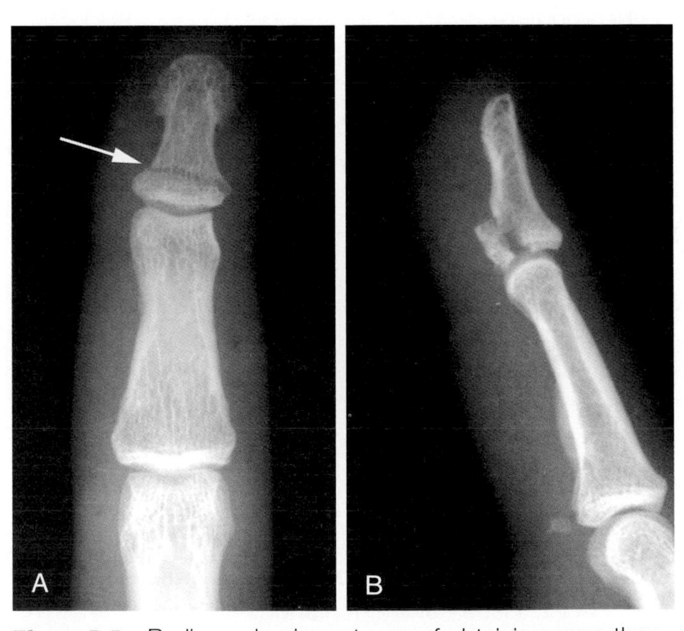

Figure 3-2 Radiography: importance of obtaining more than one view. **A**, Posteroanterior radiograph of the finger demonstrates a transverse fracture of the distal phalanx that does not appear to involve its articular surface (*arrow*). **B**, Corresponding lateral view reveals intra-articular extension and mild distraction along the fracture line.

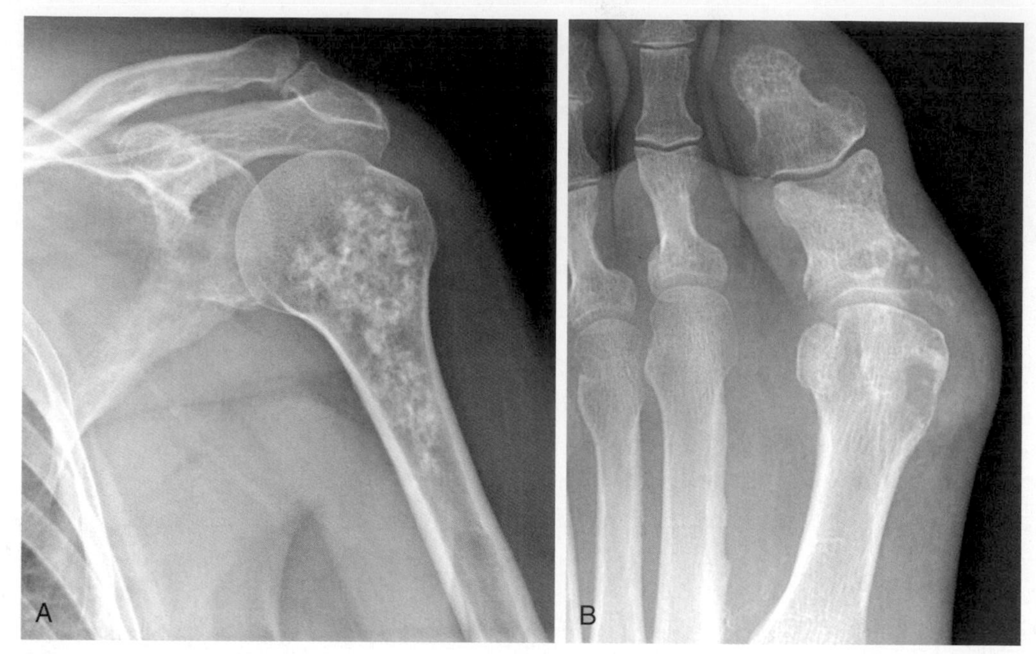

Figure 3-3 Radiography: tumor and arthritis. **A**, Frontal view of the shoulder reveals a coarse, sclerotic intramedullary lesion within the proximal humerus, compatible with a chondroid neoplasm, most likely an enchondroma. **B**, Posteroanterior radiograph of the foot demonstrates classic findings of gout involving the first metatarsophalangeal joint including large marginal and para-articular erosions, calcific densities in the adjacent soft-tissue tophus, and relative sparing of the joint space.

- Evaluation of bone pathology (fracture, tumor, arthritis, osteomyelitis, metabolic bone disease) (Fig. 3-3)
- Assessment of orthopaedic hardware and fracture healing (Fig. 3-4)

Weaknesses
- Pathology of the medullary cavity (bone contusion, occult fracture, medullary tumor) (Fig. 3-5)
- Soft-tissue pathology
- Uses ionizing radiation

Computed Tomography
- Technique: An x-ray source is rotated around the patient, who is lying on a moving gantry, resulting in image "slices" in the transaxial plane.
- The data from these slices can then be viewed as axial images or used to create reformatted images in any plane (typically sagittal and coronal planes).
- Can be combined with IV contrast, which results in increased density (enhancement) in vessels and hypervascular tissues owing to its iodine content

Strengths
- Tomographic depiction of anatomy allowing for two- and three-dimensional reformatted images (Fig. 3-6)

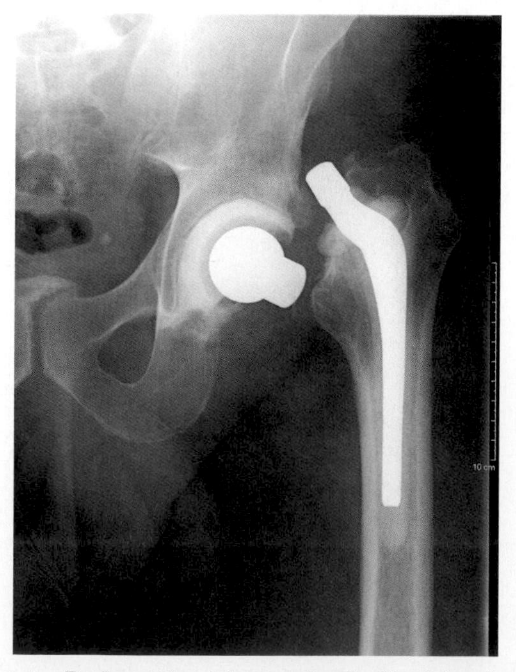

Figure 3-4 Radiography: joint prosthesis. Frontal radiograph of the left hip shows prosthetic discontinuity of the femoral component at the junction of its head and neck with resulting superolateral migration of the proximal femur.

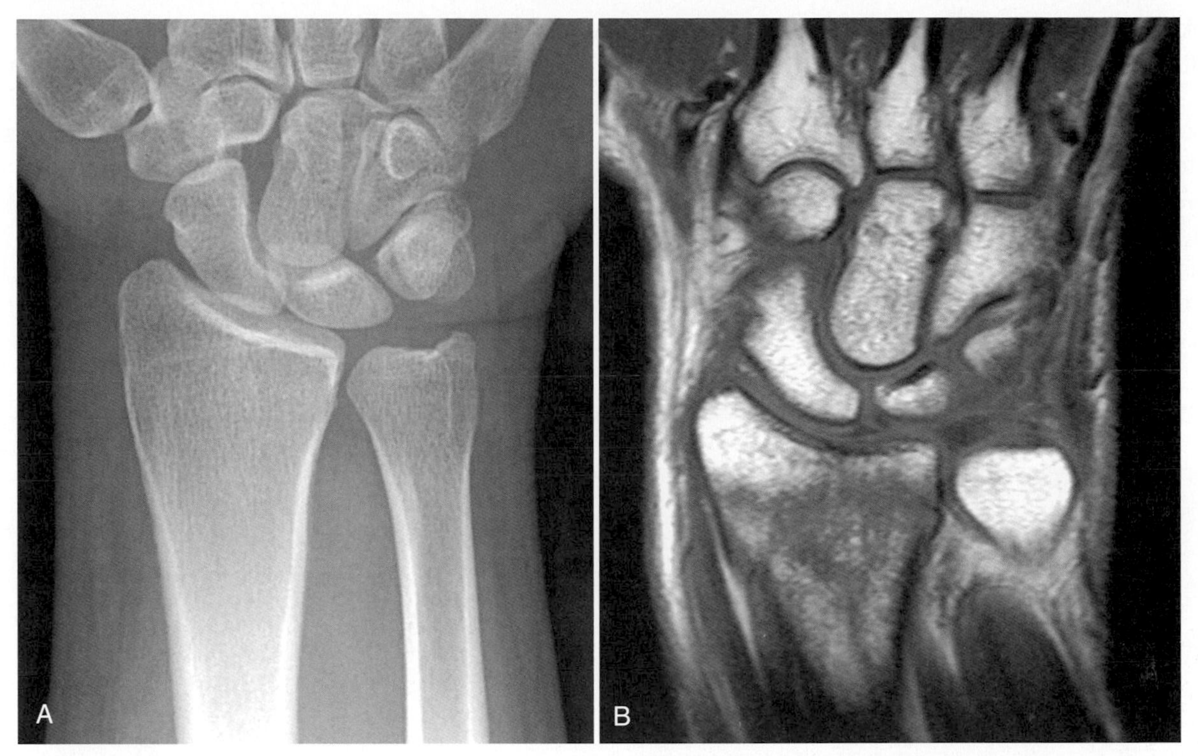

Figure 3-5 Radiography: occult fracture. **A**, No discrete fracture is evident on this posteroanterior view of the wrist obtained after injury. **B**, Coronal T1-weighted magnetic resonance image reveals numerous nondisplaced, low signal intensity fracture lines within the distal radius.

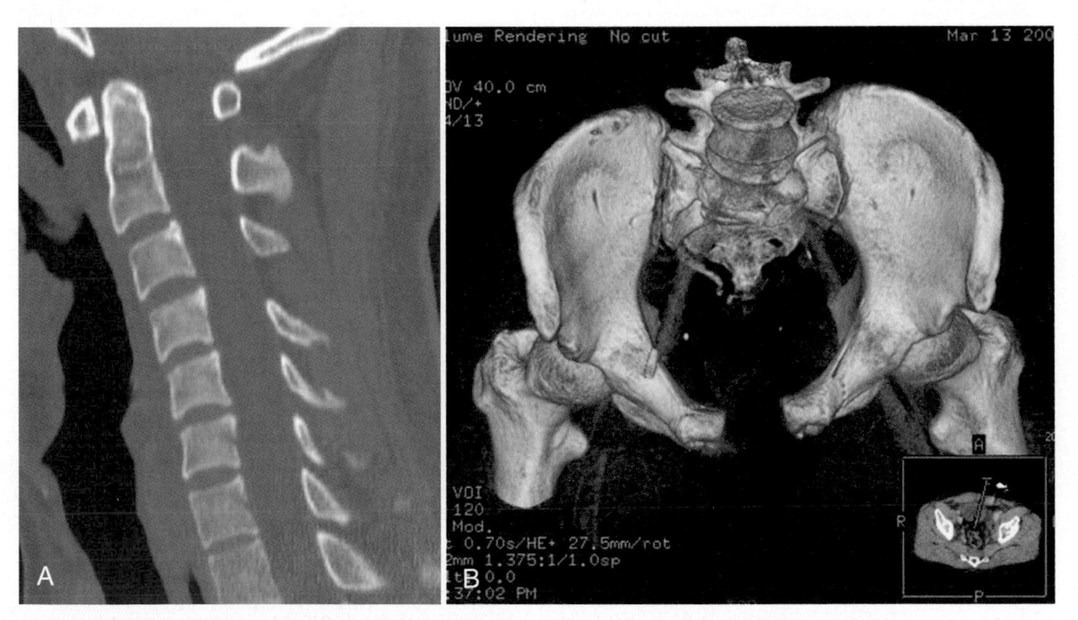

Figure 3-6 Computed tomography: reformatted images. **A**, Thin-slice computed tomography images obtained in the axial plane were combined to create this two-dimensional sagittal reconstructed image of the cervical spine. **B**, A three-dimensional reformatted image of the pelvis depicts prominent diastasis of the symphysis pubis and less prominent widening of the right sacroiliac joint.

- Depiction of complex fractures, especially those involving the spine and flat bones (pelvis and scapula) (Fig. 3-7)
- Evaluation of fracture healing
- Postoperative evaluation of the degree of fusion or hardware complications (Fig. 3-8)
- Can be combined with intrathecal or intra-articular contrast (computed tomography myelography and computed tomography arthrography, respectively) (Fig. 3-9)

Weaknesses

- Fracture detection in the setting of significant osteopenia (Fig. 3-10)
- Although computed tomography produces much better soft-tissue contrast than radiographs, it is not as good as that obtained with magnetic resonance imaging.
- Uses ionizing radiation (unlike ultrasonography and magnetic resonance imaging)

Radionuclide Scanning

- Technique: A bone-seeking radioactive material is injected intravenously (typically technetium-99m

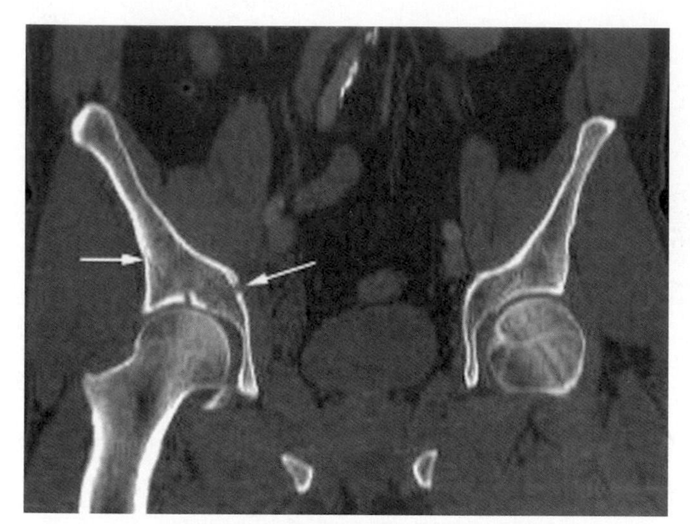

Figure 3-7 Computed tomography: complex fractures. Coronal, two-dimensional reformatted image from a computed tomography scan of the pelvis demonstrates an essentially nondisplaced, comminuted right acetabular fracture (*arrows*).

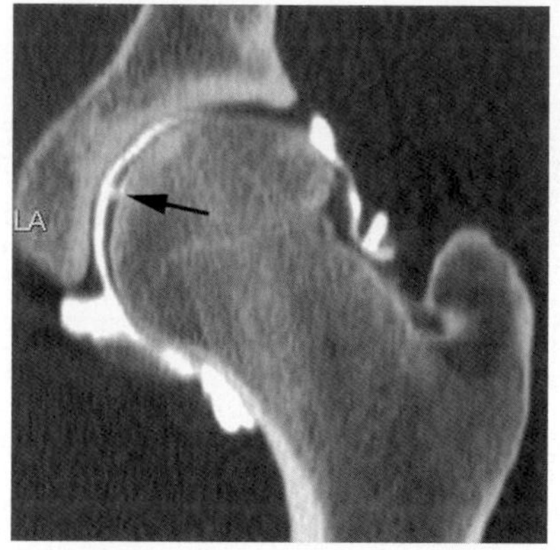

Figure 3-9 Computed tomography arthrogram. Coronal reformatted image from a computed tomography arthrogram of the left hip reveals a small cartilage flap along the medial femoral head (*arrow*).

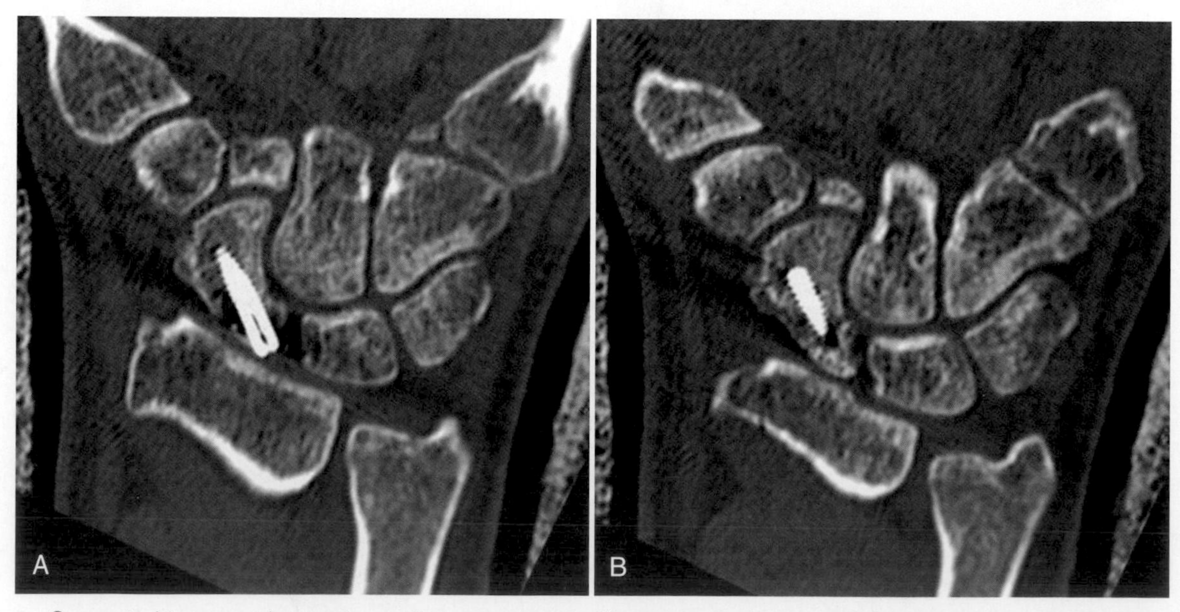

Figure 3-8 Computed tomography: postoperative assessment. Ajacent coronal reformatted images of the wrist reveal a nondisplaced scaphoid fracture transfixed with a surgical screw. Note the lack of metal-related artifact.

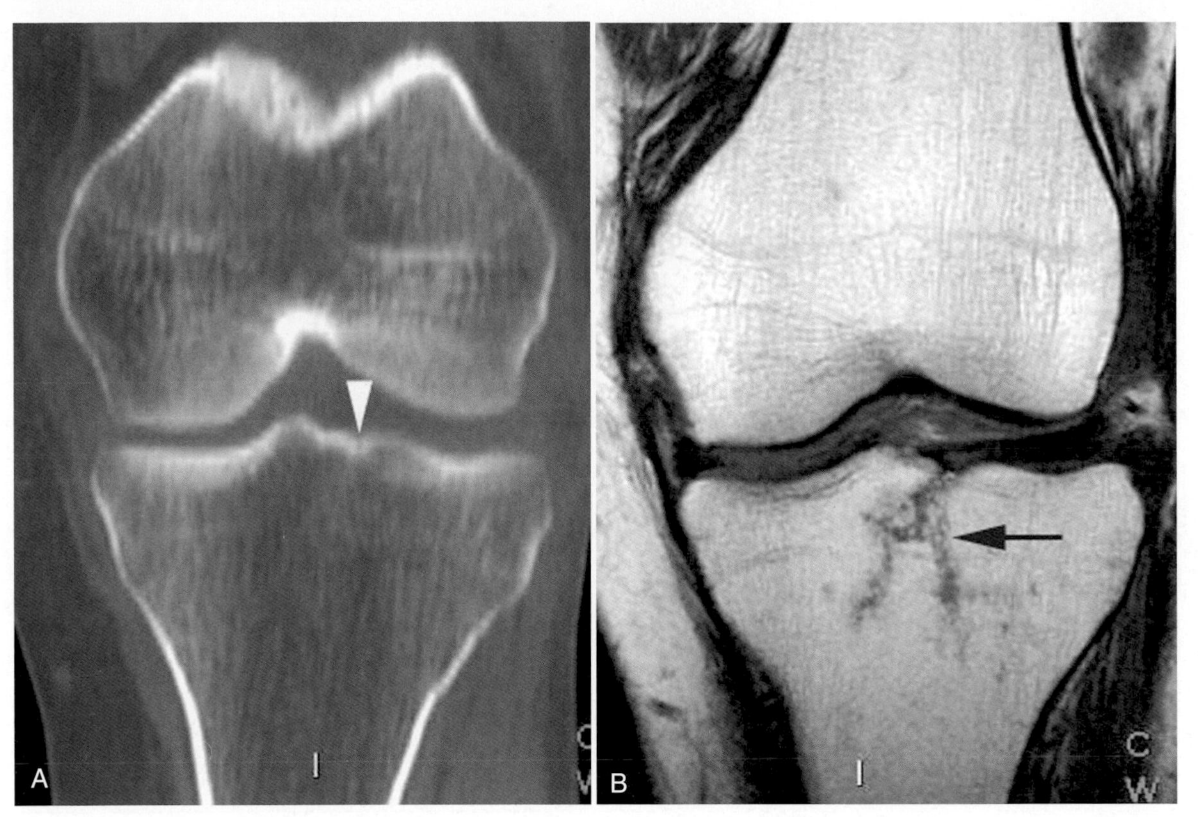

Figure 3-10 Computed tomography versus magnetic resonance imaging for a tibial plateau fracture. **A**, Coronal reformatted computed tomography image of the knee reveals a very small cortical lucency (*arrowhead*) in the tibial plateau at the site of a nondisplaced fracture that is much better demonstrated on a coronal T1-weighted magnetic resonance image (**B**).

diphosphonate, a phosphorous analog that is taken up in areas of increased bone turnover such as tumor, infection, and fracture), and the patient is scanned 4 to 6 hours later, at which time whole-body images may be obtained.

- More localized, "spot" images may also be acquired in areas of specific clinical concern, and the use of single-photon emission tomography technology can produce tomographic images in the axial, sagittal, and coronal planes.
- Positron emission tomography scanning uses a metabolically active tracer, typically ^{18}F-fluorodeoxyglucose, a glucose analog that is taken up in tissues proportional to glucose utilization.
    - Pathologic processes typically show increased metabolic activity and increased ^{18}F-fluorodeoxyglucose uptake.
    - This modality also has theoretical value for the evaluation of a variety of neoplastic, infectious, and inflammatory conditions of the musculoskeletal system. Although promising results have been reported for some indications, the number of studies has been limited to date, and further investigation is needed.

Strengths

- Whole-body imaging allows rapid assessment of the entire skeleton; this is the study of choice to evaluate possible skeletal metastases.
- Provides physiologic information regarding the activity of a bone lesion (Fig. 3-11)
- High sensitivity

Weaknesses

- Relatively low specificity
- Any process resulting in increased bone turnover (infection, tumor, fracture) may result in a focus of increased activity.
- False-negative examinations may occur in the initial 24 to 48 hours, especially in elderly patients.
- Insensitive for detecting multiple myeloma (plain radiographs are actually better for this purpose)
- Poor soft-tissue evaluation
- Produces ionizing radiation

Ultrasonography

- Technique: Sound waves are passed into tissue via a hand-held transducer, and the image is produced based on the pattern of returning waves.

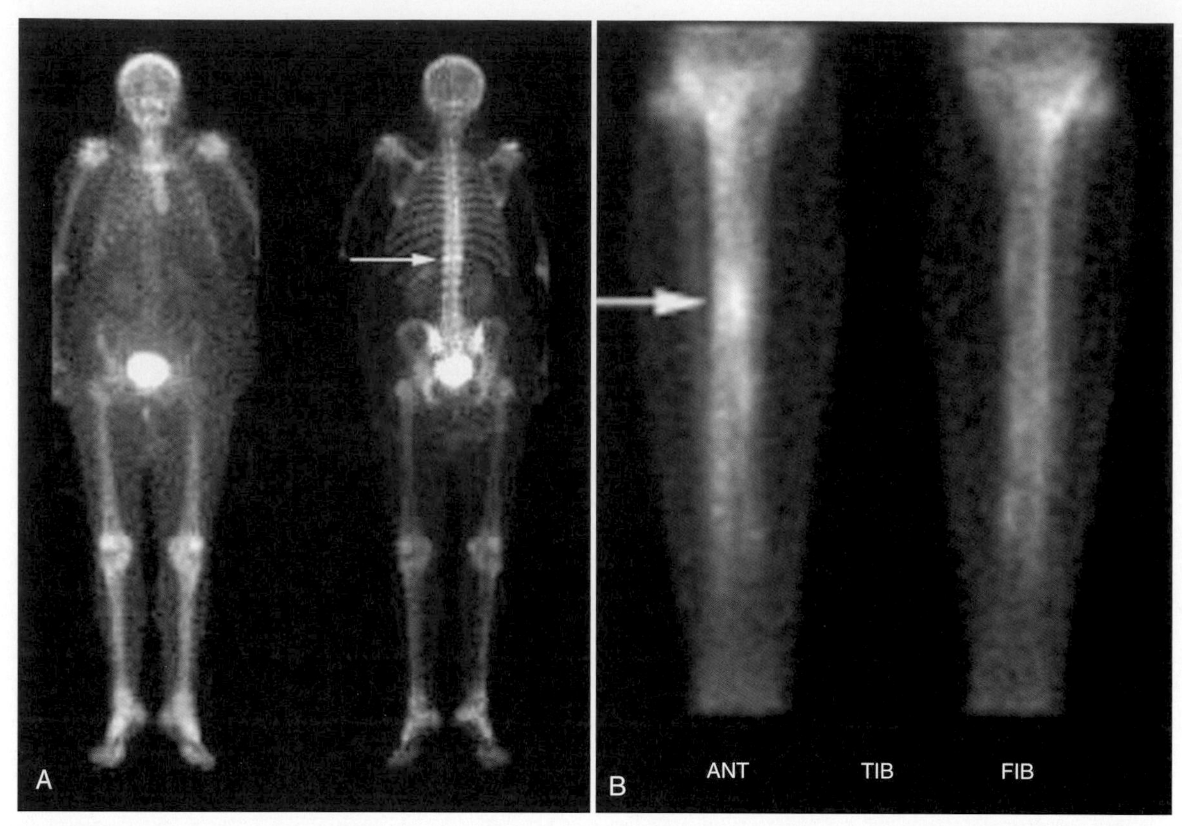

Figure 3-11 Bone scan. **A**, Anterior and posterior whole body bone scan images reveal focal uptake at the thoracolumbar junction (*arrow*) at the site of a pathologic fracture related to a vertebral metastasis. **B**, Spot images of the lower legs from a bone scan in a different patient show abnormal uptake in the right mid-tibia at the site of a stress fracture (*arrow*).

- Tissues can be assessed in a dynamic, real-time fashion or on static images.
- Best if used for a specific clinical question (e.g., tendon laceration, evaluation of a soft-tissue mass, foreign body detection)
- Vascularity and flow dynamics can be assessed with Doppler ultrasound imaging.

Strengths

- Allows anatomic and dynamic functional evaluation of musculoskeletal tissues (e.g., tendon function, developmental dysplasia of the hip) (Fig. 3-12)
- Determining whether a soft-tissue mass is of a cystic or solid nature
  - Cystic masses appear as anechoic (black) structures with a sharp posterior wall and enhanced through transmission (owing to the lack of sound reflectors within the homogeneous fluid) (Fig. 3-13).
- Assessing the vascularity of a lesion
- Real-time guidance for percutaneous interventional procedures
- Foreign body detection (Fig. 3-14).
- No ionizing radiation

Weaknesses

- Limited assessment of deeper tissues and bone
- Relatively time-consuming and very operator dependent
- Limited field of view

Magnetic Resonance Imaging

- Technique: Magnetic resonance imaging is based on the fact that hydrogen protons within the body (most abundant in water and fat) will act like small bar magnets. The patient is placed in a strong magnetic field and a small percentage of protons will align with the field.
- Energy, in the form of radio waves, is added to the tissue causing some of the protons to shift to a higher-energy state. When the radiofrequency source is turned off, the protons will relax back to their resting state and in the process release energy, again in the form of radio waves, which are detected and used to create the magnetic resonance image.
- The protons resonate differently in different tissues based primarily on two tissue-specific factors called T1 and T2, and scanning parameters can be set to

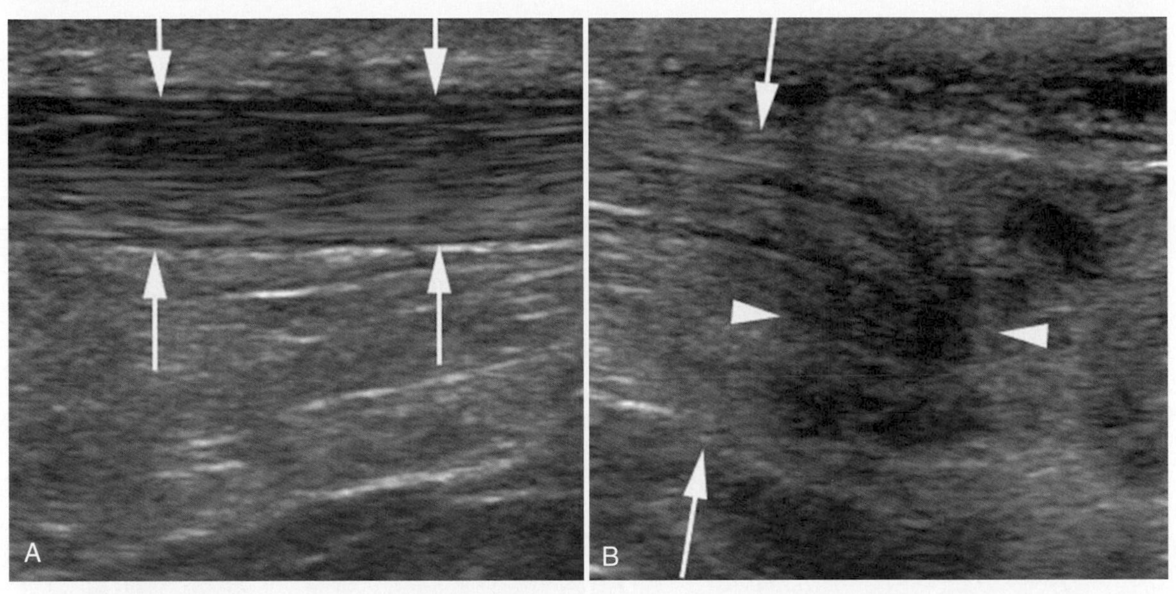

Figure 3-12 Ultrasonography: tendons. **A**, Longitudinal sonogram of a normal Achilles tendon (*arrows*). **B**, Longitudinal scan of the Achilles tendon in a different patient demonstrates diffuse thickening of the tendon (*arrows*) and an area of high-grade partial tearing (*arrowheads*).

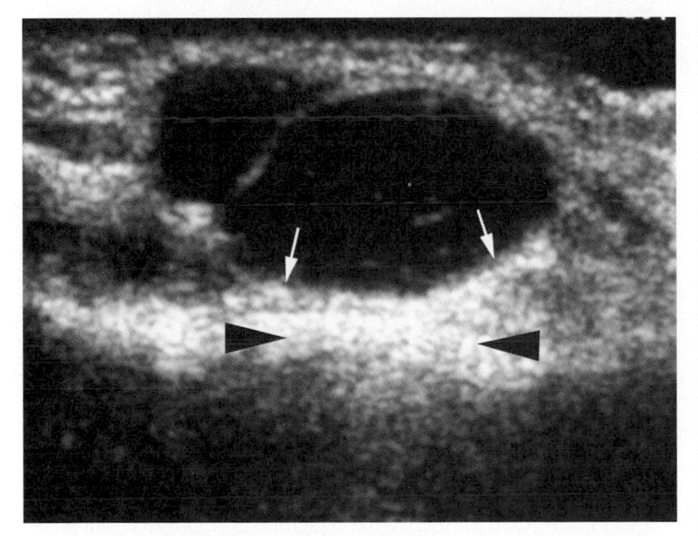

Figure 3-13 Ultrasonography: ganglion cyst. Ultrasound scan of the finger reveals a small, bilobed ganglion cyst. Note the lack of internal echoes, sharp posterior wall (*arrows*), and enhanced through transmission (*arrowheads*), all of which are typical sonographic characteristics of a cyst.

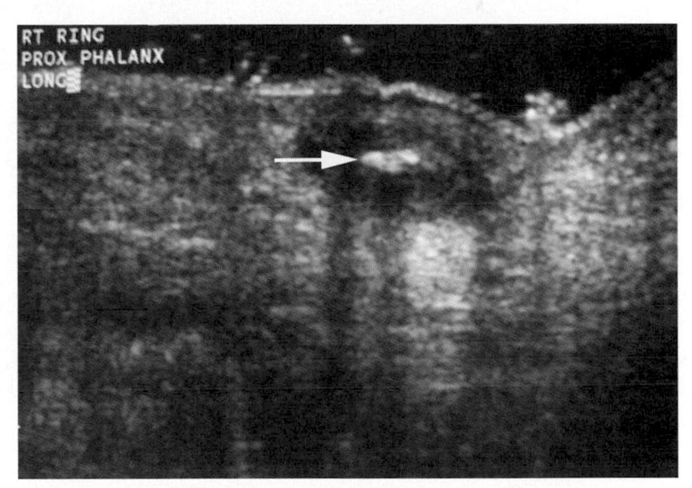

Figure 3-14 Ultrasonography: foreign body. A small, echogenic foreign body (*arrow*) and surrounding hypoechoic (dark) reactive tissue is identified on this longitudinal sonogram of the finger.

emphasize either factor, thereby producing T1-weighted and T2-weighted images, respectively.

- Each tissue displays a specific signal intensities on T1-weighted and T2-weighted images, allowing some degree of tissue characterization (Table 3-1 and Fig. 3-15).
- Using special techniques, the high signal from fat can be suppressed during scanning, thereby producing a fat-saturated image. This is especially useful for demonstrating marrow pathology on "fat-saturated"

TABLE 3-1 *Tissue Characterization on Magnetic Resonance Images*

Tissue	T1	T2
Fluid	Dark	Bright
Fat	Bright	Intermediate
Tendon/ligament	Dark	Dark
Air	Black	Black

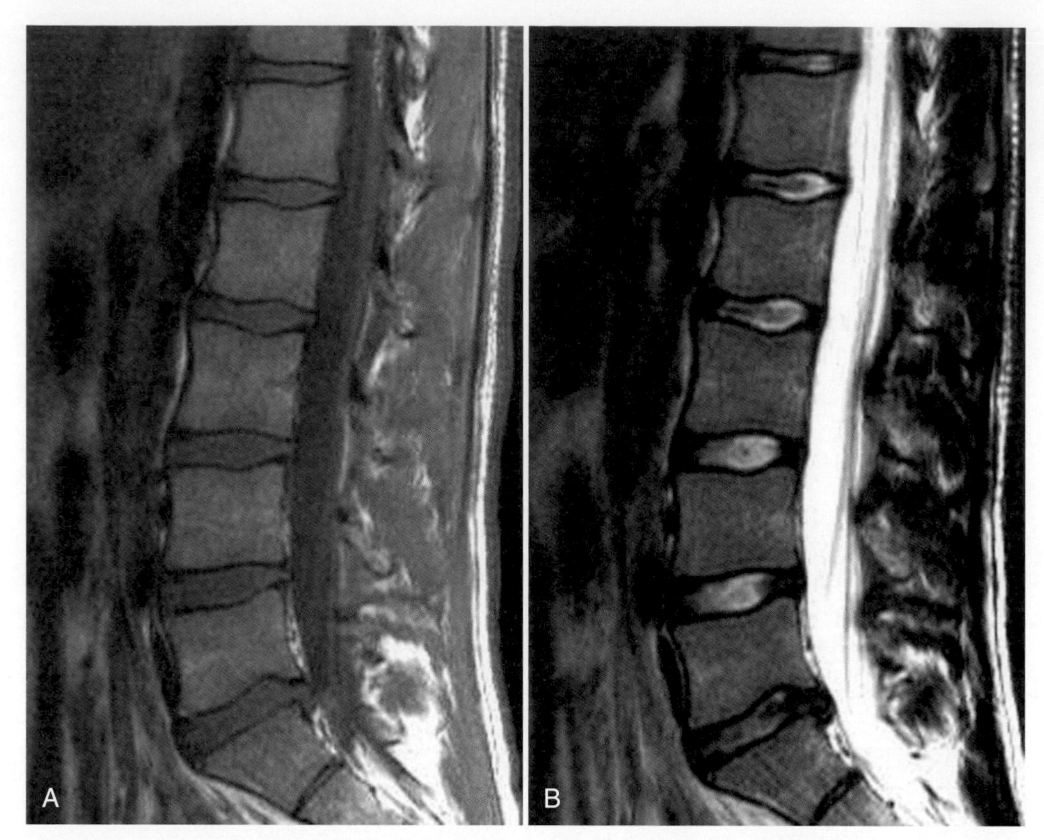

Figure 3-15 Magnetic resonance imaging: T1- and T2-weighted images. Sagittal T1-weighted (**A**) and T2-weighted (**B**) images of the lumbar spine illustrate the characteristic signal characteristics of fluid. Note the low signal intensity of the cerebrospinal fluid on the T1-weighted image and bright signal on the T2-weighted scan.

T2-weighted images, and areas of tissue enhancement after intravenous contrast administration on fat-saturated T1-weighted images (because gadolinium contrast results in increased T1 signal) (examples are shown in Figures 3-17, 3-18, and 3-20).

- Because of the strong magnetic field involved, contraindications to magnetic resonance imaging include the presence of a cardiac pacemaker, a metallic foreign body in the orbit, certain vascular aneurysm clips and cochlear implants, a metallic fragment (e.g., bullet) of unknown composition near a vital structure (e.g., spinal cord, heart), among other items. As a result, each patient should undergo a thorough screening process prior to scanning.

Strengths

- Images can be obtained in any plane and provide superb soft-tissue contrast, anatomic detail, and simultaneous demonstration of bones and soft tissues. As a result, it is the best single modality for evaluating most types of musculoskeletal pathology (Figs. 3-16 to 3-18).
- The most sensitive modality for detecting marrow pathology (neoplastic marrow infiltration, bone contusion, occult fracture, tumor) (Fig. 3-19)
- The test of choice for evaluating neurologic deficits related to spinal trauma or neoplasm
- Can be combined with gadolinium-based contrast agents injected either intravenously (to highlight tissues with increased vascularity) or directly into a joint (magnetic resonance arthrography) (Figs. 3-20 and 3-21)
- No ionizing radiation

Weaknesses

- Fractures of the posterior elements of the spine are difficult to detect with MRI.
- Assessment of fracture healing
- Hardware (depending on type, may produce severe artifact, obscuring adjacent tissues) (Fig. 3-22)

Imaging Algorithms

- Please see Figures 3-23 to 3-27.

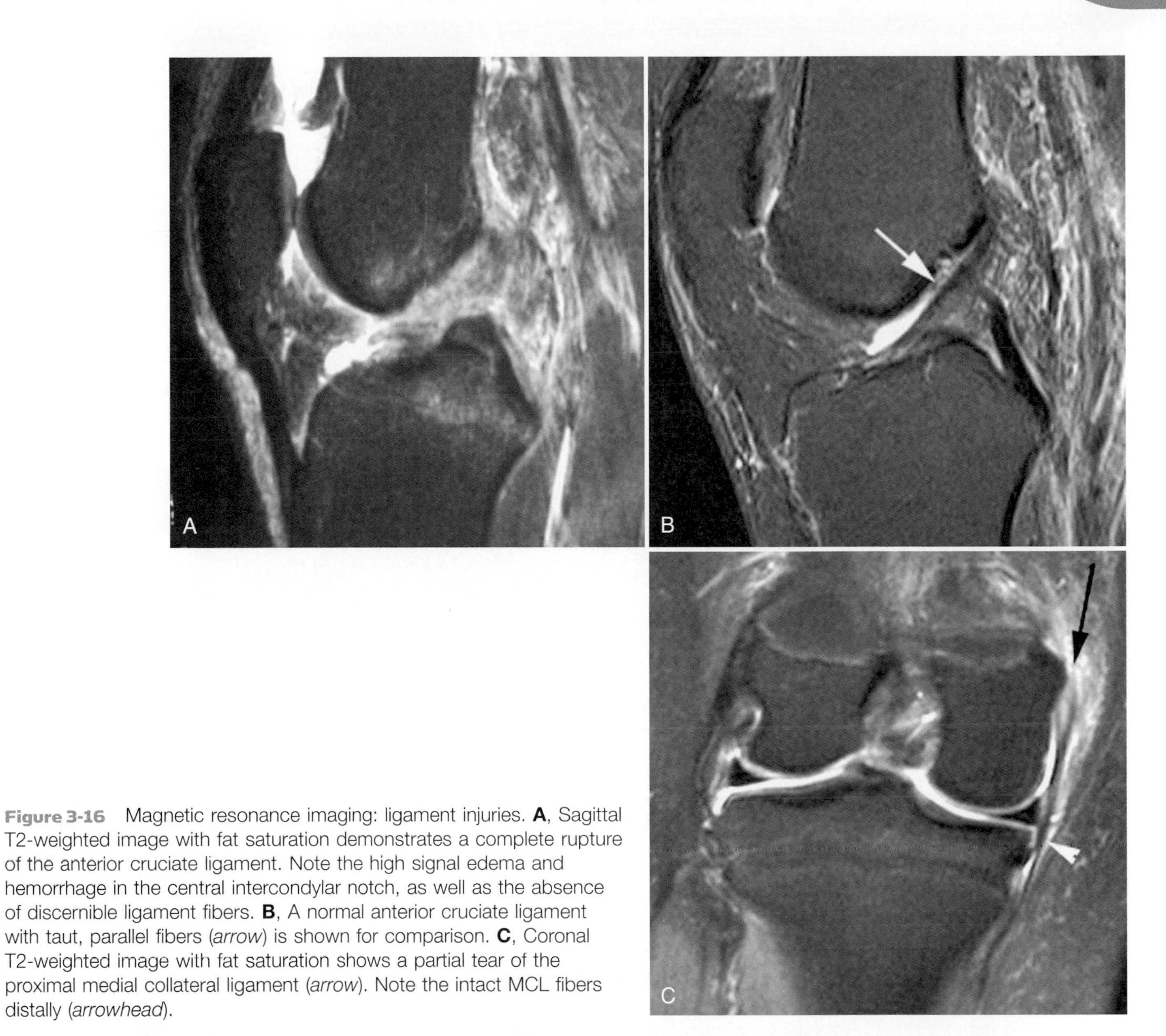

Figure 3-16 Magnetic resonance imaging: ligament injuries. **A**, Sagittal T2-weighted image with fat saturation demonstrates a complete rupture of the anterior cruciate ligament. Note the high signal edema and hemorrhage in the central intercondylar notch, as well as the absence of discernible ligament fibers. **B**, A normal anterior cruciate ligament with taut, parallel fibers (*arrow*) is shown for comparison. **C**, Coronal T2-weighted image with fat saturation shows a partial tear of the proximal medial collateral ligament (*arrow*). Note the intact MCL fibers distally (*arrowhead*).

Figure 3-17 Magnetic resonance imaging: bone tumor. **A**, Anteroposterior radiograph of the pelvis reveals subtle lucency in the right acetabulum (*arrow*) that could be potentially missed owing to the degree of diffuse osteopenia. Coronal T1-weighted (**B**) and

Continued

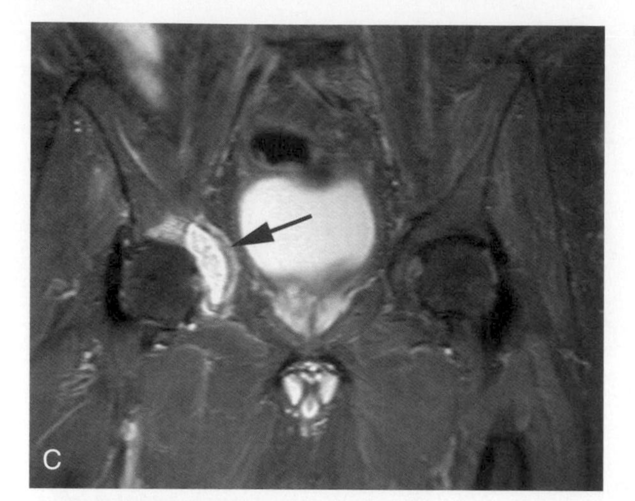

Figure 3-17, cont'd fat-saturated T2-weighted (**C**) images demonstrate the lesion to much better advantage (*arrows*).

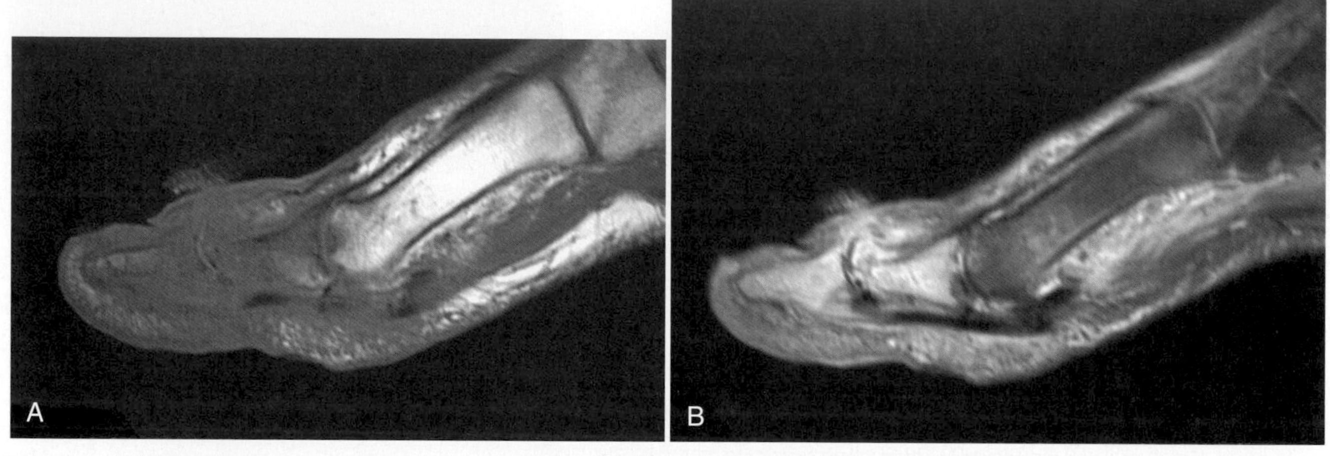

Figure 3-18 Magnetic resonance imaging: osteomyelitis. Sagittal T1-weighted (**A**) and T2-weighted (**B**) images of the foot reveal abnormal, fluid-like signal throughout the marrow of the proximal and distal phalanges of the great toe compatible with osteomyelitis in this diabetic patient who had an adjacent cutaneous ulcer.

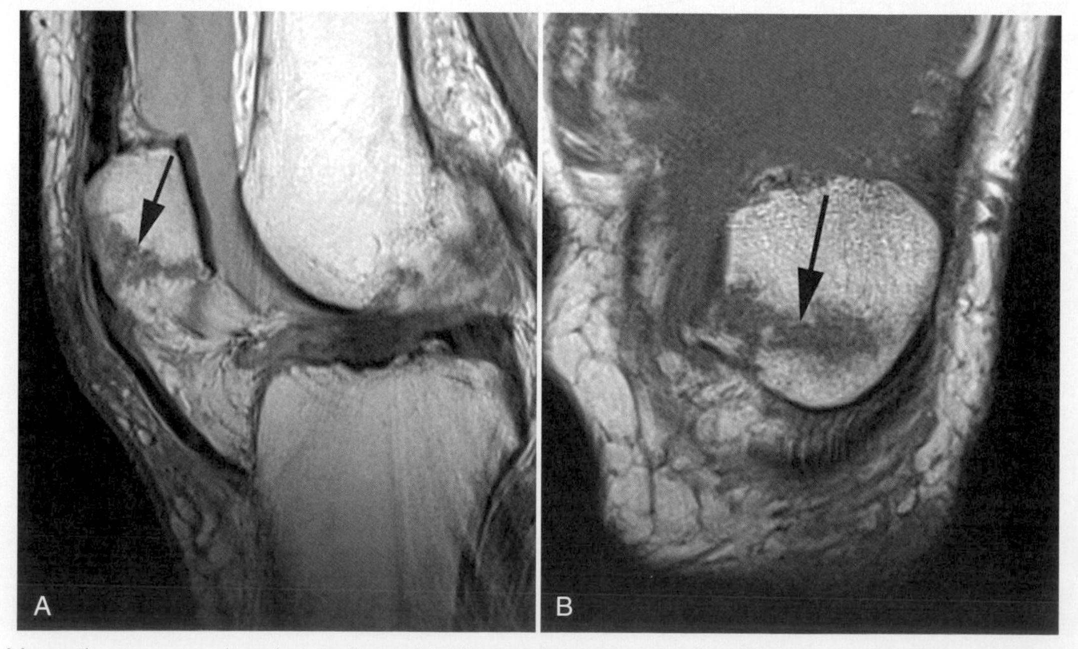

Figure 3-19 Magnetic resonance imaging: radiographically occult fracture. Sagittal (**A**) and coronal (**B**) T1-weighted images of the knee reveal a nondisplaced fracture in the lower pole of the patella (*arrows*). The fracture was not visible on radiographs. (This is the same patient as in Figure 3-1.)

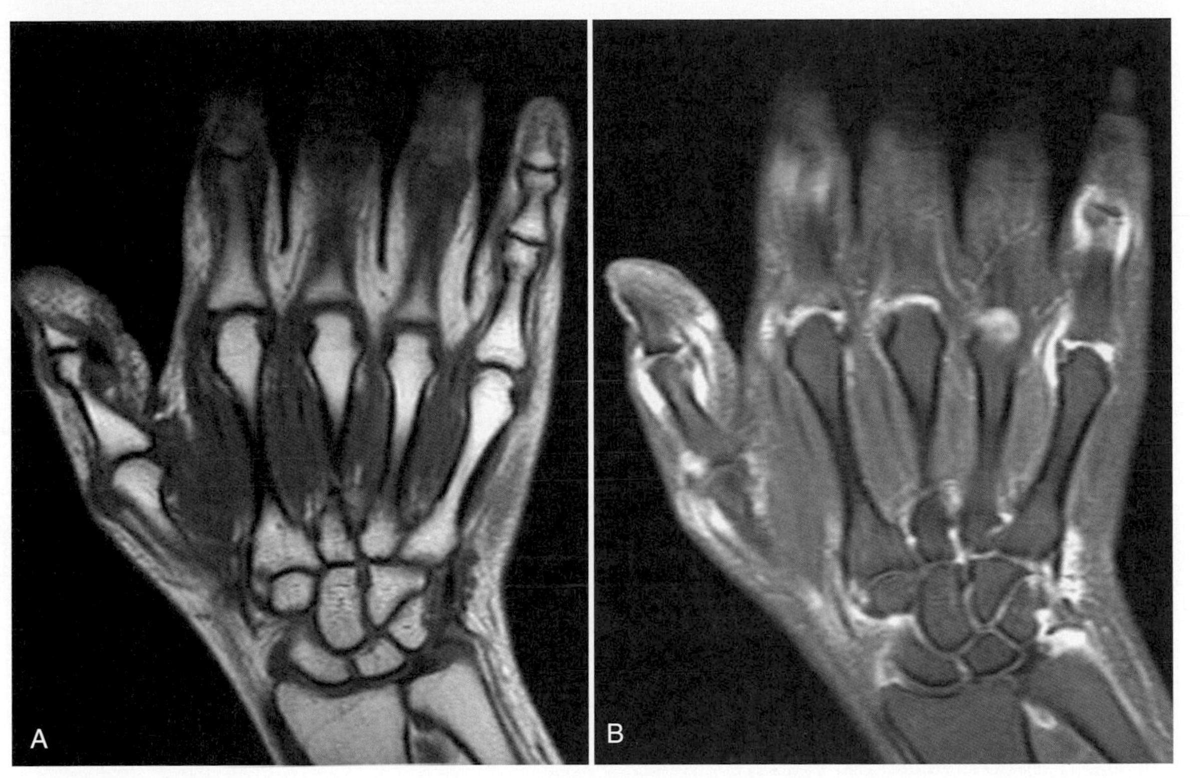

Figure 3-20 Magnetic resonance imaging: Use of intravenous contrast. **A**, Coronal T1-weighted image before intravenous contrast administration shows no abnormality. **B**, Coronal T1-weighted fat-saturated postcontrast image demonstrates prominent synovial enhancement throughout the joints of the hand and wrist, compatible with an inflammatory (rheumatoid) arthritis.

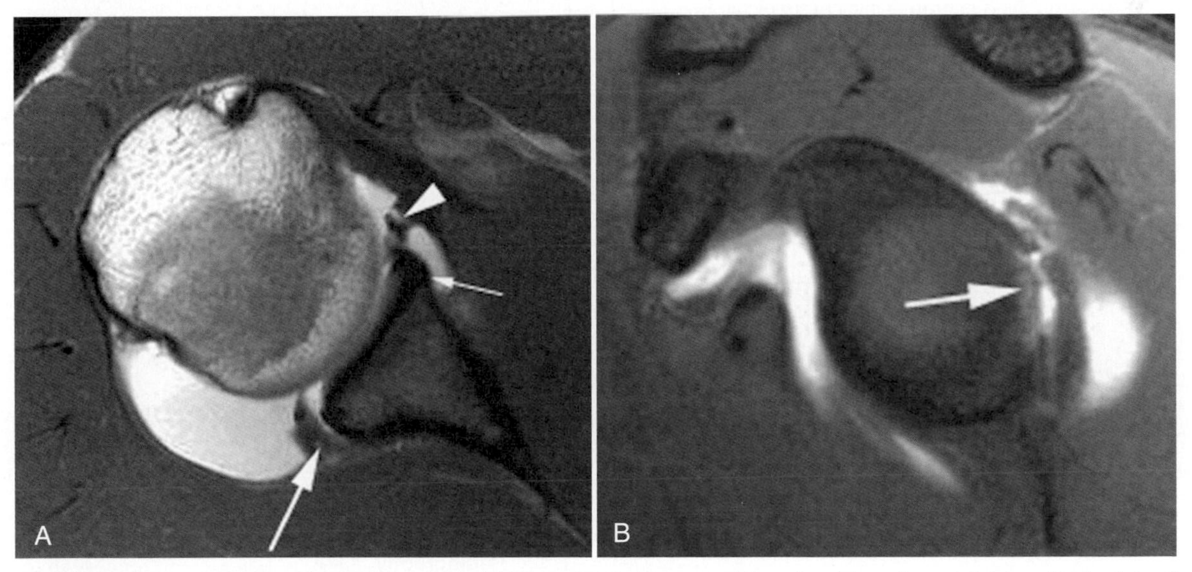

Figure 3-21 Magnetic resonance arthrography. **A**, Axial T1-weighted image of the shoulder after an intra-articular injection of a dilute gadolinium solution reveals a posterior labral tear (*large arrow*). Note also the normal labrum (*small arrow*) and middle glenohumeral ligament (*arrowhead*) anteriorly. **B**, Oblique sagittal T1-weighted image with fat saturation confirms the posterior labral tear (*arrow*).

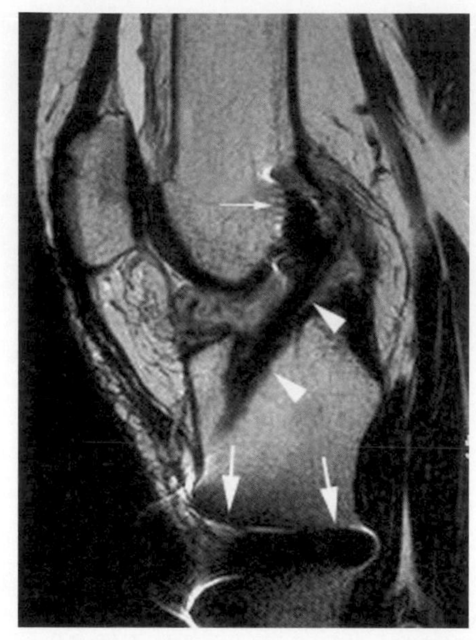

Figure 3-22 Magnetic resonance imaging: metal artifact. Sagittal T2-weighted image of the knee after anterior cruciate ligament reconstruction demonstrates the normal anterior cruciate ligament graft (*arrowheads*) as well as prominent low signal artifacts related to associated metal hardware (*arrows*). Note how these partially obscure and distort adjacent tissues.

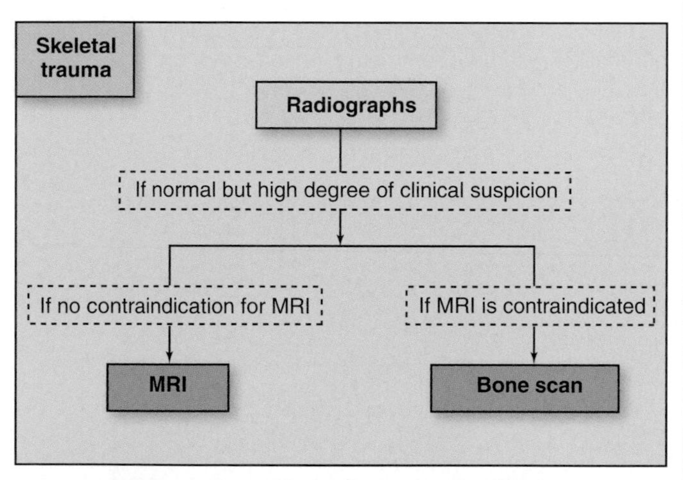

Figure 3-23 Skeletal trauma algorithm.

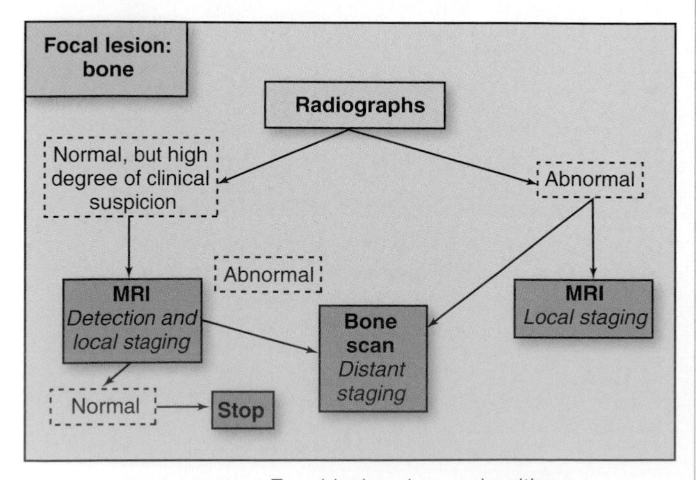

Figure 3-24 Focal lesion: bone algorithm.

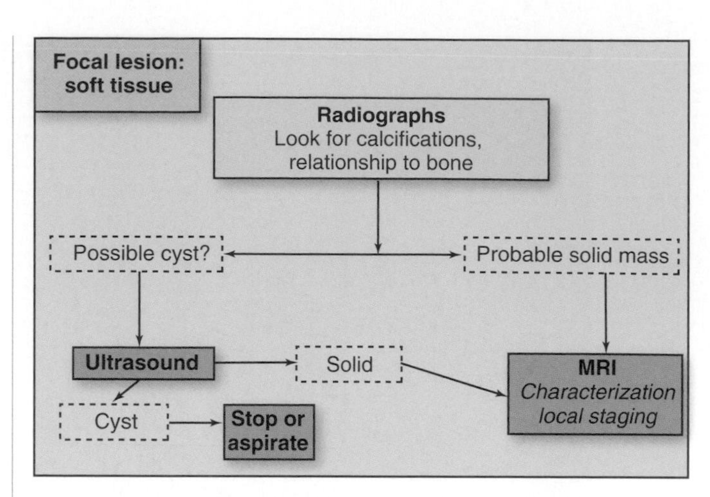

Figure 3-25 Focal lesion: soft-tissue algorithm.

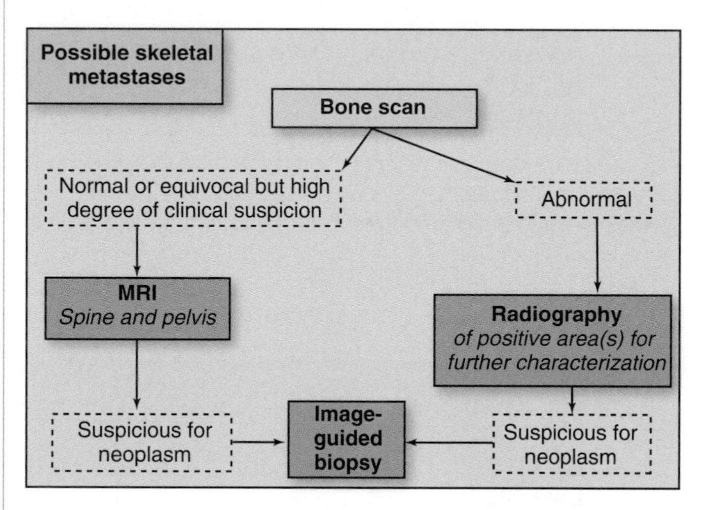

Figure 3-26 Possible skeletal metastases algorithm.

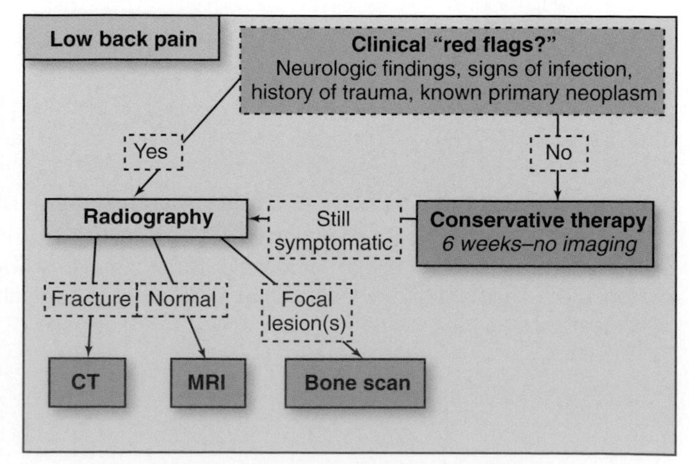

Figure 3-27 Low back pain algorithm.

Suggested Reading

- Ahn JM, El-Khoury GY: Role of magnetic resonance imaging in musculoskeletal trauma. Top Magn Reson Imaging 2007;18:155–168.
- Chaipat L, Palmer WE: Shoulder magnetic resonance imaging. Clin Sports Med 2006;25:371–386.
- Duet M, Pouchot J, Liote F, Faraggi M: Role for positron emission tomography in skeletal diseases. Joint Bone Spine 2007;74:14–23.
- Geijer M, El-Khoury GY: MDCT in the evaluation of skeletal trauma: Principles, protocols, and clinical applications. Emerg Radiol 2006;13:7–18.
- Ilaslan H, Sundaram M: Advances in musculoskeletal tumor imaging. Orthop Clin North Am 2006;37:375–391.
- Imhof H, Mang T: Advances in musculoskeletal radiology: Multidetector computed tomography. Orthop Clin North Am 2006;37:287–298.
- Khoury V, Cardinal E, Bureau NJ: Musculoskeletal sonography: A dynamic tool for usual and unusual disorders. AJR Am J Roentgenol 2007;188:W63–W73.
- Lalam RK, Cassar-Pullicino VN, Tins BJ: Magnetic resonance imaging of appendicular musculoskeletal infection. Top Magn Reson Imaging 2007;18:177–191.
- Love C, Din AS, Tomas MB, et al: Radionuclide bone imaging: An illustrative review. Radiographics 2003;23:341–358.
- Mhuircheartaigh NN, Kerr JM, Murray JG: MR imaging of traumatic spinal injuries. Semin Musculoskelet Radiol 2006;10:293–307.
- Papp DR, Khanna AJ, McCarthy EF, et al: Magnetic resonance imaging of soft-tissue tumors: Determinate and indeterminate lesions. J Bone Joint Surg Am 2007;89A(Suppl 3):103–115.
- Sanders TG, Miller MD: A systematic approach to magnetic resonance imaging interpretation of sports medicine injuries of the knee. Am J Sports Med 2005;33:131–148.
- Vande Berg B, Malghem J, Maldague B, Lecouvet F: Multi-detector CT imaging in the postoperative orthopedic patient with metal hardware. Eur J Radiol 2006;60:470–479.

Chapter 4 Sports Pharmacology

Mark Bouchard

Key Concepts

- Athletes commonly use medications for nutritional supplementation, pain relief, asthma, and contraception.
- Older athletes frequently have common medical conditions that require medications that may adversely affect performance.

Epidemiology

- Survey of Sydney Olympians (2000) about medication use: 78% took some form of medication in the previous 3 days. These included vitamins, 51%; nonsteroidal anti-inflammatory drugs, 26%; minerals, 21%; amino acids, 13%; alternative medications, 11%; oral contraceptives, 9%; and asthma medications, 5%. Twenty percent of athletes took five or more medications.
- This survey brought out concerns about inappropriate dosing of nonsteroidal anti-inflammatory drugs (the use of several concomitantly as well as too high and too low dosing regimens). Also, there was concern about the overuse of beta-agonists for asthma and the underuse of controller medications for asthma such as inhaled corticosteroids.

Analgesics

- Nonsteroidal anti-inflammatory drugs
  - For athletes, one of the most commonly used classes of medication: 25% of Olympic athletes (see previously), 75% of high school football players
  - Theoretic risk of healing delay in soft-tissue injuries
  - Fair evidence of healing delay in fractures
  - Renal dysfunction potentiated by dehydration leading to the risk of renal failure
  - Gastrointestinal bleeding: more than 20,000 deaths annually due to nonsteroidal anti-inflammatory drug use in the United States
  - Coronary thrombosis: Several cyclooxygenase-2 inhibitors were taken off the market due to increased rates of acute coronary events. Nonselective nonsteroidal anti-inflammatory drugs were also mentioned by the U.S. Food and Drug Administration as possibly aggravating symptoms in those athletes with asthma
  - No ergolytic effects noted
- Acetaminophen
  - No ergolytic effects noted
  - May be hepatotoxic at higher doses (>4 g/day), potentiated by alcohol
- Opioids
  - Decreased psychomotor performance due to prolonged reaction time and sedation
  - Constipation due to decreased gut motility
  - Addiction potential
  - Use banned by World Anti-Doping Agency (WADA)

Oral Contraceptives

- Used for treating amenorrhea, oligomenorrhea, and dysmenorrhea, and for contraception
- Concerns for female athletes include fluid retention, weight gain, nausea, headache, and risk of deep vein thrombosis
- Possibility of decrease in VO_{2max} (maximal oxygen consumption) in elite female athletes
  - Decrease of 4.7% in VO_{2max} in small study of triphasic oral contraceptives versus placebo (Lebrun and colleagues)
  - Decrease of 6% in VO_{2max} in study with low-dose oral contraceptive for oligomenorrheic athletes versus regularly menstruating athletes (Rickenlund and colleagues)
  - The cited studies were small, and larger studies are needed to confirm results.

Antibiotics

- May be overused in some athletic populations (i.e., National Football League study of St. Louis Rams concerning methicillin-resistant *Staphylococcus aureus* outbreak published in the *New England Journal of Medicine* in 2005)

- Sixty percent of players had taken antimicrobials during the previous year
- 2.6 antimicrobial prescriptions per player during preceding year was 10 times the national average
- Fluoroquinolones and tendon ruptures: many reported cases of tendon injury
  - Occurs more commonly with pefloxacin than ciprofloxacin, but seen with all fluoroquinolones
  - Achilles tendon rupture most common
  - Fifty percent of ruptures occurred within first 6 days of treatment
  - Rare event: 1 to 3 cases per 1000 patient-years

Stimulants/Sympathomimetics

- Stimulants: amphetamine, dextroamphetamine, methylphenidate
  - Commonly used by student athletes for attention-deficit/hyperactivity disorder
  - Stimulants are controversial in terms of performance enhancement.
  - Ergogenic effects include enhanced concentration, increased alertness, decreased pain, decreased fatigue, and increased aggression.
  - Concerns are due to decreased thermoregulation leading to increased risk of heatstroke and dehydration. Misuse is also associated with sudden death.
  - Addiction potential
  - Prohibited by WADA
- Sympathomimetics: phenylephrine, pseudoephedrine, synephrine
  - Side effects include tachycardia, palpitations, anxiety, insomnia, and possible predisposition to heat stress.
  - Monitored by WADA, but not prohibited
- Ephedrine alkaloids: banned in February 2004 by the U.S. Food and Drug Administration due to cases of acute myocardial infarction, stroke, heatstroke, and death

Antihistamines

- Commonly used in over-the-counter cold remedies, which include diphenhydramine, chlorpheniramine, loratadine, cetirizine, and fexofenadine
- Ergolytic effects include somnolence and decreased psychomotor performance.
- No known effects on strength and endurance
- Corticosteroid nasal sprays are more effective for allergic rhinitis and do not have the previously mentioned side effects.

Antihypertensives

- Hypertensive athletes should be screened for supplement use such as sympathomimetics, anabolic steroids, alcohol, and other recreational drugs.
- β-Blockers
  - Ergolytic
  - This class attenuates the heart rate and blood pressure response to exercise and decreases tidal volume, thus increasing respiratory rate. Thermoregulation and lipolysis are also impaired.
  - Nonselective β-blockers are more ergolytic than β_1-selective agents. In one study, 25 runners underwent three separate 10-km time trials. The results were 36 minutes with placebo, 39 minutes with atenolol, and 41 minutes with propranolol.
  - Impairment increases with the fitness of the athlete. Elite athletes may experience as much as a 15% decrease in $\dot{V}O_{2max}$.
  - No known effect on strength training
  - Banned by WADA in several sports including shooting sports, wrestling, skiing/snowboarding, and sailing
- Calcium channel blockers: diltiazem and verapamil
  - Ergolytic
  - Decrease the heart rate response to exercise
  - May decrease myocardial contractility
- α-Blockers
  - Probably ergolytic
  - Decrease peripheral vascular resistance, which can lead to orthostatic hypotension and reflex tachycardia
- Angiotensin-converting enzyme inhibitors and angiotensin receptor blockers
  - First-line agents to treat hypertension in competitive athletes
  - Minimal cardiac effects
  - May potentiate hyperkalemia and renal insufficiency
- Diuretics
  - Potassium depletion leading to arrhythmias
  - Transient decrease in plasma volume, which may predispose to hypovolemia and increased risk of heat illness
  - Many are banned by WADA due to their use as masking agents in drug screening.

World Anti-Doping Agency

- The WADA Web site (www.wada-ama.org/en) has the latest list of prohibited drugs and therapeutic use exemption forms.

Doctors are men who prescribe medicines of which they know little, to cure diseases of which they know less, in human beings of whom they know nothing.

Voltaire

Suggested Reading

- Anderson RL, Wilmore JH, Joyner MJ, et al: Effects of cardio-selective and nonselective beta-adrenergic blockade on the performance of highly trained runners. Am J Cardiol 1985;55: 149D–150D.
- Armstrong LE, Costill DL, Fink WJ: Influence of diuretic-induced dehydration on competitive running performance. Med Sci Sports Exerc 1985;17:456–461.
- Chick TW, Halperin AD, Gacek EM: The effect of antihypertensive medications on exercise performance: A review. Med Sci Sports Exerc 1988;20:447–454.
- Ciocca M: Medication and supplement use by athletes. Clin Sports Med 2005;24:719–738.
- Corrigan B, Kazlauskas R: Medication use in athletes selected for doping control at the Sydney Olympics (2000). Clin J Sport Med 2003;13:33–40.
- Eichner R: Ergolytic drugs in medicine and sports. Am J Med 1993;94:205–211.
- Lebrun CM, Petit MA, McKenzie DC, et al: Decreased maximal aerobic capacity with use of a triphasic oral contraceptive in highly active women: A randomized controlled trial. Br J Sports Med 2003;37:315–320.
- Rickenlund A, Carlström K, Ekblom B, et al: Effects of oral contraceptives on body composition and physical performance in female athletes. J Clin Endocrinol Metab 2004;89:4364–4370.

Chapter 5 Impairment and Disability

Lucien Parrillo and William Dexter

General Considerations

- Workers' compensation is a system of social insurance that provides some form of entitlement to workers in the event of an occupational injury.
- These laws are the result of a historic compromise in which the employee gives up the right to sue his or her employer for negligence in exchange for the employer's agreement to pay the cost of medical care and to compensate the worker for time lost from work.
- To be compensable, an injury must usually "arise out of and in the course of employment." A work injury that activates or aggravates a preexisting condition is also compensable.
- Although workers' compensation in most countries is embedded in their social security system, the United States is unique in that workers' compensation has essentially no link with the Social Security system.

Impairment versus Disability

- Impairment is a rating of anatomic and/or functional loss.
- Physicians may be asked to assess the degree of impairment using the most current American Medical Association *Guides to the Evaluation of Permanent Impairment* (Fig. 5-1).
- Using this rating, nonmedical professionals determine the level of disability.
- Disability, unlike impairment, depends on the job tasks and one's ability to compete in the open job market. For example, the loss of a distal phalanx results in the same impairment rating in a concert pianist and in a plumber, but the disability is much greater for the musician.
- Thus, impairment does not always imply disability, and, as a result, it is important to realize that these concepts are separate entities.
- Insurers may request physicians to provide work restrictions (i.e., no overhead lifting for someone with rotator cuff tendonitis) in order to match impairment to a specific job.
- In some situations, exact physical capabilities/restrictions are best determined by a detailed analysis called a functional capacity evaluation.
- Functional capacity evaluations are completed by occupational medicine physicians or physical therapists and focus on patients' bodily movements specific to their job tasks and their ability to perform these duties adequately.
- If a workers' compensation dispute results in litigation, an unbiased physician may be asked to evaluate the worker, acting as an independent medical examiner.
- The independent medical examiner's judgment is usually the final opinion for the worker and often determines the outcome of the claim. The independent medical examiner's evaluation is usually a single visit, and he or she does not assume any responsibility for medical care of the worker.
- The independent medical examiner's report includes an exhaustive history and physical examination and lists the diagnosis, cause of injury, prognosis, maximal medical improvement status, impairment rating, and work capacity and an opinion on clinical management.

Disability Classification

- Most injuries in the workplace involve the musculoskeletal system and are the result of traumatic events, repetitive-motion disorders, or other ergonomic factors.
- Payment benefits awarded to workers or their families are based on the degree and duration of the disability and are divided into six categories.

Permanent Total Disability

These workers are so disabled that they will never be able to perform any work duties in any capacity for the rest of their lives.

- Most states compensate these workers with approximately 85% to 90% of their average take-home wages.

- Although few states limit the duration of payments, most provide compensation for the rest of the injured worker's life.
- Some states may also provide additional funds for the employee's dependents.

Temporary Total Disability

This category encompasses the greatest number of workers. These individuals are expected to recover with proper treatment but are unable to work for an unspecified length of time. Figure 5-2 depicts a graph showing the percentage of workers who return to work for every week that they are away from work.

- Although minimal and maximal limits apply, as much as two thirds of gross or 80% of take-home wages is awarded to the worker until he or she is able to return to work or reaches maximal medical improvement.
- Instilled in this type of compensation is a mandatory waiting period, and compensation is paid retroactively if they are unable to work for a known number of days.
    - This waiting period is designed as an incentive to return to work after less severe injuries.

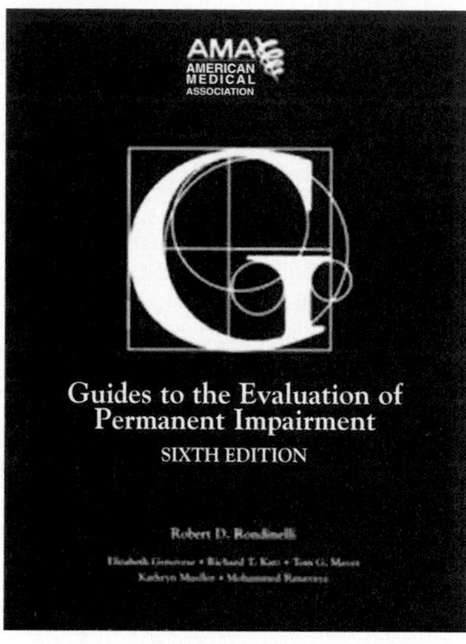

Figure 5-1 The sixth edition of the *AMA Guides to the Evaluation of Permanent Impairment*. Chicago: American Medical Association Press, 2008.

Permanent Partial Disability

These workers have lost some ability to compete in the open job market and are compensated for losses in future earnings.

- The types of injuries compensated fall into two categories: scheduled injuries (e.g., loss of a limb, loss of an eye) or nonscheduled injuries (e.g., low back injury or carpal tunnel syndrome).
- Scheduled injuries are compensated according to a fixed schedule that varies from state to state, and payment is provided for a specified length of time.
- Nonscheduled injuries are compensated weekly based on a wage loss replacement percentage. This figure is derived from the difference between wages earned before and after injury. However, some states reward nonscheduled permanent partial disability as a percentage of the total disability benefits.

Temporary Partial Disability

This category consists of workers who are injured to a degree that they are unable to perform their usual duties, but are still capable of working at some job during their treatment.

- The injured worker is compensated for the difference between wages earned before the injury and those earned while disabled, usually at 70% of the difference.

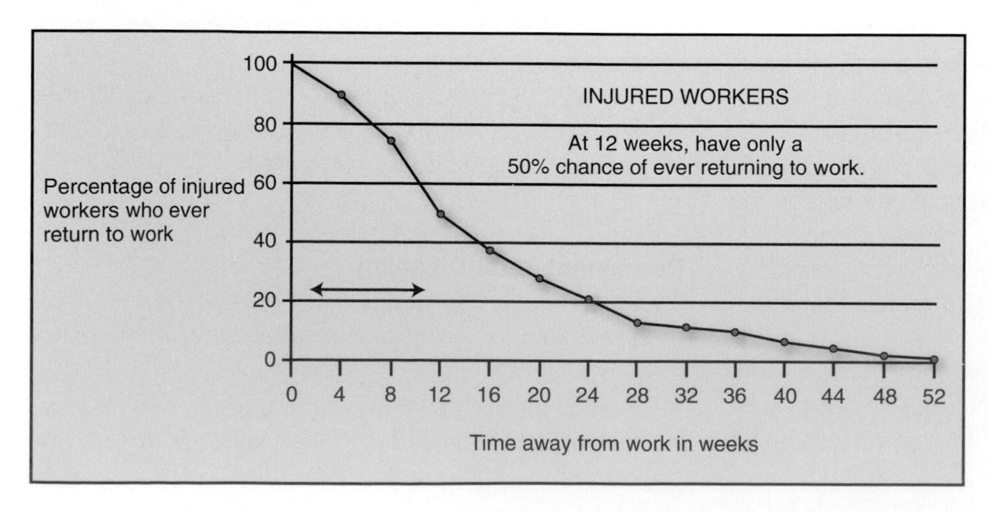

Figure 5-2 Graph showing the percentage of workers who return to work for every week that they are away from work. (Adapted from LaDou J [ed]: Current Occupational & Environmental Medicine, 4th ed. New York: McGraw-Hill Medical, 2007.)

Vocational Rehabilitation Benefits

Some level of rehabilitation, be it physical or psychological, is provided to return the injured worker to gainful employment.

Survivors' Benefits

Dependent survivors of employees killed on the job are paid death benefits under workers' compensation. The method/size of payment varies widely from state to state.

Suggested Reading

- Bernacki EJ: Factors influencing the costs of workers' compensation. Clin Occup Environ Med 2004;4:v–vi, 249–257.
- Harris I, Mulford J, Solomon M, et al: Association between compensation status and outcome after surgery. JAMA 2005;293:1644.
- LaDou J (ed): Current Occupational & Environmental Medicine, 4th ed. New York: McGraw-Hill Medical, 2007.
- Wind H, Gouttebarge V, Kuijer PP, Frings-Dresen MH: Assessment of functional capacity of the musculoskeletal system in the context of work, daily living, and sport: A systematic review. J Occup Rehabil 2005;15:253–272.
- Wind H, Gouttebarge V, Kuijer PP, et al: The utility of functional capacity evaluation. Int Arch Occup Environ Health 2006;79:528–534.

Chapter 6 Rehabilitation

Jeffrey G. Jenkins

Key Concepts

- Within a medical context, rehabilitation can be defined as a process by which the patient strives to achieve his or her full physical, social, and vocational potential.
- A formal medical rehabilitation program is most commonly employed after an individual has experienced a loss of function due to an injury or disease process or as a side effect of necessary medical treatment (e.g., surgery).
- For rehabilitation to be successful, it is crucial that the patient, physician, and therapist(s) involved in the case share the same clearly defined functional goals; treatment will be directed toward the achievement of these goals.
- Although medical professionals provide direction and guidance during rehabilitation, the patient plays the most important active role in the program.
- The patient also needs to give frequent feedback regarding effectiveness of interventions and any detrimental effects of treatment so that the rehabilitation plan and functional goals can be modified as needed throughout the rehabilitation process.
- Therapeutic exercise, physical modalities, and orthotic devices are the main components of a medical rehabilitation program for patients with musculoskeletal dysfunction.
- Physical therapists are trained to identify, assess, and work with the patient to alleviate acute or prolonged movement dysfunction. Most physical therapists employ a combination of therapeutic exercise, physical modalities, manual manipulation, and massage to achieve the treatment goals.
- Occupational therapists are trained to identify, assess, and work with the patient to alleviate functional deficits in the areas of self-care, vocational, and avocational activities.

Therapeutic Exercise

- In most cases, therapeutic exercise should be taught and supervised, particularly during early stages, by a physical therapist.
- Occupational therapists are specifically trained to supervise exercises directly related to self-care, vocational, and avocational activities and are appropriate to refer to in these cases.
- Major categories of exercise include muscle strengthening (strength training), range of motion (flexibility), and neuromuscular facilitation.

Strength Training

- Both high-resistance/low-repetition and low-resistance/high-repetition techniques exist and can be effective.
- High-resistance techniques are generally considered more effective and efficient in building strength.
- Low-resistance techniques are useful during injury or when training for highly repetitive tasks.
- The most important factor in increasing strength in either case is to exercise muscle to the point of fatigue.
- Observed effects of strength training occur primarily due to neuromuscular adaptations, specifically, improvement in the efficiency of neural recruitment of large motor units.
- Additional increases in muscle strength result from muscle hypertrophy, an actual enlargement of total muscle mass and cross-sectional area.

Flexibility Training

- Flexibility generally describes the range of motion present in a joint or group of joints that allows normal and unimpaired function.
- Flexibility can be defined as the total achievable excursion (within limits of pain) of a body part through its range of motion.
- Flexibility training is an important aspect of most therapeutic exercise regimens.
- Flexibility training seeks to achieve a maximal functional range of motion and is most typically accomplished by stretching.
- Three categories of stretching exercises have been employed

- Passive stretching
  - Employs a therapist or other partner who applies a stretch to a relaxed joint or limb
  - Requires excellent communication and slow, sensitive application of force
  - Very efficient means of flexibility training
  - Should be performed in the training room or in a physical or occupational therapy context
  - Potentially increases risk of injury when performed without due caution
- Static stretching
  - A steady force for a period of 15 to 60 seconds is applied.
  - Easiest and safest type of stretching
  - Associated with decreased muscle soreness after exercise
- Ballistic stretching
  - Employs the repetitive, rapid application of force in a bouncing or jerking maneuver
  - Momentum carries the body part through the range of motion until muscles are stretched to their limits.
  - Less efficient than other techniques because muscle contracts during these conditions to protect from overstretching
  - A rapid increase in force can cause injury.
  - This type of stretching has been largely abandoned as a training technique.

Neuromuscular Facilitation

- Seeks to improve function through improved efficiency of the interplay between the nervous and musculoskeletal systems
- Neuromuscular facilitation techniques in flexibility training
  - Isometric or concentric contraction of the musculotendinous unit followed by a passive or static stretch
  - Prestretch contraction of muscle facilitates relaxation and flexibility.
  - Examples include hold-relax and contract-relax techniques.

Plyometrics

- Performance of brief explosive maneuvers consisting of an eccentric muscle contraction followed immediately by a concentric contraction
- This technique is primarily employed in the training of athletes.
- Example: depth jumps from boxes
- Should be approached with caution under the supervision of a trained therapist and begun at an elementary level
- Some studies demonstrate a decreased risk of serious injury during sports activity among athletes who receive plyometric training (e.g., reduction in the incidence of knee injuries in female athletes participating in a jump training program).

Proprioception

- Background
  - Proprioceptive deficits have been shown to result from and predispose to injury.
  - Impairment of joint proprioception is believed to influence the progressive joint deterioration associated with both rheumatoid arthritis and osteoarthritis.
  - Proprioceptive exercises seek to improve joint position sense and thereby prevent injury.
  - For example, a tilt or wobble board is commonly employed after ankle ligamentous injury to reduce the incidence of recurrence.

Exercise Prescription

- A prescription for therapeutic exercise with a therapist should always include the following components
  - Diagnosis
  - Frequency of treatment (i.e., number of sessions per week)
  - Specific exercises required
  - Precautions (includes restrictions on weight bearing and limb movement, as well as identification of significant tissue damage or other factors that may interfere with performance of specific exercises)
  - Contraindicated exercises or modalities (should include any specific motions, positions, or modalities that should be avoided to ensure appropriate tissue healing and patient safety without incurring further injury)
- Ideally, individual exercises are further defined by
  - Mode: specific type of exercise (e.g., closed chain quadriceps strengthening)
  - Intensity: relative physiologic difficulty of the exercise (this is often best described in terms of the patient's rating of perceived exertion, ranging from very light to very hard)
  - Duration: length of an exercise session
  - Frequency: number of sessions per day/week
  - Progression: increase in activity expected over the course of training

Modalities: Heat, Cold, Pressure, Electricity

- Physical agents: use of physical forces to produce beneficial therapeutic effects

Heat

Superficial Heat Application

- Hot packs (hydrocollator)
  - Transfer of heat energy by conduction
  - Application: Silicate gel in a canvas cover
  - When not in use, these packs are kept in thermostatically controlled water baths at 70°C to 80°C.
  - Used in terry cloth insulating covers or with towels placed between the pack and the patient for periods of 20 to 30 minutes
  - Advantages: low cost, easy use, long life, and patient acceptance
  - Disadvantages: difficult to apply to curved surfaces
  - Safety: One should never lie on top on the pack, as it is more likely to cause burns. Towels should be applied between the skin and the hydrocollator pack.
- Heat lamps
  - Heat primarily by the conversion of radiant energy to heat (i.e., the direct application of photons to living tissue leading to heat production)
  - Application: simple to use but requires some attention to avoid injuries or burns
  - In practice, therapeutic temperatures are usually obtained when the heat sources are approximately 50 cm from the skin.
  - Long-term use may produce a permanent brownish discoloration.
- Paraffin baths
  - Heat primarily by conduction: liquid mixture of paraffin wax and mineral oil
  - Helpful in the treatment of scars and hand contractures
  - Temperatures (52°C to 54°C) are higher than those of hydrotherapy (<40°C to 45°C) but are tolerated well due to the low heat capacity of the paraffin/mineral oil mixture and a lack of convection.
  - Treatments may include dipping, immersion, or, occasionally, brushing onto the area of treatment.
  - Safety: Burns are the main safety concern with paraffin treatment.
  - Visual inspection is important: The paraffin bath should have a thin film of white paraffin on its surface or an edging around the reservoir.

Diathermy (Deep Heating)

- Deep heating agents (diathermies) raise tissue to therapeutic temperatures at a depth of 3.5 to 7 cm.
  - Use for analgesic effects, decreasing muscle spasms, enhancing local blood flow, increasing collagen extensibility
- Deep heating modality: ultrasound (US)
  - US is defined as sound waves at a frequency above the threshold of human hearing (frequencies > 20 kHz). US uses sound waves to heat tissues. A wide range of frequencies are potentially useful, but in the United States, most machines operate between 0.8 and 1 MHz.
  - US penetrates soft tissue well and bone poorly; the most intense heating occurs at the bone–soft tissue interface.
  - Treatments are relatively brief (7 to 10 minutes) and demand the constant attention of the therapist/technician.
  - The typical intensity for application is 0.8 to 1.5 W/cm^2.
  - US indications
    - — Tendonitis and bursitis
    - — Muscle pain and overuse
    - — Contractures
    - — Inflammation and trauma
    - — Scars and keloids
    - — Fractures: Low-intensity US (e.g., 30 mW/cm^2) accelerates bone healing and is approved by the U.S. Food and Drug Administration for the treatment of some fractures.
  - The relative effectiveness of US treatment over that of other conventional approaches is unknown.
  - US is typically avoided in the acute stages of an injury due to concerns that it may aggravate bleeding, tissue damage, and swelling.
  - Phonophoresis
    - — US may be used to deliver medication into tissues. The active substance is mixed into a coupling medium, and US is used to drive (phonophorese) the material through the skin.
    - — Corticosteroids and local anesthetics are most frequently used in the treatment of musculoskeletal conditions.
    - — Results of clinical studies are conflicting.

- US contraindications
  - Fluid-filled areas (i.e., eye and the pregnant uterus)
  - Growth plates
  - Inflamed joints
  - Acute hemorrhages
  - Ischemic tissue
  - Tumor
  - Laminectomy site
  - Infection
  - Implanted devices such as pacemakers and pumps
  - US is relatively contraindicated near metal plates or cemented artificial joints because the effects of localized heating or mechanical forces on prosthesis–cement interfaces are not well known.

Therapeutic Cold

- Sometimes referred to as cryotherapy
- Superficial only
- Used for analgesic effects, reduction of muscle spasm, decreasing inflammation, decreasing muscle spasticity/hyperactivity, vasoconstriction (reduction in local blood flow and associated edema)
- Ice massage used for treatment of localized, intense musculoskeletal pain (e.g., lateral epicondylitis)
- General indications
  - Acute musculoskeletal trauma
  - Pain
  - Muscle spasm
  - Spasticity
  - Reduction of metabolic activity
- General contraindications and precautions
  - Ischemia
  - Insensitivity
  - Cold intolerance
  - Raynaud's phenomenon and disease
  - Severe cold pressor responses
  - Cold allergy
- Methods of application
  - Ice packs and compression wraps are most common.
  - Sessions typically last 20 to 30 minutes.
  - Ice massage is a vigorous approach suitable for limited portions of the body. A piece of ice is rubbed over the painful area for 7 to 10 minutes.
  - Iced whirlpools cool large areas vigorously.
  - Vapocoolant and liquid nitrogen sprays produce large (as much as 20°C), rapid decreases in skin temperature and are used at times to produce superficial analgesia as well as in spray and stretch treatments.
- Trauma application
  - Cooling applied soon after trauma may decrease edema, metabolic activity, blood flow, compartmental pressures, and tissue damage and accelerate healing.
  - Rest, ice, compression, and elevation are the mainstays of treatment.
  - Cyclic ice application is often recommended (e.g., 20 minutes on, 10 minutes off or 30 minutes on, 2 hours off) for 6 to 24 hours.
- Contrast baths
  - Two water-filled reservoirs, warm (43°C) and cool (16°C); alternate soaks; duration varies according to treatment protocol
  - Used for desensitization and vasogenic reflex effects
  - Mostly used on hands or feet; typical indications include rheumatoid arthritis and sympathetically mediated pain (reflex sympathetic dystrophy)

Traction

- Technique used to stretch soft tissues and to separate joint surfaces or bone fragments by the use of a pulling force
- Based on available medical evidence, therapeutic use of spinal traction is generally limited to the cervical spine.
- The efficacy of lumbar traction is controversial.
- Traction has been shown to lengthen the cervical spine by 2 to 20 mm.
- Decreases muscle spasm, possibly by inducing fatigue in the paravertebral musculature
- May decrease neuroforaminal narrowing and associated radicular pain
- The patient should be positioned in 20 to 30 degrees of cervical flexion during traction to optimize the effect on the neural foramina.
- Therapeutic benefit is usually obtained with 25 pounds of traction (this includes the 10 pounds required to counterbalance the weight of the head).
- The duration of a treatment session is typically 20 minutes.
- The best results are obtained when a trained therapist administers manual traction in a controlled setting.
- Home cervical traction devices can be used (these typically employ a pulley system over a door, and a bag filled with ≥20 pounds of sand or water).
- Home cervical traction devices should not be used without previous training and observation by a trained therapist or physician.

- Heat (hot packs) is helpful in decreasing muscle contraction and maximizing the benefit of treatment.
- Contraindications
  - Cervical ligamentous instability resulting from rheumatoid arthritis, achondroplastic dwarfism, Marfan syndrome, or previous trauma
  - Documented or suspected tumor in the vicinity of the spine
  - Infectious process in the spine
  - Spinal osteopenia
  - Pregnancy
- Cervical spinal traction should not be administered with the neck in extension, particularly in patients with a history of vertebrobasilar insufficiency.

Therapeutic Massage

- Causes therapeutic soft-tissue changes as a direct result of the manual forces exerted on the patient by a trained therapist
- Specific techniques can be helpful for musculoskeletal patients
  - Deep friction massage
    - Used to prevent and break up adhesions after muscle injury
    - Friction is applied transversely across muscle fibers or tendons
  - Soft-tissue mobilization
    - Forceful massage performed with the fascia and muscle in a lengthened position
    - Effective as an adjunct to passive stretching in the treatment and prevention of contractures
  - Myofascial release
    - Applies prolonged light pressure specifically oriented with regard to fascial planes
    - Typically combined with passive range of motion techniques to stretch focal areas of muscle or fascial tightness
- Contraindications
  - Should not be performed over malignancies, open wounds, thrombophlebitis, or infected tissues

Electricity

- Transcutaneous electrical nerve stimulation is the most common treatment.
  - Most common direct therapeutic application of electrical current
  - Used for its analgesic properties
  - The unit uses superficial skin electrodes to apply small electrical currents to the body.
  - Theorized to provide analgesia via the gate control theory of pain, in which stimulation of large myelinated afferent nerve fibers blocks the transmission of pain signals by small, unmyelinated fibers (C, A delta) at the spinal cord level
  - Signal amplitudes generally do not exceed 100 mA.
  - With initiation of treatment, transcutaneous electrical nerve stimulation use is typically taught and monitored by a physical therapist. Once the patient is competent and confident in using the device (electrode placement, stimulator settings, duration of treatments), the unit can be used independently, outside the medical or therapy setting.
  - Common indications include posttraumatic/postsurgical pain, diabetic neuropathic pain, chronic musculoskeletal pain, peripheral nerve injury, sympathetically mediated pain/reflex sympathetic dystrophy, and phantom limb pain.
- Iontophoresis
  - Uses electrical fields to drive therapeutic agents through the skin into underlying soft tissue
  - Treatments in the musculoskeletal patient population typically employ anti-inflammatory agents and/or local anesthetics.
  - Conditions commonly treated include plantar fasciitis, tendinitis, and bursitis.
  - Most physical therapists are trained in this technique, although not all have access to the necessary equipment.
  - It is worth noting that, in most cases, injection enables a more efficient delivery of a greater concentration of the therapeutic agent in question.
- Electrical stimulation
  - At higher intensities than those used in transcutaneous electrical nerve stimulation, electrical stimulation can be used to maintain muscle bulk and strength.
  - This technique can be useful for immobilized limbs and for paretic muscles after nerve injury.
  - Evidence does not suggest, however, that electrical stimulation can strengthen otherwise healthy muscle.
  - Relative contraindications to electrical stimulation include demand cardiac pacemakers, congestive heart failure, pregnancy, skin sensitivity to electrodes, and actively healing wounds near the stimulation site. Stimulation over the carotid sinus is also highly discouraged due to the propensity for vagal response.

Orthoses

- An orthosis is an external device that is worn to restrict or assist movement. Examples include braces and splints.

- Orthoses are typically prescribed and used for one or more of the following reasons
  - To rest the body part: reduce inflammation, prevent further injury
  - To prevent contracture: minimize loss of range of motion in a joint or limb
  - To correct deformity: typically in conjunction with therapy or surgery
  - To promote exercise: encourage strengthening of certain muscles and/or correct muscle imbalances
  - To substitute for lost function
- Orthoses can be subdivided into static and dynamic devices.
  - Static orthoses keep underlying body parts from moving, thereby encouraging rest and healing while preventing or minimizing deformity.
  - Dynamic orthoses have internal or external power sources that encourage restoration and/or control of joint movements.
- Orthoses are named for the body parts that they incorporate, for example, ankle-foot orthosis and wrist-hand orthosis.
- Prescriptions for orthotics should include the type (defined by incorporated limb segments/body parts) and a static/dynamic classification. If a dynamic orthosis is to be used, the prescription should specifically identify the motion(s) to be assisted or inhibited.
- Prefabricated, off-the-shelf orthotics can be effectively employed in the treatment of most orthopaedic injuries. Frequently encountered examples include knee and ankle braces prescribed for ligamentous injury or wrist splints used by patients with carpal tunnel syndrome.
- In special populations (examples include hand trauma, nerve injury, partial limb loss, severe deformity), orthoses should be custom fitted by an orthotist or an appropriately trained occupational therapist.
- Orthotic use should generally be restricted to injured or dysfunctional limbs. Prophylactic bracing of joints is a controversial subject.
- Indications for orthoses include
  - Trauma (e.g., fracture, joint sprain)
  - Surgery (e.g., tendon repair, joint reconstruction)
  - Nerve injury
  - Painful disorders (e.g., rheumatoid arthritis, carpal tunnel syndrome)
- Orthoses and sports
  - There is no compelling evidence in the literature to support the use of prophylactic knee bracing in football players. In fact, both the American Academy of Pediatrics and the American Academy of Orthopaedic Surgeons have advised against the routine use of prophylactic knee bracing in football, in part due to data that actually showed an increase in anterior cruciate ligament injuries in brace wearers.
  - There is some evidence that use of a semirigid ankle orthosis can decrease the risk of ligamentous injury in athletes, particularly those with a history of sprain.

When to Refer

- To a significant extent, the primary physician's own personal comfort level in managing a rehabilitation program determines the need for referral. However, some indications for referral include
  - Patient's inability to progress functionally with the current therapy regimen
  - Suboptimally controlled acute or chronic pain
  - Painful or functionally disabling spasticity
  - Neuromuscular or musculoskeletal comorbidities (e.g., stroke, spinal cord injury, cerebral palsy, multiple sclerosis, rheumatoid arthritis, fibromyalgia, and chronic pain syndromes) that can compound functional deficits and/or complicate the process of progressing toward functional goals

Patient Instructions

- Your active participation in the rehabilitation process is the most important factor in determining the success of the program.
- Be involved in the formulation of the functional goals for your rehabilitation program.
- Follow physician and physical therapist instructions as closely as possible.
- Give feedback to care providers as to the effectiveness of interventions as well as any side effects of treatment.
- Do not persist in performing exercises or in using modalities that worsen your symptoms or condition without checking with your physician.

Considerations in Special Populations

- Hand injuries
  - Whenever possible, a rehabilitation program for hand or wrist dysfunction should involve evaluation and treatment of the patient by a certified hand therapist. Certified hand therapists are

occupational and physical therapists with at least 5 years of experience in hand therapy who have demonstrated advanced clinical skills in upper quarter rehabilitation and have passed a certification examination.
    - Swelling will occur after any surgery or injury to the hand. Orthoses can potentially aggravate edema, and their use must be carefully monitored during this stage of rehabilitation to prevent loss of function.
- Sensory deficits
    - For obvious reasons, physical modalities and orthotic devices should be employed with great caution in patients with sensory deficits. Orthotic pressure over insensate areas must be minimized, and cryotherapy of these areas is contraindicated.
- Pregnancy
    - The safety of some physical modalities, including transcutaneous electrical nerve stimulation and electrical stimulation, has not been established in patients who are pregnant. Therapeutic US is definitely contraindicated over the low back and abdomen of a pregnant woman.
- Diabetes
    - Many diabetic patients will experience a decrease in blood glucose levels when beginning a new therapeutic exercise regimen. Levels should be monitored closely and medications adjusted as necessary to avoid hypoglycemia.
- Elderly
    - Where possible, therapeutic exercise modalities prescribed for elderly patients should be chosen to minimize stress on the bones and joints.
- Pain
    - Pain is not a contraindication to therapeutic exercise, physical modalities, or the use of orthotic devices. However, significant worsening of pain or onset of new pain after initiation of treatment demands further investigation and/or referral.

Suggested Reading

- Alfano AP: Physical modalities in sports medicine. In O'Connor FG, Sallis RE, Wilder RP, St. Pierre P (eds): Sports Medicine: Just the Facts. New York: McGraw-Hill, 2005, pp 405–411.
- American Society of Hand Therapists (ASHT), Splint Nomenclature Task Force: Splint Classification System. Garner, NC: ASHT, 1991.
- Hennessey WJ: Lower limb orthoses. In Braddom RL (ed): Physical Medicine and Rehabilitation, 3rd ed. Philadelphia: Saunders, 2007, pp 343–367.
- Brault JS, Kappler RE, Grogg BE: Manipulation, traction, and massage. In Braddom RL (ed): Physical Medicine and Rehabilitation, 3rd ed. Philadelphia: Saunders, 2007, pp 437–457.
- Patel AT, Garber LM: Upper limb orthotic devices. In Braddom RL (ed): Physical Medicine and Rehabilitation, 3rd ed. Philadelphia: Saunders, 2007, pp 325–341.
- Wilder RP, Jenkins J, Seto C: Therapeutic exercise. In Braddom RL (ed): Physical Medicine and Rehabilitation, 3rd ed. Philadelphia: Saunders, 2007, pp 413–436.

Chapter 7 Special Populations: Geriatrics

Alfred Cianflocco and Emily Harold

Key Concepts

- By 2030, approximately 20% of the U.S. population will be older than 65 years of age (Fig. 7-1).
- With the increasing elderly population, every health care worker should be familiar with both the physiologic changes associated with aging as well as the common musculoskeletal conditions.
- Research has proven that regular exercise in the elderly population confers many health benefits; however, only 30% of people age 65 to 74 exercise for at least 20 minutes 3 days per week, and this percentage decreases to 20% by 75 years of age.
- There is a decline in athletic performance with aging that can be attributed to multiple factors including underlying disease states, physiologic changes associated with aging, and difficulty maintaining optimal training.
- Although physiologic changes occur with aging, the capacity for the elderly to exercise and improve strength, endurance, flexibility, and performance is maintained.
- Exercise is safe in the elderly population and provides numerous health benefits.
- An exercise prescription is one way for physicians to support healthy lifestyles in the elderly.

Physiologic Changes Associated with Aging

- Decrease in maximal heart rate by 6 to 10 beats per decade
- Decrease in Vo_{2max} (maximal oxygen consumption) by 5% to 15% per decade after age 25
- Older adults have a higher blood pressure and systemic vascular resistance both at rest and at exercise.
- A decrease in thoracic mobility and lung compliance creates a decrease in vital capacity (30% to 50% by age 70) with an increase in residual volume and forced residual capacity.
- Decrease in plasma volume and red blood cells
- Decline in coordination, balance, and reaction time
- Impaired vision, hearing, and short-term memory
- Decrease in bone mineral density with losses as high as 3% per year in postmenopausal women and 0.5% per year in men older than 40 years
- Development of sarcopenia with an average 30% reduction in strength from age 50 to age 70 secondary to atrophy of type II muscle fibers
- Decrease in tensile strength and increased stiffness of tendons and ligaments
- Weakening of articular cartilage and a decrease in elastic properties of intervertebral discs

Common Orthopaedic Conditions in the Elderly

- Elderly athletes experience fewer acute traumatic injuries than younger athletes during competition. However, the elderly population has a high rate of falls, which affects one in three individuals older than the age of 65 and results in moderate to severe injuries in approximately 25% of cases.
- Osteoarthritis is the most common musculoskeletal condition in the elderly population; studies attempting to associate osteoarthritis in the older patient with high rates of strenuous activity as a young adult have conflicting results.
- Secondary to the decrease in tensile strength and increase in stiffness of ligaments and tendons during aging, the elderly are more likely to present with tendonosis including rotator cuff strains, medial epicondylitis, and Achilles tendinitis.
- Elderly patients are also more likely to have degenerative meniscus tears because of age-related collagen changes.
- Muscle strains are also common secondary to a decrease in flexibility.

Benefits of Exercise in the Elderly

- Endurance training is associated with lower fasting and postprandial plasma insulin levels and improved insulin sensitivity.

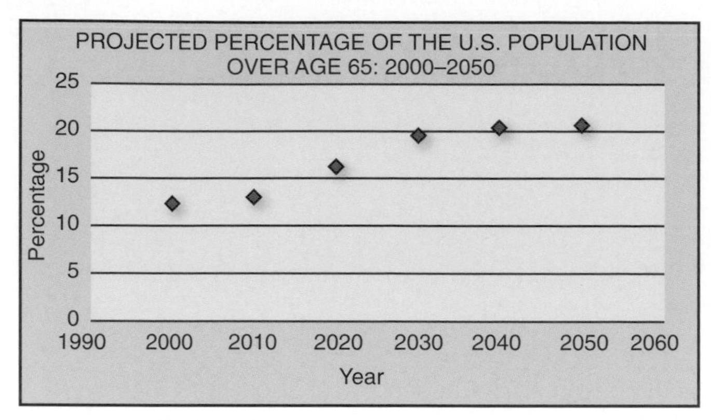

Figure 7-1 Projected percentage of the U.S. population older than age 65, 2000–2050.

- Light to moderate exercise training has been shown to decrease systolic blood pressure by as much as 10 mmHg.
- Exercise programs that include walking, flexibility exercises, and strength exercises have been shown to significantly reduce the number of falls in the elderly.
- The Iowa 65+ Rural Health Study showed an inverse relationship between daily walking and self-reported depressive symptoms in 3000 elderly followed over a 10-year period.
- Weight-bearing exercise has been shown to attenuate bone density loss in several studies.
- Improvement in osteoarthritis pain with adherence to a regular exercise program has been demonstrated in randomized, controlled trials.

Promoting Safe Exercise

- Physical exertion may trigger either sudden death or a myocardial infarction in individuals with underlying heart disease, especially if they normally lead a sedentary lifestyle.
- In order to promote safe exercise, preparticipation screening should be performed to assess for cardiovascular risk factors prior to initiating or continuing an exercise program.
- In 2001, the American Heart Association published screening guidelines to help guide physicians in the evaluation of elderly individuals either beginning or continuing an exercise program (Box 7-1).
- In addition to the American Heart Association guidelines, the 26th Bethesda Conference has guidelines regarding participation in various athletic endeavors in the setting of known cardiac abnormalities.
- After passing a preparticipation physical examination, one should ensure that the exercise program chosen is consistent with that individual's neurologic and physical capabilities. Modifications may be necessary based on underlying conditions (i.e., water aerobics for those with severe knee osteoarthritis instead of jogging).
- Proper nutrition must be maintained for optimal performance. Hydration is especially important secondary to a decrease in thirst perception with age.

BOX 7-1 *American Heart Association Guidelines for Preparticipation Screening*

All men older than 45 years of age or women older than 55 years of age who have at least one or more of the following risk factors should undergo exercise stress testing:

Total cholesterol >200 mg/dL
Low-density lipoprotein >130 mg/dL
High-density lipoprotein <35 mg/dL for men and <45 mg/dL for women
Systolic blood pressure >140 mmHg
Diastolic blood pressure >90 mmHg
Current or recent cigarette smoking
Diabetes mellitus
History of myocardial infarction or sudden cardiac death in a first-degree relative younger than 60 years old

In addition, any athlete with symptoms suggestive of underlying coronary disease or who is older than 65 years in the absence of symptoms should undergo exercise stress testing.

BOX 7-2 *Exercise Prescription*

An exercise prescription should include the recommended frequency, intensity, type, time, and progression of exercise.

Five to seven times per week
30 minutes either at one time or in two separate sessions
Moderate as judged by ability to carry on a conversation and/or at 50% to 60% of maximum heart rate
Increase daily exercise time by 10 minutes every week until at a maximum of 60 minutes per day

Exercise Prescriptions

- After cardiac clearance, an exercise prescription is an excellent way to promote a healthy lifestyle in an elderly patient.
- An exercise prescription should include the recommended frequency, intensity, type, time, and progression of exercise (Box 7-2).
- Exercise prescriptions should also take underlying conditions into account such as avoiding high-impact activities in individuals with osteoarthritis.

Patient Instructions

- As individuals age, a regular exercise program with both aerobic, flexibility, and strength components provides numerous health benefits.
- A preparticipation screening should be done before initiating an exercise program to ensure safety and assess for cardiac risk factors.

Suggested Reading

- Agency for Healthcare and Quality, Centers for Disease Control and Prevention: Physical activity in older Americans: Benefits and strategies, 2002. Available at: www.ahrg.gov/ppip/activity.htm. Accessed March 15, 2006.
- Chen A, Mears S, Hawkins R: Orthopaedic care of the aging athlete. J Am Acad Orthop Surg 2006;13:407–416.
- Hagberg J, Graves J, Limacher M, et al: Cardiovascular responses of 70- to 79-year-old men and women to exercise training. J Appl Physiol 1989;66:2589–2594.
- Hersey W, Graves J, Pollock M, et al: Endurance exercise training improves body composition and plasma insulin responses in 70- to 79-year-old men and women. Metabolism 1994;43:847–854.
- Kannus P, Niittymaki S, Jarvinen M, Lehto M: Sports injuries in elderly athletes: A three-year prospective, controlled study. Age Ageing 1989;18:263–270.
- Kaplan FS, Hayes WC, Keaveny TM, et al: Form and function of bone. In Simon SR (ed): Orthopaedic Basic Science. Rosemont, IL: American Academy of Orthopaedic Surgeons, 1994, pp 127–184.
- Kasch FW, Boyer JL, Van Camp S, et al: Cardiovascular changes with age and exercise: A 28-year longitudinal study. Scand J Med Sci Sports 1995;5:147–151.
- Lynch N, Ryan A, Evans J, et al: Older elite football players have reduced cardiac and osteoporosis risk factors. Med Sci Sports Exerc 2007;39:1124–1130.
- MacRae PG, Feltner ME, Reinsch S: A 1-year exercise program for older women: Effects on falls, injuries, and physical performance. J Aging Phys Act 1994;2:127–142.
- Maharam L, Bauman P, Kalman D, et al: Master athletes. Sports Med 1999;28:273–285.
- Maron B, Araujo C, Thompson P, et al: Recommendations for preparticipation screening and the assessment of cardiovascular disease in master athletes. Circulation 2001;103:327–334.
- Maron BJ, Mitchell JH (eds): 26th Bethesda Conference: Recommendations for determining eligibility for competition in athletes with cardiovascular abnormalities. J Am Coll Cardiol 1994;24:845–899.
- Mazzeo R, Cavanagh P, Evans W, et al: ACSM position stand on exercise and physical activity for older adults. Med Sci Sports Exerc 1998;30:992–1008.
- McDermott A, Mernitz H: Exercise and older patients: Prescribing guidelines. Am Fam Physician 2006;74:437–444.
- Menard D, Stanish WD: The aging athlete. Am J Sports Med 1989;17:187–196.
- Mobily KE, Rubenstein LM, Lemke JH, et al: Walking and depression in a cohort of older adults: The Iowa 65+ Rural Health Study. J Aging Phys Act 1996;4:119–135.
- Ogawa T, Spina R, Martin W, et al: Effects of aging, sex, and physical training on cardiovascular responses to exercise. Circulation 1992;86:494–503.
- Powell AP: Issues unique to the master athlete. Curr Sports Med Rep 2005;4:335–340.
- Prasad A, Popovic Z, Arbab-Zadeh A, et al: The effects of aging and physical activity on Doppler measurements of diastolic function. Am J Cardiol 2007;99:1629–1636.
- Roddy E, Zhang W, Doherty M, et al: Evidence-based recommendations for the role of exercise in the management of osteoarthritis in the hip or knee—the MOVE consensus. Rheumatology 2005;44:67–73.
- Rogers M, Hagberg J, Martin W III, et al: Decline in VO2max with aging in master athletes and sedentary men. J Appl Physiol 1990;68:2195–2199.
- Siscovick DS, Weiss NS, Fletcher RH, et al: The incidence of primary cardiac arrest during vigorous exercise. N Engl J Med 1984;311:874–877.
- Trappe S, Costill D, Vukovich M, et al: Aging among elite distance runners: A 22-year longitudinal study. J Appl Physiol 1996;80:285–290.
- U.S. Department of Commerce: Bureau of the Census: Current Population Reports: Statistical Abstract of the United States: 2000. Washington, DC: U.S. Government Printing Office, 2001, p 42.
- Yamakazi SY, Ichimura S, Iwamoto J, et al: Effect of walking exercise on bone metabolism in postmenopausal women with osteopenia/osteoporosis. J Bone Miner Metab 2004;22:500–508.

Chapter 8 Special Populations: Disabled

Alfred Cianflocco and Emily Harold

Key Concepts

- A disability as defined by the World Health Organization is a condition (either mental or physical) that limits the ability of a person to perform an activity in the range considered normal for a human being.
- Almost 50 million Americans have some type of disability according to 2000 U.S. Census data.
- Musculoskeletal diseases are some of the major causes of disability in the United States and the world.
- The benefits of a regular exercise program can be obtained by those with disabilities, but 56% of people with disabilities lead predominantly sedentary lives compared with just 34% of their peers without disabilities.
- Physicians who have disabled patients must encourage physical activity while being mindful of both the limitations of the disability and common injury patterns either unique to the disability or the result of the activity type.
- Physicians must also be aware of societal and environmental factors that hinder the activities of disabled persons and provide tools to eliminate obstacles as necessary.

Background

- A disabled sports program was begun for wheelchair athletes in the 1950s and 1960s.
- The first Paralympic games were held in Rome in 1960. The Paralympics were games established for athletes with either a physical disability or visual impairment.
- The Special Olympics began in 1960 and has since grown to involve more than 1 million athletes in 150 different countries. The games are for those athletes with mental retardation regardless of physical ability.
- The Rehabilitation Act of 1973 aided in bringing physical activity programs to most disabled people regardless of participation in competitive sports.
- Currently, there are a myriad of programs promoting physical activity for the disabled including the Special Olympics, the United States Association of Blind Athletes, the National Wheelchair Athlete Association, the National Association of Sports for Cerebral Palsy, and Healthy Lifestyles.
- In addition, the Centers for Disease Control and Prevention have recently sponsored several programs aimed at improving physical fitness and promoting healthy lifestyles for disabled persons.

Musculoskeletal Disabilities

- Several different types of disabilities exist (Box 8-1).
- Musculoskeletal disabilities are among the most common types and involve everything from back pain to rheumatoid arthritis to muscular dystrophy.
- The burden to the health care system from musculoskeletal disabilities worldwide is significant and is growing. In the United States alone, one in seven people have restricted movement from a musculoskeletal disease.
- The Bone and Joint Decade was established worldwide to help prevent musculoskeletal disability and improve the quality of life for those with musculoskeletal disease.

Common Injuries in the Disabled

- According to data from the Special Olympics, the injuries sustained in disabled individuals were no different from those sustained in their nondisabled peers.
- Over a 4-year period, the Special Olympics Hawaii had 90 medical tent visits from 2326 athletes; 52 were for musculoskeletal injuries, with the majority being abrasions, muscle strains, and sprains. The remaining 38 visits were medical and included headaches, gastrointestinal discomfort, epistaxis, and heat illness.
- When a physician performs a preparticipation physical examination on a disabled athlete, abnormalities that predispose to injury should be identified.
  - The relationship of Down syndrome to atlantoaxial instability requires that all Down syndrome athletes obtain lateral cervical spine films in both flexion and extension as well as neutral: the atlantodens

BOX 8-1 *Types of Disabilities*

Visual impairment	Osteoarthritis
Hearing impairment	Traumatic brain injury
Mental retardation	Limb loss
Autism	Depression
Spinal cord injuries	Dementia
Cerebral palsy	Stroke
Muscular dystrophy	Addiction
Multiple sclerosis	Diabetes mellitus
Chronic pain	Obesity

This is a partial list. The definition of disability encompasses any condition that prohibits an individual from performing an activity in the range considered normal for a human being.

interval must be less than 5 mm. If the radiographs are abnormal, then participation in contact sports is precluded.

- All traumatic paraplegic or quadriplegic athletes should undergo a stress test before participation in high-demand sports (i.e., basketball, track).
- The athlete should be examined for any skin abnormalities including pressure sores. If pressure sores are present, the athlete cannot compete.
- If an athlete has a spinal cord injury, he or she will be at increased risk of both hypothermia and hyperthermia secondary to autonomic dysreflexia. The athlete should be counseled regarding these conditions.
- Other medical conditions should be carefully documented. These include seizure disorders, congenital and acquired cardiovascular disease, visual problems, and allergies.

Treatment

- Following a preparticipation physical, physical activity should be encouraged for all individuals with disabilities as it has been demonstrated to improve overall health.
- Disabled athletes have higher self-esteem, experience more satisfaction and happiness in life, and are better educated than their nonathletic disabled peers.
- Disabled athletes also have less weight gain than their sedentary peers, resulting in a lower incidence of diabetes mellitus and heart disease.
- In a recent study, a disabled patient's attitude toward physical activity was the strongest predictor of future physical activity.
- A strong support system has been shown to limit an individual's disability.
- Multidisciplinary care involving physical therapists, physicians, social workers, occupational therapists, and others has been shown to improve pain and function in such chronic conditions as back pain and fibromyalgia.

Patient Instructions

- A disability should not preclude an individual from obtaining the benefits of living a healthy lifestyle.
- There are several Web sites and community programs that can help provide access to services offered to help people with a disability.
  - www.nod.org (National Organization on Disability)
  - www.paralysis.org (funded by the Centers for Disease Control and Prevention to improve the lives of those with paralysis)
  - www.ncpad.org (National Center on Physical Activity and Disability)
- Disabled athletes derive the most benefit from a multidisciplinary approach to their disability.

Suggested Reading

- Batts KB, Glorioso JE, Williams MS: The medical demands of the special athlete. Clin J Sports Med 1998;8:22–25.
- Birrer R: The Special Olympics athlete: Evaluation and clearance for participation. Clin Pediatr 2004;43:777–782.
- Brooks P: The burden of musculoskeletal disease—a global perspective. Clin Rheumatol 2006;25:778–781.
- Carmona R: Disability and Health 2005: Promoting the Health and Well-Being of People with Disabilities. Rockville, MD: Department of Health and Human Services, Centers for Disease Control and Prevention, 2005.
- European Action Towards Better Musculoskeletal Health: A Public Health Strategy to Reduce the Burden of Musculoskeletal Conditions. A Bone and Joint Decade Report. Lund, Sweden: The European Bone and Joint Health Strategies Project, 2004.
- Fox PL: Environmental modifications in the homes of elderly Canadians with disabilities. Disabil Rehabil 1995;17:43–49.
- Gordon NF, Gulanic M, Costa F, Fletcher G, et al: Physical activity and exercise recommendations for stroke survivors: An American Heart Association scientific statement. Circulation 2004;109:2031–2041.
- Ivey F, Ryan A, Hafer-Macko C, et al: Treadmill aerobic training improves glucose tolerance and indices of insulin sensitivity in disabled stroke survivors: A preliminary report. Stroke 2007;38:2752–2758.
- Ivey FM, Hafer-Macko CE, Macko RF: Exercise rehabilitation after stroke. NeuroRx 2006;3:439–450.
- Kosma M, Ellis R, Cardinal B, Bauer J, McCubbin J: The mediating role of intention and stage of change in physical activity among adults with physical disabilities: An integrative framework. J Sport Exerc Psychol 2007;29:21–38.

- Lerman J, Sullivan E, Barnes D, Haynes R: The Pediatric Outcomes Data Collection Instrument (PODCI) and functional assessment of patients with unilateral upper extremity deficiencies. J Pediatr Orthop 2005;25:405–407.
- Platt L: Medical and orthopaedic conditions in Special Olympics athletes. J Athletic Train 2001;36:74–80.
- Price MJ, Campbell IG: Effects of spinal cord lesion level upon thermoregulation during exercise in the heat. Med Sci Sport Exerc 2003;35:1100–1107.
- Pueschel SM, Scola FH, Perry CD, Pezzullo JC: Atlanto-axial instability in children with Down syndrome. Pediatr Radiol 1981;10:129–132.
- Tanji JL: The preparticipation exam: Special concerns for the Special Olympics. Physician Sportsmed 1991;19:61–68.
- United States Bone and Joint Decade, 2007: Available at: www.usbjd.org. Accessed October 16, 2007.
- U.S. Department of Health and Human Services: The Surgeon General's Call to Action to Improve Health and Wellness of Persons with Disabilities. Rockville, MD: U.S. Department of Health and Human Services, Office of the Surgeon General, 2005.
- Vallaint PM, Bezzubyk I, Daley ME: Psychological impact of sport on disabled athletes. Psychol Rep 1985;56:923.
- Ward MM, Leigh JP: Marital status and the progression of functional disability in patients with rheumatoid arthritis. Arthritis Rheum 1993;36:581–588.
- Warms C, Belza B, Whitney J: Correlates of physical activity in adults with mobility limitations. Family Community Health 2007;30:s5–s16.
- Weigl M, Cieza A, Cantista P, Stucki G: Physical disability due to musculoskeletal conditions. Best Pract Res Clin Rheumatol 2007;21:167–190.
- World Health Organization: The Burden of Musculoskeletal Conditions at the Start of the New Millennium. Technical Report Series 919. Geneva: World Health Organization, 2003.
- World Health Organization: International Classification of Functioning, Disability and Health: ICF. Geneva: World Health Organization, 2001.

Chapter 9 Special Populations: Pediatrics

Nancy M. McLaren

Key Concepts

- At least 44 million American young people of all ages participate in organized sports today.
- Over the past several decades, the model of youth sports has shifted from the school playground and neighborhood activities to organized sports.
- Youth sports are now more competitive than previously. Many children play at competitive levels at younger ages, often specialize in a single sport at younger ages, and may even follow a year-round cycle of practice and events for that sport.
- Sports-related injuries are (1) increasing among young people, (2) the leading cause of all injuries in adolescents, and (3) the leading reason for adolescent visits to health care providers. The majority of these injuries relate to the specific developmental issues of children and/or to overtraining or other overuse.
- Skeletal growth and the physiologic and psychological changes of puberty can each affect which sports activities adolescent athletes choose and how well they perform.
- There is growing recognition of the value of training and conditioning programs for young athletes. Well-designed and supervised training programs are increasingly common and are safe for all youth athletes, including prepubertal children.
- Primary care providers should encourage appropriate physical activities for their young patients and should provide anticipatory guidance to parents on developmentally appropriate sports and activity levels for their patients, with a goal of choosing activities that are fun, safe, and rewarding.
- Providers should be involved with parents and athletes to assess young people's "sports readiness," that is, their cognitive, social, and motor development, to determine whether they can meet the demands of the specific sport and level of competition that they desire.

Trends in American Youth Sports

- Participation in highly organized youth sports is now pervasive in the United States.
- Over the past several decades, the numbers of children and adolescents involved in formal youth sports have nearly doubled (Table 9-1). Although the relative increase in female participants has been greater than that in male participants, males still outnumber females in absolute numbers.
- The marked increase in female participation is in part a function of Title IX, a 1972 federal law that mandated equal athletic facilities and programs for females and males. In concert with other societal changes, Title IX has led to a greater acceptance of girls and women in competitive sports and the ascension of female sports figures as role models.
- For many children, parents, and communities, the athletic focus has shifted away from the recreational component of physical activity to that of organized weekly sports practices, games, and tournaments.
- There is increasing competition in youth athletics and earlier participation and intensity of training for more competition-level sports.
- The most frequently cited reasons for younger children's participation in organized sports are to have fun, learn new skills, test abilities, and experience excitement. Receiving individual awards, winning games, and pleasing others are ranked lower.
- A recent troubling trend in sports activities for children and youths is the specialization in one sport at ever-younger ages. This specialization can limit development of various physical and mental athletic skill sets.

Sports Injuries

- Sports injuries are the most common type of injury in adolescents, and sports-related injury is the

TABLE 9-1 *Numbers of High School–Age American Boys and Girls Involved in Organized Sports*

Group	1971	2006
Boys	3,500,000	4,321,000
Girls	380,000	3,021,000
Total	3,880,000	7,342,000

leading reason for adolescent visits to primary care providers.
    - Ongoing rapid changes in height, weight, muscle growth, and strength affect flexibility, coordination, balance, and power.
- However, the highest incidence of sports-related pediatric injuries is in the 5- to 14-year age group.
    - Children ages 5 to 14 are less coordinated, have slower reaction times, and are less proficient than older children and adults in assessing and avoiding the risks of sports.
    - Immature epiphyses in children and younger adolescents are weaker than the surrounding muscles and ligaments, and therefore significant stress to the skeleton is more likely to cause a traumatic fracture than a sprain.
    - Recently noted increases in injury frequency, especially with overuse injury, seem to be related to the increased specialization, intensity, and year-round athletic activity of ever-younger athletes.
- Injury risk is greatest when athletes begin a sports season in poor physical condition and then have rapid increases in activity over short periods. Injury risks are also greater when athletes play above their skill level and/or their age level. Finally, athletes who deprive their bodies of rest time and time to adapt to the increased demands of their sport are at increased risk of injury.

Growth and Maturation

- Preparedness for particular sports, capabilities for training, and skills development are all directly related to age-specific maturation in children's neuromuscular, cardiovascular, and cognitive systems.
- By age 6 years, most children have acquired sufficient physical skills to participate in some organized sports.
- Gaining experience in a variety of sports is important for children, especially at younger ages, to enable them to acquire a mix of skill sets and to keep physical activity interesting and fun.

Developmental Levels and Readiness for Sports at Various Prepubertal Ages

- Selection of appropriate athletic activities for children should be guided by knowledge of the developmental skills and limitations of specific age groups.

Ages 3 to 5 Years

- Focus should be on learning basic skills such as running, swimming, tumbling, throwing, and catching.
- Direct competition should be avoided; fun play should be emphasized.

Ages 6 to 9 Years

- Children have a short attention span and limited memory development and do not easily make rapid decisions; they need simple and flexible rules and short instruction times.
- Sports should continue to focus on developing fundamental skills with limited emphasis on direct competition.
- To learn additional fundamental skills and work toward a transition to direct competition, sports like swimming, running, and gymnastics can be tried.

Ages 10 to 12 Years (Prepubertal Years)

- Children can now compete in activities for which they have mastered the basic skills; they are able to learn more complex motor skill patterns.
    - Can accept increasing emphasis on game tactics and strategy
    - Successful mastery of new skills closely linked to child's self-esteem
- They have the cognitive, social, and emotional maturity to handle modest competitive pressure and complex skill sports such as football, basketball, soccer, and field hockey.
- Flexibility and joint hypermobility are increased, which increases the risk of glenohumeral and patellar subluxation and dislocation.
- Muscle strength, speed, and skills are usually nearly equal in boys and girls until age 10 to 11 years, and sports activities can still be coeducational due to these similarities.
- Capacities for both aerobic and anaerobic exercise are beginning to increase.

Athletic and Sports Issues of Puberty

- Girls generally begin their pubertal changes at approximately 10 years of age, approximately 2 years before boys.

- Many changes occurring during puberty can affect children's athletic performance. The exact timing of these changes can be affected by genetics, endocrine function, nutritional status, and amounts and types of exercise.
- By age 12 to 13 years, pubertal differences start to affect the skill and strength involved in sports, and, depending on the sport, these differences may affect whether girls and boys should continue to play and compete together.

Physiologic Changes of Puberty

- Increasing aerobic capacity, as reflected in greater maximum oxygen uptake ($\dot{V}O_{2max}$), is due to increases in pulmonary ventilation and cardiac output and to more efficient extraction and use of oxygen by muscle.
- The capacity for anaerobic metabolism is also increasing, allowing short, intense bursts of activity.
- These increases allow longer and more intense periods of exercise to be tolerated.
- The downside of these physiologic changes is that although pubertal children are less limited by body fatigue and can thus exercise longer, they are also more capable of overexercising, which can lead to overuse injuries.

Skeletal Changes of Puberty

- Changing body contours during early puberty can lead to physical awkwardness, which may be associated with increased chances of injury, especially in early adolescence when new skills have not caught up with new capacities and new growth.
- During early puberty, bone mineral density begins to increase in both boys and girls.
- The calcium needs of all adolescents are great during puberty due to the deposition of calcium into rapidly growing bone.
  - Adolescents accrue 40% of their eventual adult bone mass during puberty.
- Recommended calcium intake for adolescents is 1300 mg/day (1500 mg/day for amenorrheic females).

Linear Growth

- Linear growth begins first in the long bones of the extremities and can contribute to a temporary clumsiness that can have an impact on the athletic performance of younger adolescents (Table 9-2). The child who previously exhibited strong skills may suddenly appear to be "all hands and feet."

TABLE 9-2 *Average Timing of Pubertal Changes in Linear Growth (Height)*

Specific Pubertal Change	Girls	Boys
Increasing height velocity begins	9 yr	11 yr
Peak height velocity and timing	9 cm/yr, at Tanner stage 2–3	10 cm/yr, at Tanner stage 3–4
Duration of growth spurt	24–36 mo	24–36 mo
Average age at complete skeletal maturity	14 yr	16 yr

- Puberty-related increases in height velocity usually begin in girls at approximately 9 years of age and in boys at approximately 11 years of age.
- The preadolescent and adolescent growth spurt, which can last for 24 to 36 months, accounts for approximately 20% of final adult height.

Weight Increases during Puberty

- Puberty-related weight increases account for approximately 50% of adult weight.
- On average, boys end up with 1.5 times the lean body mass and one half the body fat of girls.

Weight Changes in Girls

- Due to increasing body fat, girls' lean body mass decreases during puberty to 75% of the total body weight.
- Girls' hip enlargement decreases their waist-to-hip ratio.
- Girls' maximum weight velocity occurs approximately 6 months before their linear growth (height) spurt.
- Higher levels of fat in young female athletes involved in sports where low body fat is valued (e.g., dancing, gymnastics, figure skating) may lead to inappropriate body image concerns.
  - Loss of self-esteem and eating disorders are a particular risk in this age group.

Weight Changes in Boys

- Higher androgen levels in boys lead to greater lean body mass, to approximately 90% of total weight.
- Muscle mass accounts for 54% of boys' body weight, making the average male athletes stronger and faster than the average female athletes.

Epiphyseal Growth Plates and Other Vulnerable Anatomic Sites

- The articular surfaces, epiphyseal growth plates, and apophyses where cartilage develops are sites of rapid cell production.
- At the epiphyseal plates and apophyses, this rapid cell production leads to bone formation and increasing bone length. By adulthood, after growth has been completed, these sites are replaced by stronger and more solid bone.
  - Until then, the epiphyseal plates are relatively weak compared with adjacent ligaments, tendons, and bone and are therefore more susceptible to injury, including fracture.
  - Fractures at these growth plates represent 15% to 30% of all childhood fractures.
- In early puberty, bone grows more rapidly than muscle and tendons, leading to a progressive loss of the flexibility of childhood. This imbalance places greater stress on bones, particularly at the epiphyseal plates, apophyses, and articular cartilage, further increasing the susceptibility to overuse injuries.
  - Tendons and tendon-apophyseal interfaces are the most common sites of growth injury in adolescent athletes.
  - Overuse injuries that can affect growth plates include osteochondritis dissecans and patellofemoral syndrome.
  - Apophysitis can include, for example, Sever's disease, Osgood-Schlatter disease, and Sinding-Larsen-Johansson disease; each is self-limited, but each may benefit from temporary reduction in activity.
  - Physeal and epiphyseal injuries include little league shoulder, little league elbow, spondylolysis, and spondylolisthesis.
- A higher incidence of various injuries, including fractures, in this age group can result from lack of skills, overuse, lack of appropriate protective equipment, improperly learned (or taught) techniques, and/or excessive performance expectations.
- Until the growth plates are closed, both males and females should avoid power lifting, which has been associated with avulsion fractures of the growth plates.
- Although stretching can be a part of any organized athletic activity in children, athletes in this pubertal group can gain particular benefit from stretching regimens, especially in the lower extremities.
- Children who are smaller and/or thinner at this age can help improve their performance and safety through adequate preparation, including regular conditioning and stretching regimens and light strength training.

Training and Conditioning

- Benefits of training and conditioning include greater muscle strength, power, and coordination and a lower risk of athletic injuries (especially knee injuries); training can improve athletic performance, increase bone density, promote weight loss, and enhance children's self-esteem.
  - Training is a noncompetitive (or less competitive) means of improving conditioning, strength, and coordination.
  - Training can promote a healthy lifestyle that can last into adulthood.
  - The purpose of all athletic training programs for young athletes should include acquisition of skills and improvement in speed, flexibility, strength, and conditioning, maintenance of good nutrition, and attention to hydration.
  - The key to successful strength training, especially for younger children, is that it should include qualified adult supervision, start with very low weights, and, most importantly, be fun.
- Adult supervisors should stress positive attitude, character building, teamwork, and safety.
  - In prepubertal children, training will increase strength and neuromuscular adaption but will not result in muscle hypertrophy. In pubescent children, increasing testosterone will result in larger muscle mass, especially with increasing weights and resistances.
- Guidelines for training include
  - No minimum age for participation in a youth resistance training program, but children need to have enough emotional maturity to accept and follow directions; this is generally possible by 7 to 8 years of age.
  - Training should include sufficient instruction in proper techniques and equipment use.
  - A reasonable goal is improvement of baseline strength and muscle tone by 40% to 50% over a 6-week period.
  - Conditioning should start at least 6 weeks before beginning a sports season.
    - — Two to three times per week on nonconsecutive days (to allow a day of rest between sessions)
    - — Warm-ups and cool downs, including stretching, should be part of each session.

- — One to 3 sets of 6 to 15 repetitions with light weights on a variety of exercises, starting with a small number of exercises
- — Gradual increase in weights, number of repetitions, and number of exercises
- — Core exercise should be supplemented by some form of cardiovascular activity for 30 to 40 minutes 3 to 4 times weekly.

Resources for Health Care Providers, Parents, and Patients

- American Academy of Pediatrics. Sports medicine. Available at: www.aap.org/sections/sportsmedicine/default.cfm. Accessed January 21, 2009.
- Hospital for Special Surgery, New York. Web site with lots of information and handouts. Available at: www.hss.edu/conditions_youth-sports.asp. Accessed January 21, 2009.
- Kraemer WJ, Flech SJ: Strength training for young athletes. Champaign, IL: Human Kinetics, 2004.
- Metzl JD, Shookhoff C: The Young Athlete: A Sports Doctor's Complete Guide for Parents. New York: Time Warner, 2002.

Suggested Reading

- American Academy of Pediatrics, Committee on Sports Medicine and Fitness and Committee on School Health: Organized sports for children and preadolescents. Pediatrics 2001;107:1459–1462.
- Benjamin HJ, Glow KM: Strength training for children and adolescents: What can physicians recommend? Physician Sports Med 2003;31:19–25.
- Brenner JS: The Council on Sports Medicine and Fitness: Overuse injuries, overtraining and burnout in child and adolescent athletes. Pediatrics 2007;119:1243–1245.
- Greydanus D, Patel D, Pratt H: Essential Adolescent Medicine. New York: McGraw-Hill, 2006.
- Metzl JD: Sports Medicine in the Pediatric Office. Elk Grove Village, IL: American Academy of Pediatrics, 2008.
- Neinstein L, Gordon CM, Katzman DK, et al: Adolescent Health Care: A Practical Guide, 5th ed. Philadelphia: Lippincott Williams & Wilkins, 2008.
- Nelson MA: Developmental skills and children's sports. Physician Sports Med 1991;19:67–79.
- Pommering TL, Kluchurosky L: Overuse injuries in adolescents. Adolesc Med 2007;18:95–120.
- Sports-related injuries among high school athletes—United States, 2005–06 school year. MMWR Morb Mortal Wkly Rep 2006;55:1037–1040.
- Strasburger VC, Brown RT, Braverman PK, et al: Adolescent Medicine: A Handbook for Primary Care. Philadelphia: Lippincott Williams & Wilkins, 2006.
- Sullivan JA, Anderson ST: Care of the Young Athlete. Oklahoma City, OK: American Academy of Pediatrics and the American Academy of Orthopedic Surgeons, 2000.

Chapter 10 Special Populations: Obesity

Alfred Cianflocco and Emily Harold

Key Concepts

- According to 2006 World Health Organization data, obesity has become a significant public health problem with nearly 300 million obese adults worldwide.
- In the United States, the percentage of adults who have a body mass index (BMI) greater than 30 has steadily increased over the past several years and is currently 31% (Fig. 10-1).
- Obesity has been implicated in many musculoskeletal conditions including knee osteoarthritis, medial epicondylitis, rotator cuff tendinitis, carpal tunnel syndrome, and postural instability.
- Obesity is also a risk factor for the development of chronic medical diseases including diabetes, hypertension, cardiovascular disease, and certain types of cancer.
- Weight loss can help treat both the musculoskeletal conditions and chronic medical diseases caused by obesity.

Demographics

- Obesity is defined by a BMI greater than 30. Overweight is characterized by a BMI between 25 and 30 (Fig. 10-2).
- The BMI is calculated with the following equation: (weight [kg]/height [m^2]).
- The percentage of adults in the United States who are obese was 31% in 2000. This was an 8% increase from survey data for the period 1988 to 1994. The percentage of overweight children ages 6 to 19 years in 2000 was 15%. This was a 4% increase when compared with survey data for the period 1988 to 1994. The percentage of overweight children in the data for the period 1966 to 1970 was less than 5%.

Obesity and Musculoskeletal Conditions

- The risk of knee osteoarthritis increases with an increasing BMI. A longitudinal study demonstrated that a BMI greater than 24.7 in patients ages 20 to 29 years predicted three times the risk of knee osteoarthritis later in life than a BMI less than 22.8 in the same group.
- While a high BMI has been associated with knee osteoarthritis, it has not been associated with hip or ankle osteoarthritis suggesting that mechanical factors cause the knee to experience greater forces during weight-bearing activities.
- In a recent retrospective review of anterior cruciate ligament reconstructions, a higher BMI significantly predicted the extent of intra-articular injury seen during arthroscopic surgery.
- In one case-control study, rotator cuff tendinitis requiring surgery was twice as likely in obese patients compared with those of normal weight. The risk increased with an increasing BMI, ranging from a 120% higher risk in moderately obese patients to a 300% higher risk in those with a BMI greater than 35.
- Obesity was found to be an independent risk factor for medial epicondylitis in women in a Finnish population study involving 5000 patients.
- Difficulty with balance has been correlated with increasing weight. It is unclear whether this increases falls in obese individuals at this time.
- Carpal tunnel syndrome is twice as likely in obese people compared with those of average weight. This is hypothesized to be secondary to increased median nerve compression by adipose tissue and altered mechanics secondary to girth.

Treatment

- Prevention of obesity will help to decrease the prevalence of many of the aforementioned musculoskeletal conditions. This is especially important for knee osteoarthritis, which affects 70% of the population older than the age of 65.
- The U.S. government created Healthy People 2010 with a goal of decreasing adult obesity to 15% by

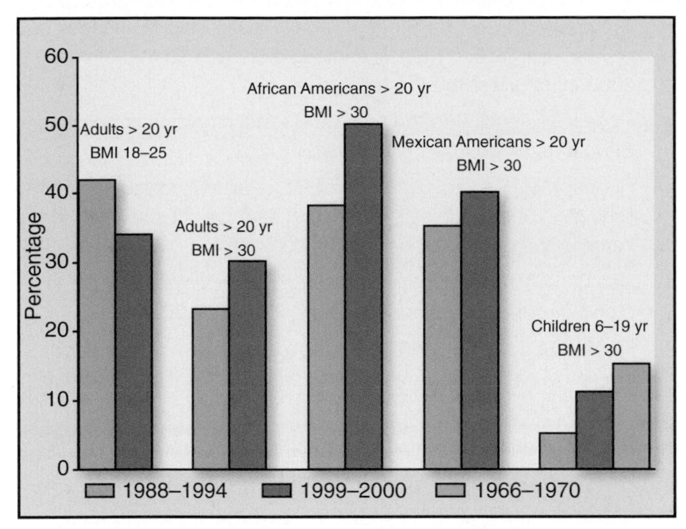

Figure 10-1 Obesity data from Healthy People 2010. BMI, body mass index.

2010 through programs based on healthy eating and exercise.

- For those individuals who are overweight or obese with knee osteoarthritis, several randomized, controlled trials have demonstrated a decrease in osteoarthritis symptoms with weight loss. The Framingham study demonstrated that a weight loss of just 11 pounds was associated with a 50% reduction in arthritis symptoms.
- A recent study demonstrated that weight loss by diet alone decreased symptoms of knee osteoarthritis.
- Physical therapy incorporating quadriceps and hip muscle strengthening has been associated with a decrease in knee osteoarthritis symptoms.
- Gastric bypass surgery has also been associated with a decrease in musculoskeletal pain likely secondary to weight loss.

BMI	19	20	21	22	23	24	25	26	27	28	29	30	31	32	33	34	35
Height	Weight (pounds)																
4'10" (58")	91	96	100	105	110	115	119	124	129	134	138	143	148	153	158	162	167
4'11" (59")	94	99	104	109	114	119	124	128	133	138	143	148	153	158	163	168	173
5' (60")	97	102	107	112	118	123	128	133	138	143	148	153	158	163	168	174	179
5'1" (61")	100	106	111	116	122	127	132	137	143	148	153	158	164	169	174	180	185
5'2" (62")	104	109	115	120	126	131	136	142	147	153	158	164	169	175	180	186	191
5'3" (63")	107	113	118	124	130	135	141	146	152	158	163	169	175	180	186	191	197
5'4" (64")	110	116	122	128	134	140	145	151	157	163	169	174	180	186	192	197	204
5'5" (65")	114	120	126	132	138	144	150	156	162	168	174	180	186	192	198	204	210
5'6" (66")	118	124	130	136	142	148	155	161	167	173	179	186	192	198	204	210	216
5'7" (67")	121	127	134	140	146	153	159	166	172	178	185	191	198	204	211	217	223
5'8" (68")	125	131	138	144	151	158	164	171	177	184	190	197	203	210	216	223	230
5'9" (69")	128	135	142	149	155	162	169	176	182	189	196	203	209	216	223	230	236
5'10" (70")	132	139	146	153	160	167	174	181	188	195	202	209	216	222	229	236	243
5'11" (71")	136	143	150	157	165	172	179	186	193	200	208	215	222	229	236	243	250
6' (72")	140	147	154	162	169	177	184	191	199	206	213	221	228	235	242	250	258
6'1" (73")	144	151	159	166	174	182	189	197	204	212	219	227	235	242	250	257	265
6'2" (74")	148	155	163	171	179	186	194	202	210	218	225	233	241	249	256	264	272
6'3" (75")	152	160	168	176	184	192	200	208	216	224	232	240	248	256	264	272	279

Figure 10-2 Body mass index (BMI) table. (Data from National Heart, Lung and Blood Institute: Clinical guidelines on the identification, evaluation, and treatment of overweight and obesity in adults: The evidence report. Bethesda, MD: NIH Publications, 1998.)

Patient Instructions

- Obesity is a risk factor for several diseases from diabetes and hypertension to knee osteoarthritis and rotator cuff tendinitis.
- A weight loss as little as 5 kg can drastically help with musculoskeletal and medical conditions caused by obesity.

Suggested Reading

- Bagge E, Bjelle A, Eden S, Svanborg A: Osteoarthritis in the elderly: Clinical and radiographic findings in 79 and 85 year olds. Ann Rheum Dis 1991;50:366–371.
- Becker J, Nora DB, Gommes I, et al: An evaluation of gender, obesity, age and diabetes mellitus as risk factors for carpal tunnel syndrome. Clin Neurophysiol 2002;113:1429–1434.
- Bowers A, Spindler K, McCarty E, Arrigain S: Height, weight, and BMI predict intra-articular injuries observed during ACL reconstruction: Evaluation of 456 cases from a prospective ACL database. Clin J Sport Med 2005;15:9–13.
- Christensen R, Astrup A, Bliddal H: Weight loss: The treatment of choice for knee osteoarthritis? Osteoarthritis Cartilage 2005;13:20–27.
- Felson DT, Zhang Y, Anthony JM, et al: Weight loss reduces the risk for symptomatic knee osteoarthritis in women: The Framingham study. Ann Intern Med 1992;116:535–539.
- Gelber AC, Hochberg MC, Mead LA, et al: Body mass index in young men and the risk of subsequent knee and hip osteoarthritis. Am J Med 1999;107:542–548.
- Gregg EW, Cauley JA, Stone K, et al: Relationship of changes in physical activity and mortality among older women. JAMA 2003;289:2379–2386.
- Hooper M: Tending to the musculoskeletal problems of obesity. Cleve Clin J Med 2006;73:839–845.
- Hooper MM, Stellato TA, Hallowell PT, et al: Musculoskeletal findings in obese subjects before and after weight loss following bariatric surgery. Int J Obes (Lond) 2007;31:114–120.
- Hue O, Simoneau M, Marcotte J, et al: Body weight is a strong predictor of postural stability. Gait Posture 2006;26:32–38.
- Messier S, Loeser R, Miller G, et al: Exercise and dietary weight loss in overweight and obese older adults with knee osteoarthritis. Arthritis Rheum 2004;50:1501–1510.
- Shaw K, Gennat H, O'Rourke P, Del Mar C: Exercise for overweight or obesity. Cochrane Database Syst Rev 2006;4: CD003817.
- Shiri R, Viikari-Juntura E, Varonen H, Heliovaara M: Prevalence and determinants of lateral and medial epicondylitis: A population study. Am J Epidemiol 2006;164:1065–1074.
- U.S. Department of Health and Human Services: CDC National Center for Health Statistics. Healthy People 2010, January 23, 2004. Available at: www.cdc.gov/nchs/about/otheract/hpdata2010/focusareas/fa19-nutrition.htm. Accessed January 19, 2009.
- Wendelboe AM, Hegmann KT, Gren LH, et al: Associations between body-mass index and surgery for rotator cuff tendinitis. J Bone Joint Surg Am 2004;86A:743–747.

Chapter 11 Special Populations: Comorbidities

Alfred Cianflocco and Emily Harold

Key Concepts

- Comorbid conditions are increasingly common in today's patient population.
- With the known health benefits of physical activity, it is the physician's responsibility to encourage exercise in all patients as part of a comprehensive treatment plan for conditions such as obesity, hypertension, diabetes mellitus, coronary artery disease, and dyslipidemia.
- The physician must be able to safely promote exercise in patients with multiple diseases.

Definition

- A comorbidity is the presence of an additional or coexisting disease with reference to an index diagnosis. For instance, when a patient is diagnosed with obesity, he or she often has comorbidities of hypertension and/or diabetes mellitus.
- The presence of comorbidities can place an individual in a higher risk category than if no comorbidities exist.
- In this chapter, common comorbid conditions are discussed in relation to how they may affect one's ability to exercise safely, as well as the beneficial effects of exercise on the comorbidity.

Diabetes Mellitus

- Diabetes can be subdivided into two groups: type 1 and type 2.

Type 1 Diabetes

- The usual onset is in childhood secondary to lack of insulin production in the pancreas.
- Exercise in individuals with type 1 diabetes is recommended to decrease macrovascular complications but has not been shown to affect glycemic control.
- American Diabetes Association guidelines for exercise in type 1 diabetes mellitus
  - In general, the goal in type 1 diabetes mellitus is to prevent hypoglycemia and hyperglycemia during exercise.
  - Blood glucose should be checked before exercise.
  - Exercise should be avoided if blood glucose is more than 250 mg/dL and ketones are present; if blood glucose is less than 100 mg/dL, carbohydrates should be ingested before exercise.
  - Carbohydrate-based foods should be readily available during exercise if needed.

Type 2 Diabetes

- Common in adults but becoming increasingly prevalent in children
- In individuals who are in the early stage of disease, exercise has been shown to prevent the onset of diabetes. In individuals in the late stages, it has been shown to decrease insulin resistance and allow better blood glucose control.
- American Diabetes Association guidelines for exercise in type 2 diabetes mellitus
  - A regular exercise program should be part of the treatment plan.
  - An exercise stress test should be performed based on any one of the criteria in Box 11-1 before beginning an exercise program.
  - Diabetics with peripheral neuropathy should abstain from activities that may cause foot blistering including jogging, prolonged walking, and stair exercises.
  - Diabetics with moderate to severe nonproliferative diabetic retinopathy or proliferative retinopathy should not perform activities that substantially increase systolic blood pressure including boxing, power lifting, and heavy competitive sports.

Hypertension

- Hypertension is the most common cardiovascular condition in competitive athletes.
- Different stages of hypertension were defined by Joint National Committee VII and are listed in Table 11-1.
- The use of antihypertensive agents may limit an athlete's exercise performance. This is especially true with β-blockers and diuretics, which should be avoided in competitive athletes.

BOX 11-1 *Exercise Stress Test*

An exercise test should be considered if the diabetic patient has at least one of the following risk factors and is going to start a workout of at least moderate intensity (50% maximum heart rate)

Age >35 years
Type 2 diabetes >10 years' duration
Type 1 diabetes >15 years' duration
Presence of any additional risk factors for coronary artery disease*
Presence of nephropathy including microalbuminuria
Peripheral vascular disease
Autonomic neuropathy
Presence of proliferative retinopathy

*Smoking, blood pressure >140/90 mmHg; total cholesterol >200 mg/dL; low-density lipoprotein >130 mg/dL; family history of myocardial infarction in first-degree relative younger than 60 years of age; high-density lipoprotein <35 mg/dL for men and <45 mg/dL for women.

TABLE 11-1 *Joint National Committee VII Guidelines*

Definition	Systolic BP	Diastolic BP
Normal	<120 mm Hg	<80 mm Hg
Prehypertension	120–139 mm Hg	80–89 mm Hg
Stage 1 hypertension	140–159 mm Hg	90–99 mm Hg
Stage 2 hypertension	>160 mm Hg	>100 mm Hg

BP, blood pressure.

- Exercise has been shown to decrease both systolic and diastolic blood pressures; these results are obtained with low- to moderate-intensity exercise for 20 to 60 minutes 2 to 3 days per week. Therefore, individuals with hypertension should engage in a regular exercise program as part of a comprehensive treatment plan.
- Recommendations for exercise in hypertensive patients are based on the Bethesda Conference guidelines, as follows:
  - Stage 1 hypertension: Patients may exercise as long as there is no evidence of heart disease or other end organ damage. Physical activities should be primarily dynamic. Frequent office visits should ensure that blood pressure is adequately controlled.
  - Stage 2 hypertension: Patients may exercise as long as their blood pressure is well controlled and no end organ damage exists. Activities such as weight lifting, boxing, and wrestling with a static component should be avoided if blood pressure is not optimally controlled.
  - End organ damage: If it is present, the severity of the damage and the activity attempted dictate the patient's ability to participate. These decisions should be made on an individual basis.

Coronary Artery Disease

- The most frequent cause of exercise-related cardiac events in adults is coronary artery disease; therefore, before beginning an exercise program, athletes should see their physician for a preparticipation evaluation.
- Individuals at risk of cardiovascular disease should undergo screening as recommended by the American Heart Association guidelines (see Box 7-1) before starting an exercise program.
- An individual is classified as having coronary artery disease if (1) a lesion in at least one major artery is documented on coronary angiography, (2) there is a history of myocardial infarction, or (3) there is a history of angina pectoris with an abnormal stress test.
- Both the American Heart Association and the American College of Sports Medicine recommend 30 minutes of physical activity most days of the week for all individuals with coronary artery disease to positively affect risk factors such as obesity, diabetes, and hypertension.
- After an athlete is diagnosed with coronary artery disease, he or she can be categorized into two separate levels of risk: mildly increased or substantially increased.
- Mildly increased risk
  - Normal or near normal ejection fraction (>50%), normal exercise tolerance for age, no exercise-induced ischemia or ventricular arrhythmias on a stress test, and no significant stenosis (>50%) in all major coronary arteries
  - Can participate in low dynamic and low/moderate static competitive sports (e.g., golf, billiards, bowling, archery, walking); re-evaluation yearly
- Substantially increased risk (any one of these factors indicates substantial risk)
  - Impaired left ventricular ejection fraction (<50%) at rest, evidence of exercise-induced ischemia or ventricular arrhythmias on a stress test, or significant stenosis (>50%) of a major coronary artery
  - Can participate in low dynamic and low static sports (e.g., golf, bowling, billiards) if able but re-evaluation needed every 6 months
- After a myocardial infarction, a patient should be enrolled in a cardiac exercise and rehabilitation program; these have been shown to reduce overall mortality by as much as 25%.

- Cardiac rehabilitation programs typically involve supervised exercise for 2 to 6 months followed by a home exercise program.
- After a rehabilitation program is completed, the individual can then be risk stratified as previously described.

Obesity

- The musculoskeletal complications of obesity are outlined in Chapter 10.
- Obesity is defined as a body mass index greater than 30. Overweight is characterized by a body mass index between 25 and 30 (see Fig. 10-2).
- Obesity is associated with increased cardiovascular mortality, diabetes, hypertension, dyslipidemia, and stroke. It also increases one's risk of gallbladder disease, sleep apnea, and a number of cancers including breast, colon, and prostate cancer.
- Advice to begin an exercise program is appropriate for all overweight individuals; the contraindications to exercise should be based on other comorbidities (e.g., diabetes, hypertension).
- A 5% to 10% weight loss reduction can help reduce the risk of developing comorbid conditions such as hypertension, knee osteoarthritis, and diabetes mellitus.

Patient Instructions

- A routine exercise program has been shown to help treat common medical conditions such as hypertension, diabetes, coronary artery disease, and obesity.
- If the previously cited underlying conditions are present, a preparticipation physical should be performed before an exercise program is begun, and instructions should be given regarding any known contraindications to exercise.

Suggested Reading

- American Diabetes Association: Diabetes mellitus and exercise. Diabetes Care 2002;25:S64–S68.
- Bauman AE: Updating the evidence that physical activity is good for health: An epidemiological review 2000–2003. J Sci Med Sport 2003;7:6–19.
- Flegal K, Graubard B, Williamson D, Gail M: Cause-specific excess deaths associated with underweight, overweight, and obesity. JAMA 2007;298:2028–2037.
- Garber CE: Section IV: Exercise testing and training for individuals with chronic disease. In Kaminsky L (ed): ACSM's Resource Manual for Guidelines for Exercise Testing and Prescription. Baltimore: Lippincott Williams & Wilkins, 2006, pp 411–528.
- MacKnight J: Exercise considerations in hypertension, obesity, and dyslipidemia. Clin Sports Med 2003;22:101–121.
- Maron B, Araujo C, Thompson P, et al: Recommendations for preparticipation screening and the assessment of cardiovascular disease in master athletes. Circulation 2001;103:327–334.
- Maron BJ, Mitchell JH (eds): 26th Bethesda Conference: Recommendations for determining eligibility for competition in athletes with cardiovascular abnormalities. J Am Coll Cardiol 1994;24:845–899.
- Thompson PD, Buchner D, Pina IL, et al: Exercise and physical activity in the prevention and treatment of atherosclerotic cardiovascular disease. Circulation 2003;107:3109–3116.

Chapter 12 Special Populations: Female Athletes

Kelly Waicus

FEMALE ATHLETE TRIAD

ICD-9 CODES

626.0	*Amenorrhea*
307.50	*Eating Disorder*
733.0	*Osteoporosis*

Key Concepts

- The female athlete trial has three inter-related conditions: low energy availability (with or without eating disorder), amenorrhea, and osteoporosis.
- For each condition, the athlete may fall somewhere on the continuum between the normal health end and the pathologic end of the spectrum.
- The prevalence of the triad is unknown; disordered eating is reported in 1% to 62% of female athletes, menstrual dysfunction in 6% to 79%, and decreased bone mineral density in 10% to 50%. There are large ranges based on type of athlete studied, diagnostic criteria, and study methodology.
- It is more common in sports in which physical appearance and/or weight are an integral part of the sport, which include events judged subjectively as well as endurance events that favor low-body-weight athletes.
- Females participating in gymnastics, figure skating, running, and diving are likely to be most at risk. Ballet dancers are also at risk for the conditions in female athlete trial.

History

- A history of amenorrhea or altered menstruation is often the first abnormality detected. It may be detected in preparticipation screening. Primary amenorrhea is defined as the absence of menses by age 15 with secondary sex characteristics present. Secondary amenorrhea is the discontinuation of menstrual cycles for more than 3 months.
- Some athletes are diagnosed only after presenting with a stress fracture, prompting further questioning and bone health investigation.
- Answers to questions about disordered eating practices, either on preparticipation screening or during a regular office visit, may be the first indication of the triad. Athletes may reveal pathologic weight control behaviors or inadequate intake based on energy output.
- Athletes with a clinical eating disorder may present with symptoms of that illness, including cold intolerance, light-headedness, constipation, and sore throat.
- Decreasing athletic performance or fatigue may be the only symptom reported.

Physical Examination

- The majority of information leading to the diagnosis of female athlete triad will be from the patient's history. The physical examination is often normal.
- There may be findings suggestive of an eating disorder, including bradycardia, hypotension (particularly orthostatic hypotension), lingual enamel erosion, parotid gland hypertrophy, Russell's sign (callus on finger from self-induced vomiting), cold/discolored hands and feet, and lanugo hair or skin dryness.
- The physical examination may be consistent with stress fracture (see Chapters 136, 163, and 195).

Imaging

- If there is concern for a stress fracture, appropriate images should be obtained (see Chapters 136, 163, and 195).
- Bone mineral density should be assessed by dual-energy x-ray absorptiometry in female patients with a history or diagnosis of a stress fracture and after a total of 6 months or more of amenorrhea, oligomenorrhea, disordered eating, or an eating disorder. Re-evaluation in 12 months is recommended for those with persistent triad symptoms.

Additional Tests

- Electrolytes, serum proteins, and liver enzymes, complete blood count with differential, erythrocyte sedimentation rate, thyroid function tests, and urinalysis should be obtained in athletes with disordered eating or a clinical eating disorder.
- Workup to exclude other causes of amenorrhea should include pregnancy test, follicle-stimulating hormone and luteinizing hormone, prolactin, and thyroid function studies.
- Consider free serum testosterone and dehydroepiandrosterone sulfate if evidence of androgen excess is seen on physical examination.
- Consider serum estradiol or a progesterone challenge test (medroxyprogesterone acetate 10 mg once daily for 7–10 days) to assess estrogen levels. Athletes with functional hypothalamic amenorrhea are likely to be hypoestrogenic and may fail to have withdrawal bleeding with the challenge test.
- Consider additional testing for primary amenorrhea based on history and physical examination.

Differential Diagnosis

- Other causes of amenorrhea include, but are not limited to, pregnancy, thyroid disease, pituitary or adrenal tumor/disease, polycystic ovarian syndrome, premature ovarian failure, and Turner's syndrome (primary amenorrhea).
- Hyperparathyroidism and excess glucocorticosteroid use may cause decreased bone mineral density and recurrent stress fractures.
- Consider other causes of low energy availability including malabsorption syndromes such as celiac disease, autoimmune disease, or malignancy.

Treatment

- A multidisciplinary treatment team should include a physician or other health care provider, a registered dietitian/nutritionist, and, for athletes with clinical eating disorders, a mental health professional specializing in these disorders.
- Modifications in diet and exercise need to be made to increase energy availability. A written contract may be necessary in athletes with eating disorders to ensure that minimal criteria are met to continue training and competition.
- Consider calcium and vitamin D supplementation.
- Adequate nutrition, optimal energy availability, and healthy body weight should be the primary focus of treatment to restore regular menses and improve bone mineral density.
- If older than 16 years of age, consider oral contraceptive pills in athletes with functional hypothalamic amenorrhea if bone mineral density is decreasing despite adequate nutrition and body weight.

Troubleshooting

- Prevention of the female athlete triad through education should be the goal of those caring for at-risk athletes. Athletes, coaches, and parents should be educated about the triad and the impact it can have on young women.
- Counseling on energy/caloric needs and nutritional requirements for the athletes' age group including calcium and vitamin D should be provided. Special attention should be given to maximizing bone mineral accrual in pediatric and adolescent athletes.
- Female athletes should be educated about the detrimental effects of amenorrhea.
- Screening is essential for early detection and intervention. The preparticipation examination is often an ideal time to screen young women. Questions regarding menstrual, diet, and exercise history should be included. Reports of amenorrhea or oligomenorrhea should be addressed and investigated. A history of disordered eating, pathologic weight control practices, or stress fracture should prompt further questioning and workup as indicated.

Patient Instructions

- Restoring optimal energy balance through good nutrition and monitoring of activity is essential to long-term bone health.
- Returning to a state of optimal energy balance is very likely to improve endurance and athletic performance.
- Absence of menstruation should not be considered a convenience, but rather an indication that the body does not have enough energy available to continue normal physiologic function. Spontaneous return of menses is an indicator of improving energy availability.

Suggested Reading

- Beals KA, Meyer NL: Female athlete triad update. Clin Sports Med 2007;26:69–89.
- Lebrun CM: The female athlete triad: What's a doctor to do? Curr Sports Med Rep 2007;6:397–404.

- Nattiv A, Loucks AB, Manore MM, et al: American College of Sports Medicine position stand. The female athlete triad. Med Sci Sports Exerc 2007;39:1867–1882.

EXERCISE AND PREGNANCY

ICD-9 CODES

V 22	*Normal Pregnancy*
V 22.1	*Pregnancy Antepartum Care*
646.90	*Complications of Pregnancy*

Key Concepts

- Recommendations for exercise during pregnancy have changed significantly in the past 20 years.
- Exercise is now considered safe for both the mother and fetus during pregnancy. Recent recommendations support initiating or continuing exercise in the majority of pregnancies.
- Exercise is likely beneficial in the prevention of gestational diabetes and is an important adjunctive therapy for treatment of mothers who do not achieve euglycemia with diet alone.
- Both absolute and relative contraindications to aerobic exercise as well as warning signs to terminate exercise during pregnancy exist.
- Changes affecting the musculoskeletal system during pregnancy make women highly susceptible to musculoskeletal discomfort.
- Concerns of the pregnant, competitive athlete include both the effects of pregnancy on the woman's competitive abilities and the effects of strenuous training on the pregnancy and fetus. Close obstetric monitoring of these athletes is essential.
- Physiologic changes that occur during pregnancy usually persist for 4 to 6 weeks postpartum but may last longer if the mother is breast-feeding.

History

- Before making recommendations regarding exercise during pregnancy, several factors should be considered including the patient's age, general physical condition, and exercise history including her prepregnancy regimen. Any history of orthopaedic injuries or musculoskeletal issues as well as risk factors for cardiovascular disease should be assessed. Other important factors include current medications, medical history including the presence of pulmonary disease or diabetes, and obstetric history.
- Patients should be aware of warning signs to stop exercise and seek medical attention (Box 12-1).

BOX 12-1 *Warning Signs to Terminate Exercise While Pregnant*

Vaginal bleeding
Dyspnea before exertion
Dizziness
Headache
Chest pain
Muscle weakness
Lower leg pain or swelling
Preterm labor
Decreased fetal movement
Amniotic fluid leakage

Adapted from the American College of Obstetricians and Gynecologists Committee Opinion No. 267

Physical Examination

- Routine obstetric visits are important for all pregnant women. With regular follow-up, problems with maternal health, fetal health, or both may be detected as early in the pregnancy as possible.
- It is important for health care providers to be aware of physical conditions that are either absolute or relative contraindications to aerobic exercise in pregnancy (Box 12-2).

Imaging

- Ultrasound imaging is likely to be performed as part of routine obstetric care. Unless problems arise, it is unlikely that other imaging studies will be needed.

Additional Tests

- The need for additional testing during the pregnancy may be determined by the patient's obstetrician.
- If warning signs occur (see Box 12-1), further workup may be pursued by the patient's primary care provider, obstetrician, or both.

Differential Diagnosis

- Problems occurring during pregnancy and associated differential diagnosis most likely will require the expertise of an obstetrician and should be referred to these health care professionals.

Treatment

- Encourage exercise during pregnancy for all women without known contraindications.

BOX 12-2 *Contraindications to Aerobic Exercise in Pregnancy: Absolute and Relative*

Absolute contraindications to exercise during pregnancy

- Hemodynamically significant heart disease
- Restrictive lung disease
- Incompetent cervix/cerclage
- Multiple gestation pregnancy at risk of premature labor
- Persistent second or third trimester bleeding
- Placenta previa after 26 weeks' gestation
- Premature labor during current pregnancy
- Ruptured membranes
- Preeclampsia-/pregnancy-induced hypertension

Relative contraindications to exercise during pregnancy

- Severe anemia
- Unevaluated maternal cardiac arrhythmia
- Chronic bronchitis
- Poorly controlled type 1 diabetes
- Extreme morbid obesity
- Extreme underweight (body mass index < 12)
- History of extremely sedentary lifestyle
- Intrauterine growth restriction in current pregnancy
- Poorly controlled hypertension
- Orthopaedic limitations
- Poorly controlled seizure disorder
- Poorly controlled hyperthyroidism
- Heavy smoking

Adapted from the American College of Obstetricians and Gynecologists Committee Opinion No. 267

BOX 12-3 *Guidelines for Exercise in Pregnancy*

Beginning Exerciser or Not Previously Active
Frequency: at least three times per week
Type: low-impact (walking, bicycling, swimming, aerobics, water aerobics)
Intensity: perceived exertion = moderately hard, heart rate 65% to 75% maximum
Duration: 30 minutes

Recreational Athlete
Frequency: three to five times per week
Type: low-impact plus previous activities such as running, tennis, cross-country skiing
Intensity: perceived exertion = moderately hard to hard, heart rate 65% to 80% maximum
Duration: 30 to 60 minutes

Elite Athlete
Frequency: four to six times per week
Type: same as above plus competitive activities depending on gestational age
Intensity: perceived exertion = hard, heart rate 75% to 80% maximum
Duration: 90 minutes

Adapted from Joy EA: Exercise in pregnancy. In Ratcliffe SC (ed): Family Practice Obstetrics, 2nd ed. Philadelphia: Hanley & Belfus, 2001, pp 81–88.

- General guidelines for exercise in pregnancy are given in Box 12-3.
- Competitive athletes need to be aware of the effects of pregnancy on athletic performance as well as the effects of high-intensity training on the pregnancy.
- Weight gain, altered center of gravity, and ligamentous laxity can all result in an inefficiency of movement and a decrease in competitive ability during pregnancy.
- The long, frequent, high-intensity workouts of most competitive athletes may increase their risk of thermoregulatory problems during pregnancy. Although there is no consensus regarding maternal exercise and fetal weight, it is likely that pregnant competitive athletes and their infants will have less weight gain during pregnancy. Such elite athletes should be monitored carefully for fetal growth.
- Finally, a small increase in uterine contractions may be seen with physical activity. Therefore, those competitive athletes with a history of preterm labor should reduce activity in the second and third trimesters.
- Avoid the use of nonsteroidal anti-inflammatory medications when treating pregnant women with musculoskeletal conditions. Cryotherapy, bracing, acetaminophen, and physical therapy may all be helpful. Most conditions are self-limited and resolve when the woman returns to her prepregnancy state.

Troubleshooting

- Although exercise is generally thought to be safe during pregnancy, there is no upper limit of exercise that has been determined as safe. Physically active women should plan to maintain, rather than drastically increase, their level of fitness during pregnancy.
- Pregnant women should be educated about the increased fluid and nutritional needs of both pregnancy and exercise as well as the dangers of heat stress.
- Pregnant patients should be counseled to avoid sports with a high potential for contact or increased risk of falling. Both scuba diving and exertion at altitudes above 6000 feet should be avoided. Women who are active at higher altitudes (below 6000 feet is thought to be safe) need to be aware of signs of altitude sickness.
- After the first trimester, pregnant women should avoid exercising in the supine position as well as motionless standing during exercise.

Patient Instructions

- Most women can exercise safely throughout their pregnancy.
- Exercising at least 30 minutes most days of the week can provide significant health benefits including preventing or treating gestational diabetes; reducing back pain, constipation, bloating, and swelling; increasing mood, energy, and posture; promoting muscle tone, strength, and endurance; and improving sleep. Regular activity may also make it easier to restore prepregnancy levels of fitness once the baby is born.
- Consult with your physician before beginning any exercise program to make sure there is no reason to limit your activity. There are many forms of exercise that are safe during pregnancy for both beginners and those who have exercised regularly before pregnancy.
- After the first trimester, avoid exercises that require you to lie on your back.
- Throughout your pregnancy, it is recommended that both contact sports and sports with a high risk of falling be avoided. Exercise above 6000 feet and scuba diving should also be avoided.

Suggested Reading

- American College of Obstetricians and Gynecologists: Exercise during pregnancy and the postpartum period. American College of Obstetricians and Gynecologists Committee Opinion No. 267. Obstet Gynecol 2002;99:171–173.
- Borg-Stein J, Dugan SA: Musculoskeletal disorders of pregnancy, delivery and postpartum. Phys Med Rehabil Clin N Am 2007;18:459–476.
- Paisley TS, Joy EA, Price RJ: Exercise during pregnancy: A practical approach. Curr Sports Med Rep 2003;2:325–330.

Chapter 13 Special Populations: Athletes

Alfred Cianflocco and Emily Harold

Key Concepts

- A very substantial portion of the population competes in athletic events at the grade school, high school, collegiate, master, recreational, and professional levels.
- A preparticipation physical examination should be performed annually in any individual competing in sporting events to ensure safe play.
- An understanding of common sport-specific injuries will aid in diagnosis of an injured athlete.
- A team physician at the event needs to be able to stabilize and triage injuries as necessary.
- Treating athletes requires knowledge of return to play guidelines.

Demographics

- An estimated 7.2 million high school students participated in sports in 2005 to 2006. These athletes accounted for 1.4 million injuries with an injury rate of 2.4 per 1000 athlete exposures (competitions or practices).
- More than 375,000 athletes compete at the collegiate level. The National Collegiate Athletic Association has an Injury Surveillance System that documents injury rates in every sport during the year (Fig. 13-1). These are reported in terms of injury per athlete exposure (one exposure is equivalent to one practice or game).
- Other data regarding competition at additional levels of sport are not readily available.

Preparticipation Examination

- A comprehensive physical designed to detect individuals who may be at high risk of injury during competition should be performed annually.
- The examination includes medical history, family history, menstrual history, history of injuries, height, weight, blood pressure, and a thorough physical examination.
- At this time, additional screening tests such as electrocardiograms and echocardiograms are not recommended except in those individuals deemed at risk of sudden cardiac death based on their history and physical examination.
- The 26th Bethesda Conference is an excellent resource for information regarding cardiac problems and clearance for participation in sports.
- The American Academy of Pediatrics is also an outstanding resource for participation questions regarding medical conditions.

Diagnosis

- Diagnosis of athletic injuries requires a history and an examination targeted to the injured area.
- If on site, one should be able to appropriately treat and refer the athlete when necessary.
- An understanding of sport-specific injuries can aid in the diagnosis.

Sport-Specific Injuries

- Injury rates vary based on sport and are substantially higher in games than practice. For full injury data from the National Collegiate Athletic Association for the years 1988 to 1989 and 2003 to 2004, see Figure 13-1.
- The following are some common injuries in selected competitive National Collegiate Athletic Association sports.
    - Football
        - — The most common injuries reported in the National Collegiate Athletic Association from 1988 to 1989 through 2003 to 2004 are knee internal derangements, ankle ligament sprains, upper leg muscle contusions, and concussions. All these injuries were more common in games than practices.
        - — In games, the rate per 1000 athlete exposures of knee internal derangement was 6.17, ankle

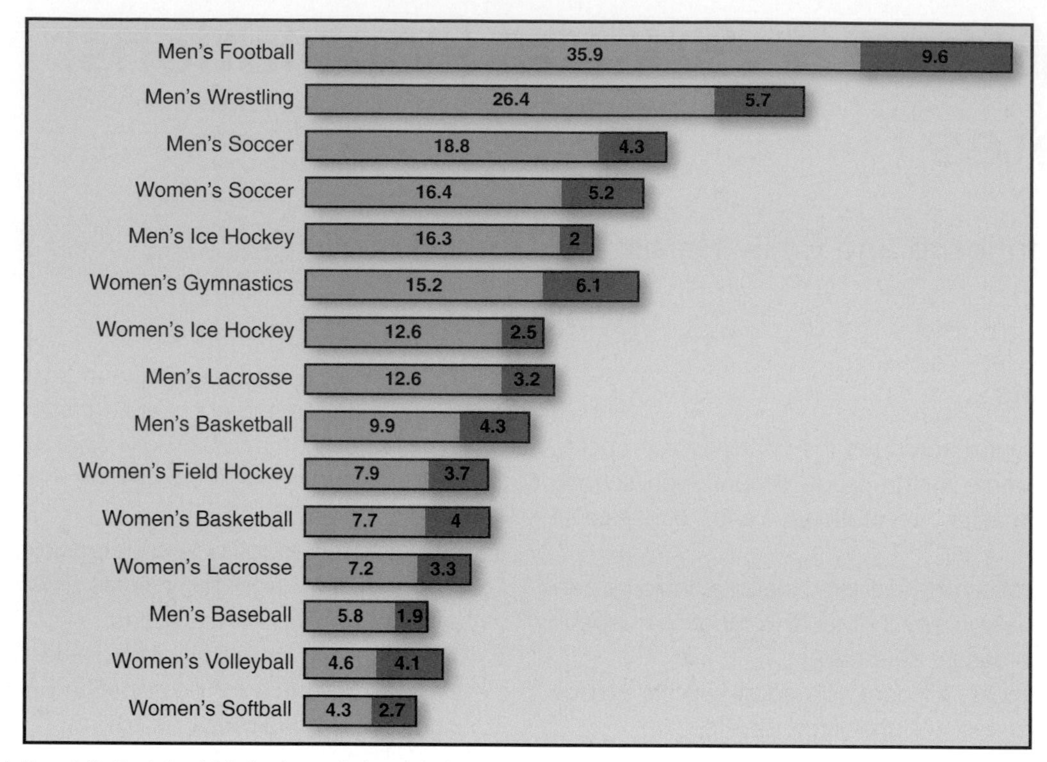

Figure 13-1 National Collegiate Athletic Association injuries per 1000 athlete exposures, 1998–1999 through 2003–2004. *Blue* indicates during games; *red* indicates injuries during practice.

sprains was 5.39, upper leg contusions was 1.27, and concussions was 2.34.

— Of the 4767 knee internal derangements reported, 45% resulted in less than 10 days of time loss. The most common knee injuries were meniscus injuries (2293), anterior cruciate ligament injuries (2159), and posterior cruciate ligament injuries (382). Of the anterior cruciate ligament injuries reported, 31% were noncontact.

- Soccer
  - — Common injuries in men's games were knee internal derangements and ankle ligament sprains, which accounted for 28% of all injuries. In men's practices, ankle ligament sprains and upper leg muscle strains accounted for 34% of all injuries.
  - — In men's games, players were four times more likely to sustain an ankle injury, six times more likely to sustain a knee injury, and more than 13 times more likely to have a concussion compared with practices.
  - — The injury rates for women's soccer over the same period were similar to those listed for men's soccer.
- Basketball
  - — Approximately 60% of injuries are to the lower extremities, with ankle ligament sprains accounting for 26% of all injuries. The next highest percentage is for knee internal derangements at 7% for men and 16% for women.
  - — The incidence of anterior cruciate ligament injuries in men's games was 0.18 per 1000 athlete exposures for the period 1988 to 2004.
  - — The incidence of anterior cruciate ligament injuries in women's games was 0.66 per 1000 athlete exposures for the period 1988 to 2004. This is approximately 3.6 times the incidence in men during the same period.
- Baseball
  - — In college baseball, approximately one fourth of all injuries were severe, resulting in more than 10 days of time loss from participation. Of these, muscle strains and tendonitis of the shoulder accounted for 30%, knee internal derangement for 13%, and ankle sprains for an additional 10%.
  - — Almost half of all injuries involved the upper extremities.

— During games, 15% of all reported injuries involved pitching and 10% involved being hit by a batted ball.

Treatment

- All injuries should be treated as outlined in accompanying chapters.
- Specific goals for return to play should also be determined and met during the course of treatment, allowing safe return to play.

Suggested Reading

- Agel J, Evans T, Dick R, et al: Descriptive epidemiology of collegiate men's soccer injuries: National Collegiate Athletic Association Injury Surveillance System, 1988–1989 through 2003–2004. J Athletic Training 2007;42:270–277.
- Agel J, Olson D, Dick R, et al: Descriptive epidemiology of collegiate women's basketball injuries: National Collegiate Athletic Association Injury Surveillance System, 1988–1989 through 2003–2004. J Athletic Training 2007;42:202–210.
- American Academy of Pediatrics, Committee on Sports Medicine and Fitness: Medical conditions affecting sports participation. Pediatrics 1994;94:757–760.
- Centers for Disease Control and Prevention: Sports-related injuries among high school athletes—United States 2005–2006 school year. Available at: www.cdc.gov/mmwr/preview/mmwrhtml/mm5538a1.htm. Accessed November 19, 2007.
- Dick R, Agel J, Marshall S: National Collegiate Athletic Association Injury Surveillance System commentaries: Introduction and methods. J Athletic Training 2007;42:173–182.
- Dick R, Ferrara M, Agel J, et al: Descriptive epidemiology of collegiate men's football injuries: National Collegiate Athletic Association Injury Surveillance System, 1988–1989 through 2003–2004. J Athletic Training 2007;42:221–233.
- Dick R, Hertel J, Agel J, et al: Descriptive epidemiology of collegiate men's basketball injuries: National Collegiate Athletic Association Injury Surveillance System, 1988–1989 through 2003–2004. J Athletic Training 2007;42:194–201.
- Dick R, Putukian M, Agel J, et al: Descriptive epidemiology of collegiate women's soccer injuries: National Collegiate Athletic Association Injury Surveillance System, 1988–1989 through 2003–2004. J Athletic Training 2007;42:278–285.
- Dick R, Sauers E, Agel J, et al: Descriptive epidemiology of collegiate men's baseball injuries: National Collegiate Athletic Association Injury Surveillance System, 1988–1989 through 2003–2004. J Athletic Training 2007;42:183–193.
- Hootman J, Dick R, Agel J: Epidemiology of collegiate injuries for 15 sports: Summary and recommendations for injury prevention initiative. J Athletic Training 2007;42:311–319.
- Kurowski K, Chandran S: The preparticipation athletic evaluation. Am Fam Physician 2000;61:2683–2690, 2696–2698.
- Mellion M, Walsh W, Madden C, et al: Team Physician's Handbook, 3rd ed. Philadelphia: Hanley & Belfus, 2002.
- National Collegiate Athletic Association (NCAA) Injury Surveillance System: Game Rate Injury Summary. NCAA Injury Surveillance. Available at: www.ncaa.org/membership/ed_outreach/health-safety/iss/GameandPractice_Comparisons/Fig2_2005.pdf. Accessed November 16, 2007.
- National Collegiate Athletic Association (NCAA): Online Resource for the NCAA. Available at www.ncaa.org. Accessed November 19, 2007.

Chapter 14 Trauma: Principles of Fracture Management

David J. Berkoff and Brian J. Finnegan

ICD-9 CODES
810–819 *Fracture of Upper Limb*
820–829 *Fracture of Lower Limb*
805–809 *Fracture of Neck and Trunk*

Key Concepts

- A fracture represents a disruption of bone continuity, either complete or partial.
- Fractures are most commonly the result of trauma.
- They can be related to an abnormal force in normal bone or a normal force in abnormal bone.
- In nontrauma patients, these can be related to overuse, osteoporosis, or diseases related to abnormal bone formation.
- Fractures can result in gross or microscopic destruction of bone matrix.
- Fractures that compromise neurovascular structures or have the potential to become open injuries must be emergently treated with immediate reduction of the fracture and/or dislocation.
- An open fracture is defined as one with a disruption of the skin overlying a fractured bone allowing contact with the external environment.
- A closed fracture has intact overlying skin.
- Lacerations or abrasions require evaluation for possible open fracture and/or joint involvement, particularly those over bony prominences.
- Accurate fracture description is important for both proper diagnosis and treatment (Table 14-1).

History

- Fractures most commonly occur from an acute traumatic injury.
- The mechanism of injury (e.g., direct blow, rotation, ground level fall) should be used to guide accurate evaluation of the injury.
- Trauma may be minor if underlying bone abnormality is present.
- Patients frequently complain of pain and loss of function typically at the site of fracture. Severity, type, and quality of pain vary widely among patients.
- Pain without obvious fracture should prompt consideration of stress fractures in the setting of repetitive trauma or in those with abnormal bone formation or osteoporosis.

Physical Examination

- Carefully inspect injury to determine skin integrity for open or closed status of fractures.
- Palpate injured area for crepitus, swelling, and deformity.
- Assess neurovascular integrity and document thoroughly both before and after any manipulation of the fractured bone.
- Fractures that result from high-energy trauma require careful evaluation for compartment syndrome, especially in the setting of crush injuries.
- Always examine the joint above and below to identify potential occult injuries.

Imaging

- Plain radiographs frequently identify acute and chronic fractures.
- Stress fractures, nondisplaced fractures, and other subtle fractures may not be visible initially and may require further radiographic evaluation either in the acute setting or during timely follow-up evaluations to fully assess bone abnormalities.
- Computed tomography can be used to further describe fractures and better identify fracture fragments, displacement, and angulation. It is also often helpful before surgical management.
- Magnetic resonance imaging is used to further identify occult fractures, stress fractures, and insufficiency fractures and to better evaluate the soft-tissue structures that surround the fractured bone.

TABLE 14-1 *Fracture Description*

Fracture Descriptor	Type	Pathologic Description
Anatomic location	Epiphyseal	End of bone
	Metaphyseal	Flared portion of bone between diaphysis and epiphysis
	Diaphyseal	Shaft of long bone
	Physeal (growth plate)	Salter-Harris classifications I–V describe fractures involving the growth plate
Orientation of fracture line	Transverse (Fig. 14-1)	Fracture perpendicular to long axis of bone
	Oblique (Fig. 14-2)	Angular fracture down long axis of bone
	Spiral (Fig. 14-3)	A complex fracture line that encircles shaft of bone (twisting fracture)
	Longitudinal	Along long axis of bone
	Segmental (Fig. 14-4)	Free-floating fracture segment bordered by fracture lines
	Torus (Fig. 14-5)	Buckling of the cortex without breaking bone on other side (pediatric)
	Greenstick (Fig. 14-6)	Fracture with disruption through one cortex while the other side remains intact (pediatric)
	Pathologic	Fracture of bone with underlying disease
Fragments	Simple	2 fragments
	Comminuted (Fig. 14-7)	>2 fragments
	Avulsion (Fig. 14-8)	Fragment of bone torn away from the main mass of bone
	Compression (Fig. 14-9)	Collapse of a bone, most often a vertebra
Position/displacement (described distal segment relative to proximal)	Nondisplaced	Anatomic alignment preserved
	Displaced (Fig. 14-10)	Fragments without usual anatomic alignment
	Angulated (Fig. 14-11)	The angle away from normal that the distal fragment makes with the proximal; frequently described relative to the apex of the fracture
	Shortened (bayonette)	Described as the number of centimeters of overlap
	Rotated	Description of distal fragment relative to proximal

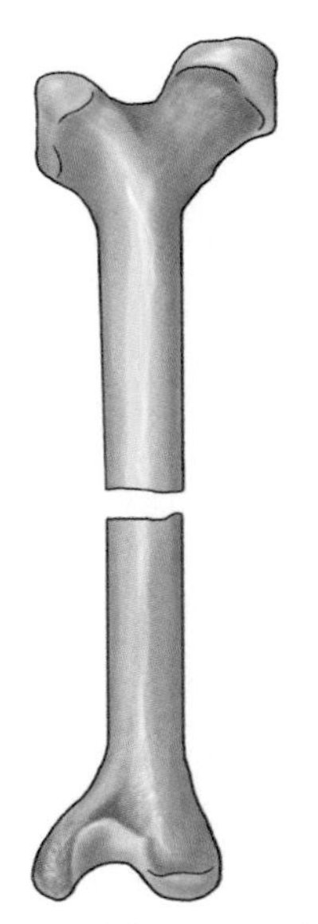

Figure 14-1 Transverse fracture.

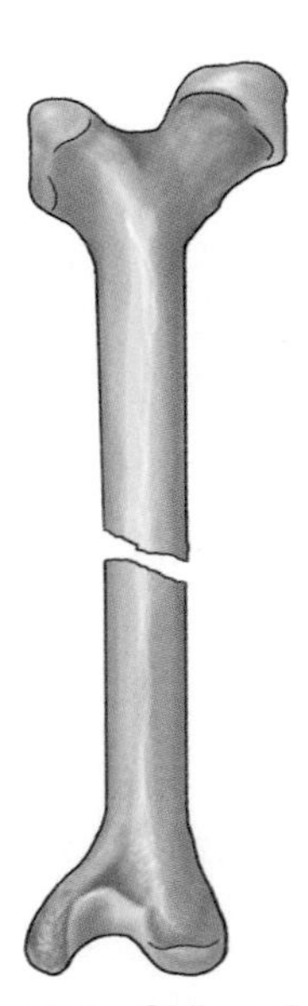

Figure 14-2 Oblique fracture.

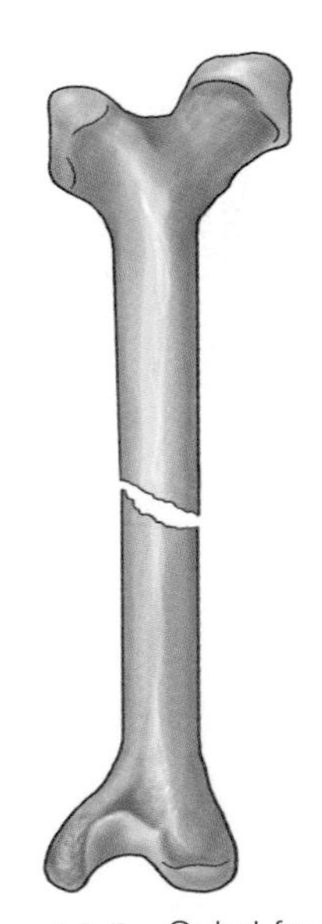

Figure 14-3 Spiral fracture.

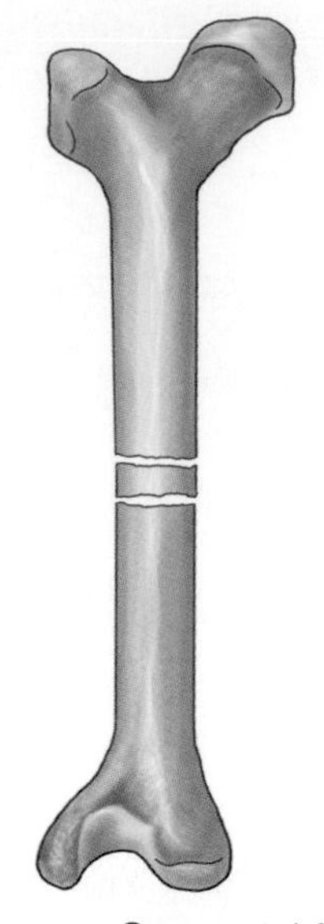

Figure 14-4 Segmental fracture.

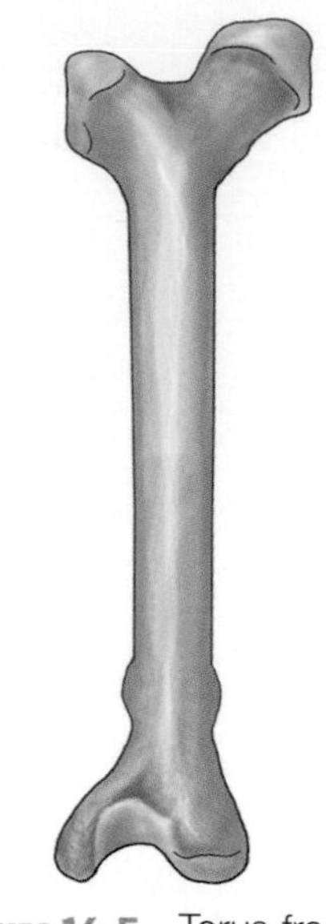

Figure 14-5 Torus fracture.

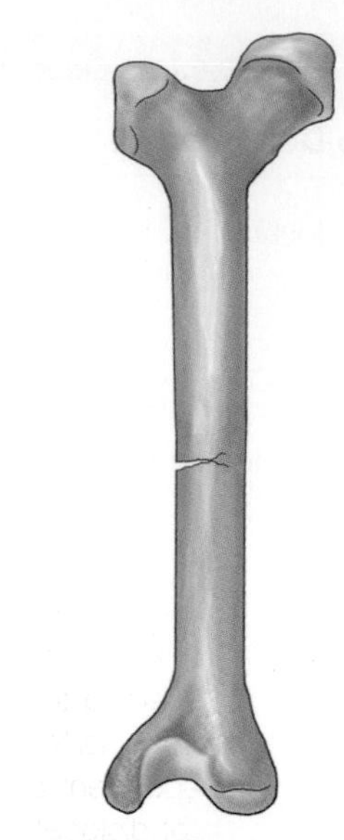

Figure 14-6 Greenstick fracture.

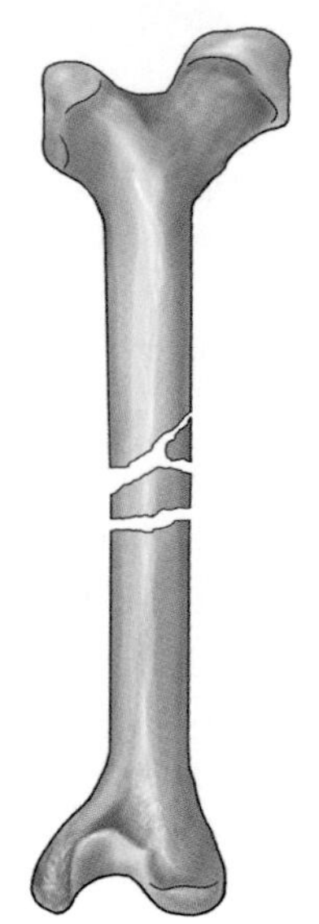

Figure 14-7 Comminuted fracture.

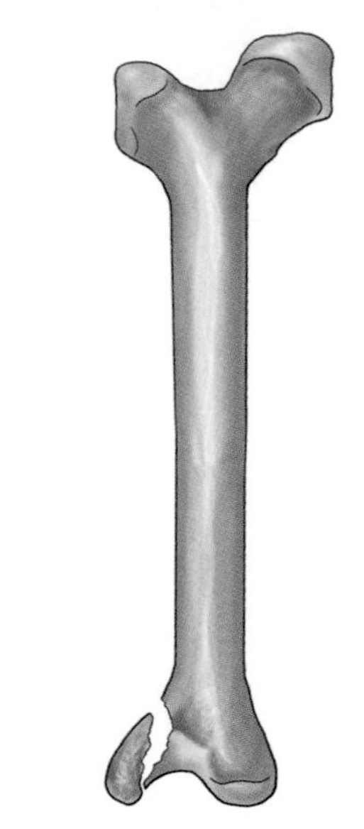

Figure 14-8 Avulsion fracture.

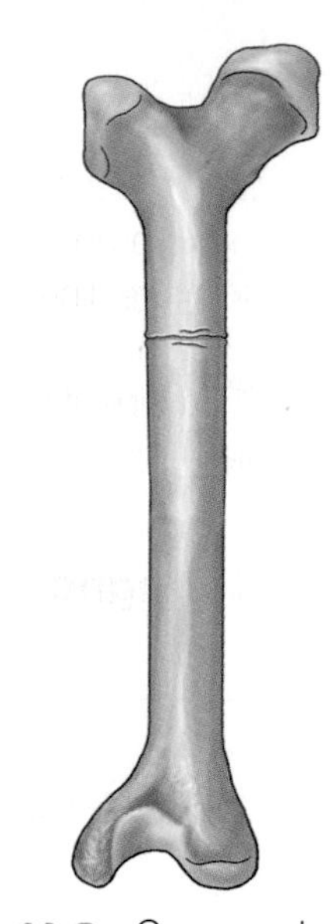

Figure 14-9 Compression fracture.

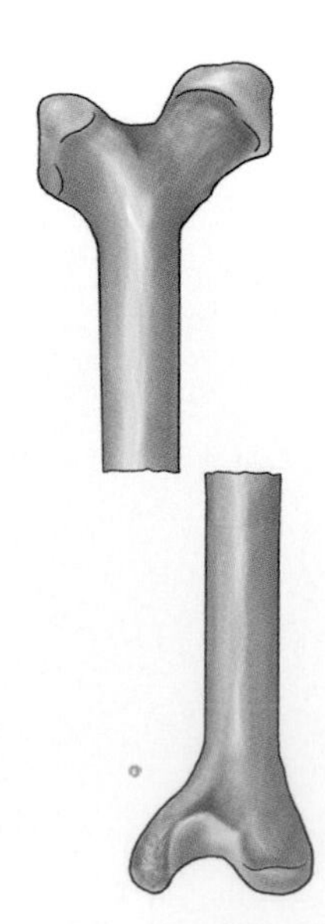

Figure 14-10 Displaced fracture.

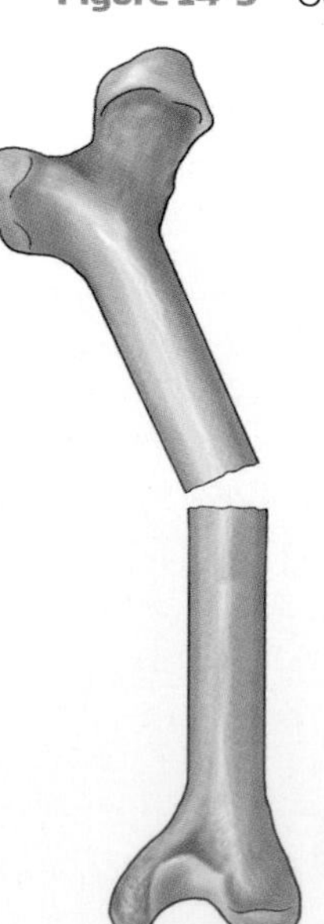

Figure 14-11 Angulated fracture.

TABLE 14-2 *Differential Diagnosis*

Diagnosis	History	Symptoms/Signs	Radiographic Evaluation
Fracture	Trauma with or without deformity	Pain, swelling, deformity, loss of function	Radiographs for uncomplicated, computed tomography or magnetic resonance imaging for complicated/operative fractures
Contusion	Direct blow to body part	Pain, swelling, ecchymosis, decreased function	Negative for fracture
Sprain	Excessive force applied to a joint causing ligamentous injury	Point tenderness, swelling, ecchymosis, minimal range of motion	May be negative or show avulsion fracture at site of ligamentous insertion, joint space widening
Strain	Overexertion or overstretching of muscle leading to damage of muscle/tendon complex	Pain, swelling, ecchymosis, decreased range of motion, palpable defect if complete disruption	Negative for fracture
Dislocation	Dependent on specific type of dislocation	Pain, gross deformity, decreased range of motion; possible neurovascular deficits	Shows disarticulation of involved bones with possible accompanying fracture

- Proper fracture description requires a consistent and logical approach and includes skin integrity, anatomic location, fracture line orientation, and displacement (see Table 14-1).
- Always obtain repeat radiographs after splinting/reducing to evaluate changes in fracture orientation.

Differential Diagnosis

- See Table 14-2.

Treatment (Fig. 14-12)

- Initial treatment should focus on accurate diagnosis to ensure proper immediate and long-term planning for fracture care.
- Pain control is essential for patient comfort and to aid in patient cooperation for splinting and/or reductions.
- Closed reduction employing traction and realignment is used for displaced fractures.
- Splinting and/or casting are used to maintain anatomic alignment in both simple fractures and those requiring reduction/relocation.
- Repeat imaging is required after reduction or splinting to assess and document post-reduction changes in bony alignment.
- Referral or consultation for further management or urgent/emergent treatment should be considered if (1) open reduction and internal fixation are required, (2) closed reduction is not possible, (3) there are open fractures, (4) neurovascular compromise is present, or (5) the severity and complexity of fracture require more definitive treatment than can initially be provided.

Troubleshooting

- Recognizing compartment syndrome due to acute injury or casting injury too tightly is imperative.
- Malunion, nonunion, stiffness, and neurovascular injury should all be comprehensively evaluated and discussed with the patient before treatment and discharge.
- The potential for long-term complications including the development of arthritis and loss of motion in a fractured joint should be discussed with the patient.

Patient Instructions

- Rest, ice, elevation, splinting, and nonsteroidal anti-inflammatory drugs
- Nonsteroidal anti-inflammatory drugs may inhibit bony healing in long bones; therefore, they should be used with a clear understanding of their role in fracture management.
- Weight-bearing status and use limitations must be clearly outlined to the patient.
- Ensure prompt and appropriate follow-up care for patients with fractures that threatened neurovascular structures, required closed or open reduction, or have been splinted or casted.
- Make patients aware of signs of possible compartment syndrome such as increasing pain, pain on

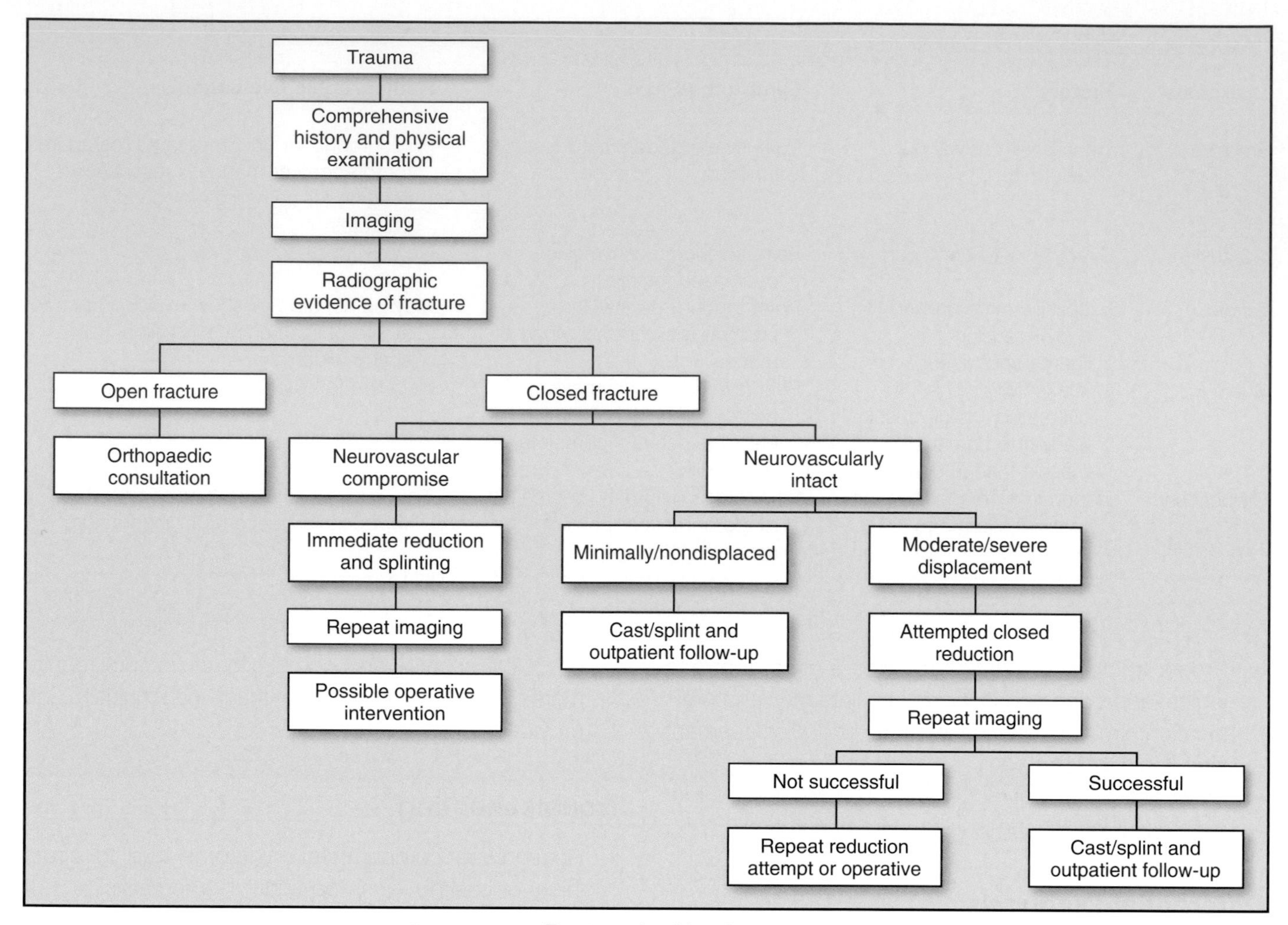

Figure 14-12 Fracture algorithm for acute trauma.

passive range of motion, pain out of proportion to injury, paresthesias, pallor, and weakness. If any of these signs are present, the patient should seek immediate orthopaedic evaluation.

Considerations in Special Populations

- Normal radiographs alone do not rule out stress fractures in sports medicine patients who are subject to repetitive impact injuries.
- In the elderly or others with osteoporosis, there may not be a defined traumatic event that precedes a fracture.
- In the pediatric population, tenderness overlying a growth plate can be a nondisplaced Salter-Harris type I fracture, which requires appropriate treatment to ensure optimal outcomes.

Suggested Reading

- Buckwalter JA: Fracture principles. In Griffen LY (ed): Essentials of Musculoskeletal Care, 3rd ed. Rosemont, IL: American Academy of Orthopaedic Surgeons, 2005, p 62.
- DeLee JC, Drez D, Jr., Miller MD (eds): DeLee and Drez's Orthopaedic Sports Medicine: Principles and Practice, 2nd ed. Philadelphia: Saunders, 2003.
- Eiff MP, Calmbach WL, Hatch RL: Fracture Management for Primary Care, 2nd ed. Philadelphia: Elsevier, 2002.
- Geiderman JM: General Principles of Orthopedic Injuries. In Marx JA, Hockberger RS, Walls RM (eds): Rosen's Emergency Medicine: Concepts and Clinical Practice, 6th ed. Philadelphia: Mosby, 2006.
- Green NE, Swiontkowski MF (eds): Skeletal Trauma in Children, 3rd ed. Philadelphia: Saunders, 2003.
- Koval KJ, Zuckerman JD (eds): Handbook of Fractures, 3rd ed. Philadelphia: Lippincott Williams & Wilkins, 2006.
- Menkes J: Initial evaluation and management of orthopedic injuries. In Tintanalli JE, Kelen GD, Stapczynski S (eds): Emergency Medicine: A Comprehensive Study Guide, 6th ed. New York: McGraw-Hill, 2003.
- Perron AD: Approach to musculoskeletal injuries. In Harwood-Nuss AL, Wolfson AB, Linder CH, et al (eds): Clinical Practice of Emergency Medicine, 4th ed. Philadelphia: Lippincott, 2005, p 1022.

Chapter 15 Trauma: Compartment Syndrome

Kevin L. Krasinski and Jeffrey R. Bytomski

ICD-9 CODES
729.9 *Compartment Syndrome, Nontraumatic*
958.8 *Compartment Syndrome, Traumatic*

Key Concepts

- Skeletal muscles are contained within distinct osseofascial compartments throughout the body.
- Compartment syndrome is caused by an increase in pressure within these relatively noncompliant compartments.
- Can be acute or chronic
- Acute compartment syndrome (ACS) is associated with progressive symptoms that can lead to permanent functional loss if not treated emergently.
- Chronic exertional compartment syndrome usually results in exercise-induced symptoms that resolve with rest.
- Elevated compartment pressures in ACS can result from internal or external factors.
  - Internal: Fluid accumulation within the compartment, secondary to hemorrhage or edema, diminishes the space available for the muscles and nerves.
  - External: Compression or traction of the limb can lead to change in the size/volume of the compartments.
- Epidemiology
  - 3.1 per 100,000 in Western populations
  - Male-to-female predominance of 10:1
  - Higher incidence in younger (<35 years old) men, which may reflect the increased muscle mass within the compartments in this population
  - Equal incidence of both high- and low-energy injuries
  - Fractures most common cause of ACS (69% of cases)
  - Can occur in both open and closed fractures
- Most common fractures
  - Tibial diaphyseal fractures (1% to 11% incidence of ACS); approximately 40% of all compartment syndromes
  - Distal radius fractures (0.25% incidence of ACS)
  - Forearm diaphyseal fractures (3% incidence of ACS)
- Etiology
  - Fractures
  - Soft-tissue trauma/crush injury
  - Vascular injury
  - Bleeding diatheses or anticoagulation leading to hemorrhage/hematoma
  - Burns, which cause soft-tissue contractures
  - Constrictive circumferential dressings/casts
  - Skeletal traction for fracture reduction
  - Fluid extravasation (e.g., intravenous fluids, contrast dye)
  - Intramedullary reaming during fracture fixation (forces blood and marrow into surrounding compartments)
  - Surgical positioning
  - Prolonged recumbent position leading to limb compression (e.g., drug overdose)
  - Reperfusion after prolonged ischemia
  - Abscess/infection
- Pathophysiology
  - Increased intracompartmental pressure results in the following progressive pathologic pathway
    - — Alteration in arteriovenous pressure gradient
    - — Diminished capillary perfusion
    - — Cellular anoxia
    - — Muscle and nerve ischemia
    - — Tissue necrosis
    - — Functional impairment of the limb
  - Vicious cycle: Elevated intracompartmental pressure leads to a reduction in venous outflow, which increases interstitial pressure and contributes to edema formation.
  - Tissue ischemia can also lead to an increase in vascular permeability and exacerbate the intracompartmental pressure elevations.

    - The innermost muscle fibers are the first to become ischemic with progression to peripheral muscle involvement in a centrifugal fashion.
    - It is the magnitude and duration of elevated intracompartmental pressure that determine the extent of muscle and nerve ischemia and necrosis.
- Locations
    - Upper extremity
        - — Shoulder girdle
        - — Arm (two compartments: anterior and posterior)
        - — Forearm (three compartments: dorsal, volar, and mobile wad)
        - — Hand (10 compartments)
    - Lower extremity
        - — Buttock
        - — Thigh (three compartments: anterior, posterior, and adductor)
        - — Leg (four compartments: anterior, lateral, superficial, and deep posterior): most common location
        - — Foot (nine compartments)
    - Spinal musculature

History

- Acute compartment syndrome is a clinical diagnosis that is supported by compartment measurement; making the diagnosis and deciding when to treat can be a challenge.
- A high clinical suspicion must be maintained so that the diagnosis is not missed.
- It is important to understand the mechanism of injury; ACS most often occurs after a traumatic event.
- Inquire about other risk factors such as age, anticoagulants, bleeding diatheses (i.e., hemophilia), or other medical comorbidities (i.e., neuropathy, hypotension, or shock).

Physical Examination

- Observation of swelling, skin discoloration, or blistering (Fig. 15-1)
- Limb compartment palpation/manual compression to estimate tension
- Active and passive motion of involved limb
- Muscle strength testing
- Evaluation of sensory function
- Assessment of vascular status
    - Close monitoring with serial examinations is critical because the development of compartment syndrome can occur over hours to days.

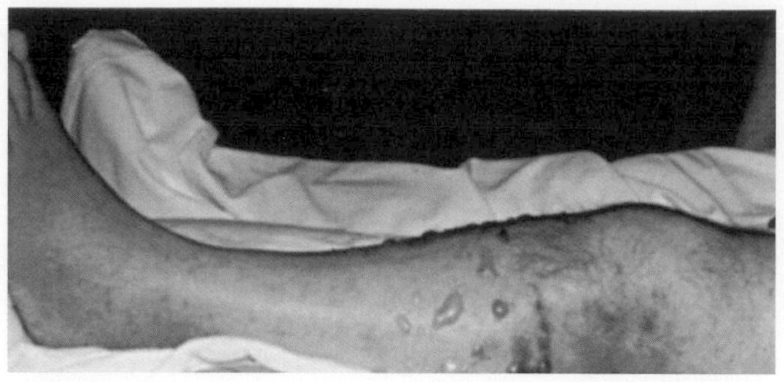

Figure 15-1 Appearance of acute compartment syndrome. (From Amendola A, Twaddle BC: Compartment syndromes. In Browner BD, Jupiter JB, Levine AM, Trafton PG [eds]: Skeletal Trauma: Basic Science, Management, and Reconstruction, 3rd ed. Philadelphia: Saunders, 2003, p 271.)

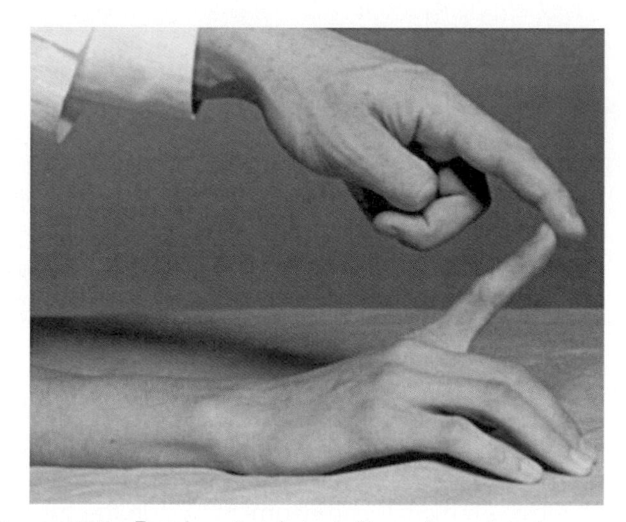

Figure 15-2 Passive stretch test. (From Amendola A, Twaddle BC: Compartment syndromes. In Browner BD, Jupiter JB, Levine AM, Trafton PG [eds]: Skeletal Trauma: Basic Science, Management, and Reconstruction, 3rd ed. Philadelphia: Saunders, 2003, p 271.)

    - The diagnosis is made by considering the entire clinical picture because no examination finding is pathognomonic.
    - Individually, the classic P signs (*p*ain, *p*ulselessness, *p*aresis/*p*aralysis, *p*aresthesias, *p*ressure, and *p*allor) can be absent or equivocal. However, together, the constellation of signs and symptoms including severe or intensifying pain, firm compartments, and sensory changes are strong indicators of an ACS.

Early Signs

- Pain
    - Pain with passive movement of the muscles in the involved compartment is one of the most sensitive signs (Fig. 15-2).

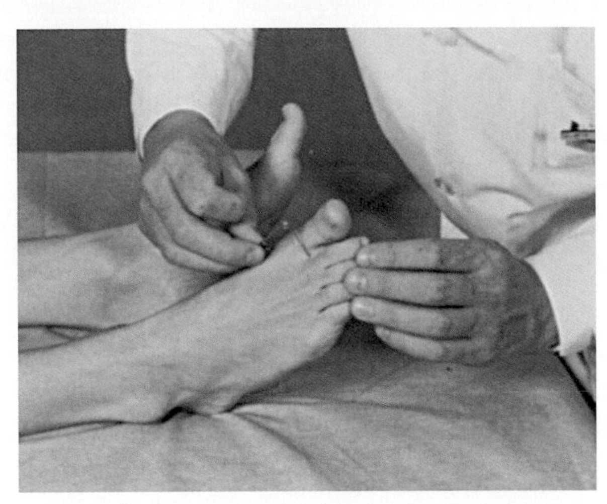

Figure 15-3 Sensory assessment of first dorsal webspace. (From Amendola A, Twaddle BC: Compartment syndromes. In Browner BD, Jupiter JB, Levine AM, Trafton PG [eds]: Skeletal Trauma: Basic Science, Management, and Reconstruction, 3rd ed. Philadelphia: Saunders, 2003, p 272.)

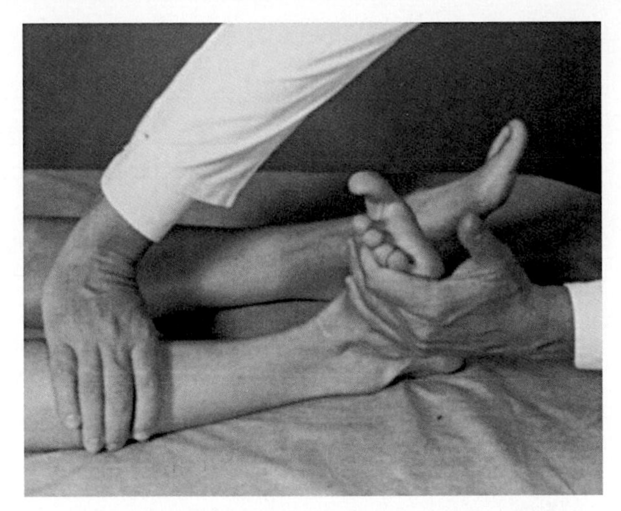

Figure 15-4 Muscle strength testing. (From Amendola A, Twaddle BC: Compartment syndromes. In Browner BD, Jupiter JB, Levine AM, Trafton PG [eds]: Skeletal Trauma: Basic Science, Management, and Reconstruction, 3rd ed. Philadelphia: Saunders, 2003, p 272.)

  - Severe or progressive pain, with an increasing narcotic requirement, is concerning for an evolving compartment syndrome.
  - It is important to remember that pain may not be elicited in the involved extremity, if the patient
    - is obtunded from head injury or intoxication
    - has received general or regional anesthesia
    - has a concomitant nerve injury
    - has other distracting injuries present
- Pressure
  - Increased tension of muscle compartments may be the only sign of an impending ACS.
  - The degree of swelling can be difficult to quantitate clinically, and the deep posterior compartment cannot be palpated, which can make this assessment subjective and unreliable.
- Paresthesias (Fig. 15-3)
  - Herald ischemia of the nerves within the involved compartments
  - Occur early because nerves are extremely sensitive to anoxia
  - Can progress to hypesthesias and later, irreversible motor and sensory loss, if early treatment is not initiated
  - Can also be present with nerve injuries and are not specific for ACS

Late Signs

- Paresis/paralysis (Fig. 15-4)
  - Etiology of extremity weakness can be difficult to distinguish from direct muscle or nerve injury or inhibition secondary to pain.
  - These signs are found in established compartment syndrome. If they are present, full recovery is doubtful.
- Pallor/pulselessness
  - A palpable pulse can be misleading.
  - Peripheral pulses and capillary refill are always found, unless a concomitant vascular injury is present.
  - The ischemia in compartment syndrome is secondary to decreased capillary perfusion, not interruption of arterial inflow.
  - If no pulses are present in the setting of ACS, consider an angiogram to look for large vessel occlusion or disruption.
  - Remember that the corollary to this is palpable pulses do not rule out a compartment syndrome.

Imaging

- Radiographs
  - To diagnose fractures
- Angiogram
  - If pulses are absent and vascular injury is suspected
- Near infrared spectroscopy, magnetic resonance imaging, scintigraphy, laser flow Doppler scan
  - No proven diagnostic utility in the setting of ACS

Additional Tests

- Compartment pressure monitoring
  - The only objective measurement is compartment pressure assessment.

- Resting compartment pressures are 0 to 8 mmHg.
- It is critical to record the compartment pressure at the level of the fracture, where the pressures are the highest. Significant pressure differences can be obtained just 5 cm from the fracture site.
- Different methods for measuring compartment pressures exist; most commonly a STIC catheter is used in acute situations (Fig. 15-5).
- In leg injuries, all four compartments must be measured; the anterior compartment is most commonly affected and the anterior and deep posterior compartments typically have the highest pressures.

- Absolute pressure
  - Traditionally, controversy had existed regarding the actual pressure at which compartment syndrome developed; pressures of 30, 40, and 50 mm Hg had been proposed as the indicators for fasciotomy.
  - These pressures were selected because they exceeded the normal capillary blood pressure of 20 to 30 mmHg.
  - However, variations in tolerance to elevated intracompartmental pressure have been observed among individuals and are believed to be secondary to differences in their systemic blood pressures.
- Pressure differential
  - Although the pressure at which ischemia of the muscle occurs has not been delineated, studies now indicate that the difference between compartment pressure and diastolic blood pressure (ΔP) determines muscle perfusion.

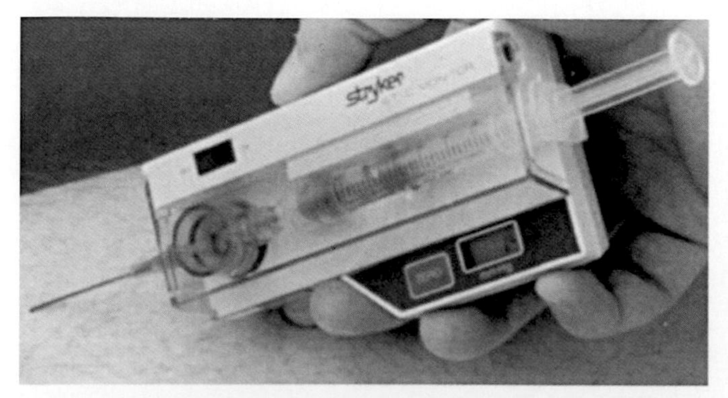

Figure 15-5 Stryker STIC catheter. (From Amendola A, Twaddle BC: Compartment syndromes. In Browner BD, Jupiter JB, Levine AM, Trafton PG [eds]: Skeletal Trauma: Basic Science, Management, and Reconstruction, 3rd ed. Philadelphia: Saunders, 2003, p 281.)

  - ΔP = (diastolic blood pressure) – (intracompartmental pressure). A difference of less than 30 mmHg has been supported in the literature as the point at which tissue perfusion pressure is compromised and fasciotomy is indicated.
  - Postischemic muscle is more vulnerable to elevation in pressures; hypoxic changes are observed at a ΔP of less than 40 mmHg.
- Laboratory studies
  - Complete blood count with differential
    - Can detect extensive blood loss/extravasation or be used as an indicator of infection
  - Chemistry panel with blood urea nitrogen/creatinine
    - To evaluate for electrolyte abnormalities and assess renal function
  - C-reactive protein/erythrocyte sedimentation rate
    - If infection suspected
  - International normalized ratio/prothrombin time and partial thromboplastin time
    - To evaluate for anticoagulant use
  - Serum myoglobin/urinalysis
    - Evaluate for rhabdomyolysis

Differential Diagnosis

- Vascular or neurogenic claudication: pain relieved with rest or pain related to position
- Venous insufficiency: leg discoloration, varicose veins, heart disease
- Deep vein thrombosis: consider duplex scan to rule out
- Lymphedema/congestive heart failure: frequently pitting is present with palpation
- Hematoma: focal swelling, history of trauma
- Neuropathy: consider if history of diabetes, other neuropathic conditions
- Tenosynovitis: pain with passive stretch and tenderness along path of tendons, focal swelling of digit
- Deep infection/abscess/pyomyositis/cellulitis/necrotizing fasciitis: history of penetrating trauma, open wound, monitor for sepsis, elevated infection markers
- Complex regional pain syndrome: chronic, mild swelling, hypersensitivity
- Stress fracture: history of repetitive athletic activity or distance running

Treatment

- At diagnosis
  - Remove compressive dressings or cast, if present.

- Maintain limb at level of heart; elevation may impede optimal limb perfusion.
- Avoid systemic hypotension.
- Supplemental oxygen assists in preventing tissue hypoxia.
- Determine rapidly whether these measures relieve symptoms of pain, pressure, or paresthesias.
- If symptoms persist, ACS must be considered and compartment pressure measurements obtained.

- Definitive: surgical fasciotomy
  - Lower leg (Figs. 15-6 and 15-7)
    — Must decompress all four compartments

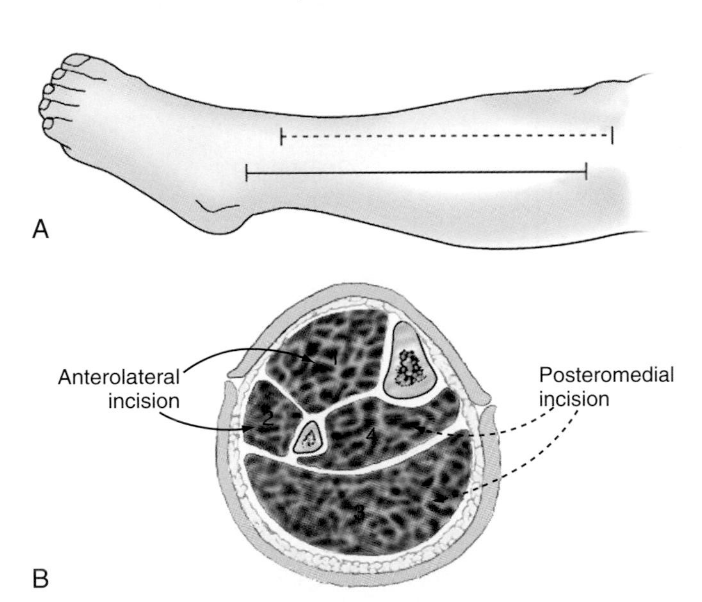

Figure 15-6 **A,** Illustration of two-incision fasciotomy technique for the lower leg. Incisions should be at least 16 cm in length. **B,** Axial diagram of the lower leg demonstrating how all four compartments can be decompressed through the two-incision technique. (Adapted from Amendola A, Twaddle BC: Compartment syndromes. In Browner BD, Jupiter JB, Levine AM, Trafton PG [eds]: Skeletal Trauma: Basic Science, Management, and Reconstruction, 3rd ed. Philadelphia: Saunders, 2003, p 286.)

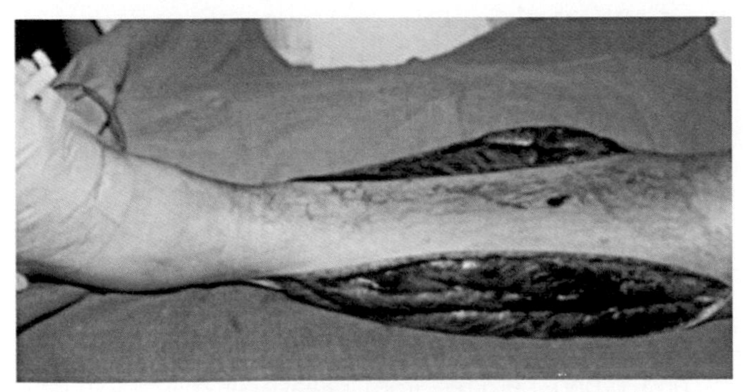

Figure 15-7 Lower extremity fasciotomy incisions. (From Amendola A, Twaddle BC: Compartment syndromes. In Browner BD, Jupiter JB, Levine AM, Trafton PG [eds]: Skeletal Trauma: Basic Science, Management, and Reconstruction, 3rd ed. Philadelphia: Saunders, 2003, p 287.)

    — One or two incision techniques are available for release.
    — Incisions 16 cm in length have been shown to be required for adequate decompression.
    — Avoid injury to the superficial peroneal nerve during anterior and lateral fascial incisions and the tibial nerve, along with the posterior tibial vessels, during release of the deep posterior compartment.
  - Thigh
    — Most often can be adequately decompressed through a single lateral incision, although a second medial incision may be necessary to release the adductor compartment if pressures are elevated there.
  - Arm
    — Anterior and posterior incisions; rarely, the deltoid muscle must be released separately
  - Forearm (Figs. 15-8 and 15-9)
    — Perform a volar incision from the wrist to the elbow first and then reassess dorsal compartment pressures.
    — Often the volar incision is enough to decompress both.
    — If the pressures remain elevated, a separate, second dorsal incision can be made.
  - Hands and feet
    — Decompression is performed through two dorsal incisions made over the second and fourth metacarpals or metatarsals.

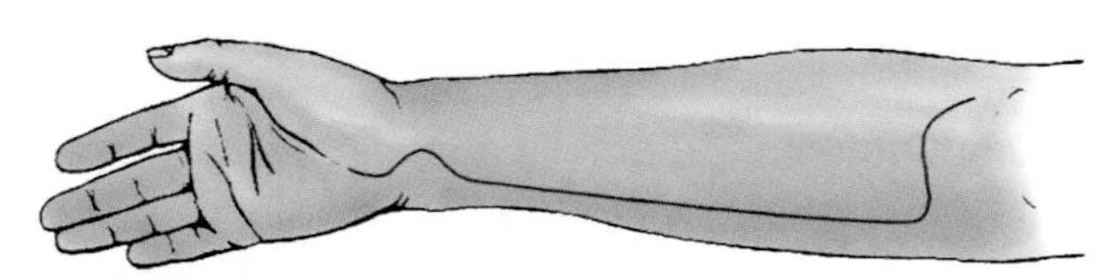

Figure 15-8 Anterior fasciotomy incision of the forearm. (Adapted from Amendola A, Twaddle BC: Compartment syndromes. In Browner BD, Jupiter JB, Levine AM, Trafton PG [eds]: Skeletal Trauma: Basic Science, Management, and Reconstruction, 3rd ed. Philadelphia: Saunders, 2003, p 283.)

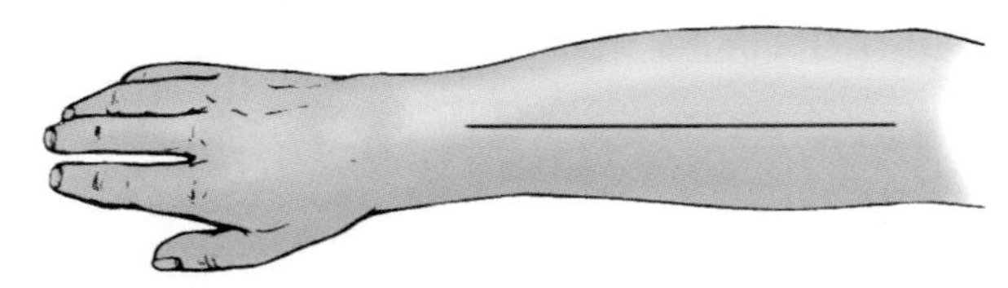

Figure 15-9 Dorsal fasciotomy incision of the forearm. (Adapted from Amendola A, Twaddle BC: Compartment syndromes. In Browner BD, Jupiter JB, Levine AM, Trafton PG [eds]: Skeletal Trauma: Basic Science, Management, and Reconstruction, 3rd ed. Philadelphia: Saunders, 2003, p 284.)

    - The foot may require a separate medial incision to adequately decompress the plantar and hindfoot compartments.
  - Management of fasciotomy wounds
    - Primary skin closure is avoided to ensure adequate compartment decompression.
    - Vacuum-assisted closure dressings are now frequently used to cover wounds and may assist in reducing tissue edema.
    - The patient must be brought to the operating room 24 to 48 hours after initial compartment release to reassess tissue viability.
    - Necrotic tissue must be débrided to reduce the risk of infection.
    - Delayed skin closure may be performed at this time if swelling has adequately resolved and approximation of the skin edges without undue tension is possible.
    - Split-thickness skin grafts may be required to cover wounds.
- Treatment algorithm (Fig. 15-10)

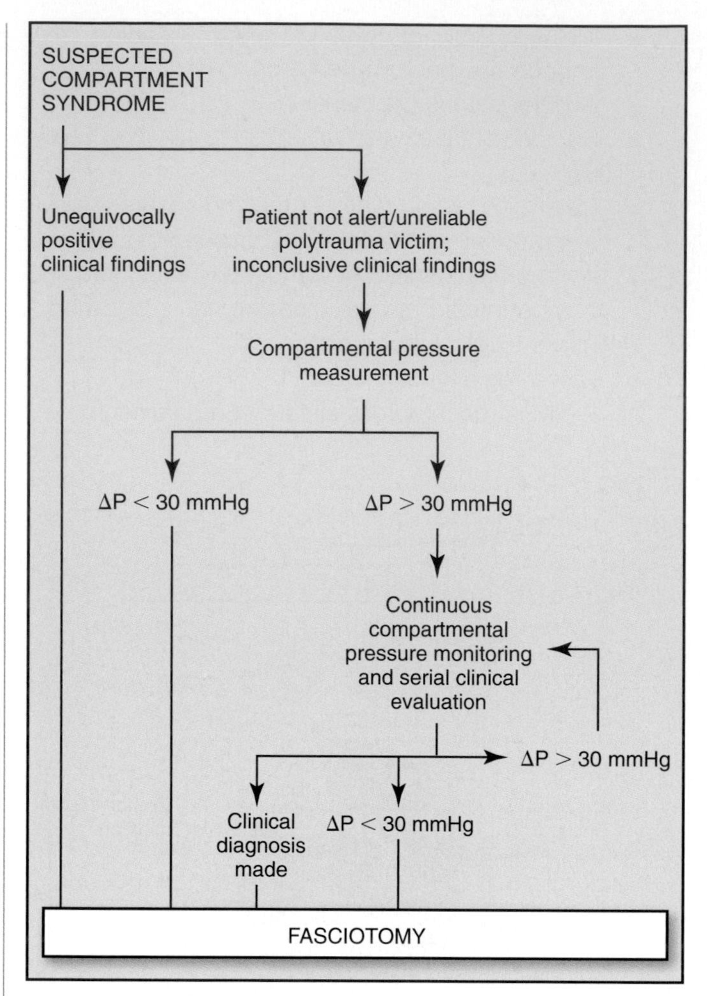

Figure 15-10 Treatment algorithm. (From Amendola A, Twaddle BC: Compartment syndromes. In Browner BD, Jupiter JB, Levine AM, Trafton PG [eds]: Skeletal Trauma: Basic Science, Management, and Reconstruction, 3rd ed. Philadelphia: Saunders, 2003, p 274.)

When to Refer

- There is no role for conservative management of ACS.
- The definitive management is surgery.
- An orthopaedic surgeon should be promptly consulted if the diagnosis of ACS is suspected based on history, physical examination, and compartment measurements, as discussed previously.

Prognosis

- Compartment syndrome is a surgical emergency.
- The ideal time for fasciotomies is within 6 hours of onset; however, it can be difficult to determine when the compartment syndrome started and the duration of ischemic insult to the tissues. Therefore, surgical decompression should be performed as soon as the diagnosis is made.
- Muscles can withstand 4 to 6 hours of anoxic insult.
- After 6 hours of the development of compartment syndrome, complete functional recovery cannot be guaranteed, and beyond 8 to 12 hours, the damage is irreversible.
- Once paralysis and sensory deficits are present, usually after 6 to 8 hours, delayed fasciotomies are not recommended because the necrotic muscle tissue becomes a medium for infection.

Complications

- Muscle necrosis
- Volkmann's ischemic contractures
- Delayed fracture healing
- Infection
- Permanent weakness or sensory loss
- Amputation for insensate or nonfunctional limb or severe infection
- Crush syndrome/reperfusion injury: acute renal failure and organ damage from release of myoglobin and other inflammatory mediators secondary to muscle necrosis; depends on the extent and duration of the compartment syndrome

Patient Instructions

- After recent extremity surgery, trauma, or placement of a circumferential cast or dressing, symptoms that should prompt patients to seek immediate medical evaluation include
  - A significant increase in pain intensity, either not alleviated by or necessitating an increasing narcotics requirement
  - Changes in sensation or presence of tingling in an extremity
  - Progressive, new onset of muscle weakness in an extremity

Considerations in Special Populations

- Pediatric patients may not be able to accurately verbalize the symptoms associated with a compartment syndrome; suspect the diagnosis if the child exhibits intensifying pain with an increasing narcotic requirement.
- Diabetics or other patients with peripheral neuropathy may not experience the pain or sensory changes that can accompany a compartment syndrome.
- In addition, patients with head injuries or those who are intoxicated may be difficult to assess clinically. They are often unable to give a history, and their examination may be unreliable. In these patients, a physician should have a low threshold for measuring compartment pressures.

Suggested Reading

- Amendola A, Twaddle BC: Compartment syndromes. In Browner BD, Jupiter JB, Levine AM, Trafton PG (eds): Skeletal Trauma: Basic Science, Management, and Reconstruction, 3rd ed. Philadelphia: Saunders, 2003, pp 268–292.
- Elliot K, Johnstone A: Diagnosing acute compartment syndrome. J Bone Joint Surg Br 2003;85B:625–632.
- Matsen FA, Sheridan GW: Fasciotomy in the treatment of the acute compartment syndrome. J Bone Joint Surg Am 1976;58A:112–115.
- McQueen M: Compartment syndrome. In Bucholz RW, Heckman JD, Court-Browne C (eds): Rockwood and Green's Fractures in Adults, 6th ed. Philadelphia: Lippincott Williams & Wilkins, 2005, pp 425–443.
- Mubarak S, Owen C: Double-incision fasciotomy of the leg for decompression in compartment syndromes. J Bone Joint Surg Am 1977;59A:184–187.
- Olson S, Glasgow R: Acute compartment syndrome in lower extremity musculoskeletal trauma. J Am Acad Orthop Surg 2005;13:436–444.
- Tornetta P, Templeman D: Compartment syndrome associated with tibial fracture. Instructional course lecture. J Bone Joint Surg Am 1996;78A:1438–1444.
- Whitesides T, Heckman M: Acute compartment syndrome: Update on diagnosis and treatment. J Am Acad Orthop Surg 1996;4:209–218.

Chapter 16 Trauma: Heterotopic Ossification

Mario Ciocca

Heterotopic ossification is the formation of lamellar bone outside the skeletal system. This may occur in the skin, subcutaneous tissue, fibrous tissue adjacent to joints, ligaments, walls of blood vessels, and skeletal muscle. New bone formation occurs in five clinical settings: genetic, neurogenic, postsurgical, distinctive reactive lesions, and post-traumatic.

Key Concepts

- First described in the late 1600s
- The true mechanism for the development of heterotopic ossification is uncertain, although four factors are thought to be necessary for its development.
  - An inciting event that may form a hematoma
  - A signaling protein (bone morphogenic protein) secreted from cells of injured tissue or inflammatory cells
  - A supply of mesenchymal cells that can differentiate into osteoblasts or chondroblasts
  - An appropriate environment for the continued production of heterotopic bone
- Post-traumatic heterotopic ossification occurs most frequently in the hip after total hip arthroplasty and also occurs frequently after open reduction and internal fixation of acetabular fractures.

History

- There has been recent trauma or surgery followed by pain and an increase in joint stiffness.
- Usually develops 3 to 12 weeks after injury

Physical Examination

- Joint erythema, warmth, edema, and limited range of motion

Imaging

- Radiographic abnormalities can be seen within 18 to 21 days but may take 4 to 5 weeks to develop and should be present by 8 weeks.
- Nuclear medicine bone scan is the most sensitive imaging modality for early heterotopic ossification and can be used to indicate whether the lesion is active or has matured. It is usually positive by 2 to 4 weeks and can be used to predict the optimal timing for surgical resection.
- Ultrasound may be able to detect heterotopic ossification sooner than radiographs.
- Magnetic resonance imaging is not typically used but can identify a nonspecific soft-tissue mass within the first few weeks. Both magnetic resonance imaging and computed tomography may be useful in the preoperative setting to help describe relationships to other structures.

Additional Tests

- Alkaline phosphatase and sedimentation rate may be elevated in the early stages.
- Alkaline phosphatase reaches 3.5 times normal at 4 weeks, peaks at 12 weeks, and normalizes when the bone matures.
- Prostaglandin E_2 excretion in a 24-hour urine collection may be increased.

Differential Diagnosis

- Clinically, the early inflammatory stage may be confused with cellulitis, deep venous thrombosis, thrombophlebitis, or osteomyelitis.
- An early lesion may be misdiagnosed as a soft-tissue osteosarcoma, whereas a late lesion may be mistaken for parosteal osteosarcoma.

Treatment

At Diagnosis (Prevention after Injury)

- Gentle range of motion within a pain-free zone
- Nonsteroidal anti-inflammatory drugs have been effective after total hip arthroplasty. The mechanism of action includes inhibition of differentiation of mesenchymal cells into osteogenic cells and suppression of the prostaglandin-mediated inflammatory response.

- Radiation
  - Has been effective prophylactically after total hip arthroplasty or resection of heterotopic ossification
  - May inhibit the differentiation of pluripotent mesenchymal cells into osteoblasts

Later (If Heterotopic Ossification Develops)

- Bisphosphonates
  - Have been effective in neurogenic heterotopic ossification
  - Mechanisms include
    - Inhibition of precipitation of calcium phosphate
    - Delaying aggregation of hydroxyapatite crystals
    - Blocking conversion of calcium phosphate into hydroxyapatite
  - May develop rebound and bone growth after discontinuation due to resumption of osteoid mineralization while osteoclast function remains suppressed
  - May need long-term treatment (at least 6 months)
- Radiation has been used in heterotopic ossification related to spinal cord injury
- Surgery
  - Indications
    - Peripheral nerve compromise
    - Pain
    - Impaired range of motion not amenable to conservative measure
- Need to combine with nonsteroidal anti-inflammatory drug and/or radiation
- Resection should be performed after maturation (12–18 months) to help avoid recurrences.

When to Refer

- Refer to surgeon for indications listed.

Troubleshooting

- Delayed treatment of an initial injury may increase the risk of developing heterotopic ossification.
- Removal of ectopic bone before maturation will often lead to an increased risk of recurrence.

Patient Instructions

- Educate patient on importance of early rest, ice, compression, and elevation and stretch treatment.
- Educate patient that earlier treatment will lead to quicker recovery and less risk of heterotopic ossification.
- Have patient inform physician if pain, swelling, and/or loss of motion persists or recurs or a mass can be felt.

Specific Clinical Entities

Myositis Ossificans

- Occurs after muscle contusion (Fig. 16-1)
- Incidence 9% to 20% and related to severity of contusion
- Most common sites: knee extensors and elbow flexors
- After trauma, a mass may appear 1 to 2 days later, reach 4 to 10 cm after 1 to 2 months, and then mature and harden. It may become smaller but rarely disappears.
- Should be suspected if pain and swelling do not resolve 4 to 5 days after a muscle contusion
- Treat contusion with rest, ice, compression, and elevation and place muscle in the stretch position
- Nonsteroidal anti-inflammatory drugs have been used to treat muscle contusions (2–6 weeks) as preventive treatment for myositis ossificans.
- Ultrasound or heat should be avoided in the acute phase of a muscle contusion.
- Refer if the patient is symptomatic with muscle atrophy and/or decreased joint motion.
- See Chapter 17 for more details.

Pellegrini-Stieda Syndrome

- Refers to ossification in the medial collateral ligament of the knee; may also involve the adductor magnus tendon (Fig. 16-2)

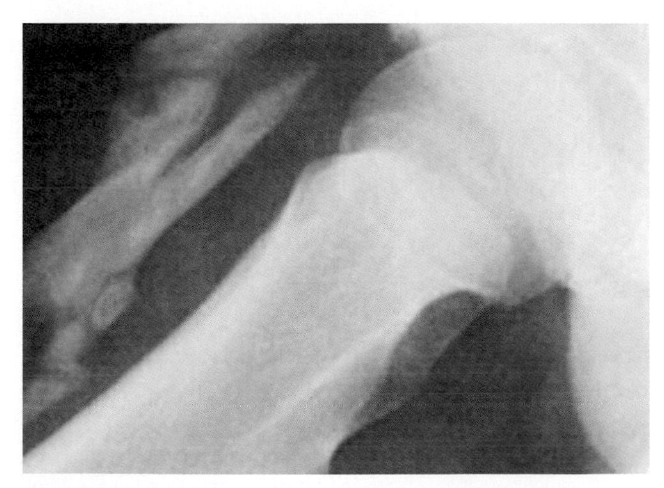

Figure 16-1 Myositis ossificans occurs after muscle contusion.

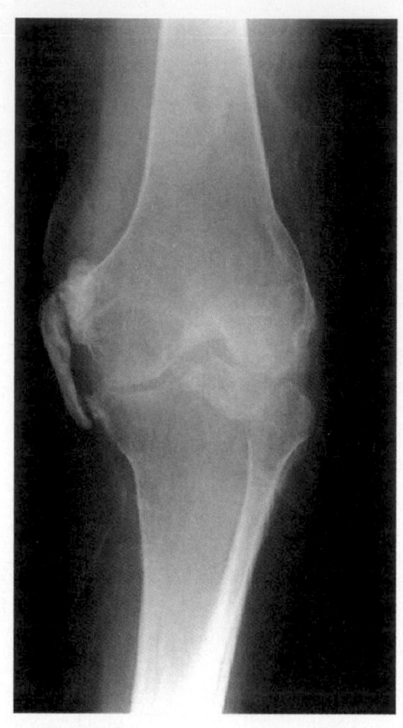

Figure 16-2 Pellegrini-Stieda syndrome refers to ossification in the medial collateral ligament of the knee and may also involve the adductor magnus tendon. (From Altschuler B: Pellegrini-Stieda Syndrome, vol. 354. Copyright 2006 Massachusetts Medical Society. All rights reserved.)

- Usually occurs near the superior medial femoral condyle
- First described in the early 1900s
- Usually develops 3 to 4 weeks after injury
- Medial side swelling, pain, stiffness, and possibly a palpable mass develop.
- May be due to direct or indirect injury
- Theories of origin include
  - Hematoma formation that later calcifies
  - Direct metaplasia of the ligament
  - An avulsion fragment with subperiosteal proliferation of bone
  - Traumatic tear of the adductor magnus tendon with periosteal new bone formation
- Ossification may occur in as many as 3% of knee injuries
- Calcification may increase in size or may eventually recede
- Surgical removal is indicated for a painful mass or a large mass that limits motion.

Heterotopic Calcification of the Elbow Ulnar Collateral Ligament

- Mainly seen in baseball pitchers
- Chronic stress leads to edema and inflammation followed by scarring, calcification, and ossification in the ligament.

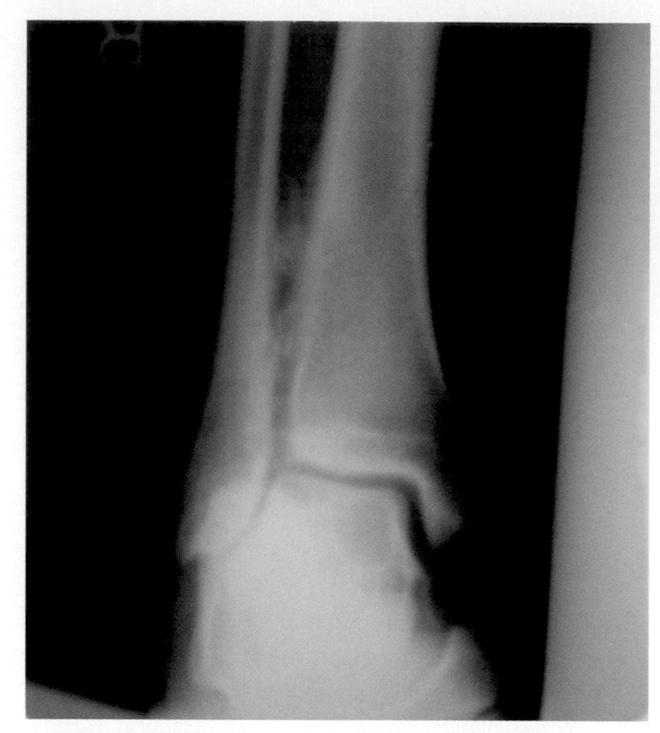

Figure 16-3 Calcification of the syndesmosis can develop as a complication of injuries to the ankle.

- Smoothly marginated and usually measures 4 to 5 mm × 1 to 2 mm
- May have associated partial or complete tear of the ligament
- Radiographs are more sensitive in detecting the calcification because magnetic resonance imaging will show the integrity of the ligament but may not detect the heterotopic ossification.

Syndesmotic Ankle Sprain

- Calcification of the syndesmosis can develop as a complication of injuries to this area (Fig. 16-3).
- Can occur whether treated conservatively or surgically
- Can be seen 3 to 12 months after injury
- Persistent pain and a palpable mass develop
- If symptomatic, can undergo operative excision, although there is a risk of recurrence

Heterotopic Ossification after Elbow Trauma

- Risk of developing is 16% to 20% with a fracture/dislocation (Fig. 16-4)
- Risk increases with fracture severity
- Most common extrinsic cause of elbow contracture
- Symptoms include pain, stiffness, sensory loss, weakness, and possibly a palpable mass.
- Usually present 6 weeks after injury

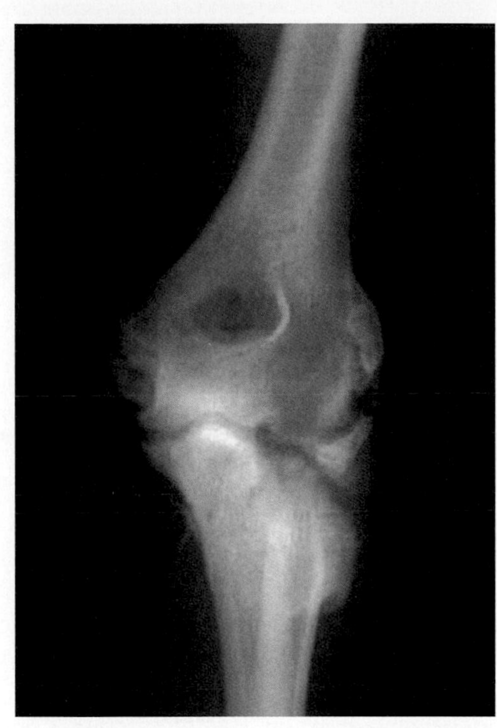

Figure 16-4 Risk of heterotopic ossification developing is 16% to 20% with a fracture/dislocation.

- Those at risk of developing heterotopic ossification may receive preventive nonsteroidal anti-inflammatory drugs or radiation after injury.
- If functionally limiting, can treat surgically combined with prophylactic nonsteroidal anti-inflammatory drugs or radiation
- Although heterotopic ossification is most commonly described after hip surgery, it has also been described after anterior or posterior cruciate ligament reconstruction, arthroscopy of the knee, multiple types of tendon injury, and traumatic, combat-related amputations.

Suggested Reading

- Beiner JM, Jokl P: Muscle contusion injury and myositis ossificans traumatica. Clin Orthop Relat Res 2002;403S:S110–S119.
- Keschner MT, Paksima N: The stiff elbow. Bull NYU Hosp Jt Dis 2007;65:24–28.
- King JB: Post-traumatic ectopic calcification in the muscles of athletes: A review. Br J Sports Med 1998;32:287–290.
- Larson CM, Almekinders LC, Karas SG, Garrett WE: Evaluating and managing muscle contusions and myositis ossificans. Phys Sportsmed 2002;30:41–44, 49–50.
- McCarthy EF, Sundaram M: Heterotopic ossification: A review. Skeletal Radiol 2005;34:609–619.
- Mulligan SA, Schwartz ML, Broussard MF, Andrews JR: Heterotopic calcification and tears of the ulnar collateral ligament: Radiographic and MR imaging findings. AJR Am J Roentgenol 2000;175:1099–1102.
- Niitsu M, Ikeda K, Iijima T, et al: MR imaging of Pellegrini-Stieda disease. Radiat Med 1999;17:405–409.
- Vanden Bossche L, Vanderstraeten G: Heterotopic ossification: A review. J Rehabil Med 2005;37:129–136.
- Wang JC, Shapiro MS: Pellegrini-Stieda syndrome. Am J Orthop 1995;24:493–497.
- Williams GN, Jones MH, Amendola A: Syndesmotic ankle sprains in athletes. Am J Sports Med 2007;35:1197–1207.

Chapter 17 Myositis Ossificans Traumatica

Jeffrey Roberts and Jeffrey R. Bytomski

Key Concepts

- Nonpenetrating trauma over a muscle complex that results in injury to muscle fiber and blood vessels, causing a muscle contusion
- For reasons not entirely understood, heterotopic bone may develop in an area of previous trauma or hematoma.
- Initially, there is tenderness, swelling, decreased range of motion, and warmth, and eventually a firm mass can be palpated.
- Radiographic evidence at 3 to 4 weeks
- Management includes rest, ice, compression, and elevation; indomethacin (or equivalent), for the anti-inflammatory effect; and knee immobilization in flexion.
- Surgical removal (if clinically necessary) performed at a minimum of 6 months from onset of trauma to ensure that heterotopic bone formation has ceased

Definition

- Myositis ossificans traumatica is calcification in a muscle group as a result of muscle injury.
- Several theories have been proposed
  - Hematoma organization involving a progressive transformation of fibrous tissue to cartilage and then bone
  - Hematoma calcification
  - Intramuscular bone formation after detachment of periosteal flaps
  - Periosteal rupture with escape and proliferation of periosteal osteoblasts within adjacent muscle tissue
  - Metaplasia of intramuscular connective tissue into cartilage and bone
  - Individual predisposition to myositis

Epidemiology

- Most common in adolescent or adult males younger than 30 years old
- Incidence is 9% to 20% after muscle contusion.
- Proximal limb muscles are frequently injured with the triceps, quadriceps, and thigh adductors having the highest prevalence of injury.

History

- Nonpenetrating trauma over a muscle complex that causes compression of the muscle against underlying bone
- Compression results in injury to muscle fiber and blood vessels, causing a muscle contusion.
- Initial injury can be accompanied by partial or complete tear of the muscle.
- Limitations of range of motion (i.e., knee flexion < 120 degrees)
- Warning signs for myositis ossificans include contusions that are unresponsive to conservative treatment within 4 to 5 days or worsening of symptoms at 2 to 3 weeks.
- Types of heterotopic bone formation
  - Flat new bone adjacent to shaft of bone
  - Mushroom-like formation of new bone that is congruent with the bone
  - Bone formation within the muscle
- Heterotopic bone formation can occur for 6 to 12 months.

Etiology

- For reasons not entirely understood, nonneoplastic proliferation of bone (heterotopic bone) can occur in the area of previous trauma or hematoma, which is characteristic of myositis ossificans.

Physical Examination

- Initially, there are tenderness, swelling, decreased range of motion, and warmth, consistent with findings associated with contusion and hematoma.
- A firm mass can later be palpated as heterotopic bone formation occurs.

- A palpable defect may be seen during the initial few weeks of injury as well.

Imaging

- Initial radiographs are used to evaluate bone injury but will not show myositis ossificans acutely.
- Radiographic demonstration of heterotopic bone formation in the area of reported trauma occurs 3 to 4 weeks after trauma.
- Follow-up radiographs can demonstrate evolution and growth of the heterotopic bone for 6 to 12 months.
- Magnetic resonance imaging
  - More specific than radiographs
  - Helpful in the workup of other causes (see "Differential Diagnosis")
- Computed tomography
  - More specific than radiographs
  - Helpful in the workup of other causes (see "Differential Diagnosis")
- Bone scan
  - Can be useful in determining whether there is still an active phase of heterotopic bone formation
  - See Figures 17-1 and 17-2.

Additional Tests

- The alkaline phosphatase level and erythrocyte sedimentation rate can be elevated but are nonspecific in the initial phase.
- Levels should return to normal soon after the initial trauma; if not, then other pathology needs to be considered.

Differential Diagnosis

- Periosteal osteosarcoma
- Parosteal osteosarcoma
- Synovial sarcoma
- Osteochondroma
- Juxtacortical chondroma
- Infection
- Muscle contusion
- Fracture
- Tendon rupture
- Growth plate avulsion

Treatment

- Rest, ice, compression, and elevation
- Nonsteroidal anti-inflammatory drugs, particularly indomethacin, which has been shown to decrease heterotopic bone formation

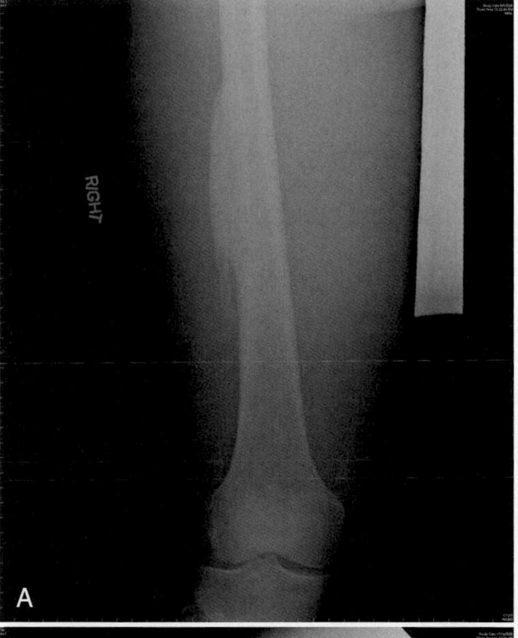

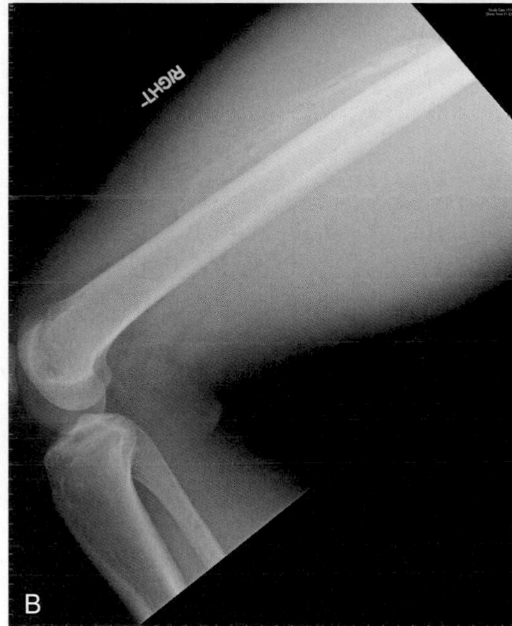

Figure 17-1 Anteroposterior (**A**) and lateral (**B**) views of myositis ossificans of the quadriceps muscle.

- Knee immobilized in flexion (minimum of 120 degrees) for 24 hours but no longer than 5 days
- Bone formation will occasionally resolve spontaneously.
- Pad area for return to play.
- Physical therapy for range of motion and strength training
- Cross-training exercises to maintain cardiopulmonary conditioning
- Surgical removal performed at a minimum of 6 months if heterotopic bone formation has ceased and the lesion is still clinically painful. Some lesions may take

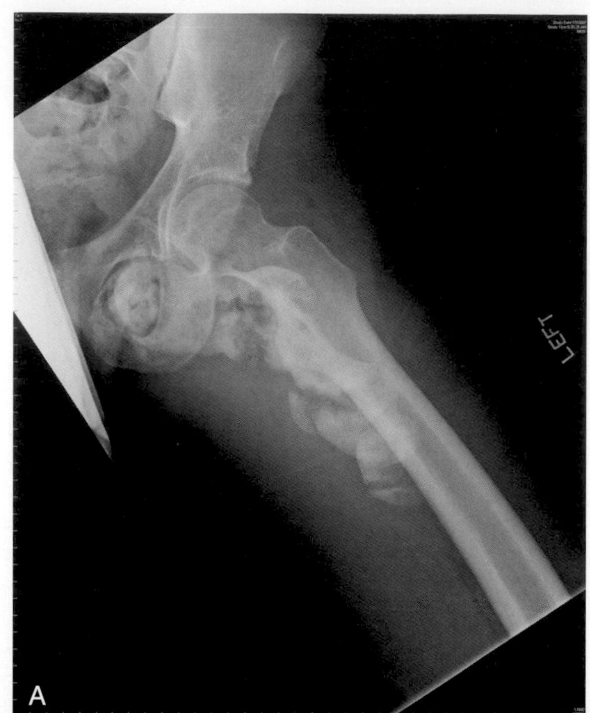

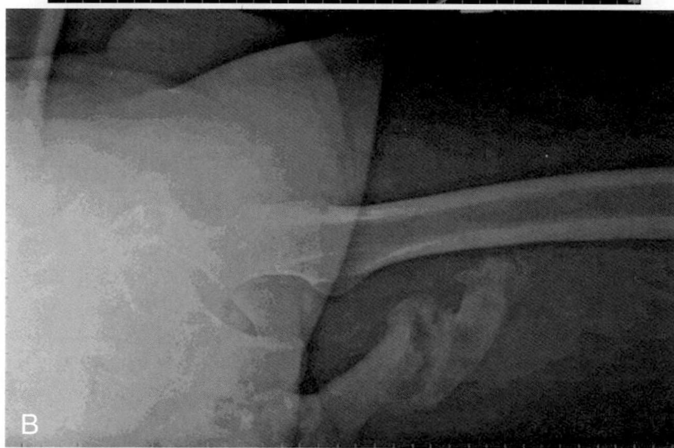

Figure 17-2 Frog leg lateral (**A**) and cross-table lateral (**B**) views of myositis ossificans of the hip extensors.

a year to mature before removal is warranted. Surgical intervention is not necessary in painless, clinically stable lesions.

When to Refer

- Patients with myositis ossificans should be followed by sports medicine physicians or physicians trained in orthopaedics.
- Contusion not resolving within 4 to 5 days or increasing symptoms over the first few weeks of injury
- After 6 to 12 months for surgical evaluation

Prognosis

- Most do well with return to activity in several weeks. The few that become chronic can have prolonged symptoms for months or longer. Surgery does very well for relief of symptoms as long as heterotopic bone formation has ceased at the time of surgery.

Troubleshooting

- Did the patient receive nonsteroidal anti-inflammatory drugs, and was the patient placed in flexion after the initial injury?
- Removal while there is still active formation of heterotopic bone results in worsening of the myositis ossificans and significant morbidity.

Patient Instructions

- Muscle contusions should initially be treated with nonsteroidal anti-inflammatory drugs, rest, ice, compression, and elevation.
- If symptoms are not improving within 4 to 5 days of injury or symptoms are worsening within the first few weeks, then the patient should seek professional assistance.

Consideration in Special Populations

- Heterotopic bone formation can occur postoperatively, especially with hip replacements.
- Congenital heterotopic bone formation (myositis ossificans progressive or fibrodysplasia ossificans progressive) can also occur. It is most common in the pediatric population (average age at onset, 5 years; range, from fetus to 25 years).

Suggested Reading

- Armfield DR, Kim D, Towers J, et al: Sports-related muscle injury in the lower extremity. Clin Sports Med 2006;25:803–842.
- Beiner JM, Jokl P: Muscle contusion injury and myositis ossificans traumatica. Clin Orthop Relat Res 2002;403S:S110–S119.
- DeLee JC, Drez D Jr, Miller MD (eds): DeLee and Drez's Orthopaedic Sports Medicine, 2nd ed. Philadelphia: Saunders, 2003.
- Järvinen TA, Järvinen TM, Kääriäinen M, et al: Muscle injuries: Biology and treatment. Am J Sports Med 2005;33:745–764.
- LaBella CR: Common acute sports-related lower extremity injuries in children and adolescents. Clin Pediatr Emerg Med 2007;8:31–34.

Chapter 18 Arthritides

Thomas S. Weber and Joseph J. Schumann

ICD-9 CODES

274.0	*Gout*
714.0	*Rheumatoid Arthritis*
715.0	*Osteoarthritis (General)*
710.0	*Systemic Lupus Erythematosus*
088.81	*Lyme Disease*
696.1	*Psoriasis*
099.3	*Reiter Syndrome*

Key Concepts (Fig. 18-1)

- As its name implies, this group of disease processes is characterized by inflammation (*tides,* plural form of *itis*) of the joint (*arthros*).
- A healthy joint such as the hip or knee is designed to move freely and painlessly due in part to the smooth surface of articular cartilage lining the bone ends and synovial fluid. The friction coefficient of these joint surfaces is similar to that of ice sliding on ice.
- Aging, trauma, infection, autoimmunity, and gravity all contribute to the breakdown of this natural state and eventually cause the patient pain and limited motion. Cadaveric studies show degenerative joint disease beginning as early as age 13.
- Osteoarthritis (OA) most commonly affects the weight-bearing joints due to several factors.
  - Cumulative trauma to joint surfaces from sprains and contusions
  - Decreased hyaluronic fluid from decreasing numbers of chondrocytes
  - Loss of hydrostatic forces leads to meniscal and articular cartilage fraying and eventual loss of cushioning between bone ends.
  - Articular cartilage loss exposes underlying bone to mechanical forces resulting in the activation of pain/sensory nerve endings in the subchondral bone.
- Acute joint pain and swelling require rapid workup as bacterial infection (septic joint) can begin joint destruction within several hours of symptoms. *Staphylococcus* and *Streptococcus* are the most commonly found organisms. Lyme disease is a subacute infection rarely causing primary joint damage.
- Rheumatoid disease causes hyperproliferation of synovial cells stemming from an autoimmune response of the body to unknown antigens. High levels of CD4+ and plasma cells infiltrate the synovium along with tumor necrosis factor and interleukins. Increased osteoclastic activity erodes and thins cortical margins of the bone ends, weakening collateral ligaments as well.
- Humans lack the enzyme uricase, which breaks down urate to a more soluble form. Gout arthritis occurs when overproducers or underexcreters of uric acid, a product of purine metabolism, accumulate excess levels of urate crystals in a joint, causing an acute inflammatory reaction.
- Pseudogout or chondrocalcinosis is characterized by idiopathic deposition of calcium or calcium pyrophosphate dihydrate crystals in the joint.
- Other autoimmune syndromes such as systemic lupus erythematosus, psoriasis, and Reiter syndrome frequently have joint inflammation as a component of the disease process. Identifying the systemic source aids in appropriate treatment of the joint(s) involved.

OSTEOARTHRITIS

History

- Morning pain is often better, and patients tend to have increased pain with prolonged walking or standing, or at the end of the day. Onset is typically gradual over weeks or months.
- Knees and hips are affected most, followed by the first carpometacarpal joint in hands and the cervical/lumbar spine as well. Ankles, the first metatarsophalangeal joint, shoulders, and hand distal interphalangeal joints also can be affected.
- There is swelling with activity; nonweight bearing usually reduces the intensity of pain.
- Trauma/overuse can exacerbate pain and disability in a previously asymptomatic joint.

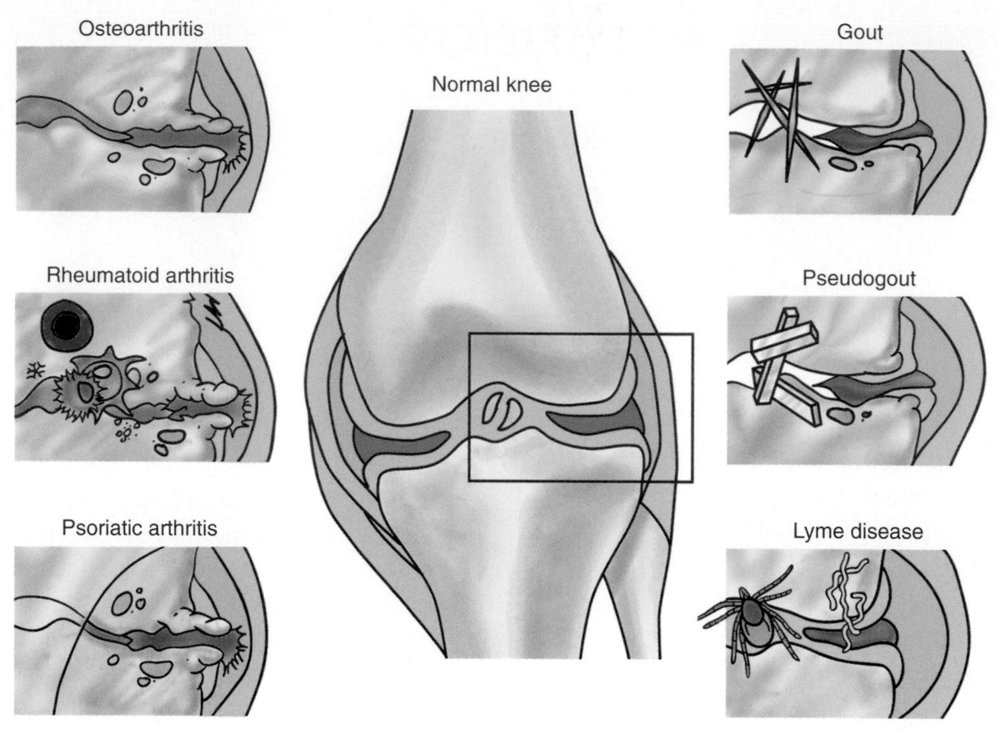

Figure 18-1 Common sources of arthritis.

- Unilateral or bilateral involvement
- The incidence increases dramatically after the sixth decade.

Physical Examination

- Vital signs
  - Usually normal (be sure to calculate body mass index to address obesity issues)
- Gait
  - Often antalgic with lower extremity joint involvement
- Joints
  - Joint effusions may or may not be present; joint deformity is common in late disease.
  - OA rarely has palpable warmth in the joint. All other causes of arthritis often are warm to the touch (always compare sides).
  - The joint range of motion is limited, with pain at the endpoints of motion. Joint lines are tender to palpation.
  - Ligamentous stability is usually unaffected in early disease; it is more common in late disease.
- In general, the hand distal interphalangeal joint involvement is OA- or psoriatic arthritis–related.
  - The physician will often palpate crepitus in the knee and shoulder in OA examination. On hip examination, pain is usually greater on internal rotation.

Imaging

- Often shows spurring, decreased joint space, calcifications, or osteochondral defects (Fig. 18-2)
- Negative radiographs do not exclude any form of arthritis.
- Magnetic resonance imaging may show severe chondromalacia and even subchondral bone edema.
- Bone scans often will have increased uptake on the edges of a joint.

Additional Tests

- No blood work or joint fluid analysis is specific for OA.

Differential Diagnosis

- Septic joint
- Meniscus degeneration or tear
- Fracture
- Joint sprain
- Osteochondritis dissecans
- Osteonecrosis
- Metastasis
- Paget's disease
- Avascular necrosis

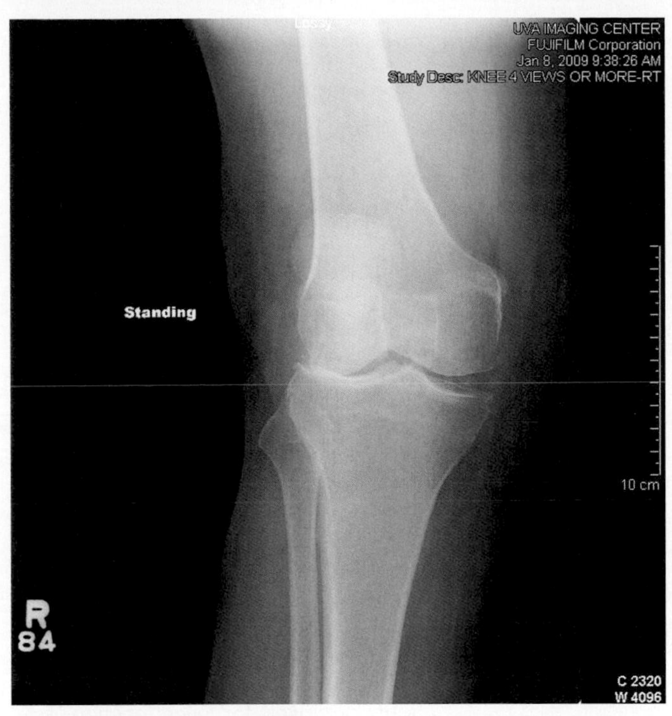

Figure 18-2 Classic radiographic findings of osteoarthritis, lateral compartment of knee.

- Sickle cell anemia
- Pigmented villonodular synovitis
- Hyperparathyroidism
- Endocarditis
- Ankylosing spondylitis
- Tuberculosis

Treatment

- Oral anti-inflammatory drugs and topical ice give effective relief in many cases.
- Weight loss is very beneficial to reduce stress across lower extremity joints.
- Physical therapy strengthens the muscle that supports the affected joint.
    - Increased muscle strength also acts as a shock absorber for the joint.
- Aquatic therapy allows for calorie-burning exercise while off-loading the joints.
- Corticosteroids via the oral route or intra-articular injections often rapidly reduce pain associated with the inflammatory response from the loss of the protective articular cartilage.
- Intra-articular viscosupplementation with hyaluronic acid derivatives is shown to reduce symptoms in mild to moderate arthritis.
- Unloader braces may assist in off-loading the medial or lateral joint space in patients with OA of the knee that is primarily limited to either the medial or lateral compartment.
- Partial and total joint replacements are generally well tolerated and effective in the shoulder, elbow, interphalangeal, hip, knee, ankle, and first metatarsophalangeal joints.
- Future directions include chondral cartilage transplantation and cartilage regeneration.

RHEUMATOID ARTHRITIS

History

- Morning pain is worse than at the end of the day, and periods of inactivity increase stiffness.
- Female-to-male incidence 3:1
- Between 1% and 3% of adults worldwide have rheumatoid arthritis (RA).
- Peak onset age 35 to 45 years; hands, wrists, and feet most commonly affected initially
- Symmetrical joint involvement, prolonged morning stiffness, general fatigue, and malaise are hallmarks of RA.
- Rash is not associated with RA.
- Gradual development of symptoms over several months
- Patients may report loss of appetite.
- Patients may have difficulty opening doors or jars due to pain or weakness in the hands.

Physical Examination

- Vital signs
    - Usually normal; may have low-grade fever
- Gait
    - May be antalgic if ankles or feet affected
- Skin
    - Subcutaneous nodules present in RA, not with psoriasis (Fig. 18-3)
- Joints
    - Metacarpophalangeal joints and proximal interphalangeal joints may be warm to the touch and swollen with thickened synovium.
    - Progressive disease shows classic ulnar deviation of metacarpophalangeal joints (Fig. 18-4).
    - The range of motion may be limited due to pain and stiffness; typically, joints have no crepitus.
    - Palpate unaffected joints to compare for subtle temperature changes.

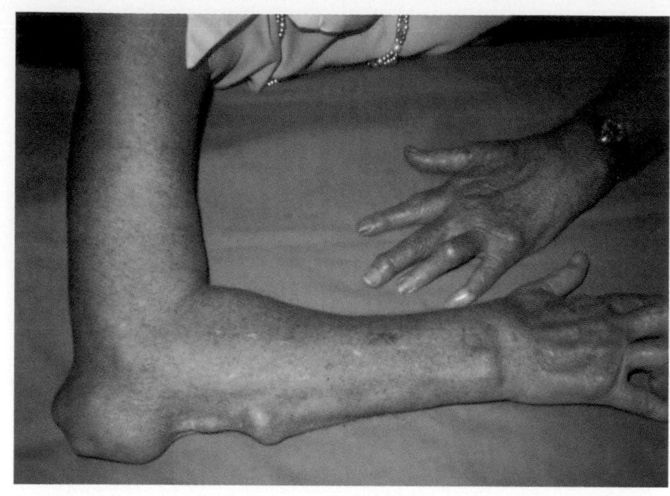

Figure 18-3 Subcutaneous rheumatoid nodules in forearm; tophaceous gouty changes of olecranon. (From Canale ST, Beaty JH [eds]: Campbell's Operative Orthopaedics, 11th ed. Philadelphia: Mosby, 2007, Fig. 70-10.)

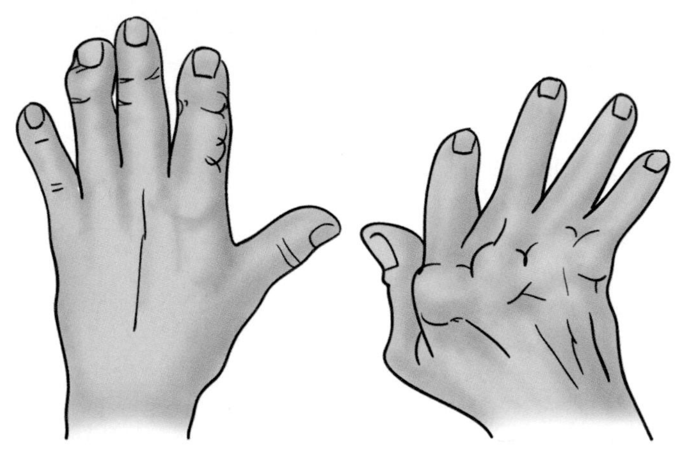

Figure 18-4 Types of arthritis affecting the hand joints. Normal left hand with ulnar deviation of the MCP joints seen in rheumatoid arthritis on the right hand.

Imaging

- Radiographs show loss of joint space and bony demineralization.
- Hand radiographs reveal classic ulnar deviation at the metacarpophalangeal joints.
- Cervical spine radiographs may demonstrate degenerative changes and vertebral body subluxations.
- Magnetic resonance imaging may show synovial hypertrophy and erosions.

Additional Tests

- Joint fluid analysis: white blood cell count greater than 5000 with elevated lymphocytes and rheumatoid factor (60%)

TABLE 18-1 *Treatment Options for Rheumatoid Arthritis*

Antirheumatoid Drugs	Comments
Nonsteroidal anti-inflammatory drugs, salicylates	Follow for gastrointestinal ulcers, decreased creatinine clearance
Corticosteroids	Used as baseline and for flare-ups, intra-articular injections helpful
Methotrexate	Most commonly used. PO or SC. 6–8 weeks for response; monitor for liver, lungs, bone marrow suppression
Hydroxychloroquine (Plaquenil)	For mild disease. Onset is 2–4 months. Monitor eyes for side effects
Entanercept (Enbrel)	TNF inhibitor: 50 mg SC weekly Onset of action 1–4 weeks Increased risk of infection from immunosuppression
Infliximab (Remicade)	TNF inhibitor: weekly IV infusions over 1–2 hours Monitor closely for fever, reaction during infusions
Adalimumab (Humira)	TNF inhibitor, SC every 2 weeks Effective monotherapy
Gold salts	Not often used due to cost and marrow suppression

TNF, tumor necrosis factor.

- Blood work: rheumatoid factor true positive in 75% of cases (increased number of false positives)
- Cyclic citrullinated peptide antibody is very specific to RA and should be used to confirm a positive rheumatoid factor.
- A complete blood count may show elevated leukocytes.
- Some patients with classic clinical findings may have seronegative disease with no positive laboratory markers.

Treatment

- Nonsteroidal anti-inflammatory drugs are commonly used for early mild cases.
- Early detection and treatment appear to lessen the severity of joint destruction in the future.
- Disease-modifying antirheumatoid drugs are the mainstay of treatment (Table 18-1).
- Joint replacement and joint fusions are often necessary for severely damaged joints.

GOUT AND PSEUDOGOUT

History

- Acute onset of symptoms
- Males 30 to 50 years at highest risk; postmenopausal females as well
- Patients report warm, swollen, exquisitely painful joint, sensitive even to light touch (bed sheets).
- First metatarsophalangeal joint (*podagra*) and knee are most commonly affected as well as the mid-foot/ankle
- Increased alcohol intake often reported within 1 to 4 days of the onset of symptoms
- Gout is often called the "great masquerader" because of subtle signs on examination. "If in doubt, think gout."
- Pseudogout presents usually after age 50, primarily in the knees and wrists.
- Symptoms typically develop more gradually than with gout, over days or weeks.
- Often follows overuse such as excessive walking.

Physical Examination

- Vital signs
  - Afebrile typically; may have increased heart rate due to pain
- Skin
  - Often inflamed, indurated over the affected joint
  - Palpable nodules (gouty tophi) on fingers, olecranon bursae, helix of ears
- Gait
  - Typically limping due to knee or toe involvement
- Joints
  - Warm to touch; may mimic infected joint (which must be ruled out)
  - In acute cases, the patient has moderate to severe pain even with light touch.
  - The range of motion is extremely limited due to pain and joint swelling.
  - No ligamentous laxity

Imaging

- Radiographs are often negative in early disease. Late disease may show oval periarticular erosions in gout (Fig. 18-5).
- Pseudogout shows classic chondrocalcinosis (linear calcium deposits in articular or meniscal cartilage) (Fig. 18-6).

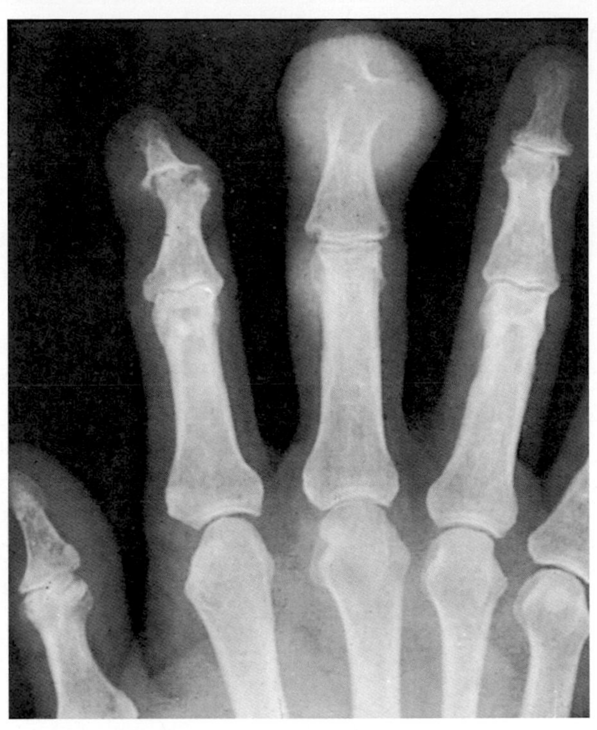

Figure 18-5 Oval erosions in chronic gout distal interphalangeal joints. (From Canale ST, Beaty JH [eds]: Campbell's Operative Orthopaedics, 11th ed. Philadelphia: Mosby, 2007, Fig. 74-33.)

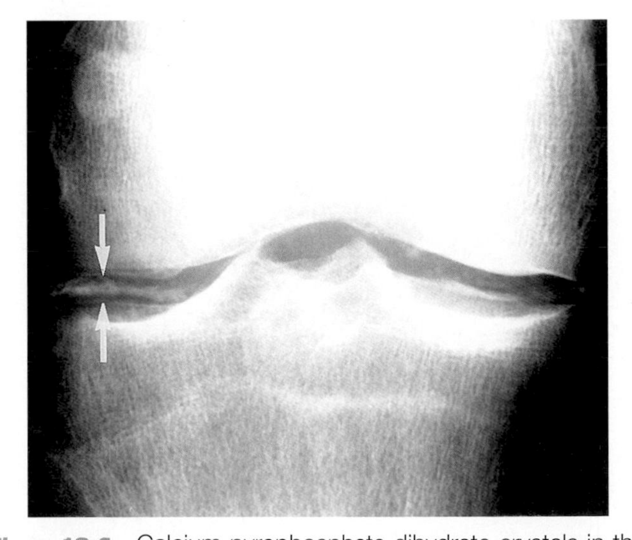

Figure 18-6 Calcium pyrophosphate dihydrate crystals in the lateral meniscus (*arrows*). (From Mettler FA Jr: Essentials of Radiology, 2nd ed. Philadelphia: Elsevier, 2004, Fig. 8-128.)

Additional Tests

- Essential to proper diagnosis (Fig. 18-7 and Table 18-2)

Treatment

- Acute treatment for both gout and pseudogout consists of oral nonsteroidal anti-inflammatory drugs or

corticosteroids. Intra-articular corticosteroid injections can be given (after sepsis is ruled out).
- Colchicine 0.6 mg two or three times daily is the standard dose.
- Colchicine must be dose adjusted for renal failure and often causes diarrhea.
- Chronic pseudogout is best managed with treatments similar to OA, with the final step being total joint replacement.
- Chronic gout is best managed with reduction/cessation of alcohol intake, avoiding purine-rich foods, weight loss, and limitation of thiazide diuretic use.
- Allopurinol (50–300 mg/day) inhibits uric acid production. It should not be started in the setting of an acute gout flare.
- Probenecid, used less often, increases uric acid excretion. It cannot be used if the patient has a history of renal insufficiency (creatinine clearance < 60), takes aspirin, or has nephrolithiasis.

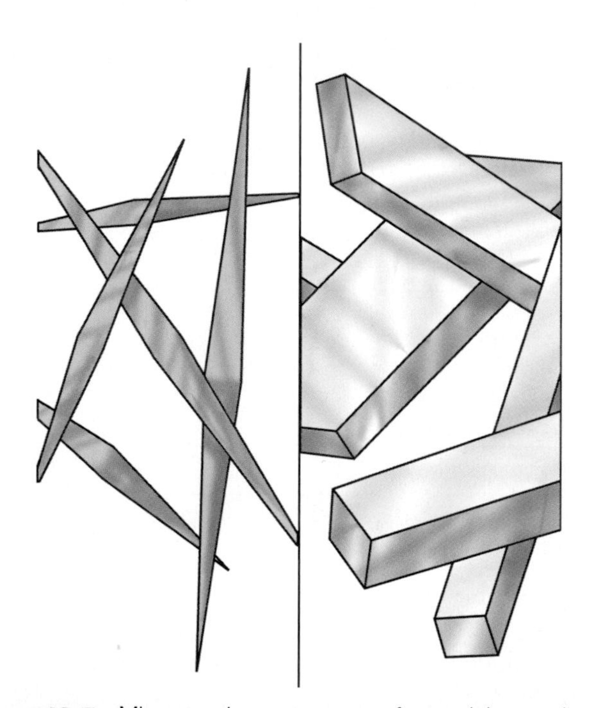

Figure 18-7 Microscopic appearance of synovial crystals from gout (*left*) and pseudogout (*right*).

LYME DISEASE

History

- A bull's-eye target rash (erythema chronicum migrans) develops in 80% of affected patients 1 to 4 weeks after the initial infection caused by the deer tick. Patients are often unaware of the link between the rash and future symptoms. *Ixodes scapularis* (deer tick) is the main vector.
- Report of flulike symptoms with body aches, fatigue, headache, and arthralgias that develop within 4 weeks of exposure
- The knee is the most common location of joint symptoms, including stiffness and swelling.
- Monoarthritis may develop weeks to months after the initial infection.
- The tick must be attached at least 36 hours to transmit infection.

Physical Examination

- Vital signs
  - May have low-grade fever
- Skin
  - Red, annular spreading rash with possible ringed appearance; not raised or palpable
- Gait
  - Often antalgic as knee is most common site of involvement
- Joints
  - Warmth, moderate joint effusion; joint lines are typically tender to the touch; range of motion limited by the size of effusion; ligamentous stability intact; no crepitus

TABLE 18-2 *Laboratory Evaluation of Common Arthritic Conditions*

	Osteoarthritis	Gout	Pseudogout
Joint fluid analysis	<2000 WBCs No organisms Negative culture	>2000 WBCs Negative birefringent crystals, yellow (needle shaped)	>2000 WBCs Positive birefringent crystals, blue (rhomboid)
Agent	Damage/loss of cartilage	Monosodium urate crystals	Calcium pyrophosphate dihydrate
Blood work	Normal WBC Normal ESR	High/normal WBC High/normal uric acid High/normal ESR	High/normal WBC Normal uric acid High/normal ESR

ESR, erythrocyte sedimentation rate; WBC, white blood cell.

Imaging

- Radiographs may show effusion but are otherwise normal in a younger patient. Preexisting arthritis may be misleading as to the source of the pain.
- Magnetic resonance imaging confirms effusion with no joint derangement.

Additional Tests

- Joint fluid analysis: white blood cell count greater than 5000, often 20,000 to 30,000; culture negative
- Polymerase chain reaction analysis for causative organism *Borrelia burgdorferi*
- Blood work: high or normal white blood cell count, high or normal erythrocyte sedimentation rate
- Antibody tests for Lyme disease: enzyme-linked immunosorbent assay (sensitive) or Western blot (specific)

Treatment

- Infection
  - Early infection: doxycycline 100 mg PO twice daily for 10 to 21 days
  - Pediatric patients and in pregnancy: amoxicillin 500 mg three times daily for 14 to 21 days
  - Late infection with neurologic or cardiac involvement: hospitalization required for monitoring of atrioventricular block
  - Ceftriaxone 2 mg/day IV for 14 to 28 days or doxycycline 200 to 400 mg/day PO in two divided doses for 14 to 28 days
- Late infection with arthritis
  - Ceftriaxone 1 to 2 g IV every 12 hours for 14 to 28 days or doxycycline 100 mg twice daily for 28 days; amoxicillin 500 mg three times daily for 28 days
- Arthritis
  - Nonsteroidal anti-inflammatory drugs, intra-articular corticosteroids, consideration of methotrexate; surgical synovectomy may be required

OTHER AUTOIMMUNE DISEASES AFFECTING THE JOINTS

Systemic Lupus Erythematosus

- Peak onset in teenage years, affects mostly females
- Malar rash common along with joint symptoms
- Joint involvement very painful, red, and swollen; not as symmetrical as RA
- Raynaud's phenomenon symptoms frequently reported by patients

Psoriatic Arthritis

- Only a small percentage of patients also report skin changes of psoriasis.
- Develops in the 30s and 40s; males and females equally affected
- Small joints of hands and feet affected the most
- May have morning stiffness similar to RA
- Spine involvement is more common than with others in this category.

Reiter Syndrome (Reactive Arthritis)

- In contrast to psoriatic arthritis, this usually affects the larger joints, knees, and hips.
- Triad of arthritis, conjunctivitis, and nongonococcal urethritis/cervicitis
- Recent infections with *Salmonella*, *Shigella*, *Campylobacter*, *Yersinia*, or *Chlamydia*
- Thought to be an autoimmune stimulus

Physical Examination

- Vital signs
  - Typically normal
- Skin
  - The malar rash of systemic lupus erythematosus mimics the shadowing of a wolf's (lupus) facial markings.
  - Psoriasis has circumscribed erythematous scaling plaques; nail pitting common (Fig. 18-8)
  - Pustular lesions on soles of feet (keratoderma blennorrhagicum) only seen in Reiter syndrome
- Gait
  - May or may not be affected
- Joints
  - Systemic lupus erythematosus
    - — Very common to have diffuse pain in the larger joints with nonspecific findings on examination
    - — May have slight warmth but nearly full range of motion; rare to have joint deformity initially
    - — Joint pain symptoms may be without physical findings in early disease.
  - Psoriasis
    - — Swollen fingers or toes seen (sausage digits)

- — The spine and sacroiliac joints can be affected with pain and limitations on range of motion testing.
- Reiter syndrome
  - — Ninety-five percent of affected patients have joint involvement.
  - — Generally in multiple joints; begins with painful knees, ankles, or toes
  - — May also have low back stiffness with testing
  - — Tendons are often painful on examination and may be swollen.

Imaging

- Radiographs may show cartilage loss and erosions as with RA.
- Reiter syndrome and psoriatic involvement can show beaklike nonmarginal syndesmophytes.
- Distal interphalangeal joints of the fingers may be affected in psoriatic arthritis, along with subluxations or fusions.

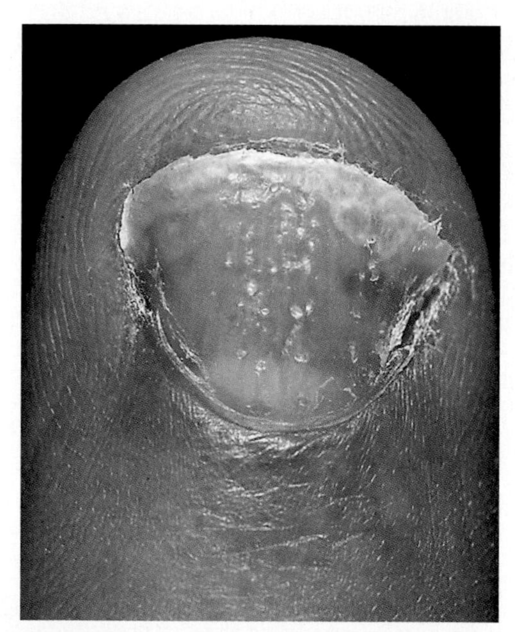

Figure 18-8 Psoriatic nail plate pitting. (From Habif TP: Clinical Dermatology, 4th ed. Philadelphia: Mosby, 2004, Fig. 8-10.)

Additional Tests (Table 18-3)

- No specific laboratory test exists for psoriatic arthritis; may be diagnosed by presence of skin lesions or exclusion of other causes
- Eighty percent of patients with Reiter syndrome are positive for HLA-B27.

Treatment

- The primary goal is controlling the autoimmune response systemically, which in turn should lessen the amount of arthritic symptoms.
- Nonsteroidal anti-inflammatory drugs and corticosteroids are mainstays of anti-inflammatory treatments.
- Immunomodulating therapies may also be appropriate for systemic lupus erythematosus or psoriatic arthritis (Table 18-4).

Troubleshooting

- Always perform arthrocentesis on a warm, swollen joint.
- Septic arthritis must be ruled out before addressing other diagnoses.
- Joint fluid should be analyzed with a Gram stain, crystals, rheumatoid factor, gonorrhea culture (chocolate agar), cell count, and cytology.
- Lyme disease is no longer endemic to only the northeastern United States; it has been diagnosed in patients throughout the United States.
- A positive rheumatoid factor test does not mean that the patient has RA; there are a high number of false-positive tests.

TABLE 18-3 *Laboratory Evaluation of Other Arthritis Etiologies*

	SLE	Psoriatic Arthritis	Reiter Syndrome
Joint fluid analysis	>2000 WBCs	>2000 WBCs	>2000 WBCs
Blood work	High ANA (>1 : 640) High anti-DS DNA, ESR, Smith AB, CBC Complement levels	Rheumatoid factor ANA CCP High/normal ESR Seronegative usually	HLA-B27 positive In 50–90%, AB titers of infectious organisms elevated ESR elevated

AB, antibody; ANA, antinuclear antibody; CBC, complete blood count; CCP, cyclic citrullinated peptide; DS, double-stranded; ESR, erythrocyte sedimentation rate; HLA, human leukocyte antigen; SLE, systemic lupus erythematosus; WBC, white blood cells.

TABLE 18-4 *Treatment of Other Immune Arthritides*

Condition	Treatment
Systemic lupus erythematosus	Oral steroids Methotrexate Joint fusions favored over replacements
Psoriatic arthritis	NSAIDs, methotrexate Sulfasalazine effective Caution oral steroids can cause plaques to become pustular TNF inhibitors
Reiter syndrome	Address bacterial infection if still present Inflammatory treatment is similar to rheumatoid arthritis

NSAIDs, nonsteroidal anti-inflammatory drugs; TNF, tumor necrosis factor.

Patient Instructions

- Provide clear advice for the patient regarding the diagnosis along with detailed instructions for treatment.
- Always address obesity issues if present.

Considerations in Special Populations

- Monitor the elderly closely for side effects of nonsteroidal anti-inflammatory drugs including gastrointestinal bleeding and renal function. Joint pain and disability have a negative effect on balance; canes and walkers are appropriately used to lessen the chance of falling.
- Ensure that the affected joint(s) in athletes are asymptomatic before patients return to play.
- Although joint pain and swelling are common in those older than 60 years of age, any joint effusion in a child requires immediate attention and investigation.

Suggested Reading

- American Academy of Orthopaedic Surgeons: AAOS Clinical Practice Guideline on Osteoarthritis of the Knee. Rosemont, IL: American Academy of Orthopaedic Surgeons, 2003.
- Cohen SB: Rheumatoid arthritis: Update on therapy. Paper presented at the American College of Rheumatology 67th Annual Scientific Meeting, Oct 23–28, 2003, Orlando, Florida.
- Eggebeen MD, Aaron T: Gout: An update. Am Fam Physician 2007;76:801–808.
- Fox MD, Robert L: Update on systemic lupus erythematosus. Paper presented at the American College of Rheumatology 67th Annual Scientific Meeting, Oct 23–28, 2003, Orlando, Florida.
- Wormser GP, Datwyler RJ, Shapiro ED, et al: The clinical assessment, treatment, and prevention of Lyme disease, human granulocytic anaplasmosis and babesiosis. Clin Infect Dis 2006;43:1089–1134.

Chapter 19 Infections (Septic Joint, Septic Arthritis, and Osteomyelitis)

Joseph Armen and Oana Panea

OSTEOMYELITIS

ICD-9 CODES
730.0 *Acute Osteomyelitis*
730.1 *Chronic Osteomyelitis*

Key Concepts

- Acute osteomyelitis is an acute infection of bone without the development of necrotic bone (sequestra). The duration is variable, but the condition usually evolves over several days to weeks.
- Chronic osteomyelitis is a long-term infection of bone with the presence of dead bone (the sequestrum). Common features include reactive bony encasement of the sequestrum (involucrum), local bone loss, and the possibility of sinus tract development if there is extension of the infection through cortical bone.
- The pathogenesis can include hematogenous spread of bacteria, contiguous spread from a soft-tissue infection, and local inoculation after surgery or trauma.
- Hematogenous spread has a biphasic distribution, occurring in children due to their unique bone anatomy and in patients older than the age of 50 who have increased risk factors for bacteremia.
- The long bones are most often involved in children. In adults, the vertebrae and sternoclavicular and sacroiliac bones are most commonly involved.
- This is a difficult disease to diagnose; testing must be tailored to the clinical scenario and may require bone biopsy for definitive diagnosis.
- When present, positive blood cultures with typical radiographic changes obviate the need for a bone biopsy.

History

- Signs and symptoms can vary with duration of disease.
  - Acute osteomyelitis
    - — Typically has an insidious onset over several days to a week with bone pain, tenderness, warmth, and swelling
    - — Fevers can be present, and pain occurs with and without movement. Complaints can be vague and nonspecific, with few constitutional symptoms.
  - Chronic osteomyelitis
    - — May be subtle with few symptoms. There may be a history of chronically developing skin changes or ulcerations, bone pain, or concomitant medical issues including diabetes and peripheral vascular disease.
    - — Easily recognized if there is a draining sinus along with recurrent pain, erythema, and swelling in someone with a known history of osteomyelitis

Physical Examination

- Acute osteomyelitis
  - Children
    - — If hematogenous in origin, abrupt onset of fever and local signs of inflammation may be present
    - — A limp or refusal to walk may be observed if the spine, pelvis, or lower extremity is involved. Pseudoparalysis may occur when the upper extremity is involved.
  - Adults
    - — Usually present with vague, nonspecific pain and few constitutional symptoms
    - — Limitation of joint motion, swelling, erythema, fever, and a symptomatic effusion may be present.
- Chronic osteomyelitis
  - External physical findings may be minimal; however, soft-tissue inflammation and tenderness may develop.

- Persistent drainage through a sinus tract or fistula, low-grade fever, chronic pain, local bone loss, and mild systemic symptoms may be present.

Imaging

- Plain radiographs
  - Acute osteomyelitis
    - — Two to three weeks are required for bone changes to be evident.
    - — The triad of soft-tissue swelling, bone destruction, and periosteal reaction is specific.
  - Chronic osteomyelitis
    - — Bone sclerosis, periosteal new bone formation, and sequestra are the primary findings.
- Ultrasonography
  - Findings may include a fluid collection adjacent to the bone and periosteal elevation by more than 2 mm with thickening.
  - Larger studies are needed to evaluate more accurately the sensitivity and specificity of this modality.
- Computed tomography
  - Accurately detects cortical destruction, periosteal reaction, intraosseous gas, and soft-tissue extension
- Magnetic resonance imaging
  - Provides anatomic detail when planning surgical débridement and identifying abscesses
  - Especially advantageous when evaluating vertebral or foot osteomyelitis
- Three-phase bone scan
  - This is the test of choice when evaluating acute osteomyelitis if plain radiographs are normal. The scan generally turns positive in 2 to 3 days.
  - Results in increased uptake in all three phases, making it useful when differentiating from cellulitis

Additional Tests

- Laboratory studies
  - Complete blood count
    - — Leukocytosis is common in acute, but not chronic, osteomyelitis.
  - Erythrocyte sedimentation rate
  - Monitoring can be useful to detect relapses.
- Cultures
  - Blood (positive in 50% of cases of acute osteomyelitis)
- Bone biopsy
  - The gold standard is an open bone biopsy with histopathologic examination and cultures.

Differential Diagnosis

- Cellulitis
- Gout
- Acute leukemia
- Bone malignancy
- Septic arthritis
- Rheumatic fever
- Bone infarct (i.e., sickle cell disease)

Treatment

- At diagnosis
  - Débridement of necrotic bone and empiric antibiotics to cover suspected organisms based on patient age, severity of disease, and comorbid conditions (Table 19-1)
  - Neurosurgical decompression is required for patients with vertebral osteomyelitis with an epidural abscess.
- Later
  - Definitive antimicrobials chosen based on culture and sensitivity results when available

TABLE 19-1 *Common Organisms in Osteomyelitis Based on Age and Chronic Conditions*

Osteomyelitis Type	Age	Likely Microorganism
Acute and chronic osteomyelitis	Newborn to 4 mo	Group A and B streptococcus, *Staphylococcus aureus*, *Enterobacter*
	4 mo to 4 yr	*S. aureus*, *Haemophilus influenzae*, *Escherichia coli*, group A streptococcus
	4 yr to adults	Group A streptococcus, *Staphylococcus epidermidis*, *Pseudomonas*, *Serratia marcescens*
Special populations	Immunocompromised	*Bartonella henselae*, *Aspergillus*, *Mycobacterium avium-intracellulare*, *Candida albicans*, anaerobes, *Mycobacterium tuberculosis*
	Sickle cell disease	*Salmonella*, *Streptococcus pneumoniae*

Data from Carek PJ, Dickerson LM, Sack JL: Diagnosis and management of osteomyelitis. Am Fam Physician 2001;63:2413–2420.

- Parenteral antibiotics are traditionally continued for 4 to 6 weeks.
- In chronic osteomyelitis, oral quinolones for 6 to 8 weeks can also be considered for susceptible organisms.

When to Refer

- Atypical infectious agents
- Difficulty in differentiating osteomyelitis from other diagnoses

Prognosis

- A good result can be expected with successful early treatment in an immunocompetent host.
- Progression to a chronic state is more common when the lower extremities are involved and in diabetics.

Troubleshooting

- The diagnosis of acute osteomyelitis cannot be excluded if the plain films are negative.
- False-positive magnetic resonance imaging results can occur with either a bone infarct or healed osteomyelitis.
- The sensitivity of a needle biopsy is especially low in the postoperative or posttrauma patient.
- The hip, pelvis, and vertebral locations tend to manifest few signs and symptoms.

Patient Instructions

- Follow your physician's instructions regarding treatment including antibiotic duration and pain medication use.
- As symptoms improve, physical therapy may be recommended to help the affected joint or limb regain function and flexibility.
- Notify your physician if symptoms persist or recur or new symptoms develop.
- Alert your physician if the drugs used for treatment produce side effects.

Considerations in Special Populations

- Sickle cell disease
  - Difficulty in differentiating bony crisis pain from osteomyelitis
  - *Salmonella* is the most common infectious organism involved.
- Diabetes
  - Underlying osteomyelitis is often missed in diabetic foot ulcers.
  - Magnetic resonance imaging is the imaging modality of choice for diabetic foot ulcers.

Suggested Reading

- Aloui N, Nessib N, Jalel C: Acute osteomyelitis in children: Early MRI diagnosis. J Radiol 2004;85:403–408.
- Burnett MW, Bass JW, Cook BA: Etiology of osteomyelitis complicating sickle cell disease. Pediatrics 1998;101:296–297.
- Carek PJ, Dickerson LM, Sack JL: Diagnosis and management of osteomyelitis. Am Fam Physician 2001;63:2413–2420.
- Gold RH, Hawkins RA, Katz RD: Bacterial osteomyelitis: Findings on plain radiography, CT, MR, and scintigraphy. Am J Roentgenol 1991;157:365–370.
- Karchevsky M, Schweitzer ME, Morrison WB, Parellada JA: MRI findings of septic arthritis and associated osteomyelitis in adults. Am J Roentgenol 2004;182:119–122.
- Lew DP, Waldvogel FA: Osteomyelitis. N Engl J Med 1997; 336:999–1007.
- Norden C, Gillespie WJ, Nade S: Infections in Bones and Joints. Boston: Blackwell Scientific, 1994.

SEPTIC ARTHRITIS

ICD-9 CODE
711.0 *Septic Arthritis*

Key Concepts

- Also referred to as infectious arthritis
- Many pathogens can be involved including bacteria, viruses, spirochetes, mycobacteria, and fungi.
- Bacterial pathogens are most significant because of their rapidly destructive nature.
- Two major classes of bacterial arthritis are gonococcal and nongonococcal.
  - Gonococcal
    - — *Neisseria gonorrhoeae*: most frequent among younger sexually active individuals
  - Nongonococcal
    - — *Staphylococcus aureus*: overall, the most common cause among adults and children older than 2 years of age
    - — Aerobic gram-negative rods: seen in the very young, the very old, intravenous drug users, and the immunosuppressed population
    - — Polymicrobial and anaerobes: usually a consequence of trauma or an abdominal infection
- There are three types of prosthetic joint infections: early, delayed, and late.

- Early
  - — Less than 3 months
  - — *S. aureus*
- Delayed
  - — Three to 24 months
  - — Coagulase-negative *S. aureus* and gram-negative aerobes
  - — Acquired in the operating room
- Late
  - — More than 24 months
  - — Due to seeding from hematogenous spread
- Joints can be infected by three mechanisms
  - Direct inoculation
  - Contiguous spread from infected periarticular tissue
  - Hematogenously
- Previously damaged joints are most susceptible.
- Articular cartilage damage due to the particular organism or host response is a major local consequence.

History

- Fever, extra-articular manifestations, and/or underlying joint disease may be present.
- Acute onset of joint pain is typical.
- Monoarticular involvement is common.
- Risk factors include history of intravenous drug use, sexually transmitted infections, prosthetic joint surgery, arthroscopy, chronic disease, and immunosuppression.

Physical Examination

- Findings can vary, but may include
  - General
    - — Fever, tachycardia
  - Inspection
    - — Erythema, rash involving the overlying skin
  - Palpation
    - — Warmth, joint effusion
  - Range of motion
    - — Pain and/or restriction of both active and passive range of motion

Imaging

- Plain radiographs
  - Evidence of demineralization may be present within days of onset.
  - Bony erosions and narrowing of the joint space followed by osteomyelitis may be seen within 2 weeks.
- Ultrasonography
  - Can be helpful in identifying joint effusions (especially of the hip) and guide needle aspirations
- Computed tomography/magnetic resonance imaging
  - Better when evaluating the sacroiliac and sternoclavicular joints along with the spine
  - Best when ruling out osteomyelitis, periarticular abscess, or other soft-tissue extensions
- Radionuclide scans
  - Helpful in identifying infections in deep-seated joints (i.e., the hip and sacroiliac joints)
  - Nonspecifically localizes other regions affected by inflammatory processes

Additional Tests

- Arthrocentesis with synovial fluid analysis (Table 19-2)
- Laboratory tests
  - Complete blood count with differential
  - Erythrocyte sedimentation rate
- Cultures
  - Blood and synovial fluid along with urethral, pharyngeal, and/or rectal if clinically indicated

TABLE 19-2 *Synovial Fluid Analysis*

Synovial Fluid	Color	Clarity	WBC (μL)	PMN (%)	Crystals	Culture
Normal	Clear	Transparent	<200	<25	Negative	Negative
Noninflammatory	Straw to yellow	Transparent	2000	<25	Negative	Negative
Inflammatory	Yellow	Translucent	2000–50,000	>70	May be positive	Negative
Septic*	Variable	Opaque	>50,000	>90	May be positive	85–95% positive†
Hemorrhagic	Red	Bloody	200–2000	50–75	Negative	Negative

*Glucose and lactate dehydrogenase levels have low sensitivity/specificity to confirm or exclude the diagnosis of septic joint.
†Eighty-five percent to 95% positive cultures for nongonococcal arthritis and 25% for gonococcal arthritis.
PMN, polymorphonuclear neutrophil; WBC, white blood cell count.

Differential Diagnoses

- Still's disease
- Rheumatic fever
- Lyme disease
- Transient synovitis
- Gout
- Pseudogout
- Osteoarthritis
- Rheumatoid arthritis
- Psoriatic arthritis
- Osteomyelitis
- Pseudoseptic reaction (after an intra-articular injection)

Treatment

- At diagnosis
  - Parenteral antibiotics
    - — Initial choice is based on clinical judgment of causative organism (Table 19-3) and is modified if necessary based on culture and sensitivity results.
  - Frequent local aspirations
    - — When synovial fluid rapidly reaccumulates and causes symptoms
  - Surgical drainage
    - — To be considered if the hip is involved and/or medical therapy fails over a 2- to 4-day period
  - Rest, immobilization, elevation, local hot compresses, and early passive and active range of motion exercises as pain tolerates
- Later
  - Physical therapy
    - — If needed to address any functional limitations or impairments
  - Frequent outpatient follow-up visits after hospital discharge
    - — Allow for early recognition of adverse outcomes or recurrences
  - Consider prosthetic replacement

When to Refer

- Failed arthrocentesis
- Joint that is difficult to aspirate (i.e., the hip and sacroiliac joints)
- Atypical infectious agents

Prognosis

- Five percent to 10% death rate, usually from respiratory complications of sepsis
- Fifty percent of adults have residual decreased range of motion and chronic pain, especially if treatment is delayed.
- Predictors of poor outcome include age older than 60, involvement of the hip or shoulders, underlying rheumatoid arthritis, positive cultures after a week of appropriate therapy, and a delay of more than 1 week before initiating treatment.

Troubleshooting

- Fever is common, but may be absent in as many as 20% or more of patients, especially if they are immunosuppressed or are taking corticosteroids or antipyretics.
- A superimposed cellulitis is a relative contraindication to arthrocentesis.
- An undiagnosed chronic monoarthritis requires arthroscopy with or without a closed synovial biopsy.
- Patients taking warfarin can undergo arthrocentesis if their international normalized ratio is less than 4.

TABLE 19-3 *Likely Infecting Organism and Empirical Antibiotic Treatment of Septic Arthritis*

Age	Likely Organism	Initial Antibiotic Regimen
Neonate	*Staphylococcus aureus,* group B streptococcus	Oxacillin + gentamicin
Child < 5 yr	*S. aureus*, group A streptococcus, *Streptococcus pneumoniae*, *Haemophilus influenzae*	Second-generation cephalosporin
5 yr to adolescence	*S. aureus*	Oxacillin
Adolescence to adulthood	*Neisseria gonorrhoeae*	Ceftriaxone
Older adults	*S. aureus*	Oxacillin or cefazolin + aminoglycoside

Data from Griffin LY (ed): Essentials of Musculoskeletal Care, 3rd ed. Rosemont, IL: American Academy of Orthopaedic Surgeons, 2005, p 115.

Patient Instructions

- Educate yourself about the disease and risk factors and seek medical attention if needed for early diagnosis and treatment.
- Sometimes treatment requires hospitalization, and patient participation in developing a treatment plan can be beneficial.
- Once the infection is under control, exercises can strengthen joints and muscles and improve the range of motion.

Considerations in Special Populations

- Pediatric
  - Negative clinical predictors include fever, non–weight bearing on the affected joint, white blood cell count greater than 12,000, and an erythrocyte sedimentation rate greater than 40.
  - Joint destruction or physeal damage is possible.
- Geriatric
  - Be aware of drug interactions between antibiotics prescribed and long-term medications.
  - Renal dosing of antibiotics should be used when appropriate.
  - Instruct patients with prosthetic joints to recognize early signs of joint infection.

Suggested Reading

- Donatto KC: Orthopedic management of septic arthritis. Rheum Dis Clin North Am 1998;24:275–286.
- Frank G, Mahoney HM, Eppes SC: Musculoskeletal infections in children. Pediatr Clin North Am 2005;52:1083–1106, ix.
- Griffin LY (ed): Essentials of Musculoskeletal Care, 3rd ed. Rosemont, IL: American Academy of Orthopaedic Surgeons, 2005, p 115.
- Mararetten ME, Kohlwes J, Moore D, Bent S: Does this patient have septic arthritis? JAMA 2007;297:1478–1488.
- Shmerling RH, Delbanco TL, Tosteson AN, Trentham DE: Synovial fluid tests. What should be ordered? JAMA 1990;264:1009–1014.
- Simon RR, Koenigsknecht SJ: Septic arthritis of the hip joint. In Emergency Orthopedics: The Extremities, 4th ed. New York: McGraw-Hill, 2001, pp 404–406.

Chapter 20 Neurovascular Disorders: Deep Venous Thrombosis

Blake Boggess and Harry C. Stafford

ICD-9 CODE
453.9 *Deep Venous Thrombosis*

Key Concepts

- Deep venous thrombosis (DVT) is a venous thromboembolism or clot that forms after the coagulation pathway has been activated.
- Incidence is one per 1000 people every year. Rates increase with age and are higher in males compared with females.
- Risk factors include Virchow's triad of venous statis with alteration in normal blood flow, vascular endothelium injury, and hypercoagulability.
- Seventy-five percent of patients with DVT have at least one risk factor (Box 20-1).
- Half of all cases of DVT occur in hospitalized patients or nursing home residents.
- Ninety percent of all pulmonary embolisms are from emboli of the proximal veins of the lower extremities.
- Upper extremity DVT is less common, but may lead to a pulmonary embolism as well.

History

- Classic symptoms are swelling, pain, and discoloration in the involved extremity.
- Obtain a complete thrombosis history including location of previous DVT, age at onset, and family history of venous thrombosis in first-degree relatives.
- Genetic defects such as factor V Leiden mutation or protein C or S deficiency
- More than 48 hours of immobilization in the previous month
- Surgery or hospital admission in the past 3 months

Physical Examination

- Inspection of the extremity may reveal
  - Ipsilateral edema
  - Erythema
- Palpation of the extremity may reveal
  - Palpable cord (reflecting thrombosed vein)
  - Increased warmth
  - Superficial venous dilation
- Homans' sign: passive dorsiflexion of the ankle elicits pain in the calf because of thrombosis in the vein
- Painful deep vein syndrome: pain with palpation along major veins of the thigh
- Phlegmasia cerulean dolens: reddish purple lower extremity from venous engorgement and obstruction
- Evaluate for signs of pulmonary embolus: tachycardia, tachypnea, low-grade fever, and cardiac examination with signs of right-sided heart strain including
  - Loud pulmonary component of second heart sound
  - Right-sided S3 heart sound increased with inspiration
  - Palpable lift over the left sternal border (right ventricular heave)
- A complete knee and ankle examination should be done to evaluate for additional pathologies.

Imaging

- Duplex ultrasonography is a combination of real-time ultrasonographic imaging with Doppler flow studies.
- Sensitivity of duplex ultrasonography for proximal vein DVT is 97% and for calf vein DVT, 73%. The negative predictive value for proximal vein DVT is 99%. Overall specificity is 95%.
- Duplex ultrasonography is also helpful to differentiate venous thrombosis from hematoma, Baker's cyst, abscess, and other causes of leg pain and edema.
- The disadvantage of duplex ultrasonography is its inaccuracy in the diagnosis of calf vein thrombosis, venous thrombi proximal to the inguinal ligament, and nonoccluding thrombi. Diagnostic accuracy is also operator dependent.
- In ambulatory outpatients with suspected DVT, duplex ultrasonography remains the initial diagnostic test of choice (Fig. 20-1).

- Two percent of patients with negative initial ultrasonography results will have positive results on reevaluation 1 week later.

Additional Tests

- D-Dimer is a degradation product of cross-linked fibrin elevated in patients with DVT.
- A negative D-dimer test result is useful for ruling out DVT, but a positive or elevated test result is insufficient to diagnose DVT because many conditions may cause false positives.
- Contrast venography: Invasive imaging test performed by injecting contrast dye in the vein to visualize a thrombus. Contrast venography is the gold standard with which noninvasive tests are compared to diagnose DVT. It is not recommended as an initial screening test due to patient discomfort and difficulty in obtaining an adequate study.
- Noninvasive tests with equal accuracy for diagnosing a DVT have reduced the need for contrast venography.
- Impedance plethysmography measures changes in blood volume of an extremity, which is directly related to venous outflow using electrical impedance.
- Impedance plethysmography has been shown to be sensitive and specific for proximal vein thrombosis, but many facilities have neither the equipment nor the skilled personnel to perform the test.
- Magnetic resonance imaging is the diagnostic test of choice for suspected iliac vein or inferior vena caval thrombosis when computed tomography venography is contraindicated or technically inadequate.
- In calf vein thrombosis, magnetic resonance imaging is more sensitive than any other noninvasive study, but expense, lack of general availability, and technical issues limit its use.
- Computed tomography venography has high sensitivity for DVT compared with duplex ultrasonography.
- The major problems with computed tomography venography are technical issues with inadequately visualized veins, artifactual interference from metal implants such as hip and knee arthroplasties, and contraindications to the administration of contrast dye.

BOX 20-1 *Risk Factors for Deep Venous Thrombosis*

Previous venous thromboembolism
History of immobilization (e.g., bed rest, recent airplane flight)
Recent surgery
History of stroke
Hormone replacement therapy or oral contraceptive use
Pregnancy or postpartum patient
History of malignancy
Obesity
Lower extremity trauma
Congestive heart failure
Hyperhomocystinemia
Disorders affecting blood viscosity (e.g., sickle cell anemia, polycythemia, multiple myeloma)

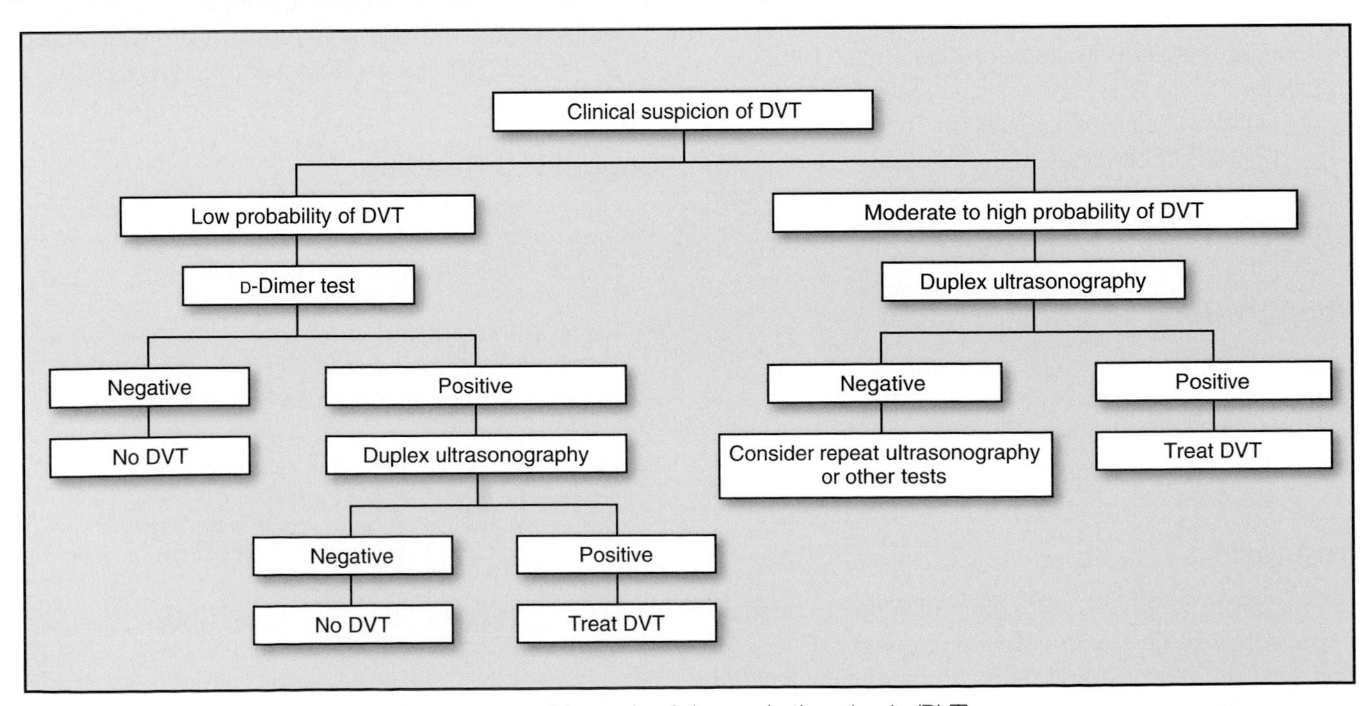

Figure 20-1 Diagnosis of deep vein thrombosis (DVT).

Differential Diagnosis

- Muscle strain/tear
- Lymphangitis
- Venous insufficiency
- Baker's cyst
- Cellulitis
- Knee injury
- Asymmetrical peripheral edema
- Hematoma
- Prolonged immobilization or limb paralysis
- Extrinsic compression of iliac vein secondary to tumor, hematoma, or abscess

Treatment

- At diagnosis
    - The goal of treatment is to stop clot propagation and prevent pulmonary embolism and clot recurrence.
    - Upon diagnosis, start anticoagulation using heparin followed by warfarin.
- Low molecular weight heparin or unfractionated heparin may be used, but low molecular weight heparin is usually preferred because dosing is fixed, it can be given once or twice daily, and laboratory monitoring is not required.
- Warfarin can be administered simultaneously with heparin with an initial dose of 5 to 10 mg/day unless contraindicated. The heparin can be discontinued on day 5 if the international normalized ratio has been therapeutic for two consecutive days. The international normalized ratio target range should be 2 to 3.
- Later
    - Duration of anticoagulation depends on the number of episodes of DVT, presence of ongoing risk factors for thromboembolism, and known thrombophilia.

When to Refer

- A referral to a cardiology, pulmonary, or anticoagulation clinic is appropriate if the physician is unable to monitor the international normalized ratio or is uncomfortable managing patients with DVT.

Prognosis

- Pulmonary embolism will occur in 50% of untreated patients with DVT within days or weeks.
- If the DVT was caused by a thrombophilic disorder, the risk of a repeat episode may be high.

Troubleshooting

- An inferior vena caval filter may be required in individuals with complications on anticoagulant therapy or recurrent thromboembolism despite adequate anticoagulation.

Patient Instructions

- When patients are traveling, they should sit in seats that allow leg extension, take hourly walking breaks, wear loose clothing, and keep hydrated. They should not cross their legs.
- Patients should also be aware that certain foods can increase or decrease the effect of warfarin (e.g., foods high in vitamin K may diminish the anticoagulant effects of warfarin).

Considerations in Special Populations

- Sports medicine
    - Athletes taking continued anticoagulation therapy should not participate in collision or contact sports.
    - Individuals involved in noncontact sports may participate after appropriate counseling.
    - If an athlete has finished a course of anticoagulation and a hypercoagulability evaluation is negative, gradual return to play may be granted with careful monitoring for recurrence.
    - Athletes who use erythropoietin are at increased risk of DVT due to increased blood viscosity.

Suggested Reading

- Fraser D, Moody A, Morgan P: Diagnosis of lower-limb deep venous thrombosis: A prospective blinded study of magnetic resonance direct thrombus imaging. Ann Intern Med 2002;136:89–98.
- Hirsh J, Lee A: How we diagnose and treat deep vein thrombosis. Blood 2002;99:3102–3110.
- Lensing A, Prandoni P, Pins M: Deep-vein thrombosis. Lancet 1999;353:479–485.
- Mateo J, Oliver A, Borrell M, et al: Laboratory evaluation and clinical characteristics of 2,132 consecutive unselected patients with venous thromboembolism—results of the Spanish Multicentric Study on Thrombophilia (EMET-Study). Thromb Haemost 1997;77:444–451.
- Meyering C, Howard T: Hypercoagulability in athletes. Curr Sports Med Rep 2004;3:77–83.
- Schulman S: Care of patients receiving long-term anticoagulant therapy. N Engl J Med 2003;349:675–683.

Chapter 21 Neurovascular Disorders: Arterial Conditions in Athletes

Mario Ciocca

Vascular injury can occur with severe traumatic injury or joint dislocation. In contrast, chronic stress or overuse may also cause either damage to the vascular system or symptoms referable to the vascular system. Although uncommon, these injuries must always be considered because a delay in diagnosis can be catastrophic.

SUBCLAVIAN ARTERY/AXILLARY ARTERY OCCLUSION

Key Concepts

- The axillary artery arises from the subclavian artery at the outer border of the first rib and courses deep to the pectoralis minor muscle.
- The subclavian artery is susceptible to compression from a cervical rib, anomalous first rib, or overdeveloped scalene muscles.
- Axillary artery occlusion develops secondary to pressure from the overlying pectoralis minor muscle in the overhead position.
- The axillary artery may also be compressed by the humerus when the shoulder is in the cocked position (Fig. 21-1).
- Can occlude in baseball pitchers when in the late cocking phase of throwing
- An axillary artery aneurysm (usually at the origin of the posterior humeral circumflex artery) or distal embolization may develop.

History

- Symptoms may include
  - Claudication
  - Fatigue
  - Night pain
  - Coolness of affected arm
  - Sudden onset of numbness, coolness, and cold intolerance in the hand may be secondary to distal embolization.

Physical Examination

- Tenderness over pectoralis minor muscle area
- May have diminished distal pulses that are usually position dependent
- Provocative tests for thoracic outlet syndrome may be positive.
- Weakness or sensory deficits are rare.

Imaging

- Radiographs may demonstrate a cervical rib, a long transverse process, or other bone abnormalities that may cause thoracic outlet syndrome.
- Noninvasive vascular tests may show compression or occlusion.
- A definitive diagnosis can be made with an arteriogram in the symptom-provoking position.

Treatment

- In the absence of complete thrombosis, aneurysm, or embolism, treatment can be conservative with strengthening of the shoulder suspensory muscles to maintain the patency of the costoclavicular triangle.
- Surgical treatment may include segmental vascular excision with primary anastomosis or bypass with a venous graft.
- Release of the pectoralis minor muscle or rib resection may also be required.

QUADRILATERAL SPACE SYNDROME

Key Concepts

- Quadrilateral space bordered by the teres minor muscle, teres major muscle, proximal humerus, and long head of the triceps muscle (Fig. 21-2)
- The posterior humeral circumflex artery arises from the distal third of the axillary artery and enters the quadrilateral space with the axillary nerve.

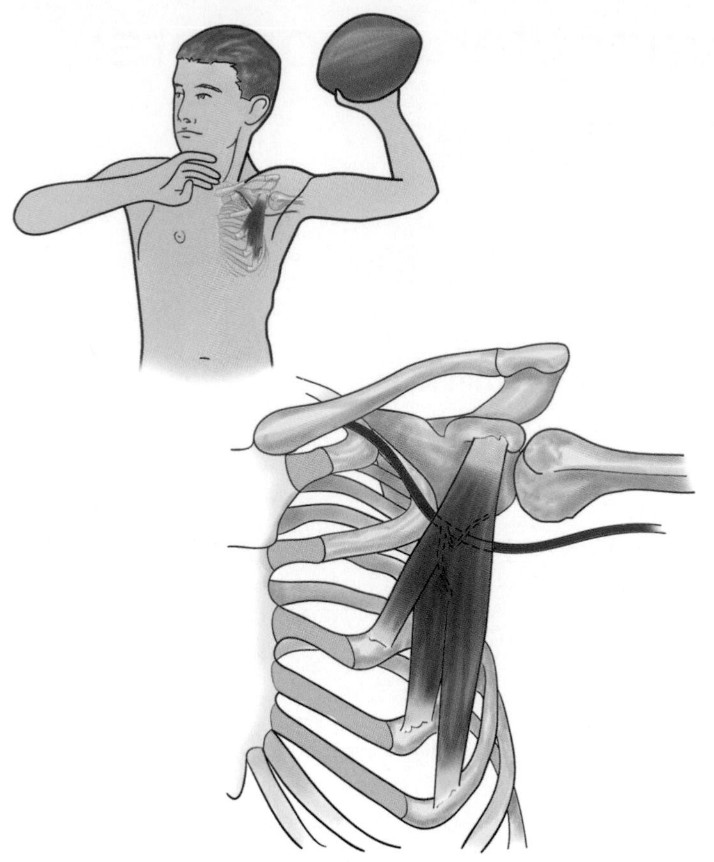

Figure 21-1 The axillary artery may also be compressed by the humerus when the shoulder is in the cocked position.

- This space is compressed when the shoulder is in the abducted and externally rotated position.
- Etiology
  - Repetitive activity can cause abnormal fibrous bands and/or muscular hypertrophy.
  - Traction on the posterior humeral circumflex artery by the pectoralis major muscle
  - Tethering of the posterior humeral circumflex artery to the proximal humerus placing it at risk of traction injury
  - Space-occupying lesions such as glenoid labral cysts
  - Glenohumeral instability
  - Symptoms may be related to compression of the axillary nerve.

History

- A typical patient is an athlete 20 to 40 years old who uses overhead throwing motions.
- Poorly localized shoulder discomfort
- May have deltoid weakness and/or atrophy
- Arm fatigue in the overhead position

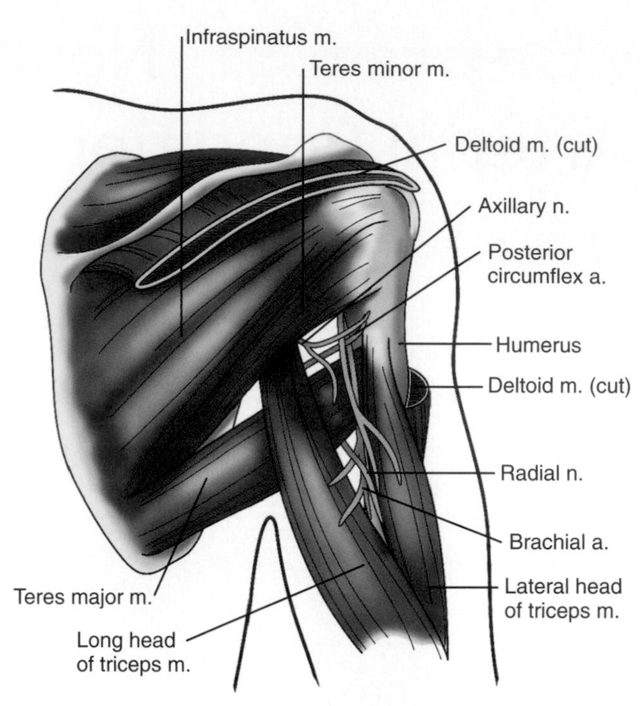

Figure 21-2 Quadrilateral space bordered by the teres minor muscle, teres major muscle, proximal humerus, and long head of the triceps muscle. a, artery; m, muscle; n, nerve.

- May have paresthesia to the lateral arm
- Possible night pain
- Throwing often affected

Physical Examination

- Localized tenderness over the quadrilateral space
- Re-creation of the pain when the shoulder is placed in forward flexion, abduction, and external rotation for 1 to 2 minutes

Imaging

- Radiographs to rule out other pathology
- Magnetic resonance imaging can rule out other causes. This procedure may also show teres minor muscle atrophy.
- Subclavian arteriography may show posterior humeral circumflex artery occlusion when the arm is abducted and externally rotated.

Additional Tests

- Magnetic resonance angiography is not useful because it is positive in as many as 80% of asymptomatic shoulders that are placed in abduction and external rotation.

Differential Diagnosis

- Cervical spine disorders
- Rotator cuff pathology
- Thoracic outlet syndrome

Treatment

- Now
  - Activity modification
  - Stretching into horizontal adduction and internal rotation
  - Rotator cuff muscle strengthening
  - Active release soft-tissue massage technique to the quadrilateral space
  - Nonsteroidal anti-inflammatory drugs
  - Corticosteroid injection
- Later (if not improved after 3–6 months)
  - Surgical decompression with release of fibrous bands via a posterior approach

ILIAC ARTERY OCCLUSION

Key Concepts

- Flow limitations may be due to lumen narrowing from endofibrotic thickening of the intima or from kinking of the vessel.
- Most often seen in highly trained cyclists but can also occur in speed skaters, runners, and triathletes
- The flow limitations will progress in 80% of patients.
- Endofibrotic lesions are thought to result from blood colliding against the vessel wall when the vessel is kinked during hip flexion.
- Endofibrotic lesions most often affect the external iliac artery, but may affect the common iliac artery and the femoral artery.
- Kinking of the artery may be caused by fixation due to a side branch of the psoas muscle, tight fibrous tissue, or excessive length of the artery.

History

- Symptoms usually develop in the mid-20s.
  - Claudication in buttock/thigh; quickly disappears at rest
  - Paresthesias of leg and plantar aspect of foot
  - Cramping at maximal effort, which may affect multiple muscles
  - Loss of power
  - Usually affects the left side but may be bilateral

Physical Examination

- Examination is usually normal.
- Auscultation of the iliac artery at rest
  - A bruit with hip extended has good specificity for flow limitation.
  - A bruit with the hip flexed is more sensitive for flow limitation.
- Auscultation after exercise is not useful because femoral bruits are heard in normal subjects.

Imaging

- Ankle brachial index normally reduced with exercise; however, insensitive for those without severe stenosis
- Echo Doppler combined with hip flexion after exercise best delineates kinking in the external iliac artery and also evaluates for intravascular lesions.
- Magnetic resonance angiography combined with hip flexion best delineates kinking in the common iliac artery. Magnetic resonance angiography can also assess excessive vessel length when the hip is extended and evaluate for intravascular lesions.
- Angiography is less useful for evaluating intravascular lesions because they are often located eccentrically.

Treatment

- Conservative
  - Reduce hours on the bike.
  - Change the cycling position to decrease hip flexion.
  - Do not actively pull the pedal upward.
- Surgical release of the iliac artery
  - Used for vessels that kink during hip flexion
  - The artery is released from the vascular sheath and the underlying surface and the vessel is left intact.
  - Psoas branches and fibrous tissue ligated
  - Low complication rate with quick return
  - Will need further treatment if vessel diameter less than 70% compared with unaffected side or kinking due to excessive vascular length
- Vascular reconstruction
  - Shortening of vessel: done for kinking due to excessive vessel length
  - Endarterectomy or replacement by venous graft
- Percutaneous transluminal angioplasty
  - May provide short-term relief
  - Generally unsatisfactory long-term outcome
- Stenting
  - Contraindicated because may induce intimal hyperplasia

POPLITEAL ARTERY ENTRAPMENT SYNDROME

Key Concepts

- The popliteal artery may be entrapped due to an anatomic variation that may include compression from an accessory medial head of the gastrocnemius muscle and an aberrant course of the popliteal artery.
  - Usually seen in sedentary males in their mid-40s who may have evidence of peripheral occlusive disease
- Another cause is functional entrapment with no anatomic variation other than a hypertrophied gastrocnemius muscle.
  - Patients are more often active females in their mid-20s without evidence of peripheral vascular disease.
- The condition may be bilateral.
- Needs to be treated early to prevent complications such as stenosis, thrombosis, and aneurysm
- Has been seen in runners, soccer players, tennis players, and weight lifters

History

- Claudication pain in the calf or anterior leg that increases with the intensity of exercise and quickly resolves when exercise stops
- Calf cramps
- Coldness of lower limb
- Paresthesia usually in tibial nerve distribution

Physical Examination

- Generally unhelpful
- May have popliteal bruit accentuated with active ankle plantar flexion or passive dorsiflexion and may increase after exercise
- Dorsalis pedis and posterior tibial artery pulses are normal in the neutral position but may diminish or disappear during passive dorsiflexion or active ankle plantar flexion.

Imaging

- Duplex ultrasonography of the popliteal artery with the ankle in dorsiflexion may reveal compression of the artery and a reduction of the velocity waves of arterial flow.
- Magnetic resonance angiography can be used to differentiate functional from anatomic entrapment.
- Angiography with the ankle in neutral position and dorsiflexion will usually establish the diagnosis.

Differential Diagnosis

- Lumbar disc disease
- Buerger's disease
- Tendinitis
- Cystic disease of the popliteal artery (mucoid cysts in the vessel adventitia, usually in men in their mid-40s)
- Popliteal artery injury due to trauma

Treatment

- Treatment is surgical with exploration of the popliteal fossa, incision of hypertrophied muscle, and small longitudinal resection and division of fascial bands.
- If the vein is damaged, vein grafting or bypassing is performed.

Suggested Reading

- Arko FR, Harris EJ, Zarins CK, Olcott C IV: Vascular complications in high-performance athletes. J Vasc Surg 2001;33:935–942.
- Aval SM, Durand P Jr, Shankwiler JA: Neurovascular injuries in the athlete's shoulder: Part II. J Am Acad Orthop Surg 2007;15:281–289.
- Baltopoulos P, Filippou DK, Sigula F: Popliteal artery entrapment syndrome anatomic or functional syndrome. Clin J Sport Med 2004;14:8–12.
- Bender MHM, Schep G, de Vries WR, et al: Sports-related flow limitations in the iliac arteries in endurance athletes. Sports Med 2004;34:427–442.
- Ehsan O, Darwish A, Edmundson C, et al: Non-traumatic lower limb vascular complications in endurance athletes: Review of the literature. Eur J Vasc Endovasc Surg 2004;28:1–8.
- Hoskins WT, Pollard HP, McDonald AJ: Quadrilateral space syndrome: A case study and review of the literature. Br J Sports Med 2005;39:e9.
- Mosley JG: Arterial problems in athletes. Br J Surg 2003; 90:1461–1469.
- Pham TT, Kapur R, Harwood MI: Exertional leg pain: Teasing out arterial entrapments. Curr Sports Med Rep 2007;6:371–375.
- Reeser JC: Diagnosis and management of vascular injuries in the shoulder girdle of the overhead athlete. Curr Sports Med Rep 2007:6:322–327.
- Schep G, Bender MHM, van de Tempel G, et al: Detection and treatment of claudication due to functional iliac obstruction in top endurance athletes: A prospective study. Lancet 2002:359:466–473.

Chapter 22 Neurovascular Disorders: Nerve Entrapment

Thomas E. Brickner

Key Concepts

- Peripheral nerve injuries due to mechanical constriction or deformation
- Pathophysiology is most often ischemic due to capillary hypoperfusion resulting from the constrictive force.
- May be due to tight anatomic passageways, space-occupying masses, external compressive forces, trauma, and inflammation
- May produce sensory and/or motor symptoms with atrophy
- Pattern of involvement is typically focal and mononeuritic
- Seddon's classification of nerve injuries (mild to severe)
  - Neurapraxia: demyelination of axon sheath
  - Axonotmesis: axonal disruption with intact epineurium
  - Neurotmesis: complete disruption

Conditions (see also Chapters 47, 65, 83, 129, and 182)

- Median nerve
  - Sites of compression: bicipital aponeurosis in antecubital fossa, between two heads of pronator teres, origin of flexor digitorum superficialis, carpal tunnel in wrist
  - Pronator syndrome
    - — Proximal, ventral forearm pain
    - — Paresthesias of radial 3.5 digits
    - — Tinel's sign at proximal forearm
  - Anterior interosseous syndrome
    - — No sensory symptoms
    - — Proximal forearm pain
    - — Abnormal, weakened pinch (OK) sign
  - Carpal tunnel syndrome
    - — Paresthesias in radial 3.5 digits
    - — Positive Tinel's and Phalen's signs at wrist
    - — Weakness in thumb abduction
- Radial nerve
  - Sites of compression: radial tunnel between heads of supinator
  - Radial tunnel syndrome
    - — Aching pain in wrist, extensor tendon group, and lateral elbow
    - — Weakness upon metacarpophalangeal extension and of extensor carpi ulnaris
- Ulnar nerve
  - Sites of compression: cubital tunnel at the posteromedial elbow, Guyon's canal in wrist
  - Cubital tunnel syndrome
    - — Aching pain at medial elbow
    - — Paresthesias of ulnar 1.5 digits
    - — Weakness of dorsal interosseous and abductor digiti minimi muscles
- Lateral antebrachial cutaneous nerve
  - Site of compression: lateral free margin of bicipital aponeurosis
  - Terminal sensory branch of musculocutaneous nerve
  - Supplies sensation over radial half of forearm
- Femoral nerve
  - Sites of compression: inguinal ligament, lumbar plexus due to mass
  - Sensory over anteromedial thigh and leg
  - Weakness of quadriceps muscle and knee jerk reflex
- Saphenous nerve
  - Site of compression: exit point of subsartorial fascia
  - Branch of femoral nerve
  - Purely sensory: knee and lower leg medially
- Lateral femoral cutaneous nerve (meralgia paresthetica)
  - Site of compression: near attachment of inguinal ligament to anterior superior iliac spine
  - Paresthesias over anterolateral thigh
- Peroneal nerve
  - Sites of compression: fibular head, anterior tarsal tunnel at ankle

- Impairment of dorsiflexion and eversion of foot
- Deep and superficial branches
  - — Deep: paresthesias of first web space
  - — Superficial: paresthesias of lateral distal leg and dorsum of foot
- Posterior tibial nerve
  - Sites of compression: popliteal fossa due to mass, posterior tarsal tunnel behind medial malleolus
  - Proximal lesion: calf pain, plantar flexion weakness
  - Distal lesion: heel and plantar foot paresthesias
- Interdigital neuroma (Morton's neuroma)
  - Site of compression: metatarsal heads
  - Pain radiating into toes
- Sural nerve
  - Site of compression: above ankle behind lateral malleolus
  - Sensory over lateral proximal foot

Imaging

- Magnetic resonance imaging
  - Identify space-occupying masses
  - Evaluate anatomy for hypertrophy, bony constrictions/spurring, anomalous structures
  - Evaluate signal change of muscles suggesting denervation atrophy
  - Visualize pathologic characteristics of nerves
    - — Focal enlargement
    - — Hyperintense signal
    - — Altered fascicular pattern
- Ultrasonography
  - Allows dynamic study for assessment of nerve compression
  - Inherent drawback is that it is operator dependent
  - Does not show pathologic changes within nerves

Diagnostics

- Electromyography (includes needle electrode examination and nerve conduction studies)
  - Detect peripheral nervous system lesions, site of pathology, severity, chronicity, and pathophysiology
  - Abnormalities may take weeks to fully develop after injury and may be completely unrevealing in mild cases.
- Nerve conduction studies
  - Measures conduction velocities, latencies, amplitude, and areas of nerve function
  - Demonstrates changes indicative of demyelination and/or axonal loss
- Needle electrode examination
  - Evaluates muscle spontaneous and intentional activity
  - Fibrillation potentials are evidence of denervation.
  - Alterations of motor unit action potentials are seen with neurogenic lesions.

Differential Diagnosis

- Tendinitis, epicondylitis, and arthritis
- Symptoms typically more localized
- Provocative testing helpful in differentiating
- Rule out other causes of neuropathies
- Endocrine/metabolic (diabetes mellitus, hypothyroidism), vasculitis, toxic, nutritional, infectious (acquired immunodeficiency syndrome), medications
  - Typically multifocal and symmetrical

Treatment (see also Chapters 47, 65, 83, 129, and 182)

- External devices such as splints and padding
- Anti-inflammatory drugs and injections
- Stretching and postural adjustments
- Activity modifications
- Surgical intervention
  - Releases, transpositions, decompressions

Suggested Reading

- Burns J, Mauermann M, Burns T: An easy approach to evaluating peripheral neuropathy. J Fam Pract 2006;55:853–861.
- Dawson DM: Entrapment neuropathies. Hosp Pract 1995;30:37–44.
- England JD, Gooch C, Werner R: Identifying entrapment and compression neuropathies. Patient Care Nurse Pract 1999;12:28–36.
- Katirji B: The clinical electromyography examination: An overview. Neurol Clin 2002;20:291–303.
- Kim S, Choi JY, Huh YM, et al: Role of magnetic resonance imaging in entrapment and compressive neuropathy: Part 1. Overview and lower extremity. Eur Radiol 2007;17:139–149.
- Wilbourn A: Electrodiagnostic testing of neurologic injuries in athletes. Clin Sports Med 1990;9:229–245.

Chapter 23 Osteoporosis and Osteopenia

Theresa Guise and Ailleen Heras-Herzig

ICD-9 CODES
733.0 *Osteoporosis*
733.9 *Osteopenia*

Key Concepts

- Osteoporosis is a skeletal disorder characterized by low bone mineral density (BMD) and poor bone quality that leads to an increased risk of insufficiency fractures.
- Primary or involutional osteoporosis refers to the normal bone loss that occurs with aging, and it can be further subdivided into type I or II osteoporosis syndrome.
- Type I osteoporosis is believed to be primarily the result of low estrogen concentration in postmenopausal women; however, an increase in certain cytokines such as interleukin-6 and tumor necrosis factor is probably a contributing factor.
- Type I osteoporosis is characterized by a disproportionate trabecular over cortical bone loss with an increased risk of Colles' fractures and vertebral compression fractures.
- Type II osteoporosis is the result of a combination of secondary hyperparathyroidism and decreased bone formation rates due to lower estrogen concentration in aging women and men.
- In 1994, the World Health Organization offered a definition of osteoporosis based on bone density measurements and history of fracture (Table 23-1). These criteria define osteoporosis as a BMD equal to or less than 2.5 standard deviations (SD) below a young adult mean value and osteopenia as a BMD greater than 1.5 SD but less than 2.5 SD below a young adult mean value.
- Based on the World Health Organization criteria, 20% to 30% of postmenopausal women in the United States have osteoporosis, and 1.3 million fractures a year are attributable to the disease.
- More recently, the International Society for Clinical Densitometry, in association with an expert panel, determined that it is appropriate to apply the World Health Organization criteria to men while using a gender-specific database.
- Using these established cutoffs, it is estimated that 1 to 2 million men have osteoporosis and 8 to 13 million men have osteopenia.

History

- Osteoporosis is considered a silent disease until an insufficiency fracture occurs. Thus, the National Osteoporosis Foundation has provided a set of guidelines to aid practitioners in identifying patients for whom BMD testing is appropriate (Box 23-1).
- The first step in assessing fracture risk is a thorough assessment of clinical risk factors (Box 23-2). The most readily recognized risk factors are increasing age and female gender.
- Other significant risk factors include a previous insufficiency fracture, previous or present glucocorticoid therapy, a family history of insufficiency fracture, low body weight, and other factors.

Physical Examination

- Osteoporosis has few diagnostic signs, but there are a number of findings that can alert the practitioner to the possibility of disease and/or increased fracture risk.
- Poor visual acuity and depth perception, decreased proprioception, decreased proximal muscle strength, and an impaired "get up and go" test are all risk factors for fall and fracture.
- Kyphotic deformity of the spine is a late sequela of vertebral fractures.

Imaging

- BMD testing remains a cornerstone of osteoporosis diagnosis and assessment of response to treatment.
- Central dual-energy x-ray absorptiometry is the standard for BMD testing. For every 1-SD decrease in

TABLE 23-1 *Defining Osteoporosis by Bone Mineral Density Based on the World Health Organization Criteria*

Category	Definition by BMD
Normal	BMD is within 1 SD of a young normal adult mean (*T* score ≥ –1)
Osteopenia	BMD is between 1 and 2.5 SD below a young normal adult mean (*T* score between –1 and –2.5)
Osteoporosis	BMD ≥ 2.5 SD below that of a young normal adult mean (*T* score ≤ –2.5)
Severe osteoporosis (established)	BMD > 2.5 SD below a young adult mean in the presence of one or more fragility fractures

Data from the World Health Organization (WHO): Assessment of fracture list and its application to screening postmenopausal osteoporosis. Technical Report series 843. Geneva: WHO, 1994.
BMD, bone mineral density; SD, standard deviation.

BOX 23-1 *Who Should Be Tested*

National Osteoporosis Foundation
- All women aged 65 and older regardless of risk factors
- Younger postmenopausal women with one or more risk factors (other than being white, postmenopausal, and female)
- Postmenopausal women who are considering therapy if BMD testing would facilitate the decision
- Postmenopausal women who present with fractures (to confirm the diagnosis and determine disease severity)

Medicare Coverage for BMD in Individuals Age 65 and Older: Bone Mass Act
- Estrogen-deficient women at clinical risk of osteoporosis
- Individuals with vertebral abnormalities
- Individuals receiving or planning to receive long-term glucocorticoid (steroid) therapy
- Individuals with primary hyperparathyroidism
- Individuals being monitored to assess the response or efficacy of an approved osteoporosis drug therapy

BMD from the young adult mean value, there is an associated two- to threefold increase in fracture risk.

- Quantitative computed tomography of the spine is another central modality for bone density measurement. The greatest advantage of this technology is that it provides a true volumetric assessment of bone density, whereas dual-energy x-ray absorptiometry only provides an areal density.
- Quantitative computed tomography has not been traditionally used in epidemiologic or longitudinal studies of treatment effect and may be best used in patients at the extremes of size or weight.
- Peripheral technologies such as peripheral quantitative computed tomography, peripheral dual-energy x-ray absorptiometry, and quantitative ultrasonography are increasingly being used for screening purposes. The World Health Organization criteria should not be applied to these measurements. It is recommended that anyone with a positive study result undergo central dual-energy x-ray absorptiometry measurement for diagnosis and posttreatment follow-up.

BOX 23-2 *Risk Factors for Osteoporotic Fractures*

Major Risk Factors in White Women
- Personal history of fracture as an adult
- History of fragility fracture in a first-degree relative
- Low body weight (<127 pounds)
- Current smoking
- Use of oral corticosteroid therapy for >3 months

Additional Risk Factors
- Premature menopause (<45 years)
- Primary or secondary amenorrhea
- Primary and secondary hypogonadism in men
- Impaired vision
- Prolonged immobilization
- Dementia
- Excessive alcohol consumption (>2 drinks/day)
- Low calcium intake
- Recent falls
- Poor health/frailty

Additional Tests

- All patients diagnosed with osteoporosis should undergo basic laboratory testing for secondary causes of osteoporosis.
- Laboratory tests should include serum calcium, phosphorus, magnesium, creatinine, parathyroid hormone, 25-hydroxy vitamin D levels, and testosterone in men.
- Other tests such as serum and urine electrophoresis to screen for multiple myeloma and screening tests for hypercortisolism and malabsorptive syndromes should be obtained in selected patients.
- Measurement of 24-hour urine excretion may be helpful in identifying calcium malabsorption or idiopathic hypercalciuria, both of which may contribute to low BMD.

Differential Diagnosis

- Osteomalacia or impaired bone mineralization may present with low BMD and fractures.
- Patients with osteoporosis may have superimposed osteomalacia due to vitamin D deficiency and/or calcium malabsorption.

- Any component of osteomalacia should be corrected before establishing other treatments for osteoporosis.

Treatment

- The management of osteoporosis is multifactorial and includes a combination of lifestyle modifications, nutritional counseling, and pharmacologic interventions.
  - Lifestyle modifications
    - All patients should pursue a combination of weight-bearing exercises and strength training.
    - Patients with severe mobility impairment should be referred for physical therapy.
    - All patients should be advised on fall prevention measures including (1) proper lighting in all rooms, (2) removal of area rugs and floor clutter, (3) use of walking devices as deemed appropriate, (4) avoidance of uneven walking surfaces.
  - Nutritional counseling
    - Patients should be counseled on adequate calcium and vitamin D supplementation.
    - Once adequate levels of vitamin D are reached, defined as a serum value of 30 ng/mL or higher, patients should consume 800 to 1200 IU of vitamin D daily.
    - All patients with osteoporosis should also get 1500 mg of elemental calcium daily through supplements and/or dietary sources.
  - Pharmacologic therapy
    - There are several general classes of medications as treatment options including hormone therapy, selective estrogen receptor modulators, calcitonin, bisphosphonates, and recombinant human parathyroid hormone (teriparatide).
    - In general, bisphosphonates and teriparatide have been shown to be most efficacious in increasing BMD and decreasing future fracture risk.
    - Of the available bisphosphonates, oral alendronate and risedronate and intravenous zoledronic acid and ibandronate are most commonly used.

      Daily oral bisphosphonates have been associated with an increased incidence of gastrointestinal side effects including heartburn and dysphagia. This increased incidence has not been observed with the weekly or monthly formulations.
    - Intravenous formulations are associated with the occurrence of flulike symptoms for the first 24 to 48 hours after medication administration. No long-term side effects have been described.
    - There have been isolated case reports of osteonecrosis of the jaw in patients treated with oral bisphosphonates for osteoporosis. Its incidence in this setting is unknown and has been estimated to be very low (0.7 cases per 100,000 person-years of exposure).
    - Teriparatide is the only anabolic agent currently approved for the treatment of osteoporosis. This agent is composed of the amino terminal portion of the human parathyroid hormone molecule (1-34). This fragment of the intact molecule binds to the parathyroid hormone 1 receptor and, when given as an intermittent daily injection, results in the recruitment of quiescent bone-forming osteoblasts and net bone formation.
    - A transient mild hypercalcemia and an increase in uric acid levels have been noted shortly after the daily injection. There is also a reported higher incidence of dizziness and leg cramps with the use of teriparatide compared with placebo.

Prognosis

- Bisphosphonates and teriparatide have been shown to decrease fracture risk at the spine by 40% to 70% and at the hip by 30% to 50%.
- Untreated patients with a history of an insufficiency fracture have almost a 50% chance of having a second fracture within 2 to 3 years of the initial event.

Troubleshooting

- Close follow-up is required to assess compliance and response to treatment.
- A dual-energy x-ray absorptiometry scan one year after treatment initiation is recommended to document the response to therapy.
- Once an adequate response is observed including an increase in BMD and a fracture-free state, then monitoring with dual-energy x-ray absorptiometry may be done every two years.
- Patients with a poor response to therapy should be rescreened for secondary causes of osteoporosis.

Patient Instructions

- Osteoporosis is a chronic condition that requires long-term follow-up and treatment.
- Adherence to treatment modalities including lifestyle, nutritional, and pharmacologic interventions is crucial for success.

Considerations in Special Populations

- The geriatric population is most commonly affected due to the normal decrease in BMD with aging.
- Other particular populations at risk include
  - Patients with rheumatologic disorders particularly those treated with glucocorticoids
  - Patients with a history of malabsorptive syndromes including celiac sprue, inflammatory bowel disease, and gastric bypass
  - Women with a history of breast cancer or men with a history of prostate cancer treated with antihormonal therapy
  - Survivors of childhood cancer
  - Female athletes with a history of amenorrhea
  - Immobilized patients

Suggested Reading

- Bilezikian JP: Osteonecrosis of the jaw—do bisphosphonates pose a risk? N Engl J Med 2006;355:2278–2281.
- Black DM, Delmas PD, Eastell R, et al: Once-yearly zoledronic acid for treatment of postmenopausal osteoporosis. N Engl J Med 2007;356:1809–1822.
- Bone HG, Hosking D, Devogelaer JP, et al: Ten years' experience with alendronate for osteoporosis in postmenopausal women. N Engl J Med 2004;350:1189–1199.
- Dawson-Hughes B, Harris SS, Krall EA, Dallal GE: Effect of calcium and vitamin D supplementation on bone density in men and women 65 years of age or older. N Engl J Med 1997;337:670–676.
- Harris ST, Watts NB, Genant HK, et al: Effects of risedronate treatment on vertebral and nonvertebral fractures in women with postmenopausal osteoporosis: A randomized controlled trial. Vertebral Efficacy with Risedronate Therapy (VERT) Study Group. JAMA 1999;282:1344–1352.
- Liberman UA, Weiss SR, Broll J, et al: Effect of oral alendronate on bone mineral density and the incidence of fractures in postmenopausal osteoporosis. The Alendronate Phase III Osteoporosis Treatment Study Group. N Engl J Med 1995;333:1437–1443.
- McClung MR, Geusens P, Miller PD, et al: Effect of risedronate on the risk of hip fracture in elderly women. Hip Intervention Program Study Group. N Engl J Med 2001;344:333–340.
- Melton L, Atkinson W, O'Fallon W, et al: Long-term fracture prediction by bone mineral assessed at different skeletal sites. J Bone Miner Res 1993;8:1227–1233.
- National Institutes of Health (NIH): NIH Consensus Development Panel on osteoporosis prevention, diagnosis and therapy. JAMA 2001;285:785–795.
- Neer RM, Arnaud CD, Zanchetta JR, et al: Effect of parathyroid hormone (1-34) on fractures and bone mineral density in postmenopausal women with osteoporosis. N Engl J Med 2001;344:1434–1441.

Chapter 24 Tumors

Theodore W. Parsons III and Michael P. Mott

Although musculoskeletal tumors are relatively rare, when encountered, the resulting anxiety over possible loss of limb or life can be substantial. A systemic approach to the evaluation of these lesions aids in providing a timely diagnosis, guides treatment options, and lessens the anxiety associated with these often challenging lesions.

Evaluation and Staging

History and Physical Examination

The history and physical examination are the first steps in generating a meaningful diagnosis. Age is an important determinant to help limit the differential diagnosis. Metastatic lesions tend to develop in older patients, whereas primary bone tumors develop in younger patients (Table 24-1).

Hallmark Symptoms

- Onset of pain is typically gradual and may be misdiagnosed as another ailment.
- Worrisome features in history include
  - Persistent pain, especially night pain
  - Non-activity–related pain and fatigue

Hallmark Signs

- Night sweats, unexpected weight loss (late feature)
- Tenderness/mass without bruising and/or antecedent trauma

Physical Examination

- Pay particular attention to any masses (firm versus soft, fixed versus mobile) and compare with the unaffected side.
- Check the entire extremity and perform a thorough neurovascular examination. Subtle changes may be present secondary to the mass effect. Note any thrill or bruits.
- Check regional lymph nodes, which are the third most common sites of metastases after the lungs and bones.

Imaging

Conventional Radiographs

- Initial step in evaluation of all lesions
  - Obtain orthogonal views (anterior-posterior and lateral) of the entire bone and adjacent joints involved.
- Note what the lesion is doing to the bone and what the bone is doing to the lesion.
  - Large lesions with loss of cortex, poor margination, and a soft-tissue mass are more likely to be aggressive than small lesions with an intact cortex, excellent margination, and no soft-tissue mass.
  - The location of the lesion within the bone also helps to narrow the differential diagnosis, with very few lesions originating in the epiphysis and more aggressive lesions typically having an epicenter in the metaphysis.

Bone Scan (BS)

- Detect bone turnover and multifocal and distant sites of bone disease
- Identify occult lesions of bone
- Some myeloma, renal cell, and thyroid carcinomas as well as lymphomas may appear cold on a BS.

Computed Tomography (CT)

- Best to determine lung metastases (the predominant site of metastatic disease) and regional adenopathy
- Excellent for evaluating bone architecture and lesional matrix production
- Best tool to evaluate for primary site of a carcinoma

Magnetic Resonance Imaging (MRI)

- High-contrast resolution allows excellent imaging of most tumors and defining anatomic details.
- Excellent for detecting and evaluating soft-tissue masses
- T1-weighted images excellent for detecting "skip" metastases within bone

TABLE 24-1 *Common Ages of Presentation*

Age (yr)	Tumor
<5	Metastatic (especially metastatic nephroblastoma and nephroblastoma)
5–30	Ewing's sarcoma
5–20	Osteosarcoma
10–25	Chondroblastoma
10–20	Osteochondroma
5–15	Simple bone cyst
10–20	Aneurysmal bone cyst
2–16	Nonossifying fibroma
20–40	Giant cell tumor
>40	Myeloma
>40	Metastatic carcinoma (breast, prostate, thyroid, kidney, lung)
>50	Chondrosarcoma
>50	Chordoma

- Excellent tool to screen spine for metastatic disease

Positron Emission Tomography

- Not routinely used in evaluation of primary bone lesions (but indications for use are growing)
- Useful for detecting metastatic or recurrent disease (particularly Ewing's sarcoma) and tumor response to chemotherapy

The information obtained from advanced imaging studies (BS, CT, MRI, positron emission tomography) tends to be complementary as it provides clues as to the behavior, anatomy, and etiology of the lesion. In some instances, all these modalities are necessary in the workup. In general

- Obtain plain radiographs
- Consider a BS for aggressive-appearing lesions or metastatic disease
- Chest CT for pulmonary metastases
- Obtain MRI whenever a soft-tissue mass or extension is expected or to evaluate the bone marrow in a particular anatomic area.
- Lesions that are bright on the T2-weighted imaging studies generally warrant concern and further evaluation.

Tumors of the Bone

The American Cancer Society reports that there were approximately 2400 cases of primary bone cancer in 2007. However, the incidence of all bone tumors and tumor-like conditions is not truly known because many benign tumors are never reported. In some instances, a lesion may go undetected until picked up incidentally secondary to radiographs being performed for an unrelated problem or trauma. Certainly any lesion that is painful or results in a pathologic fracture requires investigation. Likewise, large lesions, lesions in critical weight-bearing areas (e.g., subtrochanteric femur), and lesions producing a periosteal reaction or soft-tissue mass require evaluation. Unless the true biological nature of a lesion is known, caution should be exercised because the radiographic appearance of benign, benign aggressive, and malignant lesions may demonstrate significant overlap.

Common Benign Bone Lesions

Osteoid Osteoma

- Osteoid osteoma is a benign lesion characterized by severe sharp, typically boring pain sometimes leading to secondary physical examination findings depending on location. These may include scoliosis (painful), limb length inequality, and synovitis/joint effusions.
- The typical age range is 10 to 30 years, and the usual locations are the long bones of the lower extremities and the posterior elements of the spine.
- A hallmark feature is night pain, often causing awakening, and marked symptomatic improvement with nonsteroidal anti-inflammatory drugs/aspirin.
- Radiographically, a small lucent lesion (<1 cm) surrounded by a variable amount of perilesional new bone (sclerosis) is observed. These lesions are "hot" on a BS, and CT or MRI is very useful in identifying the nidus of the lesion.
- Although these lesions may be managed medically with long-term nonsteroidal anti-inflammatory drugs, surgical treatment to remove the nidus (curettage, drilling, or burring) is often employed. More recently, less invasive thermal ablation (radiofrequency ablation) has been used with great success and is the preferred method in many institutions. The prognosis is generally very good.

Osteoblastoma

- Osteoblastoma is a benign bone-forming tumor occurring in the second decade with a predilection for the spine (posterior elements) and long bones.
- Most patients present with progressive pain.
- Radiographically, these lesions are geographic and radiolucent, with a thin rim of sclerotic, reactive bone (unlike osteoid osteomas). There may be mineralization within the lesion. Hot on a BS, these are larger and more aggressive appearing than osteoid osteoma.
- Treatment includes extended intralesional curettage with adjuvant treatment (e.g., phenol, liquid nitrogen,

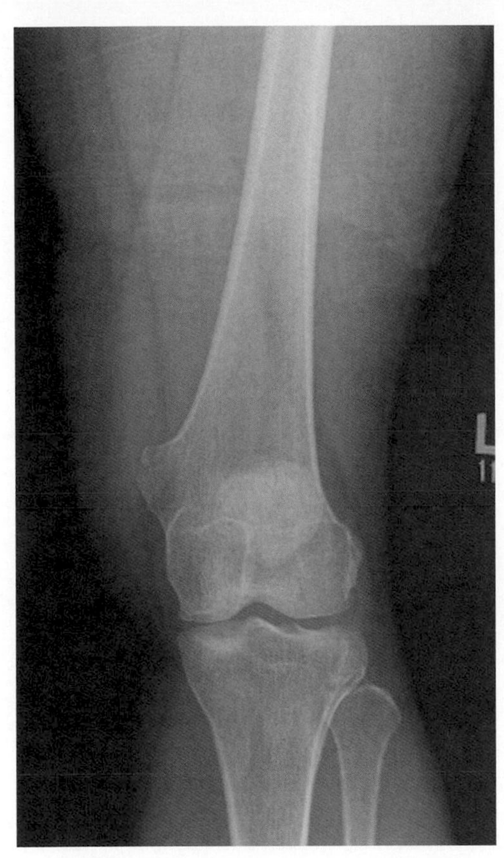

Figure 24-1 Osteochondroma of the distal femur. The lesion shares the cortex with the host bone and is classically metaphyseal in location.

argon beam) and grafting of the defect. En bloc excision may be necessary in aggressive or recurrent lesions. Recurrence rates vary from 10% to 20%.

Osteochondroma

- Osteochondroma is a benign cartilage-forming tumor also known as an osteocartilaginous exostosis. These lesions are most often single but may be multiple and part of the multiple hereditary exostosis syndrome, an autosomal dominant condition.
- These lesions can present at any age, but are most often noted in the young adult.
- Radiographically, the lesions are broad based (sessile) (Fig. 24-1) or stalk-like (pedunculated) with continuation/communication of the base of the lesion with the underlying (normal) bone.
- The pathologic cap of the lesion is composed of cartilage, generally thin (<1 cm) and often difficult to visualize on plain radiographs.
- Treatment varies from observation of asymptomatic lesions to excision of lesions causing mechanical symptoms.
- These lesions may slowly grow until skeletal maturity and, rarely, transform into a malignancy, a secondary

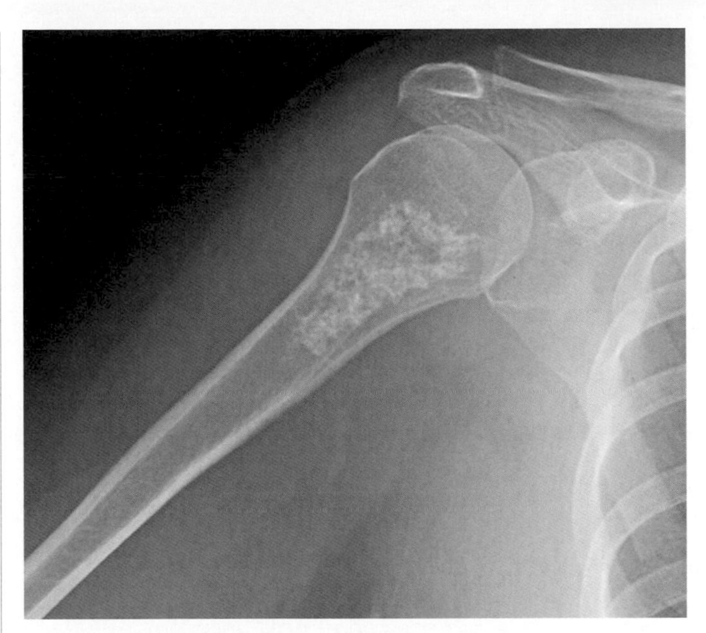

Figure 24-2 Enchondroma of the proximal humerus demonstrating classic speckled (popcorn) calcification without evidence of endosteal erosions.

chondrosarcoma. Any growth after cessation of skeletal maturity or increasing size of the cartilage cap is a cause for concern and may indicate malignant transformation.

Enchondroma

- Enchondroma is a benign cartilage tumor located within the medullary cavity of the bone.
- Found in almost any bone, the most common location is the hand where slightly more than one third originate (the thumb is typically spared).
- These lesions are generally identified in the third and fourth decades.
- Radiographs reveal a circumscribed lesion with good margination. Speckled calcifications, minimal endosteal thinning, and (very) mild bone expansion may be found (Fig. 24-2).
- These lesions can be part of a genetic syndrome, multiple enchondromas/Ollier's disease, which is an inborn error of metabolism.
- Malignant transformation can occur, and worrisome features include progressive cortical scalloping, increasing size, cortical breakthrough, and a soft-tissue mass.
- Bone scans can be hot in both benign and malignant lesions and cannot reliably be used to predict biological behavior.
- Treatment typically consists of serial observation to document lack of biological activity or, in some instances, curettage and grafting.

Chondroblastoma

- Chondroblastoma is a benign but locally aggressive bone tumor typically found in the epiphysis of long bones, most often around the knee, proximal humerus, and proximal femur.
- These lesions generally present in the second and third decades.
- They can be difficult to see and a delay in diagnosis is not uncommon.
- This benign lesion can rarely metastasize to the lung.
- Radiographs reveal a destructive epiphyseal lesion with a thin sclerotic rim, often with stippled or punctate calcification with its epicenter located within the epiphysis and occasionally extending into the metaphysis.
- Treatment consists of an extended curettage and grafting. Recurrences are not uncommon (up to 30%).

Giant Cell Tumor

- Giant cell tumor of the bone typically affects patients in their third and fourth decades, with a slight female predominance, and occurs at the ends of the long bones, most commonly around the knee.
- The typical symptom reported is pain, often of a long-standing nature.
- Rarely, these lesions may metastasize to the lungs.
- Radiographs reveal a lytic, metaphyseal/epiphyseal lesion that typically extends to the subchondral surface of the bone (Fig. 24-3). The lesions are generally contained within the bone, but may have a more aggressive appearance with extension into the soft tissue.
- Treatment is generally intralesional curettage with an adjuvant treatment (chemical/thermal ablation) to extend the margin of tumor kill, followed by defect reconstruction with cement, bone graft, and/or bone graft substitutes. Improved surgical techniques, combined with adjuvant therapies, have helped to improve on historically high local recurrence rates.

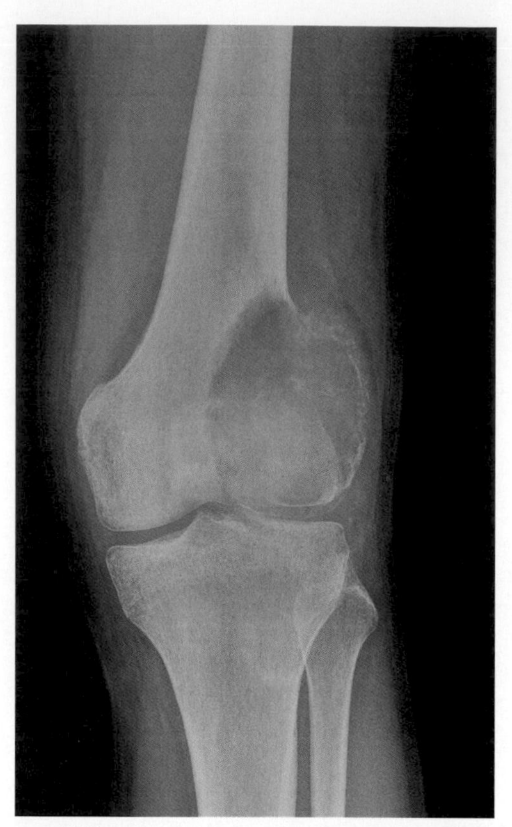

Figure 24-3 Giant cell tumor with pathologic fracture in distal femur. Lytic, geographic lesion in subchondral location is classic presentation.

Malignant Lesions of the Bone

Osteosarcoma (OSA)

- In the skeletally immature patient, OSA is the most common primary malignancy of the bone and is two to three times more common than Ewing's sarcoma.
- Typically, OSA affects adolescents in the second decade of life, with a slight male predominance.
- The knee is the most commonly involved site (distal femur > proximal tibia) followed by the proximal humerus.
- OSA is also seen in patients older than 60 years in whom it is usually associated with underlying conditions such as Paget's disease or previous irradiation.
- OSA is generally divided into three subtypes: classic (central), parosteal (parallel to the bone), and periosteal (arising from the periosteum).
- Radiographically, classic OSA lesions (Fig. 24-4) consist of a mixed picture of bone formation and destruction and may lead to a "sunburst" appearance with bone spicules forming at a right angle to the main mass and triangular elevation of the periosteum at the edge of the lesion (Codman's triangle). Hot on a BS, these lesions are best visualized on MRI. The entire bone should be imaged with MRI to rule out the presence of a skip lesion in the marrow.
- Treatment consists of neoadjuvant chemotherapy followed by wide (margin free of tumor) resection and further chemotherapy. The 5-year survival rate is generally 70% to 80%.
- Local recurrence is approximately 10%, and metastases are primarily manifest in the lungs.
    - Parosteal OSA is a low-grade lesion that presents with a very heavily mineralized mass on plain radiographs that appears to be "stuck on the bone." It is commonly found at the knee on the posterior

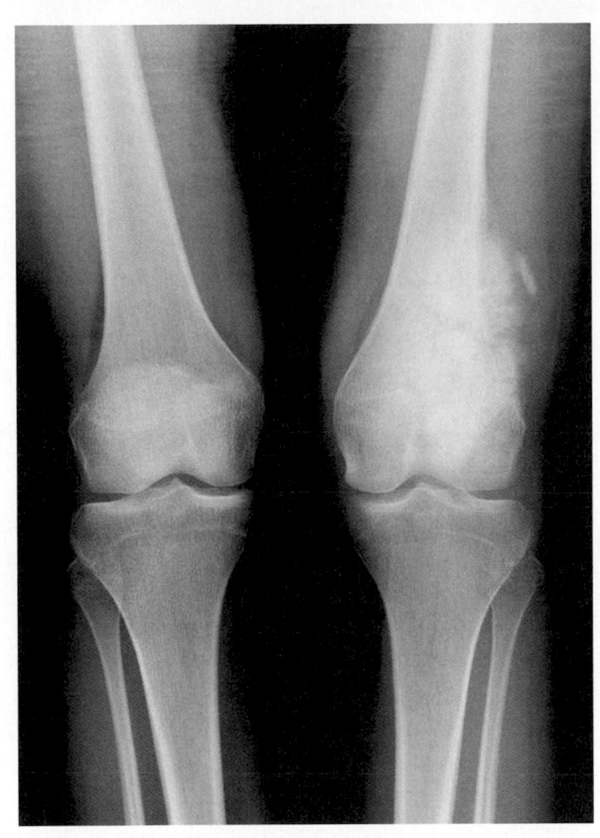

Figure 24-4 Distal femoral osteosarcoma with blastic appearance and lateral soft-tissue mass with mineral density, Codman's triangles, and sunburst appearance.

aspect of the distal femur. A very insidious onset is noted, with the major symptom reported being a progressive loss of knee flexion.

- Periosteal OSA is a somewhat more aggressive lesion, has a proclivity for the tibia, and appears radiographically as spicules of bone erupting out of the periosteum.

Chondrosarcoma

- Chondrosarcoma is a malignant primary bone tumor consisting of malignant cartilage cells. These lesions may be primary where they occur de novo within a bone or secondary where they arise from a preexisting lesion such as an enchondroma or osteochondroma.
- Most lesions present in patients older than 50 years of age, with the pelvis, ribs, femur, and proximal humerus being the most common locations.
- Radiographically, these are destructive lesions that generally contain rings and arcs or "popcorn" calcifications and can often be quite large.
- Intramedullary lesions (within the bone) demonstrate endosteal scalloping, cortical thinning (Fig. 24-5), and even cortical breakthrough with a soft-tissue mass.

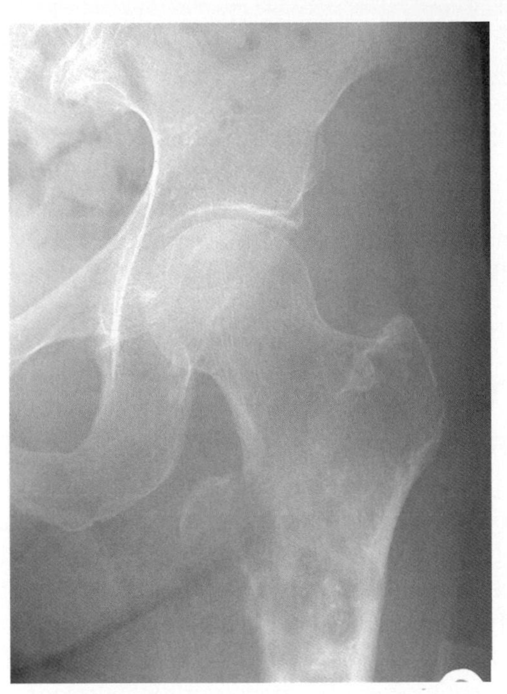

Figure 24-5 Chondrosarcoma of the proximal femur with pathologic fracture of the lesser trochanter. Note the mineral density within the lesion and the destruction of the cortex.

- These lesions are hot on a BS and best visualized with CT or MRI.
- Chondrosarcoma is relatively insensitive to chemotherapy and radiation, and, as such, the mainstay of treatment is wide resection with tumor-free margins. An excellent prognosis is anticipated for low-grade lesions (5-year survival rate of 90%), but the prognosis becomes progressively poorer with higher grade and undifferentiated and dedifferentiated lesions.

Ewing's Sarcoma Family of Tumors

- The Ewing's sarcoma family of tumors is made up of malignant round cell neoplasias (Ewing's sarcoma, primitive neuroectodermal tumor, and others) with a proclivity for the young.
- Approximately 80% of cases present in patients younger than 20 years of age.
- The clinical presentation may mimic that of osteomyelitis with fever, pain, swelling, anemia, leukocytosis, and elevated sedimentation rate. Common locations include the femur, pelvis, and scapula.
- Radiographically, the Ewing's sarcoma family of tumors present as diffuse, permeative lesions with modest destructive features that often incite excessive periosteal new bone formation that leads to an "onion skinning" or "hair on end" appearance. These lesions are very hot on a BS. A soft-tissue mass, often very large, is generally present and best seen on MRI.

- Treatment consists of a multimodality approach employing chemotherapy and radiation or surgical resection to the primary site depending on the location (and anticipated morbidity of local control). The overall prognosis is an approximately 70% survival rate at 5 years. Given the young age at presentation, late relapses and a second malignant neoplasm are not uncommon.

Soft-Tissue Tumors

Although the true incidence of soft-tissue lesions overall is not clearly reported, benign soft-tissue lesions are far more common than malignant soft-tissue lesions, at a ratio of approximately 100:1. Nonetheless, the treating physician should maintain an appropriate index of suspicion when evaluating any soft-tissue mass because most clinical problems arise when the possibility of malignancy is never entertained. Evaluation of these lesions includes a careful history and physical examination, appropriate imaging (typically plain radiographs and an MRI), and histologic evaluation as appropriate. If any question as to the diagnosis then exists—and certainly in the case of most lesions larger than 5 cm—a biopsy should be performed.

A comprehensive discussion of soft-tissue lesions is beyond the scope of this chapter. However, the most common benign and malignant soft-tissue lesions are briefly presented.

Benign Soft-Tissue Lesions

Lipoma

- Lipomas are common, benign soft-tissue lesions of mature white adipocytes.
- Although there are many different subtypes (e.g., angiolipoma, spindle cell lipoma, pleomorphic lipoma), the most common lesion is the superficial or subcutaneous lesion noted in middle-aged or older adults.
- These lesions are typically slow growing, are completely asymptomatic, and, with the exception of deeper lesions, typically are less than 5 cm in size.
- Often patients will indicate that the lesion has been present for many years.
- Plain radiographs demonstrate a radiolucent lesion in the soft tissue that very rarely may include subtle mineralization. CT and MRI are typically diagnostic of the lesion, as the mass follows the homogeneous characteristics (signal attenuation on CT, signal intensity on MRI) of subcutaneous fat. Intramuscular lesions may show some internal stranding within the fatty lesion that, when prominent, may raise concern for low-grade liposarcomas, as does gadolinium enhancement.
- Treatment of these benign lesions generally includes observation or marginal excision if the patient is anxious about the presence of the mass, is concerned about cosmesis, or if function is impaired. Most lipomas can be easily removed surgically because they tend to be rather well circumscribed.

Hemangioma

- Hemangiomas are common benign vascular malformations that have a wide variety of subtypes (e.g., epithelial, endothelial) and can affect any portion of the vascular system (arterial or venous).
- They are present in all age groups (although most commonly in children) and can present in a cutaneous, subcutaneous, or intramuscular location.
- These vascular malformations can be localized or diffuse and often slowly expand with time. The most common presentation is a deep, cavernous lesion.
- These lesions may be minimally symptomatic, often wax and wane in size, particularly with activity, and on examination are soft and pliable.
- Plain radiographs may reveal small mineral densities (phleboliths) in long-standing lesions. MRI reveals a lesion with indistinct margins, often infiltrative into the surrounding musculature, with bright signal areas on T1-weighted sequences (fatty areas) and a more diffuse, "bag of worms" bright appearance on T2-weighted sequences (dilated venous channels) (Fig. 24-6).
- Treatment is generally observation or symptomatic care. Percutaneous sclerosis of these lesions has shown promise. Surgical excision of certain lesions may be indicated.

Peripheral Nerve Sheath Tumor

- These benign lesions in peripheral nerves of adults have a variety of presentations, the most common of which are schwannoma (neurilemmoma) and neurofibroma.
  - A schwannoma typically presents as a painless mass (occasionally there is evidence of nerve irritation on examination, such as a positive Tinel's sign) on the flexor surfaces of the extremities, although they can present at any site.
  - A neurofibroma generally presents as an isolated lesion associated with a peripheral (or cranial) nerve, or there may be multiple lesions (usually plexiform, often large) in patients with neurofibromatosis. These lesions are typically asymptomatic but may undergo malignant degeneration.

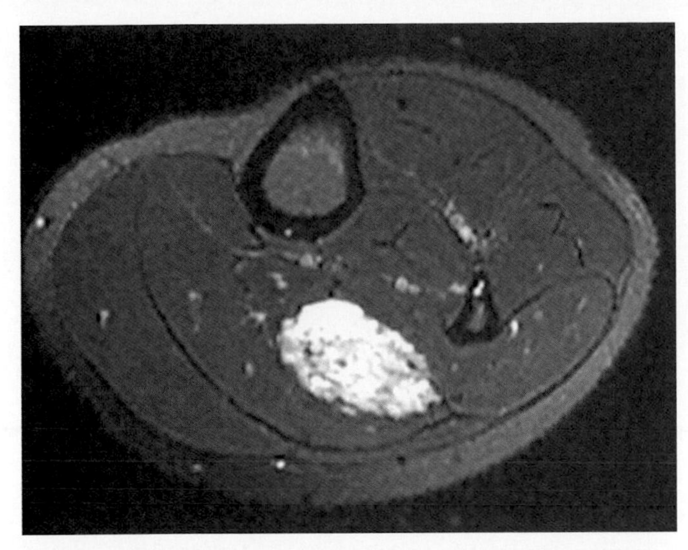

Figure 24-6 T2-weighted magnetic resonance image of the leg demonstrating a lesion consisting of a collection of bright, lobular vessels with areas of flow void, consistent with hemangioma. T1-weighted images often show fatty areas within the mass.

- MRI is the imaging study of choice and typically shows a fusiform lesion with the nerve entering and exiting the lesion or closely juxtaposed to the lesion. The T1-weighted image often shows an intermediate signal and a homogeneous mass surrounded by a rim of high signal fat, often referred to as the split fat sign. The T2-weighted image shows an inhomogeneous lesion, often with a higher signal at the periphery and less intensity toward the center (or in several central areas), often referred to as the target sign.
- Treatment of a primitive neuroectodermal tumor generally involves excision of the tumor. In the case of a schwannoma, the nerve can generally be spared. A neurofibroma, however, generally involves multiple fascicles, and excision may sacrifice the nerve, resulting in a neural deficit. Recurrence after excision is rare.

Fibromatoses

- Fibromatoses, although benign, are nevertheless locally aggressive and infiltrative in nature.
- As superficial lesions, they present in the palm (Dupuytren's disease) and the plantar fascia (Ledderhose's disease). Palmar lesions are generally not symptomatic but can result in contractures of the digits.
- Plantar lesions generally present in the non–weight-bearing portion of the foot, may be symptomatic, but typically do not result in contractures.
- As deep lesions, they are referred to as intra- or extra-abdominal desmoid tumors, which can be solitary or multiple, firm, fixed, and slow growing and typically are quite locally invasive. Common locations include the shoulder girdle, chest wall, arm, and thigh.
- Plain radiographs may reveal a soft-tissue density but are generally nonspecific. Long-standing lesions juxtaposed to bone may result in bone remodeling or in frank invasion of the cortex. MRI reveals a lesion that varies between well circumscribed and infiltrative in nature. T1-weighted images are generally isointense to muscle but with areas (spots or flecks) of low signal intensity (dense fibrous areas) within the lesion. T2-weighted images are intermediate in signal intensity but still retain the areas of low signal intensity within the lesion.
- Treatment of palmar lesions, if necessary, includes resection and release of significant contractures at the proximal interphalangeal or metacarpophalangeal joints. Plantar lesions should be treated conservatively unless they are large and very symptomatic, because recurrence is likely if the lesion is not widely resected. Deep desmoid lesions are far more difficult to treat. Wide surgical resection of primary (and recurrent) lesions has long been the mainstay, but adjuvant radiation therapy, hormonal manipulation, and even chemotherapy for recurrent or aggressive lesions have all been reported.

Malignant Soft-Tissue Lesions

High-Grade Pleomorphic Sarcoma (High-Grade Spindle Cell Sarcoma)

- This broad classification of high-grade malignant neoplasia includes lesions previously classified as malignant fibrous histiocytoma, fibrosarcoma, and malignant fibrous xanthoma.
- These are undifferentiated, pleomorphic, aggressive sarcomas found in adults and presenting as deep, firm, enlarging, and eventually painful masses.
- This group of sarcomas collectively represents the most common types of sarcoma in adult patients older than 40 years of age.
- They occur most often in the lower limb.
- Radiographs are nonspecific and reveal a soft-tissue density that obliterates normal fat/fascial lines. MRI is also nonspecific but generally reveals a soft-tissue mass that invades the surrounding tissues (Fig. 24-7), but usually does not encircle neurovascular bundles (rather tends to displace them). These lesions are usually very bright on T2-weighted images.
- Treatment is wide resection of the lesion with adjuvant therapy, typically radiation. Prognosis is poor; typically, the 5-year survival rate is approximately 50%.

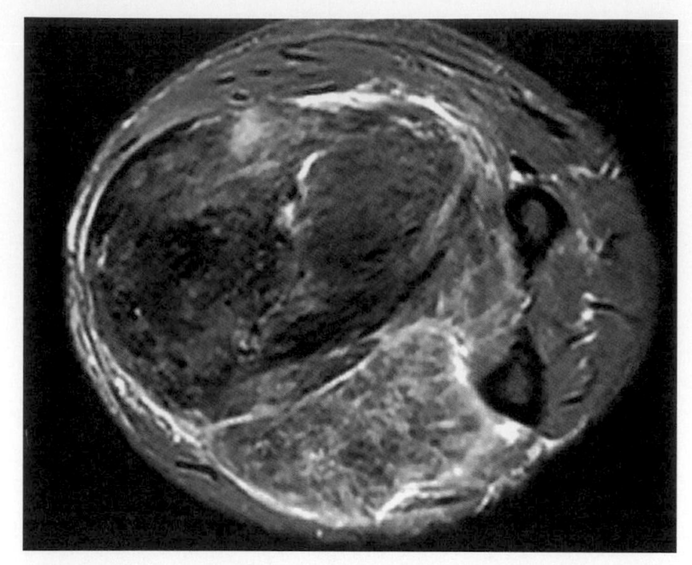

Figure 24-7 T2-weighted magnetic resonance image demonstrating a high-grade soft-tissue sarcoma of the forearm. Note the centripetal growth of the lesion as it expands in the limb.

Liposarcoma

- Liposarcoma is the second most common soft-tissue sarcoma and generally presents in middle-aged and older adults (peak in the fourth and fifth decades).
- They are typically deep lesions, most often presenting as a painless mass in the deep thigh.
- There are multiple subtypes that range from low-grade to very high grade, aggressive lesions. The most common subtype is the well-differentiated (low-grade) lesion, followed by the myxoid (slightly higher grade) subtype.
- Liposarcoma may metastasize to the retroperitoneum or arise there as a primary lesion.
- Plain radiographs reveal a soft-tissue mass that obliterates tissue planes and possibly evidence of mineralization within the lesion. MRI appearance is similar to other high-grade soft-tissue tumors, although there may be evidence of a fatty signal in part of the mass.
- Treatment includes marginal resection in low-grade lesions and wide local excision and radiation in higher-grade lesions. Prognosis ranges from a 5-year survival rate of nearly 100% in low-grade lesions to approximately 50% in high-grade lesions.

Rhabdomyosarcoma

- Rhabdomyosarcoma is the most common sarcoma in children younger than 15 years of age, particularly the embryonal and alveolar subtypes. The pleomorphic subtype is more common in adults.
- This tumor of striated muscle is most common in the head and neck and genitourinary tract, but may present in the extremities as a deep, enlarging mass (usually in older children or adults).
- Imaging is nonspecific as with all soft-tissue sarcomas.
- Treatment includes chemotherapy (this lesion tends to be chemosensitive) and wide resection. Prognosis is variable but tends to be good overall, with a 5-year survival rate of approximately 75%.

Synovial Cell Sarcoma

- Synovial cell sarcoma is the fourth most common soft-tissue sarcoma and generally presents in young adults (15–35 years of age) as an enlarging, often painless mass in the lower extremities or less often in the shoulder girdle or upper extremity.
- These lesions are slow growing and may often be present for years before diagnosis.
- Imaging may reveal calcification in the mass, either by plain radiographs or CT. MRI may reveal a cystic appearance to the lesion, and fluid/fluid levels are not uncommon. These lesions often appear well circumscribed, which belies their malignant nature.
- Treatment includes wide resection with adjuvant radiation. Prognosis is generally poor, with a 5-year survival rate of approximately 50% and a 10-year survival rate of approximately 25%.

Tumors of Uncertain Origin/ Tumor-like Conditions

Simple Bone Cyst

- Simple bone cysts (solitary bone cyst, unicameral bone cyst) are benign intramedullary lesions filled with serous or serosanguineous fluid.
- Most lesions present in children (first two decades), with the proximal humerus and proximal femur as the most common locations. Adults may present with pelvic or calcaneal lesions. These may be found serendipitously or may present with a pathologic fracture.
- Radiographs show a central, lytic, and well-demarcated lesion of the metaphysis, often abutting the physis. The lesion may show limited expansion (width of the physis) and often reveals cortical thinning. A BS typically shows minimal uptake. MRI confirms a cystic lesion.
- Treatment can be observation, injection of steroids or marrow substitutes, or curettage and bone grafting. The prognosis is excellent, although lesions can recur.

Aneurysmal Bone Cyst

- Aneurysmal bone cyst is a benign cystic lesion of bone composed of blood-filled spaces separated by soft-tissue septae.
- These lesions appear in all age groups but are most common in the first two decades.
- Although present in virtually any bone, they arise commonly in the metaphysis of the long bones (tibia, femur, humerus) and in the posterior elements of the spine.
- Pain and swelling are common presentations, and spine lesions may demonstrate neurologic symptoms (nerve compression). These lesions can arise de novo or secondarily to other lesions (giant cell tumor, osteoblastoma, chondroblastoma, fibrous dysplasia).
- Plain radiographs reveal a lytic, usually eccentric, expansile lesion that is typically well marginated. Expansion into the soft tissue is common, but a thin bony rim around the lesion is generally present. These lesions are hot on a BS and on MRI show the classic, multilobulated lesion (multiple septae) with fluid/fluid levels.
- Treatment is extended intralesional curettage (with or without adjuvant treatment) and bone grafting. Prognosis is very good, with recurrence of approximately 5% to 10% in appropriately treated lesions.

Fibrous Dysplasia

- Fibrous dysplasia is a benign fibro-osseous lesion that can occur in one (monostotic, most common) or multiple (polyostotic) bones. Most lesions appear in the head, but may also be seen in the long bones of the lower extremities.
- The lesions are usually asymptomatic, but pain and pathologic fractures are not uncommon. Endocrine abnormalities (including McCune-Albright syndrome) are well-known associations with the polyostotic form.
- Radiographs reveal a nonaggressive, geographic lesion with the typical ground glass appearance, often with mild expansion of the bone and thinning of the cortex. Long-standing lesions of the proximal femur may result in deformity (shepherd's crook). A BS is generally warm. MRI and CT are rarely warranted but will demonstrate a central lesion with intermediate to high signal on T2-weighted images and minimal surrounding edema.
- Treatment is observation or surgical stabilization in symptomatic lesions or lesions at risk of fracture. Prognosis is excellent.

Eosinophilic Granuloma

- Eosinophilic granuloma is part of the spectrum of lesions that constitute Langerhans cell histiocytosis, a neoplastic proliferation of Langerhans cells.
- This lesion occurs most commonly in those younger than 30 years of age, but can present at any age. Most common sites are the skull, femur, and pelvis. Vertebral body lesions may present with collapse (vertebra plana) and neurologic symptoms.
- Most lesions present with pain and swelling, although they may be asymptomatic in the adult.
- The radiographic appearance is highly variable, but typically shows lytic, geographic, well-marginated lesions, often with periosteal new bone formation. MRI is nonspecific but shows a high signal T2-weighted lesion with significant surrounding edema.
- Treatment can include observation, injection of steroids, simple curettage, and low-dose radiation. Prognosis is good for eosinophilic granuloma, but can be very poor in the more widespread, systemic conditions of Hand-Schüller-Christian disease and particularly Letterer-Siwe disease.

Paget's Disease

- Paget's disease is a common lesion seen in adults older than age 50 (~5% of individuals are older than age 55), but the actual prevalence is unclear.
- Although almost any bone can be affected, the pelvis, spine, skull, femur, and tibia are the most common locations.
- The disease can be monostotic or polyostotic, and although often asymptomatic, pain, deformity, and arthritic symptoms can be present. The bone pathology results from increased bone resorption and synchronous bone formation, the etiology of which is unclear.
- Radiographs are typically characteristic, with sweeping involvement of the affected bone, which includes coarse, purposeful trabeculae; thickened cortex; enlargement of the bone; and lytic/blastic changes in the bone (Fig. 24-8). The advancing blade or flame of resorption is a common finding in long bones and presents as osteoporosis circumscripta in the skull. This lesion is very hot on a BS, and MRI generally shows a moderately increased T2-weighted signal, with a low to moderately low T1-weighted appearance.
- Treatment is generally observation, but bony changes may require surgery for progressive skeletal deformity or pathologic fracture or joint arthroplasty for symptomatic joints. Medical treatment includes calcitonin or, more recently, bisphosphonates to slow the

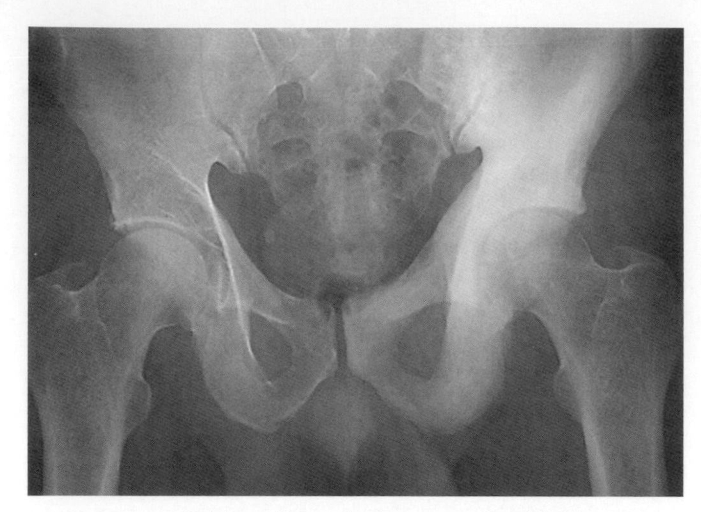

Figure 24-8 Pelvic radiograph demonstrating blastic appearance of the hemipelvis with thickening of the cortex and enlargement of the bone in long-standing Paget's disease.

resorptive process. Prognosis is generally very good, but the risk of sarcomatous degeneration is a real concern (~5% to 10%), and pagetic sarcoma has a very poor survival rate (<5%) at 5 years.

Suggested Reading

- Bullough PG: Orthopaedic Pathology, 4th ed. St. Louis: Mosby, 2003.
- Fischgrun JS (ed): Orthopaedic Knowledge Update 9. Rosemont, IL: American Academy of Orthopaedic Surgeons, 2007.
- Schwartz HS (ed): Orthopaedic Knowledge Update: Musculoskeletal Tumors 2. Rosemont, IL: American Academy of Orthopaedic Surgeons, 2007.
- Weiss SW, Goldblum JR: Enzinger and Weiss's Soft Tissue Tumors, 5th ed. St. Louis: Mosby, 2008.

Chapter 25 Pain Management: Acute Pain

Maria Nguyen and Robin J. Hamill-Ruth

ICD-9 CODES

Codes vary by location of the pain

338 *Pain, Not Classified Elsewhere*
307.89 *Pain, Other*
338.19 *Other Acute Pain*

Key Concepts

- The joint is richly innervated with pain receptors in the capsule, ligament, menisci, periosteum, and subchondral bone. Acute injury, repetitive stress, and surgery can cause myofascial, joint, and peripheral nerve damage.
- Pathophysiology of acute pain starts with peripheral nociceptor activation by mechanical, chemical, or thermal stimulation. Then faster-conducting A delta fibers and slower-conducting C fibers transmit the noxious peripheral stimulation to the central nervous system.
- The myelinated A delta fiber has a quicker onset but short-lived sharp pain.
- The unmyelinated C fiber has a delayed onset, which is perceived as a dull sensation that is more sustained.
- Repetitive noxious stimuli can intensify the release of mediators (e.g., bradykinin, prostaglandins, substance P) that enhance nociceptive output, which ultimately leads to peripheral and central sensitization (wind-up).
- Preemptive analgesia is essential, especially for perioperative and postoperative pain control to reduce the likelihood of wind-up of pain pathways leading to hyperalgesia and allodynia.

History

- Trauma or surgery is the most common initiating event.
- A detailed pain history includes onset, location, duration, and quality (burning, aching, stabbing) of pain, and aggravating and alleviating factors.

Physical Examination

- Perform a thorough physical examination focusing on the area of pain.
- Look for discoloration or edema.
- Perform range of motion, if applicable, looking for possible instability or laxity.
- Perform an in-depth neurologic examination including sensory and motor examinations.

Imaging

- Plain radiograph if bone fracture suspected
- Magnetic resonance imaging if meniscal, ligamentous, or soft-tissue injury suspected

Additional Tests (If Applicable)

- Complete blood count
- C-reactive protein, erythrocyte sedimentation rate

Differential Diagnosis

- Bone fracture
- Ligamentous injury
- Meniscal injury
- Myofascial pain
- Nerve injury/entrapment
- Ischemia
- Abscess
- Hematoma
- Infection
- Sympathetically mediated pain

Treatment

- Nonsteroidal anti-inflammatory drugs
- Tramadol (weak μ-agonist, inhibits the reuptake of serotonin and norepinephrine)
- Opiates
  - Start with short-acting agents such as oxycodone/acetaminophen or hydrocodone/acetaminophen. Do not exceed 4 g/day of acetaminophen (APAP)

with a patient with a normal liver. If liver disease does exist or medication will be used for more than a few days, decrease to less than 4 g/day or avoid intake depending on the degree of liver function.

- If the patient takes eight doses of oxycodone/APAP or hydrocodone/APAP per day, consider supplementing with a long-acting agent for smoother analgesic coverage and decreased risk of acetaminophen toxicity (e.g., methadone, sustained-release morphine, sustained-release oxycodone).
  - — To calculate the conversion from a short-acting opioid to a long-acting opioid, first calculate the total 24-hour opioid use.
  - — For an equivalent opioid in the sustained-release preparation, divide by 2 for a 12-hour preparation or the entire dose for a 24-hour preparation and then reduce the dose by 25% to 50%.
  - — Give 10% to 20% of the sustained-release dose in an immediate-release preparation to be used for breakthrough pain as needed.
  - — For conversion from an immediate-release opioid to a different sustained-release opioid, the conversion of oral medications is 7.5 mg hydromorphone = 10 mg methadone = 20 mg oxycodone = 30 mg hydrocodone = 60 mg morphine.
  - — For example, 40 mg oxycodone/acetaminophen per day = 10 mg methadone twice daily. Decrease by 25% → 5 mg three times daily, with two oxycodone doses of 5 mg/day for breakthrough.
- Local infiltration of local anesthetic
- Intra-articular infiltration of local anesthetic
- Blockade of peripheral nerve or plexus with local anesthetic
- Neuraxial blocks (i.e., spinal, epidural) with local anesthetic, opiate, and/or α_2-agonists
- Muscle relaxants
- Neuropathic agents (tricyclic antidepressants and antiepileptic drugs; see Chapter 26)
- α_2-Agonists (i.e., clonidine, dexmedetomidine)
- *N*-methyl-D-aspartate antagonists (i.e., ketamine, dextromethorphan)
- Heat
- Ice
- When to refer?
  - If complex regional pain syndrome I or II is suspected, refer the patient to a pain management physician.
  - A chronic pain patient before new injury who is difficult to manage secondary to opioid tolerance will benefit from a pain management referral.
- Prognosis varies widely depending on the type of injury.

Troubleshooting

- If pain is out of proportion to injury or type of surgery, look for other causes such as complex regional pain syndrome or compartment syndrome.
- Patient could be tolerant of opioids if taking them at home, so recheck medication history.
- Patient is not absorbing the medication secondary to bowel abnormalities (e.g., short gut syndrome, previous bowel surgery)
- If the patient does not have the enzyme to metabolize the drug (e.g., codeine metabolizes to morphine), try a different drug.

Patient Instructions

- Comply with physician instructions.
- Supplement medications with positioning, heat, cold, and/or a transcutaneous electrical nerve stimulator unit.

Considerations in Special Populations

- Geriatric patients tend to be more sensitive to medications. Decrease the dose accordingly.

Suggested Reading

- Gottschalk A, Wu CL, Ochroch EA: Current treatment options for acute pain. Expert Opin Pharmocother 2002;3:1599–1611.
- Kelly DJ, Ahmad M, Brull SJ: Preemptive analgesia I: Physiological pathways and pharmacological modalities. Can J Anaesth 2001;48:1000–1010.
- Jackson JL, O'Malley PG, Kroenke K: Evaluation of acute knee pain in primary care. Ann Intern Med 2003;139:575–588.
- MacPherson RD: The pharmacological basis of contemporary pain management. Pharmacol Ther 2000;88:163–185.
- McDougall JJ: Arthritis and pain: Neurogenic origin of joint pain. Arthritis Res Ther 2006;8:(6):220–229.

Chapter 26 Pain Management: Chronic Pain

Meenakshi Bindal and Sheryl Johnson

Key Concepts

Epidemiology

- Prevalence in adults ranges from 2% to 40%, with a median prevalence of 15%.
- In 2003, more than 40 million people were affected with chronic musculoskeletal pain.
- In the United States, 0.5 to 1 million spine surgeries and 2 to 5 million interventional procedures are done each year.
- More than 400 million workdays are lost each year secondary to chronic pain.
- Approximately 70 million physician office visits and 130 million outpatient, hospital, and emergency department visits are evaluations for spine and musculoskeletal disorders.
- Between $45 and $54 billion are spent annually on compensation costs, lost wages, and lost productivity.
- The majority of the cost is due to disability compensation, reduced productivity, and lost tax revenue.
- Chronic pain patients' annual health care costs, excluding surgical procedures, range from $500 to $35,400, with an average of $12,900 to $18,833.

Definitions

- Pain is described as an unpleasant sensory and emotional experience arising from actual or potential damage to tissue.
- Pain is difficult to study because it is subjective, with variability among individuals or even within individuals across time and situations.

Types of Pain

- Neuropathic
  - Caused by nerve injury
    - — Peripheral or central
- Nociceptive
  - Caused by activation of nociceptors
    - — Somatic
    - — Cancer
    - — Postoperative
- Sympathetic (see Chapter 28)
- Acute pain
  - Short-lived and associated with injury to the body that improves after the body heals
  - Serves an evolutionary function by which the body warns us of actual or potential tissue damage
  - Is often associated with autonomic symptoms such as tachycardia, sweating, hypertension, and vasoconstriction
- Chronic pain
  - Lasts 6 months or more or persists beyond the course of acute disease or a reasonable healing period
  - Not amenable to usual pain control
  - Pain where healing may never occur
  - Serves no evolutionary function, but contributes to the development and persistence of debility
  - Usually not associated with hyperactivity of the autonomic system
- Suffering
  - Not synonymous with pain
  - Can occur as a result of chronic pain when it affects a patient's occupational, physical, emotional, and spiritual life negatively
  - Makes treating chronic pain more difficult because it is complex and multifaceted and more amenable to multidisciplinary management
- Comorbidities
  - Psychopathology
    - — Psychiatric illnesses or psychological symptoms can be preexisting problems or can be a result of chronic pain.
    - — Depression and anxiety can be associated with chronic pain.
    - — Addiction in the setting of chronic pain can complicate the evaluation and treatment of the presenting complaint.
  - Medical illness
    - — Significant medical comorbidities are common and may limit treatment options (medications, interventions, physical therapies).

Treatment

- Multidisciplinary care is the mainstay of treatment for optimal outcomes, including pharmacologic treatments, interventions (i.e., injections), surgery, rehabilitation, and psychological treatments.
- Active participation for the patient is very important for successful treatment and outcome.
- The overall treatment goal is improvement in function.

History

- Location: discrete and localized versus diffuse and generalized (diagrams that the patient completes may be helpful)
- Onset: how and when the pain began
    - Sudden
    - Gradual
    - Rapid
- Inciting injury
- Duration
- Intensity
    - Visual analog scale: patients place mark on a 100-mm continuous line between "no pain" and "worst pain imaginable"
    - Verbal numeric rating scale: 0 (no pain) and 10 (worst pain imaginable)
- Character
    - Helpful to distinguish between different types of pain
        - Burning or electric shocks consistent with neuropathic pain
        - Cramping classically describes nociceptive visceral pain.
- Associated symptoms
    - Weakness
    - Loss of function of the involved limb
    - Numbness
    - Bowel or bladder incontinence
- Aggravating and alleviating factors
    - Positional or activity changes (e.g., sitting, standing, lifting, bending, walking)
    - Association with weather changes
    - Association with stressors such as job loss, divorce, death in the family, domestic abuse
    - Association with change in mood
- Previous treatment including effects on function
    - Medications
    - Procedures
    - Physical therapy
    - Occupational therapy
    - Chiropractic manipulation
    - Acupuncture
    - Psychological interventions
- Personal or family history of substance abuse
- Family history of chronic pain
- Assess for secondary gain
    - Job dissatisfaction
    - Involved in litigation
    - Currently on or applying for disability
- Assess for impact of pain on social, physical, occupational, and sexual function and overall quality of life

Physical Examination

- Vital signs (typically not elevated with chronic pain as they are in acute pain)
- General appearance
- Affect
- Gait
- Posture
- Skin rashes
- Muscular symmetry
- Muscle atrophy
- Range of motion including spinal flexion, extension, rotation
- Strength testing
- Neurologic evaluation for light touch and pinprick
- Evaluation of reflexes
- Provocative maneuvers (e.g., Spurling's test evaluating for nerve root disorder, straight-leg-raise evaluation for lumbosacral nerve root lesion, Patrick's sign evaluating for sacroiliac joint pain or intra-articular hip pathology)
- Psychological evaluation, including signs of nonorganic pain

Imaging

- The need for imaging depends on the chronic pain complaint, and appropriate imaging varies significantly. Such imaging studies can include
    - Plain radiographs
    - Computed tomography
    - Magnetic resonance imaging
    - Bone scans
    - Myelography
        - Injection of radiocontrast medium into the intrathecal space followed usually by computed tomography to assess for structural abnormalities of spinal nerves

- Discography
  - Using fluoroscopic guidance to inject the nucleus pulposus with contrast medium to obtain structural and anatomic information about the disc
  - Provides subjective information if the disc is the source of pain

Additional Tests

- Electromyography/nerve conduction velocity studies to evaluate for radiculopathy, plexopathy, polyneuropathy
- Vascular studies (e.g., arterial Doppler scan, ankle-brachial index) to evaluate for vascular insufficiency and claudication

Treatment

- Multimodality treatment is the mainstay of therapy in the specialty of pain management.
  - Combination therapy is more effective than a single approach for long-term improvement.

Pharmacologic Treatment

- The World Health Organization analgesic ladder guidelines
  - Step 1: nonopioid ± adjuvant drug
    - For mild to moderate pain, use acetaminophen, aspirin, nonsteroidal anti-inflammatory drugs, adjuvant drugs
  - Step 2: opioid for mild to moderate pain ± nonopioid ± adjuvant drug
    - For pain that persists beyond Step 1, add opioids (e.g., codeine, hydrocodone)
  - Step 3: opioid for moderate to severe pain ± nonopioid ± adjuvant drug
    - For pain that persists beyond Step 2, add opioids (e.g., morphine, oxycodone, hydromorphone)
- Adjuvant medications
  - Antidepressants for neuropathic pain treatment and/or mood enhancement
    - Tricyclic antidepressants (e.g., amitriptyline, imipramine)
    - Serotonin norepinephrine reuptake inhibitors (e.g., venlafaxine, duloxetine)
    - Serotonin selective reuptake inhibitor (e.g., fluoxetine, paroxetine)
  - Anticonvulsants for neuropathic pain treatment (e.g., gabapentin, pregabalin, carbamazepine, topiramate)
  - Antispasmodics (e.g., cyclobenzaprine, tizanidine, baclofen)

Interventions

- Epidural steroid injections for lumbar or cervical radicular pain
- Facet injections (intra-articular or medial branch blocks) for axial pain
- Joint injections including sacroiliac, hip, shoulder joint injections
- Bursa injections
- Trigger point injections for myofascial pain
- Sympathetic blocks for sympathetically mediated pain
- Intrathecal pumps for pain unresponsive to maximal conservative measures
- Spinal cord stimulators for pain unresponsive to maximal conservative measures
- Vertebroplasty or kyphoplasty
- Surgery for appropriate pathology

Rehabilitation and Nonpharmacologic Modalities

- Physical therapy
- Aquatic or land-based exercises
- Heat/cold modalities
- Massage
- Acupuncture
- Chiropractic manipulation
- Transcutaneous electrical nerve stimulator unit
- Psychological interventions
- Psychotherapy, cognitive-behavioral therapy

When to Refer

- Persistent pain nonresponsive to traditional measures

Prognosis

- Varies considerably depending on pathology and comorbidities
- Importance of prompt evaluation and treatment of pain can be demonstrated in relation to low back pain.
- Eighty percent to 90% of low back pain cases will resolve in 6 weeks regardless of treatment.
- Five percent to 10% of patients will have persistent back pain.
- Return-to-work statistics for those with a back injury are shown in Table 26-1.

TABLE 26-1 *Return-to-Work Statistics for Those with a Back Injury*

Time Away from Work (mo)	Probability of RTW (%)
≤6	<50
12	<12
≥24	<1

RTW, return to work.

Troubleshooting

- Educate patients that the goal may not include 100% pain relief. Reduction of pain and improved function are more typical and reasonable goals with chronic pain.
- Educate patients that their participation in the treatment plan is essential.

Patient Instructions

- Follow physician instructions regarding medication doses and titration schedules to help minimize side effects and improve patient safety.
- Encourage patient participation in the treatment of pain, including weight loss and smoking cessation if applicable, participation in physical therapy followed by a regular exercise routine, and psychological treatments.

Considerations in Special Populations

- Careful titration of medications is important in the elderly to account for age-related changes in kidney function and a higher predisposition to cognitive changes.
- Pediatric patients with chronic pain require special attention because it may be difficult to obtain an accurate history and assessment of pain. This is also a population that has been historically undertreated.
- Patients with a history of substance abuse who have chronic pain need more careful monitoring of prescriptions and may need the assistance of an addiction specialist.
- Patients with psychiatric comorbidities may benefit from a psychiatric consultation.

Suggested Reading

- Abdi S, Datta S, Trescot A, et al: Epidural steroids in the management of chronic spinal pain: A systematic review. Pain Physician 2007;10:185–212.
- Allegrante JP: The role of adjunctive therapy in the management of nonmalignant pain. Am J Med 1996;101:33S.
- Boswell MV, Shah RV, Everett CR, et al: Interventional techniques in the management of chronic spinal pain: Evidence-based practice guidelines. Pain Physician 2005;8:1–47.
- Chou R, Huffman LH: Nonpharmacologic therapies for acute and chronic low back pain: A review of the evidence for an American Pain Society/American College of Physicians clinical practice guideline. Ann Intern Med 2007;147:492–504.
- Leigh JP, Markowitz S, Fahs M, et al: Occupational injury and illness in the United States. Estimates of costs, morbidity, and mortality. Arch Intern Med 1997;157:1557–1568.
- Manchikanti L, Staats PS, Singh V, et al: Evidence-based practice guidelines for interventional techniques in the management of chronic spinal pain. Pain Physician 2003;6:3–80.
- Rogers M: Development of interdisciplinary spinal interventional pain centers. Pain 2003;6:527–535.
- Trescot AM, Boswell MV, Sairam AL, et al: Opioid guidelines in the management of chronic non-cancer pain. Pain Physician 2006;9:1–40.
- Verhaak PF, Kerssens JJ, Dekker J, et al: Prevalence of chronic benign pain disorder among adults: A review of the literature. Pain 1998;77:231–239.
- Warfield CA, Bajwa ZH: Principles and Practice of Pain Medicine. New York: McGraw-Hill, 2004, pp 55–68.
- Waters D, Sierpina VS: Goal-directed health care and the chronic pain patient: A new vision of the healing encounter. Pain Physician 2006;9:353–360.

Chapter 27 Pain Management: Fibromyalgia

Maria Nguyen and Robin J. Hamill-Ruth

ICD-9 CODE
729.1 *Fibromyalgia*

Key Concepts

- Fibromyalgia is a chronic pain syndrome characterized by diffuse pain and somatic symptoms.
- Somatic manifestations may include fatigue, disturbed sleep, cognitive dysfunction, and psychological distress.
- The American College of Rheumatology diagnostic criteria for fibromyalgia include
  - Widespread pain bilaterally and above and below the waist
  - 11 out of 18 specified tender points on digital palpation (Fig. 27-1)
- The pathophysiology is unknown.
  - Possible mechanisms include central sensitization, aberrant descending inhibitory pathways, decreased neurotransmitters (serotonin and dopamine), abnormality in the hypothalamus-pituitary axis, and/or psychiatric comorbidities that may predispose the patient to fibromyalgia.
- The prevalence is 2% in the general population.
- Fibromyalgia affects women more commonly than men.
- The goal of pharmacologic and nonpharmacologic therapy is to restore sleep.
- Use opioid analgesics sparingly, if at all.
  - Prescribing should depend on evidence of increased activity.
  - There are no data to support use of high-dose opioids for fibromyalgia.

History

- Pain
  - Described as deep aching pain that is perceived as arising from muscles or joints (joint stiffness)
- Fatigue
  - Occurs in 80% to 90% of fibromyalgia patients
- Disordered sleep
  - Nonrestorative sleep
  - Multiple factors that contribute to poor sleep include pain, restless legs syndrome, light sleepers, and emotional distress.
  - Paresthesia and subjective swelling
  - Subjective swelling mainly in the joints and soft tissues without clinical evidence
- Associated disorders
  - Chronic fatigue syndrome
  - Irritable bowel syndrome
  - Dysautonomia
  - Cognitive dysfunction
  - Tension-type headache
  - Migraine headache
  - Temporomandibular joint disorder
  - Primary dysmenorrhea
  - Posttraumatic stress disorder
  - Interstitial cystitis
  - Multiple chemical sensitivity
  - Restless legs syndrome
- Psychological disorders
  - Maladaptive coping mechanisms may lead to depression and anxiety.
  - More prevalent in fibromyalgia patients than the general population

Physical Examination

- Elicit trigger points with digital palpation by applying 4 kg of force bilaterally to these areas.
  - Insertion of nuchal muscles into occiput
  - Upper border of trapezius muscle, mid-portion
  - Muscle attachments to upper medial border of scapulae
  - Anterior aspects of C5–C7 intertransverse spaces

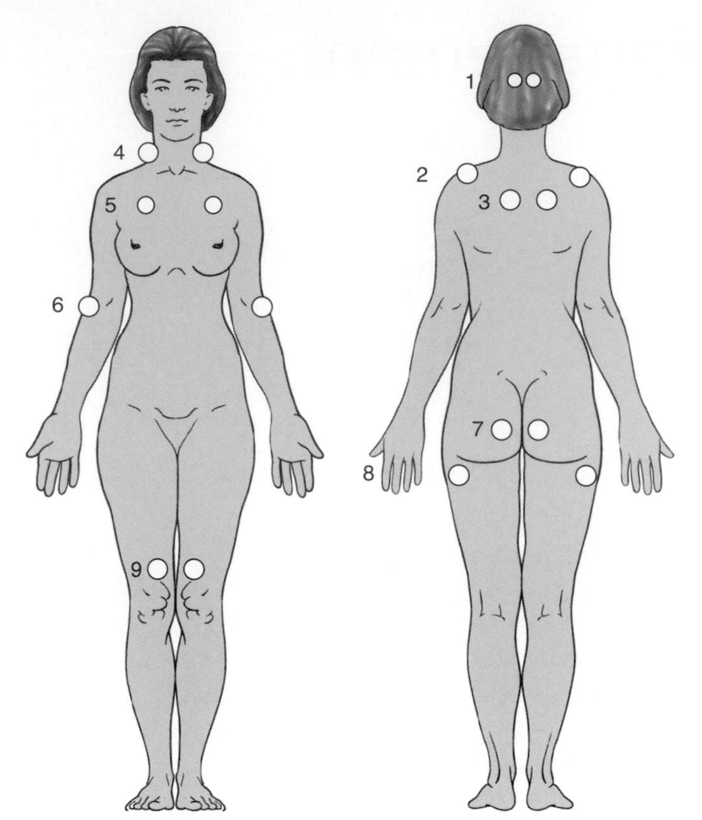

Figure 27-1 American College of Rheumatology diagnostic criteria for fibromyalgia include widespread pain bilaterally, which is above and below the waist in 11 out of 18 specified tender points on digital palpation. The tender points include (1) insertion of nuchal muscles into occiput; (2) upper border of trapezius muscle, mid-portion; (3) muscle attachments to upper medial border of scapulae; (4) anterior aspects of C5–C7 intertransverse spaces; (5) second rib space approximately 3 cm lateral to the sternal border; (6) muscle attachments to lateral epicondyle; (7) upper quadrant of gluteal muscles; (8) muscle attachments just posterior to greater trochanter; (9) medial fat pad of knee proximal to joint line.

  - Second rib space, approximately 3 cm lateral to the sternal border
  - Muscle attachments to lateral epicondyle
  - Upper quadrant of gluteal muscles
  - Muscle attachments just posterior to greater trochanter
  - Medial fat pad of knee proximal to joint line
- Palpate joints examining for other pain generators.
- Look for signs of connective tissue disorder.
- Thorough neurologic examination including strength, sensory, reflexes, cranial nerves
- Abdominal examination (looking for irritable bowel syndrome)

Imaging

- The diagnosis is based on the history and clinical examination.
- Imaging is not helpful except to exclude other diagnoses.

Additional Tests

- Complete blood count
- Complete metabolic panel
- Thyroid-stimulating hormone
- Sleep study if clinically indicated (sleep apnea, disturbed sleep patterns)
- Erythrocyte sedimentation rate
- C-reactive protein
- Rheumatoid factor
- Antinuclear antibody
- Lyme disease screening

Differential Diagnosis

- Muscle disorder
- Muscle strain
- Polymyalgia rheumatica
- Temporal arteritis
- Hypothyroidism
- Rheumatoid arthritis
- Lyme disease
- Connective tissue disorder

Treatment

- Exercise
- Sleep hygiene (counsel on caffeine, tobacco, alcohol cessation)
- Tricyclic antidepressants
- Anticonvulsants (pregabalin)
- Selective serotonin reuptake inhibitors
- Serotonin-norepinephrine reuptake inhibitors
- Muscle relaxants
- Tramadol (other opiates have not proven to be efficacious)
- Cognitive-behavioral therapy, self-regulation techniques

When to Refer

- If symptoms do not improve after a reasonable trial of exercise and pharmacologic therapy, refer the patient for rheumatology or pain management.

Prognosis

- With sleep restoration, the symptoms improve or eventually abate.

Troubleshooting

- Rule out rheumatologic disorders, connective tissue disease, or significant spine pathology.

Patient Instructions

- Comply with physician instructions.
- Improve sleep hygiene; restoring sleep quality is essential.

Considerations in Special Populations

- In patients unresponsive to all interventions, consider referral to a psychiatrist to evaluate for underlying depression.

Suggested Reading

- Abeles AM, Pillinger MH, Solitar BM, Abeles M: Narrative review: The pathophysiology of fibromyalgia. Ann Intern Med 2007; 146:726–734.
- Bennett R: Myofascial pain syndromes and their evaluation. Best Pract Res Clin Rheumatol 2007;21:427–445.
- Clauw DJ: Fibromyalgia: Update on mechanisms and management. J Clin Rheumatol 2007;13:102–109.
- Goldenberg DL: Pharmacological treatment of fibromyalgia and other chronic musculoskeletal pain. Best Pract Res Clin Rheumatol 2007;21:499–511.
- Yunus MB: Role of central sensitization in symptoms beyond muscle pain, and the evaluation of a patient with widespread pain. Best Pract Res Clin Rheumatol 2007;21:481–497.

Chapter 28 Pain Management: Complex Regional Pain Syndrome

Maria Nguyen and Robin J. Hamill-Ruth

ICD-9 CODES
337.21 *Upper Extremity*
337.22 *Lower Extremity*

Key Concepts

- Complex regional pain syndrome (CRPS) I and II, formerly known as reflex sympathetic dystrophy and causalgia, respectively
- CRPS is a neuropathic, chronic pain syndrome following an initiating event that persists with peripheral and central manifestations that are out of proportion to the initial injury (Fig. 28-1).
- CRPS II is associated with a known nerve injury; it otherwise shares clinical manifestations similar to those of CPRS I.
- The pathophysiology is unknown; suggested mechanisms include damage to afferent nerve pathways leading to reorganization of central pain pathways.
- International Association for the Study of Pain diagnostic criteria
    - Noxious event that initiated the immobilization (not required for diagnosis)
    - Disproportionate pain, allodynia (sensitivity to light touch), or hyperalgesia (increased response to painful stimulus)
    - Edema, changes in skin blood flow, or abnormal sudomotor activity in the region of pain
    - No other condition can account for the degree of pain and dysfunction (diagnosis of exclusion).
- More commonly affects females than males (2:1 ratio)
- The average age at onset is 38 years, but it can occur at any age.
- Associated with increased cerebrospinal fluid levels of inflammatory mediators including tumor necrosis factor and interleukin-6
- Early intervention is key. If CRPS is possible and the patient is not improving with treatment, refer to pain management for a diagnostic sympathetic block.

History

- Inciting event or immobilization (can occur without known noxious event)
- Unilateral extremity manifestations (rarely will spread to another extremity)
- Pain
    - Allodynia and hyperalgesia
    - Passive and active movement of the affected region can be extremely painful, leading to guarding.
- Motor changes
    - Loss of function of affected region
    - Wasting and weakness
    - Tremor and dystonia can occur
- Autonomic changes
    - Edema
    - Temperature changes
    - Color changes
    - Sweating
- Dystrophic changes
    - Skin changes such as thinning with a shiny appearance or flaky, thickened skin
    - Hair changes include abnormally coarse hair or a decrease in density of hairs.
    - Nails can become thickened.
    - Osteoporosis secondary to disuse
    - Sudeck's atrophy with loss of bone mineral content

Physical Examination

- Inspect the area carefully and compare it with the unaffected side.
- Note changes to the skin, hair growth, and nails.
- Compare muscle tone and bulk.
- Test range of motion, strength, and reflexes.
- Check sensation with light touch and pinprick.
- Check temperature sensitivity with ice or alcohol pad.
- Place skin temperature probes to affected and unaffected sides to compare temperature differences.

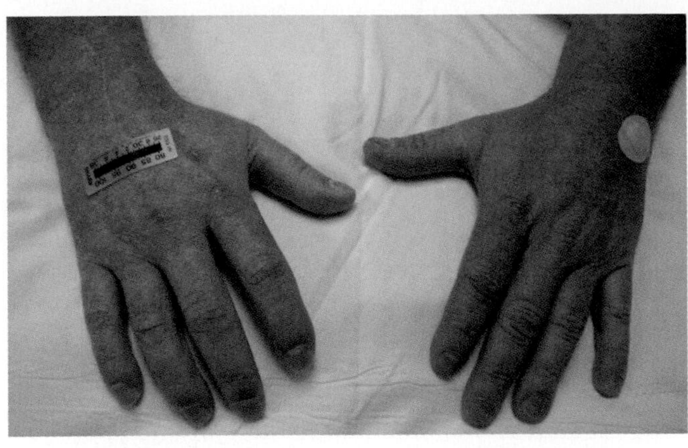

Figure 28-1 Complex regional pain syndrome.

Imaging

- None
- Bone scans are often abnormal, but nonspecific.

Additional Tests

- Diagnostic tests for sympathetically mediated pain include regional sympathetic blocks performed by interventional pain management physicians.
- Stellate ganglion blocks for the upper extremity
- Lumbar sympathetic blocks for the lower extremity
- Intravenous sympatholytic infusions such as phentolamine and bretylium to the affected extremity
- Intravenous regional blocks
- Electromyography
- Vascular studies

Differential Diagnosis

- Infection
- Hypertrophic scar
- Bone fragments
- Neuroma
- Central nervous system tumor
- Syrinx
- Peripheral vascular disease
- Lymphedema
- Fibromyalgia

Treatment

- Sympathetic blocks and intravenous sympatholytics for sympathetically mediated pain
- Start physical and occupational therapy early; it can be performed in conjunction with the sympathetic blocks (if sympathetically mediated) to maximize efficacy. The goal is to normalize function.
- Antiepileptic drugs are used effectively for neuropathic pain, and results are promising with CRPS.
- Antidepressants (e.g., amitriptyline)
- α_1-Adrenergic antagonists for sympathetically mediated CRPS
- Topical analgesics
- Opiates
- Desensitization therapy
- Implantable devices are considered if patients fail conventional therapy.
  - Spinal cord stimulation
  - Peripheral nerve stimulation
  - Deep brain stimulation
  - Intrathecal drug delivery systems

When to Refer

- Early recognition and referral to pain management specialists for aggressive treatment and intervention

Prognosis

- The prognosis is difficult to predict. Patients often have a remitting-relapsing course.

Troubleshooting

- If pain is out of proportion to the type of injury or surgery, then CRPS should be suspected, and referral to pain management should not be delayed.

Patient Instructions

- Comply with physician and physical therapist instructions.
- Frequent follow-ups to ensure that the current therapy is beneficial. Modifications may be necessary.

Suggested Reading

- De Mos M, de Bruijn AG, Huygen FJ, et al: The incidence of complex regional pain syndrome: A population-based study. Pain 2007;129:12–20.
- Harden RM, Bruehl SP: Diagnosis of complex regional pain syndrome: Signs, symptoms, and new empirically derived diagnostic criteria. Clin J Pain 2006;22:415–419.
- Janig W, Baron R: Complex regional pain syndrome: Mystery explained? Lancet Neurol 2003;2:687–697.
- Mekhail N, Kapural L: Complex regional pain syndrome type I in cancer patients. Curr Pain Headache Rep 2000;4:227–233.

- Pappagallo M, Rosenberg A: Epidemiology, pathophysiology, and management of complex regional pain syndrome. Pain Pract 2001;1:11–20.
- Reinders MF, Dijkstra PU, Geertzen JH, et al: Complex regional pain syndrome type I: Use of the International Association for the Study of Pain diagnostic criteria defined in 1994. Clin J Pain 2002;18:207–215.
- Schott GD: Complex regional pain syndrome. Pract Neurol 2007;7:145–157.
- Teasdall RD, Smith BP, Koman LA: Complex regional pain syndrome. Clin Sports Med 2004;23:145–155.

Chapter 29 Pain Management: The Use of Opioids for Chronic Pain

Sheryl Johnson

Key Concepts

- Opioid therapy is the first-line treatment for acute pain associated with orthopaedic injuries as well as moderate to severe pain related to chronic musculoskeletal conditions, cancer, human immunodeficiency virus/acquired immunodeficiency syndrome, and advanced medical illness of other types.
- The role in chronic nonmalignant pain (CNMP) is evolving and remains controversial.
- In CNMP, in contrast to acute pain or pain in terminal illness, the treatment is potentially long term, without an identifiable endpoint.
- The measure of success in the treatment of CNMP with opioids is improvement in function.
- Typically, opioids are used as adjunctive or second-line agents in CNMP, after nonopioid treatments have failed to provide adequate relief and the patient continues to have moderate to severe pain.
- Nonopioid options include such therapies as nonsteroidal anti-inflammatory drugs, acetaminophen, antidepressants, anticonvulsants, behavior modification, physical therapy, modalities such as transcutaneous electrical nerve stimulation, therapeutic nerve blocks, and surgery directed at the source of pain.
- There is a large body of literature supporting the concept that pain is undertreated even in the setting of cancer, acquired immunodeficiency syndrome, and pain at the end of life. Long-term treatment with opioids for a portion of patients with CNMP may improve function and quality of life.
- Concerns about opioids for CNMP include tolerance, addiction, diversion, and significant side effects.
- Recently, the possibilities of opioid-induced hyperalgesia and negative hormonal effects are being investigated in patients receiving opioids on a long-term basis.
- More research is needed to better define the role of long-term opioid use in the setting of CNMP.

History

- Many medical conditions can present with chronic pain, and the history of patients with CNMP thus varies significantly.
- The medical history should document the nature and intensity of the pain; modifying and exacerbating factors; associated symptoms; current and past treatments; comorbidities; the effect of the pain on physical, occupational, social, and psychological function; the personal and family history of substance abuse; a review of previous records and studies; and a medical indication for the use of opioids.

Physical Examination

- The physical examination varies significantly with the pain reported.
- The physical examination should be complete, with a focus on the area of the pain reported by the patient.
- Include a sensory examination to evaluate for nerve injury, entrapments, and evidence of complex regional pain syndrome.

Imaging

- Often there is a poor correlation between imaging findings and patient-reported pain.
- The need for imaging is variable, but can include plain radiographs, magnetic resonance imaging, computed tomography, bone scans, and other tests.

Additional Tests

- Electrophysiologic testing (e.g., electromyography and nerve conduction studies) can be a useful tool for the evaluation of some types of pain such as radicular symptoms and possible neuropathies.

- Vascular studies may be appropriate for pain that may be related to vascular disease.
- Laboratory tests for specific disease processes may help determine the etiology of some types of pain (e.g., evaluating for diabetes, hepatitis, pancreatitis, nutritional deficiencies, and rheumatologic conditions).
- Psychological assessments, using both interviews and specific tests (e.g., Pain Disability Index, Beck Depression Inventory, and Coping Strategies Questionnaire) can be helpful in determining factors that may put the patient at lower or higher risk of problems associated with long-term opioid therapy.

Treatment

- Decision phase
  - Establish a pain diagnosis.
  - Evaluate current pain severity.
  - Review previous treatments, including the adequacy of medication trials and previous adverse reactions to drugs and therapies.
  - Weigh risks and benefits, with consideration of factors such as alternatives, comorbidities, risk of abuse, and diversion. A personal history of drug abuse, a family history of substance abuse, and a history of legal problems are factors related to an increased risk of problems with long-term opioid use.
- Initiation phase
  - If a trial of opioids appears appropriate, provide the patient with education about the medication.
  - With the patient's input, define clear functional goals for the opioid therapy with the understanding that the therapy may not be continued if these goals are not met.
  - Informed consent is strongly advised for all patients undergoing a trial of opioids.
    - — There is a wide variation of the form (verbal or written) and information provided. Typically, this includes restricting the patient to receiving opioids from only one physician and pharmacy, mandating appropriate use of the medications and avoidance of sedating and illicit substances, and explaining that random urine drug screens should be expected by the patient.
    - — It often also describes reasons that the opioids may be discontinued.
    - — These agreements have not shown proven efficacy, but they may be effective educational tools (a sample opioid agreement is found at www.painmed.org/clinical_info/guidelines.html).
  - In opioid-naïve patients or in patients with minimal previous opioid exposure, short-acting, low-dose opioids are recommended to establish the opioid requirement. The medication can be prescribed on an as-needed basis or scheduled around the clock, depending on the pain severity and pattern.
  - In patients with significant renal and/or hepatic dysfunction, the chosen drug, dose, and schedule must be adjusted accordingly (e.g., avoid morphine in patients with renal disease.)
  - If a patient responds well to short-acting opioids without significant side effects, long-acting or sustained-release formulations in appropriately scheduled doses are generally thought to be the standard of care.
    - — The use of these agents helps to avoid the uneven "rollercoaster" pattern of pain control seen with short-acting agents.
    - — The appropriate dose of long-acting agents can be calculated by the use of the short-acting medications. For example, in a patient taking oxycodone/acetaminophen 5 mg/325 mg, 2 tablets 4 times daily, the total oxycodone dose is 40 mg. Sustained-release oxycodone 20 mg twice daily could replace the short-acting medication.
  - Short-acting medications can be used for breakthrough pain, in addition to the longer-acting agents.
  - Avoid the use of
    - — Meperidine (poor absorption; toxic metabolite may cause seizures, especially with renal dysfunction)
    - — Propoxyphene (poor efficacy; toxic metabolite that can lead to central nervous system and cardiac toxicity, particularly with renal dysfunction)
    - — Mixed μ-agonist/antagonists (e.g., butorphanol) (ceiling effect of medication, can cause withdrawal from μ-agonists)
    - — Other sedating medications such as benzodiazepines, sedatives, and hypnotics that can additively or synergistically cause oversedation and serious adverse events including death
- Titration phase
  - Continue nonopioid treatments
  - Titrate by increases of 10% to 50% of the dose, waiting 4 to 5 half-lives between increases.

- If the medication is not well tolerated or analgesia is inadequate, consider an opioid rotation.
- Calculate the total daily dose of the opioid.
- Use equianalgesic charts to estimate the dose of another drug.
- Reduce the documented dose by 30% to 50% to account for incomplete cross-tolerance between opioids.
- Reassess frequently to monitor for effectiveness and side effects and adjust the dosage appropriately.
- If methadone is being considered, a consultation with a physician very familiar with the drug is imperative to avoid overdosing and other serious adverse events.
  - Due to significant individual metabolic variability and nonlinear dose conversion for methadone, a simple equianalgesic chart is not appropriate for the use of methadone.

- Stable phase
  - Maintain on a stable dose, with monthly visits for refills.
  - Random urine drug screens are highly recommended to monitor compliance.
  - Continue other therapies and consider referrals as appropriate to alleviate pain using nonopioid strategies.
  - Document the analgesic response, side effects, aberrant behavior, and function in relation to the opioid therapy on a regular basis.
  - Manage opioid-related side effects, particularly constipation.

When to Refer

- Consider a surgical consultation if the pathology related to the pain may respond to surgical intervention.
- Consider a psychiatric consultation for patients with problems such as significant anxiety or depression.
- Consider a referral to an addictionologist if substance abuse appears to be a problem.
- Other referrals may be appropriate depending on the pain.

Prognosis

- There are few controlled studies on the effectiveness of opioids for CNMP. The existing literature is flawed and/or with limited validity. The use of opioids for CNMP continues to be an area of controversy.

Troubleshooting

- Side effects of opioids are common and include constipation, nausea, vomiting, sedation, pruritus, respiratory depression, and tolerance.
  - Consider an opioid rotation as individual responses to opioids are highly variable, and often a patient will respond well to one opioid even after significant side effects with another.
  - Treatment of side effects is well documented in the medical literature and is beyond the scope of this chapter.
- Addiction is a feared problem with these medications, although the risk is thought to be low in patients without a personal history or family history of substance abuse.
  - Continued careful monitoring of all patients taking long-term opioid therapy is essential to identify signs or symptoms of addiction.
  - Examples of problematic behavior are injecting oral formulations, obtaining prescription drugs from nonmedical sources, drug-related deterioration in function at work or home, repeated self-escalation in dosing, and concurrent use of alcohol or illicit substances. Sometimes the evidence is much more subtle and difficult to detect.
  - In patients with a personal history of substance abuse or dependence, a concerning family history of such issues, and/or evidence of problematic behavior in a patient taking chronic opioids, a referral to an addictionologist is prudent.
- Evidence of behaviors such as prescription tampering and diversion are illegal activities and should be dealt with accordingly.
- Failure of the opioid medications to produce an analgesic response, and more importantly a functional benefit, should prompt the prescribing physician to strongly consider tapering and discontinuing the opioid therapy.

Patient Instructions

- The patient should be given clear instructions about how to take the medications.
- The risk, benefits, and expectations of opioid prescription are outlined in opioid agreements/consents and should be thoroughly reviewed at the initiation of opioid therapy and periodically as appropriate.

Considerations in Special Populations

- As with most medications, extra caution should be taken in the elderly population, with consideration of lower doses at initiation and slow titration schedules.
- Because of the potential toxicity associated with this class of medication, opioids should be prescribed only in settings in which the patient or his/her caretaker is able to understand and carefully follow the instructions and notify the prescribing physician of problems or questions.
- As above, in patients with a history of substance abuse, long-term opioid therapy, if initiated, should be initiated with caution and ideally with the consultation of an addictionologist regarding addiction treatments, prudent drug selection, frequent follow-up, and urine drug screens.
- Caution should be used when prescribing opioids to patients with both significant medical and psychological comorbidities.

Suggested Reading

- Fishman SM, Kreis PG: The opioid contract. Clin J Pain 2002;18:S70–S75.
- Heit HA, Gourlay DL: Urine drug testing in pain medicine. J Pain Symptom Manage 2004;27:260–267.
- Hojsted J, Sjogren P: An update on the role of opioids in the management of chronic pain of nonmalignant origin. Curr Opin Anesthesiol 2007;20:451–455.
- Mahajan G, Fishman SM: Major opioids in pain management. In Benzon HT, Raja SN, Molloy RE, et al (eds): Essentials of Pain Medicine and Regional Anesthesia, 2nd ed. Philadelphia: Elsevier, 2005, pp 94–112.
- Michna E, Ross EL, Hynes WL, et al: Predicting aberrant drug behavior in patients treated for chronic pain: Importance of abuse history. J Pain Symptom Manage 2004;28:250–258.
- Model policy for the use of controlled substances for the treatment of pain, 2004. Available at: www.fsmb.org/pdf/2004_grpol_Controlled_Substances.pdf. Accessed January 21, 2009.
- Passik SD, Kirsh KL: Opioid therapy in patients with a history of substance abuse. CNS Drugs 2004;18:13–25.
- Shalmi C: Opioids for nonmalignant pain: Issues and controversy. In Warfield CA, Bawa ZH (eds): Principles and Practice of Pain Medicine, 2nd ed. New York: McGraw-Hill, 2004, pp 601–611.

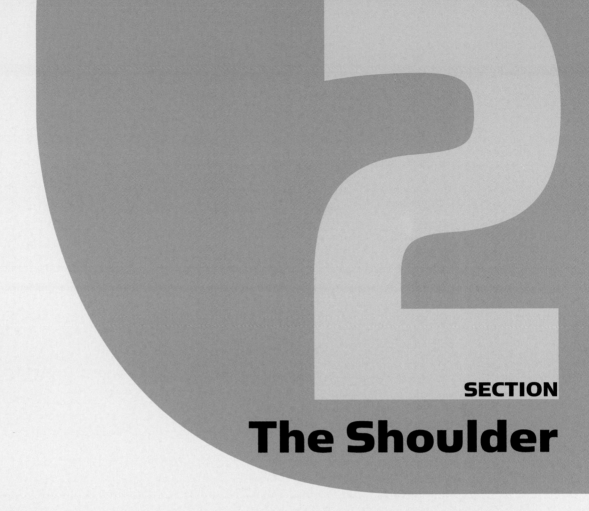

SECTION

2 The Shoulder

Chapter 30 Overview of the Shoulder

Robert Dimeff and Jason Brayley

Key Concepts

- Shoulder problems account for a significant percentage of musculoskeletal disorders with which the primary care provider is presented.
- The anatomy of the shoulder and range of motion within the glenohumeral joint can make this part of human anatomy a significant diagnostic challenge for the primary care provider.
- Diagnosis and appropriate treatment can easily be attained with knowledge of the relevant anatomy and proper correlation with historical information presented at the time of evaluation.

Bones

Clavicle

- S-shaped bone with convex anterior border medially and concave anterior border laterally
- The only bone to connect the upper extremity to the axial skeleton
- It stabilizes the glenohumeral joint and upper extremity anteriorly and protects the medial brachial plexus.
- Eighty percent of fractures occur at the medial and lateral junction secondary to weakness in this area.

Scapula

- Flat triangular bone composed of the body, spine, acromium, glenoid fossa, scapular neck, and coracoid process
- Provides numerous sights for muscular attachment
- Neurovascular structures travel along the inferomedial surface.
- Overlies the posterolateral aspect of thorax between second and seventh ribs

Proximal Humerus

- Nearly spherical humeral head
- One third has articular cartilage directed medially, superiorly, and posteriorly
- Articulates with the glenoid fossa of the scapula
- The greater and lesser tuberosities are sights for muscular insertion of the supraspinatus and subscapularis muscles, respectively.
- The intertubercular groove between the tuberosities houses the long head of the biceps tendon.
- The head is inclined 130 to 150 degrees in relation to shaft, with 20 to 30 degrees of retroversion.

Joints and Ligaments

Sternoclavicular Joint

- Only articulation between upper limb and axial skeleton
- This joint has ball and socket qualities, although it is the least stable of all major joints.
- Allows clavicle 35 degrees of elevation, 35 degrees of forward/backward motion, and 50 degrees of rotation
- Intra-articular disc and costoclavicular, interclavicular, and sternoclavicular ligaments provide stability.

Acromioclavicular Joint

- Only articulation between clavicle and scapula
- Transmits forces from extremity to axial skeleton and supports upper extremity, allowing 40 degrees of rotation
- Superior and inferior acromioclavicular ligaments control anterior and posterior stability, providing principal restraints to axial and posterior translation.
- Coracoclavicular ligaments include the trapezoid and conoid ligaments, providing anterior and posterior scapular rotation, respectively.

Glenohumeral Joint

- Greatest mobility of all joints, although stability sacrificed to maintain range of motion
- Stability conferred by interaction of bony, ligamentous, and muscle constraints
- Superior/inferior translation of 0.3 mm; 5 mm of anterior/posterior translation
- Glenoid
  - Bony base from lateral scapula

- Thicker peripheral articular cartilage allows concavity compression effect to enhance stability.
- Labrum
  - Ring of dense fibrous triangle-shaped tissue that deepens glenoid by 2.5 mm, with thickening of periphery to increase joint congruity and stability
  - Attachment site of the glenohumeral ligaments and long head of the biceps tendon
- Glenohumeral capsule
  - Twice the surface area of the humeral head
  - Lined with synovium, although has limited joint fluid volume, resulting in negative intra-articular pressure
  - Acts as "check rein" for glenohumeral articulation when placed under tension near extremes of range of motion

Glenohumeral Ligaments

- Composed of the superior, medial, and inferior glenohumeral ligaments
- Collagenous thickening of the shoulder capsule provides static stability to the glenohumeral joint.
- Assists in controlling anterior/posterior and superior/inferior translation of the humerus
- Primary stabilizer at extremes of shoulder motion

Coracohumeral Ligament

- Static suspensory function for the humeral head and glenoid with arm at side
- Provides restraint to inferior translation and reinforces rotator cuff interval

Coracoacromial Ligament

- Contributes to the roof of the glenohumeral joint

Transverse Humeral Ligament

- Connects the greater and lesser tuberosities
- Maintains the long head of the biceps tendon in the intertubercular groove

Scapulothoracic Articulation

- Provides for movement of scapula on chest wall, although not a true joint

Muscles

- Rotator cuff muscles
  - Includes the supraspinatus, infraspinatus, teres minor, and subscapularis muscles
  - Primary active stabilizers of the glenohumeral joint
  - Active contraction of these muscles compresses the humeral head within the glenoid.
  - Table 30-1 provides a summary of relevant shoulder musculature.

Neurovascular Structures and Bursae

Brachial Plexus

- Originates as roots from the anterior and primary divisions of cervical nerves 5 through 8 and thoracic nerve 1
- Divides further into upper, middle, and lower trunks

TABLE 30-1 *Major Muscles of the Shoulder Region*

Muscle	Action on Shoulder
Supraspinatus	Initiates shoulder abduction, depresses humeral head with deltoid contraction, compresses humeral head within glenoid
Infraspinatus	Primary external rotator of shoulder. Upper fibers abduct, lower fibers adduct.
Teres minor	External rotation and adduction
Subscapularis	Internal rotation; assists with abduction, adduction; flexion and extension depending on arm position
Biceps brachii	Flexion of shoulder and elbow, primary supinator of forearm
Coracobrachialis	Flexion and adduction
Pectoralis major	Flexion, adduction, and internal rotation
Pectoralis minor	Draws scapula forward and downward
Subclavius	Draws shoulder downward and forward
Deltoid	Primary mover of shoulder; abducts; anterior fibers flex and internally rotate shoulder; posterior fibers extend and externally rotate shoulder
Triceps brachii	Extends elbow; long head extends and adducts shoulder
Teres major	Adducts, extends, and internally rotates
Serratus anterior	Rotates scapula; stabilizes and draws scapula forward
Rhomboids	Draw scapula medially; depress shoulder
Levator scapulae	Elevate and rotate scapula
Latissimus dorsi	Extends, adducts, and internally rotates
Trapezius	Raises, lowers, rotates, and adducts scapula

- Trunks then form the anterior and posterior divisions, which lead to the medial, lateral, and posterior cords.
- The cords give rise to the terminal branches of the musculocutaneous, median, ulnar, radial, and axillary nerves.

Axillary Artery

- The subclavian artery becomes the axillary artery at the first rib.
- Multiple major branches from the axillary artery supply the shoulder region.
- The axillary artery becomes the brachial artery at the lower border of the teres major tendon.

Bursae

- Function as lubrication sacs to decrease friction between musculoskeletal structures
- Include the subacromial, subdeltoid, subscapular, biceps, and scapulothoracic bursae

Shoulder Biomechanics

- Result of four joints moving synchronously and simultaneously
- The humerus moves twice as fast and far as the scapula.
- Humeral motion ranges
  - Abduction, 180 degrees; adduction, 45 degrees
  - Flexion, 160 degrees; extension, 45 degrees
  - Internal rotation, 90 degrees; external rotation, 100 degrees
- Scapula
  - Elevation and depression, protraction, and retraction
- Sternoclavicular joint
  - Anterior/posterior, 35 degrees; elevation, 35 degrees; rotation, 45 degrees
- Acromioclavicular joint
  - Rotation, 20 degrees; first 20 degrees and last 40 degrees of arm elevation
- Scapulothoracic joint
  - None during first 60 degrees of flexion and 30 degrees of abduction, synchronous with glenohumeral joint, 3 degrees of glenohumeral motion for each 2 degrees of scapulothoracic motion
- Glenohumeral joint
  - Two thirds of abduction and forward flexion, nearly all adduction and extension, all rotation
  - The pattern of motion is a combination of gliding and rolling.
  - During the first 90 degrees of elevation, the clavicle tips upward 35 degrees at the sternoclavicular joint; beyond this point, scapular rotation depends on hinging of as much as 20 degrees at the acromioclavicular joint.
  - Stability is conferred by the interaction of bony, ligamentous, and muscular constraint systems that control the movement of the instant center of motion of the glenohumeral joint.
- Glenohumeral stability
  - Static
    - — Includes bone (glenoid and humerus), labrum, glenohumeral ligaments, glenohumeral joint capsule, concavity-compression, finite joint volume.
  - Dynamic
    - — Passive muscle bulk and physical barrier, muscular contraction providing compressive force to joint surface and stiffening of joint capsule
    - — Muscular contraction also provides restraint to the glenohumeral joint and redirects the joint reactive force to the center of the glenoid.

History

- The examiner should attempt to discern the following before examining the shoulder:
  - Symptom onset: acute or chronic
  - Quality and severity of symptoms
  - Activities that aggravate or relieve symptoms
  - Presence of night, exertional, or radiating pain
  - Paresthesias, "dead arm," or weakness
  - Looseness, slipping sensation, shoulder popping out of joint
  - Muscle atrophy or fatigue
  - Clicking, catching, grinding, grating
  - Edema, cyanosis, coolness
  - Trauma or overuse factors
- Other relevant historical information includes age, occupation, handedness, general medical health and medications, presence of connective tissue diseases, sports demands, loss of throwing velocity or accuracy, workers' compensation issues, and pending litigation.

Physical Examination

- A thorough examination of the shoulder should include the following:
  - Inspection: atrophy, swelling, discoloration
  - Range of motion: symmetrical, compensatory changes
  - Palpation: focal tenderness, deformities
  - Strength: assessed throughout the upper extremity, upper back, and neck

TABLE 30-2 *Specialized Physical Examination Components of the Shoulder*

Test	Physical Maneuvers	Likely Diagnosis if Positive Test
Neer impingement sign	Arm forcibly flexed to overhead position	Subacromial impingement of humerus against coracoacromial arch
Cross arm test	Forward elevation to 90 degrees with active adduction	Acromioclavicular joint arthritis
Hawkins impingement sign	Forward flexion of the shoulder to 90 degrees with internal rotation	Impingement of supraspinatus tendon
Sulcus sign	Inferior traction of the arm by pulling on elbow or wrist	Widened sulcus consistent with inferior instability
Apley scratch test	Patient touches inferior and superior aspects of opposite scapula	Loss of range of motion secondary to rotator cuff disorder
Apprehension test	Arm is abducted to 90 degrees and externally rotated; anterior force applied to humerus	Anterior glenohumeral instability
Relocation test	Posterior force applied with arm in position of the apprehension test	Improvement of pain consistent with anterior instability
Yergason test	Elbow flexed to 90 degrees with resisted forearm supination	Biceps tendonitis or biceps instability
Speed's maneuver	Elbow flexed 20–30 degrees with humerus flexed to 60 degrees	Biceps tendonitis if pain with resisted forward flexion of arm
Spurling's test	Spine extended with head rotated to affected shoulder while axially loaded	Cervical nerve root disorder
Drop sign	Arm abducted 90 degrees, externally rotated until resistance met, patient holds	Rotator cuff tear likely if unable to hold external rotation
Lift-off test	Patient places hand on lower back, attempts to lift off	Pain or inability represents subscapular muscle disorder
O'Brien's test	Arm forward flexed to 90 degrees, arm adducted 10–15 degrees, downward force, patient resists	Possible anterior superior labral tear if more pain with thumb down than palm up
Jerk test	Arm abducted to 90 degrees and internally rotated, axial load placed on humerus and arm then adducted	Sudden jerk likely represents humeral head sliding off glenoid

- Assessment of impingement and stability
- Neurovascular examination: sensation and reflexes
- Evaluation of the ipsilateral elbow and neck
- Table 30-2 provides a description of specific physical examination components.

Suggested Reading

- Bahk M, Keyurapan H, Tasaki A, et al: Laxity testing of the shoulder. Am J Sports Med 2007;35:131–144.
- Baker CL, Merkley M: Clinical evaluation of the athlete's shoulder. J Athletic Train 2000;35:256–260.
- Ebell M: Diagnosing rotator cuff tears. Am Fam Physician 2005;71:1587–1589.
- McFarland EG, Selhi H, Keyurapan H: Clinical evaluation of impingement: What to do and what works. J Bone Joint Surg Am 2006;88A:432–441.
- Myers TH, Zemanovic JR, Andrews JR: The resisted supination external rotation test. Am J Sports Med 2005;33:1315–1320.
- Quillen DM, Wuchner M, Hatch R: Acute shoulder injuries. Am Fam Physician 2004;70:1947–1954.
- Woodward TW, Best TM: The painful shoulder. Part I. Clinical evaluation. Am Fam Physician 2000;61:3079–3089.

Chapter 31 Anterior Shoulder Instability

Elizabeth Rothe and William Dexter

ICD-9 CODES
718.81 *Shoulder Joint Instability*
831.00 *Shoulder Dislocation*
718.31 *Recurrent Shoulder Dislocation*
718.21 *Pathologic Shoulder Dislocation*

Key Concepts

- Instability is defined as excessive translation of the humerus over the glenoid surface to the point that it is symptomatic.
- The degree of instability can vary (e.g., microinstability, subluxation, dislocation).
- The glenohumeral joint is predisposed to instability because it is shallow, allowing for increased range of motion.
- Both static (glenoid fossa, labrum, joint capsule, ligaments) and dynamic (rotator cuff, long head of the biceps muscle, deltoid muscle) stabilizers are needed to improve the stability of the glenohumeral joint.
- The least stable position of the shoulder is abduction with external rotation.
- Most anterior instability is caused by subluxation or anterior dislocation.
- Anterior dislocation causes traumatic instability, often with a Bankart lesion (avulsion of the anterior capsule–labral complex below the midline of the glenoid and may include a bony avulsion). Dislocation may also be associated with a Hill-Sachs lesion (injury to the posterolateral aspect of the humeral head).
- If a Hill-Sachs lesion covers more than 30% of the articular surface, it may contribute to recurrent dislocations and instability.
- Comorbidities include capsular tearing or stretching, rotator cuff tears (primarily in older patients with primary dislocations), and axillary nerve injuries.
- Chronic, repetitive microinjury, as in the overhead throwing athlete, can result in acquired anterior instability from stretching of the joint capsule or recurrent microsubluxation of the glenohumeral joint.
- Suspect microinjury in any throwing athlete who reports pain in the shoulder; he or she should be examined for instability of the glenohumeral joint.
- Anterior dislocation and instability are more common in men than in women.
- Rates of anterior instability after a primary dislocation vary from 17% to 100%.
- Rates of instability are higher in patients younger than 20 years old and decrease with age but may increase again in the elderly as a result of increasing rotator cuff problems.

History

- The diagnosis of anterior instability is primarily clinical.
- The patient may complain of shoulder discomfort with contact and overhead activities, often without any restriction of range of motion.
- There may be a vague "dead arm" sensation secondary to stretch of the brachial plexus during subluxation.
- A history of dislocation or subluxation is helpful in making the diagnosis.
- Because there are cases of anterior instability that are not frankly traumatic, a throwing history or a history of joint laxity is also important to obtain.
- A history of Marfan syndrome or other hyperlaxity condition in the athlete or immediate family is important to document.

Physical Examination

- The physical examination should include inspection for any swelling or malformations, palpation for tenderness and regions of anesthesia in axillary nerve distribution, active and passive range of motion, strength, and neurovascular testing, as well as specific tests to assess for instability.
- A decrease in mobility in anterior dislocation is primarily from pain versus an anatomic restriction. The

strength of the shoulder girdle and arm should be tested and any weaknesses noted.

- The apprehension test is done with the patient supine or sitting with shoulder abducted and externally rotated to 90 degrees. Forward pressure is applied to the posterior humeral head. Pain or apprehension indicates a positive test. This test may also be positive in patients with primary impingement and becomes more specific when only apprehension, not pain, is used as a positive indicator.
- Jobe's apprehension-relocation test is done after a positive apprehension test. Posterior force is applied to the anterior humeral head, which alleviates the pain. Patients with primary impingement will not experience pain relief.
- A load and shift test and a crank test have also been shown to predict labral tears, common in anterior instability.
- The load and shift test is done with the patient supine, while the proximal humeral head is moved anteriorly, posteriorly, and inferiorly to assess glenohumeral joint movement. Excessive translation or sensation of subluxation when compared with the opposite side indicates a positive test.
- The crank test is done with the shoulder abducted to 90 degrees and internally rotated with an axial load. Pain, catching, or grinding indicates a positive test.

Imaging

- An initial radiograph is important to diagnose a bony Bankart or Hill-Sachs lesion.
- Obtain anteroposterior radiographs of the shoulder in neutral rotation (assess the lower rim of the glenoid) and internal rotation (assess impaction of the humeral head, or Hill-Sachs lesion), an axillary view in external rotation at 90 degrees, and a profile glenoid view to detect glenoid lesions.
- Computed tomography is an excellent tool for the diagnosis of bony lesions, but may not be necessary if radiographs are negative. Computed tomography may help confirm the presence of a very small humeral fracture or inferior glenoid lesions.
- Magnetic resonance imaging is useful in detecting labral lesions and in assessing a nonbony Bankart lesion.
- Magnetic resonance arthrography is superior to magnetic resonance imaging in diagnosing labral tears.
- Arthrography or arthroscopy can visualize labral or glenohumeral ligament injuries.
- Arthroscopy is done only after all other imaging is negative but the clinical history is still highly suspicious. Direct visualization of anatomic damage indicative of anterior instability can be obtained, and it may be possible to fix the damage concurrently.

Differential Diagnosis

- Impingement, rotator cuff problems, labral tears, bicipital tendinitis, bursitis, and acromioclavicular joint injuries
- Osteoarthritis or rheumatoid arthritis should be considered.
- Consider septic arthritis if there is an associated fever.
- Adhesive capsulitis of the shoulder can present with pain and a severely limited range of motion, which differentiates it from anterior instability.
- Unusual diagnoses such as thoracic outlet syndrome should be considered if a cervical rib is discovered, whereas cervical radiculopathy or brachial neuritis can refer pain to the shoulder.
- Other causes of referred pain to the shoulder include biliary disease, blood or gas in the peritoneal cavity, a subphrenic abscess, splenic trauma, cancer, apical lung diseases, angina pectoris, or an acute myocardial infarction.

Treatment

- After a dislocation, it is unclear whether or for how long a shoulder should be immobilized.
- Traditionally, a sling is used for 1 to 6 weeks, and it can be removed when the pain has subsided and strength is improved.
- A nonsurgical approach is taken with primary dislocators older than 20 years old who are not elite athletes or in patients with atraumatic anterior instability.
- Initial management consists of rehabilitation. This typically starts with isometric exercises with an emphasis on the grip and the biceps, triceps, and deltoid muscle groups. The athlete is advanced to isotonic and range of motion exercises.
- Scapular stabilization exercises help stabilize the glenohumeral joint.
- Surgery for primary dislocation is often not addressed until after immobilization, adequate rehabilitation, and a trial of a return-to-play regimen. Depending on age and function, surgery may be addressed sooner.
- Recurrence of dislocation is less frequent with surgery than without it.
- Surgical repair of anterior instability is traditionally done via an open approach, but recent studies show that arthroscopic repair can be as effective.

- Contraindications to arthroscopic repair include large glenoid or Hill-Sachs defects.

When to Refer

- Referral to an orthopaedic surgeon should be considered in those younger than 20 years old, in recurrent dislocators, or in those with large Hill-Sachs lesions or other serious comorbid injuries to the shoulder.

Prognosis

- Factors that affect the prognosis include age (younger patients are more likely to have instability), family history of recurrent instability, bony Bankart lesion, and Hill-Sachs lesion (prognosis worsens proportionally with the size of the Hill-Sachs lesion).
- Other lesions predisposing to anterior instability include SLAP (superior labrum, anteroposterior) tear, humeral avulsion of the glenohumeral ligaments, and anterior labroligamentous periosteal sleeve avulsions.

Patient Instructions

- Return-to-play timing can range from weeks to months depending on the age of the patient, the intensity and dedication to rehabilitation, and the level of the initial injury.
- Ideal criteria for return to play include little or no pain and nearly normal range of motion, strength, functional ability, and sport-specific skills.
- Although there is no solid evidence of their efficacy, there are several commercial braces that are available to limit abduction and external rotation in the apprehensive patient or in the patient who does not quite meet all the previously stated criteria.
- A rehabilitation program before return to play is essential.
- For chronic dislocators, surgery to correct a contributing defect may be needed before return to play. For acquired anterior instability, rehabilitation is often needed, and the above criteria for return to play are applicable.

Suggested Reading

- Backer M, Warren RF: Glenohumeral instability in adults. In DeLee JC, Drez D, Miller M (eds): DeLee and Drez's Orthopaedic Sports Medicine: Principles and Practice, 2nd ed. Philadelphia: Saunders, 2003.
- Fischer AM, Dexter WW: How evidence-based is our examination of the shoulder? In MacAuley D, Best T (eds): Evidence-Based Sports Medicine, 2nd ed. Malden, MA: Blackwell, 2007, pp 303–326.
- Luime JJ, Verhagen AP, Miedema HS, et al: Does this patient have an instability of the shoulder or a labrum lesion? JAMA 2004;292:1989–1999.
- McCarty EC, Ritchie P, Gill HS, McFarland EG: Shoulder instability: Return to play. Clin Sports Med 2004;23:335–351.
- Walch G: Chronic anterior glenohumeral instability. J Bone Joint Surg Br 1996;78B:670–677.

Chapter 32 Posterior Shoulder Instability

Marc De Jong

Key Concepts

- The term *posterior shoulder instability* encompasses a spectrum of disorders, from recurrent symptomatic subluxations to acute traumatic dislocation.
  - Subluxation: excessive posterior movement of the humeral head without completely escaping the glenoid rim; usually reduces spontaneously (Fig. 32-1)
  - Dislocation: the humeral head is forced out of the glenoid cavity
- Nonacute posterior instability is often divided into three groups
  - Recurrent posterior subluxation
  - Recurrent posterior dislocation
  - Painful shoulder when placed in a position of posterior instability (forward elevation, adduction, internal rotation)
- Approximately 50% of patients with symptomatic recurrent posterior instability will have an inciting injury.
- Up to 5% of all patients presenting with shoulder instability possess an element of posterior instability.
- Posterior instability is more commonly a subluxation rather than a true dislocation.
- Traumatic posterior instability most often occurs with a posterior force directed to the arm in a position of posterior instability.
  - Also associated with seizures, high-energy trauma, and electrocution
- Only 2% to 5% of all shoulder dislocations are posterior.
- Posterior dislocations are often overlooked.
  - High clinical suspicion and appropriate imaging will minimize missed diagnoses.
  - Dislocations diagnosed more than 6 weeks from the traumatic event are considered chronic.
  - An overlooked posterior dislocation may lead to chronic range of motion loss.
- An acute posterior dislocation may self-reduce unless accompanied by a fracture of the humeral head.
- Posterior instability is often associated with an abnormal posteroinferior capsular ligament, poor rotator cuff function, and/or posterior labral lesions.
- The shape of the glenoid surface, namely, the lack of a normal concavity or glenoid hypoplasia, can increase the risk of shoulder instability of any variety.

History

- It is important to distinguish traumatic from atraumatic instability, determine activities or positions that reproduce symptoms, and assess voluntary versus involuntary instability.
  - Patients with voluntary instability need to be further evaluated as potential habitual (willful) dislocators; may be associated with psychogenic conditions and secondary gain
- Patient-reported symptoms may vary greatly depending on the preceding conditions—most importantly, traumatic versus atraumatic instability.
  - Mild discomfort with sport-specific exertion to severe pain and deficient range of motion with inability to perform activities of daily living
  - Pain is often diffuse.

Physical Examination

- In an atraumatic presentation, range of motion and strength testing may be unremarkable.
- With symptomatic recurrent subluxation, pain and/or instability can be reproduced by placing the arm in the vulnerable position of forward flexion, adduction, and internal rotation.
- Patients with atraumatic posterior instability will often demonstrate a posterior dimple sign, a small skin indentation found over the posterior shoulder, 1 cm

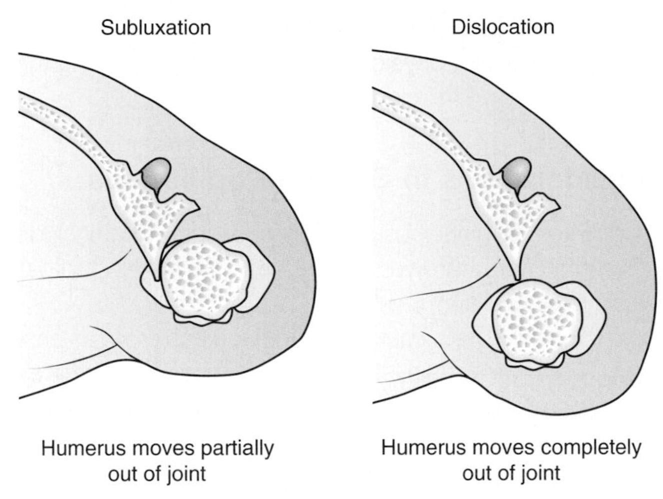

Figure 32-1 Posterior instability.

medial and inferior to the posterior angle of the acromion.
- When evaluating for posterior laxity, keep in mind that as many as 65% of female athletes and 50% of male athletes without a history of pain or trauma may possess posterior subluxation on examination.
- Tests for recurrent instability include the apprehension, sulcus sign, and jerk tests.
- Patients should be evaluated for generalized ligamentous laxity.
  - Elbow hyperextension greater than 10 degrees
  - Genu recurvatum greater than 19 degrees
  - Thumb sign: ability to touch both thumbs to the ipsilateral forearm
- Traumatic presentation may lack obvious physical deformity.
- The affected arm is often positioned in adduction and internal rotation across the abdomen.
- Forward flexion, external rotation, and forearm supination are often severely limited.
- A prominent coracoid may be found with a posterior fullness from the displaced humeral head.
- Pain may involve the long head of the biceps muscle, the rotator cuff, and the periarticular musculature.
- The severity of posterior instability is based on the degree of translation of the humeral head in relation to the glenoid.
  - Grade 0: no detectable translation
  - Grade 1+: humeral head movement up to but not over the glenoid rim
  - Grade 2+: translation over the rim with spontaneous reduction
  - Grade 3+: locked dislocation upon removal of the translating force

Imaging

- Posterior dislocation can be overlooked if only anteroposterior views are obtained. It is important to obtain lateral view(s) as well.
- Lateral view options: axillary lateral, trans-scapular, Y view
- The West Point view, a modified axillary view, and the Stryker notch view serve as more specific options to assess for bony abnormalities of the glenoid (e.g., Bankart lesions) and the humeral head (e.g., Hill-Sachs deformities), respectively.
- Pain associated with acute dislocations can make standard axial views difficult; apical oblique, Velpeau, or modified axial radiographs are often possible to obtain while the patient's arm is still in a sling.
- If appropriate axillary views are not possible, CT scan is indicated to make the diagnosis.
- MRI with arthrography may be used for more detailed assessment of the soft tissues, with attention given to the possibility of a reverse Bankart lesion, associated with traumatic dislocations.
  - Reverse Bankart lesion: tear of the posteroinferior aspect of the capsulolabral complex
- Glenoid morphology can be assessed with CT or MRI; the best detail may be found in using CT with intra-articular contrast.

Differential Diagnosis

- Rotator cuff injury
- Impingement
- Labral tear
- Glenohumeral arthritis
- Suprascapular and long thoracic nerve entrapment/palsies
- Scapular winging (may be found along with posterior instability)
- A chronic posterior dislocation may be interpreted as a frozen shoulder.

Treatment

- At diagnosis
  - Avoid any painful or inciting activities and motions.
  - Acute dislocations will often require reduction under anesthesia.
- Later
  - Atraumatic instability and first-time dislocators: rehabilitation with emphasis on the rotator cuff

(particularly external rotators), posterior deltoid muscle, and periscapular musculature
- Educate patients to avoid voluntary dislocation.

When to Refer

- Failure to reduce an acute dislocation
- Axillary nerve injury
- Failure to improve with 6 months of therapy; recurrent pain or dislocations
- Nonoperative treatment may be attempted for posterior dislocations that are diagnosed within 6 weeks of injury and have a humeral head defect of less than 20%.
  - Guided reduction in a closed manner with the necessary level of sedation may be required.

Prognosis

- Sixty-five percent to 80% of patients can be treated nonsurgically.
- Risks for recurrent instability and failed nonsurgical treatment include a traumatic event (especially in the presence of a reverse Bankart lesion), younger age, and increased time from onset to diagnosis.

Troubleshooting

- With traumatic dislocation, be aware of possible brachial plexus lesions or fractures of the humeral surgical neck, tuberosities, or glenoid rim.
- Voluntary recurrent posterior instability is classically associated with psychogenic disorders and secondary gain.

Patient Instructions

- A full return to activity and long-term function is more likely with dedication to physical therapy and home rehabilitation programs.
- Avoid any voluntary dislocation.
- Do not attempt physical exertion directly involving the affected arm until cleared.

Considerations in Special Populations

- Athletes at higher risk of posterior instability include weight lifters, throwers, racket sport athletes, football players, and swimmers.
  - Return-to-play guidelines include achieving at least 90% of normal strength and motion as well as performing the sport-specific activity without pain.
- Patients older than 40 years with a traumatic injury are prone to rotator cuff tears.
- In patients who are elderly, have limited disability, or have low functional expectations, nonsurgical rehabilitation is typically the standard of care.

Suggested Reading

- Antoniou J, Harryman D: Posterior instability. Orthop Clin North Am 2001;32:463–473.
- Millett PJ, Clavert P, Hatch GF 3rd, Warner JJ: Recurrent posterior shoulder instability. J Am Acad Orthop Surg 2006;14:464–476.
- Petersen S: Posterior shoulder instability. Orthop Clin North Am 2000;31:263–274.
- Robinson C, Aderinto J: Posterior shoulder dislocations and fracture-dislocations. J Bone Joint Surg Am 2005;87A:639–651.
- Steinmann S: Posterior shoulder instability. Arthroscopy 2003;19(1 Suppl):102–105.

Chapter 33 Multidirectional Shoulder Instability

Marc De Jong

Key Concepts

- Classically defined as shoulder instability in all directions; commonly used to encompass bidirectional instability as well (Fig. 33-1)
- Diagnostic criteria, specificity of physical examination findings, and treatment recommendations are somewhat variable.
- The term *laxity* refers to the ability to sublux or dislocate the joint, whereas the term *instability* is reserved for situations in which the laxity is also symptomatic.
- May be classified as congenital, single traumatic onset, or recurrent microtrauma
  - Congenital cases often present at an earlier age and are commonly bilateral
  - Microtraumatic, overuse injuries are common in the athletic population.
- Increased shoulder laxity may be an independent risk factor for symptomatic instability.
- The primary pathologic issue seems to be generalized laxity of the shoulder capsule (Fig. 33-2).
  - Other contributing factors include deficient shoulder proprioception and muscle control; biomechanical abnormalities; and irregular bony, labral, and ligamentous anatomy.
- It is possible, although rare, for multidirectional instability to be present in the absence of hyperlaxity; this may be found in an individual with multiple traumatic events leading to instability in multiple directions.

History

- The onset of symptoms may or may not be related to an injury or recurrent traumatic events.
- Chief symptoms reported are often vague, including pain, fatigue, and sense of apprehension.
  - A presenting symptom of actual instability is less common.
- Voluntary dislocators can demonstrate instability on their own, in either one or multiple directions; this usually develops before skeletal maturity and is less commonly associated with trauma.
- Atraumatic instability may be associated with connective tissue disorders such as Marfan syndrome or Ehlers-Danlos syndrome
- Symptoms are common in the mid-range of shoulder range of motion and may affect activities of daily living.
- Associated with repetitive overhead activities including swimming, gymnastics, and baseball pitching
  - Athletes may present with indistinct symptoms of decreased performance, lack of confidence in shoulder function, or painful execution of shoulder activity.

Physical Examination

- The examination should start with the contralateral shoulder for comparative laxity and for enhanced patient understanding.
- The presence of multidirectional instability should be evaluated after traumatic dislocation of any nature, when pain allows.
- Tests for recurrent instability include apprehension testing, the sulcus sign, and the jerk test.
- Shoulder laxity testing should include the anterior and posterior drawers.
- Assessment for generalized ligamentous laxity should be performed
  - Elbow hyperextension greater than 10 degrees
  - Genu recurvatum greater than 19 degrees
  - Thumb sign: ability to touch both thumbs to the ipsilateral forearm
- The presence of laxity alone on physical examination is not sufficient to diagnose multidirectional instability, as subluxation of the humeral head on the glenoid rim should be symptomatic (on examination and during activity) for further treatment to be considered.

Imaging

- Standard radiographs for multidirectional instability may include scapular anteroposterior with external rotation of the humeral head, true anteroposterior with

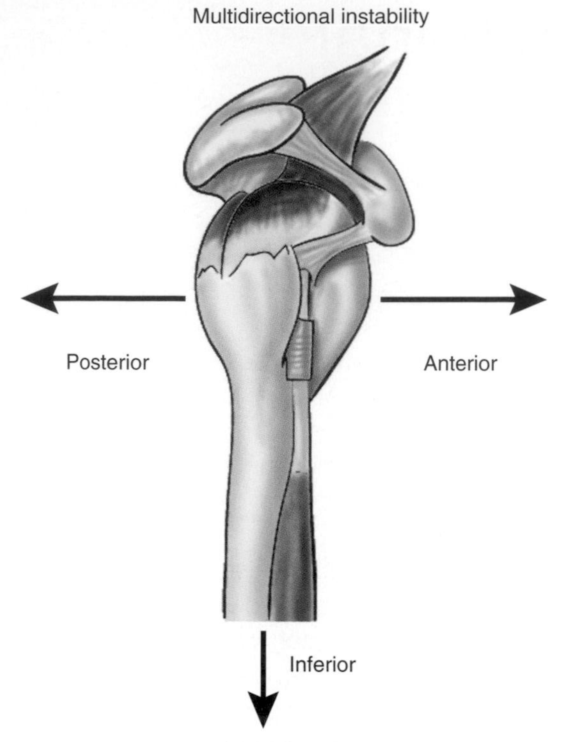

Figure 33-1 Multidirectional instability.

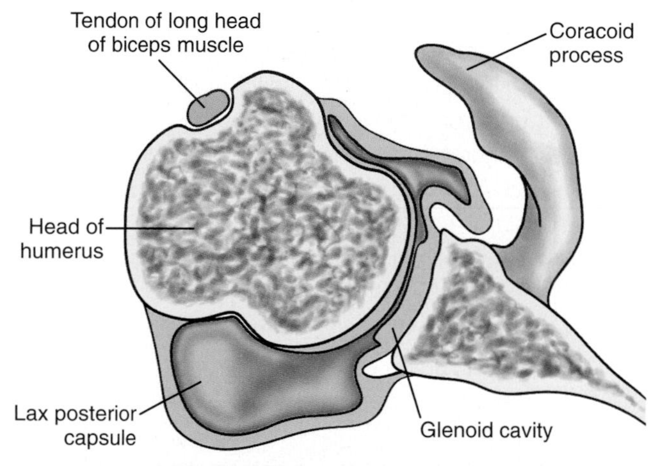

Figure 33-2 Axial view of shoulder anatomy depicting excessive laxity of posterior capsule.

internal rotation, West Point, and Stryker notch views.
  - West Point and Stryker notch views are more sensitive to assess for bony abnormalities of the glenoid (e.g., Bankart lesion) and the humeral head (e.g., Hill-Sachs lesion), respectively.
- Normal radiographs do not exclude a diagnosis of multidirectional instability.
- Computed tomography may be used for detailed evaluation of bony anatomy, which may be appropriate after traumatic events.
- Magnetic resonance imaging with arthrography may be considered for further assessment of a labral injury, if suspected.

Differential Diagnosis

- Rotator cuff injury
- Impingement
- Labral tear
- Suprascapular and long thoracic nerve entrapment/palsies
- Cervical radiculopathy
- Scapular winging
- Glenohumeral or acromioclavicular arthritis

Treatment

- At diagnosis
  - Relative rest and activity modification to aid pain control
  - Temporary use of nonsteroidal anti-inflammatory drugs for pain control
  - Gentle, pain-free range of motion therapy is encouraged.
- Later
  - Rehabilitation that emphasizes strengthening and improved tone and coordination of the deltoid, rotator cuff, pectoralis major, and periscapular musculature
  - Important to incorporate assessment and correction of abnormal scapular motion
  - Reconditioning, particularly in athletes, should include core training.

When to Refer

- Failure to improve with 6 to 12 months of therapy with recurrent pain or dislocations
  - Some recent studies have noted that individuals treated successfully without surgery tend to demonstrate significant improvement within 3 months of rehabilitation.
  - Axillary nerve injury
  - Surgery is commonly deferred in patients who have not reached full skeletal maturity.

Prognosis

- As many as 20% of patients may require surgical intervention.

- Surgical correction holds better promise for athletes with single shoulder involvement, whereas bilateral repairs are less successful.
- Patients of high school and college age may fare worse than an older patient population, although it is unknown whether this is due to higher physical demands or a natural history of improvement of instability with age.
- Voluntary dislocators are typically poor surgical candidates.
- When surgery is indicated, an inferior capsular shift repair is usually the intervention of choice.
  - Isolated thermal capsulorrhaphy has largely fallen out of favor.

Troubleshooting

- Preceding trauma should be properly evaluated for the presence of fractures.
- Rarely, secondary bursitis or tendonitis may cause difficulty in rehabilitation efforts.
  - Treat with oral nonsteroidal anti-inflammatory drugs or a subacromial corticosteroid injection.

Patient Instructions

- Full return to activity and long-term function is more likely with dedication to physical therapy and home rehabilitation programs.
- Avoid any voluntary dislocation.
- Do not attempt physical exertion of the affected arm until properly cleared.

Considerations in Special Populations

- Return-to-play guidelines for athletes have been more thoroughly studied in anterior dislocation; recommendations include achieving at least 90% of normal strength and motion as well as performing sport-specific activity without pain.
- Athletes who use overhead throwing motions, particularly pitchers, with instability require extra attention to rehabilitation of lower extremity and core musculature as an element of their return to activity.
- Less common in older populations; nonsurgical treatment is standard

Suggested Reading

- Choi C, Ogilvie-Harris D: Inferior capsular shift operation for multidirectional instability of the shoulder in players of contact sports. Br J Sports Med 2002;36:290–294.
- Gerber C, Nyffeler R: Classification of glenohumeral joint instability. Clin Orthop Relat Res 2002;400:65–76.
- Levine W, Prickett WD, Prymka M, et al: Treatment of the athlete with multidirectional shoulder instability. Orthop Clin North Am 2003;32:475–484.
- Misamore G, Sallay PI, Didelot W, et al: A longitudinal study of patients with multidirectional instability of the shoulder with seven- to ten-year follow-up. J Shoulder Elbow Surg 2005;14:466–470.
- Remia L, Revalin RV, Lemly KS, et al: Biomechanical evaluation of multidirectional glenohumeral instability and repair. Clin Orthop Relat Res 2003;416:225–236.
- Richards R: The diagnostic definition of multidirectional instability of the shoulder: Searching for direction. J Bone Joint Surg Am 2005;85A:2145–2146.

Chapter 34 The Overhead Throwing Athlete

John R. Hatzenbuehler and William Dexter

Key Concepts

- The overhead throw involves complex motions through the shoulder, elbow, and wrist.
- Proper mechanics involve distribution of energy through a kinetic chain from the lower extremity push-off, to pelvic and torso rotation, and into elbow extension and shoulder rotation.
- Lower extremity propulsion and body rotation produce 50% of the velocity of a throw.
- Weak leg and core strength necessitates increased shoulder forces to achieve high velocities. This places the thrower at increased risk of injury.
- Extreme forces placed on the shoulder and elbow during repetitive throws often cause microtrauma to the surrounding soft tissues leading to overuse injuries.
- A football pass differs from a baseball pitch
  - Decreased range of motion
  - Lower joint forces
  - Lower velocity
- Football injuries are typically from trauma; baseball injuries are typically due to overuse.
- The throw is generally divided into six phases
  - Wind-up
  - Early arm cocking (stride)
  - Late arm cocking
  - Arm acceleration
  - Arm deceleration
  - Follow-through
- Wind-up and early arm cocking phases
  - These stages use very little energy.
  - The wind-up phase begins with the throw initiation and ends as the stride leg moves toward the target (Fig. 34-1A and B).
  - The early arm cocking phase (or stride phase) begins with the stride and ends when the foot contacts the ground (see Fig. 34-1C).
  - The hind foot pushes off, and the pelvis and torso rotate to move the thrower toward the target.
  - Almost no injuries occur during the early phases of throwing.
- Late arm cocking phase
  - Begins as the stride foot contacts the ground and ends as shoulder internal rotation begins (Fig. 34-2A)
  - Maximal external rotation occurs.
  - The inferior glenohumeral ligament and the long head of the biceps muscle prevent anterior translation of the humeral head.
  - The rotator cuff muscles contract to center the humeral head on the glenoid.
  - Strong valgus forces applied to medial elbow

Pathology

- Extreme external rotation can cause anterior laxity of the glenohumeral joint capsule leading to instability and impingement.
- Internal impingement syndrome: anterior instability during external rotation causes the rotator cuff tendons and the labrum to be pinched between the greater tuberosity of the humeral head and the posterosuperior glenoid.
- Internal impingement may lead to a variety of problems
  - Rotator cuff tendon fraying
  - Chondromalacia of the humeral head
  - Superior labrum anteroposterior lesions/tears
- Glenohumeral internal rotation deficits caused by posterior capsular tightness can also contribute to internal impingement.
- Glenohumeral internal rotation deficits should be suspected if internal rotation range of motion is decreased in the throwing arm compared with the nonthrowing arm (Fig. 34-3).
- The etiology of glenohumeral internal rotation deficits is unknown.
- Anterior laxity can increase strain on the biceps tendon causing bicipital tendonitis (see Chapter 31).
- The elbow placed in a maximal valgus position can cause medial elbow pain if an underlying pathology is present.

- Acceleration phase
  - Most forceful phase
  - Begins with shoulder internal rotation and ends with ball release (see Fig. 34-2B)
  - Large rotational torque placed on the soft tissues of the shoulder
  - Elbow extension begins, causing increased elbow forces.
  - Ulnar collateral ligament is under maximal valgus stress, preventing elbow instability.

Pathology

- Subacromial impingement may occur as the humerus is internally rotated (see Chapter 38).
- Younger pitchers typically have internal impingement, whereas older pitchers tend to have subacromial impingement.
- Extreme elbow forces cause medial tension and posterior/lateral compression injuries.
- Medial injuries
  - Ulnar collateral ligament damage (see Chapter 62)
  - Medial epicondyle apophysitis (little league elbow)
  - Flexor-pronator mass strain
  - Ulnar neuritis (see Chapter 65)
- Lateral and posterior compression injuries
  - Valgus extension overload syndrome, excessive compressive force of olecranon in the olecranon fossa; should be considered especially with range of motion deficits
  - Olecranon osteophyte formation secondary to valgus extension overload syndrome causing posterior olecranon impingement
  - Osteochondritis desiccans lesions of the capitellum or radial head (see Chapter 57)

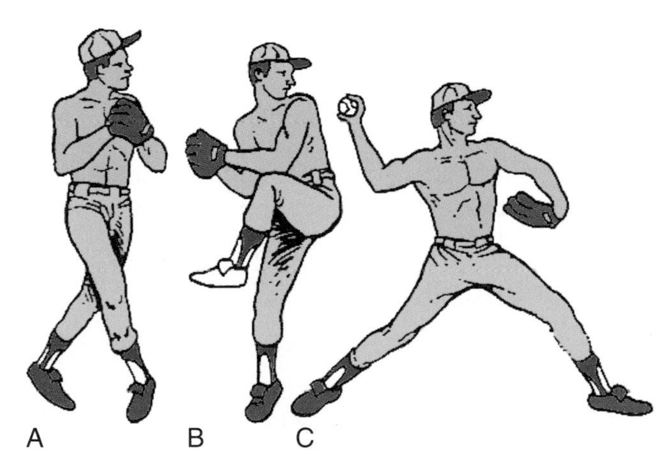

Figure 34-1 The sequence of motion of the early phases of throwing from throw initiation (**A**), to the windup (**B**), and then into the early cocking phase (**C**). (Adapted from Park S, Loebenberg ML, Rokito AS, Zuckerman J: The shoulder in baseball pitching: Biomechanics and related injuries—part 1. Bull Hosp Joint Dis 2002–2003;61:68–79.)

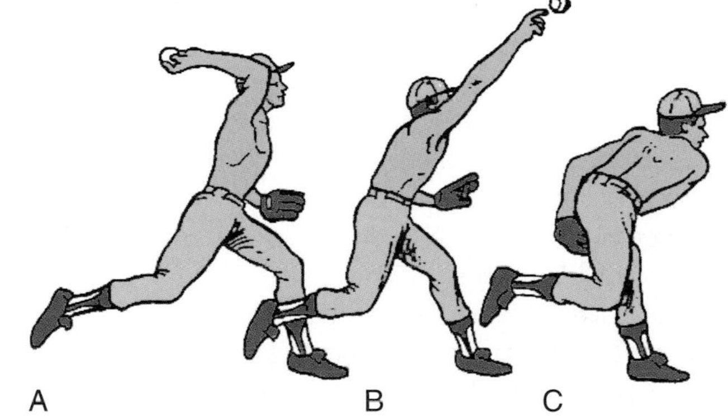

Figure 34-2 The sequence of motion of the late phases of throwing from the late cocking phase (**A**), to the acceleration phase (**B**), and ending with the deceleration phase and follow-through (**C**). (Adapted from Park S, Loebenberg ML, Rokito AS, Zuckerman J: The shoulder in baseball pitching: Biomechanics and related injuries—part 1. Bull Hosp Joint Dis 2002–2003;61:68–79.)

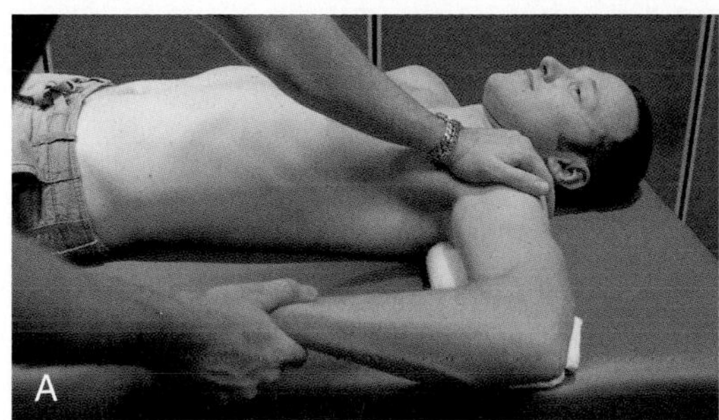

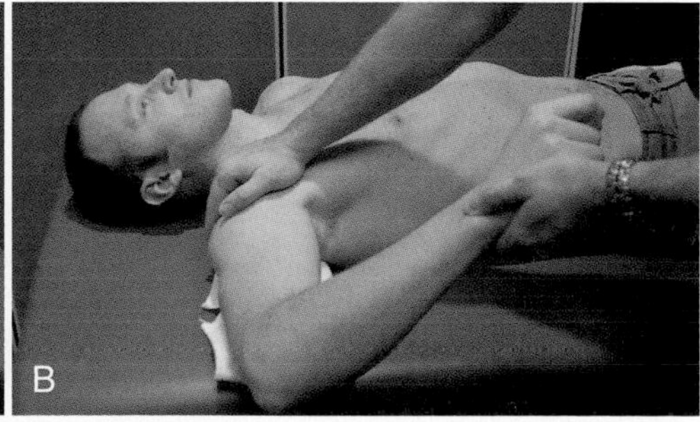

Figure 34-3 The physical examination of a right-handed throwing patient with glenohumeral internal rotation deficit. **A,** The left side depicts normal left shoulder glenohumeral internal rotation. **B,** The right side shows an approximately 30-degree internal rotation limitation of the right shoulder.

  - Intra-articular loose bodies
  - Olecranon apophysitis or triceps tendon avulsion
- Deceleration phase
  - Begins at ball release and ends when shoulder reaches maximal internal rotation (see Fig. 34-2C)
  - Dissipates excess energy from acceleration phase
  - Rotator cuff muscles contract to oppose internal rotation and glenohumeral distraction.
  - Large traction force applied to the long head of the biceps to decelerate extending elbow
- Laxity can develop in the posterior shoulder capsule as microtears occur during resisted glenohumeral distraction.
- Posterior laxity produces instability and painful glenohumeral subluxation (see Chapter 32).
- Eccentric rotator cuff forces may eventually lead to tears (see Chapter 39).
- Tears may occur even in the absence of impingement.
- Because the long head of the biceps muscle attaches to the superior labrum, repetitive traction can produce superior labrum anteroposterior lesions as the labrum is pulled off the glenoid (see Chapter 35).
- Superior labrum anteroposterior lesions often occur concomitantly with rotator cuff tears.
- Forceful hyperextension of the elbow can lead to anterior capsule strains.
- Excessive elbow extension may also produce avulsion injuries of the lateral epicondyle apophysis.
- Follow-through phase
  - Begins at maximal shoulder internal rotation and ends when thrower returns to a balanced stance (see Fig. 34-2C)
  - Arm adducted across the body
  - The body flexes and a long follow-through path helps dissipate deceleration force.
  - No primary injuries occur during this phase; however, the thrower may experience elbow pain if posterior impingement is limiting full elbow extension.

Treatment

- At diagnosis
  - In most cases, activity modification/limit throwing
  - Formal physical therapy
    - — Disease-specific exercises (see related chapters)
    - — Preservation of full shoulder and elbow range of motion
    - — Biomechanical and kinetic chain evaluation imperative
- Later
  - May need adjustment in throwing motion
    - — Formal throwing assessment to identify poor mechanics is recommended.
  - Maintenance strengthening program to prevent muscular fatigue
  - Glenohumeral internal rotation deficits treatment focused on restoring internal rotation
    - — Affected arm abducted 90 degrees and externally rotated 90 degrees, and elbow flexed 90 degrees; contralateral arm applies internal rotation force to throwing arm to stretch out contracted posterior glenohumeral ligament

Troubleshooting

- Weak core and lower extremity strength increases shoulder and elbow stress leading to frequent injury.
- Evaluating the complete kinetic chain for abnormalities can provide insight into the cause of the injury.
- Following pitch count restriction will help prevent many overuse injuries.
- Resting between throwing episodes is essential to avoid repetitive soft-tissue microtrauma.

Patient Instructions

- Follow defined pitch count restrictions, which are provided according to age.
- Learning proper throwing mechanics will help avoid increased shoulder and elbow strain, which can lead to injury.
- Notify a physician early if a problem occurs to limit serious injury.

Suggested Reading

- Ahmad C, El Atttrache N: Valgus extension overload syndrome and stress injury of the olecranon. Clin Sports Med 2004; 23:665–676.
- Cain E, Dugas R, Wolf R, Andrews J: Elbow injuries in throwing athletes: A current concepts review. Am J Sports Med 2003; 31:621–635.
- Jobe C, Coen M, Screnar P: Evaluation of impingement syndrome in the overhead-throwing athlete. J Athletic Train 2000;35:293–299.
- Meyers J, Laudner KG, Pasquale MR, et al: Glenohumeral range of motion deficits and posterior shoulder tightness in throwers with pathologic internal impingement. Am J Sports Med 2006; 34:385–391.

- Park P, Loebenberg ML, Rokito AS, Zuckerman J: The shoulder in baseball pitching: Biomechanics and related injuries—part 1. Bull Hosp Joint Dis 2002–2003;61:68–79.
- Park P, Loebenberg ML, Rokito AS, Zuckerman J: The shoulder in baseball pitching: Biomechanics and related injuries—part 2. Bull Hosp Joint Dis 2002–2003;61:80–88.
- Zheng N, Fleisig G, Barrenine S, Andrews J: Biomechanics of pitching. In Hung G, Pallis JM (eds): Biomechanical Engineering Principles in Sports. New York: Kluwer Academic/Plenum Publishers, 2004, pp 209–256.

Chapter 35 Superior Labral Injuries

Kevin deWeber

Key Concepts

- Superior labral injuries are commonly described as SLAP (superior labral tears anteroposterior direction) tears and are located at the superior aspect of the glenoid labrum in the shoulder joint.
- The incidence in the general population is unknown; it is present in 6% of shoulders that undergo arthroscopy for pain.
- Anatomy of the superior labrum
  - Anatomic variations exist and can consist of simply a fold attached circumferentially to the glenoid rim or a partially separated meniscal structure (Fig. 35-1); the tissue is more fibrous than cartilaginous.
  - The biceps tendon enters the shoulder joint anterosuperiorly, and its fibers blend into the superior labrum before it inserts on the supraglenoid tubercle.
- Injuries can take the form of fraying of the superior labrum, torn flaps of labrum, partial detachments of the biceps tendon insertion, or combinations of the above.
- Classification of these injuries is confusing, with as many as 10 subtypes based on appearance during arthroscopy, but four classic types are most commonly found (Fig. 35-2). Classification is probably best simplified to
  - Injuries in which the biceps tendon anchor is intact
  - Those in which the biceps anchor is detached from the labrum (Fig. 35-3)

History

- Patients report pain deep in the shoulder, often increased with overhead activities.
- Patients may have mechanical symptoms such as increased popping, catching, and grinding.
- Throwing athletes and swimmers are at high risk but often cannot point to a specific time of injury.
- Injuries can occur by several mechanisms.
  - Acute injuries from falling on an outstretched arm, motor vehicle accidents, and forceful traction (e.g., dislocations, pulling on a heavy object, waterskiing injuries)
  - Chronic injuries in throwing athletes, probably due to repetitive stress on the biceps anchor during the follow-through phase of the throw when forces are greatest
- Increased index of suspicion in patients with persistent shoulder pain despite conservative treatment of other shoulder injuries such as acromioclavicular joint pain, impingement syndrome, rotator cuff tendinitis, and bicipital tendinitis

Physical Examination

- Diagnosis of superior labral injuries by physical examination is difficult due to poor sensitivity and specificity of the physical findings.
- Several diagnostic maneuvers have been described in the literature, but none are considered accurate enough to be used as the sole basis of diagnosis.
- The most commonly performed tests are
  - Active compression (O'Brien's) test
    - The patient forward flexes the arm 90 degrees with the elbow in full extension, adducts 10 to 15 degrees, and internally rotates the arm so that the thumb points downward.
    - Have the patient resist downward pressure by the examiner on the arm, and note the level of pain.
    - Repeat the downward pressure with the palm now supinated, and again note the level of pain.
    - The test is positive if pain is reduced or eliminated when the arm is in the supinated position compared with the internally rotated position (Fig. 35-4).
  - Anterior slide (Kibler's) test
    - The patient puts hands on hips with thumbs pointing backward, and the examiner applies an axially directed force through the humerus from the elbow toward the anterosuperior shoulder, using the other hand on the anterior aspect of the shoulder as counterpressure.

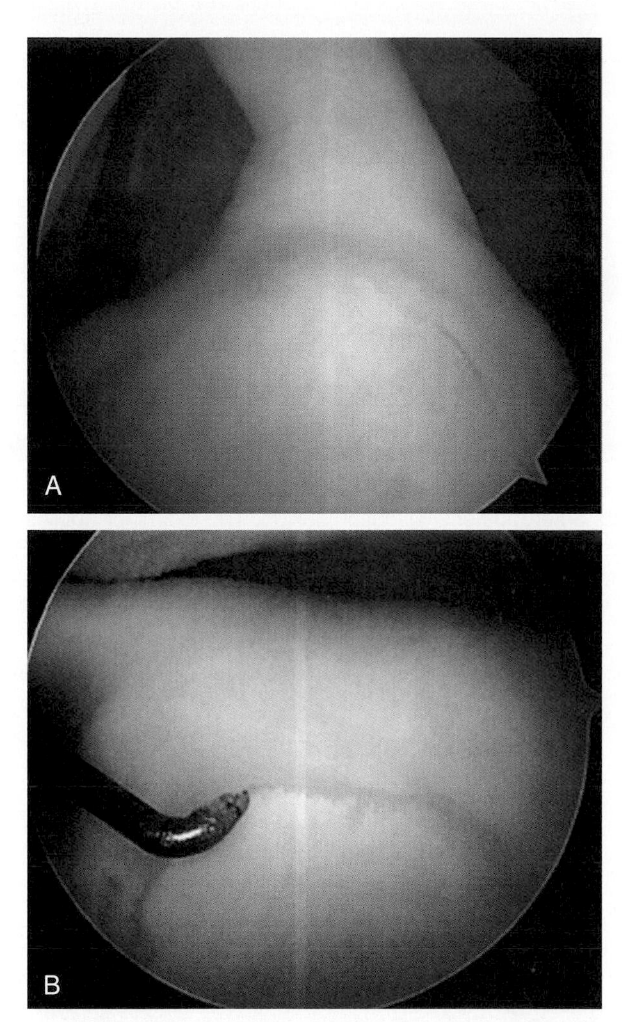

Figure 35-1 Arthroscopy picture of two common types of glenoid labrum. **A,** Labrum continuous with articular cartilage. **B,** Labrum has a meniscus-like structure. (From DeLee JC, Drez D Jr, Miller MD [eds]: DeLee and Drez's Orthopaedic Sports Medicine, 2nd ed. Philadelphia: Saunders, 2003, p 1047, Fig. 21K-2.).

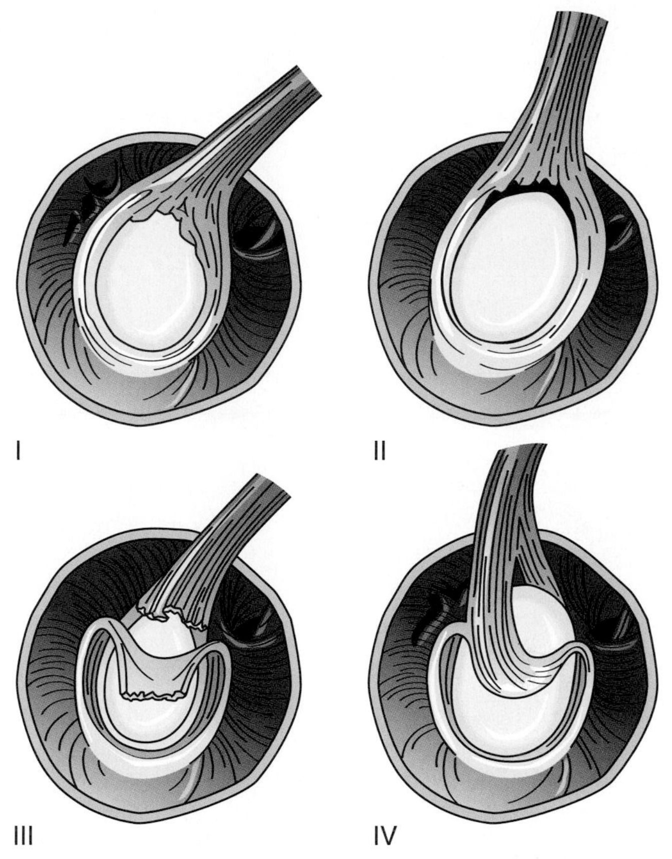

Figure 35-2 Original Snyder classification of SLAP (superior labral tears anteroposterior direction) lesions. Types II and IV involve detachment of the biceps anchor. (Adapted from Snyder SJ, Karzel RP, Del Pizzo W, et al: SLAP lesions of the shoulder. Arthroscopy 1990;6:274–279, Fig. 21K-8.)

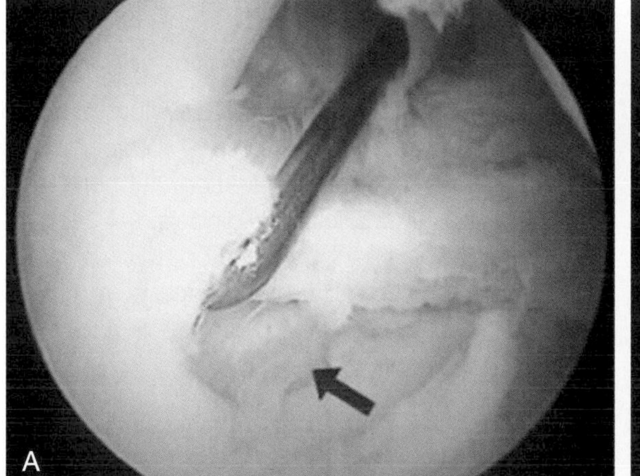

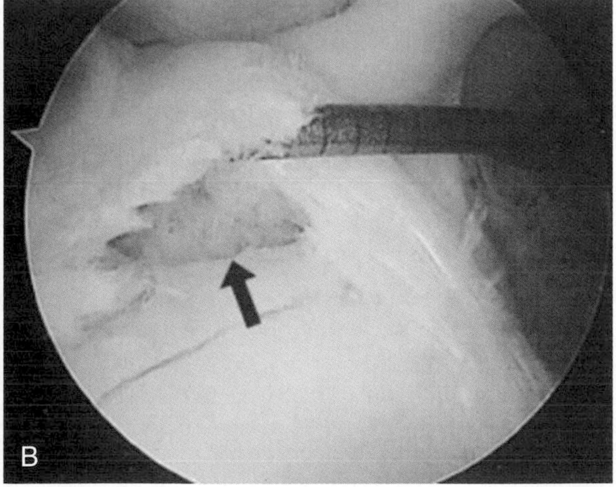

Figure 35-3 Biceps anchor is detached from the labrum. (From DeLee JC, Drez D Jr, Miller MD [eds]: DeLee and Drez's Orthopaedic Sports Medicine, 2nd ed. Philadelphia: Saunders, 2003, p 1051, Fig. 21K-10.)

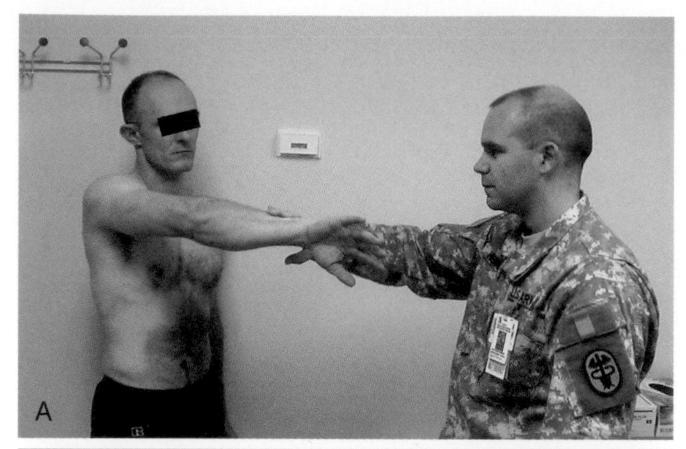

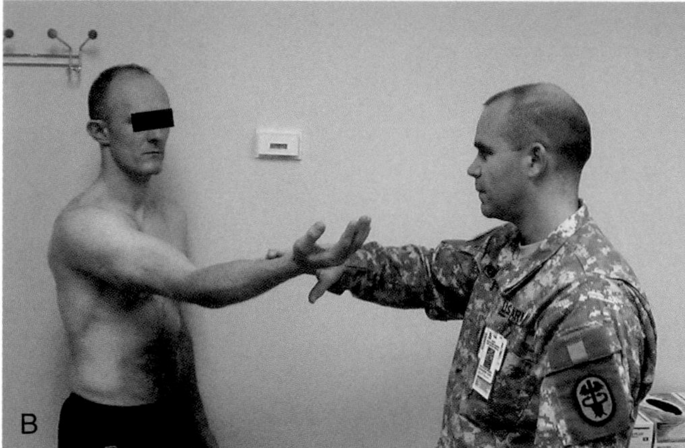

Figure 35-4 **A,** Part 1 of O'Brien's test. The patient resists downward pressure and notes the level of pain produced. **B,** Part 2 of O'Brien's test. The patient resists downward pressure and notes the level of pain produced. If pain in this second position is less than in the first position, the test is considered positive.

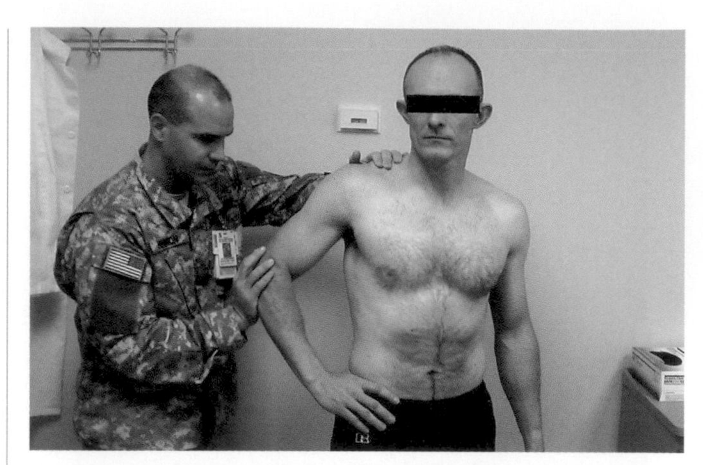

Figure 35-5 Anterior slide test for a SLAP (superior labral tears anteroposterior direction) lesion. The examiner applies pressure through the humerus; pain is suggestive of a SLAP lesion.

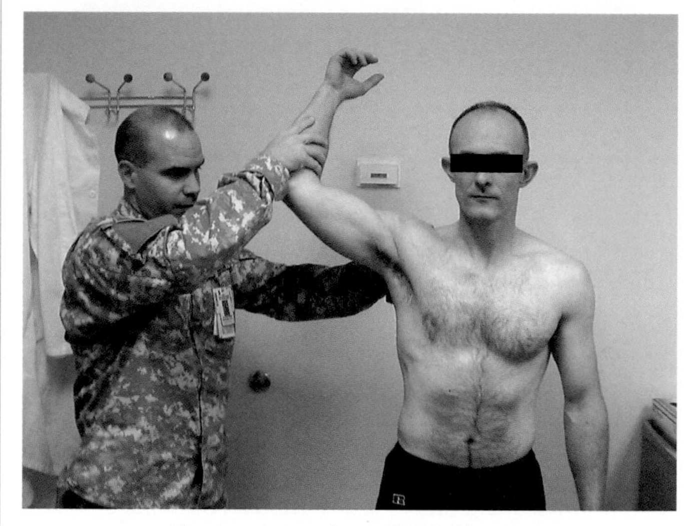

Figure 35-6 The crank test for a SLAP (superior labral tears anteroposterior direction) lesion. The examiner applies pressure axially through the humerus as the arm is internally and externally rotated. Pain or a painful click is suggestive of a SLAP lesion.

    — The test is positive if this elicits pain or popping (Fig. 35-5).
  - Crank test
    — With the patient standing, the examiner elevates the arm to 160 degrees in the scapular plane and applies an axial force through the humerus as the glenohumeral joint is passively rotated internally and externally.
    — The test is positive if this elicits pain or reproduces mechanical symptoms (Fig. 35-6).
- Clinicians should become familiar with several diagnostic maneuvers. Although they are not completely accurate, if one or more is positive, it should raise the suspicion of this injury and prompt further evaluation.

Imaging

- Plain radiography is usually normal but can be useful after acute trauma to rule out concomitant bony injuries and in chronic pain to evaluate for coexistent osseous pathologies such as acromioclavicular or glenohumeral joint degeneration, abnormally hooked acromion, and calcific tendinosis.
- Gadolinium-enhanced MRI or MR arthrography are preferred. Each modality has approximately 80% sensitivity and 98% specificity. There is suboptimal sensitivity with nonenhanced MRI.

Additional Tests

- There are no additional tests, but arthroscopy is the gold standard for diagnosis; often superior labral inju-

TABLE 35-1 *Differential Diagnosis*

Condition	Differentiating Feature	Chapter Reference
Rotator cuff tendinitis	May have tenderness focused on lateral shoulder just distal to acromion; impingement signs most prominent	38
Rotator cuff tear	May have pain with empty can maneuver and tenderness just distal to acromion, in addition to impingement signs	39
Anterior or posterior labral tears	Symptoms more commonly reproduced by maneuvers placing stress on the anterior labrum (apprehension test) or posterior labrum (posterior drawer test)	N/A
Acromioclavicular joint pathology	Localized tenderness over acromioclavicular joint; usually no mechanical symptoms; pain with cross-chest adduction	42–44
Shoulder instability	May have positive test(s) for instability or history of dislocation	31–33

ries are discovered during arthroscopy for chronic shoulder pain due to other causes.

Differential Diagnosis (Table 35-1)

- Almost 90% of patients with superior labral injuries have other coexisting shoulder injuries. The most common are
  - Rotator cuff tendinitis or tears
  - Shoulder instability and Bankart lesions
  - Bicipital tendinitis
  - Acromioclavicular joint degeneration
  - Glenohumeral joint degeneration

Treatment

- At diagnosis
  - Initiate a supervised rehabilitation program including rotator cuff and scapular stabilizer muscle strengthening, increased shoulder flexibility, and gradual return to activities.
  - Judicious use of analgesics may be worthwhile, although they have no healing properties.
  - There is no proof of efficacy of conservative management in healing superior labral injuries, but it is often helpful to improve function and will aid in preparation for surgical treatment, if needed.
- Later
  - Surgery is usually needed if pain or dysfunction persists.

When to Refer

- Pain that persists despite 3 months of conservative therapy
- Earlier referral is indicated for high-level athletes or high-demand laborers whose rapid return to participation is necessary.

Prognosis

- After surgical repair, throwing athletes can return to full activity after approximately 7 months.
- Nonthrowing athletes can return to their sports about four months after surgery.

Troubleshooting

- During conservative treatment, close follow-up is warranted to monitor progress.
- The inaccuracy of physical examination and suboptimal sensitivity of nonenhanced MRI make this a commonly missed diagnosis, so a high index of suspicion is needed.

Patient Instructions

- Proper rehabilitation will increase range of motion and strength, thereby improving function in activities; consistency and dedication are paramount.
- Regular follow-up is important to monitor progress and to facilitate referral if progress is not adequate.
- Superior labral injuries involve tissue with poor vascularity, making healing slow and incomplete in many cases and necessitating surgery in a high percentage of patients.

Suggested Reading

- Barber FA, Field LD, Ryu KN: Biceps tendon and superior labrum injuries: Decision-making. J Bone Joint Surg Am 2007;89A:1844–1855.

- Jones GL, Galluch DB: Clinical assessment of superior glenoid labral lesions. Clin Orthop Relat Res 2007;45:45–51.
- Kim TK, Queale WS, Cosgarea AJ, McFarland EG: Clinical features of the different types of SLAP lesions: An analysis of one hundred and thirty-nine cases. J Bone Joint Surg Am 2003;85A: 66–71.
- Maffet MW, Lowe WR: Superior labral injuries. In DeLee JC, Drez D Jr, Miller MD [eds]: DeLee and Drez's Orthopaedic Sports Medicine, 2nd ed. Philadelphia: Saunders, 2003.
- Waldt S, Burkart A, Lange P, et al: Diagnostic performance of MR arthrography in the assessment of superior labral anteroposterior lesions of the shoulder. AJR Am J Roentgenol 2004;182: 1271–1278.

Chapter 36 Biceps Tendon Injury

Robert G. Hosey and Kyle Smoot

ICD-9 CODES
727.6 *Rupture of Tendon, Nontraumatic*
727.62 *Tendons of Biceps (Long Head)*
726.12 *Bicipital Tenosynovitis*

Key Concepts

- Proximal biceps tendon injuries
  - Rupture
    - — Ninety-six percent of biceps ruptures involve the proximal long head of the biceps tendon, 3% the distal head, and 1% the short head.
    - — Most common in older individuals (ages 40–60 years), affecting more men than women
    - — Biceps tendon weakness and resultant predisposition for rupture are caused by an inflammatory process from subacromial impingement or biomechanical microtrauma.
    - — Most ruptures result in a characteristic "Popeye" muscle appearance.
  - Bicipital tendinitis
    - — An overuse syndrome caused by repetitive overload of the biceps tendon from elbow flexion and supination; often occurs with impingement syndrome (Figs. 36-1 and 36-2)

History

- Proximal biceps tendon rupture: Most patients recall a single acute injury with an audible "pop" noted by the patient. Others may report pain with overhead activities, elbow flexion and supination activities, or more vague anterior shoulder pain. Rest pain and night pain can also be associated with later progression of the disease. Pain may also be compounded by concomitant impingement syndrome or rotator cuff tendinitis.
- Bicipital tendinitis: May present as anterior shoulder pain that increases with activity involving flexion and/or supination at the elbow

Physical Examination

- Inspection: Evaluate for "Popeye" appearance of biceps muscle caused by retraction of the long head biceps tendon distally (Fig. 36-3). "Popeye" muscle can be elicited with Ludington's test (see "Special Tests"). Ecchymosis may be noted if injury is relatively acute.
- Palpation: Bony palpation of the sternoclavicular joint, acromioclavicular joint, acromion, greater tuberosity, coracoid process, and spine of scapula should be part of any examination of the patient presenting with shoulder pain. Soft-tissue palpation should include palpation of the long and short heads of the biceps muscle, the rotator cuff muscles, and the anterior and posterior capsules.
  - With bicipital tendinitis, point tenderness with palpation of long head tendon at the bicipital groove
- Range of motion: Both passive and active range of motion of the shoulder and elbow should be evaluated. In the acute setting, it may be limited secondary to pain.
- Neurovascular examination: Sensation and distal pulses of the upper extremity should be evaluated.

Special Tests

- Speed's test: Weakness with resisted forward flexion and supination indicates pathology of the long head of the biceps muscle.
- Yergason's test: The elbow is flexed at 90 degrees with the forearm in pronation with active resistance against supination. Palpation of the tendon at the bicipital groove while performing Yergason's test evaluates for tendon stability in the bicipital groove.
- Ludington's test: Patient places both hands behind head with interlocking fingers, flexing biceps muscles

Imaging

- Radiographs: Anteroposterior and axillary views are typically negative but should be obtained to evaluate

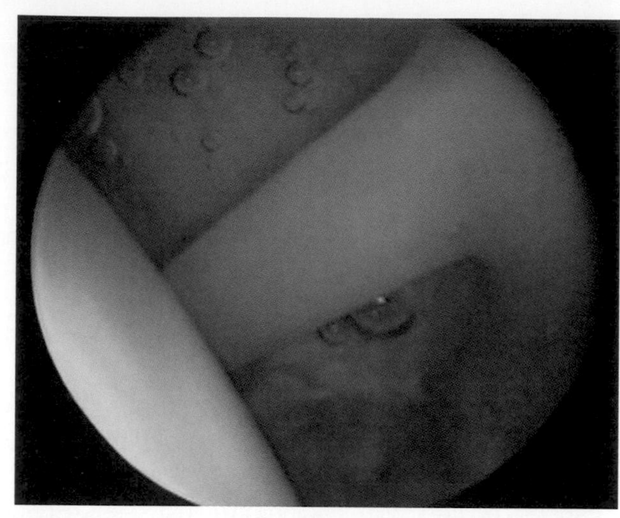

Figure 36-1 Arthroscopic view showing normal-appearing biceps tendon.

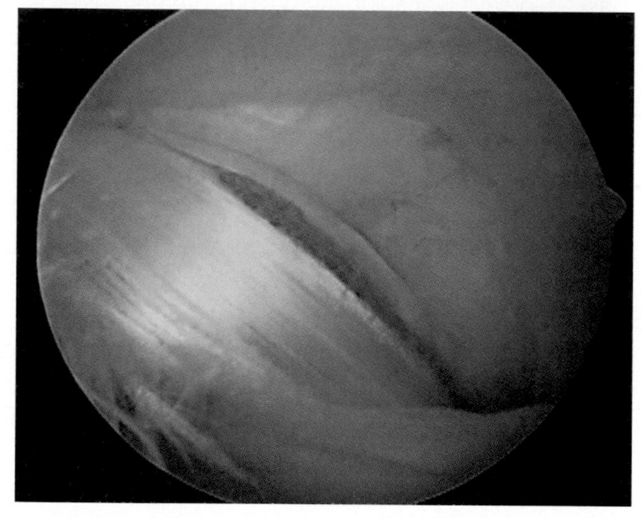

Figure 36-2 Arthroscopic view showing biceps tendinopathy and inflammation.

for acromioclavicular joint or glenohumeral bony pathology.

- Magnetic resonance imaging should be considered in young athletes and patients with persistent pain to evaluate for intra-articular pathology (associated superior labral anteroposterior lesion) as well as to evaluate for accompanying rotator cuff tear.
- Magnetic resonance imaging arthrogram can increase sensitivity of diagnosing biceps pathology; however, it is more invasive and requires experienced personnel to administer and interpret the study.
- Musculoskeletal ultrasonography for the diagnosis of biceps pathology is technically challenging and not universally available but may offer the potential for less invasive, more cost-effective, and more convenient definitive diagnosis. A recent prospective study comparing ultrasonography with arthroscopy in the diagnosis of the long head of the biceps tendon showed 100% specificity and 96% sensitivity for a diagnosis of subluxation or dislocation. Ultrasonography also was successful in diagnosing complete tears, but was not useful for diagnosing partial thickness tears.

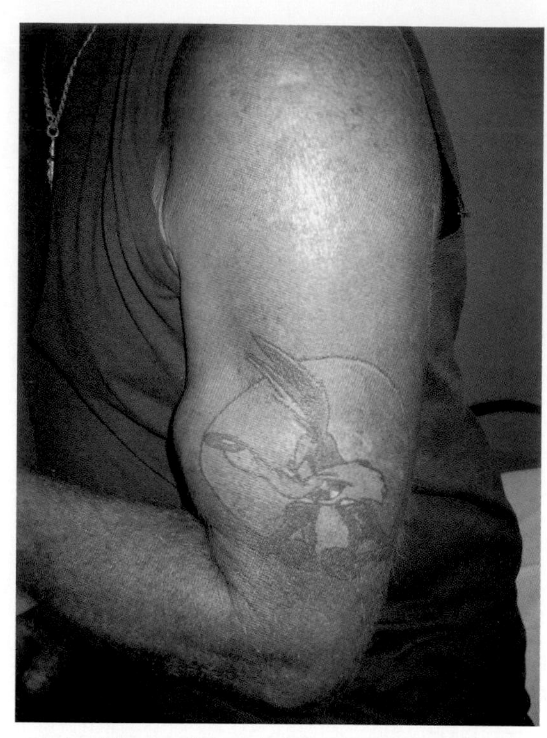

Figure 36-3 "Popeye" muscle seen in proximal biceps tendon rupture. (From Johnson DL, Mairs SD [eds]: Clinical Sports Medicine. St. Louis: Mosby, 2006, p 237.)

Differential Diagnosis

- Proximal biceps tendon rupture: biceps tendinitis, dislocated biceps tendon, distal biceps tendon rupture, glenohumeral arthritis, impingement syndrome, rotator cuff tear, pectoralis major rupture
- Bicipital tendinitis: bicipital bursitis, biceps tendon rupture, brachialis muscle tear, anterior capsule tear, lateral antebrachial cutaneous nerve compression syndrome

Treatment

- Proximal biceps tendon rupture
  - At diagnosis
    - — Relative rest with or without immobilization, control of inflammation with nonsteroidal anti-inflammatory drugs, and ice

- Biceps tendinitis
  - Relative rest, ice, nonsteroidal anti-inflammatory drugs if not otherwise contraindicated, activity modification, selected injection with informed consent of complication of tendon rupture in refractory cases.
- Later
  — Treatment is dependent on patient age and level of physical activity. Rupture of the biceps tendon usually responds to physical therapy. Conservative measures generally result in restored full range of motion and acceptable strength, with the expectation of some residual deformity. Studies have documented as much as a 20% loss of supination strength with conservative management.
  — Surgical tenodesis remains a subject of debate. A patient-centered approach including the patient's symptoms, occupation or recreational activity, and acceptance of the cosmetic deformity produced by the injury should be considered. Ideal time for repair is 2 to 3 weeks post-injury. Open surgical techniques have been well described in the past; however, arthroscopic techniques involving suture anchors, screw fixation, and screw fixation with biceps tensioning into a bony tunnel have been more recently supported.

When to Refer

- It is reasonable to consider surgical intervention for selected patient populations such as competitive athletes and young manual laborers. More recently, surgical correction has been advocated for the active patient of any age who requires high-demand supination and flexion forces. In these cases, surgical referrals should be expeditious, within 1 to 2 weeks.

Prognosis

- Generally, both conservatively and operatively managed patients do well. Research has found no difference between patients managed operatively and nonoperatively.
- In biceps tendinitis, the prognosis is generally good, depending on patient adherence to treatment.

Troubleshooting

- Counsel the patient regarding the expectations of conservative management versus the risks and benefits of surgical intervention.
- Follow-up is necessary after a trial of conservative management to address patient concerns for biceps functioning and the impact on daily life and cosmetic concerns.
- Counsel the patient regarding the expected time frame to recovery with either conservative management or surgical intervention.
- Patients undergoing local injections for conservative management for bicipital tendinitis should be provided informed consent regarding the risk of tendon rupture.

Patient Instructions

- Physical therapy for proximal biceps tendon rupture should be directed at restoring range of motion and strength.

Considerations in Special Populations

- In overhead throwing athletes, the biceps is active in deceleration of the arm and may become inflamed or lead to labral pathology from overuse if rotator cuff muscles are weak.
- Underhand throwers are at risk of biceps tendon strain but typically do not experience career-ending injuries.
- In the geriatric population, tenotomy is a reasonable treatment option after the patient has been counseled and accepts the possible deformity if the long head retracts into the arm.

Suggested Reading

- Ahmad CS, El Attrache NS: Arthroscopic biceps tenodesis. Orthop Clin North Am 2003;34:499–506.
- Aldridge JW, Bruno RJ, Strauch RJ, Rosenwasser JP: Management of acute and chronic biceps tendon rupture. Hand Clin 2000;16:497–503.
- Armstrong A, Teefey SA, Wu T, et al: The efficacy of ultrasound in the diagnosis of long head of the biceps tendon pathology. J Shoulder Elbow Surg 2006;15:7–11.
- Mariani EM, Rand JA: Subcapital fractures after open reduction and internal fixation of intertrochanteric fractures of the hip. Report of three cases. Clin Orthop Relat Res 1989;245:165–168.
- O'Conner PJ, Rankine J, Gibbon WW, et al: J Clin Ultrasound 2005;33:53–56.
- Phillips BB, Canale ST, Sisk TD, et al: Ruptures of the proximal biceps tendon in middle-aged patients. Orthop Rev 1993;22:349–353.
- Sethi N, Wright R, Yamaguchi K: Disorders of the long head of the biceps tendon. J Shoulder Elbow Surg 1999;8:644–654.

Chapter 37 Pectoralis Major Muscle Rupture

M. Brennan Royalty and Robert G. Hosey

ICD-9 CODES

840.9 *Sprain and Strain of Joint and Adjacent Muscles—Unspecified Site of Shoulder and Upper Arm*

905.8 *Late Effects of Musculoskeletal and Connective Tissue Injuries—Late Effect of Tendon Injury*

Key Concepts

- Pectoralis major muscle injuries are increasingly common in athletics. Typically, these injuries occur in males and are associated with power maneuvers such as weight lifting or tackling in rugby and American football.
- Patients present acutely with pain, swelling, and weakness of shoulder adduction and internal rotation.
- Management of the injury includes surgical and nonsurgical treatment. For the athlete, research indicates that surgical treatment offers the most complete recovery (Fig. 37-1).

History

- The patient is typically involved in power sports such as weight lifting, rugby, and football, or activities with significant risk of rapidly increasing shoulder abduction forces on the joint such as rodeo, windsurfing, and sailing.
- Injury is most common, however, in weight lifters performing bench-press exercises; injury typically occurs during the eccentric/contraction phase.
- Football players and rugby athletes may describe an anterior blow to the shoulder.
- The patient reports acute onset of burning pain experienced during sudden forceful overload of a maximally contracted pectoralis muscle.
- Patients may describe a "popping" sensation at the time of injury.
- Weight lifters may report a recent significant increase in maximum weight pressed, as in a "max-out" test or an athletic performance evaluation.
- With the exception of one documented case in a woman, injuries are limited to the male population.
- The patient expresses weakness of internal rotation and adduction.

Physical Examination

- In the acute setting, the patient reports pain on the affected side and supports the affected limb with the opposite arm.

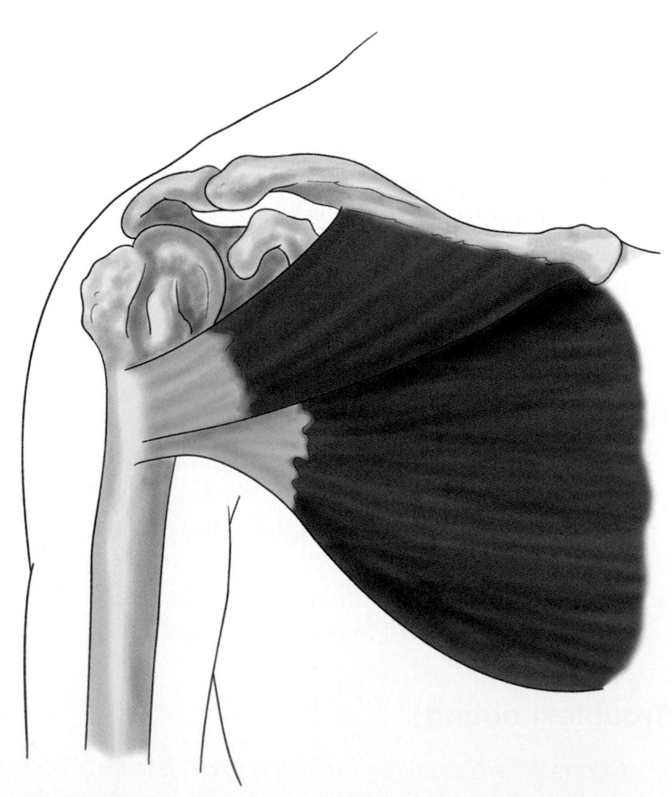

Figure 37-1 Anatomic representation of the pectoralis major muscle from its sternal and clavicular origins to its insertion at the humerus.

- Swelling of the anterior chest or axilla is commonly present.
- Ecchymosis of the anterior chest occurs with tears at the sternal or clavicular origin of the pectoralis major muscle; lateral chest ecchymosis is present with insertional tears at the humerus.
- Asymmetrical webbing of the affected axilla is observed from the loss of the anterior wall musculature.
- A retracted pectoralis muscle often is noted medially with a distal defect near the axilla.
- Tenderness to palpation is present along the anterior axillary fold and anterior chest.
- Weakness is noted with internal rotation and shoulder adduction.
- Resisted movements of the affected arm produce pain and accentuate the abnormal anatomic position of the retracted muscle.
- Chronic tears often present with marked asymmetry of the affected side (Fig. 37-2).

Imaging

- Radiographs are most often negative; however, bony avulsions at the humeral insertion may be identified.
- Magnetic resonance imaging is most useful in identifying the location and extent of pectoralis major muscle injury. T2-weighted imaging best shows acute tears, whereas T1-weighted imaging best reveals chronic injuries.
- Imaging usually reveals a complete tear of the muscle at the humeral or musculotendinous insertion with occasional preservation of anterior-proximal fibers. Tears at the clavicular or sternal origin are infrequent (Table 37-1).

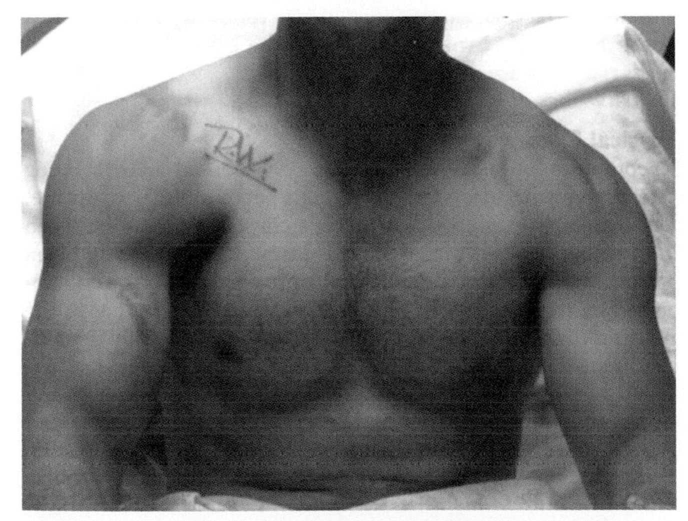

Figure 37-2 Patient with acute pectoralis major muscle rupture illustrating the asymmetry of the axilla and anterior chest as well as the webbed axillary fold.

Treatment

- Immediate
  - Rest to prevent additional injury
  - Ice for swelling control
  - Nonsteroidal anti-inflammatory drugs or non-nonsteroidal anti-inflammatory analgesics for pain
  - Arm sling for comfort
- Acute phase
  - Complete assessment for surgical intervention by an orthopaedist
  - Continue the use of ice, anti-inflammatory medications, and comfort measures.
  - Nonsurgical treatment may be appropriate in the sedentary individual.
- Late phase
  - Postsurgical care typically requires daily protection with an arm sling for approximately 6 to 8 weeks.
  - Pendulum shoulder movements, along with exercises to maintain the musculature of the forearm and hand, are initiated immediately after surgery.
  - Physical therapy progresses through increasing range of motion, isometric contraction, and resistance exercises.
  - Modified, sport-specific, noncontact activities can often begin at approximately 20 weeks.

Prognosis

- Recent studies indicate that surgical repair of both acute and chronic pectoralis muscle tears provides superior results with respect to both strength and pain control compared with nonoperative treatment.

TABLE 37-1 *Differential Diagnosis for Pectoralis Major Muscle Rupture*

Condition	Differentiating Feature
Pectoralis muscle strain	Ecchymosis and palpable defect absent
Biceps tendon injury	Pain and weakness with elbow flexion; muscle defect present in arm
Bench-presser's shoulder	Pain is insidious in onset and located medial to coracoid
Shoulder impingement syndrome	Pain with overhead movement in an athlete with repetitive activities
Chest contusion	No defect present on resisted shoulder adduction
Costochondral separation or sprain	Weakness of internal rotation and shoulder adduction is absent
Rib fracture	Pain with inspiration

- Complete return of strength, as graded by isokinetic testing, is reported with surgical repair.
- Range of motion is typically regained with either operative or conservative management.
- Long-term activity modification may be required for patients opting for nonsurgical treatment.
- Complete recovery from surgical procedures and return to full athletic participation are typically possible in 5 to 6 months.

When to Refer

- Patients require referral to an orthopaedic surgeon immediately to begin the process of assessing the location and extent of injury.
- Referral to a surgeon with particular expertise in shoulder surgery may be appropriate.

Troubleshooting

- Specific risks and benefits of surgical intervention must be discussed with the patient.
- A close follow-up with the surgeon is essential to prevent surgery-associated infection.
- Sustained physical therapy is required to ensure a complete range of motion and return to presurgery strength.
- Associated pectoral nerve injury may slow functional rehabilitation in the injured patient.
- Injury- or surgery-associated atrophy of neighboring rotator cuff muscles requires a comprehensive pectoral- and shoulder-strengthening program.
- Injuries to the unaffected side can occur as a result of compensatory use after surgery.

Patient Instructions

- Immediately stop exercises involving the affected limb with an acute injury.
- Apply ice to control swelling and pain.
- Use over-the-counter analgesics for pain control.
- Refrain from stretching the affected limb.
- Contact the primary care provider or sports medicine specialist for a full evaluation.
- Follow the physician's and physical therapist's instructions throughout the surgical and rehabilitation periods.

Considerations in Special Populations

- Weight lifters, especially power lifters, are at increased risk of injury secondary to maximized lifting goals.
- The use of anabolic steroids can weaken muscle and tendon fibers, making soft-tissue tears more likely.

Suggested Reading

- Aarimaa VA, Rantanen J, Heikkila J, et al: Rupture of the pectoralis major muscle. Am J Sports Med 2004;32:1256–1262.
- Hanna CM, Glenny AB, Stanley SN, Caughey MA: Pectoralis major tears: Comparison of surgical and conservative treatment. Br J Sports Med 2001;35:202–206.
- McEntire J, Hess WE, Coleman S: Rupture of the pectoralis major muscle. J Bone Joint Surg Am 1972;54A:1040–1047.
- Ohashi K, El-Khoury MD, Albright J, Tearse D: MRI of complete rupture of the pectoralis major muscle. Skeletal Radiol 1996;25(7):625–628.
- Quinlan JF, Molloy M, Hurson BJ: Pectoralis major tendon ruptures: When to operate. Br J Sports Med 2002;36:226–228.
- Schepsis AA, Grafe MW, Jones H, Lemos M: Rupture of the pectoralis muscle: Outcome after repair of acute and chronic injuries. Am J Sports Med 2000;28:9–15.
- Zvijac J, Schurhoff M, Hechtman KS, Uribe J: Pectoralis major tears: Correlation of magnetic resonance imaging and treatment strategies. Am J Sports Med 2006;34:289–294.

Chapter 38 Shoulder Impingement Syndrome

Marifel Mitzi F. Fernandez and Robert G. Hosey

Key Concepts

- Impingement or compression of the rotator cuff tendons in the subacromial space between the lateral aspect of the acromion and the humeral head
- May result in rotator cuff tendonitis/tendinopathy, subacromial bursitis, and degenerative rotator cuff tears
- Congenital or degenerative changes involving the overlying acromioclavicular joint may further contribute to the development of subacromial impingement syndrome.
- Most symptoms resolve with conservative management in the absence of other pathology.
- Surgical management is acromioplasty (open or arthroscopic)/subacromial decompression (Fig. 38-1).

History

- Insidious onset of throbbing or aching pain of the anterolateral shoulder
- Usually no history of acute injury
- Painful range of motion, marked increase with overhead activity
- Night pain; pain when sleeping on the affected side
- No radicular symptoms or sensory deficits

Physical Examination

- Inspection: Usually no visible shoulder abnormalities or asymmetry compared with opposite side
- Palpation: Tenderness on compression of subacromial space (below lateral edge of the acromion)
- Range of motion: Overall preserved, but pain reported on forward flexion and in mid-range of abduction (70–130 degrees, the "painful arc of abduction"); internal rotation is most difficult due to pain
- Strength testing: Usually equal to opposite side; there may be apparent strength loss due to pain with resisted abduction/external or internal rotation if there is accompanying rotator cuff tendonitis
- Neurovascular testing normal
- Special tests: Positive impingement tests: Neer and Hawkins signs (Figs. 38-2 and 38-3)

Imaging

- Radiographs
  - Posteroanterior, lateral, axillary Y, and scapular outlet views to evaluate acromioclavicular and glenohumeral joints, acromion type, presence of osteoarthritis or osteophyte formation (Fig. 38-4)
- Magnetic resonance imaging
  - If there are suspected rotator cuff or labral tears in acute injury or cases in which there is no improvement with conservative management
  - May need contrast studies to fully evaluate labral tears (Fig. 38-5)

Additional Tests

- Radiograph of cervical spine if cervical pathology is suspected in patients with vague neck and shoulder pain; may show degenerative changes on plain radiographs
  - Further evaluation and management depends on the severity of symptoms
- Neer impingement test
  - Decrease in impingement symptoms after injection of 1% lidocaine in the subacromial space

Differential Diagnosis

- Please see Table 38-1.

Treatment

- At diagnosis
  - Nonsteroidal anti-inflammatory drugs
  - Ice on affected area after activity
  - Activity modification
  - Physical therapy for stretching/range of motion
  - Rotator cuff strengthening and scapular stabilization

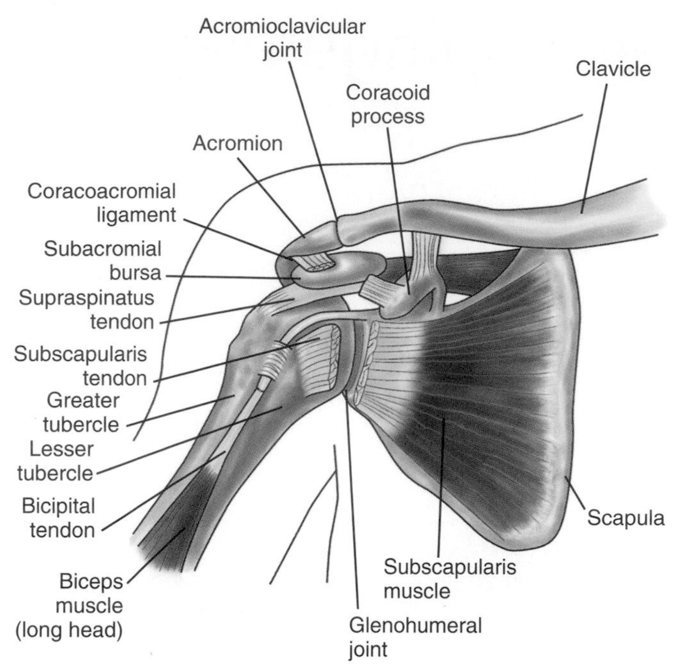

Figure 38-1 Anterolateral shoulder anatomy. (Adapted with permission from Anna Francesca Valerio, MD.)

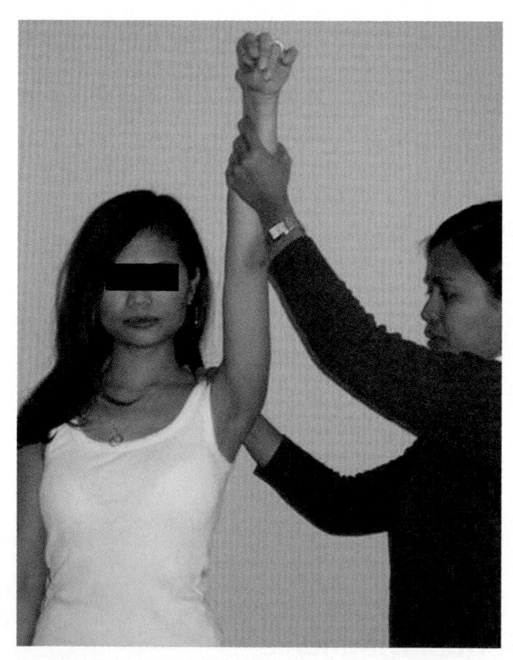

Figure 38-2 Neer sign. Pain with passive forward elevation of affected arm to 180 degrees.

- For mild symptoms, it is acceptable to give the patient a home exercise program.
- Formal referral to physical therapy is recommended for moderate to severe symptoms.
- Follow-up in 4 to 6 weeks
- Later
    - In addition to the treatments previously listed, subacromial corticosteroid injection may be offered, depending on the patient's progress.

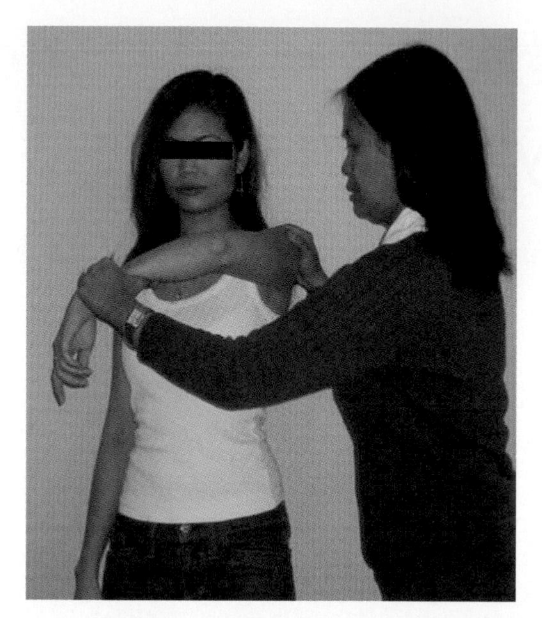

Figure 38-3 Hawkins sign. Pain is reproduced with passive flexion of the affected arm at 90 degrees and flexion of the elbow at 90 degrees. The arm is then internally rotated.

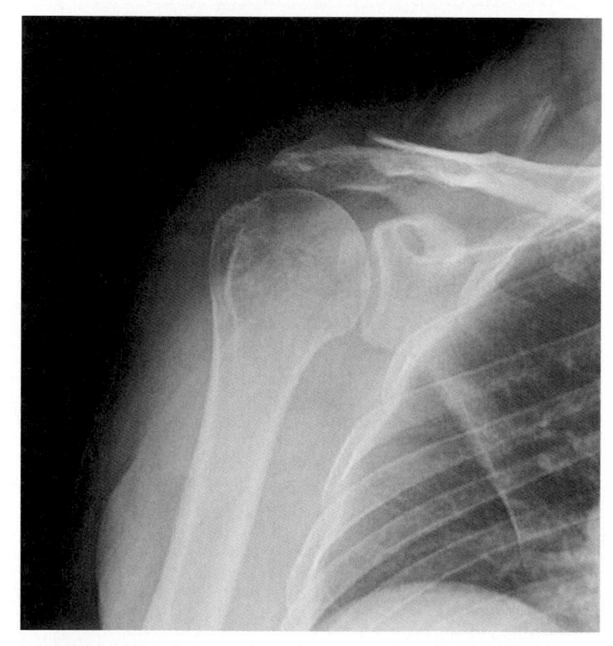

Figure 38-4 Type III acromion and arthritic changes in a patient with chronic subacromial impingement symptoms.

- Continue physical therapy and home exercises.
- Follow-up in 4 to 6 weeks.

When to Refer

- Persistence or worsening of pain despite 4 to 6 months of conservative therapy
- Magnetic resonance imaging findings of massive rotator cuff and/or labral tears
- Coexisting cervical disc disease/radiculopathy

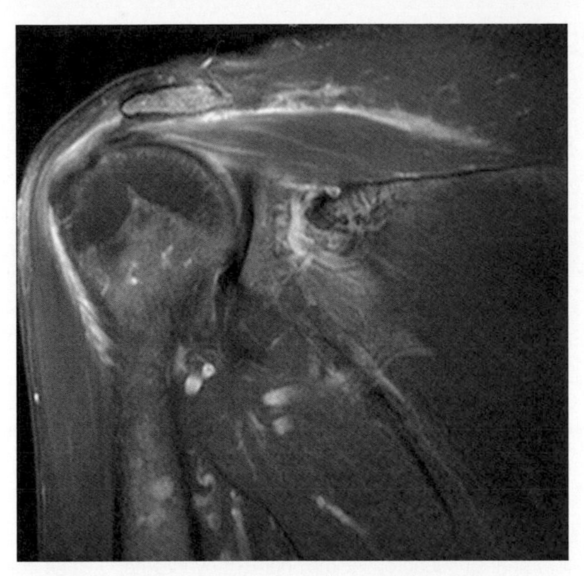

Figure 38-5 Increased fluid signal and disruption of supraspinatus tendon fibers in an elderly patient with shoulder impingement and degenerative rotator cuff tendon tear.

Prognosis

- Good with conservative therapy, in the absence of other shoulder/neck pathology

Troubleshooting

- Internal impingement is a condition found in overhead or throwing athletes in whom the posterior superior capsule of the shoulder is impinged when the arm is in the abducted and externally rotated position as in the cocking phase of throwing. This results from overall excessive laxity of the capsule as a function of repetitive throwing or overhead activities.
- A neck examination should also be performed to rule out cervical pathology.

TABLE 38-1 *Differential Diagnosis*

Condition	History	Physical Examination Findings	Treatment
Impingement syndrome	Gradual onset; pain with overhead movement; pain mostly on anterolateral shoulder; night pain	Positive impingement signs (Hawkins and Neer); ROM and strength usually normal	First line: NSAIDs and physical therapy; subacromial cortico-steroid injection and subacro-mial decompression as a last resort
AC joint pathology (arthritis, sprain)	Fall on affected side (sprain); pain on anterior shoulder near clavicle	Pain on direct palpation of AC joint; positive cross-arm adduction test; ROM may be normal	First line: NSAIDs and physical therapy; AC joint corticoste-roid injection may be done
Rotator cuff tear	Pain in anterolateral shoulder; history of trauma in acute tears; evaluate for cuff tear in elderly patients with a history of shoulder dislocation	Positive drop arm test; decreased strength testing on involved muscle group; decreased ROM	NSAIDs and physical therapy; may need surgery, especially with profound weakness
Labral tear (SLAP)	History of trauma (hyperextension injury or dislocation) or fall on outstretched arm; may also result from overuse injuries in throwing athletes; pain with overhead activity; clicking, catching symptoms	Positive O'Brien's test; may have physical examination findings similar to rotator cuff pathology; there is no one special test that is specific for labral pathology	Physical therapy; may need surgery if symptomatic
Frozen shoulder (adhesive capsulitis)	Stiffness, inability to move shoulder; pain at rest and with minimal movement, difficult to localize	Limited ROM, both active and passive	Physical therapy for mobilization/ROM; may need surgery if physical therapy fails
Cervical disc disease/ radiculopathy	Vague neck pain (upper trapezius muscle) and shoulder pain; pain radiating down arm	Pain with neck ROM testing; may have weakness of affected shoulder/arm; positive Spurling's maneuver if with nerve compression	NSAIDs, oral steroids, physical therapy; may need surgery for severe symptoms/nerve compression or if physical therapy fails

AC, acromioclavicular; NSAIDs, nonsteroidal anti-inflammatory drugs; ROM, range of motion.

Patient Instructions

- Avoid overhead activities in the acute phase.
- Modify activity, if necessary, to adapt to work or sport.
- Take anti-inflammatory medications as needed for pain.
- Physical therapy exercises may cause more pain in some cases, which may be alleviated by a subacromial corticosteroid injection.
- Continue using ice after rotator cuff strengthening exercises.
- With the chronic nature of impingement syndrome, it is important to continue exercises at home even after reduction or resolution of symptoms.

Considerations in Special Populations

- In the athletes who use overhead throwing motions, glenohumeral and scapular stabilization, in addition to rotator cuff strengthening exercises, is key to the management of internal impingement symptoms.
- In the elderly patient, if there is no improvement after several weeks of conservative therapy, evaluation for rotator cuff tears is suggested.

Suggested Reading

- Almekinders L: Impingement syndrome. Clin Sports Med 2001;20:491–504.
- Anderson B, Roberts M: Shoulder impingement syndrome. UpToDate 2007.
- Biglani L, Levine W: Current concepts review: Subacromial impingement syndrome. J Bone Joint Surg Am 1997; 79A:1854–1868.
- Cain EL Jr, Meis RC: Internal impingement. In Johnson DL, Mair SD (eds): Clinical Sports Medicine. Philadelphia: Mosby, 2006, pp 227–234.
- Codsi M: The painful shoulder: When to inject and when to refer. Cleve Clin J Med 2007;74:473–488.
- Koester M, George M, Kuhn GM: Shoulder impingement syndrome. Am J Med 2005;118:452–455.
- Morrison DS, Frogameni AD, Woodworth P: Non-operative treatment of subacromial impingement syndrome. J Bone Joint Surg Am 1997;79A:732–737.
- Natsis K, Tsikaras P, Totlis T, et al: Correction between the four types of acromion and the existence of enthesophytes: A study on 423 dried scapulas and review of the literature. Clin Anat 2007;20:267–272.

Chapter 39 Rotator Cuff Tear

Scott D. Mair

ICD-9 CODES
726.10 *Rotator Cuff Syndrome*
727.61 *Complete Rupture of the Rotator Cuff*

Key Concepts

- Rotator cuff tears may result from acute trauma, but more commonly develop insidiously due to chronic overuse or chronic tissue degeneration.
- The most consistent risk factor for the development of a rotator cuff tear is advancing age.
- Rotator cuff tears may be partial or full thickness (completely detached from the bony insertion).
- Full thickness rotator cuff tears are uncommon in patients younger than age 40, whereas they are present in approximately half of the population older than age 70.
- Partial thickness tears more commonly start on the articular (glenohumeral) side of the rotator cuff, but can be present on the bursal (subacromial) side.
- In younger patients, partial thickness rotator cuff tears are most commonly seen in athletes who use overhead throwing motions.
- Etiologic factors
  - Tendon degeneration
  - Trauma
  - Glenohumeral instability or dislocation
  - Inflammatory disease
  - Scapulothoracic dysfunction

History

- Common symptoms are pain and/or weakness.
- The majority of patients cannot recall a specific injury or relate their symptoms to a minor traumatic event.
- In younger patients, higher-energy trauma is more likely to be the cause of symptoms.
- Acute shoulder dislocation in patients older than the age of 40 results in a rotator cuff tear in approximately 25% of cases.
- Pain is most common over the anterior and lateral shoulder, radiating down over the deltoid muscle.
- Pain radiating below the elbow can occur, but should alert the physician to consider a cervical radiculopathy.
- Pain frequently occurs with use of the arm.
- Night pain is common.
- Symptoms of weakness are common with large or massive tears, particularly when they occur acutely.

Physical Examination

- Inspection may reveal atrophy of the supraspinatus or infraspinatus muscle bellies on the scapula, suggesting a chronic process.
- Passive range of motion is usually preserved in patients with a rotator cuff tear, although frozen shoulder (with resultant loss of active and passive range of motion) can occur concomitantly.
- Active range of motion may be diminished due to pain or weakness.
- Weakness to elevation in the scapular plane is frequently present with larger tears.
- Weakness to external rotation is common if the tear extends into the infraspinatus muscle, and with massive tears the patient may not be able to maintain the arm in position after passive external rotation.
- An increase in passive external rotation suggests a complete tear of the subscapularis muscle.
- Abnormal liftoff or belly press test results indicate involvement of the subscapularis muscle.
- Examination for biceps and acromioclavicular joint pathology should be done to evaluate for associated pathology.
- Cervical spine examination is required.

Imaging

- Routine shoulder radiographs include anteroposterior, supraspinatus outlet, and axillary views. Special views of the acromioclavicular joint may be added.
- Radiographs frequently show subacromial spurs, along with greater tuberosity sclerosis, cysts, or excrescence.

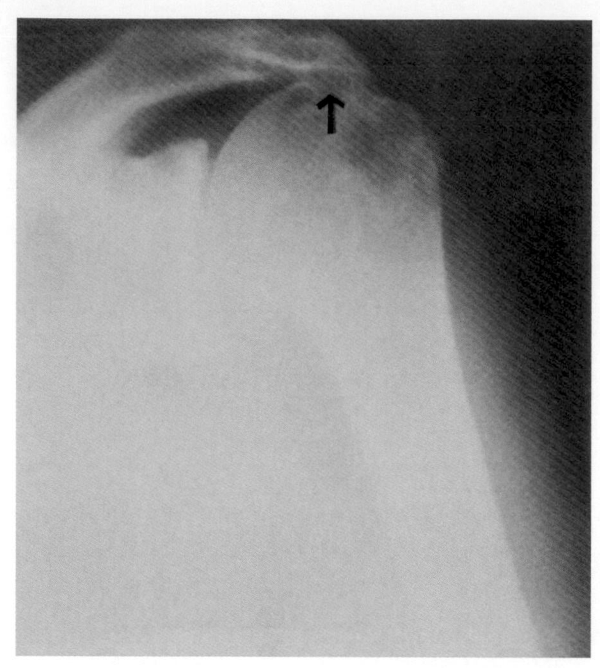

Figure 39-1 The most important radiographic finding is elevation of the humeral head *(arrow)* in relation to the glenoid.

- The most important radiographic finding is elevation of the humeral head related to the glenoid (Fig. 39-1). This is indicative of a massive tear, usually chronic.
- Magnetic resonance imaging is very effective for evaluating the rotator cuff (Fig. 39-2). Information regarding partial or full thickness tears, size and location of tears, and biceps pathology is obtained.
- The degree of muscle atrophy on magnetic resonance imaging offers clues to chronicity of the tear and whether repair is possible.

Additional Tests

- Diagnostic subacromial lidocaine injection may help in allowing a better examination for range of motion and strength once pain is eliminated.

Differential Diagnosis

- Subacromial impingement
- Acromioclavicular joint arthrosis
- Adhesive capsulitis
- Glenohumeral arthritis
- Cervical radiculopathy

Treatment

Partial Thickness Tears

- At diagnosis
  - Conservative treatment is usually effective
  - Nonsteroidal anti-inflammatory drugs

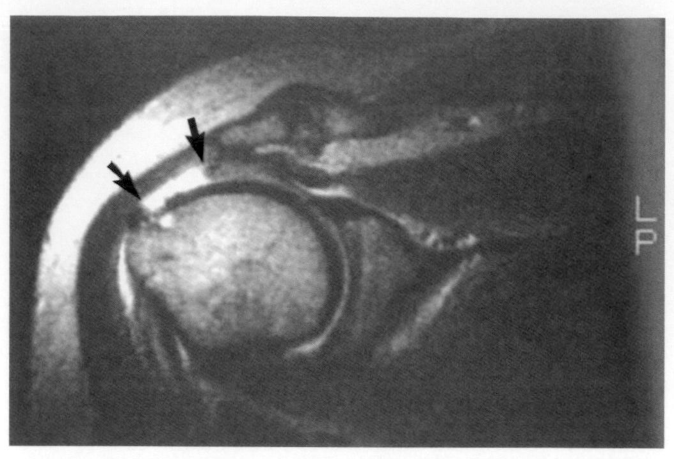

Figure 39-2 Magnetic resonance imaging is very effective for evaluating the rotator cuff. *Arrows* show the defect in the supraspinatus tendon.

  - Physical therapy
    — Modalities
    — Rotator cuff and periscapular strengthening
  - Subacromial corticosteroid injection
- Later
  - For persistent symptoms (>6 months), arthroscopy is considered.
    — Arthroscopic subacromial decompression
    — Less than 50% partial cuff thickness: arthroscopic débridement
    — More than 50% partial cuff thickness: arthroscopic or open rotator cuff repair

Full Thickness Tears

- In older patients and/or chronic tears, conservative management as above is often effective.
- In acute traumatic tears or in patients younger than 60 years, early surgical repair is considered.
- Repair involves suturing of cuff tissue back to the tuberosity.
- Repair can be done arthroscopically (Figs. 39-3 and 39-4) or with open surgery.

When to Refer

- Partial thickness tears not responding to conservative measures
- Documented full thickness tears if they are acute; are in younger patients; or are refractory to conservative treatment

Prognosis

- Partial thickness tears: approximately 90% respond well to nonoperative measures

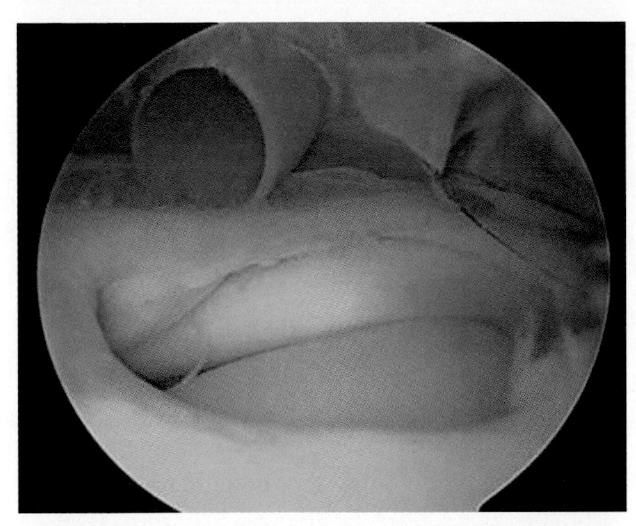

Figure 39-3 Arthroscopic view of a rotator cuff tear.

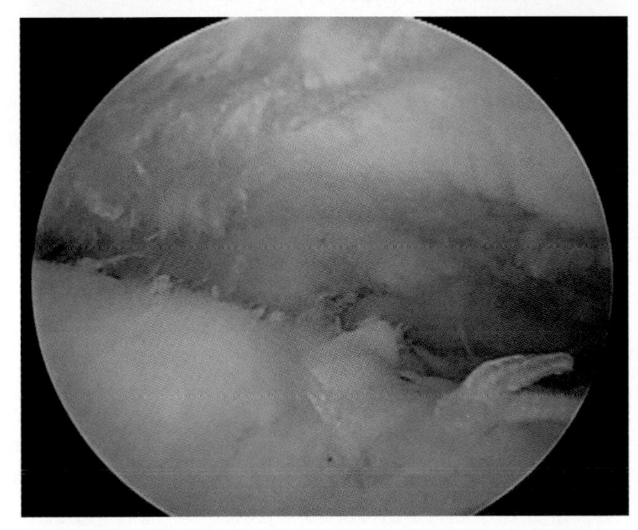

Figure 39-4 View of the same patient from Fig. 39-3 after rotator cuff repair.

- Surgical results in those with persistent pain after conservative treatment: 76% to 88% good or excellent results
- Full thickness tears: dependent on patient age and activity level, size, and chronicity of tear
- Repairable tears show more than 90% patient satisfaction in most studies.

Troubleshooting

- Rotator cuff disease can frequently be managed nonoperatively, and physical therapy is an essential part of this treatment course.
- Elevation of the humeral head on radiographs suggests a chronic, irreparable rotator cuff tear.
- Patients should receive no more than three subacromial injections over the course of one year.

Patient Instructions

- Follow physician and physical therapy instructions with regard to activities, exercises, and restrictions.
- Home-based exercises are vital to overall management and should be performed regularly and correctly.
- In patients with partial thickness or small full thickness rotator cuff tears, an acute event resulting in increased pain or weakness should be evaluated by a physician because enlargement of the tear may have occurred and may result in a change in management.

Considerations in Special Populations

- Partial thickness rotator cuff tears in young overhead athletes are frequently treated more aggressively with arthroscopic evaluation and management.
- Rotator cuff tears are ubiquitous in geriatric patients. They are usually well tolerated or respond to conservative treatment.
- Massive irreparable rotator cuff tears with significant symptoms can be treated surgically with tendon transfers or a shoulder replacement designed for this problem (reverse shoulder prosthesis).

Suggested Reading

- Ainsworth R, Lewis JS: Exercise therapy for the conservative management of full thickness tears of the rotator cuff: A systematic review. Br J Sports Med 2007;41:200–210.
- DeFranco MJ, Bershadsky B, Ciccone J, et al: Functional outcome of arthroscopic rotator cuff repairs: A correlation of anatomic and clinical results. J Shoulder Elbow Surg 2007; 16:759–765.
- Jost B, Pfirrmann CW, Gerber C, Switzerland Z: Clinical outcome after structural failure of rotator cuff repairs. J Bone Joint Surg Am 2000;82A:304–314.
- Mantone JK, Burkhead WZ Jr, Noonan J Jr: Nonoperative treatment of rotator cuff tears. Orthop Clin North Am 2000;31:295–311.
- McConville OR, Iannotti JP: Partial-thickness tears of the rotator cuff: Evaluation and management. J Am Acad Orthop Surg 1999;7:32–43.
- O'Holleran JD, Kocher MS, Horan MP, et al: Determinants of patient satisfaction with outcome after rotator cuff surgery. J Bone Joint Surg Am 2005;87:121–126.
- Tempelhof S, Rupp S, Seil R: Age-related prevalence of rotator cuff tears in asymptomatic shoulders. J Shoulder Elbow Surg 1999;8:296–299.
- Wolf BR, Dunn WR, Wright RW: Indications for repair of full-thickness rotator cuff tears. Am J Sports Med 2007;35:1007–1016.
- Wolff AB, Sethi P, Sutton KM, et al: Partial-thickness rotator cuff tears. J Am Acad Orthop Surg 2006;14:715–725.

Chapter 40 Glenohumeral Disorders

Robert G. Hosey and Jayesh Patel

GLENOHUMERAL ARTHRITIS

Key Concepts

- Primary glenohumeral osteoarthritis involves multiple degenerative changes to the glenohumeral joint.
- Clinically, glenohumeral osteoarthritis is defined by progressive loss of motion with increased pain due to loss of articular joint space and humeral head enlargement due to osteophyte formation.
- The pathophysiology can be divided into two distinct categories: primary and secondary.
  - The etiology of primary osteoarthritis is idiopathic but can be attributed to some form of remote trauma that leads to alteration of the biomechanics of the shoulder.
  - Secondary causes include but are not limited to
    - — Trauma
    - — Joint instability
    - — Previous joint surgery
    - — Infection
    - — Gout
    - — Osteonecrosis
    - — Inflammatory arthritis such as rheumatoid disease
    - — Sickle cell disease, and other metabolic diseases
- Most patients present between their fourth and fifth decades.

History

- There is no true classic presentation for shoulder osteoarthritis.
- Most patients report limited function or motion with activities of daily living rather than pain.
- If night pain is present, it is typically positional.
- Patients usually present with stiffness in the morning that improves with activity.
- It is crucial to obtain a good medical history including surgeries, medications including nonsteroidal anti-inflammatory drugs and steroid injections, and whether a trial of physical therapy has been done.

Physical Examination

- Examine the neck for cervical motion and signs of radiculopathy. Perform Spurling's test, which includes extending, laterally flexing, and rotating the neck to the affected side with axial compression. This is a sign of neuroforaminal stenosis causing nerve root compression.
- Observation of the muscle contours looking for muscle atrophy and inequalities in the level and distance between the shoulders and scapulae.
- Assessment of range of motion is done in both the supine and sitting positions. Patients usually have limited motion in all planes.
- Strength testing, paying attention to rotator cuff strength, which is usually preserved
- Motor and sensory examination

Imaging

- Plain radiographs are diagnostic.
  - An anteroposterior view (Fig. 40-1) is used to evaluate the humeral head, extent of cartilage loss, and presence of osteophytes. It is also important to check for medial glenoid bone loss and loss of subacromial humeral space.
  - An axillary view (Fig. 40-2) is used to evaluate the status of the posterior glenoid because osteoarthritis of the glenohumeral joint generally causes posterior glenoid erosions and overall malalignment of the shoulder joint.
- Computed tomography (Fig. 40-3)
  - May be needed to assess glenoid bone loss in anticipation of possible shoulder replacement or reverse shoulder arthroplasties

Differential Diagnosis

- Rotator cuff disease
- Acromioclavicular osteoarthritis
- Rheumatoid arthritis
- Cervical radiculopathy
- Osteonecrosis
- Shoulder dislocation

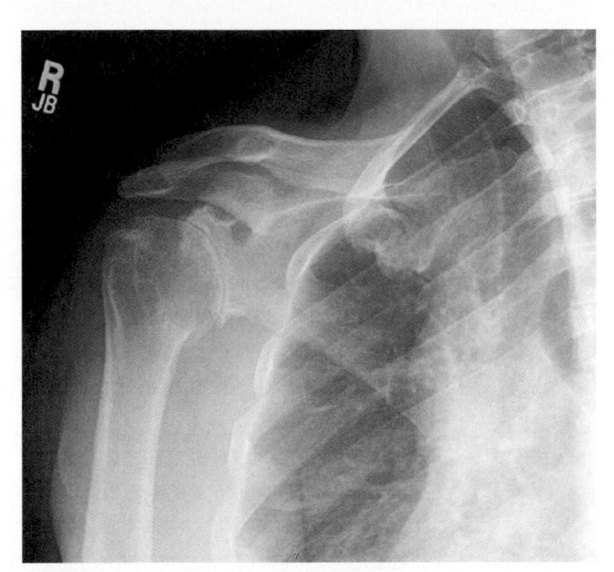

Figure 40-1 Anteroposterior view of the right shoulder showing glenohumeral osteoarthritis.

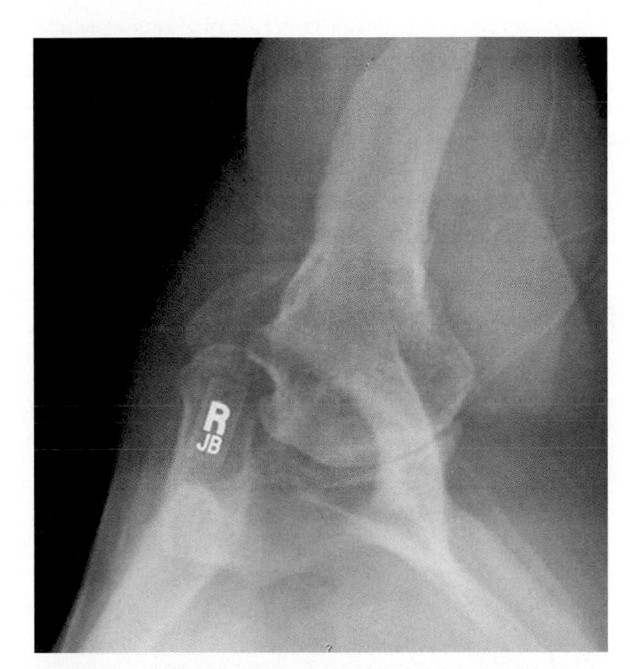

Figure 40-2 Axillary lateral view of the right shoulder showing enlargement of the humeral head and osteophyte formation.

Treatment

- Early stages
  - Medications including nonsteroidal anti-inflammatory drugs, glucosamine, and chondroitin sulfate
  - Activity modifications aimed at decreasing repetitive activities, especially overhead motion activities
- Physical therapy to focus on strengthening and improving range of motion; caution must be used if there is severe joint incongruity

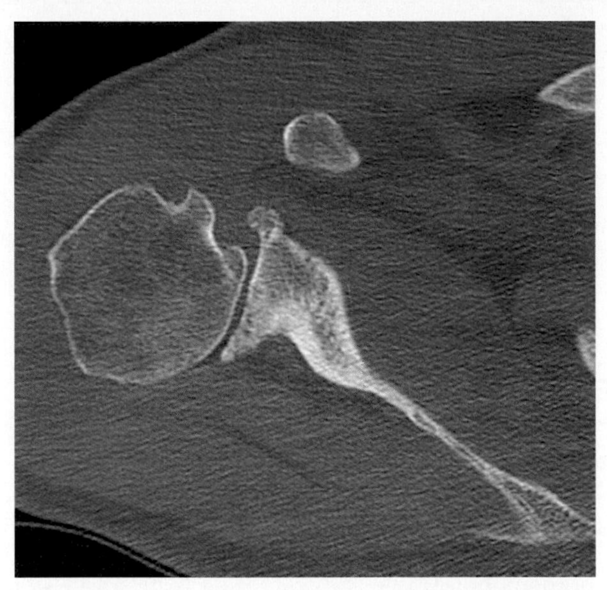

Figure 40-3 Computed tomography scan of right shoulder showing glenoid erosion.

- Late stages
  - Intra-articular corticosteroid injections may be tried for pain palliation.

When to Refer

- Patients failing conservative treatment with increased pain and loss of function
- Surgical options are limited, but do include arthroscopic and/or open joint débridement, arthrodesis, and/or arthroplasty/joint replacement.

Troubleshooting

- Counsel patient on the chronic nature and steady worsening of this condition.
- Counsel that surgery may help with pain, but function will be limited.
- Patient may not receive more than three glenohumeral corticosteroid injections in any given year.

Patient Instructions

- Taking anti-inflammatory medications as needed is important.
- Continuing daily activities and home exercises help prolong function.
- Avoiding use of narcotics is important.

Considerations in Special Populations

- This is a chronic disease primarily affecting the geriatric population.

- Treatment principles are the same regardless of age or level of function.
- Young patients should try to defer the need for surgery as long as possible given the complications and need for revision surgeries.
- Patients with rotator cuff tears and glenohumeral osteoarthritis are limited in their options, but good candidates can have reverse shoulder arthroplasties.

GLENOHUMERAL AVASCULAR NECROSIS

Key Concepts

- Osteonecrosis or avascular necrosis of the humeral head refers to the disruption of blood flow to the humeral head.
- Second only to femoral head osteonecrosis in incidence in humans
- Avascular necrosis has been divided into four causes:
  - Mechanical vascular interruption
  - Thrombosis and embolism
  - Injury to or pressure on a vessel wall
  - Venous occlusion
- The ascending branch of the anterior circumflex humeral artery is the major blood supply to the humeral head and is the main vessel that is disrupted in this disease.
- There are multiple causes of this vascular disruption.
  - Trauma: fracture, dislocation, surgery
  - Corticosteroid use
  - Alcohol use
  - Dysbarism (changes in ambient pressure)
  - Sickle cell disease
  - Systemic diseases: Gaucher's disease, systemic lupus erythematosus, rheumatoid arthritis
  - Idiopathic
  - Radiation

History

- Patients usually present with generalized shoulder pain.
- This pain is present at night, but is not necessarily positional.
- Pain is typically worse with increasing activities.
- Patients occasionally report hearing an audible click with range of motion.
- Patient's medical history is extremely important and will often provide clues to the diagnosis of avascular necrosis.

Physical Examination

- Typically decreased range of motion in all planes with associated pain

Imaging

- Plain radiographs can be negative in the early disease stages. Five stages have been identified.
  - Stage I: no changes on radiographs
  - Stage II: humeral head remains spherical but has increased sclerosis
  - Stage III: subchondral collapse, crescent sign
  - Stage IV: collapse of articular surface (Fig. 40-4)
  - Stage V: osteoarthritis that includes the glenoid
- Magnetic resonance imaging demonstrates early changes in the humeral head before radiographic changes can be visualized and stage I can be identified.
- Bone scans can be helpful, but are less useful than magnetic resonance imaging.

Additional Tests

- Laboratory work including complete blood count with differential and complete metabolic panel.

Differential Diagnosis

- Same as for osteoarthritis

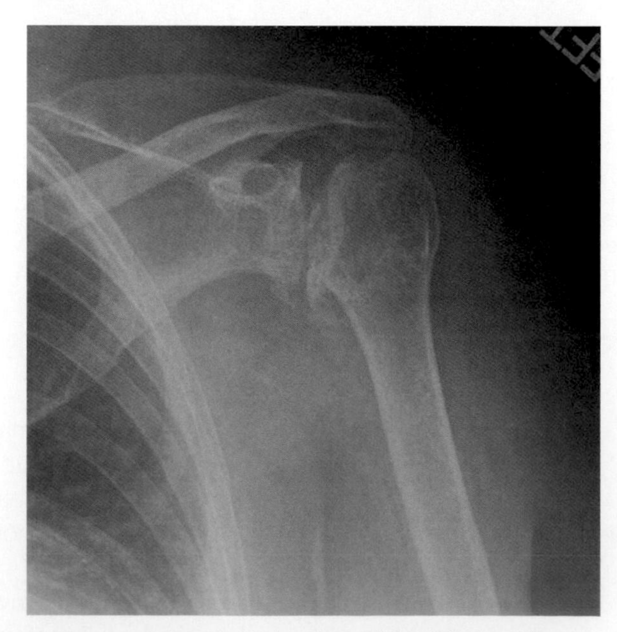

Figure 40-4 Anteroposterior view of the left shoulder showing severe humeral head avascular necrosis.

Treatment

- Treat any underlying causative disease if possible.
- Nonsurgical options are the same as for osteoarthritis of the glenohumeral joint and can be tried with stage I and II disease.

When to Refer

- Patients should be referred once this diagnosis is made to discuss potential options for surgical intervention.

Prognosis

- This is a severe progressive disease.
- Pain control and maintenance of function are mainstays of treatment.
- Data have shown that 3 years after diagnosis, 45% of patients with stage IV and 21% of those with stage V disease had good function that did not require arthroplasty.

Troubleshooting

- Treating underlying diseases can slow or even improve the progression of osteonecrosis.
- Educate patients about stopping the use of offending agents such as alcohol.

Patient Instructions

- Follow physician instructions to try to preserve function and prevent progression of disease.

Considerations in Special Populations

- Those patients who need continued steroid use need to be monitored closely and may need operative intervention.

Suggested Reading

- Boileau R, Sinnerton R, Chuinard C, Walch G: Arthroplasty of the shoulder. J Bone Joint Surg Br 2006;88B:562–575.
- Brems J: Management of Osteoarthritis of the Shoulder. OKU Shoulder and Elbow 2. Rosemont, IL: American Academy of Orthopaedic Surgeons, 2002, pp 257–266.
- Cusher M, Friedman R: Osteonecrosis of the humeral head. J Am Acad Orthop Surg 1997;5:339–346.
- Johnson L III, Galatz L: Osteonecrosis and Other Noninflammatory Degenerative Diseases of the Glenohumeral Joint. OKU Shoulder and Elbow 2. Rosemont, IL: American Academy of Orthopaedic Surgeons, 2002, pp 267–274.
- Sperling J, Steinmann S, Cordasco F, et al: Shoulder arthritis in the young adult: Arthroscopy to arthroplasty. Instr Course Lect 2006;55:67–74.

Chapter 41 Adhesive Capsulitis (Frozen Shoulder)

John M. MacKnight

ICD-9 CODE
726.0 *Adhesive Capsulitis*

Key Concepts

- Adhesive capsulitis, commonly referred to as frozen shoulder
- Progressive loss of active and passive glenohumeral motion resulting from contraction of the glenohumeral synovial capsule (Fig. 41-1)
- The pathophysiology is poorly understood and may be inflammatory; recent data have implicated cytokines and matrix metalloproteases in the development of pathologic changes in the synovium.
- Primary adhesive capsulitis is idiopathic; insidious onset of shoulder pain leads to avoidance of use and a slowly progressive decline in shoulder motion and functional ability.
- Secondary adhesive capsulitis may be associated with
  - Trauma
  - Immobilization
  - Diabetes
  - Thyroid disease
  - Autoimmune diseases (rheumatoid arthritis, scleroderma)
  - Myocardial infarction or stroke
  - Chronic lung disease or lung cancer
  - Cervical radicular disease
- Prevalence in the general population is 2%.
- Seventy percent of patients are female; there is a 20% to 30% incidence of future involvement of the opposite shoulder.
- Peak incidence is in the fifth and sixth decades of life.

History

- Stages 1 and 2 (painful "freezing" phase)
  - Symptoms present from weeks to months
  - Aching shoulder pain is present at rest and sharp pain occurs at the extremes of range of motion (ROM).
  - Progressive loss of motion in internal rotation, forward flexion, and abduction
  - The majority of motion loss in the first 3 months is secondary to painful synovitis; loss of motion after 3 months is primarily due to capsular contraction and loss of capsular volume.
- Stage 3 (adhesive phase)
  - Symptoms present for 9 to 14 months
  - Prominent stiffening of the shoulder with significant loss of ROM
  - Patients often report a history of an extremely painful phase that has resolved, resulting in a relatively pain-free but stiff shoulder.
- Stage 4 (resolution or thawing phase)
  - Characterized by slow, steady recovery of ROM resulting from capsular remodeling in response to use of the arm and shoulder.
- Prominent night pain may be present, particularly early in the earlier stages.

Physical Examination

- Patients in stages 1 and 2 have pain on palpation of the anterior and posterior capsules with radiating pain to the deltoid insertion.
- Evaluation of active and passive ROM should be performed.
  - Active and passive forward flexion, abduction, internal rotation (measured by having the patient place the thumb to the highest point possible on the spinous process), and external rotation are measured and recorded with the patient standing.
  - Passive glenohumeral motion is measured with the patient supine; scapulothoracic motion is constrained by manual pressure on the acromion.
- As able, a complete general shoulder examination, as described previously, should be attempted to evaluate for additional pathologies.
- Cervical spine examination (see Chapter 110)

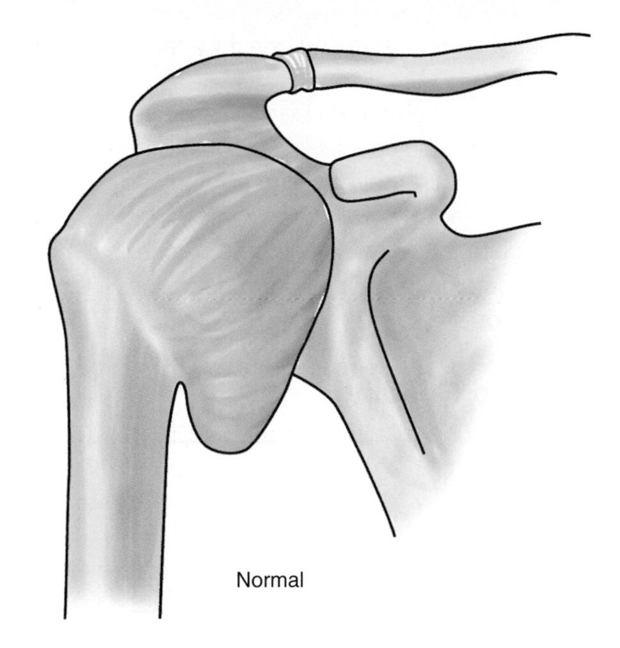

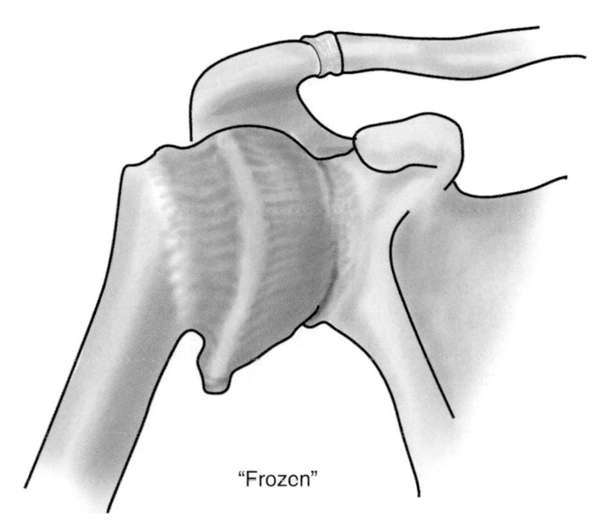

Figure 41-1 Fibrosis and contraction of the glenohumeral synovium.

Imaging

- Radiographs are typically negative but should be obtained to evaluate for significant rotator cuff disease, glenohumeral arthritis, or calcific tendinitis.
- Routine radiographic evaluation should include anteroposterior views in internal and external rotation and axillary and outlet views.
- Disuse osteopenia may be seen.
- If the diagnosis of adhesive capsulitis remains in question, MRI may be performed to evaluate for significant rotator cuff or labral cartilage pathology.
- MRI should not be pursued routinely in the adhesive capsulitis patient.
- Shoulder arthrography has been largely replaced by MRI, if warranted.

Differential Diagnosis

- Significant rotator cuff impingement or tear
- Labral tear
- Acromioclavicular osteoarthritis
- Cervical radiculopathy

Treatment

- At diagnosis (in early stages, when shoulder is acutely painful)
  - Primary early goal is relief of pain
    - — Nonsteroidal anti-inflammatory drugs (NSAIDs)
    - — Other analgesics
    - — Oral corticosteroids
  - Activity modification/relative rest
  - Formal physical therapy
    - — Gentle joint mobilization
    - — Modalities to assist with pain control and inflammation including transcutaneous electrical nerve stimulation, iontophoresis, phonophoresis, cryotherapy, moist heat, ultrasound, hydrotherapy
  - Glenohumeral corticosteroid injection (stages 1 and 2 only)
    - — May be performed under fluoroscopic guidance
    - — Multiple studies demonstrate efficacy, particularly when initiated early in the treatment course
- Later, once pain-free
  - Aggressive physical therapy for passive and active restoration of ROM
  - Graded return to full function as symptoms allow

When to Refer

- Patients in whom full ROM has not been restored despite multiple injections and in whom a completed course of aggressive physical therapy has failed
- Treatment considerations for refractory cases
  - Closed manipulation of glenohumeral joint under regional or general anesthesia
  - Arthroscopic release and synovectomy

Prognosis

- Five- to 10-year follow-up: 39% had full recovery, 54% had clinical limitation without functional disability, and 7% had functional limitation

- Fifty percent of patients with frozen shoulder may have some degree of pain and stiffness an average of 7 years after onset of the disease.
- Outcome is generally favorable even if surgical manipulation is required.
- Spontaneous remission and restoration of ROM take an average of 30 months.

Troubleshooting

- Only pain-free shoulders should undergo aggressive physical therapy.
- Close follow-up is essential to ensure compliance with the management program and to limit the overall time of shoulder dysfunction.
- Counsel patients regarding the chronic nature of this condition and the expected time frame to recovery.
- Counsel that surgery, if necessary, carries a risk of fracture and neurologic injury.
- Patients should receive no more than three glenohumeral corticosteroid injections over the course of 1 year.

Patient Instructions

- Follow physician and physical therapist instructions closely with respect to the type and quantity of shoulder activities that are acceptable.
- Home-based exercises are vital to overall management and should be performed diligently and regularly.
- Aggressively manage pain per physician directions.

Considerations in Special Populations

- Those caring for geriatric patients will encounter this condition commonly and should be vigilant for its potential presence in any geriatric patient with shoulder pain.
- Treatment principles will be the same as outlined previously, although special care should be taken to place the patient in a physical therapy setting appropriate for his or her physical abilities/limitations.
- Appreciate that any manipulative or surgical management carries a greater risk of morbidity in the geriatric population.

Suggested Reading

- Dias R, Cutts S, Massoud S: Frozen shoulder. Br Med J 2005;331:1453–1456.
- Hannafin JA, Chiaia TA: Adhesive capsulitis: A treatment approach. Clin Orthop Relat Res 2000;372:95–109.
- Iannotti JP, Kwon YW: Management of persistent shoulder pain: A treatment algorithm. Am J Orthop 2005;34(12 Suppl):16–23.
- Meislin RJ, Sperling JW, Stitik TP: Persistent shoulder pain: Epidemiology, pathophysiology, and diagnosis. Am J Orthop 2005;34(12 Suppl):5–9.
- Moskowitz RW, Blaine TA: An overview of treatment options for persistent shoulder pain. Am J Orthop 2005;34(12 Suppl):10–15.
- Reeves B: The natural history of the frozen shoulder syndrome. Scand J Rheumatol 1976;4:193–196.
- Shaffer B, Tibone JE, Kerlan RK: Frozen shoulder: A long-term follow-up. J Bone Joint Surg Am 1992;74A:738–746.
- Sheridan MA, Hannafin JA: Upper extremity: Emphasis on frozen shoulder. Orthop Clin North Am 2006;37:531–539.
- Siegel LB, Cohen NJ, Gall EP: Adhesive capsulitis: A sticky issue. Am Fam Physician 1999;59:1843–1852.

Chapter 42 Acromioclavicular Joint Injuries

Scott D. Mair

ICD-9 CODES

831.04 *Closed Dislocation of the Acromioclavicular Joint*

840.00 *Acromioclavicular Joint, Sprains and Strains*

Key Concepts

- A common term for injury to the acromioclavicular (AC) joint is a separated shoulder.
- Along with the sternoclavicular joint, the AC joint links the upper extremity to the axial skeleton.
- Stability of the AC joint is provided by two major ligament complexes.
  - AC ligaments and the joint capsule provide anteroposterior stability.
  - Coracoclavicular (CC) ligaments (conoid and trapezoid ligaments) provide vertical stability.
- The most frequent cause of AC joint injury is a fall or blow to the shoulder with the arm adducted.
- The energy of such an injury forces the acromion downward and medially, injuring first the AC ligaments and then the CC ligaments.

History

- Pain usually develops immediately after acute injury.
- Symptoms are well localized to the AC joint.
- With more severe injuries, symptoms may radiate over the trapezius muscle.
- Classification (Rockwood)
  - Type I: sprain of AC ligaments, no injury to CC ligaments
  - Type II: rupture of AC ligaments, sprain/partial tear of CC ligaments
  - Type III: rupture of both AC and CC ligaments
  - Type IV: rupture of AC and CC ligaments, posterior displacement of clavicle
  - Type V: rupture of AC and CC ligaments, more than 100% displacement of distal clavicle
  - Type VI: clavicle displaced under the coracoid (very rare)

Physical Examination

- Acute injury may present with swelling and deformity at the AC joint.
- Tenderness is present directly at the AC joint.
- Active range of motion (ROM) may be diminished secondary to pain.
- By classification type
- I: tenderness, no deformity, minimal or no swelling
- II: tenderness, mild deformity, minimal swelling
- III: patient presents with arm held adducted at the side, obvious deformity at the AC joint, pain with shoulder ROM, especially with abduction
- IV: findings similar to those for type III, with posterior displacement of the clavicle
- V: severe deformity, the clavicle often not manually reducible due to penetration of deltotrapezial fascia (Fig. 42-1)
- VI: very rare, may present with neurovascular injury

Imaging

- Patient should be upright to see deformity.
- Routine radiographs are shoulder anteroposterior (Fig. 42-2), axillary, and outlet views.
- Assessment for type IV injury (posterior displacement) is made on the axillary view.
- On a single anteroposterior view showing both shoulders, type III and V AC separation is differentiated by measuring the CC distance. If the distance is more than doubled (100% greater) compared with the normal shoulder, it is type V (Fig. 42-3).
- Weighted views are generally not helpful.
- Cross-arm adduction view helps evaluate for instability; if the acromion slides under the clavicle on this view, surgery may be required.

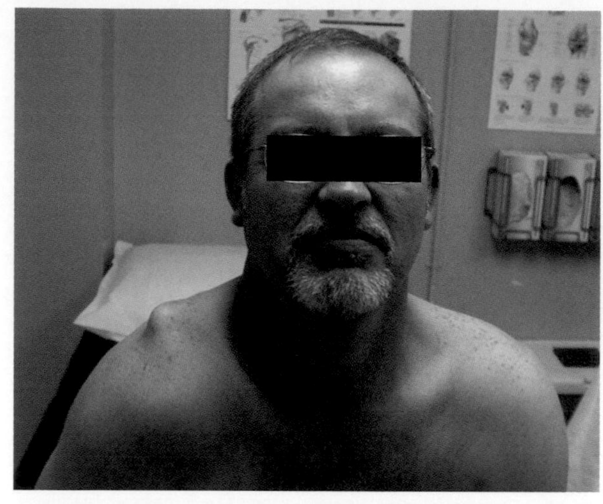

Figure 42-1 Patient with a chronic type V acromioclavicular injury with obvious deformity of the right shoulder.

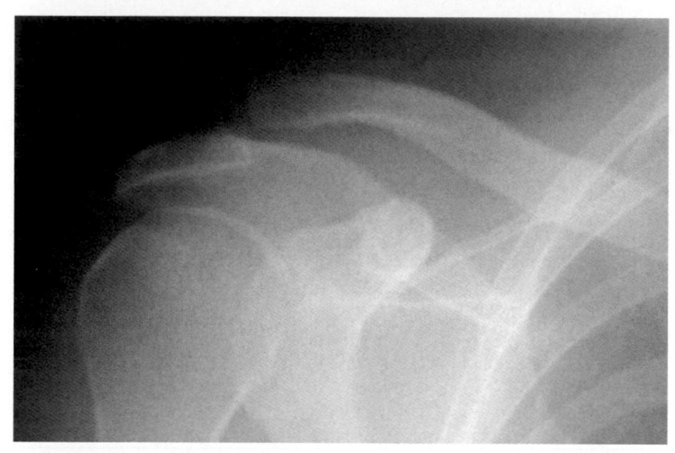

Figure 42-2 Anteroposterior view showing a type III acromioclavicular separation.

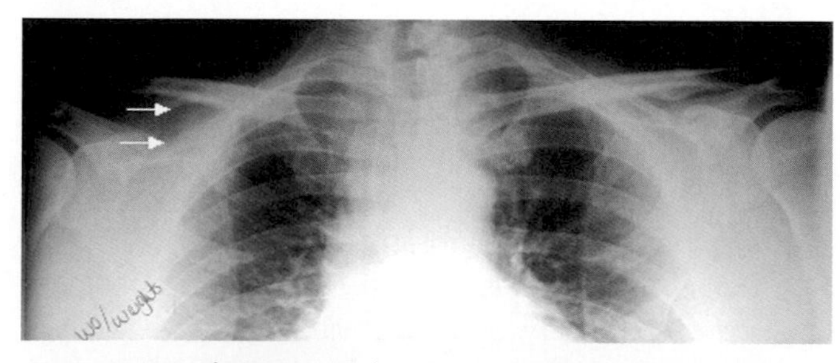

Figure 42-3 Anteroposterior view of both shoulders with a greater than 100% increase in the coracoclavicular distance of the affected shoulder with a type V injury (*arrows*).

- Magnetic resonance imaging is not necessary unless concomitant injury to other structures is suspected.

Differential Diagnosis

- Superior labral injury
- Distal clavicle fracture

Treatment

- At diagnosis
  - The majority of AC joint injuries can be effectively treated without surgery.
  - Treatment is dictated by the injury classification.
  - Type I, II, and III injuries are managed nonoperatively.
  - Sling for comfort
  - Nonsteroidal anti-inflammatory drugs
  - Modalities such as iontophoresis
  - Relative rest from sports activities
- Later
  - ROM as comfort allows; progress to strengthening rotator cuff and periscapular muscles
  - Corticosteroid injection considered for persistent symptoms
  - Type IV, V, and VI injuries are treated with early surgery to reduce the deformity and reconstruct the CC ligaments.
  - In type III injuries, if pain persists longer than 3 months, surgical reconstruction is considered.

When to Refer

- Type IV, V, and VI injuries
- Type III injuries in overhead throwers
- Patients with symptoms that persist longer than 3 to 4 months

Prognosis

- It has been reported that 9% of type I injuries and 23% of type II injuries will have some persistent symptoms with nonoperative management.
- Type III injuries result in an average 17% deficit in bench press strength compared with the uninvolved extremity.
- Approximately 10% of type III injuries eventually need surgery.
- Surgical results are predictably good (>90%) if reduction is maintained for the first few months. Various surgical methods have been described with variable failure rates.

Troubleshooting

- Careful radiographic evaluation for posterior displacement (type IV) or greater than 100% displacement (type V) is crucial in determining appropriate management.

- Average time out of sports is
  - Type I: 1 week
  - Type II: 2 to 4 weeks
  - Type III: up to 6 weeks

Patient Instructions

- Shoulder ROM can be advanced as tolerated.
- In more severe injury, a period in a sling is often necessary before initiating ROM exercises.
- Return to sports is delayed until full ROM and strength are regained.

Considerations in Special Populations

- In overhead throwers (quarterbacks, baseball players), early surgery for type III injuries is often performed to restore proper throwing mechanics.
- In a low-demand geriatric patient, type IV and V injuries may be treated nonoperatively, often with good results.

Suggested Reading

- Bergfeld JA, Andrish JT, Clancy WG: Evaluation of the acromioclavicular joint following first- and second-degree sprains. Am J Sports Med 1978;6:153–159.
- Bradley JP, Elkousy H: Decision making: Operative versus nonoperative treatment of acromioclavicular joint injuries. Clin Sports Med 2003;22:277–290.
- Schlegel TF, Burks RT, Marcus RL, Dunn HK: A prospective evaluation of untreated acute grade III acromioclavicular separations. Am J Sports Med 2001;29:699–703.
- Spencer EE Jr: Treatment of grade III acromioclavicular joint injuries: A systematic review. Clin Orthop Relat Res 2007; 455:38–44.
- Taft TN, Wilson FC, Oglesby JW: Dislocation of the acromioclavicular joint: An end-result study. J Bone Joint Surg Am 1987;69A:1045–1051.
- Tibone J, Sellers R, Tonino P: Strength testing after third-degree acromioclavicular dislocations. Am J Sports Med 1992;20: 328–331.

Chapter 43 Acromioclavicular Degenerative Joint Disease

Michael Simpson and Thomas M. Howard

Key Concepts

- Acromioclavicular (AC) joint osteoarthritis is the most common cause of AC pain.
- The AC joint is a small, diarthrodial joint that is formed by the acromion (part of the scapula) and the distal end of the clavicle (collar bone).
- The joint has a small surface area that is at risk of arthritis (wearing of the cartilage in the AC joint) due to significant forces acting across it.
- Osteoarthritis of the AC joint can be an isolated cause of anterosuperior shoulder pain, or it can be a contributor to the development of subacromial impingement.
- AC arthritis results from an acute or chronic repetitive injury due to
    - Long-term overhead activities
    - Sports such as tennis, swimming, pitching, volleyball, and weight lifting
    - Heavy labor
    - Complication of an AC ligament injury such as AC separation
- AC osteoarthritis is commonly seen on radiographs or magnetic resonance imaging studies in asymptomatic patients.
- AC arthritis is more common in patients older than 60, and the incidence doubles after age 80.

History

- Pain in the superior or anterior part of the shoulder
- Pain is worse with overhead, flexed, or adducted positions of the shoulder.
- Lifting activities exacerbate the pain.
- The patient has a history of AC separation or frequent trauma to the shoulder.
- Unrelenting pain with continued activity
- History of chronic repetitive activity and/or recent increase in use of the affected shoulder

Physical Examination

- Pain and/or crepitus of AC joint with passive or active overhead activity
- Positive cross-arm adduction test with pain at AC joint
    - This test is done with the arm elevated forward to 90 degrees with hyperadduction applied across the sternum while the examiner palpates the AC joint (Fig. 43-1).
- A diagnostic injection with 1 to 3 mL lidocaine with a 25-gauge needle into the AC joint can be helpful to isolate pain to the AC joint.
- A complete shoulder examination should be performed to rule out impingement syndrome, adhesive capsulitis, and glenohumeral arthritis.

Imaging

- Typical findings on a radiograph of the AC joint include joint narrowing, osteophyte formation, sclerosis, and subchondral cysts (Fig. 43-2).
- If the diagnosis is in doubt, magnetic resonance imaging can be helpful to rule out other causes of shoulder pain.
- The routine use of ultrasonography or computed tomography is not needed to evaluate the AC joint.
- Studies show little correlation between radiographic studies and physical examination findings for the AC joint.
- Recent data have shown that the presence of bone marrow edema in the medial acromion, lateral clavicle, or both on T2-weighted magnetic resonance images did correlate with a symptomatic AC joint.

Differential Diagnosis

- Please see Table 43-1.

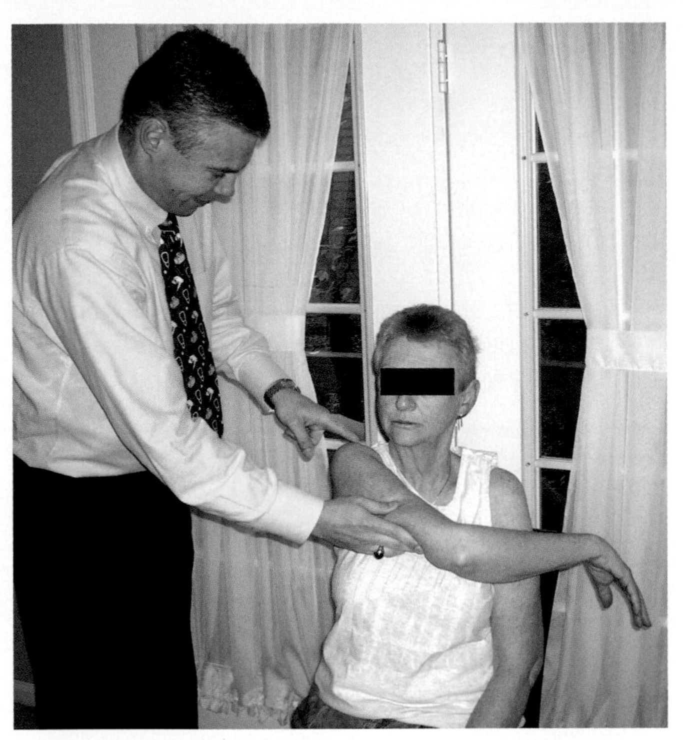

Figure 43-1 Positive cross-arm adduction test with pain at acromioclavicular joint.

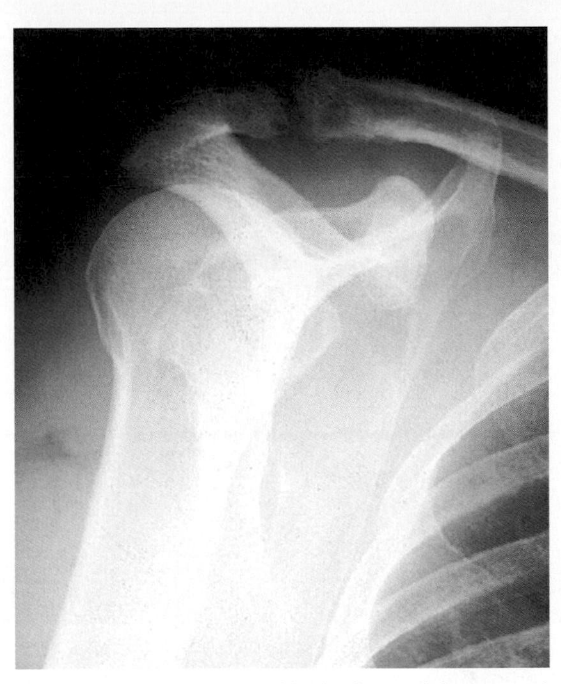

Figure 43-2 Typical radiographic findings of the acromioclavicular joint include joint narrowing, osteophyte formation, sclerosis, and subchondral cysts.

TABLE 43-1 *Differential Diagnosis of Acromioclavicular Pain*

Condition	Location of Pain	Differentiating Feature
Rotator cuff tendonosis/strain/tear	Superolateral	Pain with abducting shoulder at 70–120 degrees (painful arc) with weakness
Biceps tendon injury	Anterior	Pain with resisted elbow flexion and supination; tenderness in bicipital groove
Glenohumeral instability	Anterior	Often as a result of shoulder subluxation or dislocation; positive apprehension sign
Primary and secondary impingement	Superolateral	Positive Neer and/or Hawkins sign; pain with overhead activity
Calcific tendonosis	Superolateral	Seen on radiograph or magnetic resonance imaging as a result of rotator cuff injury
Glenohumeral arthritis	Superolateral and/or posterior	Rest pain, stiffness, and crepitus on movement
Acromion or distal clavicle fracture	Superior	Seen on radiograph as a result of trauma
Glenohumeral labral tear	Anterior	Seen in throwers or overhead motion athletes; positive O'Brien's test
Acromioclavicular osteolysis	Superior	Pain in acromioclavicular joint; most common in weightlifters
Cervical spine disease	Variable	Neck pain; positive Spurling's test
Thoracic outlet syndrome	Generalized	Intermittent pain, weakness, and neurovascular symptoms; positive Roos test
Adhesive capsulitis	Anterior	Active and passive range of motion of the glenohumeral joint is greatly restricted
Suprascapular neuropathy	Posterior	Pain and weakness with wasting of infraspinatus muscle
Referred pain (angina, Pancoast's tumor, gallbladder)	Variable; axillary pain is usually not from the shoulder	Constant pain not associated with shoulder movement; systemic symptoms; pain aggravated by deep inspiration

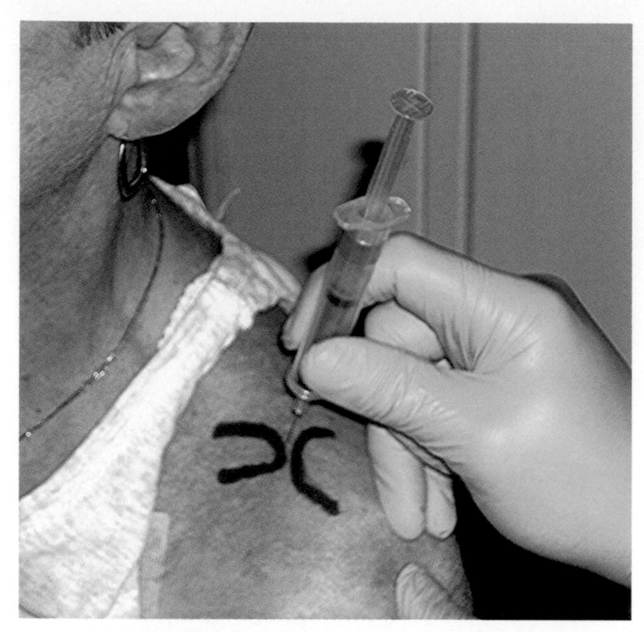

Figure 43-3 Corticosteroid injection into the acromioclavicular joint from a superoanterior approach and directed inferiorly.

Treatment

- Symptomatic/pain relief with nonsteroidal anti-inflammatory drugs and/or hot and cold compresses
- Activity modification when symptomatic to avoid overhead activities and weightlifting, such as bench press, dips, and push-ups
- Physical therapy to correct muscle imbalance and maintain range of motion
- Corticosteroid injection into the AC joint from a superoanterior approach and directed inferiorly (Fig. 43-3)
- Surgery can be considered if conservative management fails.
    - This includes the Mumford procedure with open resection of the distal clavicle.
    - A quicker recovery can be achieved if this is done arthroscopically with preservation of the superior capsule and overlying fascia, which are important stabilizing structures of the AC joint.

When to Refer

- Refer patients with refractory pain, those unwilling to accept activity modifications, and those with a poor response to steroid injections.

Troubleshooting

- Counsel regarding the chronic nature of this condition and expected time frame to recovery or deterioration.
- Patient should receive no more than three AC joint corticosteroid injections over the course of 1 year.
- Risks of steroid injection into the joint include atrophy of the fat pad, discoloration of the overlying skin, and steroid flare.

Patient Instructions

- AC arthritis is often due to constant overhead lifting. This activity should be avoided while the patient is symptomatic.
- Most cases of AC arthritis can be managed conservatively with rest, nonsteroidal anti-inflammatory drugs, and physical therapy, and avoidance of overhead activities.

Considerations in Special Populations

- Sports involving arm loading, such as gymnastics, weight lifting, and swimming, increase the risk of AC arthritis.
- Workers performing tasks involving static loading of the arms and vibration, such as foremen, bricklayers, and jackhammer operators, have an even greater risk of AC arthritis compared with athletes in sports cited previously.

Suggested Reading

- Bonsell S, Pearsall AW IV, Heitman RJ, et al: The relationship of age, gender, and degenerative changes observed on radiographs of the shoulder in asymptomatic individuals. J Bone Joint Surg Br 2000;82B:1135–1139.
- Cadet E, Ahmad C, Levine W: The management of acromioclavicular joint osteoarthrosis: Debride, resect, or leave it alone. Instr Course Lect 2006;55:75–83.
- Charron K, Schepsis A, Voloshin I: Arthroscopic distal clavicle resection in athletes. Am J Sports Med 2006;35:53–58.
- Ernberg LA, Potter HG: Radiographic evaluation of the acromioclavicular and sternoclavicular joints. Clin Sports Med 2003;22:255–275.
- Fukuda K, Craig EV, An KN, et al: Biomechanical study of the ligamentous system of the acromioclavicular joint. J Bone Joint Surg Am 1986;68A:434–440.
- Neer CS II: Impingement lesions. Clin Orthop Relat Res 1983;173:70–77.
- Neviaser RJ, Neviaser TJ: Observations on impingement. Clin Orthop Relat Res 1990;254:60–63.

- Petersson CJ, Gentz CF: Ruptures of the supraspinatus tendon: The significance of distally pointing acromioclavicular osteophytes. Clin Orthop Relat Res 1983;174:143–148.
- Rabalais RD, McCarty E: Surgical treatment of symptomatic acromioclavicular joint problems: A systematic review. Clin Orthop Relat Res 2007;455:30–37.
- Stein BE, Wiater JM, Pfaff HC, et al: Detection of acromioclavicular joint pathology in asymptomatic shoulders with magnetic resonance imaging. J Shoulder Elbow Surg 2001;10: 204–208.
- Tallia AF, Cardone DA: Diagnostic and therapeutic injection of the shoulder region. Am Fam Physician 2003;67:1271–1278.

Chapter 44 Acromioclavicular Osteolysis

Michael Simpson and Thomas M. Howard

Key Concepts

- Acromioclavicular (AC) osteolysis of the shoulder can be traumatic; however, atraumatic causes are more common.
- Systemic disease should always be considered in the differential diagnosis.
- Repetitive loading of the AC joint is thought to be the precipitating factor leading to inadequate bone formation and remodeling; normal bone remodeling cannot occur due to continued stress on the joint.
- Atraumatic osteolysis has become more common because of the increased popularity of weight lifting.
- Early diagnosis and treatment can increase the chance of success with conservative measures. This approach has been shown to reverse the osteolysis process and result in various degrees of healing.
- A delayed diagnosis usually results in a permanently widened AC joint with varying degrees of pain and mechanical dysfunction.

History

- Most commonly seen in males with a long history of strength training
- Weight lifting, football, swimming, and throwing activities are other causes of overuse.
- Osteolysis can also result from acute trauma or repetitive minor trauma to the AC joint.
- Pain in the AC joint begins insidiously and may occur only with the precipitating activity, most notably with bench presses, military presses, and dips.
- Most commonly unilateral but can also be bilateral
- As osteolysis progresses, the pain may persist for several days after the activity.

Physical Examination

- Pain and/or crepitus of the AC joint with passive or active overhead activity
- Positive cross-arm adduction test with pain at AC joint
  - This test is done with the arm elevated forward to 90 degrees with hyperadduction applied across the sternum while the examiner palpates the AC joint.
- A diagnostic injection with 1 to 3 mL lidocaine with a 25-gauge needle into the AC joint can be helpful to isolate pain to the AC joint.
- A complete shoulder examination should be performed to rule out impingement syndrome, adhesive capsulitis, and glenohumeral arthritis.
- Range of motion and strength are normal.

Imaging

- Diagnosis can be confirmed with radiographs or a bone scan.
- Radiographs show lucency, osteopenia, and osteophytes at the distal clavicle (Fig. 44-1).
- In later stages, tapering down of the distal clavicle and widening of the AC joint may be seen.
- A bone scan will show increased uptake at the distal clavicle and may precede radiographic findings.
- Magnetic resonance imaging of the shoulder can be helpful for ruling out other causes of shoulder pain and is effective at revealing soft-tissue swelling, subchondral cysts, cortical thinning, bone marrow edema, and synovial hypertrophy.

Differential Diagnosis

- Acromioclavicular arthritis
- Undiagnosed clavicle fracture
- Osteoid osteoma
- Other etiologies showing lysis or erosion of the distal clavicle: multiple myeloma, metastasis, scleroderma, hyperparathyroidism, infection, rheumatoid arthritis, rickets, spinal cord injury, and progeria

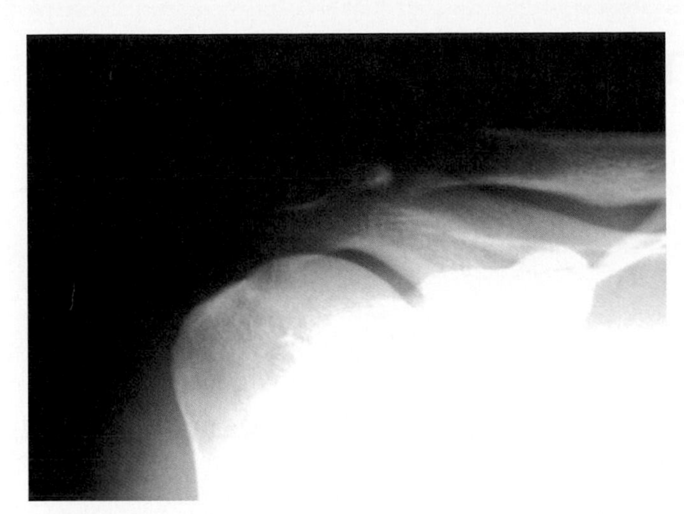

Figure 44-1 Radiograph of acromioclavicular osteolysis.

Treatment

- Symptomatic pain relief with nonsteroidal anti-inflammatory drugs and/or hot and cold compresses
- Activity modification to eliminate lifting exercises and aggravating activities can alleviate symptoms and prevent progression.
- Physical therapy does not offer any proven benefit but is helpful to maintain the range of motion and strengthen the surrounding musculature.
- Resumption of activity even after 1 year may exacerbate symptoms.
- Distal clavicle excision (Mumford procedure [open] or arthroscopy) may be performed if conservative therapy fails.
- Arthroscopic distal clavicle excision can allow patients to return to activities more rapidly and is the preferred method.

When to Refer

- Refer patients with refractory pain who are not improving despite several months of conservative treatment.

Troubleshooting

- Counsel regarding the chronic nature of this condition and expected time frame to recovery.
- Patient should receive no more than three AC corticosteroid injections over the course of 1 year.
- Risks of steroid injection into the joint include atrophy of the fat pad, discoloration of the overlying skin, and steroid flare.

Patient Instructions

- Avoid exacerbating activities, especially bench presses, military presses, and dips.
- Pain in the AC joint may persist as long as 1 year after activities stressing the AC joint.
- To prevent osteolysis, limit upper extremity weight lifting and avoid lifting very heavy weights.

Suggested Reading

- Auge WK, Fischer RA: Arthroscopic distal clavicle resection for isolated atraumatic osteolysis in weight lifters. Am J Sports Med 1998;26:189–192.
- Cahill BR: Atraumatic osteolysis of the distal clavicle: A review. Sports Med 1992;13:214–222.
- Charron KM, Schepsis AA, Voloshin I: Arthroscopic distal clavicle resection in athletes. Am J Sports Med 2006;35:53–58.
- Gajeski BL, Kettner NW: Osteolysis of the distal clavicle: Serial improvement and normalization of acromioclavicular joint space with conservative care. J Manipulative Physiol Ther 2004;27:480–488.
- Hawkins BJ, Covey DC, Thiel BG: Distal clavicle osteolysis unrelated to trauma, overuse, or metabolic disease. Clin Orthop Relat Res 2000;370:208–211.
- Kassarjian A, Llopis E, Palmer WE: Distal clavicular osteolysis: MR evidence for subchondral fracture. Skeletal Radiol 2007;36:17–22.
- Scavenius M, Iversen BF: Nontraumatic clavicular osteolysis in weight lifters. Am J Sports Med 1992;20:463–467.

Chapter 45 Sternoclavicular Injuries

Thomas E. Brickner

Key Concepts

- Pathophysiology may be acute traumatic injury or arthritic condition
- Mechanism of injury is either a direct blow to the medial clavicle or an indirectly transmitted force from posterolateral shoulder compression
- Motor vehicle accidents and sports injuries are most common causes
- Sternoclavicular (SC) dislocations represent less than 1% of all joint dislocations and only 3% of all upper extremity dislocations.
- Anterior dislocations are more common than posterior dislocations (10–20 : 1).
- Posterior dislocations are associated with intrathoracic or superior mediastinal injuries in up to 30% of cases.

Anatomy

- Diarthrodial, saddle-type joint with less than half the clavicular endplate articulating with the sternum (Fig. 45-1)
- High degree of motion during the first 90 degrees of arm elevation
- Depends on ligamentous structures, both periarticular and extra-articular, for support (Fig. 45-2)
- Periarticular ligaments include the intra-articular disc ligament, the interclavicular ligament, and the capsular ligaments
    - Posterior capsular ligament is the most important anterior-posterior stabilizer
- Extra-articular ligament is the costoclavicular ligament and connects the first rib and medial clavicle
    - Resists cephalad and caudad displacement of the clavicle

History

- Pain at the SC joint, especially with shoulder motion, arm elevation, or lateral compression
- Patients with posterior dislocations may complain of dysphagia, dyspnea, dysphonia, or paresthesias if posteriorly located structures are injured.
- Late compression of vital structures may still occur if posterior dislocations are left unreduced.
- Mechanical symptoms with pain and clicking may occur if intra-articular disc is torn

Physical Examination

- Swelling, pain, and possible palpable defect overlying the SC joint

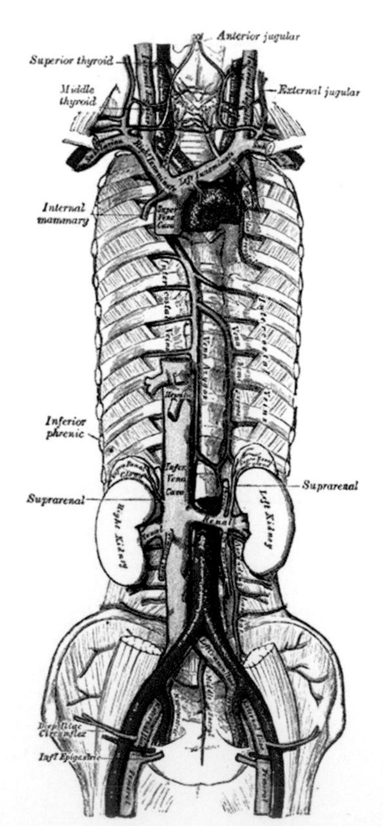

Figure 45-1 Vascular anatomy of the superior media stinum. (From Gray H: Gray's Anatomy of the Human Body, 20th ed. Philadelphia: Lea & Febiger, 1918. Image 577.)

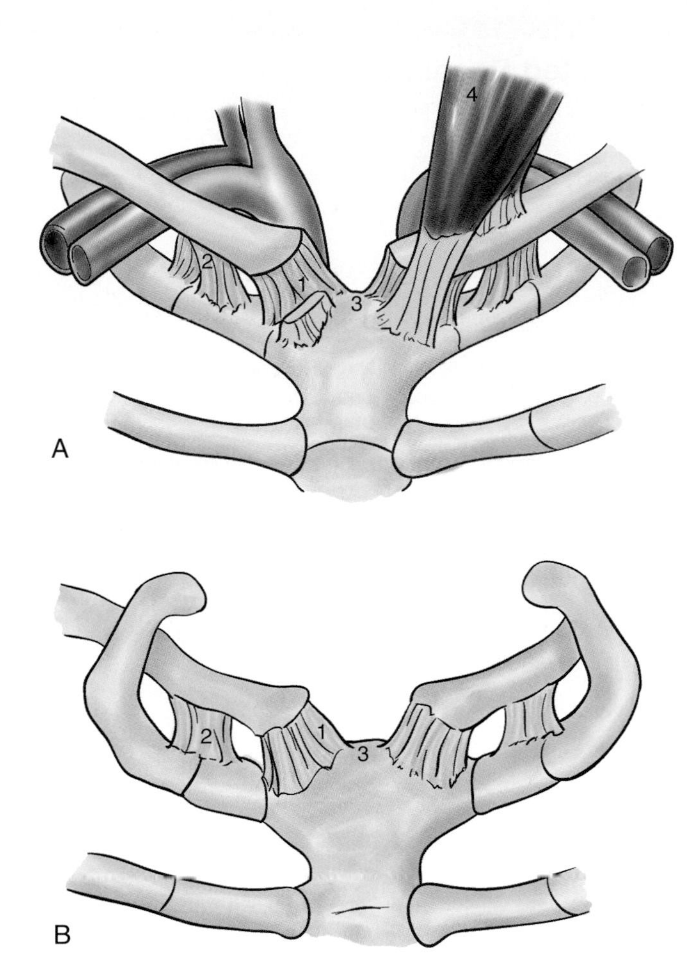

Figure 45-2 Anatomy of the sternoclavicular joint from anterior (**A**) to posterior (**B**) views. The structures are (1) anterior capsule (in part A) and posterior capsule (in part B), (2) costoclavicular ligament, (3) interclavicular ligament, and (4) the sternocleidomastoid tendon. (Adapted from Spencer EE, Kuhn JE, Huston LJ, et al: Ligamentous restraints to anterior and posterior translation of the sternoclavicular joint. J Shoulder Elbow Surg 2002;11:43–47, with permission.)

- Increased translation compared to uninjured side with manual stressing
- Paresthesias and decreased peripheral pulses of upper extremity, if associated with retroclavicular arterial damage
- Vascular engorgement of upper extremity, if venous structures compromised
- Drooling, if esophagus is compressed
- Dyspnea and stridor, if lungs and/or trachea damaged

Imaging

- Anterior-posterior, lateral chest radiograph for routine surveillance
- Serendipity view with radiograph beam projected 40 degrees cephalad
    - Raised clavicular end indicative of anterior displacement
    - Depressed clavicular end indicative of posterior displacement
- Computed tomography scan recommended for confirmation of posterior dislocations and evaluation of mediastinal and thoracic structures

Differential Diagnosis

- Contusion or fracture of sternum or clavicle
- Sternocleidomastoid strain

Treatment

Anterior Dislocations

- At diagnosis
    - Ice, analgesia
    - Grade I: Immobilize with figure-of-eight bandage or sling for 1 to 2 weeks
    - Grade II: Immobilize for 3 to 6 weeks
    - Grade III: Closed reduction followed by immobilization for 4 to 6 weeks
- Later
    - Grade III injuries often remain unstable after initial treatment but have little long-term functional impairment.
    - Open reduction with stabilization and possible medial clavicular resection reserved for chronic symptoms with instability or cosmetic concerns

Posterior Dislocations

- Closed reduction as soon as possible
- General anesthesia or heavy sedation may be needed.
- Abduction-traction technique is primary method
    - Rolled towel between scapula in supine position
    - Abduct arm to 90 degrees; apply traction and gently extend
    - Pull medial clavicle forward, if necessary.
- Adduction-traction technique
    - Position as above
    - Adduct arm and apply downward traction and downward pressure on shoulder
- After reduction, immobilize in figure-of-eight bandage or sling and swathe for 4 to 6 weeks.
- Physical therapy and active shoulder exercises after 3 weeks
- Open reduction indicated if closed reduction is unsuccessful

Troubleshooting

- Open exploration may be needed for chronic symptoms of pain, grating, or instability.
- If resection of the medial clavicle is necessary, then it is recommended to either preserve or reconstruct the costoclavicular and capsular ligaments.
- Strongly advised to avoid hardware across the SC joint for fixation due to the risk of migration and potential damage to mediastinal structures

Considerations in Special Populations

- Physeal injury is more likely than a true SC dislocation in younger age groups.
- Medial clavicular epiphysis is last to ossify (18–20 years old), and does not fuse to shaft of clavicle until 23 to 25 years old.

Suggested Reading

- Bicos J, Nicholson G: Treatment and results of sternoclavicular joint injuries. Clin Sports Med 2003;22:359–370.
- Garretson R, Williams G: Clinical evaluation of injuries to the acromioclavicular and sternoclavicular joints. Clin Sports Med 2003;22:239–254.
- Gove N, Ebraheim N, Glass E: Posterior sternoclavicular dislocations: A review of management and complications. Am J Orthop 2006;35:132–136.
- Kuzak N, Ishkanian A, Abu-Laban R: Posterior sternoclavicular joint dislocation: Case report and discussion. Can J Emerg Med 2006;8:355–357.
- Renfree K, Wright T: Anatomy and biomechanics of the acromioclavicular and sternoclavicular joints. Clin Sports Med 2003;22:219–237.

Chapter 46 Scapulothoracic Problems

Kelly Waicus

SCAPULOTHORACIC BURSITIS (SNAPPING SCAPULA SYNDROME)

ICD-9 CODES

726.0 *Scapular Bursitis Not Otherwise Specified*
955.7 *(Injury to) Other Specified Nerve(s) of Shoulder Girdle and Upper Limb*
352.4 *Disorders of Accessory (11th) Nerve*
353.5 *Neuralgic Amyotrophy, Parsonage-Aldren-Turner Syndrome*
862.8 *Thoracic Nerve Injury*

Key Concepts

- Snapping scapula syndrome may also be referred to as scapulothoracic bursitis, scapulothoracic crepitus, superior scapular syndrome, retroscapular pain, washboard syndrome, and retroscapular creaking.
- The scapula has no true synovial characteristics, but maintains its function through dynamic muscular control. Its anatomic configuration allows for smooth gliding motions along the thoracic wall.
- Dyskinesis (alteration of the normal motion or position of the scapulothoracic joint) can be caused by pain or muscle weakness, inflexibility, or imbalance.

History

- A snapping, grinding, or popping sound is heard with scapulothoracic movement. Symptoms vary from one or several snaps to frank crepitus.
- Pain with increasing shoulder activity, although some patients report no pain
- May have posterior shoulder fatigue before onset of symptoms
- May have history of repetitive, forceful, overhead sports or activities (swimming, pitching, gymnastics, weight training, and football) or history of trauma
- May have nonspecific pain under the scapula

Physical Examination

- May have asymmetry of the scapulae (slight depression of dominant extremity is within normal limits)
- Scapular winging may be present.
- Poor posture with anterior head position and rounded shoulders may contribute to the condition.
- The patient may have trapezius, levator scapulae, or pectoralis minor muscle tightness contributing to faulty scapular mechanics. A higher or more anterior supine resting shoulder position indicates a tight pectoralis minor muscle.
- Assess for weakness of scapular muscles including trapezius, rhomboid, serratus anterior, latissimus dorsi, levator scapulae, rotator cuff, and deltoid muscles (see Chapter 30).
- Rule out cervical spine radiculopathy with Spurling's test.
- Evaluate for glenohumeral impingement (see Chapter 38) and instability (see Chapter 33) as both conditions may cause excessive scapular muscle compensation and fatigue.
- Evaluate for a faulty scapulothoracic joint. Decreased glenohumeral motion with increased movement and/or protrusion of the scapula may be seen.
- Palpation of the medial scapular border may elicit pain at the superomedial or inferomedial bursa (Fig. 46-1).

Imaging

- Radiographs should include both anteroposterior and scapular/tangential Y views.
- If radiographs are negative, consider a computed tomography scan for better bony visualization.
- Fluoroscopy may be helpful to visualize symptoms during shoulder motion.
- If computed tomography does not reveal a bony etiology, magnetic resonance imaging may be used to

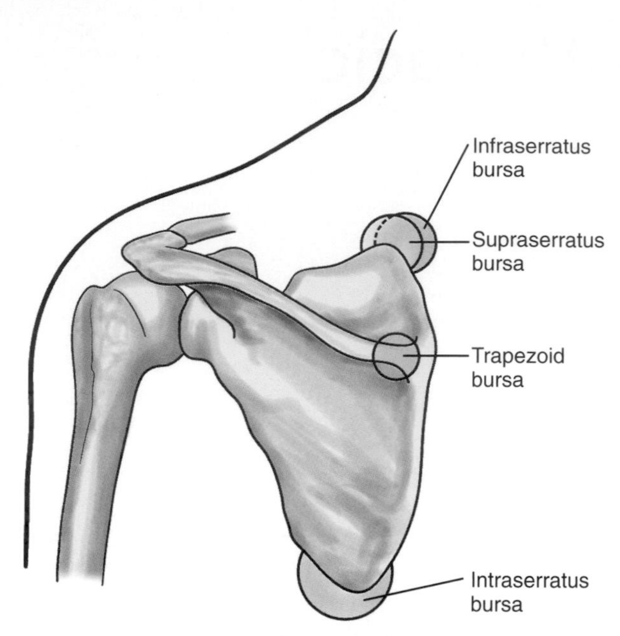

Figure 46-1 Periscapular bursae.

define a soft-tissue etiology such as an inflamed bursa.

Additional Tests

- If scapular winging is present, electromyography and nerve conduction velocity studies may help determine whether there is neurologic injury (see "Winging of the Scapula" section).

Differential Diagnosis

- Abnormalities of bone, muscle, or a bursa involved in scapulothoracic movement can all be causes of snapping scapula syndrome (Box 46-1).
- Underlying problems with the cervical spine or glenohumeral joint may be the primary cause.

Treatment

- For patients with soft-tissue abnormalities, focus initial treatment on a 3- to 4-month commitment to a physical therapy program concentrating on strengthening muscle weakness, stretching tight muscles, and correcting postural faults.
- Nonsteroidal anti-inflammatory medications, ultrasound, and electrical stimulation may help with initial pain control.
- For patients who fail initial conservative treatment or those who have focal symptoms at either the superomedial or inferomedial border of the scapula, injection of a corticosteroid/anesthetic agent combination can be both diagnostic and therapeutic (Figs. 46-2 and 46-3).
- If all conservative measures fail, surgical options should be considered.
- Patients with definitive bony abnormalities should be referred for surgical evaluation.

BOX 46-1 Causes of Snapping Scapula Syndrome

Bony Abnormalities
Scapula
- Exostoses or spurs
- Osteochondromas
- Scapular tubercle of Luschka (bony or fibrocartilaginous protrusion at the superior angle of the scapula)
- Anterior angulation of the superior angle of the scapula
- Fractures (acute or healed)
- Sprengel's deformity (congenital undescended scapula)

Rib
- Tumors
- Abnormal angulations
- Fractures (acute or healed)

Vertebrae
- Omovertebral bone (abnormal cervical transverse process)
- Scoliosis or thoracic kyphosis

Soft-tissue Abnormalities
Superomedial, inferomedial, or subscapular bursitis
Shoulder muscle atrophy
- Serratus anterior atrophy secondary to long thoracic nerve palsy
- Subscapularis atrophy secondary to glenohumeral fusion

Skeletal muscle intrafascicular fibrosis due to chronic inflammation
Subscapular elastofibroma

Other
After first rib resection for thoracic outlet syndrome
Tuberculosis or syphilitic lesions

Adapted from Carlson HL, Haig AJ, Stewart DC: Snapping scapula syndrome: Three case reports and an analysis of the literature. Arch Phys Med Rehabil 1997;78:506–511.

Troubleshooting

- A diagnostic workup to rule out bony abnormality or elastofibroma (especially in younger overhead athletes) should be undertaken early in the course of treatment to identify those who might benefit from early surgical intervention.
- Patients with nerve injuries may fail conservative management if the muscle is unable to be recruited for strengthening exercises; consider electromyography/nerve conduction velocity studies for evaluation.

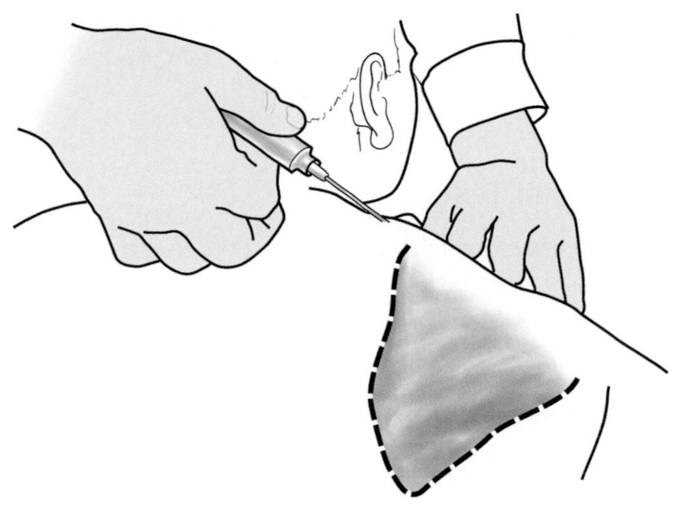

Figure 46-2 Injection of a superomedial bursa.

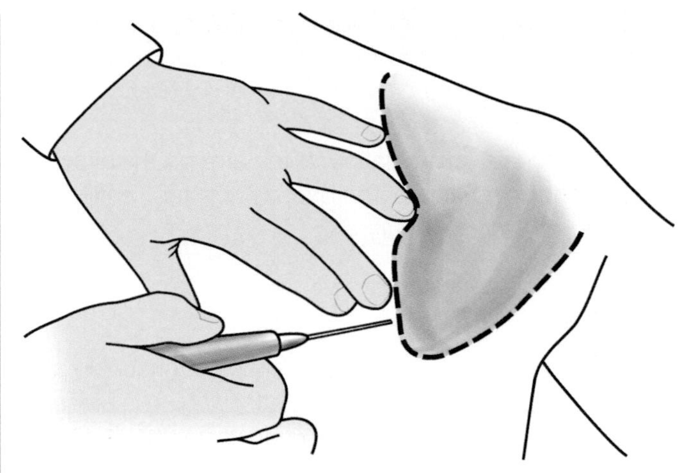

Figure 46-3 Injection of an inferomedial bursa.

- Scapulothoracic crepitus is not always pathologic. Asymptomatic individuals should be reassured, but also warned that, over time, repetitive snapping of the scapula may become painful.

Patient Instructions

- Most cases of snapping scapula syndrome resolve or improve with 3 to 4 months of physical therapy.
- Try to avoid repetitive activities that reproduce snapping and pain.
- Do not intentionally cause scapular snapping because this may eventually lead to pain in an otherwise asymptomatic individual.

WINGING OF THE SCAPULA (WINGED SCAPULA)

Key Concepts

- Although winging of the scapula is generally associated with serratus anterior muscle dysfunction due to long thoracic nerve injury, many other causes have been reported.
- Winging is defined as the prominence of the medial (vertebral) border of the scapula, but the winged scapula may also be rotated or displaced medially or laterally.
- Winging can be either static (present at rest) or dynamic (noted with active or resisted movement of the shoulder and arm).
- Static winging is due to a fixed deformity of the scapula, spine, ribs, or shoulder.
- Dynamic winging is caused by a neuromuscular disorder.

History

- Scapular winging may be asymptomatic.
- Commonly reported symptoms include pain (usually posterior) and weakness about the shoulder, particularly with overhead activity.
- Patients may have difficulty with arm elevation, particularly with prolonged activity.
- Repetitive or stressful activity may produce clicking and/or popping.
- Patients with static winging may report a posterior "lump" with or without discomfort while supine.
- A history of neck, shoulder (axilla), or thoracic surgery; a direct blow to the shoulder; or prolonged or repetitive trauma or strain may be present.
- Symptoms may develop after a compression or stretch injury to the neck, shoulder, or arm.
- Spontaneous severe pain followed by onset of weakness after a few days is suggestive of amyotrophic brachial neuralgia (Parsonage-Aldren-Turner syndrome).

Physical Examination

- Shoulder asymmetry and atrophy of the affected muscle may be noted.
- Prominence of the medial border (winging) at rest may be noted (static winging).
- Winging may become present or increase with active arm forward elevation or abduction or with slow lowering of the arm from the forward elevated position.
- Active range of motion may be limited in forward elevation or abduction above the horizontal position.
- Assess passive range of motion to rule out adhesive capsulitis or impingement.

- Having the patient lean forward against a wall in the push-up position may magnify the scapular winging.
- Examination of the cervical spine is necessary to rule out cervical disease (see Chapter 110).
- Neurovascular examination of the arm on the affected side should evaluate for brachial plexus, peripheral nerve, or vascular injury.

Imaging

- Plain radiographs of the cervical spine, shoulder, and thorax should be obtained. If static winging is present, include scapular/tangential Y views in the shoulder series.
- Computed tomography or magnetic resonance imaging to rule out scapular or disc lesion/pathology

Additional Tests

- Electromyography and nerve conduction velocity studies will help to confirm and clarify neurologic causes of scapular winging.

Differential Diagnosis

- Please see Table 46-1.

TABLE 46-1 *Differential Diagnosis*

Etiology	Findings
Serratus anterior weakness/palsy (long thoracic nerve injury, avulsion, or congenital absence of serratus anterior)	Winging accentuated with push-up against wall (Fig. 46-4)
Trapezius weakness/palsy (spinal accessory nerve injury, congenital absence of trapezius)	Causes scapular winging and elevation; winging accentuated by arm abduction at shoulder level (Fig. 46-5)
Rhomboid weakness (dorsal scapular nerve or C5 nerve root injury)	Winging accentuated with slow lowering of the arm from forward elevation
Amyotrophic brachial neuralgia (Parsonage-Aldren-Turner syndrome)	Spontaneous onset of severe shoulder girdle pain with onset of weakness and winging of the scapula after a few days
Facioscapulohumeral dystrophy	Onset of weakness in the second decade of life; weakness of multiple muscle groups causes severe winging and inability to elevate arm >90 degrees; asymmetry of facial muscles
Skeletal deformity (scoliosis) or solitary, localized lesion of the scapula, rib, or clavicle	Static winging, deformity noted on physical examination or imaging studies
Congenital or postinjection fibrosis of the deltoid	Abduction or flexion contracture and static winging
Degenerative or inflammatory joint disease of the shoulder	Abduction or internal rotation contracture; evidence of joint disease on imaging studies

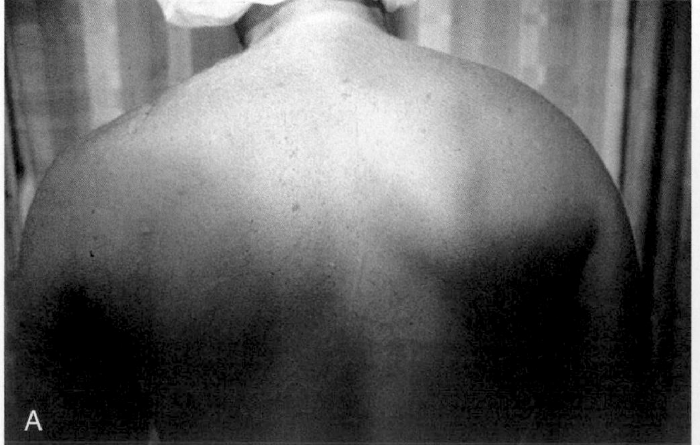

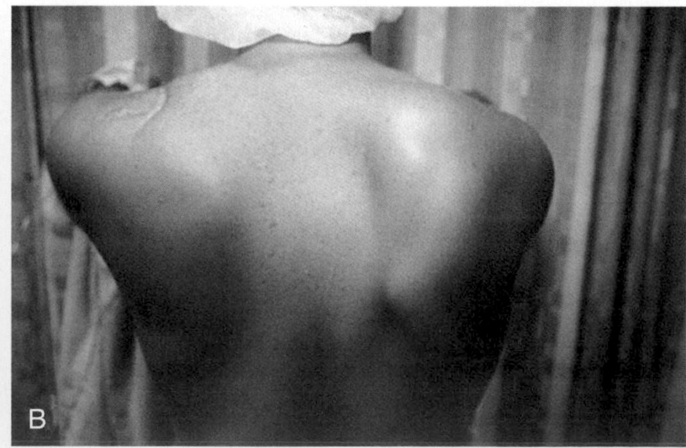

Figure 46-4 Scapular winging associated with long thoracic nerve injury and serratus muscle palsy. **A**, The scapula assumes a superomedial position at rest. **B**, Winging is accentuated with elevation of the arms. (Reprinted with permission from Kuhn JE: Scapulothoracic crepitus and bursitis in athletes. In DeLee JC, Drez D, Jr, Miller MD [eds]: DeLee and Drez's Orthopaedic Sports Medicine, 2nd ed. Philadelphia: Saunders, 2003, p 1009.)

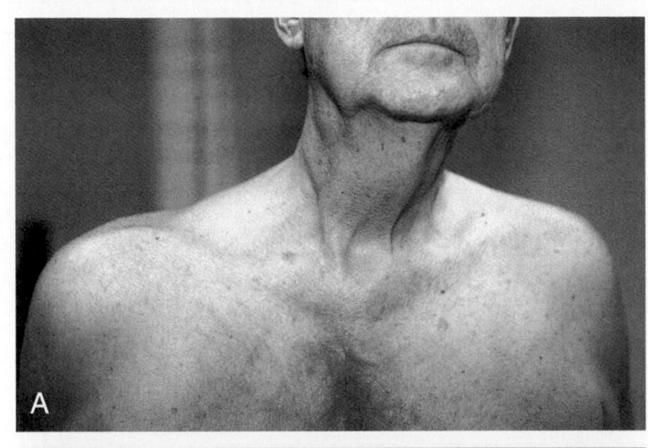

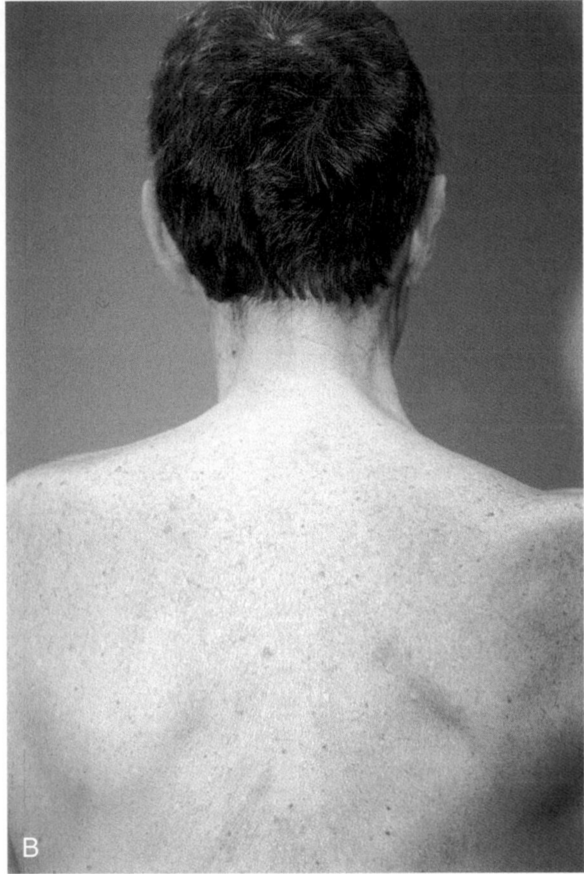

Figure 46-5 Scapular winging associated with spinal accessory nerve injury and trapezius muscle palsy. **A**, Anterior view. **B**, Posterior view. The scapula assumes a depressed and laterally deviated position. (Reprinted with permission from Kuhn JE: Scapulothoracic crepitus and bursitis in athletes. In DeLee JC, Drez D, Jr, Miller MD [eds]: DeLee and Drez's Orthopaedic Sports Medicine, 2nd ed. Philadelphia: Saunders, 2003, p 1009.)

Treatment

- Treatment depends on the cause of scapular winging.
- Acute serratus anterior and trapezius muscle palsies often resolve spontaneously.
- Begin early range of motion and strengthening exercises to prevent contractures and strengthen the remaining functional shoulder muscles to maintain function.
- Modify activity if repetitive use is a contributing or causative factor.
- Use of a shoulder/scapular cup type of brace or sling may help to stabilize the scapula and reduce pain in the early stages of treatment.
- Patients with a neurologic etiology should have baseline electromyography at 3 months post-injury to evaluate for denervation with follow-up studies at 6-week intervals to follow return of nerve function.
- Patients with a history of penetrating trauma or surgery followed by immediate, complete deficit should be referred for possible surgical exploration and repair/graft.
- Consider surgical referral in motivated, active patients if nerve function does not return within 1 year. Surgeons may choose to observe for as long as 2 years post-injury before recommending surgical treatment.
- Refer patients with skeletal or bony lesions for surgical evaluation.
- Patients with congenital abnormalities or progressive muscular dystrophies should be referred for possible surgical scapular stabilization to improve function and cosmetic appearance.

Troubleshooting

- Consider early surgical referral for acute injury with complete disability or patients with penetrating or surgical causes of muscle paralysis. Early referral will increase the chance of a successful exploration and repair or graft of a transected nerve.

Patient Instructions

- The majority of cases of acute serratus anterior and trapezius muscle palsies as well as Parsonage-Aldren-Turner syndrome resolve spontaneously. It may take 6 months to 2 years for full return of function.
- Compliance with physical therapy and recommended bracing will help maintain current function and prevent future disability.
- Avoid repetitive activities that may have caused or continue to aggravate your condition.

Suggested Reading

- Carlson HL, Haig AJ, Stewart DC: Snapping scapula syndrome: Three case reports and an analysis of the literature. Arch Phys Med Rehabil 1997;78:506–511.

- Duralde XA: Evaluation and treatment of the winged scapula. J South Orthop Assoc 1995;4:38–45.
- Fiddian NJ, King RJ: The winged scapula. Clin Orthop Relat Res 1984;185:228–236.
- Manske RC, Reiman MP, Stovak ML: Nonoperative and operative management of snapping scapula. Am J Sports Med 2004;32:1554–1565.
- Wiater JM, Bigliani LU: Spinal accessory nerve injury. Clin Orthop Relat Res 1999;368:5–16.
- Wiater JM, Flatow EL: Long thoracic nerve injury. Clin Orthop Relat Res 1999;368:17–27.

Chapter 47 Neurovascular Entrapment

John P. Colianni and William Dexter

ICD-9 CODES
353.0 *Thoracic Outlet Syndrome*
955.7 *Suprascapular Nerve Entrapment*
955.7 *Long Thoracic Nerve Entrapment*
955.7 *Quadrilateral Space Syndrome*

THORACIC OUTLET SYNDROME

Key Concepts

- Thoracic outlet syndrome refers to symptoms of neurologic or vascular compression along the neurovascular bundle from the cervicothoracic region to the axilla.
- The lower trunk of the brachial plexus and the subclavian artery and vein pass through several potentially compressing spaces.
- Moving laterally from the midline, these spaces include
  - The region between the anterior and middle scalene muscles and their attachment to the first rib
  - The costoclavicular area defined by the clavicle, the first rib, and the superior portion of the scapula
  - The pectoralis minor space formed by the undersurface of the pectoralis minor tendon insertion and the coracoid process
- Risk factors for entrapment include
  - Presence of a cervical rib
  - Presence of a space-occupying lesion (including lymphadenopathy or tumor)
  - Slender body type with a long neck and droopy shoulders, often described in females with a "swan" neck
- May commonly present with coexistent carpal tunnel syndrome

History

- Presenting symptoms often are vague but may include pain, numbness, weakness, and a sensation of swelling in the affected arm.
- Neurogenic etiologies often present with paresthesias in the medial hand and forearm regions on the affected side.
- Vascular etiologies may additionally present with pallor or cyanosis, distended surface veins, and cool temperature of the affected arm.
- Symptoms often are exacerbated by overhead activity.
- Obesity or large pendulous breasts may distort posture and increase risk for syndrome.

Physical Examination

- Complete general shoulder and cervical spine examination
- Complete neurovascular examination of the upper extremity
- Additional special examination maneuvers intended to decrease the costoclavicular space
  - Adson's maneuver
    - — With the patient in a seated position, the examiner palpates the radial pulse of the affected arm.
    - — The affected arm is then brought to at least 90 degrees of abduction, the neck is fully extended, the head is turned toward the affected side, and the patient is asked to perform a Valsalva maneuver.
    - — The test result is considered positive if the radial pulse is diminished or absent.
    - — The maneuver may also reproduce the patient's symptoms.
  - Modified Adson's test
    - — Performed as in Adson's maneuver; however, with the patient's head turned away from the affected side
    - — The test result is positive if the radial pulse is diminished or absent.
  - Roos test
    - — The patient's arms are placed in 90 degrees of abduction and are externally rotated, and the elbows are flexed.

- — The patient is then asked to repeatedly clench and unclench his or her fists.
  - — A positive test result occurs with the reproduction of symptoms.
- Costoclavicular maneuver
  - — The patient is asked to thrust his or her shoulders posteriorly and inferiorly, similar to an exaggerated military attention pose.
  - — The test result is positive if the radial pulse is diminished or absent.
- Hyperabduction-extension test
  - — The patient's extended arms are brought overhead in nearly full abduction.
  - — If the patient's symptoms are reproduced, the test result is considered positive.

Imaging

- Plain radiographs of the cervical spine and anteroposterior radiograph of the chest
  - Useful to evaluate for cervical rib, prominent C7 transverse process, or space-occupying lesion; however, these studies are usually normal

Additional Tests (If Applicable)

- Traditional angiography or magnetic resonance angiography
  - Consider if a vascular cause is strongly suspected.
- Nerve conduction studies
  - Useful to evaluate for other diagnoses in the differential diagnosis, including carpal tunnel syndrome, cubital tunnel syndrome, and cervical radiculopathy
- Cervical spine and upper thoracic magnetic resonance imaging
  - Used to rule out a spinal cord process

Differential Diagnosis

- Cervical radiculopathy
- Brachial plexus injury
- Cubital tunnel syndrome
- Carpal tunnel syndrome
- Space-occupying lesion of the costoclavicular space, tumor (e.g., Pancoast's syndrome), or bulky lymphadenopathy
- Peripheral neuropathy
- Chronic regional pain syndrome
- Hypothyroidism
- Cervical spinal cord tumor
- Syringomyelia

Treatment

- At diagnosis
  - Conservative measures include
    - — Physical therapy
    - — Posture training
    - — Shoulder and rib cage elevation exercises
    - — Myofascial release
    - — Strain-counterstrain techniques
    - — Home exercise program instructions
    - — Sleep position adjustments to prevent arm abduction at night
    - — Overhead activity restrictions until symptoms resolve
    - — Vocational modifications to prevent extended overhead activity
    - — Appropriately supportive bra, if indicated
    - — Pain control regimen for neuropathic pain (if needed)
    - — Tricyclic antidepressants
    - — Anticonvulsants
- Later
  - Graded return to regular activity
  - Maintain home exercise program as established in physical therapy

When to Refer

- Surgical consultation should be obtained for excision of symptomatic cervical rib
- Surgical consultation indicated for possible first rib excision if conservative measures fail
- Surgical intervention should be considered for patients presenting with unrelenting sensory loss, disabling pain, or muscle wasting

Prognosis

- Conservative measures often provide relief in 50% to 90% of patients, usually within 6 weeks.
- The surgical failure rate for primary operations is 28%.
- Operative complications can include brachial plexus injury.

Troubleshooting

- Carpal tunnel syndrome may be coexistent and should be treated appropriately before surgery for thoracic outlet syndrome.
- Carefully exclude proximal or distal disorders, including cervical disc lesion and elbow nerve entrapment.

- Consider imaging to exclude space-occupying lesions.
- For recalcitrant cases, be certain that all aggravating factors are eliminated including improper vocational activities or sleep positions.
- Encourage adherence to a home exercise regimen.

SUPRASCAPULAR NERVE ENTRAPMENT

Key Concepts

- The suprascapular nerve innervates the supraspinatus and infraspinatus muscles.
- Suprascapular nerve entrapment often occurs at the site of the suprascapular notch where the nerve passes beneath the superior transverse scapular ligament.
- Another potential site of entrapment is at the level of the spinoglenoid ligament where the nerve courses beneath the scapular spine.
- Previous shoulder injury, repetitive overuse, or posterior labral tear may lead to the development of a posterior ganglion cyst and nerve impingement via the mass effect.
- Often associated with repetitive overhead activities, with most case reports involving competitive volleyball players; participants of tennis, baseball, basketball, weight lifting, or other overhead sports or occupations are also at risk

History

- Patient presents with insidious onset of posterior shoulder pain or dull ache, often in dominant arm
- Pain is exacerbated by overhead activity.
- Alternatively, patients may present with the symptom of shoulder weakness.

Physical Examination

- Complete general shoulder and cervical spine examination
- Complete neurovascular examination of the upper extremity
- Inspection of the supraspinatus and infraspinatus muscles may reveal atrophy.
- Diminished strength to resisted arm abduction may suggest supraspinatus muscle weakness.
- Diminished strength to resisted external rotation of the arm may suggest infraspinatus muscle involvement.
- Cross-adduction test
  - The examiner adducts the affected arm across the patient's chest. A reproduction of the pain may be elicited with this maneuver as the suprascapular nerve is stretched against the suprascapular transverse ligament.
- Tinel's sign or pain with palpation of the suprascapular notch may be present.

Imaging

- Plain radiography of the shoulder and cervical spine
  - Usually normal; however, testing useful to evaluate for other disorders
- Magnetic resonance imaging of the shoulder
  - May demonstrate muscle changes associated with nerve injury including decreased muscle bulk, fatty infiltration, and signal intensity differences
  - Potentially helpful in evaluating for other disorders in the differentia diagnosis

Additional Tests (If Applicable)

- Electrodiagnostic studies
  - Nerve conduction studies
  - Electromyography
    - — Consider these modalities for diagnostic confirmation and localization of the lesion.

Differential Diagnosis

- Cervical radiculopathy
- Shoulder or acromioclavicular joint disorder
- Ganglion cyst associated with labral tear
- Rotator cuff tear
- Chronic regional pain syndrome

Treatment

- At diagnosis
  - Conservative measures include
    - — Overhead activity restrictions
    - — Physical therapy
      - — Scapular stabilization program
      - — Flexibility program for surrounding muscles of glenohumeral joint
    - — Injection of local anesthetic into the suprascapular notch may increase the ability to participate in rehabilitation if pain is the main symptom.
- Later
  - Introduction of rotator cuff strengthening program
  - Graded return to activity once symptoms resolve

When to Refer

- Surgical consultation is warranted if the entrapment is associated with trauma.
- Consider surgical consultation if there is no improvement with conservative treatment after 6 months.

Prognosis

- Most patients will improve with conservative measures alone; however, the prognosis is not well known.
- Operative treatment results in improvement of functional impairments and relief of pain for most patients.

Troubleshooting

- Overhead activity restriction is vital to improvement.
- Counsel the patient that resolution may take 6 to 12 months.
- Counsel the patient that surgery, if necessary, carries a risk of nerve or vascular injury.
- Close follow-up is warranted to ensure compliance with a management program and to limit the duration of activity restrictions.

LONG THORACIC NERVE ENTRAPMENT

Key Concepts

- The long thoracic nerve innervates the serratus anterior muscle group.
- Compression or entrapment can occur after repetitive exercise or trauma when the shoulder girdle depresses the long thoracic nerve against the second rib.
- Particular populations affected include weight lifters, new military recruits carrying heavy backpacks, backstroke swimmers, and football players.
- Trauma associated with motor vehicle accidents, chiropractic manipulation, and recent thoracic or breast surgery has also been implicated.

History

- Patients may present without symptoms.
- Patients may report shoulder pain due to impingement from incomplete scapular stabilization.

Physical Examination

- Complete shoulder examination
- Complete neurovascular examination of the upper extremity
- Scapular winging may be noted during arm flexion or after instructing the patient to press the outstretched arm against a wall.
- No associated sensory changes

Imaging

- Usually not indicated unless coincident trauma

Differential Diagnosis

- Avulsion of the nerve root
- Trapezius muscle dysfunction
- Brachial plexus neuropathy

Treatment

- At diagnosis
  - No overhead or exacerbating activity
  - A sling may provide support and prevent discomfort if pain is a component of presentation.
  - Physical therapy
    - — General shoulder strengthening program
    - — Resistance exercises for serratus anterior muscle
- Later
  - Graded return to activity once symptoms and scapular winging resolve

When to Refer

- Neurologic consultation warranted if no improvement with conservative treatment or after 6 weeks

Prognosis

- Prognosis for recovery is good unless the nerve has been completely severed by trauma.

Troubleshooting

- No exacerbating activity is vital to improvement.
- Close follow-up is warranted to ensure compliance with the management program and to limit the duration of activity restrictions.

QUADRILATERAL SPACE SYNDROME

Key Concepts

- The quadrilateral space is defined by the area bordered by the teres minor muscle superiorly, the teres

major muscle inferiorly, the long head of the triceps muscle medially, and the surgical neck of the humerus laterally.
- The axillary nerve and posterior humeral circumflex artery pass through the quadrilateral space, a potential site of neurovascular entrapment.
- The axillary nerve innervates the teres minor and deltoid muscles and terminates as the superior lateral cutaneous nerve of the arm.
- Entrapment can occur with compression to the area, hypertrophy of muscular quadrilateral space boundaries, repetitive motion, shoulder dislocation, or fractures of the surgical neck of the humerus.
- Activities that have been associated with this syndrome include throwing sports including football, swimming, and rowing.

History

- Patients report posterior shoulder pain and paresthesias over the lateral arm in the distribution of the superior lateral cutaneous nerve of the arm.
- Patients often note shoulder weakness, especially with forward flexion and abduction of the arm corresponding to poor deltoid function.
- Overhead arm activity may exacerbate pain.
- The patient may report intermittent claudication symptoms in the upper extremity.
- Index of suspicion is raised if previous shoulder dislocation, subluxation event, or direct trauma to lateral shoulder

Physical Examination

- Complete general shoulder and cervical spine examination
- Complete neurovascular examination of the upper extremity
- Special attention should be given to testing the sensation in the lateral shoulder and upper arm; diminished or absent sensation is suggestive of nerve entrapment.
- Point tenderness may be noted overlying the quadrilateral space.
- Active range of motion testing may reveal deficits in the first 30 degrees of arm abduction and forward flexion, which is associated with a weakened or denervated deltoid muscle.
- Diminished strength to resisted external rotation may be associated with a weakened or denervated teres minor muscle.
- Placing the affected arm in full forward flexion and/or abduction with external rotation of the humerus may reproduce the patient's pain.

Imaging

- Routine radiographs of the shoulder including internal and external rotation views
  - Evaluate for fracture or evidence of dislocation including bony Bankart or Hill-Sachs lesion.
- Magnetic resonance imaging of the shoulder
  - Helpful to rule out other possibilities in differential diagnosis
  - May show findings of teres minor muscle and/or deltoid muscle denervation including fatty infiltration and decreased muscle bulk

Additional Tests (If Applicable)

- Subclavian arteriography with the arm in abduction and external rotation
  - May demonstrate posterior humeral circumflex artery compression or injury in settings of trauma or other acute presentations

Differential Diagnosis

- Cervical radiculopathy
- Brachial plexus injury
- Thoracic outlet syndrome
- Shoulder impingement syndrome
- Rotator cuff tear

Treatment

- At diagnosis
  - Conservative therapy including
    - — Rest and restriction from any exacerbating activity
    - — Routine treatment for fracture or dislocation as indicated
    - — Analgesics as appropriate
    - — Early gentle range of motion exercises to prevent shoulder contracture
- Later
  - Physical therapy
    - — Range of motion exercises for deltoid, rotator cuff, and periscapular muscles
    - — Increase resistance once symptoms of entrapment have abated.
    - — Regular home exercise program once cleared by physician

- Graded return to activity once asymptomatic and full function returns

When to Refer

- Surgical consultation is warranted if there has been no improvement after 3 to 6 months.
- Consider surgical consultation for decompression in settings of trauma, especially direct blows to the quadrilateral space.
- Athletes who use overhead throwing motions may benefit from referral for surgical decompression at the time of diagnosis.

Prognosis

- Most patients respond to conservative management; however, prognosis data are limited.
- The expected period of recovery is within 3 to 6 months of conservative management.
- Athletes who use overhead throwing motions may take longer to recover full function given the high biomechanical demands placed on the deltoid muscle and shoulder.

Troubleshooting

- Close-interval follow-up is important to assess recovery and grade the return to activity recommendations.
- Patients may regain full arm abduction before entrapment is fully healed by increased use of the supraspinatus muscle.
- It is important that a patient not progress to unrestricted activities until full nerve function is recovered.

Patient Instructions

- Follow physician and physical therapist instructions closely regarding activity restrictions.
- A home exercise program established during physical therapy is a key to improvement and must be completed regularly.
- Surgery may be indicated if conservative measures do not improve symptoms.

Suggested Reading

- Cummins C, Messer T, Nuber G: Suprascapular nerve entrapment. J Bone Joint Surg Am 2000;82A:415–424.
- Hoskins W, Pollard H, McDonald A: Quadrilateral space syndrome: A case study and review of the literature. Br J Sports Med 2005;39:e9.
- Nichols A: The thoracic outlet syndrome in athletes. J Am Board Fam Pract 1996;9:346–355.
- Reeser J: Diagnosis and management of vascular injuries in the shoulder girdle of the overhead athlete. Curr Sports Med Rep 2007;6:322–327.
- Woodward T, Best T: The painful shoulder: Part I. Clinical evaluation. Am Fam Physician 2000;61:3079–3088.

Chapter 48 Proximal Humerus Fractures

Peter S. Johnston, Brandon D. Bushnell, and Timothy N. Taft

ICD-9 CODES

812.0 *Upper End, Closed*
812.01 *Surgical Neck*
812.02 *Anatomic Neck*
812.03 *Greater Tuberosity*
812.09 *Other: Head and Upper Epiphysis*
812.1 *Upper End, Open*
812.10 *Upper End, Unspecified Part*
812.11 *Surgical Neck*
812.12 *Anatomic Neck*
812.13 *Greater Tuberosity*
812.19 *Other*

CPT CODES

23620 *Closed Treatment of Greater Humeral Tuberosity Fracture; without Manipulation*
23600 *Closed Treatment of Proximal Humeral (Surgical or Anatomical Neck) Fracture; without Manipulation*
23630 *Open Treatment of Greater Humeral Tuberosity Fracture, with or without Internal or External Fixation*
23615 *Open Treatment of Proximal Humeral (Surgical or Anatomical Neck) Fracture, with or without Internal or External Fixation, with or without Repair of Tuberosity(ies)*
23616 *Open Treatment of Proximal Humeral (Surgical or Anatomical Neck) Fracture, with or without Internal or External Fixation, with or without Repair of Tuberosity(ies); with Proximal Humeral Prosthetic Replacement*

Key Concepts

- In patients older than 65 years, proximal humerus fracture is the third most common fracture after hip and distal radius fractures.
- Three percent of all upper extremity fractures
- Females older than 50 years are at highest risk.
- Isolated greater tuberosity fractures are more common in younger individuals.
- The degree of fragment displacement predicts the risk of injury to the anterior humeral circumflex and arcuate arteries and thus the risk of potential avascular necrosis of the humeral head.
- Usually managed nonoperatively with good functional results

History

- Proximal humerus fractures primarily result from indirect force (fall on an outstretched arm) or a direct blow to the shoulder.
- Contributing factors: bone quality (typically osteoporotic in elderly), history of falls, medical comorbidities, syncopal event
- Patients report pain with movement of extremity, but it can be minimal.
- Patients may experience numbness or tingling in the extremity. Usually self-limited, benign, and not found in any anatomic pattern, it can be associated with a brachial plexus stretch or other nerve injury.
- If a patient experiences loss of consciousness, bilateral injuries, or an associated posterior dislocation, a seizure disorder or electric shock may have been involved in the injury.
- Elderly patients often require a workup for the reason for their fall, which may include heart disease, stroke, and metabolic abnormalities.

Physical Examination

- The upper extremity is often held close to the chest wall, supported by the contralateral hand.
- Painful range of motion and pseudoparalysis (inability to move the arm due to pain from the fracture) may obscure the motor examination.
- Swelling and thick soft-tissue coverings usually obscure bony deformity, but it may be more apparent in more slender patients.
- Ecchymosis can last as long as 2 to 4 weeks and often moves into a dependent position.

- Injuries to the neck, chest, and head must be excluded, especially in the setting of high-energy trauma.
- Perform a careful neurovascular examination with particular attention to axillary nerve function (sensation in the lateral "sergeant's patch" distribution and full motor function of the deltoid muscle) as well as function of the distal upper extremity. The axillary patch is the most commonly injured structure with a proximal humerus fracture.

Pathomechanics

- Deforming forces of fragments
  - Shaft translated anteriorly and medially by the pectoralis major muscle
  - Greater tuberosity translated posteriorly/superiorly by supraspinatus and infraspinatus muscle
  - Lesser tuberosity translated medially by subscapularis muscle
  - Younger patients tend to have minimally displaced fractures or more comminution of dense bone due to higher-energy trauma.
  - Older patients, with decreased bone density, typically have greater fracture displacement even with lower-energy trauma.

Imaging

- Adequate imaging is essential for complete evaluation.
  - True anteroposterior (Grashey) view of the shoulder with internal and external rotation views
  - Scapular Y view
  - Axillary lateral view (extremely important in cases involving possible surgery)
- A computed tomography scan can be performed to further characterize the fracture and should be obtained if glenoid involvement or a possible split of the humeral head is suspected.

Classification

- Neer classification (Fig. 48-1)
  - Based on the number of parts, wherein each part is defined as a fragment with displacement of more than 1 cm and/or angulation of more than 45 degrees
- A valgus-impaction pattern is associated with a better prognosis than the classic four-part fracture due to a better chance of maintenance of the vascular supply.

Treatment

- Nonoperative
  - Mainstay of treatment for most proximal humerus fractures with generally good results
  - Acceptable for minimally displaced fractures not meeting Neer criteria of less than 1 cm of displacement and 45 degrees of angulation
  - May be more appropriate in the elderly or debilitated patient with low functional demands
  - Treatment course
    - — Initial treatment: non-weight bearing in a sling, encouraging active elbow and hand motion
    - — At 2 weeks: Obtain a radiograph to ensure that the fracture has not displaced and begin passive motion as tolerated as well as active pendulum exercises.
    - — At 4 to 6 weeks: If radiographs demonstrate maintenance of alignment, begin active motion as tolerated.
    - — At 2 to 3 months: Confirm radiographic and clinical healing, and then begin aggressive range of motion exercises, capsular stretching, and periscapular muscle stretching and active strengthening.
- Operative
  - Indications are dependent on fracture displacement; bone quality; patient's age, work, and functional demands; overall medical condition; and the presence of other fractures in the multitrauma patient.
  - Goals of surgery are to restore anatomic relationships with attention to rotator cuff musculature and articular congruity, while maintaining the vascular integrity of the anatomic head.
  - Two-part fractures
    - — Anatomic neck: rare fracture pattern, but with a high risk for osteonecrosis
      - — Open reduction/internal fixation in younger patients versus hemiarthroplasty (shoulder prosthesis) in elderly patients
    - — Surgical neck: indicated with impaction and more than 45 degrees of angulation
      - — Closed reduction and percutaneous pinning versus open reduction and internal fixation
    - — Greater tuberosity: displacement greater than 5 mm
      - — Open reduction and internal fixation versus intraosseous suture fixation
    - — Can be arthroscopically assisted and may involve rotator cuff repair

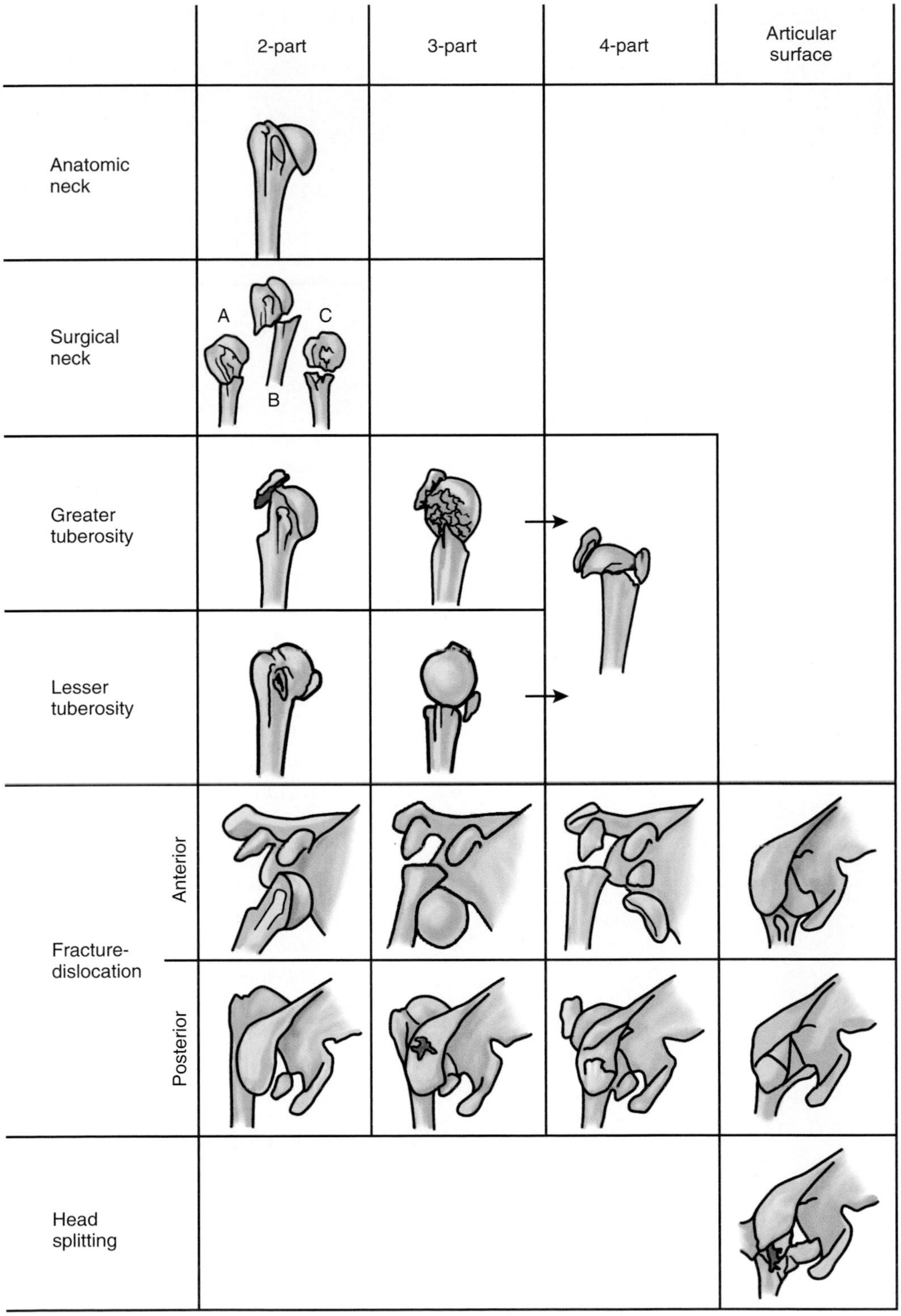

2-part
3-part
4-part
Articular surface
Anatomic neck
Surgical neck
A
B
C
Greater tuberosity
Lesser tuberosity
Fracture-dislocation
Anterior
Posterior
Head splitting

Figure 48-1 Neer classification: accepted method for the classification of proximal humerus fractures, based on the number of parts displaced more than 1 cm or more than 45 degrees.

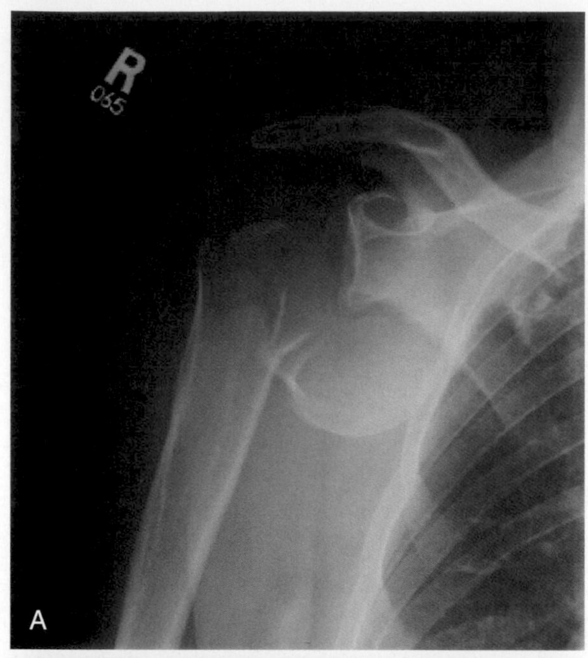

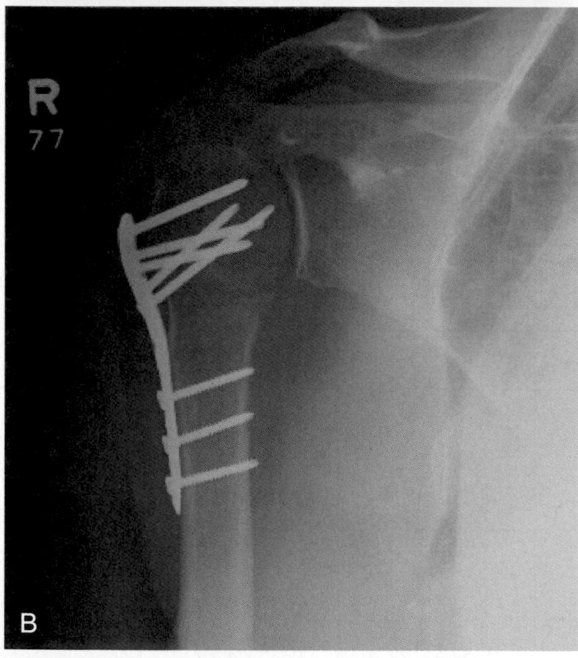

Figure 48-2 **A**, Four-part proximal humerus fracture-dislocation. **B**, Appearance after open reduction and internal fixation.

- Two-part fractures
  - Displaced, unstable fractures require open reduction and internal fixation versus intraosseous suture fixation in most cases.
  - Elderly patients may require hemiarthroplasty or total shoulder arthroplasty.
- Four-part fractures (Fig. 48-2)
  - More urgent treatment is indicated in younger patients to reduce the risk of osteonecrosis.

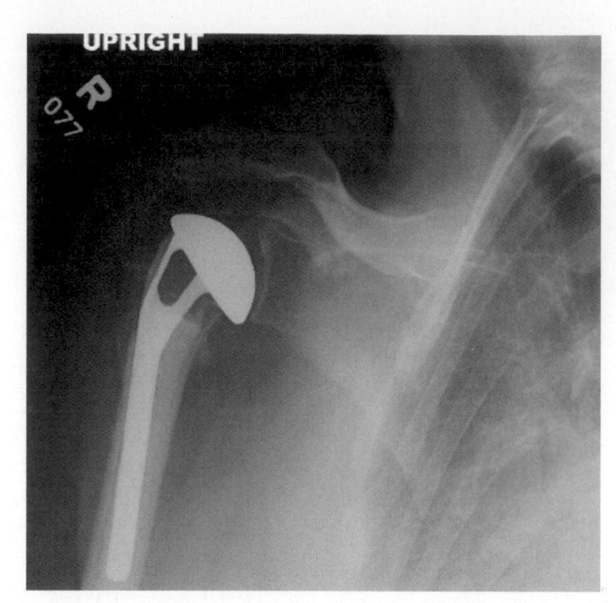

Figure 48-3 Proximal humerus fracture treated with hemiarthroplasty.

  - Open reduction and internal fixation with locking plate versus transosseous suture technique
  - Hemiarthroplasty (Fig. 48-3) versus total shoulder arthroplasty in elderly patients
  - Valgus impacted fractures are unique because the medial soft-tissue hinge and vascular supply are maintained; usually treated with closed reduction and percutaneous pinning versus nonoperative management
- Articular surface fractures
  - Common in posterior shoulder dislocations and associated with severe glenoid impaction
  - Surgery is usually indicated, often consisting of open reduction and internal fixation versus hemiarthroplasty.

Differential Diagnosis

- Acute rotator cuff tear: superior displacement of humeral head radiographically; magnetic resonance imaging confirms examination findings
- Clavicle fracture: deformity over clavicle, confirmed radiographically
- Acromioclavicular separation: deformity at the acromioclavicular joint, confirmed radiographically
- Calcific tendinitis: acute exacerbation, rotator cuff calcification seen radiographically, relieved with nonsteroidal anti-inflammatory drugs

Additional Tests

- Magnetic resonance imaging: most effective method for evaluating soft-tissue injuries, i.e., rotator cuff tear

When to Refer

- If the clinician believes that the fracture is displaced to a degree requiring surgical fixation as based on the Neer classification and if the patient's overall health, including functional demands, makes the patient an appropriate candidate

Troubleshooting

- The patient should be counseled on benefits and risks of surgery.
  - Benefits
    — Fracture stabilization and decreased pain allow early joint mobilization.
    — Anatomic reduction restores rotator cuff dynamics and articular congruity.
  - Risks
    — Bleeding, infection, and neurovascular injury (axillary nerve is at risk in most approaches to the proximal humerus)
    — Failure of fixation, malunion, nonunion, and avascular necrosis of the humeral head
    — Shoulder stiffness can be seen after surgical management (prevented by early mobilization and aggressive physical therapy postoperatively).

Suggested Reading

- Hodgson S: Proximal humerus fracture rehabilitation. Clin Orthop Relat Res 2006;442:131–138.
- Neer CS: Four-segment classification of displaced proximal humeral fractures. AAOS Instr Lect 1975;24:160–168.
- Nho SJ, Brophy RH, Barker JU, et al: Management of proximal humeral fractures based on current literature. J Bone Joint Surg Am 2007;89A(Suppl 3):44–58.
- Rees J, Hicks J, Ribbans W: Assessment and management of three- and four-part proximal humeral fractures. Clin Orthop Relat Res 1998;353:18–29.
- Vallier HA: Treatment of proximal humerus fractures. J Orthop Trauma 2007;21:469–476.

Chapter 49 Humeral Shaft Fractures

Conor Regan, Brandon D. Bushnell, and Timothy N. Taft

ICD-9 CODES
812.2 *Fracture of Shaft or Unspecified Part, Closed*
812.3 *Fracture of Shaft or Unspecified Part, Open*

Key Concepts

- The humeral shaft is usually fractured as a result of a direct blow; the type of fracture depends on the amount of energy imparted by the impact.
- Shaft fractures can be transverse, oblique, spiral, or segmental.
- Because union rates average approximately 90% to 95% with nonoperative methods alone, nonoperative treatment is overwhelmingly preferred.
  - Operative treatment results in a similar rate of ultimate healing but exposes the patient to greater risk of complications.
- Fragment displacement depends on the location of the fracture.
  - Above the pectoralis major muscle, the proximal fragment is abducted and externally rotated by the muscles of the rotator cuff and the distal fragment is displaced medially and proximally by the pectoralis major and deltoid muscles, respectively.
  - Between the insertion of the pectoralis major muscle and the deltoid tuberosity, the proximal fragment is pulled medially by the pectoralis major, teres major, and latissimus dorsi muscles, whereas the distal fragment is pulled laterally and proximally by the deltoid muscle.
  - Distal to the deltoid tuberosity, the proximal fragment is abducted by the deltoid muscle and the distal fragment is pulled medially and proximally by the biceps and triceps muscles.
- The Holstein-Lewis fracture is located in the distal one third of the humeral shaft.
  - A fracture here has a relatively higher likelihood of radial nerve entrapment because it pierces the lateral intermuscular septum and is relatively tethered.
- See Figure 49-1 for the AO classification of humeral shaft fractures.

Etiology

- The incidence of humeral shaft fractures increases with age from 14.5/100,000 per year in the 5th decade of life to 60/100,000 per year in the 9th decade of life.
- As age increases, the etiology of fracture changes from high-energy trauma in the young to overwhelmingly low-impact trauma, such as a simple fall, in the elderly.
- Humeral shaft fractures in the young are often part of multiple traumas as a result of their mechanisms.

Physical Examination

- Patients will usually present with pain, swelling, deformity, and a shortened extremity.
- It is important to perform a thorough neurovascular examination of the injured extremity before and after reduction attempts due to the vulnerability of the radial nerve.
- Abrasion continuity with a joint space can be determined by injecting sterile saline into the joint.

Imaging

- Anteroposterior and lateral radiographs are often all that are necessary to diagnose the fracture.
- Reserve magnetic resonance imaging or computed tomography for suspected pathologic fracture.
- Contralateral humerus radiographs can be used for preoperative planning.

Treatment

Nonoperative

- Closed treatment can be tolerated for most fractures of the humeral shaft because nonoperative treatment results in acceptable healing as much as 90% of the time.
- Malunion of 20 to 25 degrees of anteroposterior angulation, 15 degrees of rotation, and 2 to 3 cm of shortening are well tolerated functionally.

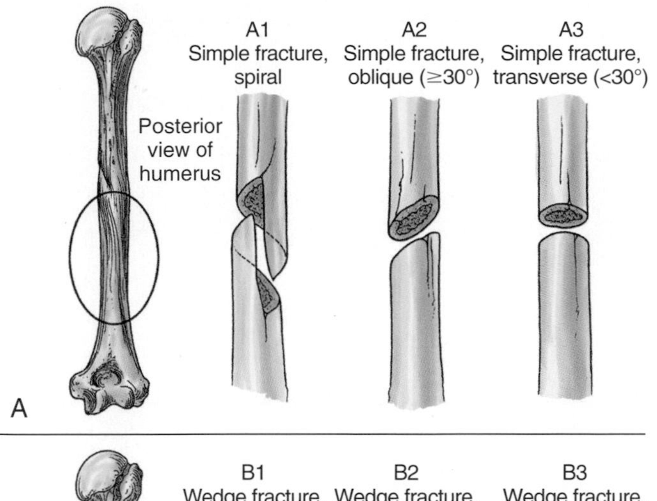

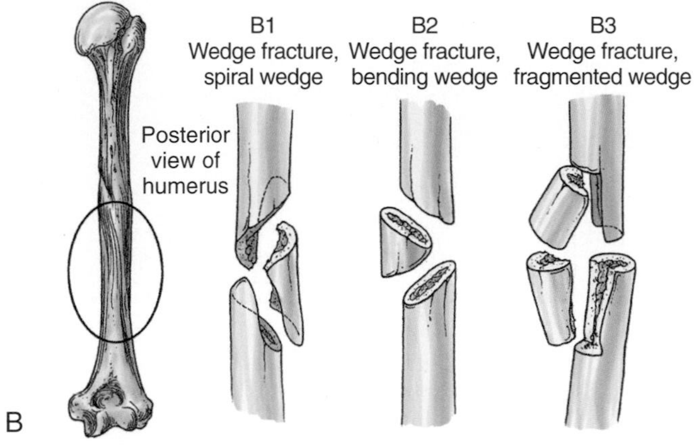

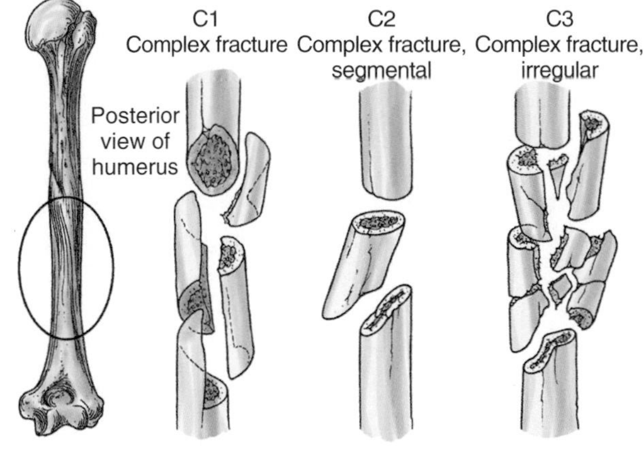

Figure 49-1 AO classification of humeral shaft fractures. **A**, Simple fracture; **B**, wedge fracture; **C**, complex fracture. (From DeFranco MJ, Lawton JN: Radial nerve injuries associated with humeral fractures. J Hand Surg [Am] 2006;31:655–663. With permission from Elsevier, 2006.)

- Hanging arm cast (Fig. 49-2)
  - Use for spiral or oblique fractures
    — Can cause nonunion with transverse fractures secondary to traction
  - Uses gravity to effect fracture reduction
  - Cast arm from axilla to wrist with the elbow at 90 degrees

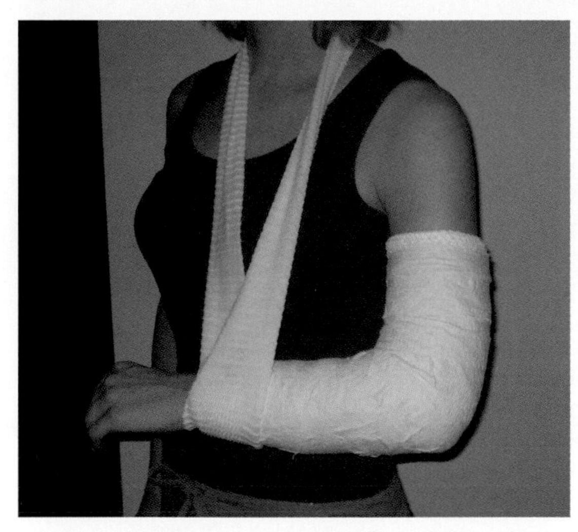

Figure 49-2 Hanging arm cast.

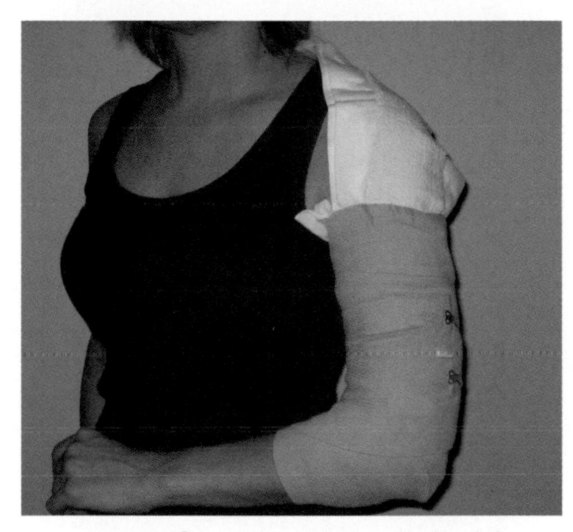

Figure 49-3 Coaptation splint applied to left arm.

  - The cast must hang free from the body to allow proper use of gravity to effect alignment.
    — The patient must also remain upright for 1 to 2 weeks for the cast to be effective.
- Coaptation splint (Fig. 49-3)
  - Offers the advantage of minimal shortening of the fracture site
  - Uncomfortable given the bulkiness of the splint
  - The splint often slips down the arm; this can be prevented by placing an extension over the shoulder.
- Velpeau or sling and swathe bandage (Fig. 49-4)
  - Can be used for nondisplaced fractures in children and the elderly

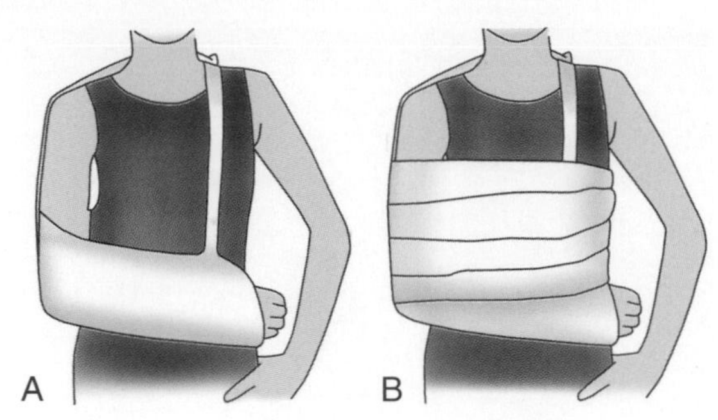

Figure 49-4 Sling (**A**) and swathe (**B**) bandage. (With permission from Kronfol R: Splinting of musculoskeletal injuries. In Rose BD [ed]: UpToDate. Waltham, MA: UpToDate, 2007.)

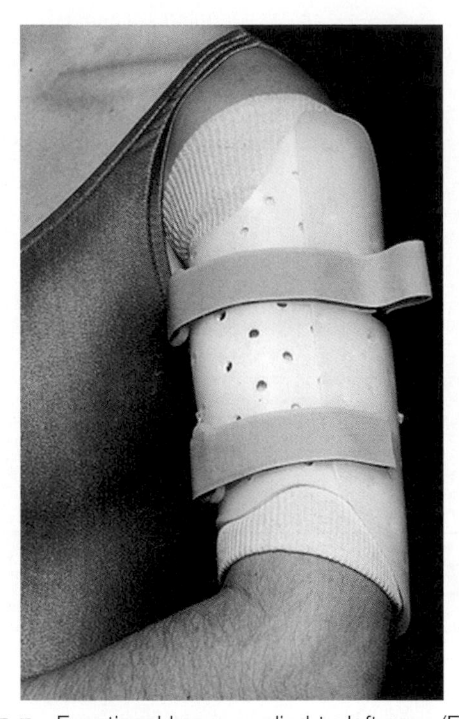

Figure 49-5 Functional brace applied to left arm. (From Sarmiento A, Zagorski JB, Zych GA, et al: Functional bracing for the treatment of fractures of the humeral diaphysis. J Bone Joint Surg Am 2000;82A:478–486. With permission from The Journal of Bone and Joint Surgery, Inc., 2000.)

- Does not aid in fracture reduction; used for comfort rather than immobilization
- Change to a functional brace or other method once acute pain subsides.

- Functional brace (Fig. 49-5)
  - Uses soft-tissue compression to effect fracture reduction
  - Cannot use if the patient has extensive soft-tissue injury or bone loss or if it is not possible to reduce the fracture by closed manipulation

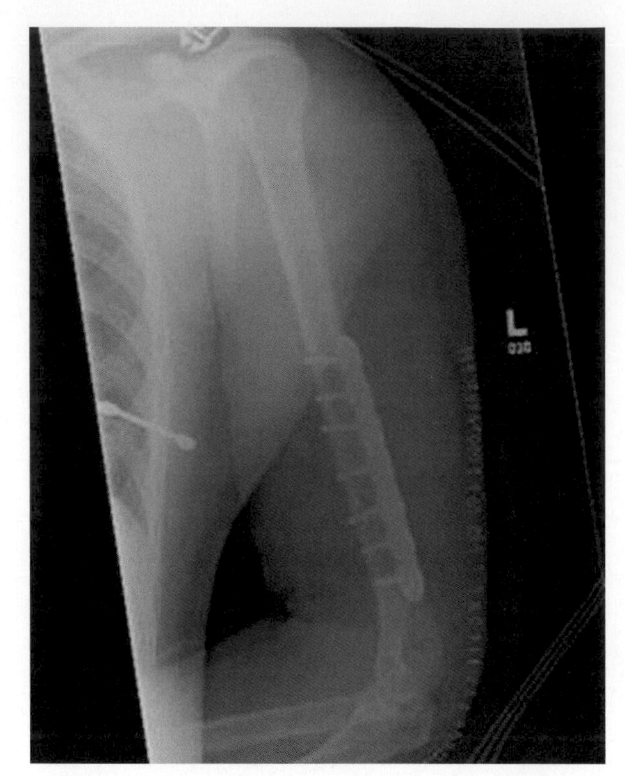

Figure 49-6 Postoperative radiograph of plate-and-screw fixation of a well-reduced humeral shaft fracture.

  - Typically applied 1 to 2 weeks after the injury when coaptation or hanging arm casts are removed
  - Worn for longer than 8 weeks

Operative

- Indications for operative management include
  - Open fracture
  - Associated neurovascular injury
  - Segmental fractures
  - Ipsilateral radius and ulna fractures (floating elbow)
  - Irreducible fractures
  - Fractures with intra-articular extension
  - Bilateral humeral fractures
  - Nerve injury after attempting closed reduction
  - Penetrating injury with radial nerve palsy
  - Pathologic fractures
  - Polytrauma
- External fixation (Fig. 49-6)
  - Use with extensive soft-tissue injury, overlying burns or compromise of the skin, or infected nonunions
  - Care must be taken with pin placement to avoid damage to the axillary artery or nerve or the neighboring tendons in the arm.

- Postoperative course
  - Range of motion exercises in the hand and wrist should be started immediately after injury as pain allows.
  - Range of motion exercises in the shoulder should begin as pain permits, starting with Codman exercises.
  - Range of motion exercises in the elbow should be active only; passive range of motion in the elbow can result in myositis ossificans.
  - Strengthening in the elbow/shoulder can begin when there is radiologic evidence of healing

Special Considerations

- Radial nerve palsy complicates between 8% and 18% of humeral shaft fractures. Classically, this occurs with a Holstein-Lewis type distal humeral shaft fracture, but the incidence is actually higher with midshaft fractures.
- Seventy percent to 90% of radial nerve palsies resolve in 3 to 4 months with conservative management.
- Exploration of the radial nerve should be performed if
  - There is no evidence of recovery at 3 to 4 months post-injury.
  - There is an open fracture with radial nerve palsy.
  - There is a penetrating mechanism of injury with immediate radial nerve palsy.
  - There is radial nerve palsy after closed manipulation of the fracture.
- Vascular injury is often a clinical diagnosis with a cold, pulseless extremity.
  - If present, the patient should be emergently taken to the operating room, the fracture stabilized, and the brachial artery repaired by a vascular surgeon. Warm ischemic time should be kept to less than 6 hours maximum.
- Refer to a specialist if there is no evidence of callus formation after approximately 12 to 16 weeks or if there is suspected radial nerve damage.

Suggested Reading

- Crenshaw A: Fractures of the shoulder girdle, arm, and forearm. In Canale ST (ed): Campbell's Operative Orthopaedics, 9th ed. St. Louis: Mosby, 1998, pp 2296–2309.
- Ekholm R, Adami J, Tidermark J, et al: Fractures of the shaft of the humerus. An epidemiological study of 401 fractures. J Bone Joint Surg Br 2006;88B:1469–1473.
- Sarmiento A, Zagorski JB, Zych GA, et al: Functional bracing for the treatment of fractures of the humeral diaphysis. J Bone Joint Surg Am 2000;82A:478–486.
- Shao YC, Harwood P, Grotz MR, et al: Radial nerve palsy associated with fractures of the shaft of the humerus, a systematic review. J Bone Joint Surg Br 2005;87B:1647–1652.
- Zuckerman JD, Koval K: Fractures of the shaft of the humerus. In Rockwood C, Green D, Bucholz RW, Heckman JD (eds): Rockwood and Green's Fractures in Adults, 4th ed. Philadelphia: Lippincott, 1996, pp 1025–1051.

Chapter 50 Scapula Fractures

Daniel S. Heckman, Brandon D. Bushnell, and Timothy N. Taft

ICD-9 CODES

811.00 *Closed Fracture of Scapula, Unspecified Part*
811.01 *Closed Fracture of Acromial Process of Scapula*
811.02 *Closed Fracture of Coracoid Process of Scapula*
811.03 *Closed Fracture of Glenoid Cavity and Neck of Scapula*
811.09 *Closed Fracture of Other Part of Scapula*
811.10 *Open Fracture of Scapula, Unspecified Part*
811.11 *Open Fracture of Acromial Process of Scapula*
811.12 *Open Fracture of Coracoid Process of Scapula*
811.13 *Open Fracture of Glenoid Cavity and Neck of Scapula*
811.19 *Open Fracture of Other Part of Scapula*

Key Concepts

- Scapula fractures comprise 3% to 5% of shoulder girdle injuries and 0.4% to 1% of all fractures.
- The mean age of patients with scapula fractures is 35 to 45 years.
- Associated injuries are common
  - Occur in 35% to 98% of patients with scapula fractures
  - Responsible for a 10% to 15% mortality rate in patients with scapula fractures
  - Many require urgent attention, leading to a delayed diagnosis of the scapular fracture
  - Incidence of injuries associated with scapula fractures
    - — Pneumothorax (11% to 55%)
    - — Pulmonary contusion (1% to 54%)
    - — Rib fracture (27% to 54%)
    - — Clavicle fracture (23% to 39%)
    - — Skull fracture (24%)
    - — Closed head injury (20%)
    - — Peripheral neurovascular injury (brachial plexus, axillary artery) (5% to 13%)
    - — Spinal cord injury (5%)

History

- Usually caused by high-energy trauma
- As many as 50% result from motor vehicle accidents
- Mechanisms of injury and associated patterns
  - Blunt trauma to posterior chest wall: scapular body fracture
  - Blunt trauma to shoulder: acromion or coracoid fracture
  - Axial loading through outstretched arm: scapular neck or intra-articular glenoid fracture
  - Glenohumeral dislocation: glenoid rim fracture
  - Traction injuries: avulsion fracture

Physical Examination

- Patient typically presents with the arm held adducted against the chest.
- The shoulder may appear flattened with a displaced scapular neck or acromion fractures.
- Swelling, abrasions, ecchymosis, tenderness, or crepitus over the scapular region
- Painful shoulder range of motion in all directions, particularly with abduction
- In patients with a high-energy mechanism of injury, a complete trauma evaluation should be performed with careful assessment for associated pulmonary or neurovascular injuries.
- Comolli's sign is a triangular swelling overlying the scapula on the posterior thorax representing a hematoma that can cause increased compartment pressures in the supraspinatus and infraspinatus muscles.

Imaging

- Multiple radiographic views are needed for accurate radiographic diagnosis of scapula fractures (Fig. 50-1).
  - True anteroposterior view of shoulder (Grashey view, tangential to glenoid)
  - Axillary lateral view to evaluate acromial and glenoid rim fractures
  - Scapular Y

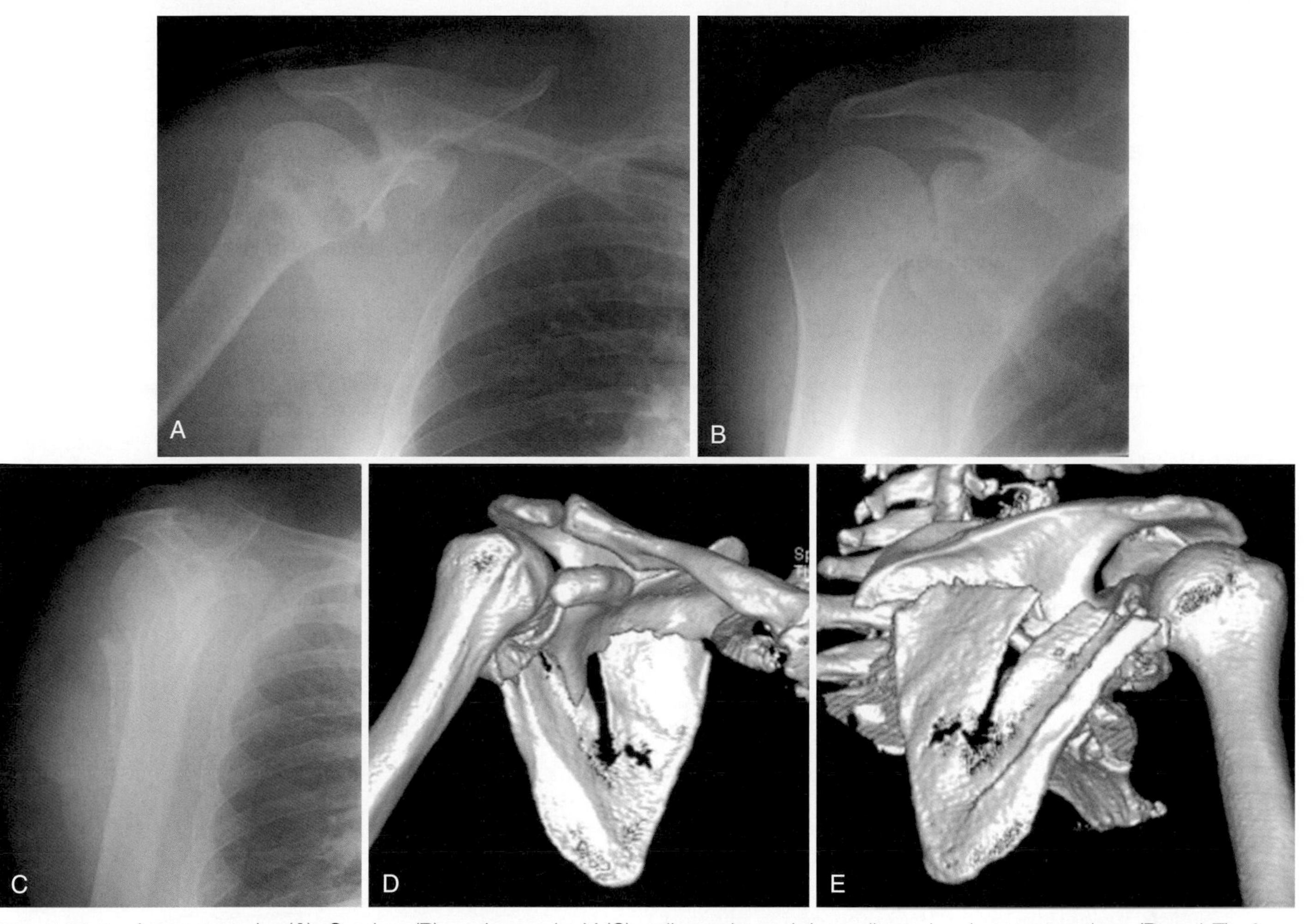

Figure 50-1 Anteroposterior (**A**), Grashey (**B**), and scapular Y (**C**) radiographs and three-dimensional reconstructions (**D** and **E**) of a computed tomography scan showing a scapular fracture involving the inferior glenoid.

  - Stryker notch (45-degree cephalic tilt) to evaluate coracoid fractures
  - Apical oblique view (Garth view) to evaluate anterior/inferior glenoid rim
  - Standing weight-bearing views to evaluate injuries of the acromioclavicular joint and coracoclavicular ligaments
  - Chest radiographs are usually obtained as part of the trauma evaluation and can identify rib fractures or other associated injuries.
- Computed tomography
  - Useful aid for evaluating intra-articular glenoid or coracoid fractures, humeral head position, and associated injuries
  - Full chest and cervical spine computed tomography scans are often performed as part of a complete multitrauma workup.

Additional Tests

- Arteriography should be performed emergently in patients with a pulseless upper extremity to identify vascular injury.
- Electromyography to assess the extent and potential recovery of associated neurologic deficits

Classification

- Scapular fractures are described by anatomic location (Zdravkovic and Damholt)
  - Type I: scapular body
  - Type II: apophyseal fractures, including acromion and coracoid process
  - Type III: fractures of the superolateral angle, including the scapular neck and glenoid

- Scapular body (49% to 89%) and scapular neck (10% to 60%) fractures are most common.

Differential Diagnosis

- Posterior rib fractures
  - Pleuritic pain
- Rotator cuff impingement or tear
  - Positive impingement tests
  - No swelling, tenderness, ecchymosis, or crepitus over scapula
- Scapulothoracic dysfunction
  - Significant traction/rotation force to upper extremity
  - Neurovascular injury is more common than with scapular fractures.

Nonoperative Treatment

- At diagnosis
  - Treatment is often affected by treatment of associated injuries.
  - Most scapular fractures can be treated nonoperatively.
  - Closed reduction usually is not possible.
  - Supportive treatment with pain medication and a sling for comfort
  - Allow weight bearing as tolerated on the affected upper extremity.
- Later
  - Early gravity-assisted range of motion is recommended during the immediate posttrauma period.
  - Progressive range of motion and strengthening exercises
  - Close radiographic follow-up of intra-articular fractures to ensure that unacceptable displacement does not occur

When to Refer

- See surgical indications

Prognosis

- Nonunion is rare, and most fractures heal within 6 weeks.
- Full functional recovery may take several months.
- Ultimately, the prognosis is excellent for most scapular fractures.

Operative Treatment

- Indications for surgical treatment
  - More than 25% of the articular surface
  - More than 10-mm displacement of articular fragment
  - More than 5-mm articular step-off
  - More than 40 degrees of angulation of scapular neck
  - Floating shoulder with concomitant clavicle and/or humeral fractures (Fig. 50-2)
  - Subacromial space impingement
  - Symptomatic nonunion/malunion
- Surgical approach (anterior or posterior) depends on fracture pattern.
- The usual treatment involves fixation with plates, screws, and/or wires.
- The benefit of surgery decreases with increasing fracture fragments.
- Nonoperative management of comminuted intra-articular fractures is considered if the humeral head remains centered on the glenoid.
- Early gravity-assisted range of motion treatment may improve fracture alignment and overall outcome.

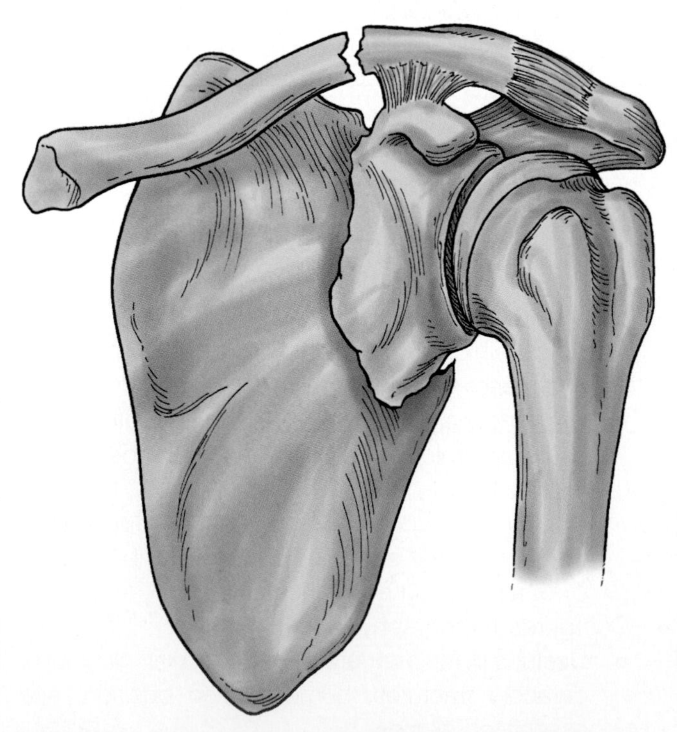

Figure 50-2 Floating shoulder consisting of fractures of the scapular neck and the clavicle. (Adapted from Canale ST [ed]: Campbell's Operative Orthopaedics, 10th ed. Philadelphia: Mosby, 2003.)

Troubleshooting

- Incomplete imaging is the most common diagnostic pitfall.
- Os acromiale
  - Rounded, unfused apophysis that can resemble an acromial fracture
  - Present in 2.7% of adults
  - Bilateral in 60% of patients with an os acromiale
- Glenoid hypoplasia
  - Can resemble an impaction fracture of the glenoid
  - Often associated with an acromial or humeral head abnormality
  - Glenoid retroversion usually also present
- Pseudorupture of the rotator cuff
  - Scapular body fractures can mimic rotator cuff tears.
  - Painful intramuscular swelling, rotator cuff weakness, and loss of active arm elevation
  - Probably due to intramuscular hemorrhage
  - Usually resolves within several weeks

Patient Instructions

- Remind patients that use of a sling is for comfort only and encourage daily use of the upper extremity out of the sling.
- Reinforce the importance of early range of motion therapy to prevent shoulder/elbow stiffness and loss of function.

Considerations in Special Populations

- Patients with high-energy mechanisms should receive a complete trauma evaluation to assess for associated injuries.
- Patients with low-energy mechanisms usually have scapula fracture patterns that are amenable to nonoperative treatment.

Suggested Reading

- Butters KP: Fractures of the scapula. In Bucholz RW, Heckman JD, Court-Brown CM (eds): Rockwood and Green's Fractures in Adults, 6th ed. Philadelphia: Lippincott Williams & Wilkins, 2006, pp 1257–1284.
- DeFranco MJ, Patterson BM: The floating shoulder. J Am Acad Orthop Surg 2006;14:499–509.
- Goss TP: Fractures of the glenoid cavity. J Bone Joint Surg Am 1992;74A:299–305.
- Goss TP: Scapular fractures and dislocations: Diagnosis and treatment. J Am Acad Orthop Surg 1995;3:22–33.
- Zdravkovic D, Damholt VV: Comminuted and severly displaced fractures of the scapula. Acta Orthop Scand 1974;45(1):60–65.
- Zlowodzki M, Bhandari M, Zelle BA, et al: Treatment of scapula fractures: Systematic review of 520 fractures in 22 case series. J Orthop Trauma 2006;20:230–233.

Chapter 51 Clavicle Fractures

James H. Rubright, Brandon D. Bushnell, and Timothy N. Taft

ICD-9 CODES

810.00 *Clavicle Fracture Not Otherwise Specified, Closed*
810.10 *Clavicle Fracture Not Otherwise Specified, Open*
810.01 *Sternal End Closed*
810.11 *Sternal End Open*
810.02 *Shaft (Middle Third) Closed*
810.12 *Shaft (Middle Third) Open*
810.03 *Acromial End Closed*
810.13 *Acromial End Open*

CPT CODES

25000 *Closed Treatment Clavicle Fracture without Manipulation*
23505 *Closed Treatment Clavicle Fracture with Manipulation*
23515 *Open Treatment Clavicle Fracture with or without Internal or External Fixation*

Key Concepts

- Clavicle fractures account for 2.5% to 5% of all fractures.
- Diagnosis is generally made by history and physical examination findings and confirmed with radiographs.
- Since the days of Hippocrates, clavicle fractures have been regarded as injuries that heal easily with excellent functional outcomes after minimal or no intervention.
- Nonunion and symptomatic malunion were thought to be rare, but recent studies show rates to be higher than historically suspected, and operative treatment is becoming more popular.

Function of the Clavicle

- Provides the only bony link between the upper extremity and the axial skeleton
- Protects underlying brachial plexus, subclavian vessels, and apical pleura
- Strut function: It acts as a strut, preventing medial migration of the shoulder girdle, thus allowing the thoracohumeral muscles to maintain their optimal working length.
- Suspensory function: With help from the trapezius muscle, the clavicle stabilizes the shoulder girdle against inferior displacement.

Classification of Fractures

- Most often grouped by which third of the bone the fracture involves: medial (proximal), middle, or lateral (distal) third (Fig. 51-1)
- Several complex systems exist, but in most clinical situations, the following system by Allman with further subdivision of group II by Neer and Craig is sufficient.
  - Group I: fracture of the middle third (70% to 80%)
  - Group II: fracture of the distal third (10% to 20%)
    - Type I: minimal displacement with fracture line between intact coracoclavicular ligaments
    - Type II: fracture line is medial to the coracoclavicular ligaments, resulting in a displaced medial segment
    - Type III: intra-articular extension into acromioclavicular joint
    - Type IV: periosteal sleeve fracture (usually children)
    - Type V: comminuted, with ligaments attached neither medially nor laterally but rather to an inferior fragment of comminution
  - Group III: fracture of the proximal third (<5%)

Fracture Biomechanics: Deforming Forces

- Medial segment
  - Displaced superiorly by sternocleidomastoid muscle
  - Displaced superiorly and posteriorly by trapezius muscle
- Lateral segment
  - Displaced anteriorly and rotated inferiorly by the weight of the arm
  - Displaced medially by the pectoralis major and latissimus dorsi muscles (acting through the humerus)

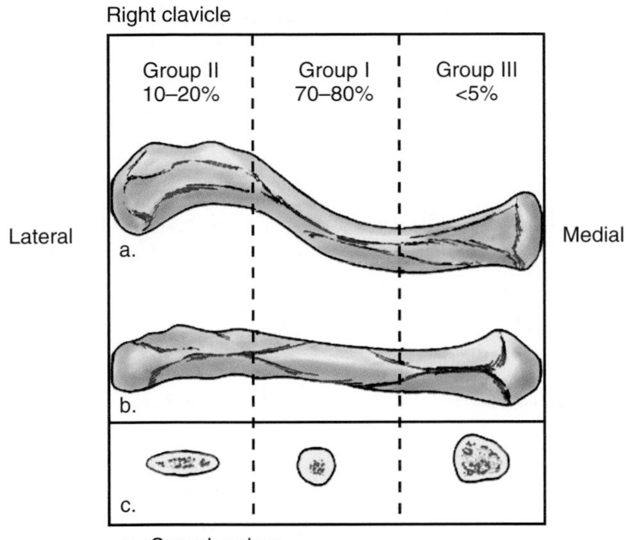

Figure 51-1 Osteology and classification of clavicle fractures. The S-shaped bone resembles its namesake, the musical symbol the clavicula. The junction of the middle and lateral thirds is the thinnest portion of the bone and is the only section of bone not reinforced by muscular or ligamentous attachments. This explains why group I fractures are the most common. Group II fractures involve the lateral third. Group III fractures involve the medial third. (Adapted with permission from Rockwood CA, Matsen FA, Wirth MA, Lippitt SB [eds]: The Shoulder, 3rd ed. Philadelphia: WB Saunders, 2004.)

- Result of these forces is often shortening and overriding of segments

History

- Common mechanisms include motor vehicle collisions, falls from height, and sports injuries.
- Approximately 90% of the time, the clavicle fails in axial loading from blows to the point of the shoulder.
- Blunt or penetrating trauma along the shaft of the bone accounts for approximately 7% of clavicle fractures (i.e., seatbelt, lacrosse or hockey stick, blunt weapon, gunshot).
- Falls onto an outstretched hand account for only 2% to 6% of all clavicle fractures.
- Medial fractures are usually the result of high-energy mechanisms, are often accompanied by significant multisystem trauma, have a high associated mortality rate (from other injuries), and predominate in males.

Physical Examination

- Look for visible or palpable deformity; tenting of the skin; localized swelling, ecchymosis, abrasions, or tenderness; relative droop or shortening of the shoulder; scapular protraction; and motion or crepitus at the fracture site.
- Include peripheral pulses, distal motor strength, and sensation testing in both arms.
- A complete secondary survey should be performed in the setting of high-energy trauma. Examine for signs and symptoms of commonly associated injuries such as brachial plexopathy, hemothorax, pneumothorax, neurovascular injury, rib fractures, and scapular neck and body fractures.

Imaging

- Upright anteroposterior view of the shoulder and the clavicle (Fig 51-2)
- Cephalad and/or caudad oblique views can help bring the image of the clavicle away from the thoracic cage
- Anteroposterior view of contralateral clavicle can help assess relative length to evaluate shortening
- Axillary view or Zanca 15-degree oblique view of the shoulder can help assess acromioclavicular joint involvement

Additional Tests

- CT scan in cases involving comminution, possible articular extension, medial fractures, and high-energy injury to the thorax
- Chest radiograph if pneumothorax is suspected
- Angiography if vascular injury is suspected

Differential Diagnosis

- Lateral third fracture: acromioclavicular separation, physeal injury
- Medial third fracture: sternoclavicular dislocation, physeal injury

Treatment

- Goals
  - Restoration of preinjury shoulder strength and motion
  - Elimination of pain
  - Minimization of deformity
- Closed reduction
  - Closed reduction before immobilization is uncommon and has not been shown to improve healing or long-term alignment of midshaft fractures in particular.

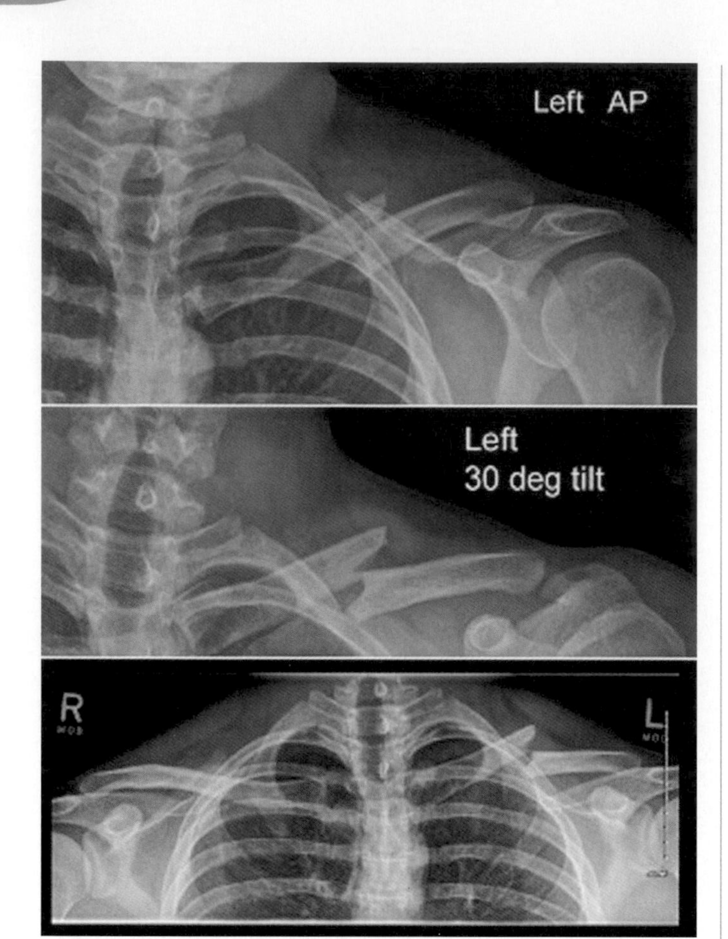

Figure 51-2 Midshaft clavicle fracture. *Top,* Note that on an anteroposterior (AP) view, the ipsilateral upper lung field, acromioclavicular joint, and sternoclavicular joint is visualized, but the fracture site is partially obscured by the rib cage and scapula. *Middle,* A cephalic tilt view brings the shadow of the clavicle fragments away from the rib cage and scapula, allowing a better view of the fracture pattern. *Bottom,* Anteroposterior view of both clavicles allows for measurement of relative shortening of the injured clavicle. Note the superiorly displaced medial fragment, inferiorly displaced lateral fragment, and overall shortening.

- Immobilization
  - Of the more than 200 described methods, sling immobilization and figure-of-eight bracing are the most common (Fig. 51-3).
  - They are equally effective in terms of union rate and speed of recovery.
  - Sling scores higher in patient comfort and satisfaction
  - Figure-of-eight bracing keeps the hand free for activity.
  - Duration is based on patient comfort and resolution of pain and motion at fracture site (typically 2–6 weeks)
- Rehabilitation
  - Usually simple home-based stretching exercises are sufficient after immobilization (or operative fixation); some cases may require formal physical therapy.
  - Overhead activity should be avoided for 4 to 6 weeks to limit rotational stress on the fracture site during healing.
  - Light duty work may begin when the patient is able to participate comfortably, depending on the job.
  - Heavy labor and athletics may begin after radiographic and clinical union, anywhere from 6 to 12 weeks.
- Group I (midshaft) fractures
  - The majority are minimally displaced or nondisplaced and are treated successfully with immobilization (see Fig 51-2).
  - Absolute surgical indications: open fracture, severe “tenting” of skin by fracture ends, vascular injury needing repair, progressive brachial plexus injury, scapulothoracic dissociation
  - Relative indications: floating shoulder, bilateral fractures, ipsilateral upper extremity fracture, multitrauma, symptomatic malunion or nonunion, neurologic disorder (head injury, seizures, Parkinson’s disease), expected prolonged bed rest, intolerance to immobilization, cosmesis
  - Controversial indications that remain to be elucidated in the literature: highly comminuted fractures, high-energy mechanism, closed fractures with more than 15 to 20 mm of shortening or more than 20 mm of displacement
  - Described open reductions with internal fixation techniques fall into two main categories
    - — Intramedullary devices (Kirschner wires, pins, screws)
    - — Plate and screw fixation (Fig. 51-4)
- Group II (distal third) fractures
  - Type I: immobilization
  - Type II: open reduction with internal fixation
  - Type III: immobilize with or without late acromioclavicular resection for arthritis
  - Type IV: immobilization
  - Type V: open reduction with internal fixation
- Group III (medial third) fractures
  - The vast majority are nondisplaced and treated with immobilization.
  - Posterior displacement that endangers neurovascular structures warrants surgical management.

When to Refer

- Group II or III fractures (far medial or far lateral)
- High-energy trauma or multiple additional injuries
- Group I fractures with possible surgical indications

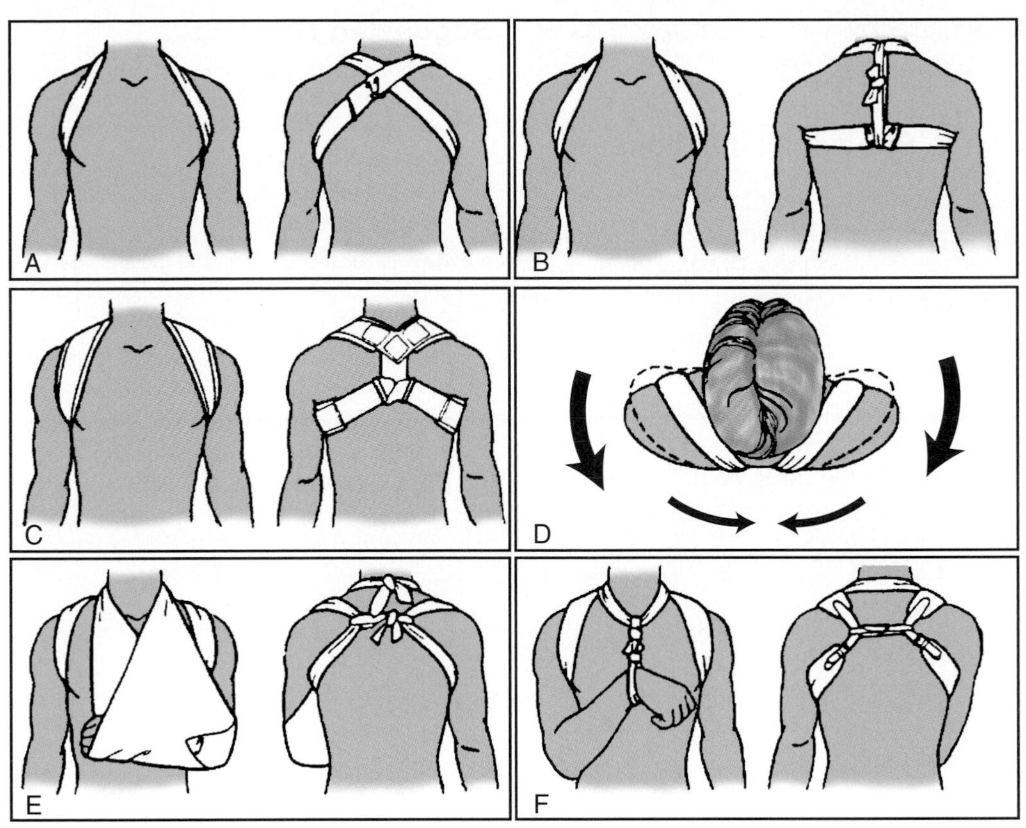

Figure 51-3 Sling and figure-of-eight bracing. Simple sling (not pictured) and figure-of-eight bracing is designed to maintain closed reduction of clavicle fractures. More than 200 combinations of sling and/or braces have been described. **A**, Padded stockinette fastened with safety pins. **B**, Stockinette not crossed in the back, but secured with a second piece of stockinette that can be tightened daily to help maintain reduction. **C**, Commercially available figure-of-eight brace. **D**, The shoulders are pulled up and backward by the figure-of-eight brace, helping to maintain reduction. **E**, A figure-of-eight brace with sling. **F**, Figure-of-eight brace with cuff and collar. (Adapted with permission from Rockwood CA, Matsen FA, Wirth MA, Lippitt SB [eds]: The Shoulder, 3rd ed. Philadelphia: Saunders, 2004.)

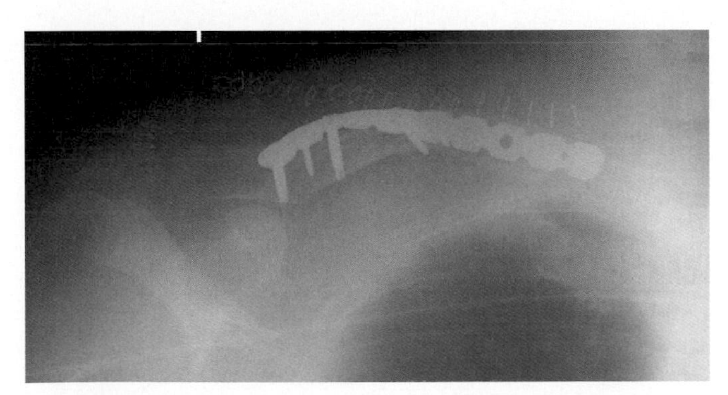

Figure 51-4 Open reduction with internal fixation using a clavicle plate. The plate is contoured to fit the shape of the clavicle.

- Nonunion or symptomatic malunion of fracture with closed treatment

Troubleshooting

- The overall nonunion rate for all clavicle fractures is approximately 7% for closed treatment, but increases to 15% or more with significant shortening, displacement, and comminution.
- Nonunion requires surgical referral.
- Malunion, if symptomatic with pain or functional disability, also merits referral.

Patient Instructions

- Warn patients undergoing closed treatment to expect mild discomfort for as long as 3 months and some degree of permanent cosmetic deformity.
- Inform patient about potential complications and long-term sequelae of operative treatment
  - Prominent hardware (pain, poor cosmesis)
  - Future operation for hardware removal (requested by 30% to 50% of patients with plate fixation)
  - Intramedullary pin migration or hardware failure
  - Neurovascular injury including permanent supraclavicular nerve numbness
  - Unsightly or painful incisional scar
  - Infection or nonunion

- Potential acromioclavicular or sternoclavicular arthrosis despite surgical fixation

Considerations in Special Populations

- Children: Nearly all clavicular fractures in children are treated nonoperatively and heal with excellent results, even with poor patient compliance. Physeal injury may result in growth-related deformity.
- Pathologic fracture of the clavicle is rare, but may occur as a result of a primary or metastatic neoplasm or postirradiation osteitis in patients undergoing radiation treatment for breast or neck carcinomas.
  - The medial clavicle is the most common site.
  - These fractures often require operative fixation.

Suggested Reading

- Canadian Orthopaedic Trauma Society: Nonoperative treatment compared with plate fixation of displaced midshaft clavicular fractures. A multicenter, randomized clinical trial. J Bone Joint Surg Am 2007;89A:1–10.
- Jeray KJ: Acute midshaft clavicular fracture. J Am Acad Orthop Surg 2007;15:239–248.
- Ring D, Jupiter JB: Injuries to the shoulder girdle. In Browner BD, Jupiter JB, Levine AM, Trafton PG (eds): Skeletal Trauma, 3rd ed. Philadelphia: WB Saunders, 2003, pp 1633–1653.
- Throckmorton T, Kuhn JE: Fractures of the medial end of the clavicle. J Shoulder Elbow Surg 2007;16:49–54.
- Zlowodzki M, Zelle BA, Cole PA, et al: Treatment of acute midshaft clavicle fractures: Systematic review of 2144 fractures. J Orthop Trauma 2005;19:504–507.

Chapter 52 Anterior Shoulder Relocation Technique

Adam W. Anz, Brandon D. Bushnell, and Timothy N. Taft

ICD-9 CODES
831.01 *Closed Shoulder Dislocation*
831.11 *Open Shoulder Dislocation*

CPT CODES
23650 *Closed Treatment with Manipulation of Shoulder Dislocation Not Requiring Anesthesia*
23655 *Closed Treatment with Manipulation of Shoulder Dislocation Requiring Anesthesia*

Key Concepts

- Most commonly dislocated joint (45% of all joint dislocations).
- Ninety-seven percent of shoulder dislocations are anterior.
- A shallow socket of the glenoid combined with a large humeral head leads to the propensity for dislocation.
- Dislocations often result in recurrent instability of the shoulder and require operative treatment.

History

- The majority of dislocations are trauma related, with sports injuries being the most prevalent.
- Anterior dislocation often results from the arm being forced into a position of abduction, external rotation, and extension.
- Posterior dislocation often results from a posteriorly directed blow with the arm in flexion and adduction.

Imaging

- Orthogonal views, usually an anteroposterior view of the shoulder (Grashey view) and a lateral axillary view, can help make the diagnosis (Fig. 52-1).
- Postreduction radiographs confirm the anatomic reduction and are critical in the evaluation of associated fractures or other bony abnormalities such as a Hill-Sachs (humeral head) or Bankart (glenoid) lesion.

Reduction

There are many described reduction techniques with documented levels of success; however, no studies have provided sufficient evidence to establish a preferred method. The care provider should be familiar with many different options and apply them as appropriate in each individual case situation.

- Traction, countertraction methods
  - Traction on the arm with concurrent countertraction on the rib cage has been established since the time of Hippocrates as a method of relocation.
  - Care should be taken to avoid too much pressure on vital neurovascular structures in the axillary recess.
- Kocher method
  - Often preferable in heavier patients, in patients older than the age of 40 years, and in dislocations older than 4 hours (Fig. 52-2)
    - — Begin with arm adducted at shoulder.
    - — Flex elbow to 90 degrees.
    - — Externally rotate arm until resistance is felt.
    - — Forward flex arm at shoulder as far as possible.
    - — Internally rotate at shoulder for relocation.
- Milch method
  - May be performed with patient supine or prone
  - Involves abduction and external rotation of the shoulder
  - Zero position maxim: At the zero position of 165 degrees of abduction, 45 degrees of forward flexion, and 90 degrees of external rotation, the scapulohumeral axis and the rotator cuff axis align, which transforms any muscular pull of the rotator cuff into an axial pull favoring reduction.
  - Supine
    - — Slowly abduct the arm at the shoulder to a goal of 165 degrees.
    - — While abducting the arm, externally rotate it.
    - — At the zero position, the cuff muscles will be relaxed (Fig. 52-3).

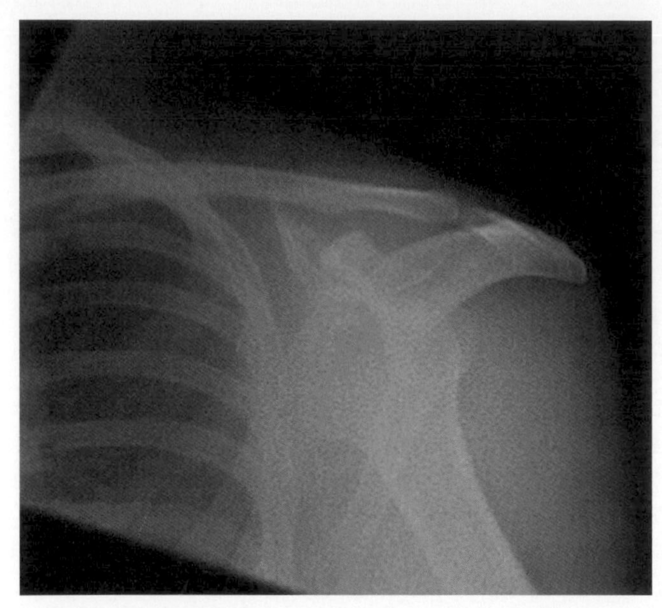

Figure 52-1 Anteroposterior radiograph of an anterior shoulder dislocation.

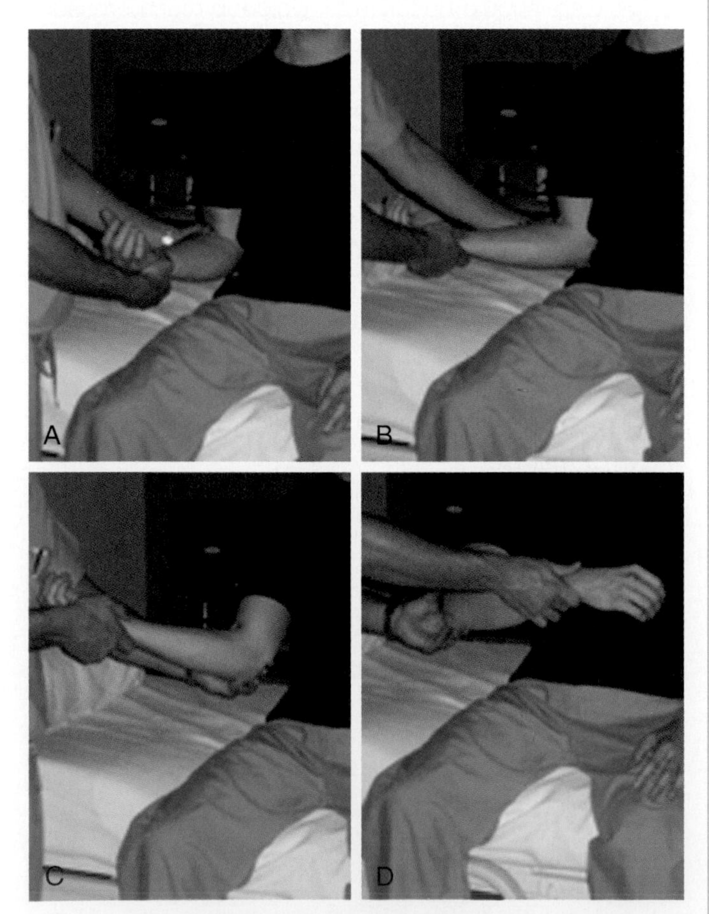

Figure 52-2 **A,** Start with adduction at the shoulder and elbow flexion. **B,** Externally rotate the arm at the shoulder. **C,** Flex the arm forward at the shoulder until resistance is felt. **D,** Internally rotate the arm at the shoulder.

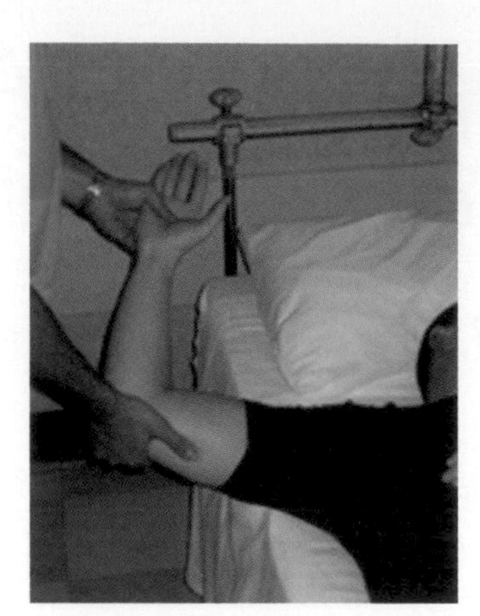

Figure 52-3 The shoulder approaches the zero position at 165 degrees of abduction, 45 degrees of forward flexion, and 90 degrees of external rotation.

  - — The humeral head can be pushed gently back over the glenoid rim.
- Prone (better for patient relaxation and surgeon control of arm) (Fig. 52-4)
  - — Position the patient lying prone with the affected arm hanging down.
  - — Allow the patient time to relax, allowing the arm to swing freely. Some will spontaneously reduce at this point.
  - — Flex the elbow to 90 degrees slowly, allowing adequate time for patient comfort. This relaxes the long head of the biceps muscle, preventing it from impeding reduction.
  - — Place the patient's hand over the dorsal forearm of the care provider and grasp the elbow with the ipsilateral hand. Longitudinal traction may be gently applied at the arm with the care provider's contralateral hand.
  - — Slowly abduct the patient's arm at the shoulder and concurrently externally rotate it.
  - — A final lift over the rim of the glenoid may be necessary.

- Scapular manipulation method
  - Position the patient lying prone with the affected arm hanging free.
  - Apply traction weights to the affected arm and allow time for the patient's muscles to relax. Some will spontaneously reduce at this point.
  - Grasp the superior-medial border of the scapula with one hand and with the other hand push the inferior tip of the scapula inferiorly and medially, creating a pivot point at the superior-medial border. Reduction should occur at this point.

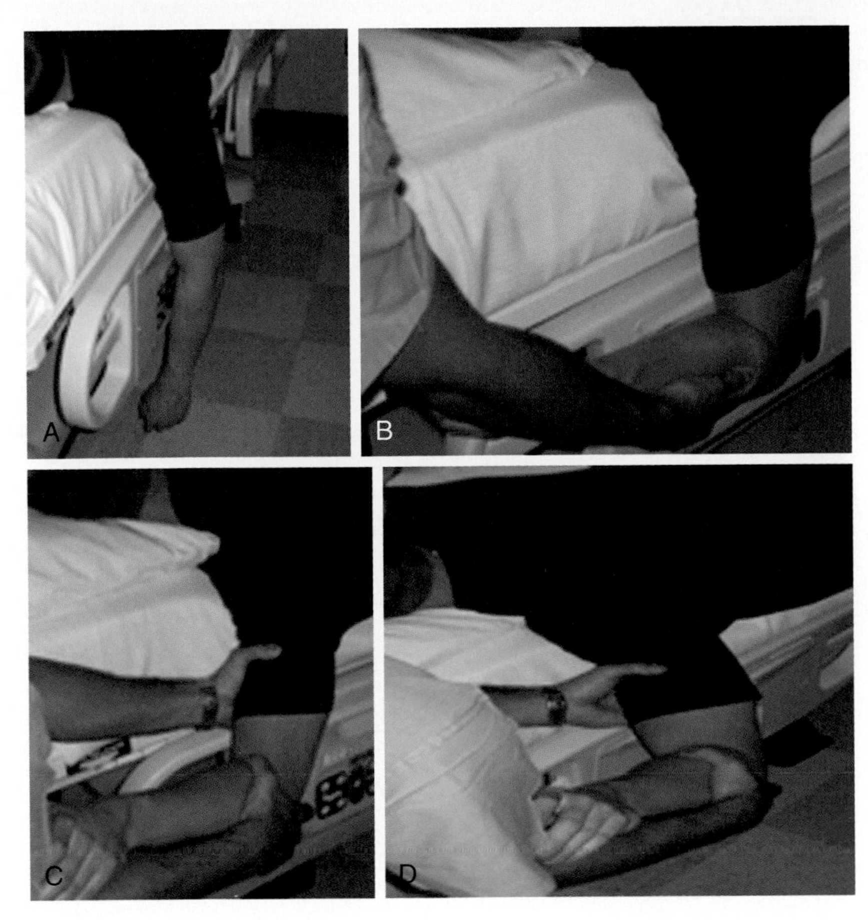

Figure 52-4 **A,** Place the patient in a prone position with the affected arm hanging. **B,** Slowly flex at the elbow to 90 degrees. **C,** Grasp with one hand at the elbow while pulling with gentle traction with the other hand. **D,** Abduct the arm and externally rotate it. A final lift into the glenoid may be necessary.

Anesthesia

- Reduction after intravenous sedation is the most common approach.
- Intra-articular local anesthesia (see Chapter 53) is also an option and has been found to shorten the emergency department stay and reduce complications with no change in success rates relative to intravenous sedation.
- Success without anesthesia has been advocated and documented by many authors, but patience is paramount when relying on time rather than medication to relax the patient and his or her muscles.

Postreduction Immobilization

- Immobilization in adduction and internal rotation with a simple sling for 3 to 5 weeks followed by rehabilitation with physical therapy is commonly used.
- Recent data suggest that immobilization in slight abduction and external rotation with a "gunslinger" type brace improves healing by tightening the anterior capsule and ligament support of the joint. This position is often not as well tolerated by patients.
- Return to heavy-duty work and athletics is permissible when the patient has regained full motion and strength relative to the uninjured side.

Recurrence

- Recurrence rates range from 30% to 100% after a primary dislocation.
- Younger male patients aged 15 to 35 years are at highest risk of recurrence.
- Older patients have a higher risk of associated rotator cuff tear.
- Open or arthroscopic surgery can decrease the risk of recurrence, and referral to an orthopaedic surgeon after initial successful reduction is mandatory.

Suggested Reading

- Beattie T, Steedman D, McGowan A, Robertson C: A comparison of the Milch and Kocher techniques for acute dislocation of the shoulder. Injury 1986;17:349–352.
- Itoi E, Hatakeyama Y, Sato T, et al: Immobilization in external rotation after shoulder dislocation reduces the risk of recurrence. A randomized controlled trial. J Bone Joint Surg Am 2007;89A: 2124–2131.

- Kuhn J: Treating the initial anterior shoulder dislocation: An evidence-based medicine approach. Sports Med Arthrosc Rev 2006;14:192–198.
- O'Connor D, Schwarze D, Fragomen A, Perdomo M: Painless reduction of acute anterior shoulder dislocations without anesthesia. Orthopedics 2006;29:528–532.
- Robinson M, Howes J, Murdoch H, et al: Functional outcome and risk of recurrent instability after primary anterior shoulder dislocation in young patients. J Bone Joint Surg Am 2006; 88A:2326–2336.

Chapter 53 Glenohumeral Joint Injection

Colin G. Crosby, Brandon D. Bushnell, and Timothy N. Taft

CPT CODE
20610 *Aspiration and/or Injection, Large Joint*

Equipment

- Sterile preparation solution: povidone-iodine, alcohol, chlorhexidine, others
- Sterile gloves: appropriate size
- Skin pretreatments (optional): ethyl chloride (cold spray) or EMLA cream
- Anesthetic needle: 25 gauge or smaller, 0.5 inch or smaller
- Anesthetic syringe: 5 mL or smaller
- Anesthetic agent: 1% or 2% lidocaine with or without epinephrine (for skin only)
- Aspiration needle: 18 or 16 gauge, 1.5 inch or larger
- Aspiration syringe: 20 mL or larger
- Injection needle: 20 to 22 gauge, 1.5 inch or larger
- Injection syringe: 10 to 20 mL
- Injection agent
  - Anesthetic options: lidocaine (1% or 2%), bupivacaine (0.25% or 0.5%), combinations
  - Steroid options: betamethasone, triamcinolone, methylprednisolone, others
  - Contrast options: various preparations for use with radiographic studies
- Sterile gauze: prepare for possible venous bleeder
- Small bandage: coverage of procedure site
- Assistant: for help with medication preparation, hand off of materials, patient positioning, other aspects
  - Choice of materials and exact procedure will vary somewhat by situation depending on the indications for the procedure, patient preferences, provider preferences, and materials available for use. Detailed discussion of these issues is beyond the scope of this chapter.

Indications

- Injection
  - Osteoarthritis
  - Rheumatoid arthritis
  - Adhesive capsulitis
  - Internal impingement
  - Labral tears/superior labral anteroposterior lesions
  - Unknown diagnosis (diagnostic injection)
- Aspiration
  - Septic arthritis
  - Crystalline arthritis (gout, pseudogout)
  - Symptomatic effusion
  - Unknown diagnosis (diagnostic aspiration)

Contraindications

- Injection
  - Septic arthritis
  - Systemic sepsis
  - Overlying skin pathology
  - Active cellulitis
  - Active osteomyelitis in the shoulder area
  - Uncontrolled coagulopathy
  - Allergy to anesthetic agents or injection agents
  - Pregnancy (injection of steroid medications)

Technique

- Informed consent is obtained and the correct shoulder is confirmed.
- With the care provider standing, the patient is placed in a seated position to bring the shoulder to an easily accessible level. The shoulder is placed in a position of internal rotation and adduction at the side.
- Anatomic landmarks for injection are identified and marked (Fig. 53-1).
- If desired, EMLA cream can be applied to the site; some delay is required for full effect.
- The skin over and around the injection site is prepared with the chosen sterile preparation solution (Fig. 53-2).
- If desired, the injection site may be treated with ethyl chloride (cold spray). The spray usually lasts only a few seconds and thus should be applied just before injection of the skin.

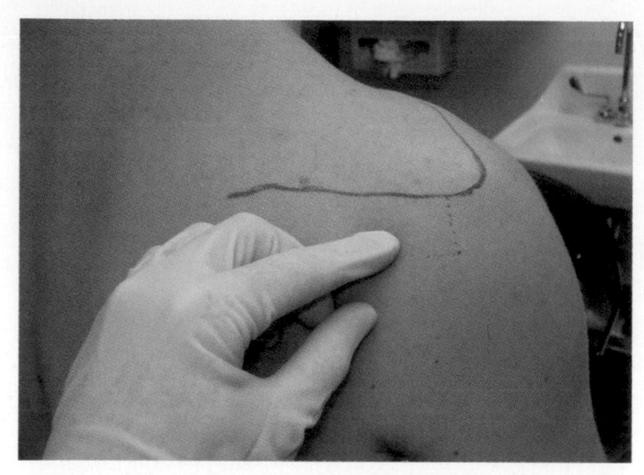

Figure 53-1 Posterior approach: identify a point 2 cm inferior and 1 cm medial to the posterolateral corner of the acromion.

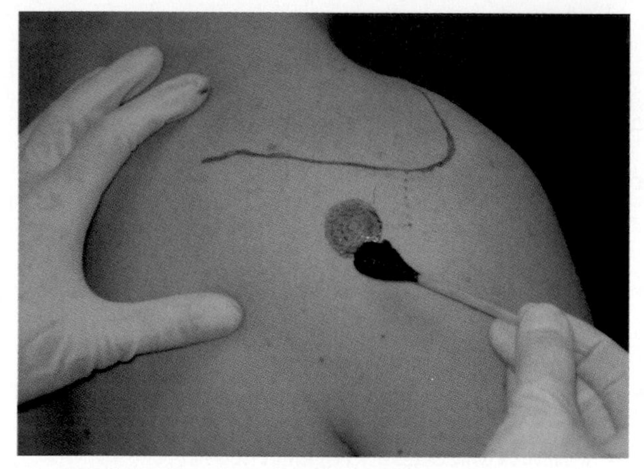

Figure 53-2 Posterior approach: sterile preparation of the injection site with Betadine (povidone-iodine).

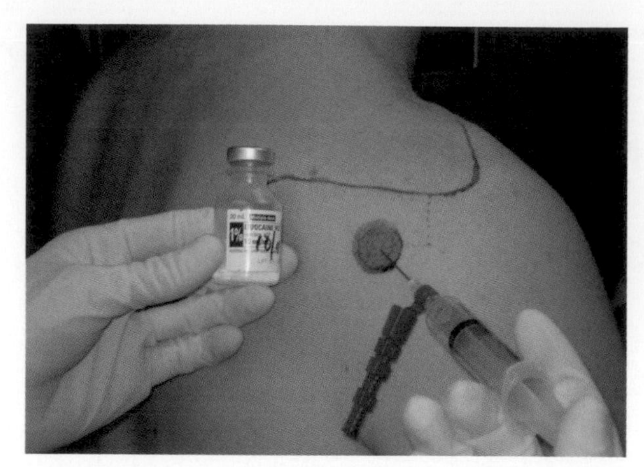

Figure 53-3 Posterior approach: skin anesthesia with 1% lidocaine.

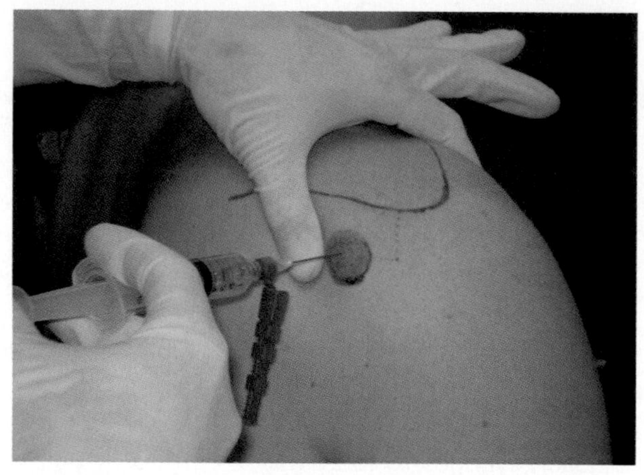

Figure 53-4 Posterior approach: injection of desired medication with the needle progressing anteromedially toward the coracoid process, using the free index finger for targeting purposes.

- Sterile gloves are used for the remainder of the procedure.
- A small needle and syringe (25 gauge, 0.5 inch or smaller, 5 mL or smaller) are loaded with a short-acting anesthetic medication (usually 1% or 2% lidocaine). A small skin wheal is raised over the site of planned injection or aspiration. Some of the deeper planned track of the needle may also be anesthetized. Adequate time is allowed for the anesthesia to reach its full effect (Fig. 53-3).
- If injection is planned, a larger needle and syringe (20–22 gauge, 1.5 inch or larger, 10–20 mL) are loaded with chosen medication(s).
- Posterior approach
  - The needle is inserted at a point 2 cm inferior and 1 cm medial to the posterolateral corner of the acromion, often identified as the soft spot (Fig. 53-4). The needle progresses anteromedially toward the coracoid process until the joint capsule is encountered. The index finger of the free hand can be placed on the coracoid process for targeting purposes. The needle then passes through the capsule with a subtle "pop."
- Anterior approach
  - The needle is inserted at a point midway between the coracoid process and the anterolateral corner of the acromion (Figs. 53-5 and 53-6). The needle progresses posteriorly in a plane perpendicular to the body until the joint capsule is encountered (Fig. 53-7). The needle then passes through the capsule with a subtle "pop."
- After entering the capsule, the joint may be aspirated. A larger syringe (20 mL or larger) provides adequate negative pressure for aspiration.
- If only injection is planned, gentle aspiration should still be performed to confirm entry into the joint rather than a vessel.

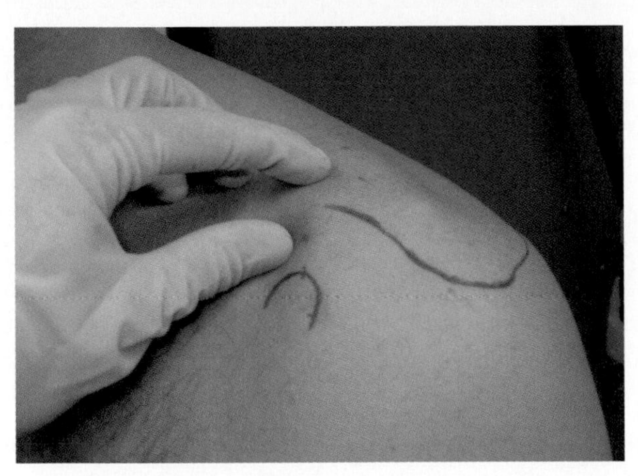

Figure 53-5 Anterior approach: identification of the coracoid process and the anterolateral corner of the acromion.

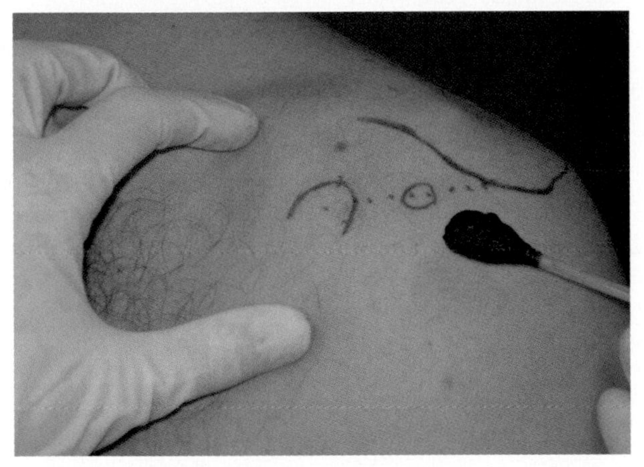

Figure 53-6 Anterior approach: marking of the injection point halfway between the coracoid process and the anterolateral corner of the acromion.

- Injection of the medication then proceeds with slow, consistent pressure. The fluid should flow readily into the joint; any increased resistance or pressure should prompt a reevaluation of location.
- After injection or aspiration, a small bandage is applied.
- All materials are appropriately disposed of, and any intra-articular specimens are appropriately handled and routed.

Special Considerations

- Care should be taken with the anterior approach to avoid injury to the brachial plexus or axillary artery.
- Needle size depends on patient size; larger patients will likely require longer needles.

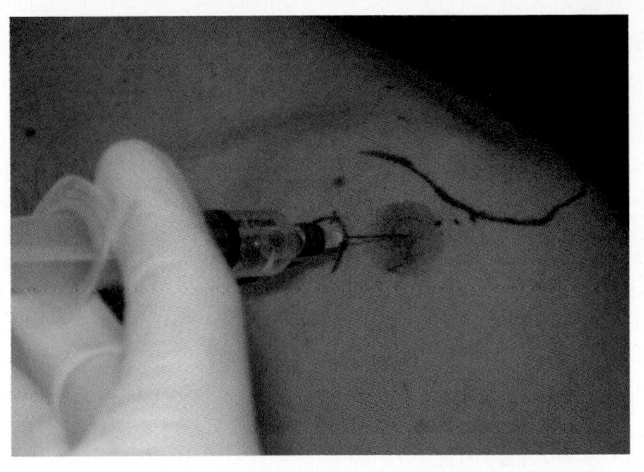

Figure 53-7 Anterior approach: needle progresses posteriorly in a plane perpendicular to the body.

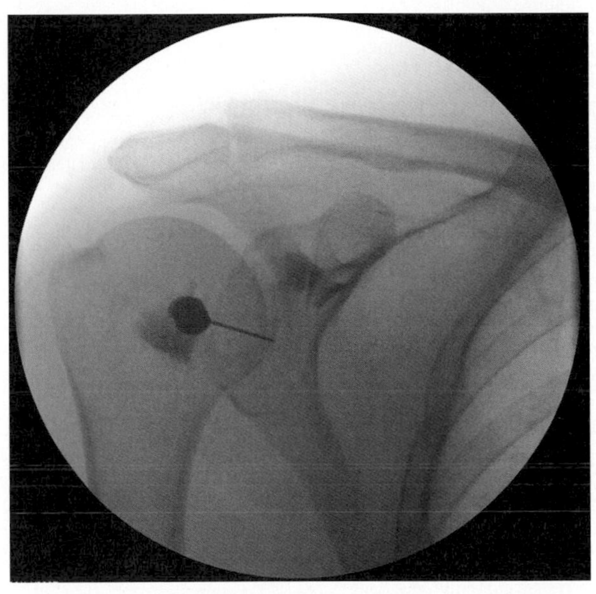

Figure 53-8 Use of fluoroscopy can aid with visualization of the injection of the glenohumeral joint.

- Injections in morbidly obese or muscular patients may be made easier by visualization with fluoroscopy or ultrasonography (Fig. 53-8).
- Complications may include systemic effects, tendon weakening or rupture, fat atrophy, muscle wasting, skin pigment changes, septic arthritis, nerve and vessel damage, steroid flare, and steroid arthropathy.
- Many clinicians recommend at least a 3-month interval between steroid injections.
- Some patients may experience a vasovagal reaction from the injection, and care should be taken to allow patients feeling light-headed or dizzy to lie down for several moments as needed.

Troubleshooting

- "Bumping" bone
  - If the needle contacts bone during the entry to the joint, the arm may be rotated to determine whether the needle is contacting the humerus or the glenoid.
  - If the needle moves with rotation of the arm, it should be directed more medially to avoid the humerus.
  - If the needle does not move with rotation of the arm, it should be directed more laterally to avoid the glenoid.
- Difficult entry
  - Fluoroscopy and ultrasonography have been shown by several studies to aid in navigating to the joint space in difficult injection cases such as in obese or very muscular patients.

Patient Instructions

- The bandage may be removed within a few hours after aspiration or injection.
- Some soreness is expected for approximately 24 to 48 hours and may be addressed with ice, heat, nonsteroidal anti-inflammatory drugs, and/or acetaminophen.
- Contact the physician immediately if any redness, warmth, increased swelling, severe increase in pain, fever, or chills develops.
- Diabetic patients should closely monitor blood glucose levels after injection of steroid medications and expect elevated levels for several days.

Suggested Reading

- DeLee JC, Drez D Jr, Miller MD (eds): DeLee and Drez's Orthopaedic Sports Medicine, 2nd ed. Philadelphia: Saunders, 2003.
- Dickson J: Shoulder injections in primary care. Practitioner 2000;244:259–265.
- Kerlan RK, Glousman RE: Injections and techniques in athletic medicine. Clin Sports Med 1989;8:541–560.
- Sauders S, Longworth S: Injection Techniques in Orthopaedics and Sports Medicine. New York: Churchill Livingstone, 2006.
- Tallia AF, Cardone DA: Diagnostic and therapeutic injection of the shoulder region. Am Fam Physician 2003;67:1271–1278.

Chapter 54 Subacromial Injection

Colin G. Crosby, Brandon D. Bushnell, and Timothy N. Taft

CPT CODE
20610 *Aspiration and/or Injection, Large Joint*

Equipment

- Sterile preparation solution: povidone-iodine, alcohol, chlorhexidine, others
- Sterile gloves: appropriate size
- Skin pretreatments (optional): ethyl chloride (cold spray) or EMLA cream
- Anesthetic needle: 25 gauge or smaller, 0.5 inch or smaller
- Anesthetic syringe: 5 mL or smaller
- Anesthetic agent: 1% or 2% lidocaine, with or without epinephrine (for skin only)
- Aspiration needle: 18 or 16 gauge, 1.5 inch or larger
- Aspiration syringe: 20 mL or larger
- Injection needle: 20 to 22 gauge, 1.5 inch or larger
- Injection syringe: 10 to 20 mL
- Injection agent
  - Anesthetic options: lidocaine (1% or 2%), bupivacaine (0.25% or 0.5%), combinations
  - Steroid options: betamethasone, triamcinolone, methylprednisolone, others
- Sterile gauze: prepare for possible venous bleeder
- Small bandage: coverage of procedure site
- Assistant: for help with medication preparation, hand off of materials, patient positioning, other aspects
- Choice of materials and exact procedure will vary somewhat by situation depending on the indications for the procedure, patient preferences, provider preferences, and materials available for use. Detailed discussion of these issues is beyond the scope of this chapter.

Indications

- Injection
  - Subacromial/subdeltoid bursitis
  - Rotator cuff impingement syndrome
  - Calcific tendonitis
  - Rheumatoid arthritis
  - Unknown diagnosis (diagnostic injection)
- Aspiration
  - Septic bursitis
  - Subacromial/subdeltoid abscess
  - Crystalline deposition diseases
  - Unknown diagnosis (diagnostic aspiration)

Contraindications

- Septic arthritis
- Septic bursitis (injection only)
- Systemic sepsis
- Overlying skin pathology
- Active cellulitis
- Active osteomyelitis in the shoulder area
- Uncontrolled coagulopathy
- Allergy to anesthetic agents or injection agents
- Pregnancy (injection of steroid medications)

Technique

- Informed consent is obtained and the correct shoulder is confirmed.
- With the care provider standing, the patient is placed in a seated position to bring the shoulder to an easily accessible level. The shoulder is placed in a position of internal rotation and adduction at the side.
- Anatomic landmarks for injection are identified and marked (Fig. 54-1).
- If desired, EMLA cream can be applied to the site; some delay is required for full effect.
- The skin over and around the injection site is prepared with the chosen sterile preparation solution (Fig. 54-2).
- If desired, the injection site may be treated with ethyl chloride (cold spray). The spray usually lasts only a few seconds and thus should be applied just before injection of the skin.
- Sterile gloves are used for the remainder of the procedure.
- A small needle and syringe (25 gauge, 0.5 inch or smaller, 5 mL or smaller) are loaded with a short-acting anesthetic medication (usually 1% or 2% lidocaine). A small skin wheal is raised over the site of planned injection or aspiration (Fig. 54-3). Some of the

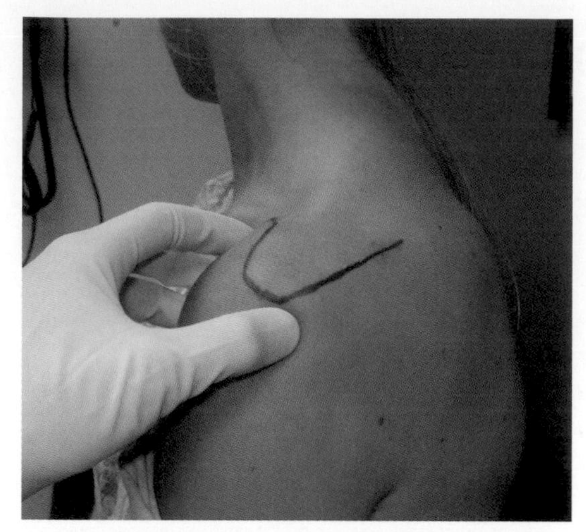

Figure 54-1 Identify the posterolateral corner of the acromion.

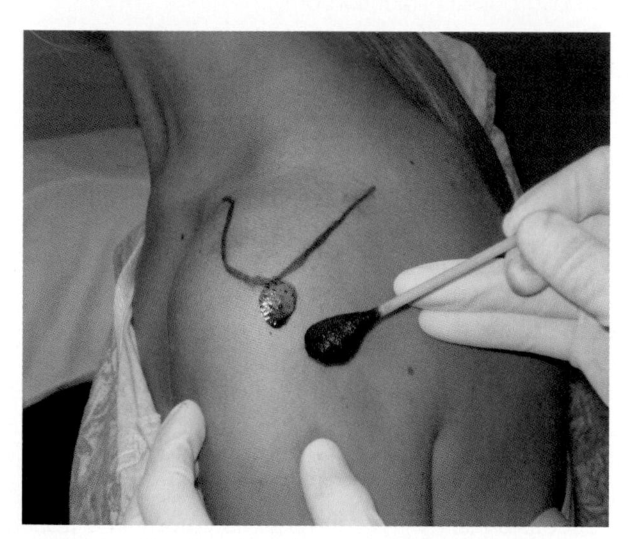

Figure 54-2 Sterile preparation with Betadine (povidone-iodine) of the injection point, just inferior to the posterolateral corner of the acromion.

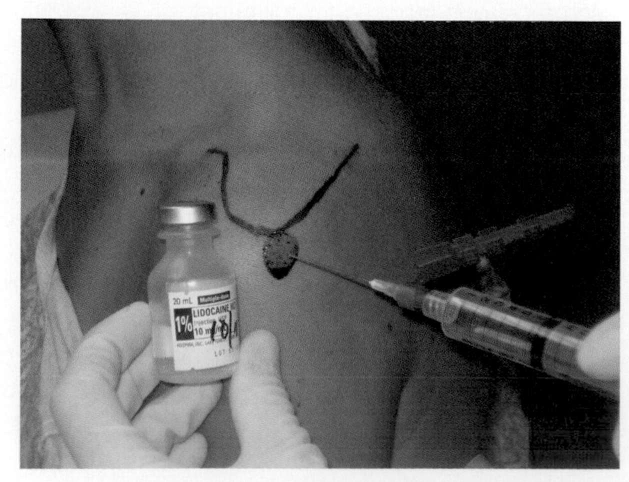

Figure 54-3 Skin anesthesia with 1% lidocaine.

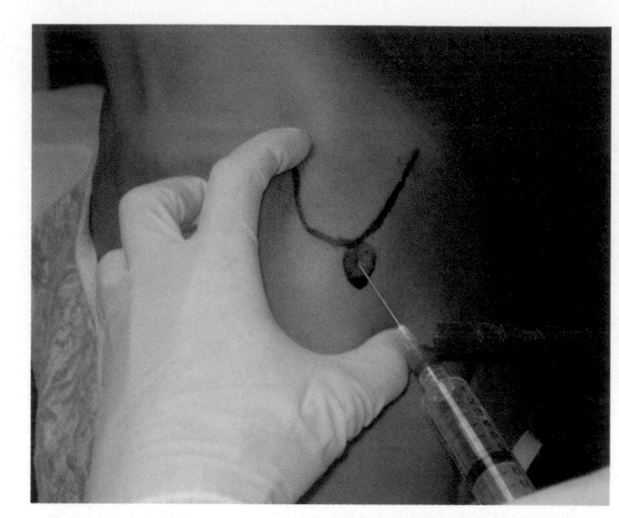

Figure 54-4 Needle advanced medially, anteriorly, and slightly superiorly.

deeper planned track of the needle may also be anesthetized. Adequate time is given for the anesthesia to reach its full effect.

- If injection is planned, a larger needle and syringe (20 to 22 gauge, 1.5 inch or larger, 10 to 20 mL) are loaded with the chosen medication(s).
- The injection point is just inferior to the posterolateral corner of the acromion, which is often easy to palpate, even in larger patients. The needle advances medially, anteriorly, and slightly superiorly into the subacromial space (Fig. 54-4).
- After entering the subacromial/subdeltoid space, the bursa may be aspirated. A larger syringe (20 mL or larger) provides adequate negative pressure for aspiration.
- If only injection is planned, gentle aspiration should still be performed to confirm that the needle has entered the bursa and not a vessel.
- Injection of the medication then proceeds with slow, consistent pressure. The fluid should flow readily into the space; any increased resistance or pressure should prompt a reevaluation of location.
- After injection or aspiration, a small bandage is applied.
- All materials are appropriately disposed of, and any intra-articular specimens are appropriately handled and routed.

Considerations

- The subacromial space can communicate with the glenohumeral joint if a rotator cuff tear exists.

- Needle size depends on patient size; larger patients will likely require longer needles.
- Complications may include systemic effects, tendon weakening or rupture, fat atrophy, muscle wasting, skin pigment changes, septic arthritis, nerve and vessel damage, steroid flare, and steroid arthropathy.
- Many clinicians recommend at least a 3-month interval between steroid injections.
- Some patients may experience a vasovagal reaction from the injection, and care should be taken to allow patients feeling light-headed or dizzy to lie down for several moments as needed.

Troubleshooting

- Difficult entry
  - Downward traction on the arm can help open the subacromial space.
- "Hooked" acromion
  - Some patients have a lateral "hook" shape to their acromion, requiring a more exaggerated inferior starting point and more superiorly directed course of the needle.

Patient Instructions

- The bandage may be removed within a few hours after aspiration or injection.
- Some soreness is expected for approximately 24 to 48 hours and may be addressed with ice, heat, nonsteroidal anti-inflammatory drugs, and/or acetaminophen.
- Contact the physician immediately if any redness, warmth, increased swelling, severe increase in pain, fever, or chills develops.
- Diabetic patients should closely monitor blood glucose levels after injection of steroid medications and expect elevated levels for several days.

Suggested Reading

- DeLee JC, Drez D Jr, Miller MD (eds): DeLee and Drez's Orthopaedic Sports Medicine, 2nd ed. Philadelphia: Saunders, 2003.
- Dickson J: Shoulder injections in primary care. Practitioner 2000;244:259–265.
- Kerlan RK, Glousman RE: Injections and techniques in athletic medicine. Clin Sports Med 1989;8:541–560.
- Sauders S, Longworth S: Injection Techniques in Orthopaedics and Sports Medicine. New York: Churchill Livingstone, 2006.
- Tallia AF, Cardone DA: Diagnostic and therapeutic injection of the shoulder region. Am Fam Physician 2003;67:1271–1278.

Chapter 55 Acromioclavicular Injection

Brian P. Scannell, Brandon D. Bushnell, and Timothy N. Taft

CPT CODE
20605 *Aspiration and/or Injection, Intermediate Joint*

Equipment

- Sterile preparation solution: povidone-iodine, alcohol, chlorhexidine, others
- Sterile gloves: appropriate size
- Skin pretreatments (optional): ethyl chloride (cold spray) or EMLA cream
- Anesthetic needle: 25 gauge or smaller, 0.5 inch or smaller
- Anesthetic syringe: 5 mL or smaller
- Anesthetic agent: 1% or 2% lidocaine with or without epinephrine (for skin only)
- Aspiration/injection needle: 20 to 22 gauge, 1 inch
- Aspiration/injection syringe: 3 to 10 mL
- Injection agent
  - Anesthetic options: lidocaine (1% or 2%), bupivacaine (0.25% or 0.5%), combinations
  - Steroid options: betamethasone, triamcinolone, methylprednisolone, others
- Sterile gauze: prepare for possible venous bleeder
- Small bandage: coverage of procedure site
- Assistant: for help with medication preparation, hand off of materials, patient positioning, other aspects
- Choice of materials and exact procedure will vary somewhat by situation depending on the indications for the procedure, patient preferences, provider preferences, and materials available for use. Detailed discussion of these issues is beyond the scope of this chapter.

Indications

- Injection
  - Osteoarthritis (Fig. 55-1)
  - Posttraumatic arthritis
  - Rheumatoid arthritis
  - Distal clavicle osteolysis
  - Unknown diagnosis (diagnostic injection)
- Aspiration
  - Septic bursitis
  - Crystalline deposition diseases
  - Unknown diagnosis (diagnostic aspiration)

Contraindications

- Septic arthritis (injection only)
- Septic bursitis (injection only)
- Systemic sepsis
- Overlying skin pathology
- Active cellulitis
- Active osteomyelitis
- Uncontrolled coagulopathy
- Allergy to anesthetic agents or injection agents
- Pregnancy (injection of steroid medications)

Technique

- Informed consent is obtained and the correct shoulder is confirmed.
- With the care provider standing, the patient is placed in a seated position to bring the shoulder to an easily accessible level. The shoulder is placed in a position of internal rotation and adduction at the side.
- Anatomic landmarks for injection are identified and marked (Fig. 55-2).
- If desired, EMLA cream can be applied to the site; some delay is required for full effect.
- The skin over and around the injection site is prepared with the chosen sterile preparation solution (Fig. 55-3).
- If desired, the injection site may be treated with ethyl chloride (cold spray). The spray usually lasts only a few seconds and thus should be applied just before injection of the skin.
- Sterile gloves are used for the remainder of the procedure.
- A small needle and syringe (25 gauge, 0.5 inch or smaller, 5 mL or smaller) are loaded with a short-acting anesthetic medication (usually 1% or 2% lidocaine). A small skin wheal is raised over the site of

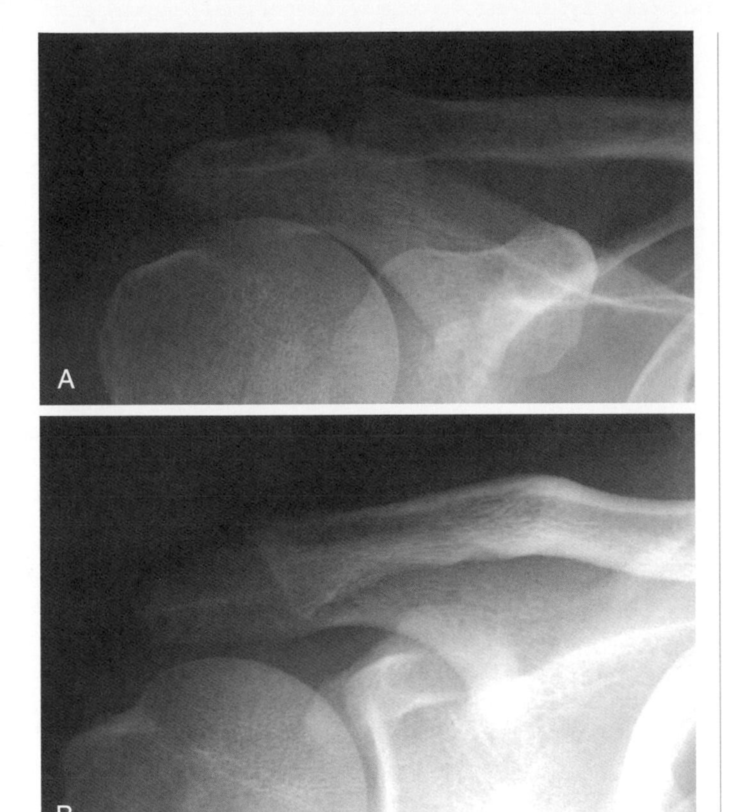

Figure 55-1 Normal acromioclavicular joint (**A**) and acromioclavicular joint with osteoarthritis (**B**). As seen here, the joint with osteoarthritis has significant narrowing and osteophyte formation, making injection much more difficult.

planned injection. Adequate time is given for the anesthesia to reach its full effect.

- If injection is planned, a larger needle and syringe (20–22 gauge, 1 inch, 3–10 mL) are loaded with the chosen medication(s).
- The injection point is identified by palpation of the clavicle lateral to its termination at the articulation with the acromion, where a slight depression can be found. Osteophytes on either side of the joint may also be palpated in some cases.
- The needle progresses inferiorly into the joint with a slight medially directed tilt (Fig. 55-4).
- A slight "pop" or change in resistance may be felt as the needle passes into the capsule.
- If only injection is planned, gentle aspiration should still be performed to confirm that the needle has entered the joint and not a vessel.
- Injection of the medication then proceeds with slow, consistent pressure. The fluid should flow readily into the space; any increased resistance or pressure should prompt a reevaluation of location. Often, only 1 to 2 mL may enter the joint.

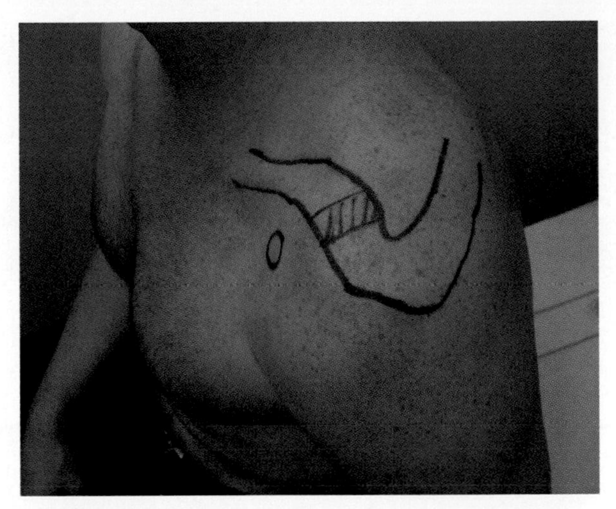

Figure 55-2 Marking bony structures to help identify the injection site.

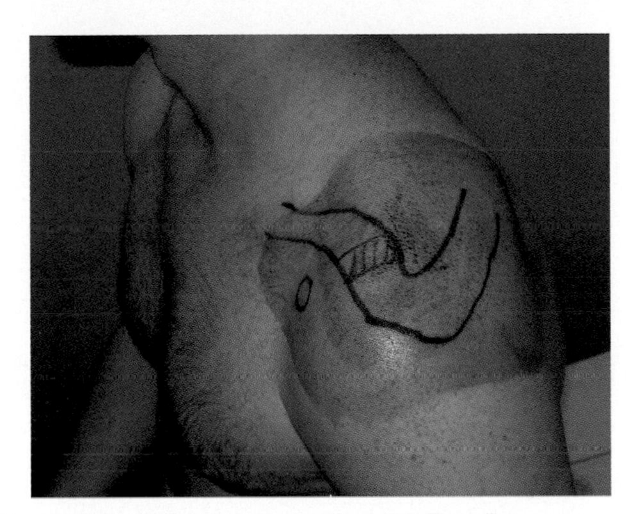

Figure 55-3 Wide skin preparation with Betadine (povidone-iodine).

- After injection or aspiration, a small bandage is applied.
- All materials are appropriately disposed of, and any intra-articular specimens are appropriately handled and routed.

Special Considerations

- The acromioclavicular joint can prove very difficult to locate in cases of severe osteoarthritis compared with a normal acromioclavicular joint secondary to joint space narrowing and osteophyte formation (see Fig. 55-1). Preprocedure radiographs with skin markers can prove quite helpful in determining the plane of the joint and facilitating a successful joint entry. The Zanca

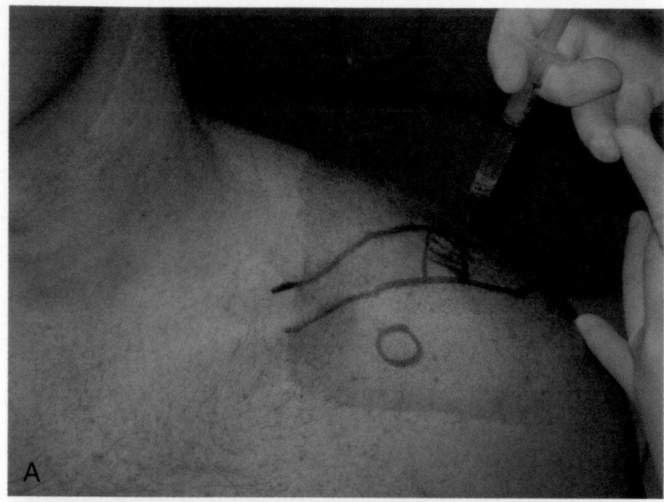

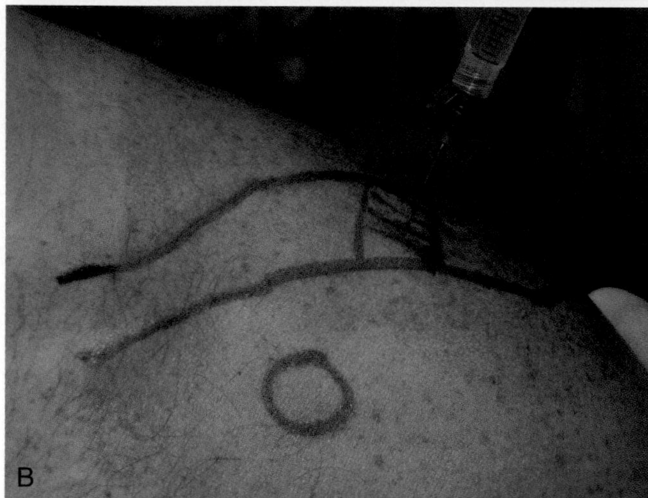

Figure 55-4 The needle is directed from superior to inferior (**A**). A slight lateral to medial tilt may assist in entering the joint (**B**).

view (anteroposterior view angled 15 degrees cephalad) is particularly useful.

- Needle size depends on patient size; larger patients may sometimes require slightly longer needles.
- Complications may include systemic effects, fat atrophy, muscle wasting, skin pigment changes, septic arthritis, nerve and vessel damage, steroid flare, and steroid arthropathy.
- Many clinicians recommend at least a 3-month interval between steroid injections.
- Some patients may experience a vasovagal reaction from the injection, and care should be taken to allow patients feeling light-headed or dizzy to lie down for several moments as needed.

Troubleshooting

- Difficult entry
  - The needle can often be "walked down the clavicle" medially to laterally until it drops into the joint. Extreme cases may require fluoroscopic guidance.

Patient Instructions

- The bandage may be removed within a few hours after aspiration or injection.
- Some soreness is expected for approximately 24 to 48 hours and may be addressed with ice, heat, nonsteroidal anti-inflammatory drugs, and/or acetaminophen.
- Contact the physician immediately if any redness, warmth, increased swelling, severe increase in pain, fever, or chills develops.
- Diabetic patients should closely monitor blood glucose levels after injection of steroid medications and expect elevated levels for several days.

Suggested Reading

- Buttaci CJ, Stitik TP, Yonclas PP, Foye PM: Osteoarthritis of the acromioclavicular joint: A review of anatomy, biomechanics, diagnosis, and treatment. Am J Phys Med Rehabil 2004; 83:791–797.
- Montellese P, Dancy T: The acromioclavicular joint. Prim Care 2004;31:857–866.
- Partington PF, Broome GH: Diagnostic injection around the shoulder: Hit and miss? A cadaveric study of injection accuracy. J Shoulder Elbow Surg 1998;7:147–150.
- Shaffer BS: Painful conditions of the acromioclavicular joint. J Am Acad Orthop Surg 1999;7:176–188.
- Tallia AF, Cardone DA: Diagnostic and therapeutic injection of the shoulder region. Am Fam Physician 2003;67:1271–1278.

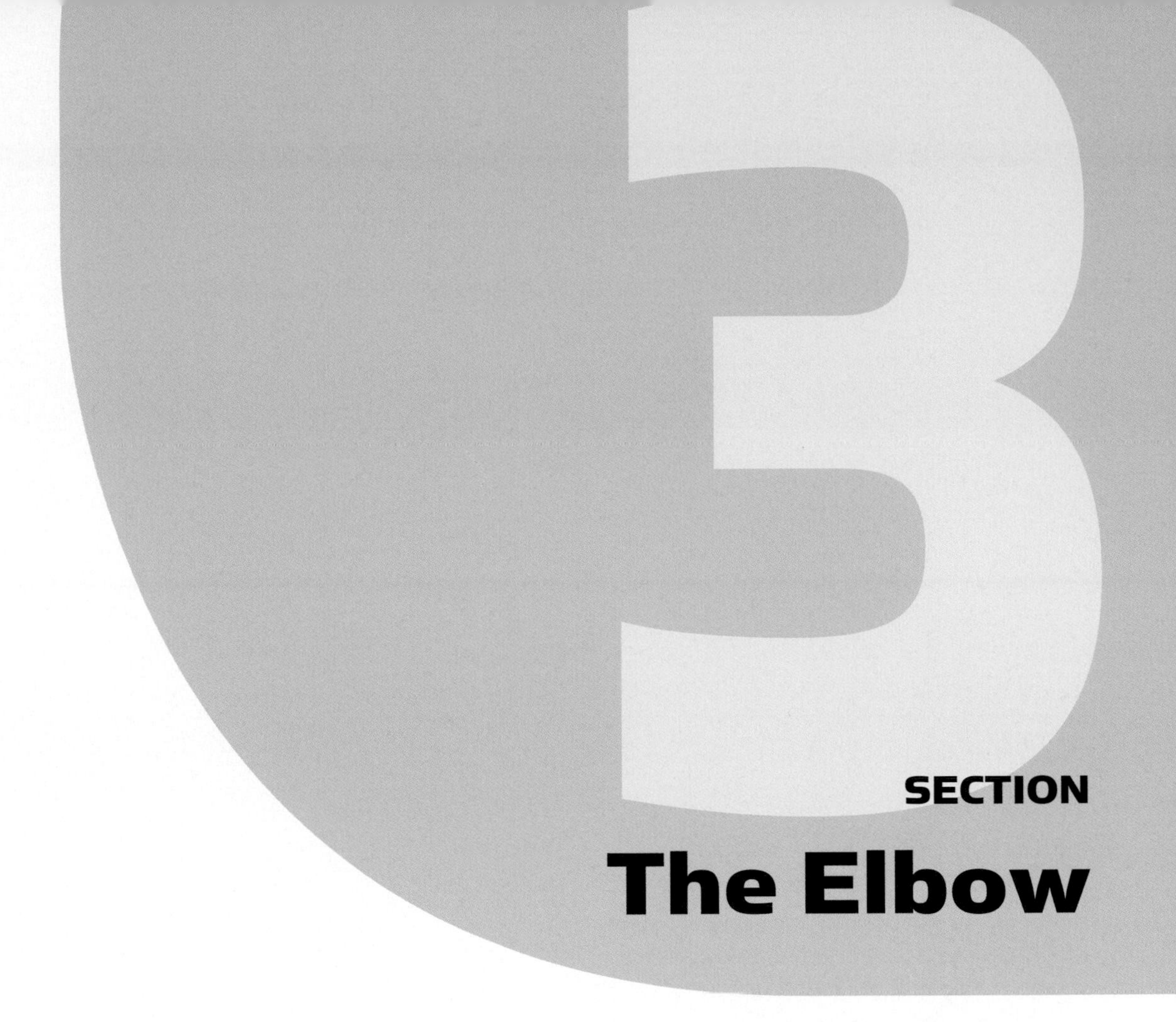

SECTION

The Elbow

Chapter 56 Overview of the Elbow

Jennifer A. Hart

Anatomy

- The elbow joint is made up of articulations between the distal humerus and the proximal radius and ulna (Fig. 56-1). These articulations allow two types of joint motion: flexion/extension and forearm rotation.

Humerus

- The articular surface of the distal humerus is composed of the trochlea and capitellum.
- The medial and lateral epicondyles are found just proximal to these structures.
- The medial epicondyle serves as an important attachment site for the ulnar collateral ligament, the common flexor tendons, and the pronator muscle.
- I he lateral epicondyle serves as an attachment site for the radial collateral ligament and the common extensor tendon.

Ulna

- The proximal ulna articulates with the trochlea to form the medial aspect of the elbow joint and also articulates with the radial head via the radial notch.
- The olecranon process is the predominant posterior bony structure that serves at the insertion point for the common distal triceps tendon.

Radius

- The radial head articulates with the capitellum in the lateral elbow joint and is also responsible for allowing pronation and supination of the forearm via its articulation with the proximal ulna.

Muscles (Box 56-1)

- Neurovascular structures (Fig. 56-2)
  - The brachial artery divides into the radial and ulnar arteries at the elbow joint, each of which further divides into small branches at the wrist.
  - The ulnar artery passes through the medial aspect of the forearm, and the radial artery passes through the lateral forearm.
  - The primary nerves located around the elbow include the ulnar (C7-T1), median (C5-T1), and radial (C5-T1) nerves.
  - The ulnar nerve passes behind the medial epicondyle and runs between the two heads of the flexor carpi ulnaris muscle.
  - The medial nerve runs beneath the pronator teres muscle on its path to the carpal tunnel at the wrist. The radial nerve divides into superficial and deep branches to provide sensation to the posterior forearm and the majority of the extensor muscles there.
- Ligaments and soft tissue (Fig. 56-3)
  - The ulnar and radial collateral ligaments are important static stabilizers of the elbow joint.
  - The ulnar (medial) collateral ligament is composed of anterior and posterior bands and functions to resist excessive valgus load to the elbow.
  - The radial (lateral) collateral ligament similarly resists varus stress at the elbow joint and actually is made up of two separate structures: the radial collateral ligament and the lateral ulnar collateral ligament.
  - The olecranon bursa lies posteriorly over the olecranon process and is frequently inflamed from direct trauma to the "point" of the elbow.

History

- A thorough history can lead to the development of an accurate and complete list of differential diagnoses that can then be refined further with physical examination and diagnostic studies.
- At the basic level, the history should include the mechanism of injury, previous similar symptoms, and pain characteristics (location, quality, severity, and radiation) (Table 56-1).

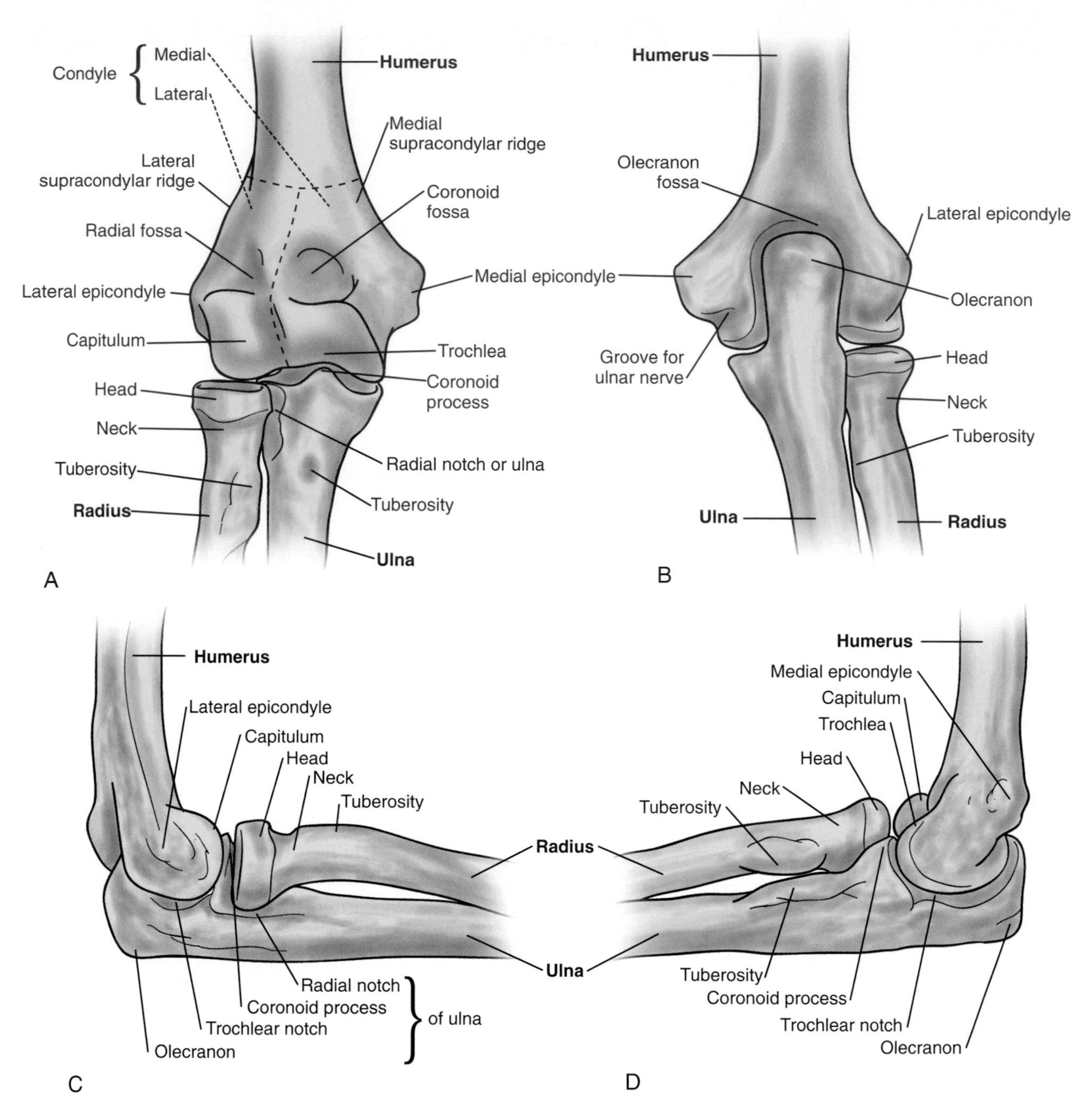

Figure 56-1 The bony anatomy of the elbow joint. In extension, anterior (**A**) and posterior (**B**) views. In 90-degree flexion, lateral (**C**) and medial (**D**) views.

BOX 56-1 *The Muscles*

Flexion
Biceps brachii
Coracobrachialis
Brachialis

Extension
Triceps brachii
Anconeus

Supination
Supinator
Biceps brachii

Pronation
Pronator quadratus
Pronator teres

Figure 56-2 The neurovascular structures of the elbow and arm (anterior view).

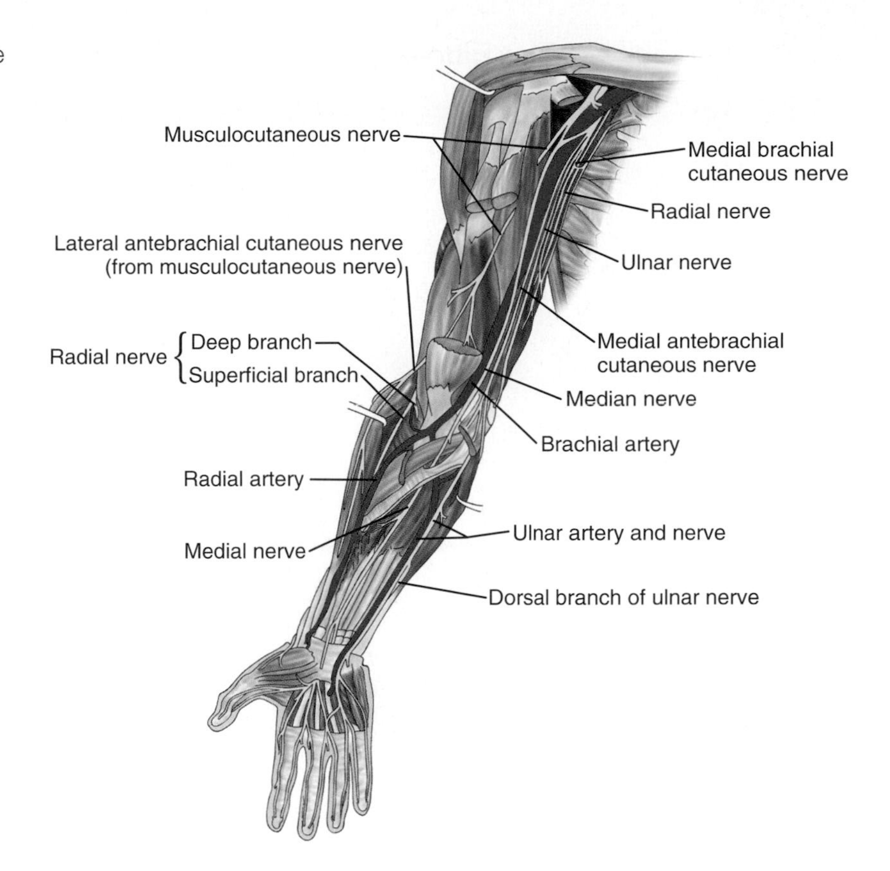

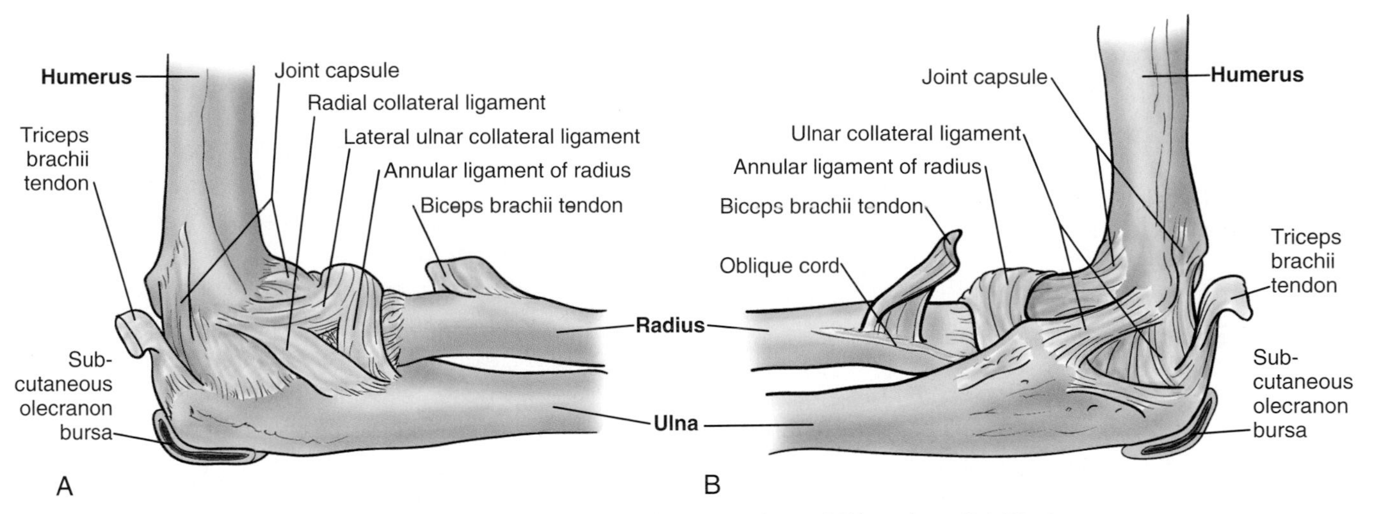

Figure 56-3 The ligaments of the elbow joint. Lateral (**A**) and medial (**B**) views.

TABLE 56-1 *History*

Fall/Trauma	Fracture
Traction injury "pulled by hand"	Nursemaid's elbow/dislocation
Night pain	Tumor/infection
Lateral overuse pain	Tennis elbow
Medial overuse pain	Golfer's elbow
Posterior traumatic pain	Olecranon bursitis
Acute loss of strength	Biceps/triceps rupture/avulsion
Locking, younger patient	Osteochondritis dissecans
Locking, older patient	Degenerative joint disease
Neurologic symptoms	Nerve entrapment

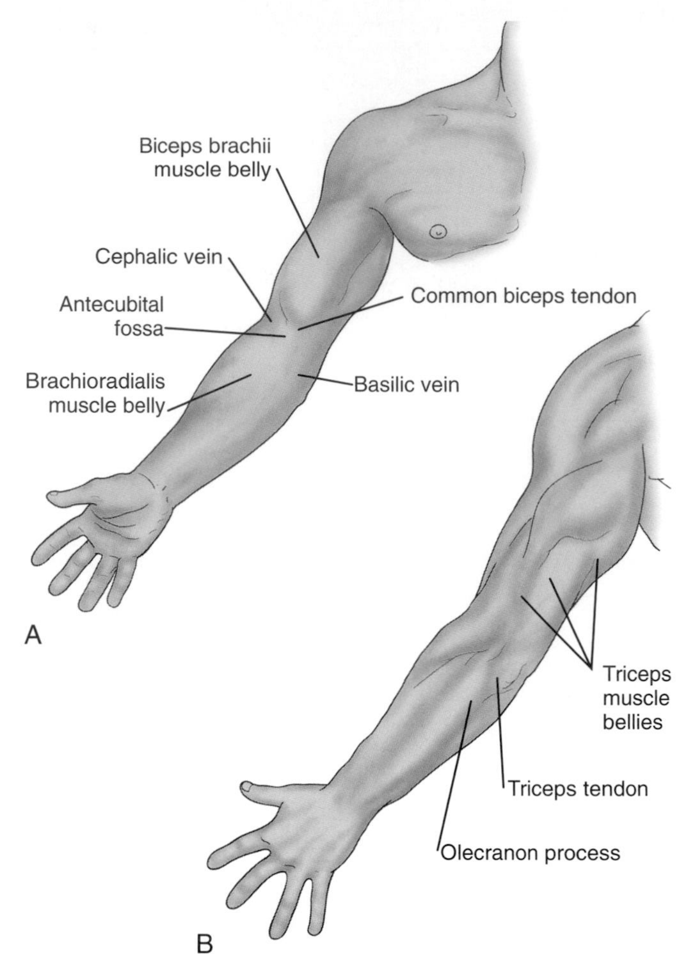

Figure 56-4 The surface anatomy of the elbow. Anterior (**A**) and posterior (**B**) views.

Physical Examination

- Inspection and palpation (Fig. 56-4)
  - Anterior elbow: Observe and palpate the antecubital fossa for masses and the biceps tendons for rupture (loss of tendon continuity and focal tenderness).
  - Posterior elbow: Palpate the tip of the olecranon for fracture/avulsion and observe any swelling in the olecranon bursa. An enlarged and erythematous area over the posterior elbow may indicate an infected bursa.
  - Medial elbow: Deformity and/or tenderness over the medial epicondyle may indicate medial epicondylitis or ulnar collateral ligament injury. A quick tap posterior to the medial epicondyle may elicit a positive Tinel's sign indicating ulnar neuropathy.
  - Lateral elbow: Deformity and/or tenderness over the lateral epicondyle may indicate tennis elbow, whereas tenderness over the radial head is suspicious for fracture.

BOX 56-2 *Strength Testing*

5: Full motion against gravity with maximum resistance
4: Full motion against gravity with moderate resistance
3: Full motion against gravity with no resistance
2: Full range of motion in gravity-eliminated position
1: No motion but muscle contraction is noted
0: No motion or muscle contraction

- Range of motion
  - Flexion/extension: 0 to 145 degrees
  - Pronation: 80 to 90 degrees
  - Supination: 85 to 90 degrees
- Strength testing (Fig. 56-5 and Box 56-2)
  - Flexion
  - Extension
  - Pronation
  - Supination
- Special tests
  - Reflexes: biceps (C5), triceps (C7) (Fig. 56-6)
  - Valgus and varus stress (Fig. 56-7)
    — Purpose: evaluation for integrity of the ulnar collateral or radial collateral ligaments
    — How to perform: Stabilize the humerus and, with the elbow slightly flexed, exert pressure on the forearm first medially (varus) and then laterally (valgus).
    — Positive: indicated by laxity or "opening" of the joint medially or laterally
  - Tinel's sign (Fig. 56-8)
    — Purpose: evaluation for cubital tunnel syndrome (ulnar nerve entrapment)
    — How to perform: Tap over the ulnar nerve as it passes by the medial epicondyle of the distal humerus.
    — Positive: indicated by reproduction of paresthesia in the ulnar nerve distribution

Imaging

- Radiography
  - The most commonly ordered plain views of the elbow joint include anteroposterior, lateral, and oblique views. Stress views may be helpful when a collateral ligament injury is suspected (Fig. 56-9).
- Magnetic resonance imaging
  - Commonly used to evaluate the soft-tissue structures such as the ligaments (Fig. 56-10)

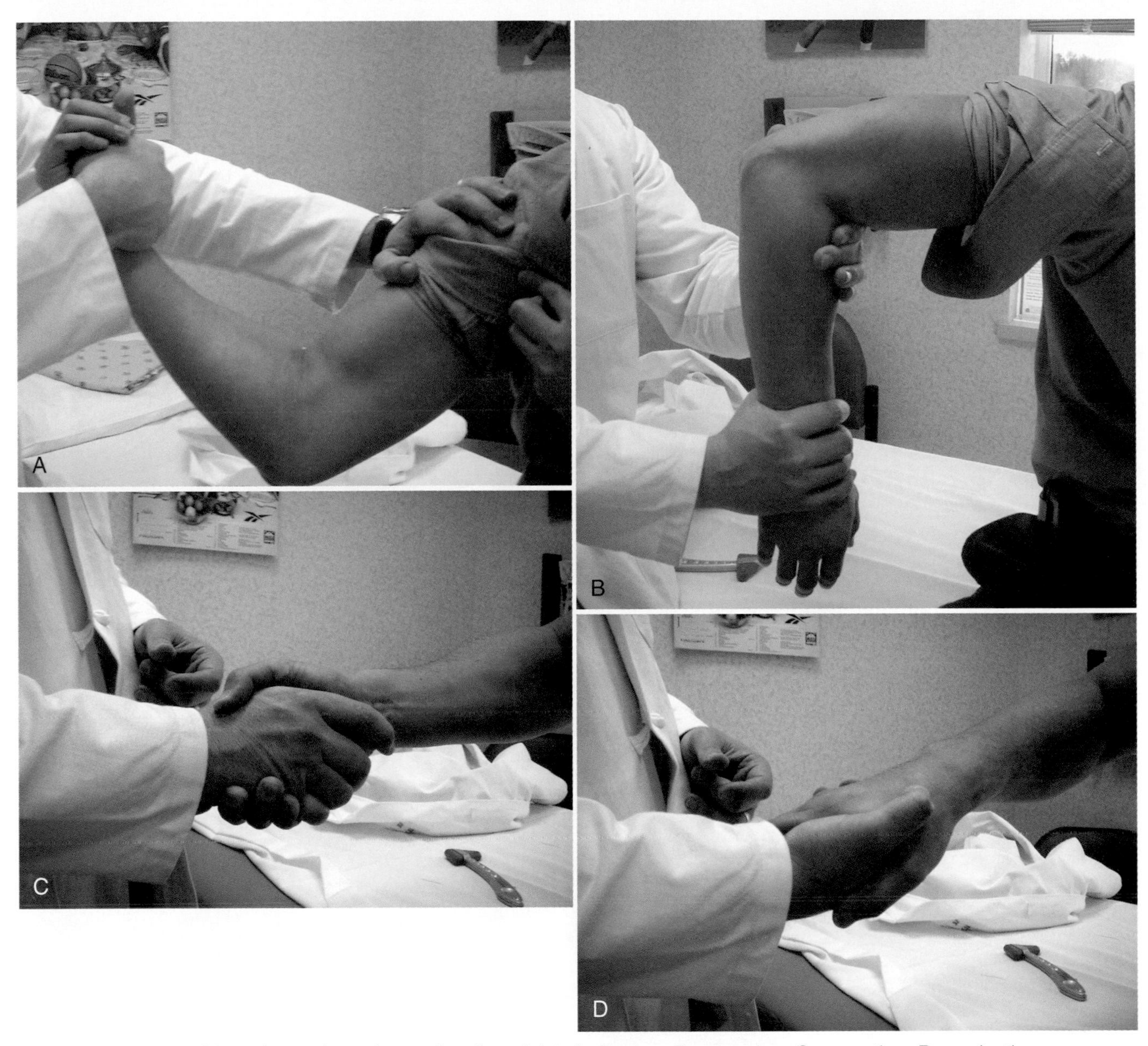

Figure 56-5 Manual muscle testing at the elbow joint. **A**, Flexion; **B**, extension; **C**, pronation; **D**, supination.

    - It is often the most helpful when combined with arthrography.
    - Other uses include evaluation of tumors, osteochondral lesions, and suspected biceps or triceps tendon ruptures.
- Computed tomography
    - Most helpful when evaluating bony problems such as complex intra-articular fractures
    - It can aid the surgeon in planning the approach and reduction of the fracture fragments.
    - It can also be useful in characterizing bony tumors seen on plain radiographs.
- Electromyography is a helpful adjunct when a patient is suspected of having a neurologic process. It can be combined with other imaging studies to localize and identify the source of the compression or injury.

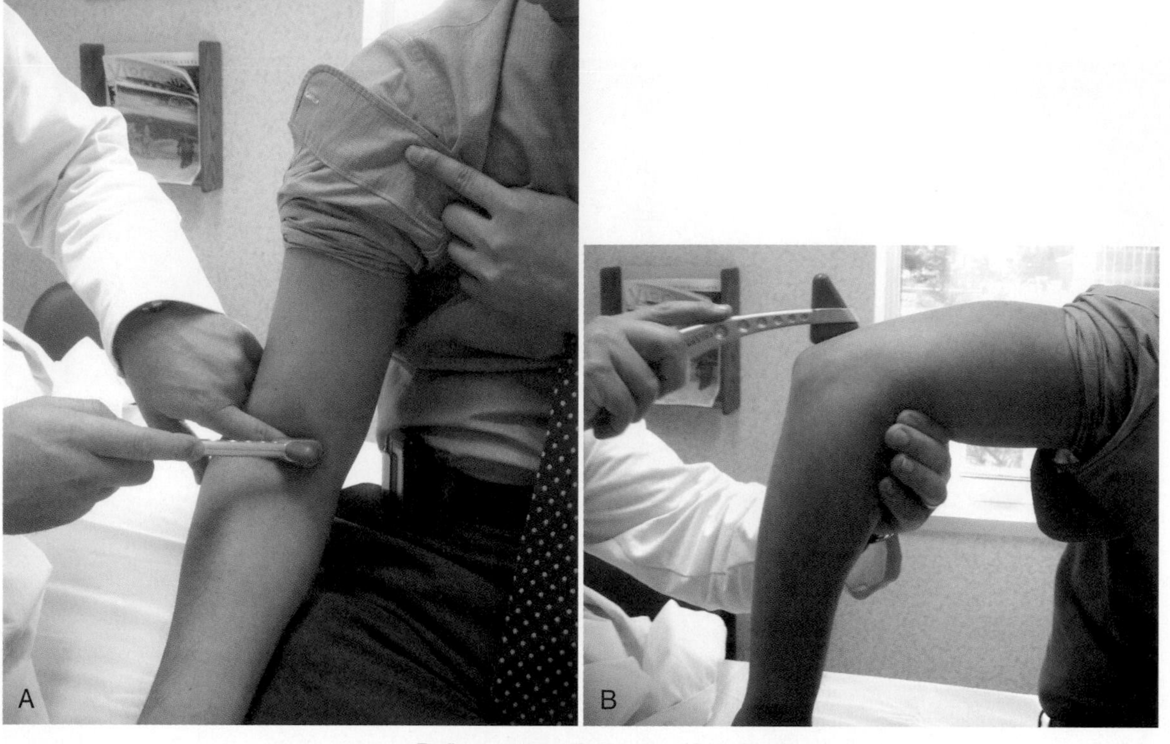

Figure 56-6 Reflex testing. **A**, Biceps (C5); **B**, triceps (C7).

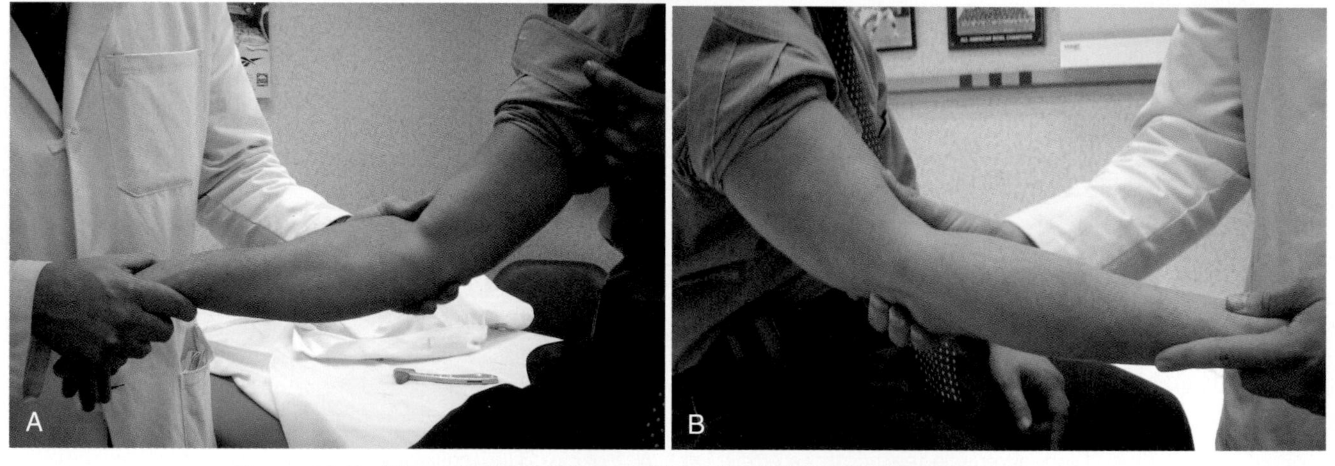

Figure 56-7 Stress testing for ligament integrity at the elbow. **A**, Valgus; **B**, varus.

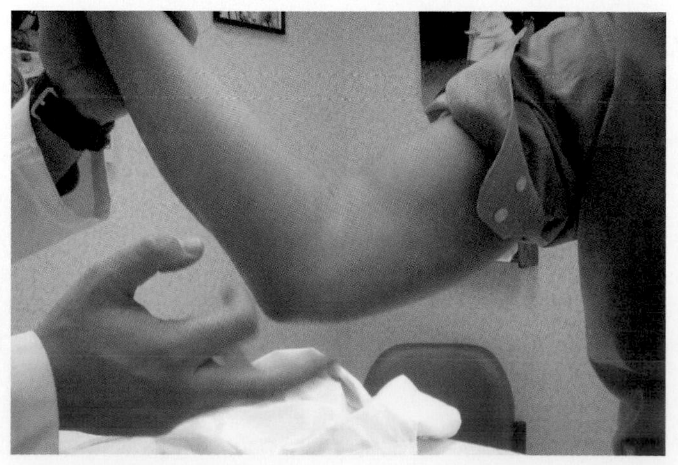

Figure 56-8 Tinel's sign for cubital tunnel syndrome (ulnar nerve entrapment).

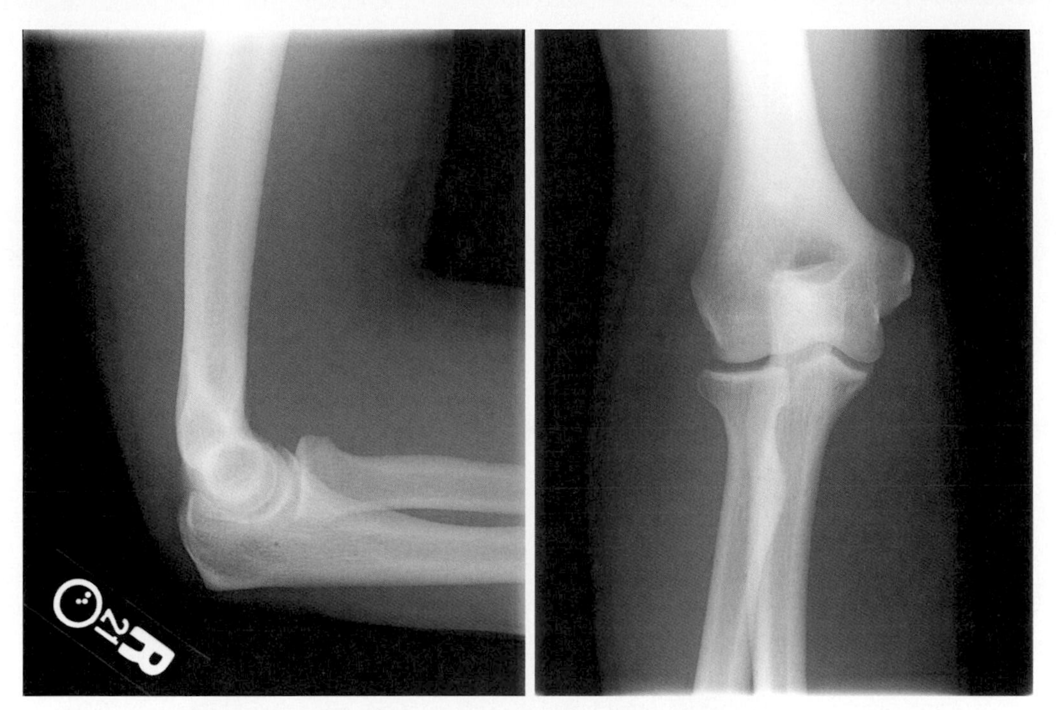

Figure 56-9 Standard radiographs of the elbow joint. **A**, Anteroposterior; **B**, lateral.

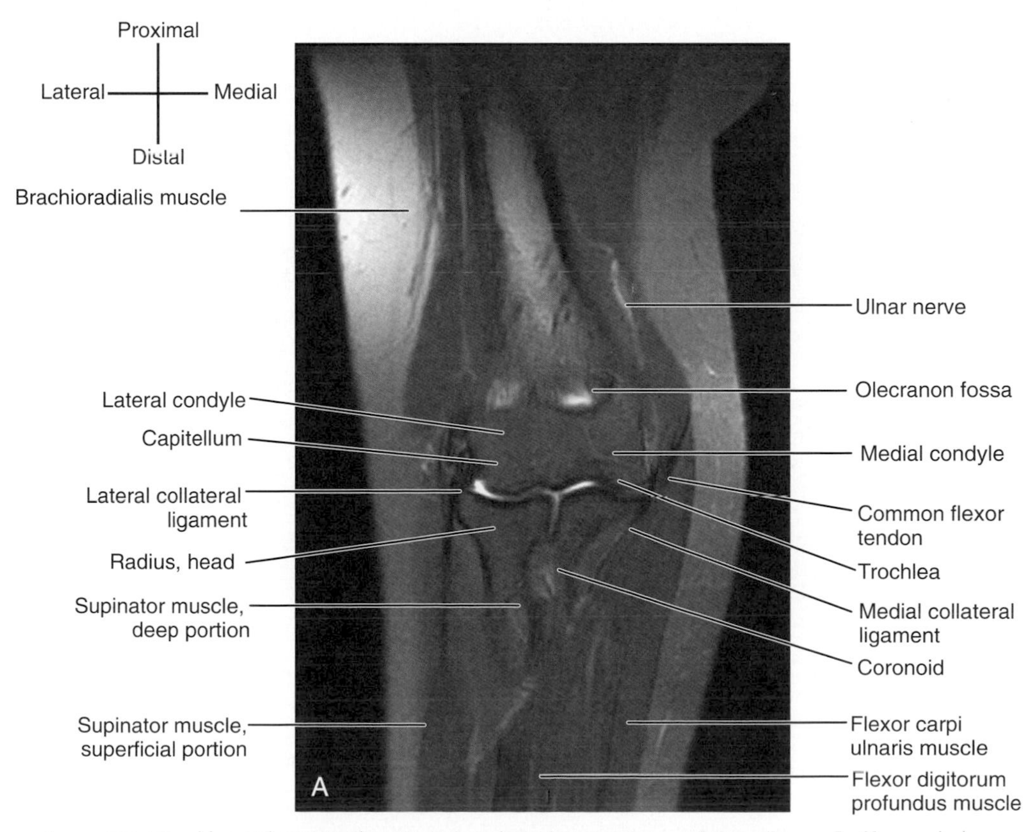

Figure 56-10 Normal magnetic resonance imaging anatomy of the elbow. **A**, Coronal view.

Continued

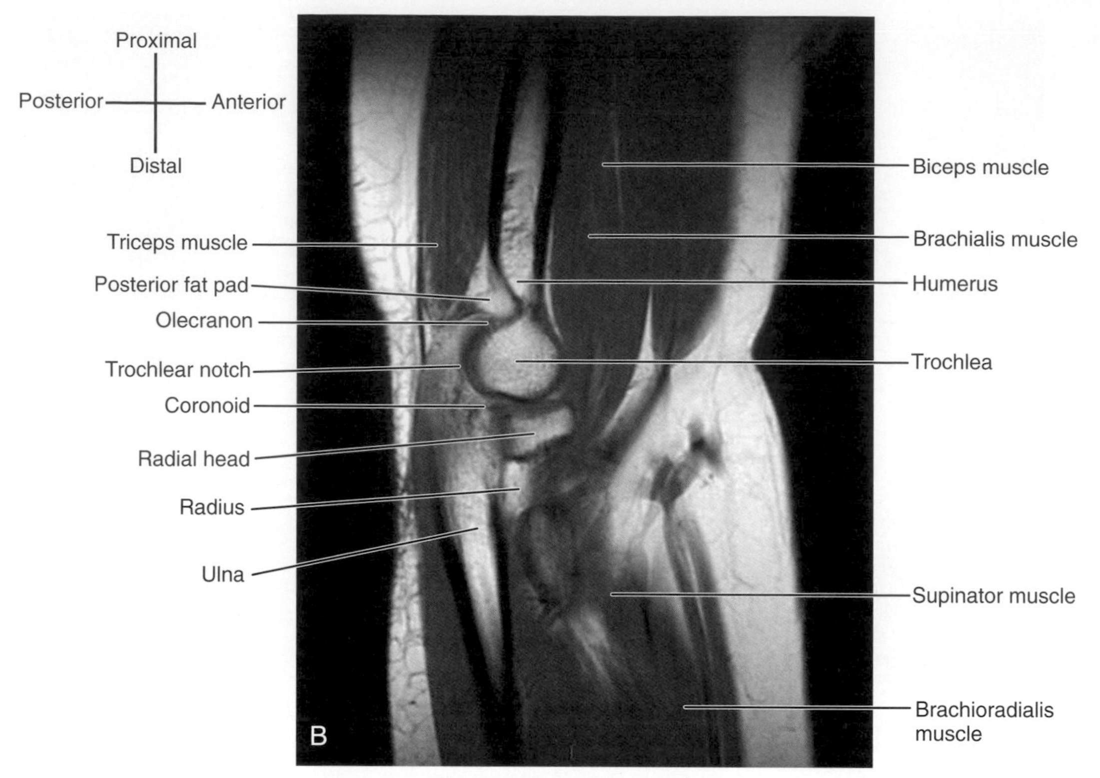

Figure 56-10, cont'd **B**, sagittal view.

Suggested Reading

- Alcid JG, Ahmad CS, Lee TQ: Elbow anatomy and structural biomechanics. Clin Sports Med 2004;23:503–517.
- Behr CT, Altchek DW: The elbow. Clin Sports Med 1997;16:681–704.
- Cain EL, Dugas JR: History and examination of the thrower's elbow. Clin Sports Med 2004;23:553–566.
- Chung CB, Chew FS, Steinbach L: MR imaging of tendon abnormalities of the elbow. Magn Reson Imaging Clin N Am 2004;12:233–245.
- Colman WW, Strauch RJ: Physical examination of the elbow. Orthop Clin North Am 1999;31:15–20.
- Fowler KAB, Chung CB: Normal MR imaging anatomy of the elbow. Radiol Clin North Am 2006;44:553–567.
- Frick MA: Imaging of the elbow: A review of imaging findings in acute and chronic traumatic disorders of the elbow. J Hand Ther 2006;19:98–113.
- Fritz FC, Breidahl WH: Radiographic and special studies: Recent advances in imaging of the elbow. Clin Sports Med 2004;23:567–580.
- Hoppenfeld S: Physical Examination of the Spine and Extremities. Norwalk, CT: Appleton & Lange, 1976.
- Miyasaka KC: Anatomy of the elbow. Orthop Clin North Am 1999;30:1–13.

Chapter 57 Chondral Injuries

Cay Mierisch

IDC-9 CODE

718.02 *Articular Cartilage Disorders Involving the Upper Arm*

Key Concepts

- Chondral lesions of the elbow may present as acute or repetitive injuries.
- Osteochondritis dissecans is a condition that may develop spontaneously or more commonly in juvenile athletes (little leaguer's elbow).
- The pathology consists of localized avascular necrosis with subsequent loss of structural support for the adjacent cartilage.
- The cause is thought to be valgus overload of the radiocapitellar joint.
- This condition is commonly found in young throwing athletes (little leaguers) and gymnasts.
- Lateral elbow joint pathology may be caused by or associated with medial collateral ligament instability.
- The typical radiologic finding is a posteromedial osteophyte of the olecranon process.
- This condition commonly leads to the development of loose bodies.
- Osteochondrosis of the capitellum (Panner's disease) is a related condition in children younger than the age of 10 years.

History

- Patients may present after acute injury.
  - Preceding injuries include elbow dislocation and periarticular fractures.
  - The mechanism most commonly reported is a fall onto the outstretched supinated hand.
- Chronic injuries leading to intra-articular pathology are commonly related to repetitive valgus stress, as seen in throwers and gymnasts.
- Patients typically report elbow pain with activity, decreased performance (throwing speed), stiffness, and swelling.
- Osteophytes and loose bodies may lead to mechanical symptoms with elbow range of motion such as locking and catching of the elbow.

Physical Examination

- Most commonly, the elbow will have lateral tenderness with crepitus over the radiocapitellar joint.
- Loss of extension with a 15- to 20-degree flexion contracture may be one of the earliest findings.
- Swelling is commonly present.

Imaging

- Plain radiographs including anteroposterior, lateral, and oblique views of the elbow may show fragmented subchondral bone, subchondral lucencies, and irregular ossification.
  - Osteophytes and loose bodies may be appreciated at later stages of the disease.
- Magnetic resonance imaging of the elbow can be helpful to detect loose bodies not visible on plain radiogaphs, avascular necrosis, and associated ligament damage.
- Elbow arthroscopy allows direct visualization and grading of osteochondritis dissecans and at the same time allows treatment of certain conditions (Table 57-1).

Differential Diagnosis

- Lateral epicondylitis: lateral tenderness and pain with passive stretch of the common extensor mechanism (see Chapter 59)
- Panner's disease: younger patients with avascular necrosis of the capitellum (see Chapter 224)
- Plica: mechanical symptoms, often a palpable catch, most commonly lateral (see Chapter 56)
- Posterolateral rotatory instability pain with pushing up from a chair (see Chapter 63)
- Synovial osteochondromatosis: multiple loose bodies without evidence of chondral injury (see Chapter 18)

Treatment

- Nonoperative treatment should be attempted for grade I and II lesions with no detachment or loose bodies.
- Treatment consists of 4 weeks of complete activity restriction, with physical therapy for strengthening and

TABLE 57-1 *Grading of Osteochondrosis Lesions*

Grade	Description	Treatment
I	Softening of cartilage	Drilling
II	Fibrillation and fissures	Drilling, removal of frayed portions to stable rim
III	Stable osteochondral fragment	Drilling and removal or fixation for larger fragments
IV	Loose but nondisplaced	Drilling or fixation of large fragments
V	Loose body	Drilling or mosaicplasty for large engaging defects

range of motion, followed by a progressive throwing program.
  - Preinjury performance levels can be reached within 3 to 4 months.
- Operative treatment is indicated after failure of conservative treatment for grade I and II lesions.
  - Operative treatment is also indicated for any patient with higher-grade osteochondritis dissecans with evidence of unstable fragments or loose bodies and progressive or fixed joint contracture.
  - Surgical treatment options include elbow arthroscopy with removal of loose bodies and contracture release, drilling of the lesions, fixation of larger fragments, and mosaicplasty for larger defects.
- The prognosis varies with the grade of disease.
- Overall surgical treatment can improve elbow range of motion and eliminate mechanical symptoms.
- The best results are accomplished after removal of isolated loose bodies with minimal morbidity and early return to full function.
- Patients should be referred for surgical treatment in the presence of mechanical symptoms or failure to progress with conservative treatment.

Troubleshooting

- Little league pitchers with chondral injury secondary to valgus overload from repetitive throwing motions are a particularly challenging group of patients to treat.
- The majority of symptomatic elbows can be treated with activity modification and periods of rest followed by gradual return to throwing.
- Unfortunately, patients and their ambitious parents are often too impatient to comply with the suggested treatment course; close supervision and reinforcement of the treatment plan may be necessary.

Suggested Reading

- Byrd JW, Jones KS: Arthroscopic surgery for isolated capitellar osteochondritis dissecans in adolescent baseball players: Minimum three-year follow-up. Am J Sports Med 2002; 30:474–478.
- DaSilva MF, Williams JS, Fadale PD, et al: Pediatric throwing injuries about the elbow. Am J Orthop 1998;27:90–96.
- Peterson RK, Savoie FH III, Field LD: Osteochondritis dissecans of the elbow. Instr Course Lect 1999;48:393–398.
- Pill SG, Ganley TJ, Flynn JM, Gregg JR: Osteochondritis dissecans of the capitellum: Arthroscopic-assisted treatment of large, full-thickness defects in young patients. Arthroscopy 2003;19:222–225.
- Takahara M, Ogino T, Sasaki I, et al: Long term outcome of osteochondritis dissecans of the humeral capitellum. Clin Orthop Relat Res 1999;363:108–115.
- Woods GW, Tullos HS, King JW: The throwing arm: Elbow joint injuries. J Sports Med 1973;1:43–47.

Chapter 58 Osteoarthritis of the Elbow

Cay Mierisch

ICD-9 CODE
715.12 *Osteoarthrosis, Localized, Primary, Upper Arm*

Key Concepts

- The elbow positions the hand in space and stabilizes the limb for prehensile activities.
- Only 1% to 2% of patients with osteoarthritis will present with elbow involvement.
- More common in male laborers
- Progressive loss of range of motion and pain
- Mechanical symptoms due to loose bodies
- Increasing functional difficulties with use of hand for activities of daily living

History

- Patients present with increasing pain and stiffness.
- Mechanical blocks to motion, clicking, and catching
- Pain with terminal extension
- Decreased range of motion often present early during the disease

Physical Examination

- Inspection
  - Swelling, deformity
  - Palpation of soft spot may allow detection of effusion.
  - Occasionally loose bodies are palpable.
- Range of motion
  - Flexion, extension, forearm rotation
  - Loss of terminal extension early in disease
  - Range of motion of 30 to 130 degrees necessary for activities of daily living
- Check for ulnar neuropathy with elbow flexion test and Tinel's sign over the cubital tunnel.

Imaging

- Plain radiographs should include anteroposterior (in extension), lateral (in 90 degrees of elbow flexion), and oblique views (Fig. 58-1).
- Findings associated with elbow osteoarthritis include
  - Posterior olecranon osteophyte
  - Radiocapitellar joint narrowing
  - Osteophytes and loose bodies
- Computed tomography with three-dimensional reconstruction
  - Road map for preoperative planning
- Magnetic resonance imaging
  - If underlying instability is suspected
  - Assessment of ligamentous integrity

Treatment

- Nonoperative
  - Activity modification
  - Nonsteroidal anti-inflammatory drugs
  - Splinting
  - Ice/heat
  - Physical therapy
  - Intra-articular injections
- Operative
  - Removal of loose bodies
  - Ulnohumeral débridement, open or arthroscopic: This procedure can improve pain and range of motion and typically allows return to heavy manual labor.
- Preexisting ulnar nerve symptoms should be addressed by concurrent ulnar nerve release/transposition.
  - Ulnar nerve symptoms are the most common but transient complication of surgical treatment
  - Total elbow arthroplasty for older low-demand patients (Fig. 58-2)
  - Will require lifetime lifting restriction
  - Usually contraindicated in the osteoarthritic population

When to Refer

- Failure of nonoperative treatment
- Elbow stiffness interfering with activities of daily living (flexion < 130 degrees); limited extension better tolerated
- Mechanical symptoms due to loose bodies

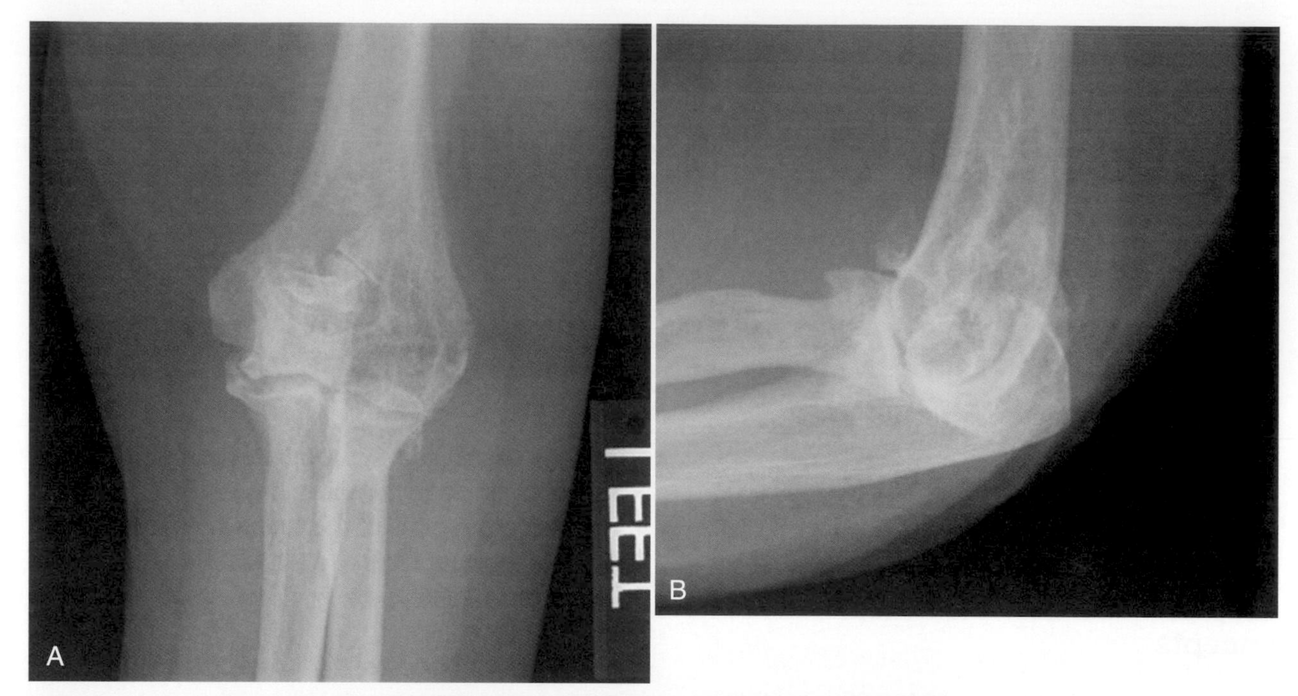

Figure 58-1 Anteroposterior (**A**) and lateral (**B**) radiographs of elbow arthritis.

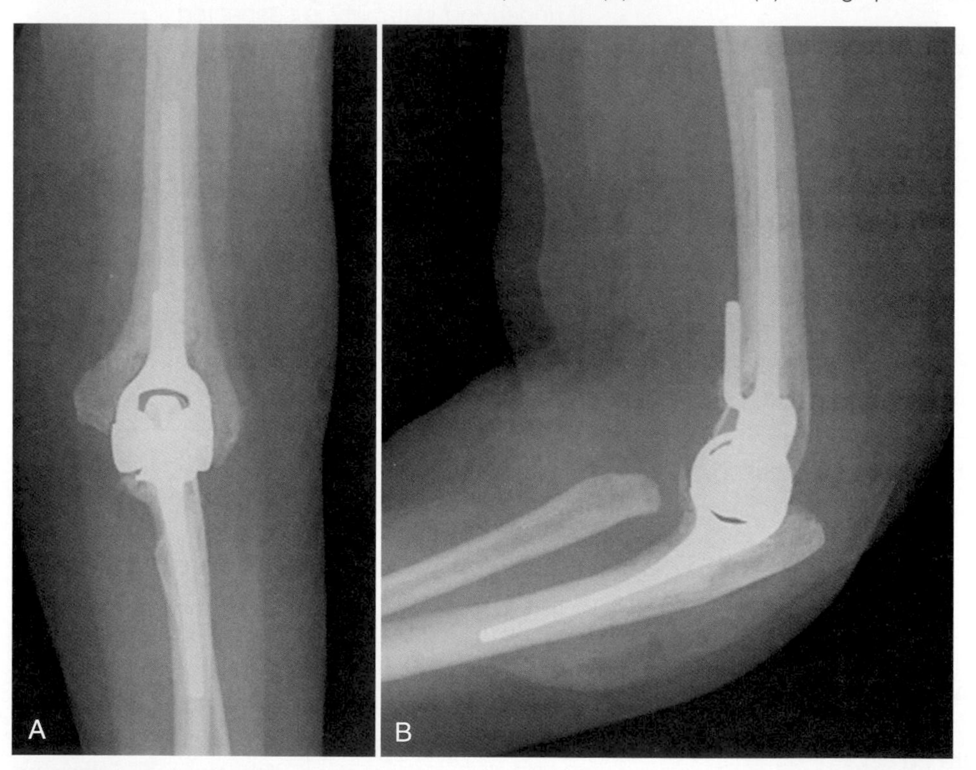

Figure 58-2 Anteroposterior (**A**) and lateral (**B**) radiographs of a total elbow arthroplasty.

Suggested Reading

- Adams JE, Wolff LH 3rd, Merten SM, Steinmann SP: Osteoarthritis of the elbow: Results of arthroscopic osteophyte resection and capsulectomy. J Shoulder Elbow Surg 2008; 17:126–131.
- Cheung EV, Adams R, Morrey BF: Primary osteoarthritis of the elbow: Current treatment options. J Am Acad Orthop Surg 2008;16:77–87.
- Cohen AP, Redden JF, Stanley D: Treatment of osteoarthritis of the elbow: A comparison of open and arthroscopic debridement. Arthroscopy 2000;16:701–706.
- Gramstad GD, Galatz LM: Management of elbow osteoarthritis. J Bone Joint Surg Am 2006;88A:421–430.
- McAuliffe JA: Surgical alternatives for elbow arthritis in the young adult. Hand Clin 2002;18:99–111.
- Morrey BF: Primary degenerative arthritis of the elbow: Treatment by ulnohumeral arthroplasty. J Bone Joint Surg Br 1992;74B: 409–413.
- Rettig LA, Hastings H 2nd, Feinberg JR: Primary osteoarthritis of the elbow: Lack of radiographic evidence for morphologic predisposition, results of operative debridement at intermediate follow-up, and basis for a new radiographic classification system. J Shoulder Elbow Surg 2008;17:97–105.
- Steinmann SP, King GJ, Savoie FH III: Arthroscopic treatment of the arthritic elbow. J Bone Joint Surg Am 2005;87A:2114–2121.

Chapter 59 Tennis Elbow (Lateral Epicondylitis)

Cay Mierisch

ICD-9 CODE
726.32 *Lateral Epicondylitis*

Key Concepts

- Lateral epicondylitis, often referred to as tennis elbow, is a tendonosis of the common extensor origin (extensor carpi radialis brevis tendon), also termed angiofibroblastic tendonosis because of its histologic appearance.
- It often is associated with tendonosis at other sites.
- It commonly coexists with nerve compression neuropathy, most commonly carpal tunnel syndrome.
- The male-to-female ratio is approximately equal.
- It typically presents as an overuse condition related to activities increasing tension in finger and wrist extensors.

History

- Patients report pain at the lateral elbow with repetitive activities requiring wrist and finger extension such as
  - Tennis
  - Repetitive lifting and gripping
  - Hammering
- The peak incidence occurs between ages 35 and 50.

Physical Examination

- Tenderness over the extensor carpi radialis brevis tendon just distal to lateral epicondyle
- Pain with resisted wrist extension/finger extension
- Pain with passive stretch of the common extensor origin (elbow extension and wrist flexion)
- Decreased grip strength
- Examine for carpal tunnel symptoms

Imaging

- Anteroposterior and lateral plain radiographs of the elbow
  - May show calcification in extensor origin
  - Will help to rule out other conditions with intra-articular pathology (arthritic conditions)
- Magnetic resonance imaging
  - Helpful to rule out associated ligamentous injury

Differential Diagnosis

- Other elbow tendonosis
  - Biceps: tenderness directly over the biceps tendon anteriorly
  - Triceps: tenderness directly over the triceps tendon posteriorly
  - Radial tunnel syndrome: numbness/tingling over radial nerve distribution (posterior forearm, dorsal hand)
- Carpal tunnel syndrome: numbness/tingling over median nerve distribution (thumb, index finger, and middle finger)
- Posterolateral rotatory elbow instability: instability with stress testing
- Intra-articular pathology
  - Arthritis: crepitus, loss of motion, radiographic changes
  - Plica: mechanical symptoms
  - Loose bodies: mechanical symptoms, may be apparent on radiographs

Treatment

- The majority of patients can be treated successfully without surgery.
- Nonoperative treatment
  - Nonsteroidal anti-inflammatory drugs
  - Activity modification
  - Counterforce bracing
  - Wrist splint (resting of wrist extensors)
  - Physical therapy (stretching, strengthening)
  - Injection with synthetic corticosteroids
- Operative treatment is recommended after failed non-operative treatment (persistent symptoms for 3 to 6 months).

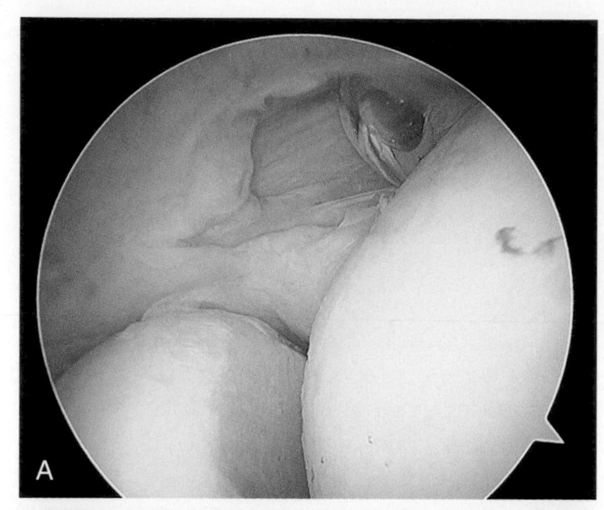

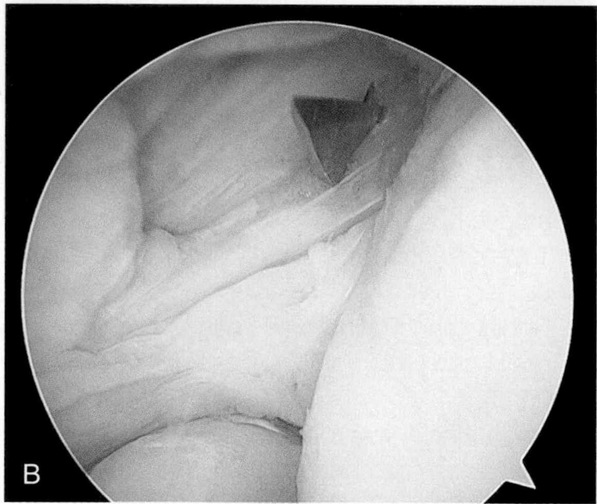

Figure 59-1 Arthroscopic appearance of lateral epicondylitis (**A**) and tennis elbow release (**B**).

- Surgical treatment consists of débridement of the common extensor origin.
- Arthroscopic and open procedures have successfully been used and have the advantage of detecting associated intra-articular comorbidities and may allow for a quicker recovery time (Fig. 59-1).
  - Patients should be referred to a specialist for consideration of surgical treatment after failure of nonoperative treatment modalities for a minimum of 3 to 6 months.

Prognosis

- Success of nonoperative treatment can be expected in as many as 90% of patients within 3 to 6 months.
- Surgical treatment results in decreased symptoms in 85% to 97% of patients; however, only 40% will be completely pain free without functional deficits.

Patient Instructions

- Patients should be instructed in activity modification and modalities, including icing, stretching, and the use of nonsteroidal anti-inflammatory drugs.

Suggested Reading

- Calfee RP, Patel A, DaSilva MF, Akelman E: Management of lateral epicondylitis: Current concepts. J Am Acad Orthop Surg 2008;16:19–29.
- Kraushaar BS, Nirschl RP: Tendinosis of the elbow (tennis elbow): Clinical features and findings of histological, immunohistochemical, and electron microscopy studies. J Bone Joint Surg Am 1999;81A:259–278.
- Nirschl RP, Ashman ES: Elbow tendinopathy: Tennis elbow. Clin Sports Med 2003;22:813–836.
- Smidt N, van der Windt DA, Assendelft WJ, et al: Corticosteroid injections, physiotherapy, or a wait-and-see policy for lateral epicondylitis: A randomised controlled trial. Lancet 2002;359:657–662.
- Szabo SJ, Savoie FH III, Field LD, et al: Tendinosis of the extensor carpi radialis brevis: An evaluation of three methods of operative treatment. J Shoulder Elbow Surg 2006;15:721–727.

Chapter 60 Golfer's Elbow (Medial Epicondylitis)

Cay Mierisch

ICD-9 CODE
726.32 *Medial Epicondylitis*

Key Concepts

- Medial epicondylitis is the most common cause of medial elbow pain.
- It is five to seven times less frequent than lateral epicondylitis.
- The pronator and flexor carpi radialis muscle origins are the most commonly involved structures originating from the medial epicondyle.
- It may be associated with ulnar neuropathy in as many as 50% of cases.
- The most common cause is occupational. A less common cause is recreational repetitive overuse leading to a degenerative tear at the flexor pronator muscle origin.
- Although medial epicondylitis is referred to as golfer's elbow, only 10% to 20% of cases are due to recreational activities.
- Acute injury may be found as the inciting event in as many as one third of patients.

History

- Patients may present with either insidious or more acute onset of medial elbow pain.
- Symptoms are activity related.
- Activities requiring repetitive wrist flexion and forearm pronation, as in golfing and throwing activities, are often associated.
- Patients may present with numbness or paresthesias in ulnar nerve distribution (small and ring fingers).
- A male predominance of 2 : 1 is reported.

Physical Examination

- Tenderness to palpation at the medial epicondyle and distally over the flexor-pronator origin
- Increased pain with resisted wrist flexion and forearm pronation
- Tinel's sign over the cubital tunnel and ulnar motor and sensory findings; elbow flexion test may be positive
- Check for associated medial elbow instability, particularly in younger throwing athletes.

Imaging

- Radiographs
  - Plain radiographs of the elbow may reveal calcification distal to the medial epicondyle.
  - Rule out arthritis or acute osseous injury of the elbow.
- Magnetic resonance imaging
  - May show degenerative changes in the flexor pronator mass
  - Assess integrity of the medial collateral ligament
  - Rule out other soft-tissue pathology

Differential Diagnosis

- Cubital tunnel syndrome: positive Tinel's sign, positive elbow flexion test
- Ulnar nerve subluxation: paresthesias and palpable anterior subluxation of the ulnar nerve (see Chapter 65)
- Snapping medial head of the triceps: mechanical snapping palpable with elbow range of motion; pain more posterior (see Chapter 56)
- Medial collateral ligament insufficiency: elbow instability, often associated with concurrent medial epicondylitis (see Chapter 62)
- Elbow arthritis: radiographic changes (see Chapter 58)
- Radiculopathy: associated with neck pain and dermatomal pain distribution (see Chapter 114)
- Medial antebrachial cutaneous nerve neuroma: positive Tinel's sign; more superficial tenderness with radiation into the ulnar aspect of the forearm (see Chapter 65)

Treatment

- Nonoperative treatment: The majority of patients with medial epicondylitis can be managed successfully nonoperatively.
  - Activity modification
  - Nonsteroidal anti-inflammatory drugs
  - Icing
  - Physical therapy
  - Corticosteroid injection for persistent symptoms
  - Flexor pronator muscle stretching and strengthening exercises after resolution of symptoms
  - Consider use of wrist splint
  - Gradual return to previous activity
- Operative treatment
  - Surgery is indicated for patients in whom nonoperative treatment fails.
  - Release of the flexor pronator origin with débridement and subsequent repair is the treatment of choice.
  - The presence of ulnar nerve symptoms is addressed by concurrent cubital tunnel release with or without ulnar nerve transposition.
  - Surgical treatment is followed by a short period of immobilization followed by early range of motion therapy and return to resisted activities within 4 to 6 weeks after surgery.

Prognosis

- Nonoperative treatment is successful in 90% to 95% of patients within 3 to 6 months.
- Good to excellent results can be expected in as many as 95% of patients after surgical release if no or only mild ulnar nerve neuropathy is present.
- Results deteriorate with severity of ulnar neuropathy.

Patient Instructions

- Patients should avoid the offending activity.
- Patients should be educated about the nonoperative treatment options, including stretching and strengthening exercises.

When to Refer

- Patients who fail to respond to nonoperative treatment within 3 to 6 months should be considered for surgical treatment and referred to an orthopaedic surgeon.

Troubleshooting

- Patients may present with subtle medial elbow instability that may be difficult to distinguish clinically from medial epicondylitis; these patients are often younger athletes, especially throwers. Magnetic resonance imaging may help to distinguish these two entities.

Suggested Reading

- Badia A, Stennett C: Sports-related injuries of the elbow. J Hand Ther 2006;19:206–226.
- Ciccotti MG: Epicondylitis in the athlete. Instr Course Lect 1999; 48:375–381.
- Eygendaal D, Safran MR: Postero-medial elbow problems in the adult athlete. Br J Sports Med 2006;40:430–434.
- Field LD, Savoie FH: Common elbow injuries in sport. Sports Med 1998;26:193–205.
- Hume PA, Reid D, Edwards T: Epicondylar injury in sport: Epidemiology, type, mechanisms, assessment, management and prevention. Sports Med 2006;36:151–170.

Chapter 61 Distal Biceps Tendon Rupture

S. Raymond Golish and César J. Bravo

ICD-9 CODES
727.69 *Nontraumatic Rupture of Other Tendon*
841.9 *Elbow Sprain*
729.5 *Elbow Pain*

Key Concepts

- Rupture of the distal biceps tendon is commonly seen in the dominant extremity of men between 40 and 60 years of age when an unexpected extension force is applied to the flexed arm.
- The rupture typically occurs at the tendon insertion into the radial tuberosity in an area of preexisting tendon degeneration; however, injury at the musculotendinous junction is reported.
- Physical examination demonstrates a palpable and visible deformity of the distal biceps muscle belly with weakness in flexion and supination.
- Risk factors include the dominant extremity, male gender, middle age, vocational activities involving high load or repetitive supination and flexion (e.g., plumber, laborer), sports (e.g., bodybuilder), and medical comorbidity (e.g., anabolic steroid use).
- Patients may experience an acute episode with an unexpected or eccentric load followed by a pop or tearing sensation in the antecubital fossa.
- The biceps brachii muscle is a supinator of the forearm and flexor of the elbow. Physical examination of the injured patient may reveal a palpable and visible deformity, weakness on supination greater than flexion, and positive provocative maneuvers.
- The distal tendon of the biceps brachii muscle crosses the antecubital fossa to insert on the radial tuberosity. The footprint and geometry of the insertion are variable.
- The tendon is proximate to numerous anatomic entities and critical structures as it crosses the fossa, including the lacertus fibrosus, the radial nerve and branches, the brachial artery and branches, and venous structures (Fig. 61-1).
- Early surgical reattachment to the radial tuberosity is recommended for optimal results, which means expedient orthopaedic referral.

History

- Patients present with a history of an acute event involving an extension/pronation load, perhaps sudden, followed by a painful pop or tearing sensation in the antecubital region.
- The ability to palpate the tendon in the antecubital fossa may indicate partial tearing of the biceps tendon.
- The event may be followed by pain, swelling, and ecchymoses; a visible deformity may be noticed as swelling subsides.
- After the acute inflammation subsides, patients may report weakness in vocational activities or sports but rarely in activities of daily living.
- Patients may report a history consistent with repetitive microtrauma from work or sporting activities before the acute event, although a history of activity-related pain is not expected.
- Activities predispose to rupture, including vocational activities involving high load or repetitive supination and flexion (e.g., plumber, laborer) and sports (e.g., bodybuilder).
- Medical comorbidity such as rheumatoid arthritis, renal failure, and anabolic steroid use may be a factor.
- In a patient with delayed (chronic) presentation, weakness is usually the main symptom rather than pain around the elbow/forearm (acute).
- Weakness may be insignificant for the sedentary or average patient engaged in activities of daily living and desk work. However, the patient at risk of the injury is often much more active at work or sports and therefore likely to be symptomatic in the same type of activities that precipitated the rupture. Cosmetic issues may precipitate presentation.

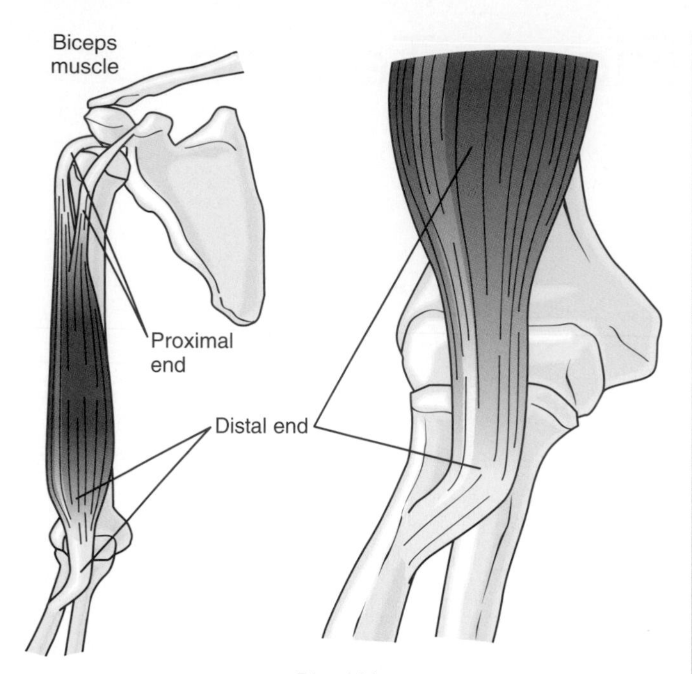

Figure 61-1 Distal biceps anatomy.

Physical Examination

- Patients present with variable swelling, ecchymoses, and tenderness to palpation in the antecubital fossa.
- Deformity presents as an accentuated upper arm anterior musculature in flexion ("Popeye" deformity).
- Comparing the contralateral side, weakness in supination much greater than in flexion is present. Specific provocative maneuvers increase the sensitivity and specificity of examination.
- The hook test involves hooking the examiner's index finger underneath the tendon from the lateral side with the elbow in 90 degrees of flexion and full supination. Sensitivity and specificity are reported to be 100% for a full tear, with superior ability to discriminate a partial from a full tear.
- The biceps squeeze test is an analog of the Thompson test for Achilles tendon rupture. The sensitivity and specificity are reported to be high, and patients who undergo successful repair exhibit return of a positive squeeze test.

Imaging

- Plain radiographs including anteroposterior, lateral, and oblique views rule out bony pathology and may show hypertrophic bone formation at the radial tuberosity.
- Magnetic resonance imaging (MRI) is the standard modality for evaluation of soft-tissue pathology in the antecubital fossa, including full and partial tears and degeneration.
- MRI technique is important, and positioning of the extremity in flexion of the elbow, abduction of the shoulder, and supination of the forearm can result in improved imaging.
- Ultrasonography is an alternative to MRI, which may be accurate and cost-effective relative to MRI.

Additional Tests

- A complete blood count and differential, erythrocyte sedimentation rate, and C-reactive protein level may be relevant for any periarticular complaint, especially in the presence of an atypical history or medical comorbidity.

Classification of Distal Biceps Tendon Ruptures

- Partial rupture
- Insertional
- Intrasubstance (elongation)
- Complete rupture
  - Acute (<4 weeks)
  - Chronic (>4 weeks) (with intact aponeurosis, tendon does not retract)
  - Intact aponeurosis (bicipital aponeurosis [lacertus fibrosus] arises from the medial aspect of the muscle belly at the junction of the musculotendinous unit and the distal biceps tendon. It passes distally and medially across the antecubital fossa, blending with the fascia overlying the proximal flexor mass of the forearm, and inserts on the subcutaneous border of the ulna)
  - Ruptured aponeurosis

Differential Diagnosis

- Please see Table 61-1.

Treatment

- At diagnosis
  - The classic technique for the repair of acute ruptures involves two incisions and a transosseous tunnel; this a modification of the Boyd-Anderson technique. Significant literature supports the two-incision technique, with or without a transosseous tunnel. Possible complications include proximal radioulnar synostosis.
  - The use of a single anterior incision and various fixation devices, including suture anchors, button fixation, interference screws, and endoscopic

TABLE 61-1 *Differential Diagnosis*

Pathology	Differentiating Examination/ Clinical Scenario
Cubital bursitis* (with and without bicipital tendinosis); biceps partial tear or degeneration	Examination, MRI
Ligament or tendon injury other than biceps (e.g., upper collateral ligament, lower collateral ligament)	Examination, MRI
Intra-articular injury (e.g., osteochondral fracture)	Examination, MRI
Bony fracture about the elbow	Radiographic analysis
Infectious or crystalline arthropathy	Lab work

*Cubital bursitis is enlargement of the bursal sac that lies between the biceps tendon and the anterior aspect of the radial tuberosity. This condition may exist in isolation or in association with a distal biceps tendon lesion. Tendon degeneration (bicipital tendinosis) without rupture may occur in isolation or in association with cubital bursitis or partial rupture.

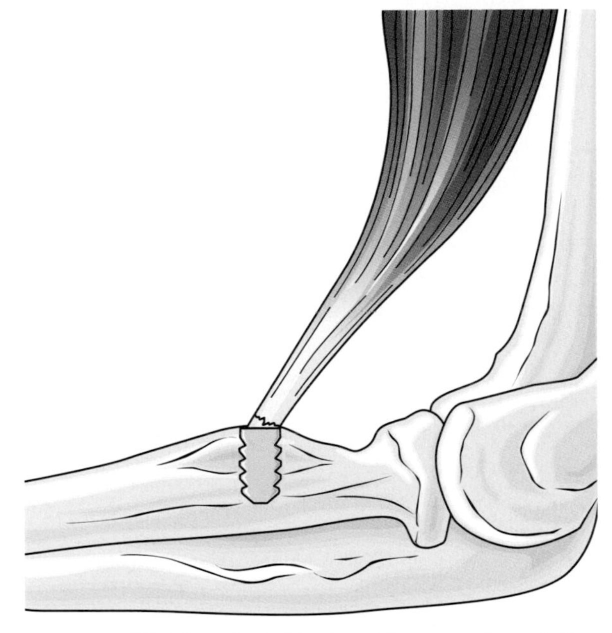

Figure 61-2 Bio-Tenodesis bioabsorble screw from Arthrex, Inc. This novel screw can be used in distal biceps repair. (Adapted from drawing courtesy of Arthrex, Inc., Naples, FL.)

methods, is favored by some surgeons (Fig. 61-2).
- Numerous biomechanical studies have been done comparing single-incision techniques with each other and with the two-incision technique. The available clinical evidence consists of retrospective series with variable follow-up.
- The inspiration behind single-incision techniques is the mitigation of complications associated with the two-incision technique and the possibility of more aggressive rehabilitation with early motion. However, all single-incision techniques have some rate of complications including posterior interosseous nerve palsy, lateral antebrachial nerve injury, and heterotopic ossification. Only a few studies have directly examined postoperative rehabilitation after device fixation through a single incision. The advantage is largely hypothetical.
- Current clinical results support suture anchors through a single incision as an alternative to the classic technique. The numerous biomechanical studies favor a button technique; however, buttons and interference screws are supported by clinical results as well.
- Partial tears represent a distinct clinical entity and may be managed conservatively or operatively.
- The patient with a chronic rupture may benefit from surgical reattachment, but proximal retraction and scarring of the muscle belly can make tendon mobilization difficult, and inadequate length of the distal biceps tendon may necessitate tendon augmentation.

- Later
  - Postoperative rehabilitation is variable, depending on the provider. Early functional range of motion is essential to avoid elbow stiffness, but range of motion and strength activities must be graduated to allow healing.
  - Rehabilitation protocol involving immediate hinged bracing starting with an extension block at 60 degrees is recommended by some. The extension block is advanced 20 degrees every 2 weeks to full extension at 6 weeks. Dynamic splinting with flexion assistance may also be used.
  - Despite variations in early management, most patients are not advanced to full strength activities until 5 to 6 months postoperatively.
  - Light strength rehabilitation may begin at 3 months.

When to Refer

- Consultation with an orthopaedist should be obtained urgently and within 2 weeks if suspicion is high.
- Typically, advanced imaging need not be obtained before referral if clinical suspicion is high. For experienced providers, the diagnosis is largely clinical and performing MRI may engender needless delay.
- If clinical suspicion is lower, an experienced nonoperative sports medicine or musculoskeletal provider may pursue further diagnosis or management. MRI may be performed to narrow the differential.

- Late presentation of chronic tears represents a difficult variant that requires operative management and frequent augmentation with tendon grafts.

Prognosis

- Excellent for acute ruptures repaired acutely

Troubleshooting

- See section on repair of distal biceps ruptures.

Patient Instructions

- At the time of an acute diagnosis, dorsal splinting with the elbow in 90 degrees of flexion and the forearm in neutral rotation is initiated.
- Parameters for emergent return should be given (e.g., pain out of proportion, pain to passive stretch, progressive tingling/numbness or weakness).
  - A referral for urgent orthopaedic follow-up should be given.
  - The necessity of urgent re-examination and possible urgent surgical care should be made clear because delayed presentation leads to more extensive surgery and poorer outcomes.
- Postoperatively, the importance of adherence to the postoperative protocol must be made clear or an increased risk of reinjury and revision surgery will result.
- The postoperative protocol may seem complex to the patient, and the protocol should be provided in writing with appropriate time points for advancement of hinged bracing, extension blocks, weight-bearing status, formal occupational therapy, strength training, and return to work or sport.

Suggested Reading

- Darlis NA, Sotereanos DG: Distal biceps tendon reconstruction in chronic ruptures. J Shoulder Elbow Surg 2006;15:614–619.
- Golish SR, Chhabra AB: Update on rupture of the distal tendon of the biceps brachii. In Green DP, Hotchkiss RN, Pederson WC, Wolfe SW (eds): Green's Operative Hand Surgery, 5th ed. Philadelphia: Churchill Livingstone, 2005, pp 1774–1776.
- John CK, Field LD, Weiss KS, Savoie FH 3rd: Single-incision repair of acute distal biceps ruptures by use of suture anchors. J Shoulder Elbow Surg 2007;16:78–83.
- Mazzocca AD, Burton KJ, Romeo AA, et al: Biomechanical evaluation of 4 techniques of distal biceps brachii tendon repair. Am J Sports Med 2007;35:252–258.
- Mazzocca AD, Spang JT, Arciero RA: Distal biceps rupture. Orthop Clin North Am 2008;39:237–249.
- Morrey BF, Askew LJ, An KN, Dobyns JH: Rupture of the distal tendon of the biceps brachii. A biomechanical study. J Bone Joint Surg Am 1985;67A:418–421.
- O'Driscoll SW, Goncalves LB, Dietz P: The hook test for distal biceps tendon avulsion. Am J Sports Med 2007;35: 1865–1869.
- Ramsey ML: Distal biceps tendon injuries: Diagnosis and management. J Am Acad Orthop Surg 1999;7:199–207.
- Schamblin ML, Safran MR: Injury of the distal biceps at the musculotendinous junction. J Shoulder Elbow Surg 2007; 16:208–212.

Chapter 62 Elbow Ligament Injuries

César J. Bravo

ICD-9 CODES

841 *Sprains and Strains of Elbow and Forearm*
841.0 *Radial Collateral Ligament Sprain and Strain*
841.1 *Ulnar Collateral Ligament Sprain and Strain*
841.2 *Radiohumeral (Joint) Sprain and Strain*
841.3 *Ulnohumeral (Joint) Sprain and Strain*
841.8 *Sprain and Strain of Other Specified Sites of Elbow and Forearm*
841.9 *Sprain and Strain of Unspecified Site of Elbow and Forearm*
718.8 *Other Joint Derangement, Not Elsewhere Classified*
Instability of Joint
Flail Joint (Paralytic)

Key Concepts

- The elbow is a highly constrained joint whose intrinsic stability is provided by both osseous and capsuloligamentous structures.
- It is composed of dynamic and static stabilizers.
  - Dynamic stabilizers include muscles that produce compressive forces across the elbow joint such as the anconeus, brachialis, and triceps muscles.
  - Static stabilizers include the lateral collateral ligament complex (LCLC), medial collateral ligament (MCL), and ulnohumeral articulation. Secondary constraints include the radial head, common flexor and extensor origins, and elbow capsule.
    - — The ulnohumeral articulation is the cornerstone of osseous stability and mobility in the flexion-extension plane.
    - — The coronoid process resists posterior subluxation in flexion.
    - — The medial facet of the coronoid imparts osseous stability to varus stress.
    - — The radial head is a secondary stabilizer to valgus loads. If the coronoid is fractured or insufficient with a concomitant MCL injury, the radial head becomes a primary stabilizer to the valgus load.
    - — The elbow is stable if its three primary static constraints (stabilizers) are whole; once disrupted, instability can ensue.
- Ligamentous complex of the elbow (Fig. 62-1)
  - Ligamentous constraints of the elbow contribute significantly to the stability of the joint.
  - Collateral ligaments are anatomically contiguous with the joint capsule.
  - Medial and lateral collateral ligaments have distinct functions.
    - — The MCL is the primary stabilizer to valgus stress.
    - — The LCLC is an important restraint to posterolateral rotatory instability of the elbow and maintains the radiocapitellar joint in contact.
  - The MCL is composed of three major bundles (some authors refer to the MCL as the ulnar collateral ligament complex): anterior (primary restraint to valgus stress within extension arc of 30 to 120 degrees), posterior, and transverse.
    - — Originates posterior to the axis of rotation and inserts onto the medial aspect of the coronoid process
    - — Full resection of the MCL leads to 6 to 8 degrees of abduction laxity with full destabilization when radial head is removed.
    - — The MCL maintains contact of the articular surface of distal articular surface with the trochlear notch of the ulna.
    - — Because the origin of the MCL is posterior to the axis of rotation of the humerus, the tautness of the ligament changes with flexion and extension of the elbow.
  - LCLC
    - — The LCLC provides rotational and varus stability and is composed of three subunits: (1) the radial collateral ligament, which provides varus stability; (2) the annular ligament, which encircles the head of the radius, stabilizing it in the radial notch; and (3) the lateral ulnar collateral ligament, which assists the annular ligament

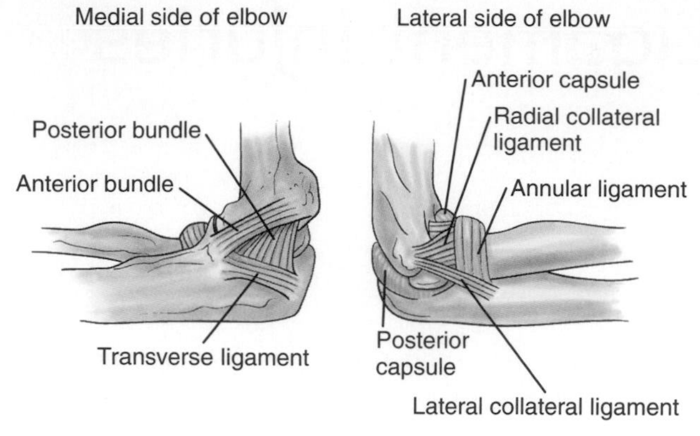

Figure 62-1 Ligaments of the elbow.

during varus stress and provides inferior rotatory stability for the humeroulnar joint.
- — Originates at the lateral humeral epicondyle and inserts into the supinator crest of the ulna
- — A cadaver study has shown that resection of both the radial collateral ligament and the lateral ulnar collateral ligament is necessary to create instability. Full instability is re-created when the extensor mass is also transected.
- — Simple dislocations can take place without injury to the anterior band of the MCL and attenuation of the LCLC (see Chapter 63).

- Two different forms of elbow instability exist with associated ligament injuries.
  - Simple instability
    - — Injury to the MCL or LCLC, specifically the lateral ulnar collateral ligament
  - Complex instability
    - — Involves both ligamentous and osseous injury
    - — Is the final common pathway of multiple distinct patterns of injury
      - — Radial head fracture and complex instability
      - — Coronoid fracture and complex instability
      - — Terrible triad injury: coronoid fracture, radial head fracture, and posterior ulnohumeral dislocation
      - — Monteggia's fracture dislocation
      - — Transolecranon fracture dislocation

History

- After documentation of handedness and the type of work performed, a history of elbow ligament injuries should include the following.
  - What is the character of the pain?
    - — Consider cervical spine or double crush neurologic injury with radiating pain.
    - — Pain in multiple joints might suggest joint disease (e.g., osteoarthritis, rheumatoid arthritis).
  - Where is the pain?
    - — Lateral elbow pain
      - — Lateral ulnar collateral ligament instability
      - — Lateral epicondylitis
      - — Radiocapitellar arthritis
      - — Radial tunnel syndrome
    - — Medial elbow pain
      - — MCL injury
      - — Flexor-pronator origin disruption
      - — Ulnar nerve compression/subluxation
      - — Snapping triceps tendon
    - — Posterior elbow pain
      - — Triceps tendinopathy
      - — Posterior impingement of olecranon spurs
    - — Anterior elbow pain
      - — Distal biceps pathology
      - — Anterior capsular strain
      - — Median nerve entrapment
      - — Primary osteoarthritis
  - Are there any exacerbating activities?
    - — Medial elbow pain during the late cocking or acceleration phase of throwing
    - — Valgus laxity may cause traction of the ulnar nerve.
  - What are the severity and duration of symptoms?
  - What is the mechanism of injury?
    - — Acute
    - — Chronic
  - Are there mechanical complaints?
    - — Loss of motion, locking, and catching
    - — Instability
- Patients with MCL deficiency usually present with increasing pain on the inside of their elbow after repetitive throwing; this is a condition typically of the overhead throwing athlete.
  - Chronic MCL insufficiency allows the medial olecranon to impinge on the olecranon fossa during terminal extension or the follow-through phase of throwing.
    - — Valgus extension overload syndrome is a spectrum of conditions occurring with progressing MCL deficiency.
      - — Posteromedial impingement of the elbow
      - — Ulnar neuropathy
      - — Increased radiocapitellar loading
      - — Radiocapitellar arthritis

- Twenty-five percent of patients also state that they have ulnar nerve sensitivity.
- Athletes with MCL injury will describe a sudden onset of symptoms including elbow pain, loss of velocity, and control.
  - Pain is greatest during the late cocking and early acceleration phase of the throwing cycle.
- Lateral ulnar collateral ligament instability is usually seen as the result of elbow dislocation or iatrogenic injury after lateral elbow surgery and can lead to posterolateral rotatory instability.
- Posterolateral rotatory instability of the elbow results from insufficiency of the lateral ligamentous and muscular support of the elbow.
  - Symptoms include locking, catching, and snapping when the elbow is extended with the forearm supinated.
  - An audible clunk can be reproduced when flexing the elbow from an extended position coupled with pronation as the joint relocates from a subluxed position.
- Posterolateral rotatory instability is not as common as medial elbow pain with laxity to valgus stress and not associated with a specific activity, such as overhead throwing.

Physical Examination (Box 62-1)

- Document motion of elbow, ligament laxity, or tenderness.
- The neck, shoulder, and wrist should be examined carefully in the patient with elbow pain.
- It is important to document the status of the ulnar nerve in patients with medial elbow pain.
- Patients with lateral collateral ligament injury usually have a variable history and some sort of injury to the elbow with or without dislocation.
- Simple abduction of the shoulder away from the body produces a varus moment to the joint.
  - Ulnar and radial ligamentous stabilities are assessed with the patient's forearm flexed at 30 degrees to unlock the olecranon from its fossa. The physician alternately applies valgus force and varus force to evaluate the area for medial or lateral laxity, pain, decreased mobility, and apprehension (i.e., sensation of impending dislocation).

Imaging

- Plain elbow radiographs
  - Valgus stress views
  - Varus stress views

BOX 62-1 *Physical Examination*

Medial Collateral Ligament Injury (Figs. 62-2 to 62-5)
Tender to palpation at the medial side of the elbow just dorsal to flexor pronator mass
Positive moving valgus stress test
Positive milking sign
Pain over radiocapitellar articulation
  Radiocapitellar arthropathy
  Capitellar osteochondral lesions
Ulnar nerve neuropathy
  Positive percussion test over the cubital tunnel
  Elbow flexion test
  Dysesthetic pain with ulnar nerve palpation
  Diminished two-point discrimination of the ring and small fingers
  Weak hand intrinsics

Lateral Collateral Ligament Complex Injury
Recurrent lateral elbow pain when elbow loaded in certain positions
  Rising from a chair
  Certain lifting activities with the involved extremity
Popping and clicking of elbow not uncommon
Patients may have a slight loss of extension
  Positive lateral pivot shift test (Fig. 62-6)
    Assesses laxity of the ulnar part of the lateral collateral ligament. This form of instability allows the humeroulnar joint to sublux, with secondary dislocation of the radiocapitellar joint. The test is performed with the patient supine. The arm to be tested is extended back over the patient's head, and the shoulder is rotated externally. While standing at the head of the table, the physician supinates the patient's forearm and simultaneously applies valgus stress, axial compression, and flexion of the elbow. Apprehension in the awake patient indicates a positive test. Displacement of the ulna from the trochlea, with radiocapitellar joint dislocation, is usually achieved only in a patient who has received general anesthesia.

- Magnetic resonance imaging of the elbow
  - Magnetic resonance imaging arthrography
    - Increases detection of partial MCL tears to 86% sensitivity
    - Better visualization of the undersurface of elbow ligaments
- Additional tests
  - Computed tomography arthrography
    - Eighty-six percent sensitive and 91% specific for complete MCL tears
  - Dynamic ultrasonography

Differential Diagnosis

- Please see Box 62-2.

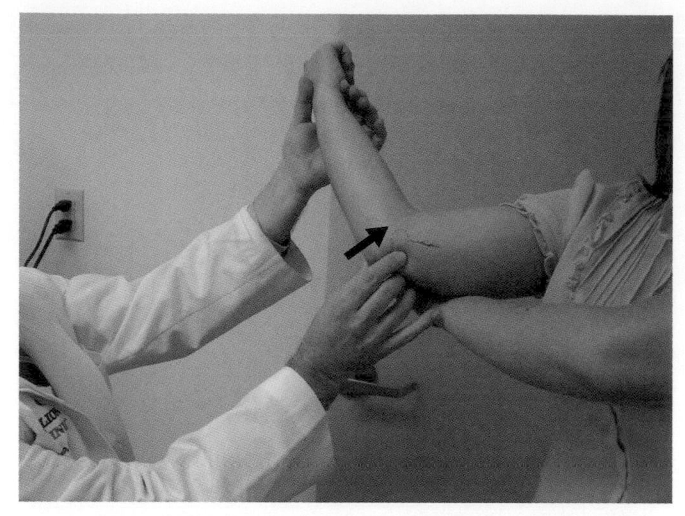

Figure 62-2 Palpation at the medial collateral ligament (MCL) with elbow flexed between 20 and 30 degrees. Tenderness with flexion may represent a tear of the MCL with or without rupture of the flexor-pronator mass (*arrow*). Tenderness over the sublime tubercle and no pain with resisted flexion or pronation suggest an isolated MCL tear.

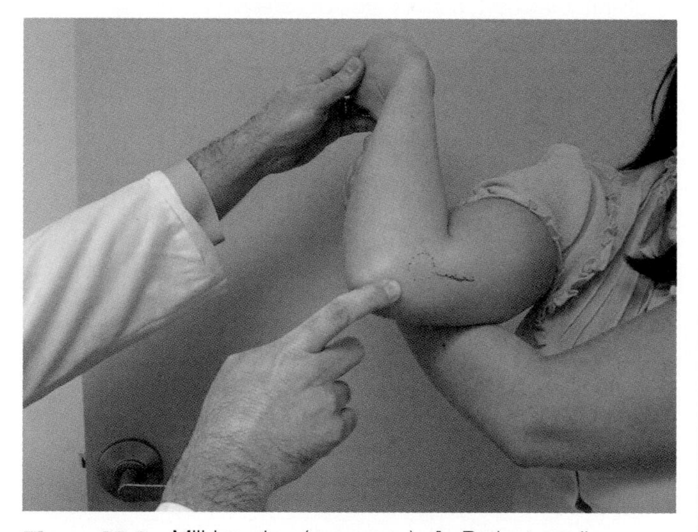

Figure 62-3 Milking sign (maneuver). **A**, Patient applies valgus stress to the elbow with the contralateral arm by grasping her thumb as shown. **B**, Safran and colleagues described a modification of this test with the patient locking the affected humerus and the examiner applying the valgus stress (see Fig. 62-2).

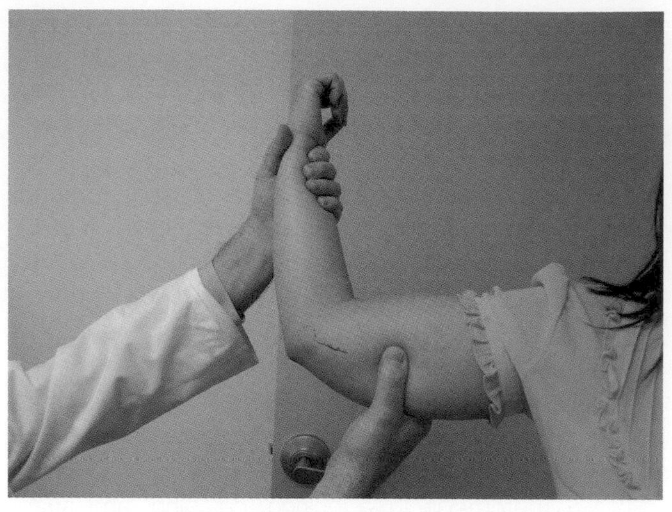

Figure 62-4 Valgus stress test. The elbow is flexed and the shoulder abducted with the humerus stabilized by the examiner and the examiner's other hand holding the wrist (or thumb), applying valgus stress at the elbow.

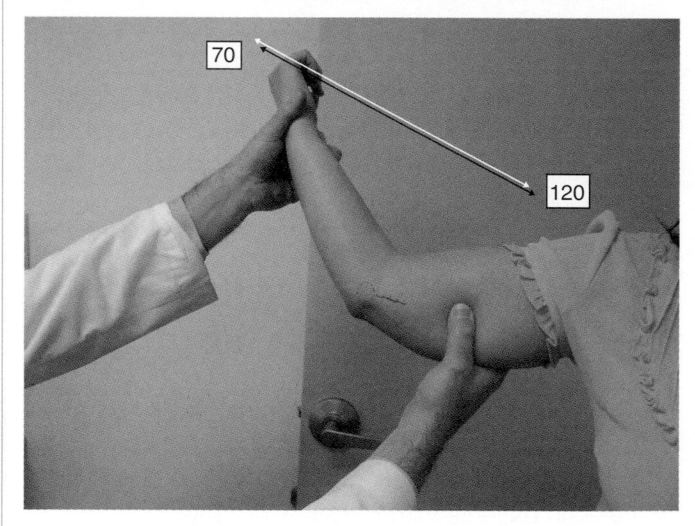

Figure 62-5 Moving valgus stress test. As described by O'Driscoll and colleagues, a valgus load is applied as the elbow is flexed and extended. A positive test is one in which pain is elicited at an elbow flexion/extension arc of 70 to 120 degrees.

Treatment

- At diagnosis
  - Treatment principles are protection, rest, ice, compression, elevation, medication, and modalities (physical therapy).
  - MCL injury
    - — Nighttime splinting for 2 to 3 months
    - — Progressive physical therapy program
    - — For patients with MCL partial tears and valgus laxity less than 2 mm, some authors recommend 6 weeks of nonoperative treatment.
    - — Nonsteroidal anti-inflammatory drugs, stretching of flexor-pronator mass/strengthening
    - — Progressive throwing program
- LCLC injury
  - — Acute
    - — Early referral for treatment
    - — Usually associated with a fracture
  - — Chronic
    - — Need for ligament reconstruction
    - — Early referral

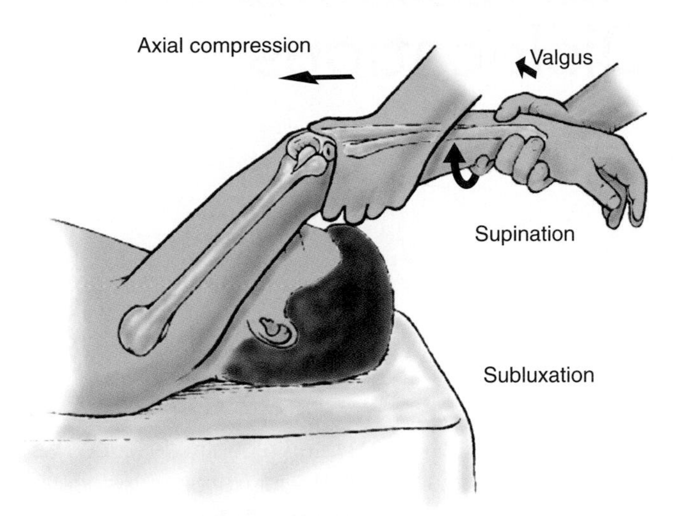

Figure 62-6 Lateral pivot shift test for posterolateral rotatory instability of the elbow. A supination valgus moment is applied during flexion, causing the elbow to subluxate maximally at approximately 40 degrees of flexion. Additional flexion causes reduction (with a palpable, visible "clunk," if successful). This test creates apprehension in the patient, who notes the sensation that the elbow is about to dislocate. (Adapted from O'Driscoll SW, Jupiter JB, King GJW, et al: The unstable elbow. Instr Course Lect 2001;50:89–102.)

BOX 62-2 *Differential Diagnosis*

Medial Elbow Pain
Elbow arthritis
Ulnar nerve neuritis
Medial epicondylitis

Lateral Elbow Pain
Chronic lateral epicondylitis: leads to attenuation of LCLC iatrogenically or multiple cortisone injections
Radiocapitellar arthritis
Radial tunnel syndrome

- Later
  - If there has been no improvement or if the diagnosis is in question, early referral to a specialist is recommended (see previously).
  - The sooner the patient sees a specialist, the better the outcome will be if surgery is required.

When to Refer

- See the treatment earlier in the chapter.

Prognosis

- Good

Patient Instructions

- Injuries to elbow ligaments may heal but usually are not normal ligaments.
- Most people with an MCL injury (complete) will notice a difference in their elbow over time, whether or not they undergo surgery.

Considerations in Special Populations

- Throwing athletes with valgus elbow laxity should be educated about the unpredictable impact of this injury.
- Those patients who choose surgery (MCL reconstruction) should be educated about the risks associated with surgery including the risk that one will be unable to return to his or her previous level of play.

Suggested Reading

- Chumbley EM, O'Connor FG, Nirschl RP: Evaluation of overuse elbow injuries. Am Fam Physician 2000;61:691–700.
- Cohen MS: Lateral collateral ligament instability of the elbow. Hand Clin 2008;24:69–77.
- Dipaola M, Geissler WB, Osterman AL: Complex elbow instability. Hand Clin 2008;24:39–52.
- Hoppenfeld S, Hutton R: Physical Examination of the Spine and Extremities. New York: Appleton-Century-Crofts, 1976, pp 35–57.
- Lyons RP, Armstrong A: Chronically unreduced elbow dislocations. Hand Clin 2008;24:91–103.
- O'Driscoll SW, Bell DF, Morrey BF: Posterolateral rotatory instability of the elbow. J Bone Joint Surg Am 1991;73A:440–446.
- O'Driscoll SW, Lawton RL, Smith AM: The moving valgus stress test for medial collateral tears of the elbow. Am J Sports Med 2005;33;231–239.
- Safran MR, Caldwell GL III, Fu FH: Chronic instability of the elbow. In Peimer CA (ed): Surgery of the Hand and Upper Extremity. New York: McGraw-Hill, 1996, pp 467–490.
- Vennix MJ, Wertsch JJ: Entrapment neuropathies about the elbow. J Back Musculoskel Rehabil 1994;4:31–43.
- Wilder RP, Guidi E: Anatomy and examination of the elbow. J Back Musculoskel Rehabil 1994;4:7–16.

Chapter 63 Elbow Dislocations

César J. Bravo

ICD-9 CODES

832.0	*Closed Dislocation of Elbow*
832.00	*Closed Unspecified Dislocation of Elbow*
832.01	*Closed Anterior Dislocation of Elbow*
832.02	*Closed Posterior Dislocation of Elbow*
832.03	*Closed Medial Dislocation of Elbow*
832.04	*Closed Lateral Dislocation of Elbow*
832.09	*Closed Dislocation of Other Site of Elbow*
832.1	*Open Dislocation of Elbow*
832.10	*Closed Unspecified Dislocation of Elbow*
832.11	*Closed Anterior Dislocation of Elbow*
832.12	*Closed Posterior Dislocation of Elbow*
832.13	*Closed Medial Dislocation of Elbow*
832.14	*Closed Lateral Dislocation of Elbow*
832.19	*Closed Dislocation of Other Site of Elbow*
729.5	*Elbow Pain*
841.9	*Elbow Sprain*

Key Concepts

- The elbow is a highly constrained joint. When dislocation of the elbow takes place, it is usually the result of a high-energy mechanism. This injury mechanism exceeds the intrinsic stability provided by the soft-tissue constraints and the anatomic articular contour of the elbow.
- Elbow dislocations occur more frequently in males than in females.
- Approximately 60% of dislocations occur in the non-dominant extremity.
- Simple elbow dislocations are those dislocations without associated fractures; those with associated fractures are termed complex dislocations.
- The classification for describing elbow dislocations is based on the direction of displacement of the forearm bones (radius and ulna) and described as posterior, anterior, lateral, medial, and divergent (Figs. 63-1 and 63-2).
- Elbow dislocations have been recently described as a spectrum of instability, from subluxation to dislocation. The three stages correspond with the pathoanatomic stages of the capsuloligamentous disruption. A perched dislocation is one in which the elbow is subluxed but the coronoid is impinged upon the trochlea (Figs. 63-3 to 63-6).
- Posterior elbow dislocations of the elbow are more common than anterior dislocations (80%). These types of dislocations are the result of an axial force applied to an extended elbow.
- Partial dislocations can occur in which either the radial head or the ulna dislocates. The radial head is less restrained than the ulna and can dislocate in conjunction with an ulnar fracture (Monteggia fracture).
- Lateral collateral ligament insufficiency is the essential lesion that results in recurrent instability.
- Cadaver studies have shown that an extension and varus moment associated with elbow dislocations results in the lateral collateral ligament being disrupted first. If further injury is transmitted to rotate the forearm, the anterior capsule and posterior capsule are disrupted. Finally, the medial ulnar collateral ligament is torn, and thus there is a complete dislocation of the elbow.

History

- The patient usually presents with a painful extremity that usually is shortened and a slightly flexed elbow.
- Radiographic evaluation of the elbow is crucial with anteroposterior and lateral views of the elbow.
- It is important to assess the mechanism of injury, hand dominance, range of motion, skin integrity around the elbow, and history of injury to the elbow.
- On the "field," reduction should not be done because of the risk of neurovascular injury without adequate sedation and analgesia.
- Early reduction is essential as this may lessen the injury to the joint or neurovascular compromise.

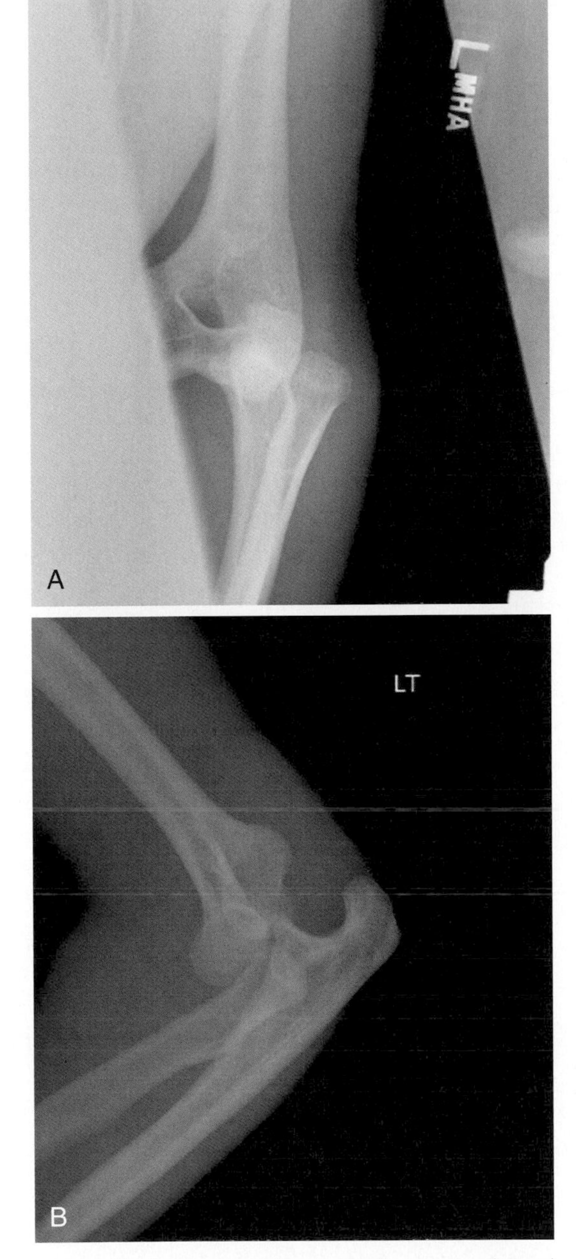

Figure 63-1 **A,** Anteroposterior view of a posterolateral dislocation. **B,** Lateral view of a posterolateral dislocation.

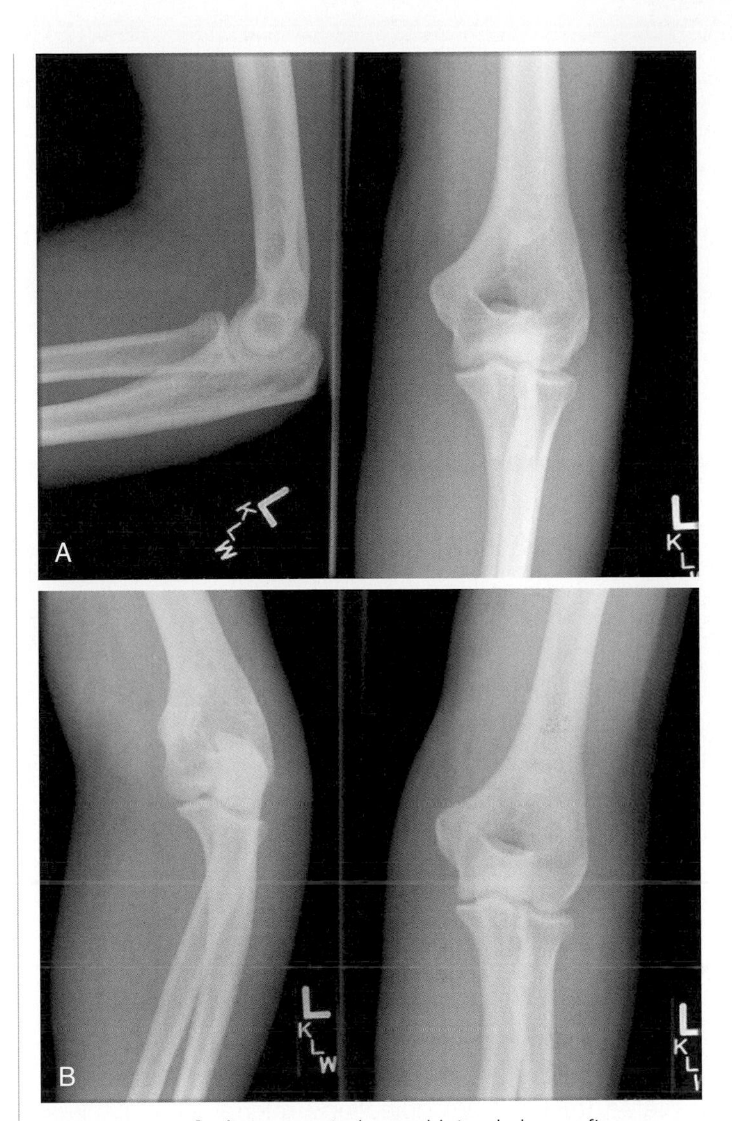

Figure 63-2 **A,** Anteroposterior and lateral views after reduction. **B,** Medial and lateral oblique views after reduction.

Physical Examination

- Diagnosis is made by clinical examination and verified with radiographs (Table 63-1).
- Need to document any open wounds that would indicate a portal of entry
- A neurovascular examination is important before and after reduction.

Imaging

- Radiographic images include anteroposterior and lateral views of the elbow, both before and after reduction.
- Postreduction radiographs assess for associated fractures and should confirm opposition of joint surfaces.
- On follow-up, we recommend oblique views of the elbow to assess for coronoid fractures, radial head fracture, and shear injuries of the capitellum that may not be recognized in anteroposterior and lateral views.

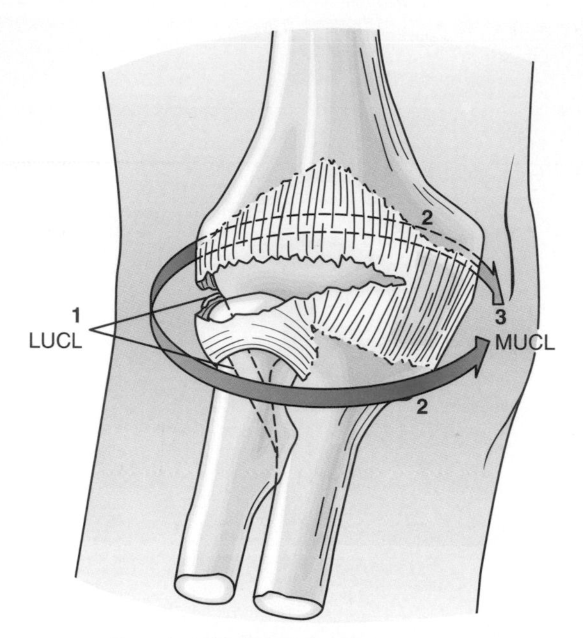

Figure 63-3 Drawing depicting the stages (1, 2, and 3) and the direction of soft-tissue injury (capsuloligamentous) seen with elbow dislocations from the lateral ulnar collateral ligament (LUCL) to the anterior/posterior capsule and finally ending with the medial ulnar collateral ligament (MUCL). (Adapted from O'Driscoll SW, Jupiter JB, King GJ, et al: The unstable elbow. Instr Course Lect 2001;50:89–102.)

Additional Tests

- Arteriogram if suspected vascular injury
- Computed tomography recommended when associated fractures are noted and referral to a specialist anticipated

Differential Diagnosis

- Please see Box 63-1.

Treatment

- Emergent referral should be made to an orthopaedic surgeon/emergency department once the patient is stabilized in the physician's office. Emergent orthopaedic consultation should be sought for all patients with elbow dislocations.
- Vascular surgery consultation may be needed in patients with possible vascular injury.
- Techniques for reduction of elbow dislocations (adequate analgesia and sedation are of paramount importance)
  - Posterior elbow dislocations
    - — Traction on the extremity with correction of medial or lateral displacement usually produces an audible "clunk" once the elbow is reduced.
    - — The second method (the Parvin method) involves placing the patient in the prone position with the humerus resting on the table and the forearm hanging perpendicular to the plane of the table. The humerus should be supported by the table, with padding or rolled towels, just proximal to the elbow joint. Five to 10 pounds of weight are applied to the wrist or the wrist is gently pulled down. Reduction should occur over a period of minutes as the muscles relax. The physician may push the olecranon into place if necessary.

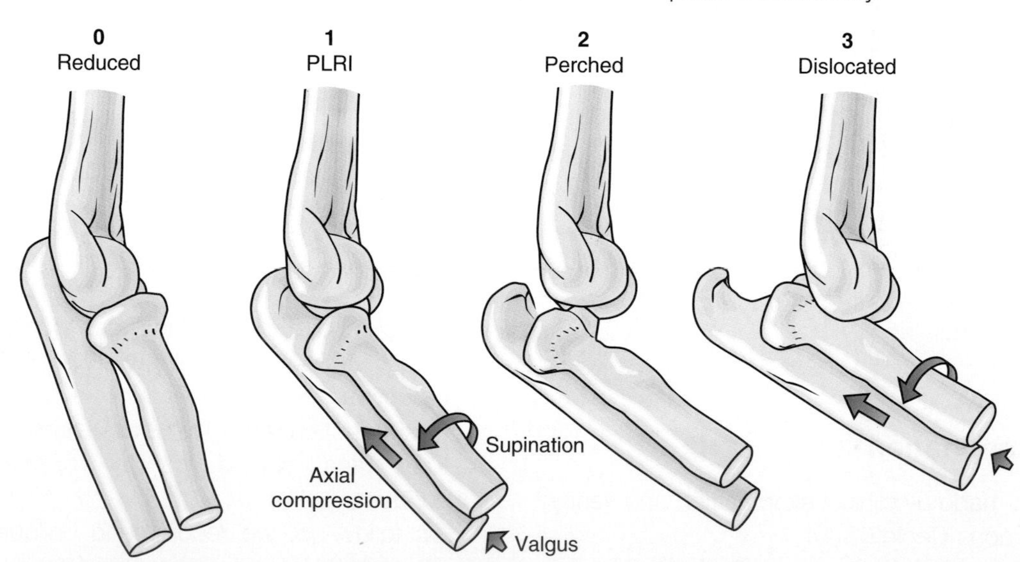

Figure 63-4 Drawing showing the spectrum of elbow instability from subluxation to dislocation. The *arrows* indicate the forces responsible for displacements. Stages 1 to 3 demonstrate the stages of capsuloligamentous disruption (see Fig. 63-1). PLRI, posterolateral rotatory instability. (Adapted from O'Driscoll SW, Jupiter JB, King GJ, et al: The unstable elbow. Instr Course Lect 2001;50:89–102.)

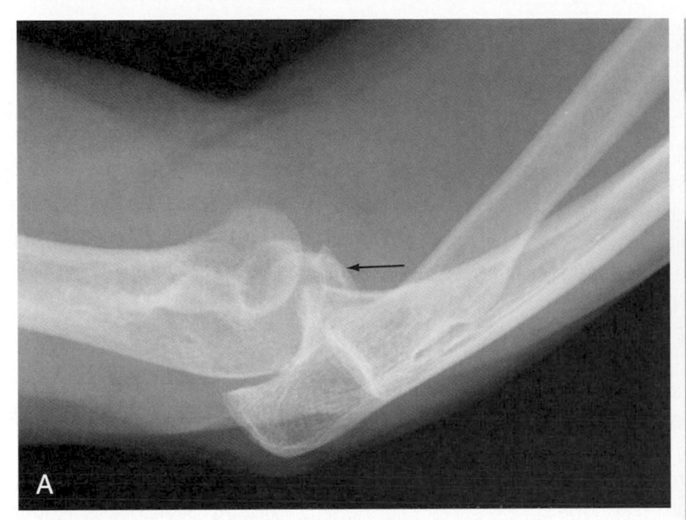

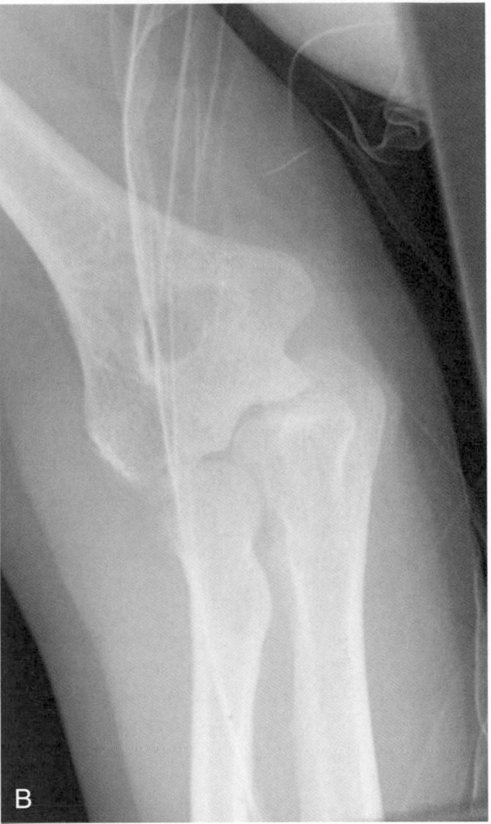

Figure 63-5 Posterior dislocation of radial head with "perching" of the ulna between the capitellum and trochlea. The patient had a coronoid fracture (*arrow*). On clinical examination, the patient was able to move the elbow. The patient was articulating within the groove between the trochlea and capitellum with the portion of the coronoid that was not fractured.

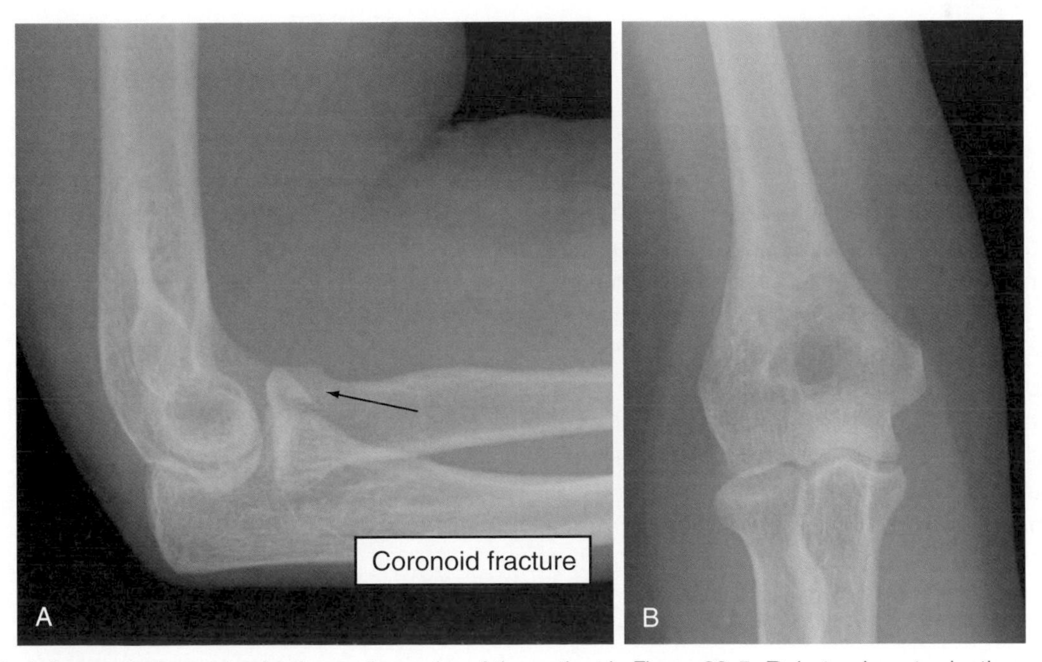

Figure 63-6 **A,** Anteroposterior postreduction radiographs of the patient in Figure 63-5. **B,** Lateral postreduction radiograph of the same patient.

TABLE 63-1 *Diagnosis Made by Clinical Examination and Verified with Radiographs*

Type of Dislocation	Clinical Presentation
Posterior elbow dislocations (see Figs. 63-1 and 63-2)	The elbow is flexed with an exaggerated olecranon; condyles of the elbow are not palpable
Anterior elbow dislocations	The elbow is held in extension and supination; the arm appears shortened; soft-tissue injury usually is severe
Lateral elbow dislocations/medial elbow dislocations	Some motion may still be maintained at the elbow joint; this is more common in lateral dislocations; motion takes place between the groove of the trochlea and capitellum (see Figs. 63-5 and 63-6)
Isolated ulnar dislocations	Cubitus varus deformity of the forearm is seen clinically; takes place when the humerus pivots around the radial head; the coronoid process may be displaced posteriorly to the humerus or the olecranon anteriorly to the humerus

BOX 63-1 *Differential Diagnosis*

Old injury to the elbow
Congenital dislocation of the radial head
Clinical examination and history
Radiographic analysis

- Anterior dislocation reduction is performed with traction on the wrist and backward pressure on the forearm. Take care to avoid hyperextension at the elbow, which may cause traction and potential injury to neurovascular structures around the elbow.
  - A postreduction neurovascular check should always be performed, as the brachial artery and the median and ulnar nerves can become entrapped with manipulation.
- A failed closed reduction is indicative of an entrapped medial epicondyle or an inverted cartilaginous flap, and the range of motion of the elbow confirms this. Range of motion should be fluid and concentric after the reduction.
- The elbow is splinted in slightly less than 90 degrees of flexion with a posterior splint for 5 to 7 days. If the elbow was stable on the postreduction examination, full unprotected motion should be started no later than 1 week. The patient is instructed to work with pronation and supination with the elbow at 90 degrees of flexion. Varus stress to the elbow is also avoided for the first 6 weeks post-injury. The patient is instructed to avoid full extension and supination.
- If forearm pronation was required to prevent extension instability, a full range of motion is allowed in a hinged brace with the forearm fully pronated. The patient may only come out of the brace for motion exercises in full pronation under the guidance of a skilled therapist. The brace is worn for 4 weeks.
- If an extension block was required, it is reduced gradually over 4 weeks. Extension blocks greater than 45 degrees require surgical intervention and early referral.
- Loss of extension between 5 and 10 degrees compared with the unaffected elbow is usually seen after this injury.
- Elbow dislocations seen after 1 week require open reduction and early referral.

Prognosis

- Good

Troubleshooting

- Fractures of the coronoid and radial head and elbow dislocation are known as the "terrible triad." Early referral is indicated for ligament reconstruction and fracture repair.

Suggested Reading

- Bucholz R, Heckman JD, Court-Brown C, et al (eds): Rockwood and Green's Fractures in Adults, 5th ed. New York: Lippincott Williams & Wilkins, 2002, pp 921–934.
- Cohen MS, Hastings H: Acute elbow dislocation: Evaluation and management. J Am Acad Orthop Surg 1998;6:15–23.
- Hobgood ER, Khan SO, Field LD: Acute dislocations of the adult elbow. Hand Clin 2008;24:1–7.
- Josefsson PO, Johnell O, Gentz CF: Long-term sequelae of simple dislocations of the elbow. J Bone Joint Surg Br 1984;69B:605–608.
- Mehta J, Bain G: Posterolateal rotatory instability of the elbow. J Am Acad Orthop Surg 2004;12:404–415.
- O'Driscoll SW, Jupiter JB, King GJ, et al: The unstable elbow. Instr Course Lect 2001;50:89–102.
- Tashjian RZ, Katarincic JA: Complex elbow instability. J Am Acad Orthop Surg 2006;14:278–286.

Chapter 64 Olecranon Bursitis

César J. Bravo

ICD-9 CODES

726.33	*Olecranon Bursitis*
729.5	*Elbow Pain*
841.9	*Elbow Sprain*
716.92	*Elbow Arthritis*

Key Concepts

- The olecranon process is the most proximal posterior eminence of the ulna located on the dorsal subcutaneous border of the elbow. Overlying this posterior eminence is the olecranon bursa. The olecranon process contains broad attachments for the triceps tendon posteriorly. The olecranon forms the greater sigmoid notch of the ulna, which articulates with the trochlea of the distal humerus.
- The olecranon bursa is a smooth sac between the loose skin and the bones of the elbow. The bursa allows the skin to move without restraint over the underlying olecranon. This prevents tissue tears by providing a mechanism for the skin to glide freely over the olecranon process. If it becomes irritated or inflamed, a condition known as bursitis develops (Fig. 64-1).
- Olecranon bursitis is inflammation of the soft tissues (bursal tissue) overlying the olecranon process and the posterior skin of the elbow. The bursa can become inflamed because of its superficial location secondary to acute trauma, infection, or repetitive shear forces across this area (i.e., student's or miner's elbow).

History

- Patients present with a swollen, painful enlargement of the posterior aspect of the elbow (e.g., goose egg appearance).
- Patients may have chronic recurrent swelling over the posterior aspect of the elbow, which in chronic cases usually is not tender.
- Frequent trauma of the swollen elbow may occur because the olecranon process overhangs farther than normal.
- Patients may report a history of isolated trauma or repetitive microtrauma (e.g., due to constant rubbing of the elbow against the table while writing).
- Onset may be sudden if the condition is secondary to infection or acute trauma.
- Onset may be gradual if olecranon bursitis is secondary to chronic irritation.
- A history of fever, marked tenderness, and overlying cellulitis coincides with a septic bursitis.
- Swelling is often the first symptom. The skin on the back of the elbow is loose, which means that a small amount of swelling may not be noticed right away. As the swelling continues, the bursa grows. This causes pain as the bursa is stretched because the bursa contains nerve endings. The swelling may grow large enough to restrict motion of the elbow.
- A history of trauma or lacerating/puncture wound needs to be documented.
- The patient's hand dominance and field of work need to be documented (i.e., student's or miner's elbow).
- Pain is located at the olecranon process, and traction osteophytes (olecranon spurs) can be seen on radiographic views, which indicate a chronic process (seen in patients with recurring bursitis).
- Reasons for olecranon bursitis
  - Trauma: A hard blow to the tip of the elbow could cause the bursa to produce excess fluid and swell.
  - Prolonged pressure: Leaning on the tip of the elbow for long periods on hard surfaces, such as a tabletop, may cause the bursa to swell. Typically, this type of bursitis would develop over several months.
  - Infection: If the tip of the elbow has an injury that breaks the skin, such as an insect bite and a scrape, bacteria may get inside the bursa and cause an infection. The infected bursa produces fluid, redness, and swelling. If the infection goes untreated, the fluid may turn to pus.
  - Medical conditions: Certain conditions such as rheumatoid arthritis and gout are associated with development of elbow bursitis.

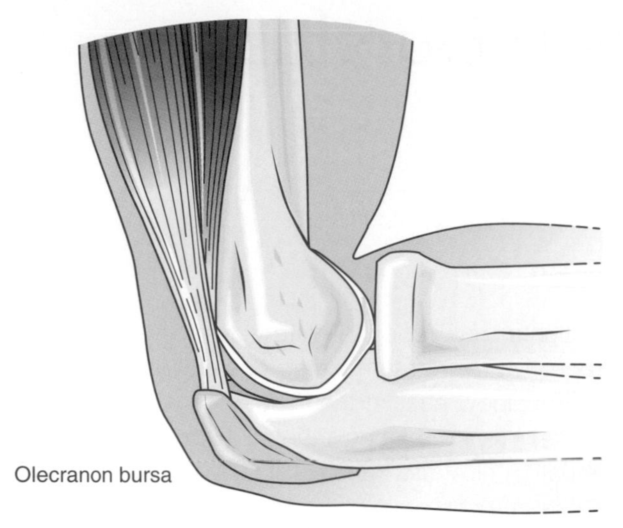

Figure 64-1 Olecranon bursa.

Physical Examination

- Swollen and painful mass on the posterior aspect of the elbow
- Need to document any open wounds that would indicate a portal of entry
- Patients with systemic inflammatory processes (e.g., rheumatoid arthritis) or crystal deposition disease (e.g., gout, pseudogout) may reveal evidence of focal inflammation at other sites.
- Patients with rheumatoid arthritis may, on inspection of the elbow, have rheumatoid nodules.
- Elbow pain during active or passive ROM may increase the clinician's suspicion of fracture of the olecranon process if there is a history of trauma.
- Loss of elbow extension against gravity would lead one to suspect a triceps rupture.
- Intra-articular pathology (e.g., septic elbow, fractures, arthritis) coincides with a painful arc of motion not usually seen in olecranon bursitis.
- It is important to try to identify the cause of the bursitis as early as possible. This is because chronic bursitis is likely to eventuate into the formation of scar tissue, which may lead to more regular flare-ups and possibly further complications in later years.

Imaging

- Radiographic anteroposterior and lateral views of the elbow
- Magnetic resonance imaging is recommended when triceps insufficiency is suspected. It also evaluates for underlying abscess or bone infection (osteomyelitis) with chronic septic bursitis.

TABLE 64-1 *Differential Diagnosis*

Pathology	Clinical Scenario/ Differentiating Examination
Triceps tendon rupture	Clinical examination by loss of elbow extension against gravity (partial rupture; magnetic resonance imaging)
Fracture of the olecranon process, radial head	Radiographic analysis
Crystalline inflammatory arthropathy (e.g., gout, pseudogout)	Pertinent laboratory work ordered
Synovial cyst of the elbow joint	Radiographic analysis

Additional Tests

- Complete blood count and differential, erythrocyte sedimentation rate, and C-reactive protein level when suspecting a septic process followed by aspiration (see section on aspiration of olecranon bursa)
- Check for rheumatoid factor to assess for rheumatoid arthritis and check the uric acid level to assess for gout.

Differential Diagnosis

- Please see Table 64-1.

Treatment

- At diagnosis
  - A nonseptic bursa can usually be treated symptomatically and the patient advised to avoid rubbing the elbow. The RICE (rest, ice, compression, elevation) protocol should be followed. Small and moderate bursae are treated by aspiration and injections of steroids followed by a compressive dressing (neoprene sleeve or elastic bandage).
  - The elbow is elevated and ice is applied. An elbow pad may be used to cushion the elbow (heelbow pad). Direct pressure to the swollen elbow should be avoided. Oral medications such as anti-inflammatories may be used.
  - If swelling and pain do not respond to these measures, then removing fluid from the bursa and injecting corticosteroid medication into the bursa is indicated.
- Later
  - Chronic bursitis, when it is recurrent and symptomatic, should be treated with an open or arthroscopic bursectomy.

When to Refer

- Consultation with an orthopaedist
  - Septic bursitis that deteriorates and does not respond to initial treatment of aspiration and culture-directed antibiotics
  - Chronic recurrent bursitis that is symptomatic
  - Suspected intra-articular elbow pathology or triceps tendon rupture
- Consultation with a physiatrist (physical medicine and rehabilitation physician) or with another qualified musculoskeletal specialist may be considered by physicians without the training, comfort, or procedural office supplies necessary for aspiration.
- Consultation with a rheumatologist may be helpful if findings are consistent with inflammatory arthropathy.

Prognosis

- Good. Recovery usually is complete. Most of the patients with olecranon bursitis respond well to treatment unless there is a persistent infection. Corticosteroid injection is usually effective in nonseptic bursitis, and long-term sequelae are unusual.

Troubleshooting

- See olecranon bursa aspiration/injection section.

Patient Instructions

- The first approach in treating olecranon bursitis should be to eliminate mechanical stress from the affected area, such as avoiding leaning on the elbow. If a repetitive activity is the cause, this activity should be stopped until the bursitis has completely healed.
- Olecranon bursitis that does not heal from rest alone or that is causing pain or discomfort may need medical intervention such as oral or topical nonsteroidal anti-inflammatory drugs or corticosteroid injections.

Considerations in Special Populations

- Patients with end-stage renal disease are more likely to develop chronic recalcitrant olecranon bursitis due to their altered immune system. Patients with gout and tophi on their elbows, as well as patients with rheumatoid arthritis with rheumatoid nodules on their elbows, are more likely to have recurrences of olecranon bursitis.

Suggested Reading

- Salzman KL, Lillegard WA, Butcher JD: Upper extremity bursitis. Am Fam Physician 1997;56:1797–1806, 1811–1812.
- Shell D, Perkins R, Cosgarea A: Septic olecranon bursitis: Recognition and treatment. J Am Board Fam Pract 1995; 8:217–220.
- Stewart NJ, Manzanares JB, Morrey BF: Surgical treatment of aseptic olecranon bursitis. J Shoulder Elbow Surg 1997;6:49–54.
- Wasserman AR, Melville LD, Birkhahn RH: Septic bursitis: A case report and primer for the emergency clinician. J Emerg Med 2007;20 [Epub ahead of print].
- Weinstein PS, Canoso JJ, Wohlgethan JR: Long-term follow-up of corticosteroid injection for traumatic olecranon bursitis. Ann Rheum Dis 1984;43:44–46.

Chapter 65 Ulnar Nerve Entrapment

César J. Bravo

ICD-9 CODES

354.2 *Lesion of Ulnar Nerve*
Cubital Tunnel
Tardy Ulnar Nerve Palsy

354.5 *Mononeuritis Multiplex*
Combinations of single conditions classifiable to 354 and 355 (e.g., ulnar tunnel at the wrist and cubital tunnel in the elbow)

For Differential

354.3 *Lesion of Radial Nerve; Acute Radial Nerve Palsy/Posterior Interosseous Nerve Palsy*

354.1 *Other Lesion of Median Nerve; Median Nerve Neuritis/Pronator Syndrome*

721.0 *Cervical Spondylosis without Myelopathy*

721.1 *Cervical Spondylosis with Myelopathy*

Key Concepts

- Cubital tunnel syndrome is compression of the ulnar nerve around the elbow.
- It is the second most common site of nerve compression in the upper extremity (carpal tunnel syndrome at the wrist is the most common).
- The ulnar nerve can be compressed in any location along its path around the elbow but is most commonly entrapped in the cubital canal (Fig. 65-1).
- Patients usually present with numbness in the ring and small fingers and weakness of intrinsic muscles of the hand.
- Symptoms are reproduced with hyperflexion of the elbow.
- Positive percussion test (Tinel's sign) at the elbow is noted.
- Ulnar claw deformity of the hand is seen with motor involvement (late presentation).
  - Hyperextension of ring and small finger metacarpophalangeal joints with hyperflexion of proximal interphalangeal joints.
- Intrinsic and extrinsic factors can compress the ulnar nerve around the elbow.
  - Intrinsic factors (e.g., perineuroma, hamartoma of the ulnar nerve)
  - Extrinsic factors (e.g., fibrous tendons, hypertrophic muscles, vascular lesions)
- Acute and chronic compression of ulnar nerve around the elbow (Table 65-1)

History

- Patient may present with ill-defined symptoms and pain on the medial aspect of the forearm.
  - Sensory symptoms may be numbness and tingling.
  - Motor symptoms range from weakness to paralysis.
- Paresthesia and numbness of the small and ring fingers are reported.
- The patient may report clumsiness with difficulty gripping, fine motor activities, and hand fatigue secondary to weak intrinsics.
- The first sensory perceptions to be lost are light touch, pressure, and vibration, and the last to be impaired are pain and temperature.
- Patient should be asked about onset of symptoms and subjective feelings of numbness (dorsal or volar aspect of hand).
- Loss of spreading fingers or thumb and inability to hold small finger together with ring finger
- Alleviating and exacerbating factors
  - Changes in skin color, temperature, texture, and moisture may result from sympathetic nervous system dysfunction
- Comorbidities (e.g., diabetes, hemophilia, gout, and generalized peripheral neuropathy, thyroid disease, and vitamin deficiency)
- Documentation of patient's handedness, occupation, and specific activities that produce symptoms.
  - Overhead elevation: thoracic outlet syndrome
  - Elbow flexion: cubital tunnel syndrome
  - Wrist flexion: ulnar tunnel syndrome (entrapment of Guyon's canal)
  - Cubitus varus or valgus deformities, medial epicondylitis, and repetitive elbow flexion/valgus stress

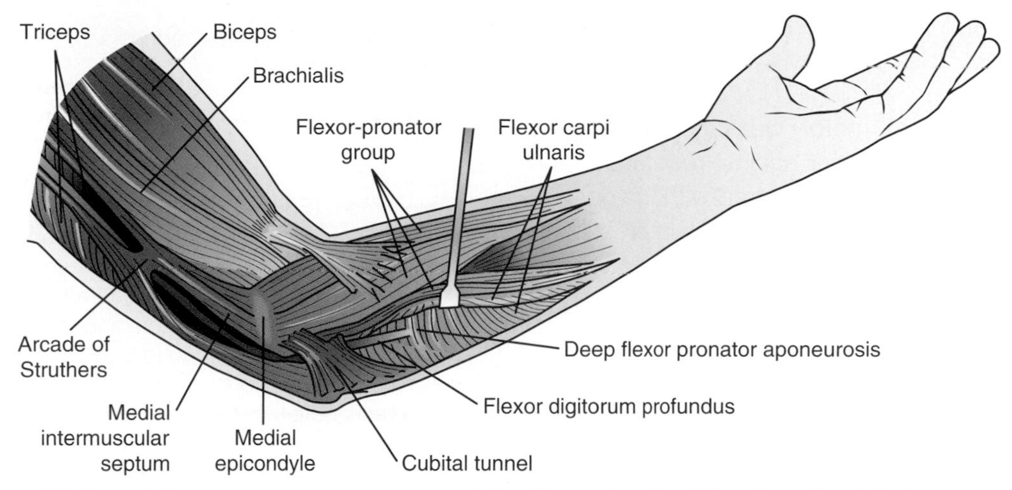

Figure 65-1 Potential sites of ulnar nerve entrapment around the elbow. Arcade of Struthers (fascial hiatus in the medial intermuscular septum as the ulnar nerve passes from the anterior to the posterior compartment, 8 cm proximal to the medial epicondyle), medial intermuscular septum, medial head of the triceps muscle, medial epicondyle, Osborne's ligament (cubital tunnel roof or retinaculum), anconeus epitrochlearis (anomalous muscle originating from the medial olecranon and inserting on the medial epicondyle), and flexor carpi ulnaris aponeurosis. Other sources of compression include tumors, ganglions, osteophytes, heterotopic ossification, and medial epicondyle nonunion.

TABLE 65-1 *Acute and Chronic Ulnar Nerve Entrapment*

Condition	Causes
Acute ulnar nerve entrapment	Fractures/dislocations of the elbow; errant placement of retractors during surgery; malpositioning of patient during surgery; open injury (knife, gunshot wound)
Chronic ulnar nerve entrapment	Cubitus valgus (late presentation of distal physeal elbow injury in children); hypertrophic callus formation of previous elbow fracture/ dislocation; ganglion cysts/tumors

during occupational or athletic activities may lead to compression of the ulnar nerve at the elbow.

Physical Examination

- Examine individual muscle strength (grades 0–5), pinch strength, and grip strength.
- Neurosensory testing should be performed in the context of both dermatomal and peripheral nerve distributions.
- Semmes-Weinstein monofilaments measure cutaneous pressure threshold, a function of large nerve fibers (the first to be affected in compression neuropathy).
- Two-point discrimination should be measured on the fingertip pulp of each digit. The inability to perceive a difference of less than 5 mm is abnormal and constitutes a late finding in compression neuropathy.
- Symptoms may include paresthesias of the two ulnar digits (ring and small fingers) and ulnar dorsal aspect of the hand.
  - Symptoms may worsen with the use of the hand requiring elbow flexion.
  - Night pain is uncommon.
- Intrinsic weakness with a positive Froment's paper sign (compensatory thumb interphalangeal flexion during pinch due to weak adductor pollicis muscle) is seen early.
- Wartenberg's sign (persistent abduction and extension of the small digit) is also seen early when the patient is asked to adduct the digits' extension caused by weakness of the third palmar interosseous and unopposed extensor digiti minimi muscles.
- Provocative tests (each test elicits worsening sensory disturbance or pain in an ulnar nerve distribution)
  - Ulnar nerve elbow compression test (patient is asked to maximally flex the elbow with reproduction of symptoms)
    - — Flexion of the elbow greater than 30 degrees narrows the shape of the cubital canal (oval to slit shape) and pressure increases as the elbow is flexed further on the nerve. Additional pressure is placed on the nerve (the medial cord origins of the ulnar nerve) with shoulder abduction.
  - Percussion test (Tinel's sign) is done by tapping posterior to the medial epicondyle.
- Clawing of ulnar digits is a severe late finding of ulnar neuropathy.

- The clinical examination is the most important aspect in establishing the diagnosis of cubital tunnel syndrome.
- The best indicator of motor weakness is resisted abduction of the index finger against resistance provided by the examiner and compared with the contralateral side to assess the first dorsal interosseous muscle.

Imaging

- Radiographic views of elbow (anteroposterior and lateral views)
- Magnetic resonance imaging of the elbow

Additional Tests

- Electromyography/nerve conduction velocity studies
  - Helpful in confirming the clinical diagnosis
  - This technique is operator dependent and has an increased rate of false negatives (approximately 50%).
  - May be enhanced by using an "inching" technique across the elbow

Differential Diagnosis

- Please see Table 65-2.

TABLE 65-2 *Differential Diagnosis*

Pathology	Clinical Scenario/ Differentiatings Examination
Cervical root impingement (C8, T1)	Magnetic resonance imaging and radicular type pain; hypoactive deep tendon reflexes
Brachial plexus impingement (lower trunk and branches)/ thoracic outlet syndrome (see section on thoracic outlet syndrome)	Chest and cervical oblique view radiographs to determine pulmonary cause of symptoms (e.g., Pancoast's tumor, presence of cervical rib); patient may present with facial pain as well as temporomandibular joint pain
Wrist ulnar nerve entrapment/ulnar tunnel syndrome (see section on ulnar tunnel syndrome)	Intact sensation at dorsum of ulnar side of the hand
Pronator syndrome	Proximal arm nerve entrapment of the median nerve, not ulnar nerve; volar forearm pain and sensory disturbances in the distribution of the palmar cutaneous branch of the median nerve

Treatment

- At diagnosis
  - Nonoperative treatment includes activity modification and almost entirely avoiding elbow flexion beyond 30 to 45 degrees for as long as 3 months.
  - Eighty percent of patients with a mild degree of compression and 30% of those with a severe degree of compression improve with the previously cited restrictions.
  - A night splint (elbow held in 45 degrees of flexion) or a towel wrapped around the elbow to prevent extreme elbow flexion is recommended.
  - During the day, critical activities that require elbow flexion are allowed.
  - Nonsteroidal anti-inflammatory drugs
- Later
  - Patients with symptoms of cubital tunnel syndrome after 3 months of nonoperative treatment and with documented neurosensory and motor evidence of abnormal ulnar nerve function and a positive Tinel's sign at the postcondylar groove of the elbow require surgical decompression. Referral at this time is appropriate.
  - Numerous surgical techniques have been described, such as in situ cubital tunnel decompression, medial epicondylectomy, and anterior ulnar nerve transposition (subcutaneous, submuscular, or intramuscular).
  - There is a high rate of recurrence of cubital tunnel syndrome (25% to 33%) with the different techniques.
    — Anterior submuscular transposition by musculofascial lengthening produces the best results, according to meta-analyses.

When to Refer

- See Treatment section.

Prognosis

- For patients with mild compression of the ulnar nerve, Dellon found that 50% achieved excellent results with nonsurgical management and almost 100% achieved excellent results with surgical intervention. For patients with moderate compression, the anterior submuscular technique yielded the best results with the least recurrence; the intramuscular technique yielded the worst results with the most recurrence.

Troubleshooting

- Congenital anomalies: The anconeus epitrochlearis muscle is an accessory muscle seen on the lateral aspect of the elbow that may lead to compression of the ulnar nerve.
  - Can only be seen during surgical decompression
- Examine patient for a subluxing ulnar nerve or prominent medial head of the triceps muscle.
- Double crush phenomenon is seen when cervical radiculopathy or proximal nerve entrapment coexists with distal nerve compression.
  - Patients need to be informed that the outcome of surgical decompression may be disappointing unless all sites of compression are released.

Patient Instructions

- Patients treated early typically have excellent relief of symptoms.
- Late presentation with progressive motor or sensory deficits decreases the likelihood of full recovery and good clinical outcome.
- Patients may have persistent symptoms due to incomplete decompression or perineural scarring.
- Injury to the posterior branch of the medial antebrachial cutaneous nerve can lead to hyperesthesia, hyperalgesia in the forearm, and a painful surgical scar.
- Subluxation of the ulnar nerve may occur with simple decompression alone.
- Injury to the medial collateral ligament of the elbow may occur as a complication of a submuscular transposition procedure.
- For individuals involved in highly-level upper extremity activities, such as a throwing sport and a job that requires lifting, a slightly extended rehabilitation period may be required.

Considerations in Special Populations

- Musicians may present with difficulty in using fingers, either as fast or for as long as they used to.
  - These include violin, guitar, flute, and piano players.
  - Symptoms tend to improve with relaxation techniques (e.g., Pilates) and changing the practice schedule.
  - Decompression is rarely required.
- People with tophaceous gout
  - Uric acid crystal deposit in tenosynovium around nerve or nerve itself
- Rheumatoid arthritis
  - Caused by proliferation of synovium and tenosynovium
  - Compression of the posterior interosseous nerve is also seen.
- Hemophiliacs
  - Predisposed to perineural, intramuscular, and intraneural bleeding

Suggested Reading

- Davis GA, Bulluss KJ: Submuscular transposition of the ulnar nerve: Review of safety, efficacy and correlation with neurophysiological outcome. J Clin Neurosci 2005;12:524–528.
- Dellon AL: Compression neuropathy. In Trumble T, Cornwall R, Budoff J (eds): Core Knowledge in Orthopaedics: Hand, Elbow, and Shoulder. Philadelphia: Mosby, 2005, pp 234–254.
- Dellon AL: Review of treatment results for ulnar nerve entrapment at the elbow. J Hand Surg [Am] 1989;14(4):688–700.
- Elhassan B, Steinmann SP: Entrapment neuropathy of the ulnar nerve. J Am Acad Orthop Surg 2007;15:672–681.
- Henry M: Modified intramuscular transposition of the ulnar nerve. J Hand Surg [Am] 2006;31:1535–1542.
- Ruchelsman DE, Lee SK, Posner MA: Failed surgery for ulnar nerve compression at the elbow. Hand Clin 2007;23:359–371, vi–vii.
- Szabo RM, Kwak C: Natural history and conservative management of cubital tunnel syndrome. Hand Clin 2007;23:311–318, v–vi.
- Zlowodzki M, Chan S, Bhandari M, et al: Anterior transposition compared with simple decompression for treatment of cubital tunnel syndrome: A meta-analysis of randomized, controlled trials. J Bone Joint Surg Am 2007;89:2591–2598.

Chapter 66 Fractures of the Distal Humerus

Rashard Dacus

ICD-9 CODES
812.41 *Supracondylar*
812.44 *Intra-articular Extension*
812.49 *Comminuted Intra-articular Extension*

Key Concepts

- Epidemiology
  - Distal humerus fractures are relatively uncommon with an incidence of roughly 6 cases per 100,000 people in the population per year.
  - Male/female distribution is nearly equal.
- Anatomy
  - The trochlea and capitellum constitute the distal articular humerus.
  - The humeral shaft divides into longitudinal medial and lateral columns.
  - The trochlea connects the columns distally at the joint.
  - The olecranon fossa is a triangular depression posteriorly.
  - The intramedullary canal tapers to end 2 to 3 cm proximal to the fossa.
  - The capitellum is part of the lateral column.
- Classification
  - Intra-articular: single column, both columns (T pattern, Y pattern, H pattern)
  - Extra-articular intracapsular: transcolumnar, high, low
  - Extracapsular: medial epicondyle, lateral epicondyle
  - Muller: type A, extra-articular; type B, single column; type C, both columns
- Goals of treatment
  - Restore articular surface, stabilize range of motion (ROM)
  - Stabilize the articular surface to the humeral shaft
- Additional findings
  - Humeral shaft fracture, olecranon or radial head fracture

History

- Symptoms: pain, inability to move elbow
- Mechanism of injury
  - Transcolumnar: axial load through forearm with elbow flexed
  - Intercondylar: axial load on olecranon with elbow flexed beyond 90 degrees

Physical Examination

- Visual inspection: edema, deformity, laceration/puncture, or ecchymosis
- Palpation: crepitus
- Range of motion: limited due to pain at elbow; always assess joints proximally and distally
- Neurologic: assess radial, median/anterior interosseous nerve, and ulnar nerve function
- Vascular: assess radial and ulnar arterial pulses; Allen's test

Imaging

- Anteroposterior and lateral elbow
- Anteroposterior and lateral humerus
- Traction views may help define fragments
- Computed tomography helpful for surgical planning or for occult fracture (Fig. 66-1)

Differential Diagnosis

- Please see Table 66-1.

Treatment

- At diagnosis
  - There is a limited role for nonoperative management of these fractures.
  - Only nondisplaced fractures may be treated nonoperatively with a long arm posterior elbow splint with the elbow in 90 degrees of flexion and the wrist in a neutral position.
  - Splint for 2 weeks.

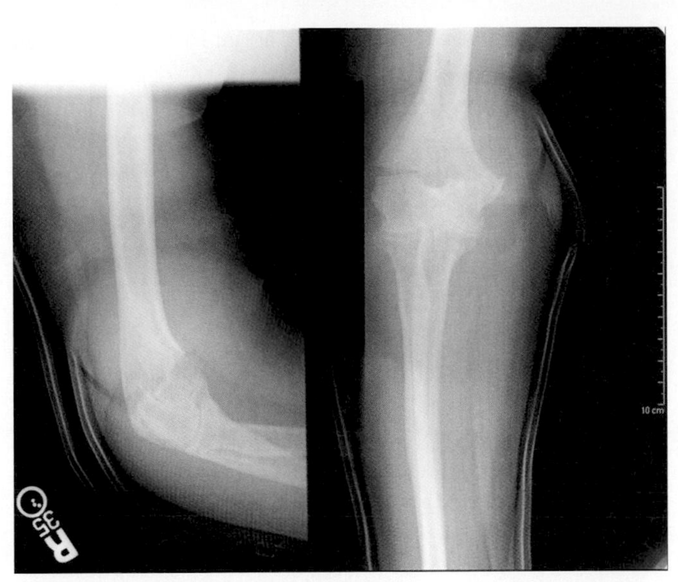

Figure 66-1 Anteroposterior and lateral radiographs of a low transverse distal humerus fracture.

TABLE 66-1 *Differential Diagnosis*

Differential Diagnosis	Differentiating Features	Chapter Reference
Elbow dislocation	Evidence of dislocation on radiographs	63
Olecranon fracture	Fracture of proximal ulna evident on radiographs	68
Triceps avulsion	Radiographs are either negative for fracture or demonstrate an avulsion fracture from the proximal ulna; inability to perform elbow extension	56

- Later
  - After 2 to 3 weeks of immobilization, recheck radiographs to monitor for displacement.
  - If reduction is maintained, transition to a hinged elbow brace and begin gentle ROM.

When to Refer

- All displaced and comminuted fractures should be placed into a long arm posterior splint as described previously and the patient referred to an orthopaedic surgeon for surgical management within 1 week of injury.
- Evidence of nerve or vascular injury requires emergent referral or consultation.
- Surgical interventions may include the following
  - Closed reduction and percutaneous pinning

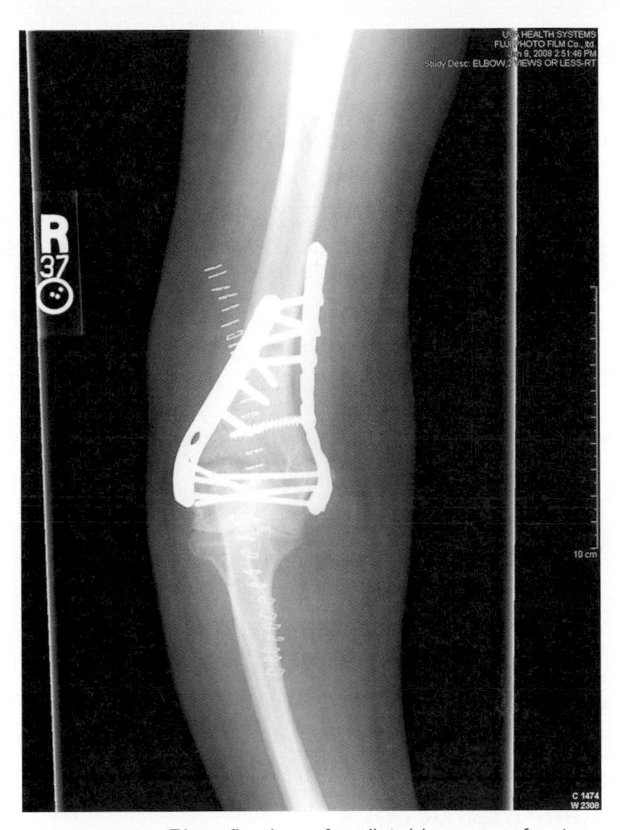

Figure 66-2 Plate fixation of a distal humerus fracture.

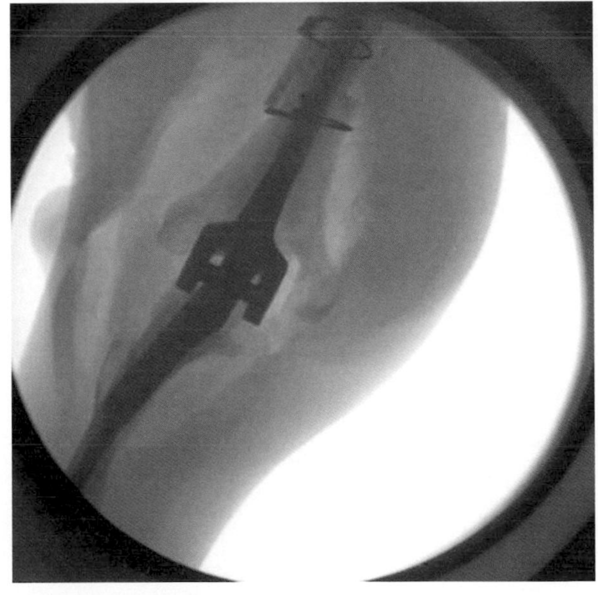

Figure 66-3 Anteroposterior radiograph of a total elbow arthroplasty.

  - Open reduction and internal fixation (Fig. 66-2)
  - Total elbow arthroplasty may be an option in the appropriate patient.
    — Comminuted fractures in osteoporotic bone
    — Preexisting elbow pathology in a low-demand patient (Fig. 66-3)

Prognosis

- Inadequate or delayed reduction, intra-articular step-offs, and prolonged immobilization can result in significant elbow stiffness and disability.
- Regardless of the treatment modality, the full elbow ROM may never be equal to the uninjured elbow, but it should be functional.
- Heterotopic ossification is commonly associated with distal humerus fractures that are treated with open reduction and internal fixation. The incidence of heterotopic ossification may be decreased by early continuous passive ROM or the use of nonsteroidal anti-inflammatory drugs (indomethacin).
- Ulnar nerve dysfunction may occur after this injury and is minimized by an ulnar nerve transposition at the time of the initial surgery.
    - Persistent ulnar nerve symptoms after open reduction and internal fixation may require secondary surgery for nerve mobilization or excision of heterotopic ossification.

Patient Instructions

- Keep splint on at all times until evaluated by orthopaedic surgeon.
- Pain medication is to be provided as indicated by presentation.
- Encourage elevation, rest, and finger ROM to decrease edema.
- Referral to an occupational or physical therapist may be necessary to promote the ROM.
- The patient may always have some elbow stiffness even after appropriate medical, surgical, and therapeutic modalities.

Suggested Reading

- Doornberg J, Lindenhovius A, Kloen P, et al: Two- and three-dimensional computed tomography for the classification and management of distal humeral fractures. Evaluation of reliability and diagnostic accuracy. J Bone Joint Surg Am 2006;88A: 1795–1801.
- Gabel GT, Hanson G, Bennett JB, et al: Intraarticular fractures of the distal humerus in the adult. Clin Orthop Relat Res 1987;216: 99–108.
- Jawa A, McCarty P, Doornberg J, et al: Extra-articular distal-third diaphyseal fractures of the humerus. A comparison of functional bracing and plate fixation. J Bone Joint Surg Am 2006;88A: 2343–2347.
- McKee MD, Jupiter JB, Division of Orthopaedics, St. Michael's Hospital, University of Toronto: A contemporary approach to the management of complex fractures of the distal humerus and their seguelae. Hand Clin 1994;10:479–494.
- Watts AC, Morris A, Robinson CM: Fractures of the distal humeral articular surface. J Bone Joint Surg Br 2007;89B: 510–515.

Chapter 67 Radial Head or Neck Fractures

Rashard Dacus

ICD-9 CODES
813.05 *Radial Head*
813.06 *Radial Neck*

Key Concepts

- Epidemiology
  - Radial head fractures account for approximately one third of all elbow fractures.
  - Fifteen percent to 20% of the time radial head and neck fractures occur simultaneously.
- Classification
  - Radial head fractures
    - Mason classification: type I, nondisplaced; type II, marginal fracture with displacement; type III, comminuted fracture of the entire radial head (Fig. 67-1)
  - Radial neck fractures
    - Acceptable alignment for radial neck fractures: 30 degrees or less of angulation and 3 mm or less of translocation
    - In adults, 45 degrees is acceptable if passive supination and pronation are 60 degrees in both directions.
- Goals of treatment
  - Pain reduction, restoration of normal forearm rotation
  - Slow the progression of arthritic change
- Additional findings
  - Evaluate for Essex-Lopresti lesion (fracture of the proximal radius causes proximal migration of the radius and subsequent ulnar positive variance resulting in wrist pain).
  - Lateral collateral ligament disruption if associated with dislocation
  - Medial collateral ligament injury
  - Chondral injury to the capitellum

History

- Symptoms: pain, limitation in elbow/forearm motion, weak grip
- Mechanism of injury
  - Radial head: fall onto outstretched upper extremity with axial load of radial head against capitellum
  - Radial neck: fall on an extended and supinated outstretched hand

Physical Examination

- Visual inspection: edema, ecchymosis
- Palpation: tenderness over the radial head
- Range of motion: Evaluate supination/pronation.
- Neurologic: Assess radial nerve function.
- Vascular: Check distal perfusion if it is associated with a dislocation.

Imaging

- Anterior and lateral views of elbow
- Greenspan: allows view of radiocapitellar joint
- Radiocapitellar (forearm neutral, beam 45 degrees cephalad)
- Computed tomography for confirmation of occult fracture or surgical planning

Differential Diagnosis

- Please see Table 67-1.

Treatment

Radial Head Fracture

- At diagnosis
  - Nondisplaced fractures with no block to motion: sling for comfort, elevation, pain control

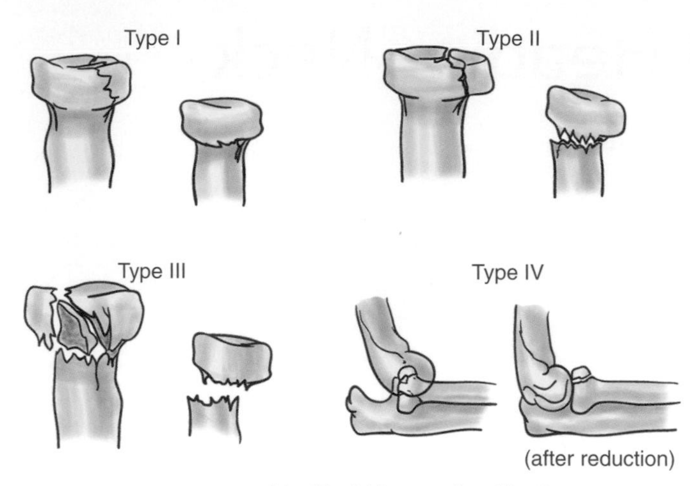

Figure 67-1 Modified Mason classification.

TABLE 67-1 *Differential Diagnosis*

Differential Diagnosis	Differentiating Features	Chapter Reference
Lateral epicondylitis	Tenderness to palpation directly over the lateral epicondyle and pain that is exacerbated by resisted wrist extension; normal radiographs	59
Posterolateral rotatory instability	Patient may report a history of dislocation or feeling of instability, clicking, or locking; positive lateral pivot shift test; magnetic resonance imaging helpful to identify injury of collateral ligaments	63
Insertional biceps tendinitis	Tenderness to palpation over distal biceps tendon at antecubital fossa; pain with resisted elbow flexion; normal radiographs	61
Radial tunnel syndrome	Tenderness to palpation over the mobile wad; normal radiographs	65

- Later
  - Recheck radiographs at 1- or 2-week intervals to evaluate for displacement.
  - Begin early range of motion exercises (within 2 weeks of injury)

Radial Neck Fracture

- At diagnosis
  - Minimally displaced fracture: Splint in 90 degrees of flexion and neutral rotation.

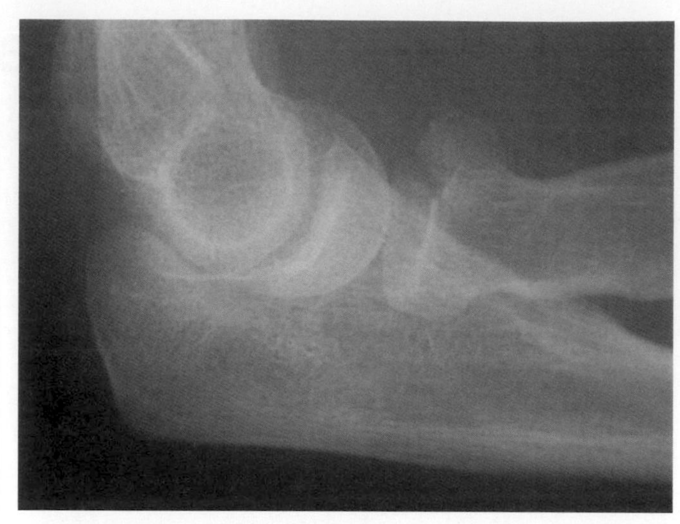

Figure 67-2 Lateral radiograph of radial head fracture.

- Later
  - Recheck radiographs to monitor for fracture displacement at 1- or 2-week intervals.
  - After 2 weeks, begin active range of motion.

When to Refer

Radial Head Fracture

- The following require operative management
  - Partial radial head fracture with block to motion
  - Partial radial head fracture with complex injury to the elbow
  - Comminuted fractures of radial head
- Operative Methods
  - Open reduction and internal fixation of the radial head (for three or fewer fragments)
  - Radial head excision (for more than three fragments)
  - Prosthetic replacement (for more than three fragments and longitudinal disruption of the forearm interosseous membrane) (Figs. 67-2 to 67-4)

Radial Neck Fracture

- Between 30 and 60 degrees of angulation or displaced: treatment can range from closed reduction under anesthesia to percutaneous Kirschner-wire fixation or open reduction and internal fixation.

Prognosis

- Patients with nondisplaced radial head and neck fractures can expect complete recovery and return of

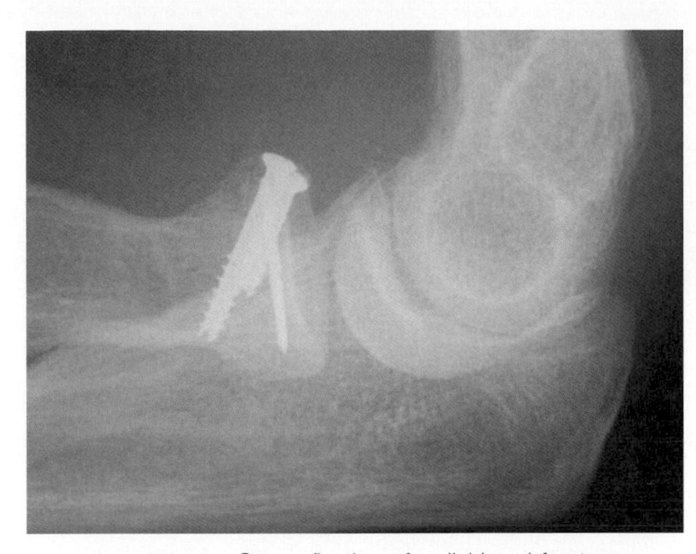

Figure 67-3 Screw fixation of radial head fracture.

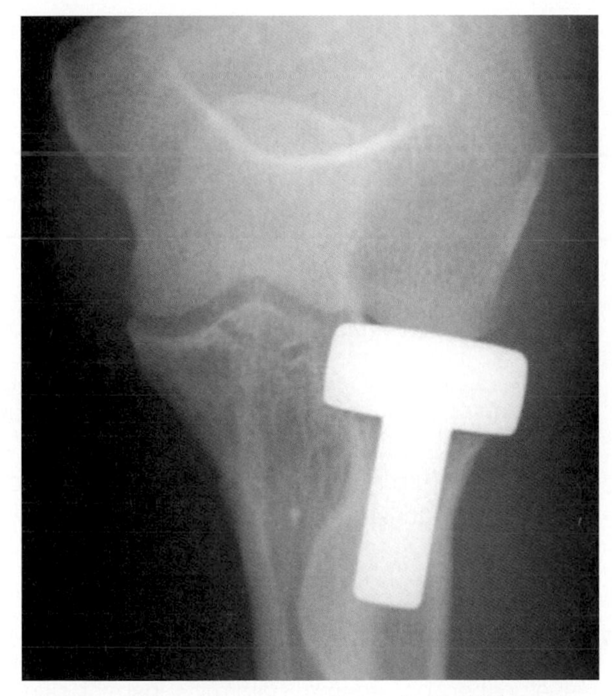

Figure 67-4 Anteroposterior radiograph of radial head replacement.

nearly full range of motion. Minimal loss of elbow extension can occur.

- Surgical treatment of displaced or comminuted fractures can significantly decrease morbidity related to range of motion. Most common complications after surgical reduction are instability, traumatic arthritis, and heterotopic ossification.

Troubleshooting

- Pain control is important in patients with acute nondisplaced fractures so that they may being early range of motion.
- It is important to recheck radiographs after a nondisplaced fracture to monitor for displacement.
- Patients presenting with a displaced radial head or neck fracture should always have a wrist evaluation to check for an Essex-Lopresti lesion. This should also be considered in patients who present with late-onset wrist pain after open reduction and internal fixation of the radial head, radial head excision, or arthroplasty.
- Chondral injuries can predispose a patient to the development of traumatic elbow arthritis.

Patient Instructions

- Encourage elevation, rest, and early motion.
- Avoid longitudinal pressure on the forearm for 6 to 8 weeks for both operative and nonoperative management.

Suggested Reading

- Goldberg I, Peylan J, Yosipovitch Z: Late results of excision of the radial head for isolated closed radial head fractures. J Bone Joint Surg Am 1986;68A:675–679.
- Koslowsky TC, Mader K, Gausepohl T, Pennig D: Reconstruction of Mason type-III and type-IV radial head fractures with a new fixation device: 23 patients followed 1-4 years. Acta Orthop 2007;78:151–156.
- Steele JA, Graham HK: Angulated radial neck fractures in children. A prospective study of percutaneous reduction. J Bone Joint Surg Br 1992;74B:760–764.

Chapter 68 Proximal Ulna Fractures

Rashard Dacus

ICD-9 CODES

813.00 *Proximal Forearm Fracture, Unspecified, Closed*
813.01 *Olecranon Process Fracture*
813.02 *Coronoid Process Fracture*
813.03 *Monteggia's Fracture*
813.07 *Proximal Ulna Fracture (Alone)*
813.10 *Proximal Forearm Fracture, Unspecified, Open*
813.11 *Olecranon Process Fracture*
813.12 *Coronoid Process Fracture*
813.13 *Monteggia's Fracture*
813.14 *Other Unspecified Fracture of the Proximal Ulna (Alone)*

Key Concepts

- Epidemiology
  - Coronoid fractures are identified in 10% to 15% of elbow dislocations.
  - As many as 30% of olecranon fractures are open.
  - Three percent to 5% have associated ulnar neuropraxia.
- Classification
  - Olecranon fractures
    - — Mayo: type I, nondisplaced or minimally displaced (<2 mm); type II, displacement of proximal fragment with stable elbow; type III, displacement of proximal fragment with instability of the ulnohumeral joint due to injury to ulnar collateral ligament; often there is an associated radial head fracture.
    - — Shatzker (fracture pattern): transverse; transverse, impacted; oblique; oblique/distal; comminuted; fracture/dislocation
  - Coronoid process fractures (usually occur in conjunction with elbow dislocation with or without radial head fracture; termed "terrible triad" if all three present)
    - — Type I: coronoid tip fracture
    - — Type II: 50% or less may be single fragment or comminuted
    - — Type III: greater than 50% of process
  - Monteggia's fracture: fracture of the proximal or middle third ulna with dislocation of the radial head
    - — Type I (most common): anterior dislocation of radial head; fracture of ulnar diaphysis
    - — Type II: posterior or posterolateral dislocation of radial head; fracture of ulnar diaphysis
    - — Type III: lateral or anterolateral dislocation of radial head; ulnar metaphysis fracture
    - — Type IV (rare): anterior dislocation of radial head; fracture of both forearm bones
- Goals of treatment
  - Articular restoration, stability, preservation of range of motion (ROM)
- Associated findings
  - Have a high suspicion for associated fractures or ligamentous injuries: Monteggia's fracture, distal humerus fracture, elbow dislocation, coronoid process fracture, radial head or neck fracture, collateral ligament injury.

History

- Symptoms: pain, inability to extend arm at the elbow, instability
- Mechanism of injury: direct blow to posterior elbow, fall on outstretched hand, or direct fall on flexed elbow

Physical Examination

- Visual inspection: edema, deformity, inspect skin for laceration/puncture
- Palpation: crepitus along posterior elbow
- Range of motion may be limited due to pain; active motion can be limited by separation of the triceps insertion from the ulnar shaft.
  - Important to assess integrity of collateral ligaments in varus and valgus stress in flexion and extension
- Neurologic: Assess motor and sensory function distal with special attention to median, ulnar, and radial nerve (posterior interosseous nerve).
- Vascular: Assess pulses and capillary refill.

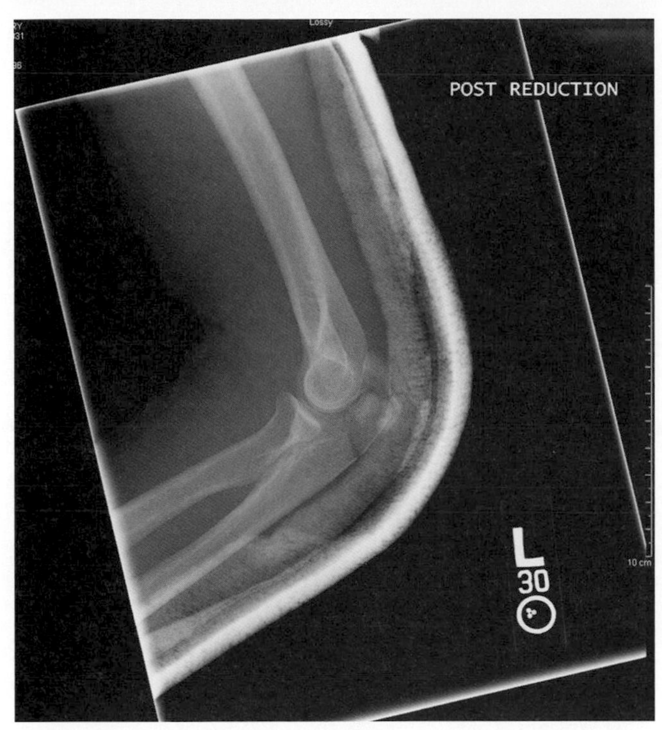

Figure 68-1 Lateral radiograph of olecranon fracture.

Imaging

- Radiographs: anteroposterior, lateral, and oblique views of the elbow
- Lateral radiograph may show displacement of coronoid process or olecranon; assess for articular involvement and comminution in this view (Fig. 68-1).

Additional Tests

- Computed tomography to assess coronoid fragment or associated distal humerus fracture

Differential Diagnosis

- Please see Table 68-1.

TABLE 68-1 *Differential Diagnosis*

Differential Diagnosis	Differentiating Feature	Chapter Reference
Olecranon bursitis	Normal radiographs; large soft-tissue swelling over posterior aspect of olecranon process	64
Bony contusion	Normal radiographs; may confirm on more advanced imaging such as magnetic resonance imaging	56
Elbow dislocation	Evidence of dislocation on radiographs or computed tomography scan; chronic dislocations may present with history of popping or clicking; perform lateral pivot shift test	63

Treatment

Olecranon Fractures

- At diagnosis
  - Nonoperative management: place into long arm posterior splint or cast with the elbow in 90 degrees of flexion, forearm neutral
- Later
  - Obtain radiographs at 2-week intervals to monitor for displacement.
  - Begin gentle ROM therapy at 3 weeks and avoid flexing the elbow past 90 degrees with the use of a hinged elbow brace.
  - May progress to full active ROM at 6 to 8 weeks

When to Refer

- Types II and III or evidence of disruption of extensor mechanism
  - Refer to orthopaedic surgeon for operative management.

Operative Methods

- Intramedullary fixation with cancellous lag screw fixation (6.5 mm versus 7 mm)
- Tension band wiring with two parallel Kirschner wires
- Plating: 3.5 mm dynamic compression plating (Fig. 68-2)

Coronoid Process Fractures

- At diagnosis
  - Nonoperative as long as the elbow is stable and there is no block to motion
  - Reduce elbow dislocation if present.
  - Splint elbow in approximately 90 degrees of flexion for 2 to 3 weeks.
- Later
  - Recheck radiographs for fracture displacement and maintenance of elbow reduction.
  - Reassess elbow for stability. If unstable, continue splinting for an additional 1 to 2 weeks. If stable, begin protected active ROM in a hinged elbow brace.

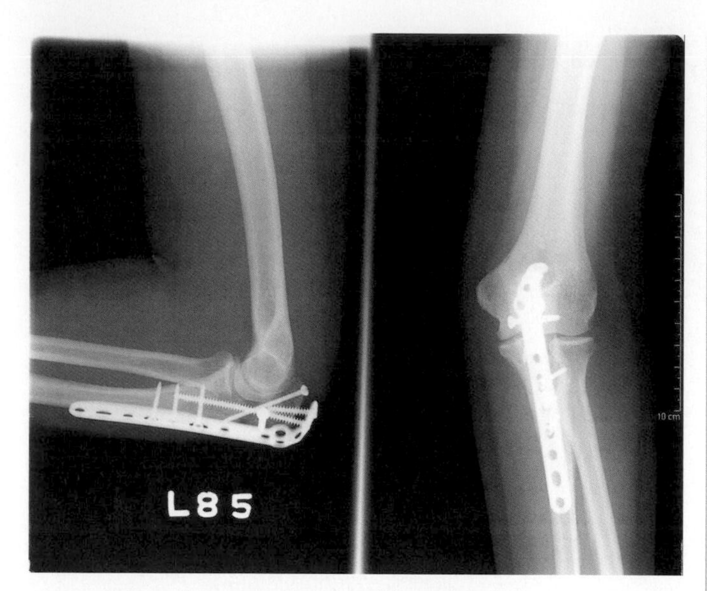

Figure 68-2 Anteroposterior and lateral radiographs of olecranon plating.

When to Refer

- Type II: Assess elbow stability; if stable, fracture may be managed as a type I; if unstable, refer for surgical management.
- Type III: All fractures considered unstable; refer for operative management.

Monteggia's Fractures

- Now
  - Attempt reduction of radial head under conscious sedation and splint in long arm posterior elbow splint.

When to Refer

- Nearly all Monteggia's fractures will require open reduction and internal fixation. Refer all fractures to an orthopaedic surgeon.

Prognosis

- Olecranon fractures: Types I and II fractures have a good prognosis and minimal loss of motion. Type III fractures have less favorable results with the most common complication being loss of ROM.
- Coronoid process fractures: Type I fractures have an excellent prognosis. Type II and III fractures frequently are associated with some loss of ROM.
- Monteggia's fractures: high incidence of injury to posterior interosseous nerve in acute setting, but this usually resolves after reduction of radial head

Troubleshooting

- When treating these fractures nonoperatively, it is important to recheck radiographs on a weekly or biweekly basis to monitor for late displacement, which can cause significant morbidity.
- Early protected ROM is essential to limit motion loss.

Patient Instructions

- Injured extremity is to be nonweight bearing for 4 to 6 weeks.
- Patients may require therapy to regain ROM.
- Potential for as much as 15 degrees of loss of extension
- Operative patients may begin ROM after suture removal.
- Olecranon process fractures may require hardware removal due to prominence (after 4–6 months).

Suggested Reading

- Hak DJ, Golladay GJ: Olecranon fractures: Treatment options. J Am Acad Orthop Surg 2000;8:266–275.
- Horner SR, Sadasivan KK, Lipka JM, Saha S: Analysis of mechanical factors affecting fixation of olecranon fractures. Orthopedics 1989;12:1469–1472.
- Murphy DF, Greene WB, Gilbert JA, Dameron TB Jr: Displaced olecranon fractures in adults. Biomechanical analysis of fixation methods. Clin Orthop Relat Res 1987;224:210–214.

Chapter 69 Radial and Ulnar Shaft Fractures

Rashard Dacus

ICD-9 CODES
813.21 *Radial Shaft, Closed*
813.22 *Ulnar Shaft, Closed*
813.23 *Radius and Ulnar Shaft, Closed*
813.31 *Radial Shaft, Open*
813.32 *Ulnar Shaft, Open*
813.33 *Radius and Ulnar Shaft, Open*

Key Concepts

- Fractures may occur as isolated single-bone fractures of the radius or ulna, both-bone fractures, or fracture-dislocations (Galeazzi's fracture).
- Deforming forces on radius
  - Proximal one third: The proximal fragment is supinated and flexed due to the biceps and supinator muscles; the distal fragment is pronated due to the pronator teres and quadratus muscles.
  - Middle one third: The proximal fragment is held in a neutral position due to the balance between the supinator and pronator teres muscles; the distal fragment is pronated by the pronator quadratus muscles.
  - Distal one third: The distal fragment of the radius is pronated and pulled toward the ulna.
- Classification
  - Transverse, oblique, spiral
  - Comminuted
  - Closed versus open
  - Proximal, diaphyseal, distal
    - — Piedmont (fracture of the junction of the middle one third and distal one third of the radius)
- Galeazzi's fracture is defined as a distal third radial shaft fracture with distal radioulnar joint dislocation.
- Goals of treatment: restore alignment, maintain forearm rotation
- Additional findings: Be aware of the potential for compartment syndrome.

History

- Symptoms: pain, edema, difficulty with motion of the wrist/fingers, pronation/supination
- Mechanism of injury: direct blow to forearm, Galeazzi's fracture, fall on outstretched hand with forearm in pronation

Physical Examination

- Visual inspection: deformity, skin integrity
- Palpation: crepitus
- Physical inspection: Assess joints proximal and distal to the injury including the elbow and distal radioulnar joint for instability.
- Range of motion: limited due to pain
- Neurologic: Assess motor and sensory function distal to site of injury.
- Vascular: palpation of radial and ulnar pulses, Allen's test, cap refill

Imaging

- Radial and ulnar fractures
  - Anteroposterior, lateral, oblique forearm (Fig. 69-1)
- Radial shaft fractures (Galeazzi variant)
  - Anteroposterior, lateral, oblique forearm (Figs. 69-2 and 69-3)
- Ulnar shaft fractures
  - Anteroposterior, lateral, oblique forearm (Fig. 69-4)

Differential Diagnosis

- Please see Table 69-1.

Treatment

Radial and Ulnar Fractures

- At diagnosis
  - Only nondisplaced fractures may be managed nonoperatively and must be monitored closely for displacement due to deforming forces.
  - Nonoperative management is generally not recommended in the adult population.

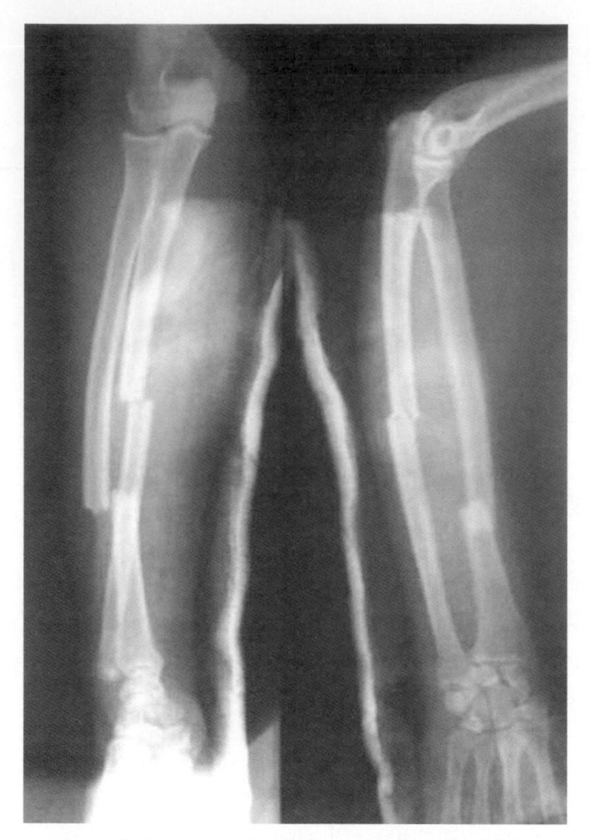

Figure 69-1 Anteroposterior (*left*) and lateral (*right*) radiographs of right both-bone forearm fracture.

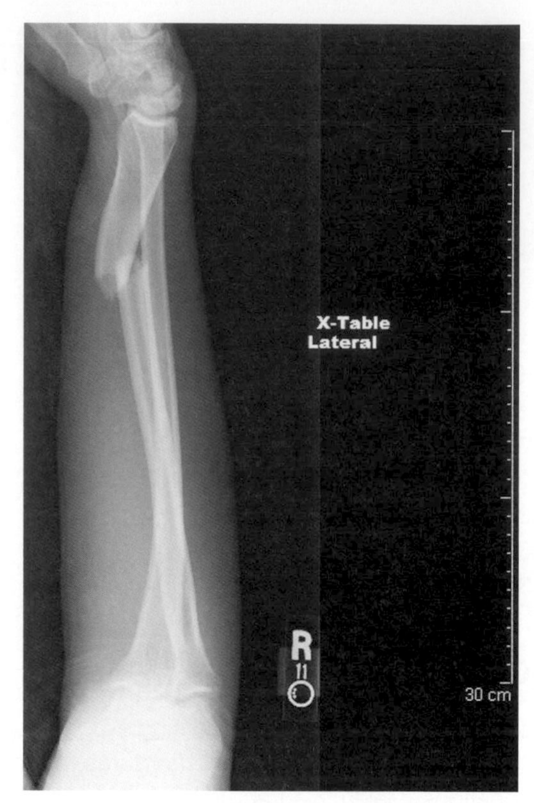

Figure 69-3 Lateral radiograph of Galeazzi's fracture.

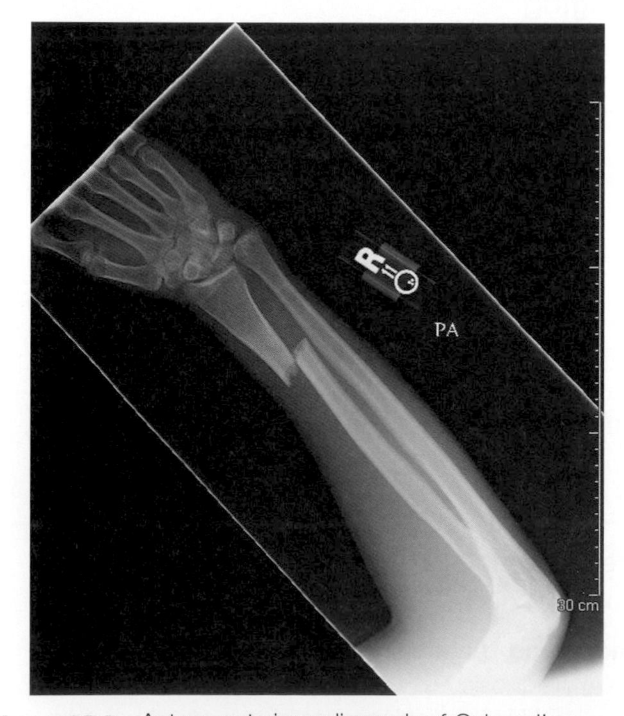

Figure 69-2 Anteroposterior radiograph of Galeazzi's fracture.

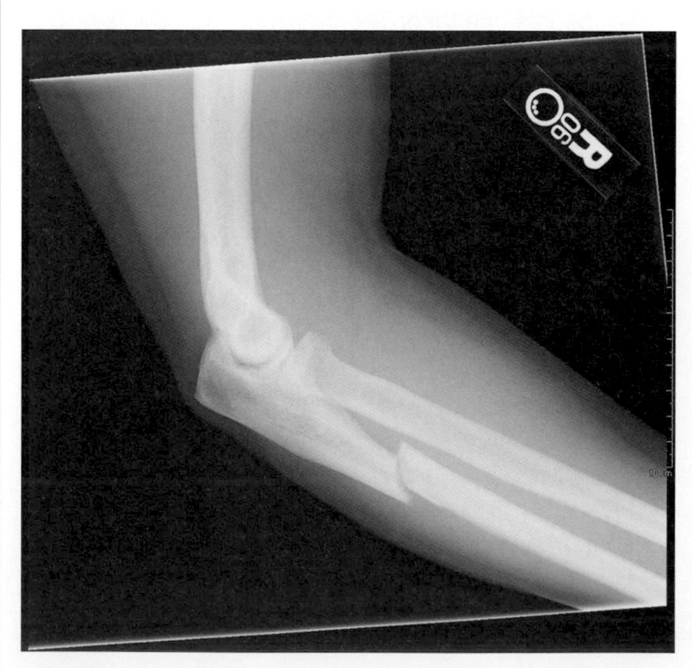

Figure 69-4 Lateral radiograph of proximal third ulnar shaft fracture.

TABLE 69-1 *Differential Diagnosis*

Differential Diagnosis	Differentiating Features	Chapter Reference
Both-bone forearm fracture	Radiographic evaluation	69
Isolated radius or ulna fracture	Radiographic evaluation	67–69

- Apply long arm posterior splint with elbow in 90 degrees of flexion and refer to orthopaedist for monitoring.

When to Refer

- All displaced and/or open fractures should be referred to an orthopaedic surgeon for operative management.
- Operative methods
  - Internal fixation, plate fixation (3.5-mm dynamic compression plate)
  - External fixation: for open injuries with gross contamination, severe soft-tissue loss, infected nonunion, or open elbow fracture-dislocation
  - Intramedullary nailing

Radial Shaft Fractures

- At diagnosis
  - Nondisplaced fractures may be managed nonoperatively. Apply a a sugar tong splint or Muenster cast if there is minimal edema.
- Later
  - Recheck radiographs at 2 weeks to monitor for displacement. Apply a Muenster cast for 4 weeks.
  - Recheck radiographs to evaluate for healing. If the fracture has healed, transition the patient into a brace for protection and begin gentle range of motion therapy.

When to Refer

- Displaced, angulated, or open fractures require open reduction and internal fixation.
- Operative methods: plating (3.5-mm dynamic compression plate) (Fig. 69-5)

Ulnar Shaft Fractures

- At diagnosis
  - Nondisplaced fractures with less than 10 degrees of angulation and less than 50% displacement of the ulnar shaft in any plane may be treated nonoperatively. Apply a sugar tong splint if edema is present or a short arm cast for 10 days.

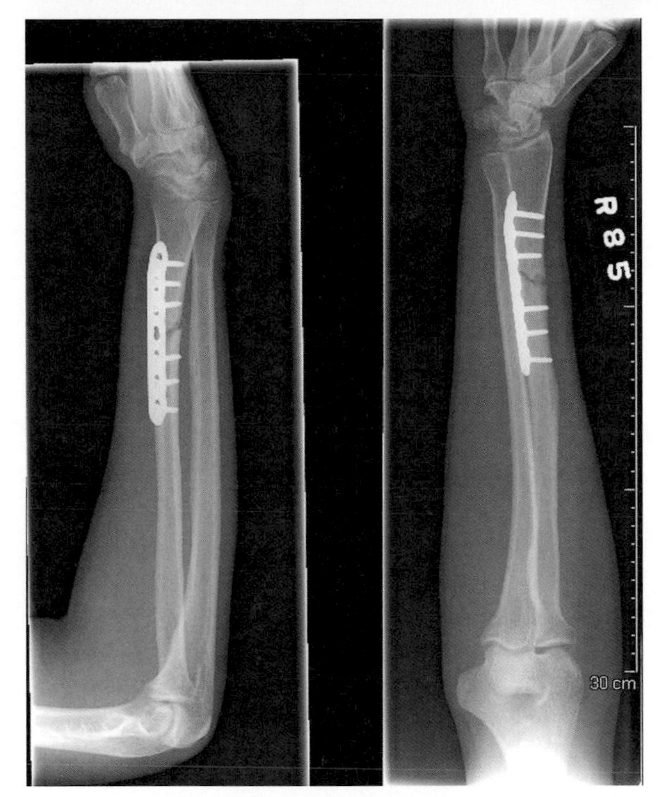

Figure 69-5 Oblique (*left*) and lateral (*right*) radiographs of plating of right distal third radial shaft

- Later
  - Recheck radiographs at 10 days and transition the patient to a short arm cast or a functional forearm brace for 4 to 6 weeks. Recheck radiographs every week for 3 weeks to monitor for displacement.

When to Refer

- Displaced fractures with more than 10 degrees of angulation or more than 50% of ulnar shaft displacement; apply a sugar tong splint and refer to an orthopaedic surgeon within 1 week of injury.
- Operative methods: plating (3.5-mm dynamic compression plate) (Fig. 69-6)

Galeazzi's Fractures

- At diagnosis
  - Attempt reduction of the distal radioulnar joint and apply a sugar tong splint. Refer to an orthopaedic surgeon for surgical reduction and fixation.

Prognosis

- Early range of motion therapy in both-bone forearm fractures results in a good functional outcome.

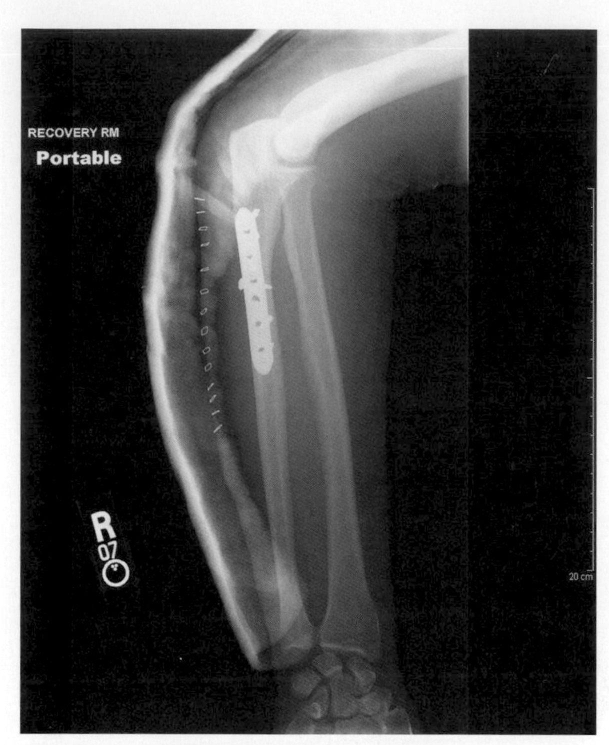

Figure 69-6 Lateral radiograph of plating of ulnar shaft with reduced radial head.

Troubleshooting

- Always assess the wrist to ensure that the radius is not shortened and the distal radioulnar joint is not disrupted.
- Always assess the elbow for instability or associated fracture.
- Always assess for compartment syndrome in the acute setting.

Considerations in Special Populations

- Athletes: Refer to an orthopaedic surgeon because operative interventions can sometimes allow earlier return to play.

Patient Instructions

- Elevate arm.
- Alert someone if there is loss of sensation, perfusion, or excessive pain.
- No weight bearing for 4 to 6 weeks

Suggested Reading

- Dymond IW: Treatment of isolated fractures of the distal ulna. J Bone Joint Surg Br 1984;66B:408–410.
- Grace TG, Eversmann WW Jr: Forearm fractures: Treatment by rigid fixation with early motion. J Bone Joint Surg Am 1980;62A:433–438.
- Mekhail AO, Ebraheim NA, Jackson WT, Yeasting RA: Anatomic consideration for the anterior exposure of the proximal portion of the radius. J Hand Surg [Am] 1996;21:794–801.
- Mih AD, Cooney WP, Idler RS, Lewallen DG: Long-term follow-up of forearm bone diaphyseal plating. Clin Orthop Relat Res 1994;299:256–258.
- Szabo RM, Skinner M: Isolated ulnar shaft fractures. A retrospective study of 46 cases. Acta Orthop Scand 1990;61:350–352.

Chapter 70 Reduction of Elbow Dislocations

Rashard Dacus

CPT CODES
24600 *Closed Reduction of Elbow Dislocation without Anesthesia*
24605 *Closed Reduction of Elbow Dislocation with Anesthesia*

Equipment

- Conscious sedation, IV analgesia, or intra-articular hematoma block (see Chapter 71)
- Stretcher or examining table
- 2- to 5-kg weight for traction is optional and may replace manual traction
- An assistant may be used to provide brachial countertraction, but this is not always necessary.
- Plaster or fiberglass splint material
- Cotton webril and/or stocking net
- 4-inch elastic bandage

Indications

- Simple (without fracture) and complex (with fracture) elbow dislocations

Contraindications

- None

Technique

- A thorough neurovascular examination should be performed and documented before reduction.
- Once the patient is sedated or the analgesic agent has taken effect, position the patient prone on the examining table with the afflicted extremity hanging over the edge.
- Parvin method
  - With the arm hanging over the edge of the table from the shoulder, apply manual downward traction (or use a 2- to 5-kg weight) from the wrist for a few minutes.
  - Place one hand on the patient's wrist and provide downward traction; place the other hand under the patient's elbow on the antecubital fossa.
  - While applying downward traction, gently push up on the antecubital fossa, lifting the elbow, and allow the olecranon to reduce into the fossa.
- Alternate method
  - Position the patient prone with the forearm only hanging from the table or stretcher.
  - Apply pressure to the medial or lateral olecranon process to correct translation as necessary.
  - Place one hand on the patient's wrist and apply downward traction and light supination to distract the coronoid from the olecranon fossa.
  - Use the other hand to apply pressure to the posterior olecranon while pronating the forearm.
  - Conclude with flexion of the elbow.
  - Reduction is achieved when a "clunk" is palpated.
- Passive range of motion to within 20 degrees of full extension implies stability; apply a posterior long arm splint with the elbow in 90 degrees of flexion and the forearm neutral.
- If the elbow is unstable through passive range of motion, re-reduce and apply a posterior long arm splint with the elbow in 90 degrees of flexion and the forearm in pronation.
- Perform postreduction neurovascular examination and document it.
- Obtain postreduction anteroposterior and lateral view radiographs.

Troubleshooting

- Ensure that the patient is adequately sedated.
- Multiple attempts or techniques may need to be used to achieve reduction.
- Always obtain postreduction radiographs.
- Avoid lateral splinting until after the lateral radiographs have been taken to better see the coronoid.

- If one cannot achicve reduction, there may be superimposed tissue or loose bodies, which may require open reduction.
- If the elbow is unstable at 90 degrees, admit the patient for operative stabilization.
- Assess the neurologic examination after reduction and document it.
- If the neurovascular examination is worsening after reduction, obtain immediate orthopaedic consult.

Complications

- Median nerve or brachial artery injury

Postreduction Management

- Observe the patient for 2 to 3 hours and recheck the neurovascular examination before discharge.
- Follow up at 1 to 2 weeks after injury and begin gentle range of motion therapy for simple elbow dislocations.
- For complex elbow dislocations, follow up within 1 week of injury. Further management depends on the fracture pattern.

Patient Instructions

- Keep the splint clean and dry.
- Do not remove the splint until the return appointment.
- Alert someone if there is loss of perfusion or sensation or if excessive pain develops.
- Loss of terminal extension after elbow dislocation is common.
- May require formal therapy to optimize range of motion

Suggested Reading

- Dürig M, Müller W, Rüedi TP, Gauer EF: The operative treatment of elbow dislocation in the adult. J Bone Joint Surg Am 1979;61A:239–244.
- Hotchkiss RN: Fractures and dislocations of the elbow. In Rockwood CA Jr, Green DP, Bucholz RW, Heckman JD (eds): Rockwood and Green's Fractures in Adults, vol. 1, 4th ed. Philadelphia: Lippincott-Raven, 1996, pp 929–1024.
- Josefsson PO, Johnell O, Gentz CF: Long-term sequelae of simple dislocation of the elbow. J Bone Joint Surg Am 1984;66A:927–930.
- O'Driscoll SW: Elbow dislocations. In Morrey B (ed): The Elbow and Its Disorders, 3rd ed. Philadelphia: Saunders, 2000, pp 409–420.
- Ross G, McDevitt ER, Chronister R: The treatment of simple elbow dislocations using an immediate motion protocol. Am J Sports Med 1999:27;308–311.

Chapter 71 Injection or Aspiration of the Elbow Joint

Cay Mierisch

CPT CODE
20610 *Aspiration and/or Injection of a Major Joint or Bursa*

Key Concepts

- Aspiration of the elbow joint allows examination of intra-articular effusions and aids in the diagnosis of multiple conditions affecting the elbow.
- Injection of the elbow allows the instillation of medication that can aid in the treatment of diseases affecting the elbow.
- The most common injection performed consists of steroid medication for arthritic conditions.

Equipment (Fig. 71-1)

- 21-Gauge needle
- 1% Lidocaine
- 10 to 40 mg triamcinolone acetonide or similar agent
- Disinfectant
- Sterile gloves
- Gauze
- Bandage

Contraindications

- Skin ulcerations
- Rash
- Adverse reaction to either medication
- Brittle diabetes mellitus

Instructions/Technique

- The preferred access to the elbow joint is through the so-called soft spot, which can be palpated posterior to the radiocapitellar joint, anterior to the olecranon.
- Use sterile technique.
- Disinfect the area on the posterolateral aspect of the elbow.
- Rest the elbow on the table in flexion with the forearm in neutral rotation and the shoulder in internal rotation while the patient is sitting on a chair.
- Palpate the lateral epicondyle and radiocapitellar joint.
- Gentle forearm rotation will aid in the identification of the radial head.
- Move the palpating finger posteriorly toward the olecranon and identify the soft spot. Effusions are commonly palpable in this area.
- Aiming the needle medially and anteriorly, enter the joint through the center of the soft spot.
- Joint fluid can then be aspirated and injection performed as indicated.

Considerations in Special Populations

- Advanced arthritic changes may make it difficult to enter the elbow joint. Fluoroscope-assisted insertion of the needle is recommended in that case.
- In very obese patients, landmarks may be difficult to identify and a fluoroscope-assisted injection may be preferable.
- Diabetic patients often react with a transient increase in the blood sugar level, which may last several days. It is important to make the patients aware of this and ask them to closely monitor the blood sugar levels.

Troubleshooting

- Patients with a history of vasovagal reactions may prefer a supine position. The elbow is positioned on a pillow with the shoulder in full external rotation and abduction.
- Injection should not encounter any resistance. If resistance is encountered, it indicates the extra-articular location of the needle tip.

Patient Instructions

- The patient needs to be informed about the risks and complications of the procedure, and verbal or written consent should be obtained.

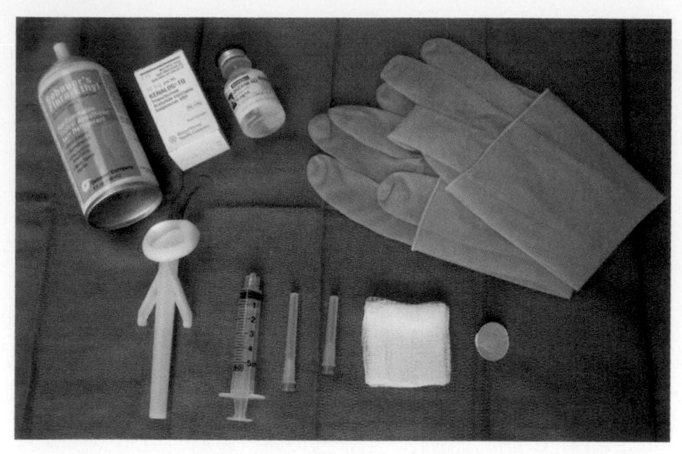

Figure 71-1 Equipment needed for injection or aspiration of the elbow joint.

- Tell the patient to expect some soreness after the local anesthetic wears off. Recommend the use of an over-the-counter pain medication to treat this, preferably a nonsteroidal anti-inflammatory drug.
- The patient should resume stretching exercises and the use of any ancillary braces.
- Symptoms should be monitored for 4 to 6 weeks, followed by re-examination.

Chapter 72 Lateral Epicondylitis (Tennis Elbow) Injection

Cay Mierisch

CPT CODE

20550 *Injection of a Tendon Sheath, Ligament, Trigger Point, or Cyst*

Key Concepts

- This procedure could also be termed tennis elbow injection.
- It often is incorrectly referred to as injection of the lateral epicondyle, but rather consists of an injection distal to the epicondyle into the common extensor origin.

Equipment

- 21-Gauge needle
- 1% Lidocaine
- 10 to 40 mg triamcinolone acetonide or similar agent
- Disinfectant
- Sterile gloves
- Gauze
- Bandage

Contraindications

- Acute infections
- Skin ulcerations
- Rash
- Adverse reaction to either medication
- Brittle diabetes mellitus

Instructions/Technique

- Use sterile technique.
- Disinfect the area on the lateral aspect of the elbow.
- Rest the elbow on the table in flexion with the forearm in neutral rotation and the shoulder in slight abduction, while the patient is sitting on a chair.
- Palpate the lateral epicondyle; it is palpable posterior to the brachioradialis muscle belly.
- Slide approximately 1 cm distal and feel the common extensor tendon; palpation in that area will typically cause tenderness and confirm the correct location.
- Insert the needle at a 45-degree angle in a distal to proximal direction aiming slightly anteriorly toward the lateral epicondyle. The radial nerve is at risk if you aim too far anteriorly.
- Ascertain that you have entered the common extensor tendon before you start the injection to avoid skin changes secondary to the steroid medication.
- Contact with bone confirms the correct depth of the needle.

Considerations in Special Populations

- In very obese patients, landmarks may be difficult to identify and a fluoroscope-assisted injection maybe preferable.
- Diabetic patients often react with a transient increase in the blood sugar level, which may last several days.
  - It is important to make the patients aware of this and ask them to closely monitor the blood sugar levels.

Troubleshooting

- Patients with a history of vasovagal reactions may prefer a supine position.
  - The elbow can be rested on a pillow next to the patient with the forearm across the patient and the shoulder in internal rotation.

Patient Instructions

- The patient needs to be informed about the risks and complications of the procedure, and verbal or written consent should be obtained.

- Tell the patient to expect some soreness after the local anaesthetic wears off.
    - Recommend the use of an over-the-counter pain medication to treat this, preferably a nonsteroidal anti-inflammatory drug.
- The patient should resume stretching exercises and the use of any ancillary braces.
- Symptoms should be monitored for 4 to 6 weeks, followed by re-examination.

Chapter 73 Medial Epicondylitis (Golfer's Elbow) Injection

Cay Mierisch

CPT CODE

20550 *Injection of Tendon Sheath, Ligament, Trigger Point, or Cyst*

Key Concepts

- This procedure is also termed golfer's elbow injection.
- The anatomic structure that is to be injected is the flexor-pronator muscle origin just distal to the medial epicondyle.

Equipment

- 21-Gauge needle
- 1% Lidocaine
- 10 to 40 mg triamcinolone acetonide or similar agent
- Disinfectant
- Sterile gloves
- Gauze
- Bandage

Contraindications

- Acute infections
- Skin ulcerations
- Rash
- Adverse reaction to either medication
- Brittle diabetes mellitus
- Previous ulnar nerve transposition

Instructions/Technique

- Use sterile technique.
- Disinfect the area on the medial aspect of the elbow.
- Rest the elbow on the table in flexion with the forearm supinated and the shoulder in external rotation, with the patient sitting on a chair.
- Palpate the medial epicondyle and the ulnar nerve.
- Ascertain that the ulnar nerve is not subluxing.
- Slide approximately 1 cm distal from the medial epicondyle and feel the common tendon of the flexor-pronator muscle group; palpation in this area will typically cause tenderness and confirm the correct location.
- Insert the needle at a 45-degree angle in a distal to proximal direction, aiming slightly anteriorly toward the medial epicondyle.
- Once in contact with the medial epicondyle, retract the needle slightly and start injecting.
- Avoid the median nerve anteriorly and the ulnar nerve posteriorly.
- Avoid injecting the skin and subcutaneous tissue to avoid skin changes secondary to the steroid medication.

Considerations in Special Populations

- In very obese patients, landmarks may be difficult to identify and a fluoroscope-assisted injection may be preferable.
- Diabetic patients often react with a transient increase in the blood sugar level, which may last several days. It is important to make the patients aware of this and ask them to closely monitor the blood sugar levels.

Troubleshooting

- Patients with a history of vasovagal reactions may prefer a supine position. The elbow is positioned on a pillow with the shoulder in full external rotation and abduction.

Patient Instructions

- The patient needs to be informed about the risks and complications of the procedure, and verbal or written consent should be obtained.
- Tell the patient to expect some soreness after the local anesthetic wears off. Recommend the use of an over-the-counter pain medication to treat this, preferably a nonsteroidal anti-inflammatory drug.
- The patient should resume stretching exercises and the use of any ancillary braces.
- Symptoms should be monitored for 4 to 6 weeks, followed by re-examination.

Chapter 74 Olecranon Bursa Aspiration/Injection

César J. Bravo

CPT CODE
20605 *Aspiration and/or Injection of Intermediate Bursa*

Key Concepts

- Olecranon bursa may become inflamed or septic, and aspiration may be indicated.
  - This is a technically reproducible technique secondary to the superficial location of the olecranon bursa.
- The bursa may become inflamed secondary to trauma, repetitive shear forces across the olecranon process, or excessive pressure along this area.
- The fluid may consist of blood in acute trauma, purulent material if infected, or thick proteinaceous fluid after repetitive injury.
- Therapeutic corticosteroid injection can be carried out once septic bursitis has been excluded.

Equipment (Fig. 74-1)

- 20-mL syringe
- 3-mL syringe for additional injection
- 18-gauge, 1½-inch needle
- 25-gauge, 1½-inch needle
- 1 mL of 1% lidocaine without epinephrine
- 1 mL of steroid solution of choice (we use 40 mg triamcinolone acetonide)
- Alcohol pads
- 3-mL Chloraprep skin applicator (chlorhexidine gluconate, 2% wt/vol; isopropyl alcohol, 70% wt/vol)
- Sterile gauze pads
- Sterile adhesive bandage
- Nonsterile, clean chuck pads
- Topical anesthetic skin refrigerant, optional (we use Gebauer's Fluro-Ethyl spray [75% wt/vol; dichlorotetrafluoroethane, 25% vol/vol ethyl chloride])

Contraindications

- Open wound with exposed olecranon
- Uncooperative patient

Instructions (Fig. 74-2)

- Patient position
  - Sitting if examining patient on hand table
  - The affected elbow is flexed to 45 degrees without maximal flexion to gain adequate access to the bursa. Too much flexion may shift fluid within the bursa making aspiration difficult.
- Landmarks
  - Point of maximum fluid fluctuance is noted at this position.
  - Usually this point is in line with the olecranon process.
- Establish sterile field
  - Have the patient wash his or her hand and elbow with soap and water before injection.
  - Use Chloraprep to establish sterile field once elbow is positioned over a nonsterile chuck pad (alcohol and povidone-iodine pads can be used to establish sterile field as alternative options).
- Anesthesia
  - Infiltrate 3 mL of 1% lidocaine into the planned area of aspiration.
  - Local anesthesia of the skin with topical vapocoolant spray before infiltration of area
- Technique
  - With sterile gloves and local anesthetic agent in place, introduce 18-gauge needle in the center of the bursa
  - Aspiration with a 20-mL syringe is performed. If a large collection of fluid is suspected, do not overtighten the needle to the syringe so that the syringe can easily be exchanged when full, leaving the needle in place.

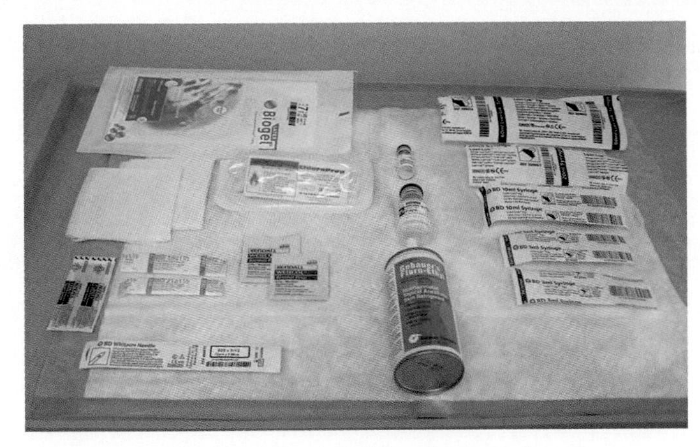

Figure 74-1 Equipment needed for olecranon bursa aspiration/injection.

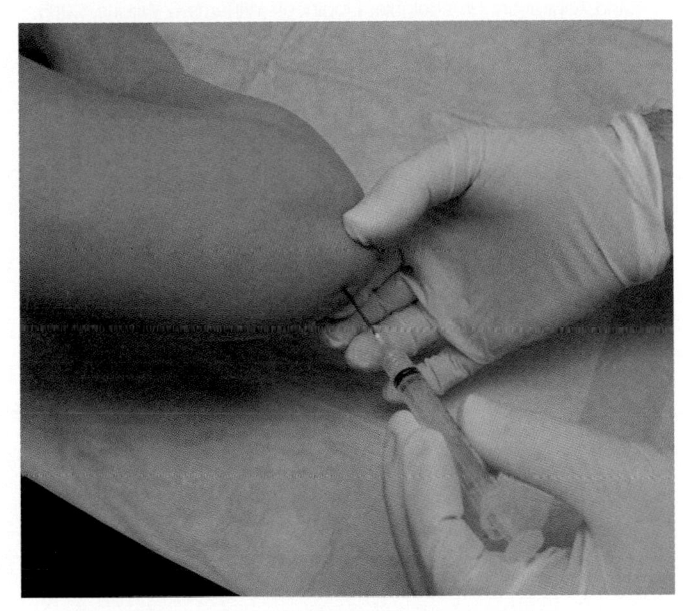

Figure 74-2 Olecranon bursa aspiration.

- If injection is planned after aspiration, grasp the hub of the needle with a hemostat or a free finger if it is not placed too tightly. Then attach the 3-mL syringe with steroid solution.
- If resistance is met, advance or withdraw the needle slightly before attempting further injection.
- Aftercare
  - Apply a sterile adhesive bandage followed by a compressive tube dressing (if compressive tube dressing is not available, an elastic bandage may also be used).
  - Re-examine the elbow after 5 minutes to confirm pain relief and no active bleeding or drainage sites.
  - Instruct the patient to avoid excessive use or heavy lifting of the elbow for the next 2 weeks.
  - Consider using a neoprene elbow sleeve or elastic compressive bandage (e.g., heelbow pad).
  - Consider re-evaluation at 2 weeks for examination and documentation of effective aspiration/injection and to be certain that no complications have arisen.

Considerations in Special Populations

- People with an active skin lesion (e.g., psoriasis, eczema) are not ideal candidates for aspiration because of increased risk of infection.
- If acute hemorrhage or septic bursitis is suspected, do not follow aspiration with a corticosteroid injection.
- Inform diabetic patients of a possible glycemic rise secondary to corticosteroid injection (usually transient and minimal).
- In dark-skinned individuals, skin hypopigmentation is more noticeable and patients should be informed of this.

Troubleshooting

- To diminish skin hypopigmentation and skin atrophy, we recommend pinching up tissue to avoid subcutaneous corticosteroid injection. This creates greater distance between the skin and actual injection site.
- Corticosteroid is used mainly for recurrent olecranon bursitis.
- Patients with gouty arthritis may have a high recurrence of bursitis and increased risk of infection secondary to multiple aspirations. These patients benefit from early referral to a specialist for open elbow bursectomy and tophi removal.
- When aspiration is done for suspected septic bursitis, send aspirate for culture and sensitivity; cell counts (white blood cell [WBC] and red blood cell); aerobic, anaerobic, fungal, and mycobacterial organisms; and crystal evaluation.
  - The leukocyte count can help determine whether the fluid is infectious or inflammatory.
  - Within synovial aspirates, WBC counts are assessed as follows:
    — A WBC count less than 200/mL is considered normal.
    — A WBC count of 200 to 2000/mL is considered noninflammatory.
    — A WBC count in the range of 2000 to 100,000/mL is considered an indication of inflammation.
    — A WBC count greater than 100,000/mL is considered an indication of a septic condition.
  - Gram stain also is helpful to determine quickly whether bacterial infection is present.

- If the Gram stain results are positive, antibiotics should be started immediately and bursal corticosteroid injection should be avoided.
- If the Gram stain results are negative or initially unavailable, antibiotics may be indicated based on the mechanism of injury, physical examination findings suggestive of infection, or the gross appearance of the aspirate.
- Gram stain can be followed by culture and sensitivity testing. The culture and sensitivity results should guide the use of antibiotics in cases of bacterial infection.
- Crystal analysis may reveal monosodium urate crystals in a patient with gout, calcium pyrophosphate crystals in a patient with pseudogout, or hydroxyapatite crystals.

Patient Instructions

- The patient is to keep the dressing in place for 48 hours.
- Some patients with corticosteroid injections may experience a flare, which improves in 48 to 72 hours and is managed with nonsteroidal anti-inflammatory drugs.
- If a patient experiences fever, chills, or exquisite pain, he or she should contact a physician immediately to rule out a septic process.

Suggested Reading (see also Chapter 64)

- McNabb JW: A Practical Guide to Joint and Soft Tissue Injection and Aspiration. Philadelphia: Lippincott Williams & Wilkins, 2005, p 133.

4

SECTION

The Wrist and Hand

Chapter 75 Overview of the Wrist and Hand

Jennifer A. Hart

Anatomy

- The wrist is made up of several articulations including the distal radioulnar joint, the ulnocarpal joint, the radiocarpal joint, and the carpometacarpal joints (Fig. 75-1).
- The hand is made up of five metacarpal bones. Each metacarpal articulates with the corresponding proximal phalanx (metacarpophalangeal [MCP] joint), which in turn articulates with the middle phalanx (proximal interphalangeal [PIP] joint), and finally the distal phalanx (distal interphalangeal joint) (Fig. 75-2).
- Of note, the thumb has no middle phalanx and, therefore, no PIP joint.
- Radius
    - The distal radius provides the majority of the proximal articular surface of the wrist joint, with the scaphoid and lunate providing the distal articular surface.
    - The styloid process forms the most lateral and distal point of the radius.
- Ulna
    - The distal ulna has a smaller distal articular surface than the proximal ulna does at the elbow.
    - The styloid process forms its most medial distal projection.
- Carpal bones
    - There are eight carpal bones that are arranged in two rows.
    - The proximal row contains the scaphoid, lunate, triquetrum, and pisiform. The distal row contains the trapezium, trapezoid, capitate, and hamate.
- Metacarpals and phalanges
    - The five metacarpal bones are triangular in cross section. Each triangle provides an important surface area for muscle attachment.
    - They articulate proximally with the distal row of carpal bones and distally with the proximal phalanx (MCP joint).
    - There are five corresponding proximal phalanges, four middle phalanges (the thumb does not include this bone), and five distal phalanges.
    - The palmar surfaces of these bones are flatter, the proximal and distal ends have a slight flare to form the articular surfaces, and the distal phalanges have a "tufted" distal end.
- Muscles (Box 75-1)
- Vascular structures
    - The wrist and hand receive their blood supply from the radial and ulnar arteries.
    - The radial artery passes through the anatomic snuffbox at the wrist and divides into the palmar carpal, dorsal carpal, and superficial palmar branches in the hand.
    - The ulnar artery is larger than the radial artery and also divides at the wrist to form the palmar carpal branch, dorsal palmar branch, dorsal carpal branch, deep palmar branch, and superficial palmar arch. The ulnar and radial arteries have an anastomosis at the wrist.
- Nerves
    - The ulnar, radial, and median nerves provide sensory and motor input to the distal upper extremity.
    - The ulnar nerve provides sensation to the ulnar side of the wrist and hand including the fifth finger and the ulnar half of the fourth finger (Fig. 75-3).
    - The median nerve innervates the majority of the palmar surface and includes the distal half of the thumb, the second finger, the third finger, and the radial half of the fourth finger (Fig. 75-4).
    - The radial nerve innervates the radial aspect of the dorsal hand (Fig. 75-5).
- Ligaments and soft tissue
    - The wrist has extensive ligamentous structures to support the joint and act as shock absorbers.
    - The triangular fibrocartilage complex is one of the more clinically significant structures and supports the radioulnar joint.

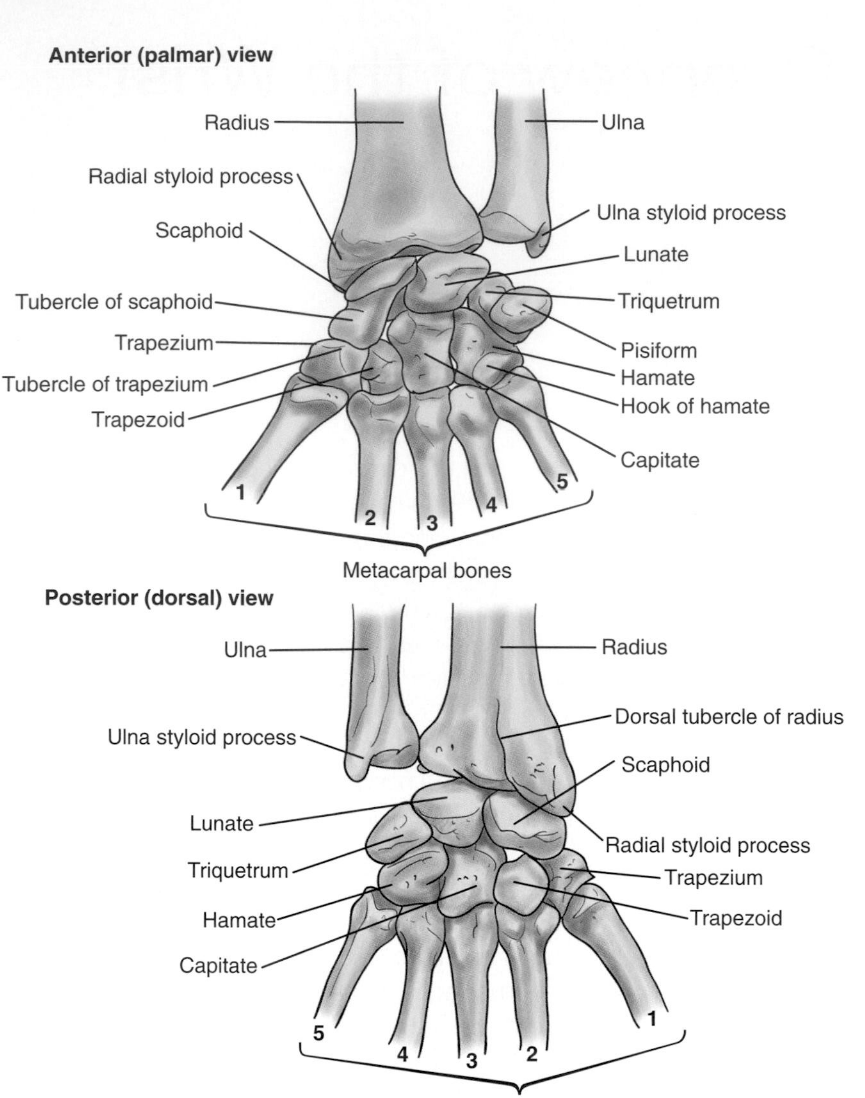

Figure 75-1 The bony anatomy of the wrist joint.

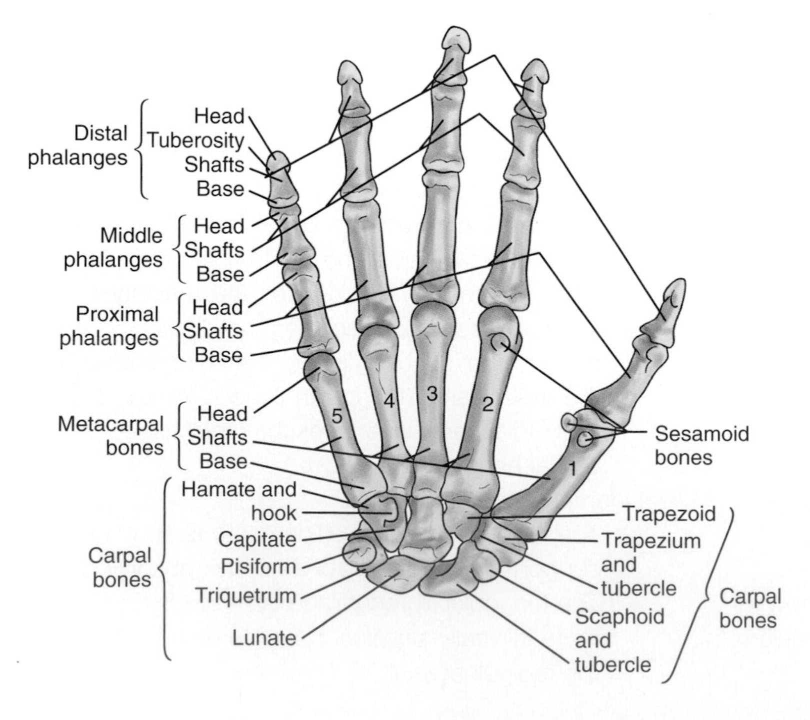

Figure 75-2 Anterior (palmar) view of the bony anatomy of the right hand.

BOX 75-1 *Muscles*

Wrist Flexors
Flexor carpi radialis
Palmaris longus
Flexor carpi ulnaris

Wrist Extensors
Extensor carpi radialis longus
Extensor carpi radialis brevis
Extensor carpi ulnaris

Finger Flexors
Flexor digitorum superficialis
Flexor digitorum profundus

Finger Extensors
Extensor digitorum
Extensor digiti minimi
Extensor indicis proprius

Thumb
Flexor pollicis longus
Abductor pollicis longus
Extensor pollicis brevis
Extensor pollicis longus

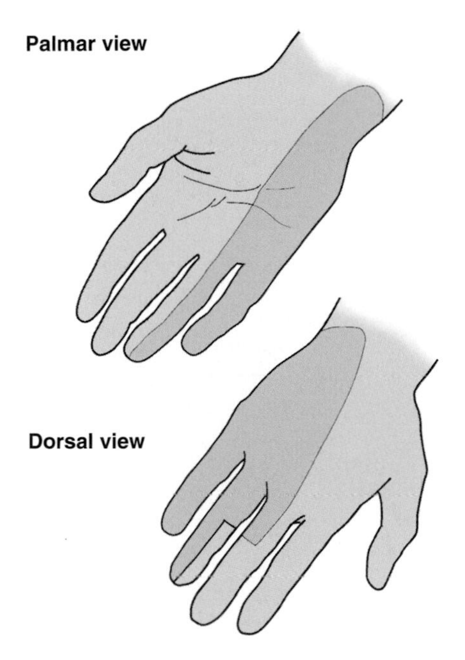

Figure 75-3 Sensory distribution of the ulnar nerve.

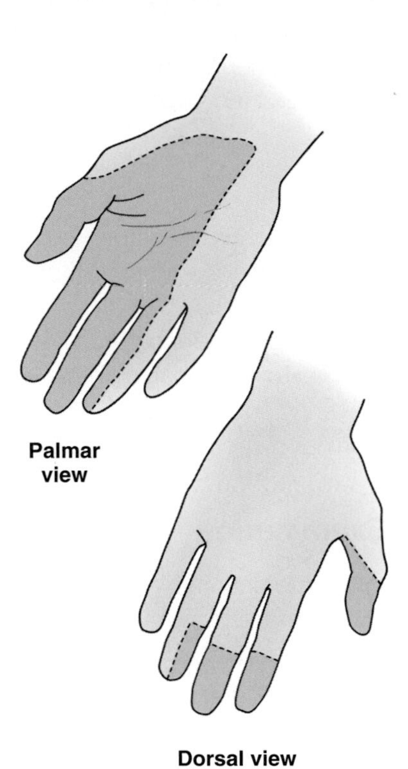

Figure 75-4 Sensory distribution of the median nerve.

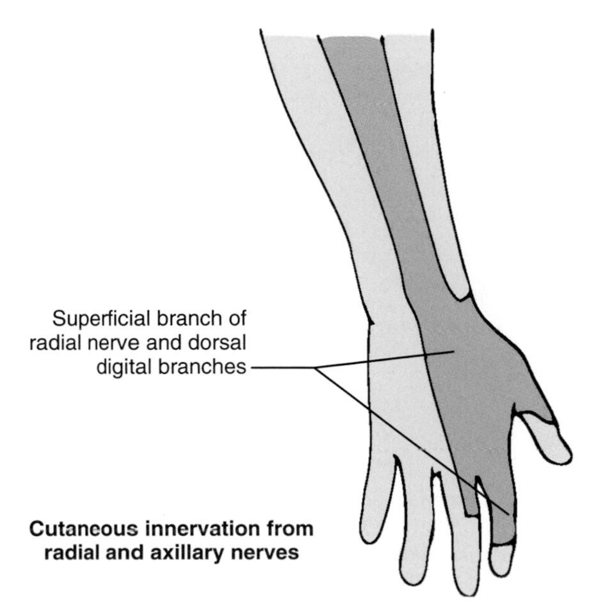

Figure 75-5 Sensory distribution of the radial nerve.

- This complex is formed by the dorsal and volar radioulnar ligaments, the triangular fibrocartilage disc, and the ulnar collateral ligament.

History

- A thorough and accurate history is the first step to defining the differential diagnosis list for each individual patient encounter.
- The history must provide accurate information regarding any trauma to the wrist or hand as well as the location, severity, and frequency of the pain and any history of similar symptoms (Table 75-1).

Physical Examination

- Inspection and palpation (Fig. 75-6)
  - Anterior wrist and hand
    — The anterior wrist and hand should be carefully evaluated for any changes in skin color, deformity, atrophy of the thenar or hypothenar muscles, and bony tenderness along the bony structures.
  - Posterior wrist and hand
    — The posterior wrist and hand should also be evaluated for skin changes, deformity, and bony tenderness.
    — In addition, special note should be taken here for rotational deformity of the fingers (often best noted by making a clenched fist) and nail bed abnormalities.

TABLE 75-1 *Pertinent History Points*

History	Possible Diagnosis
Fall/trauma	Fracture
Numbness/paresthesia	Nerve entrapment
Night pain	Tumor/infection
Cold intolerance/skin color change	Raynaud's phenomenon
Smoking history	Buerger's disease
Developing mass osteoarthritis	Depuytren's contracture, ganglion cyst

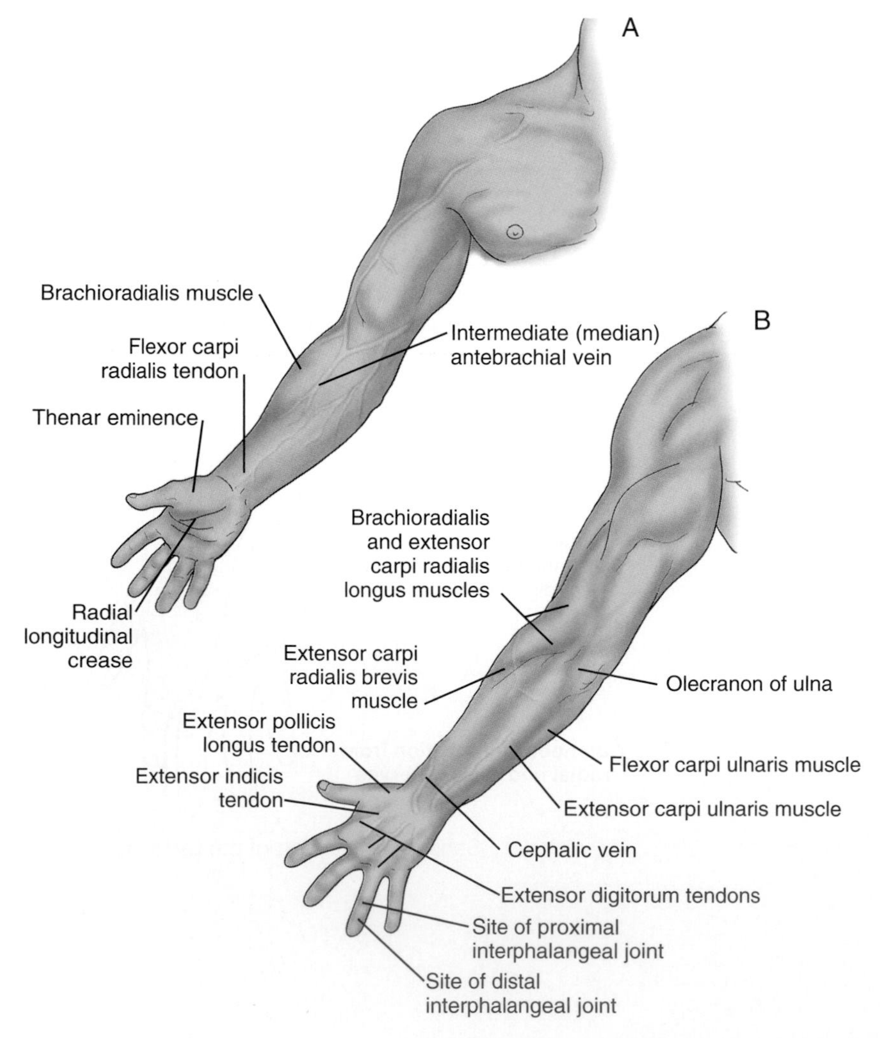

Figure 75-6 Surface anatomy of the wrist and hand. **A**, Anterior; **B**, posterior.

- Range of motion
  - Wrist flexion: 80 degrees
  - Wrist extension: 70 degrees
  - Radial deviation: 20 degrees
  - Ulnar deviation: 30 to 45 degrees
  - Finger (MCP) flexion: 90 degrees
  - Finger (MCP) extension: 30 to 45 degrees
  - Thumb (MCP) flexion: 50 degrees
  - Thumb (MCP) extension: 0 degrees
  - Thumb abduction: 70 degrees
  - Thumb adduction: 0 degrees
- Strength testing
  - Wrist flexion (Fig. 75-7A)
  - Wrist extension (see Fig. 75-7B)
  - Finger flexion (see Fig. 75-7C)
  - Finger extension (see Fig. 75-7D)
  - Finger abduction (see Fig. 75-7E)
  - Finger adduction (see Fig. 75-7F)
  - Opposition (see Fig. 75-7G)
- Special tests
  - Phalen test (Fig. 75-8)
    - — Purpose: evaluation for carpal tunnel syndrome
    - — How to perform: Passively flex the patient's wrist and hold it in that flexed position to try to reproduce the symptoms of numbness and paresthesia in the thumb and index finger.

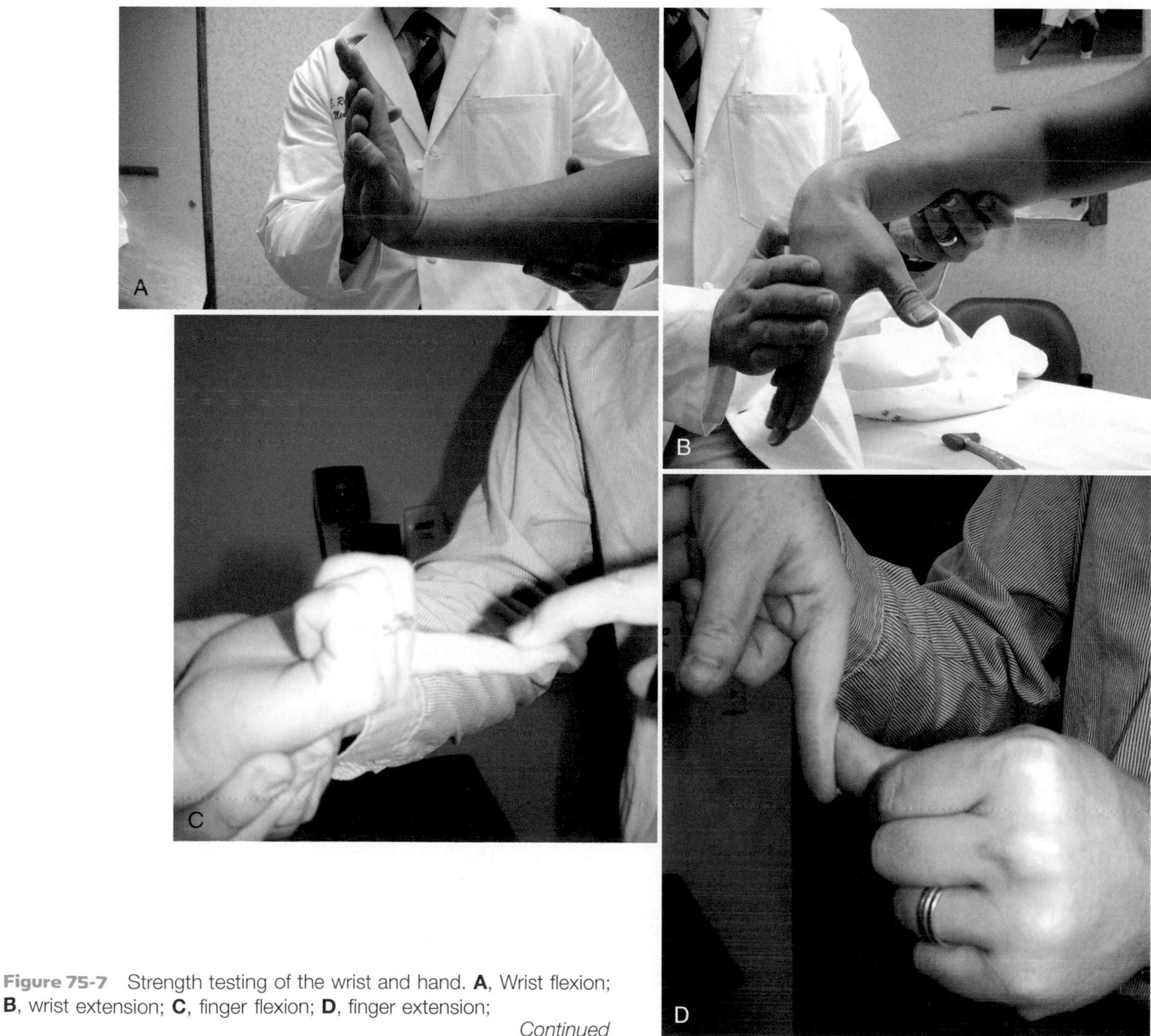

Figure 75-7 Strength testing of the wrist and hand. **A**, Wrist flexion; **B**, wrist extension; **C**, finger flexion; **D**, finger extension;

Continued

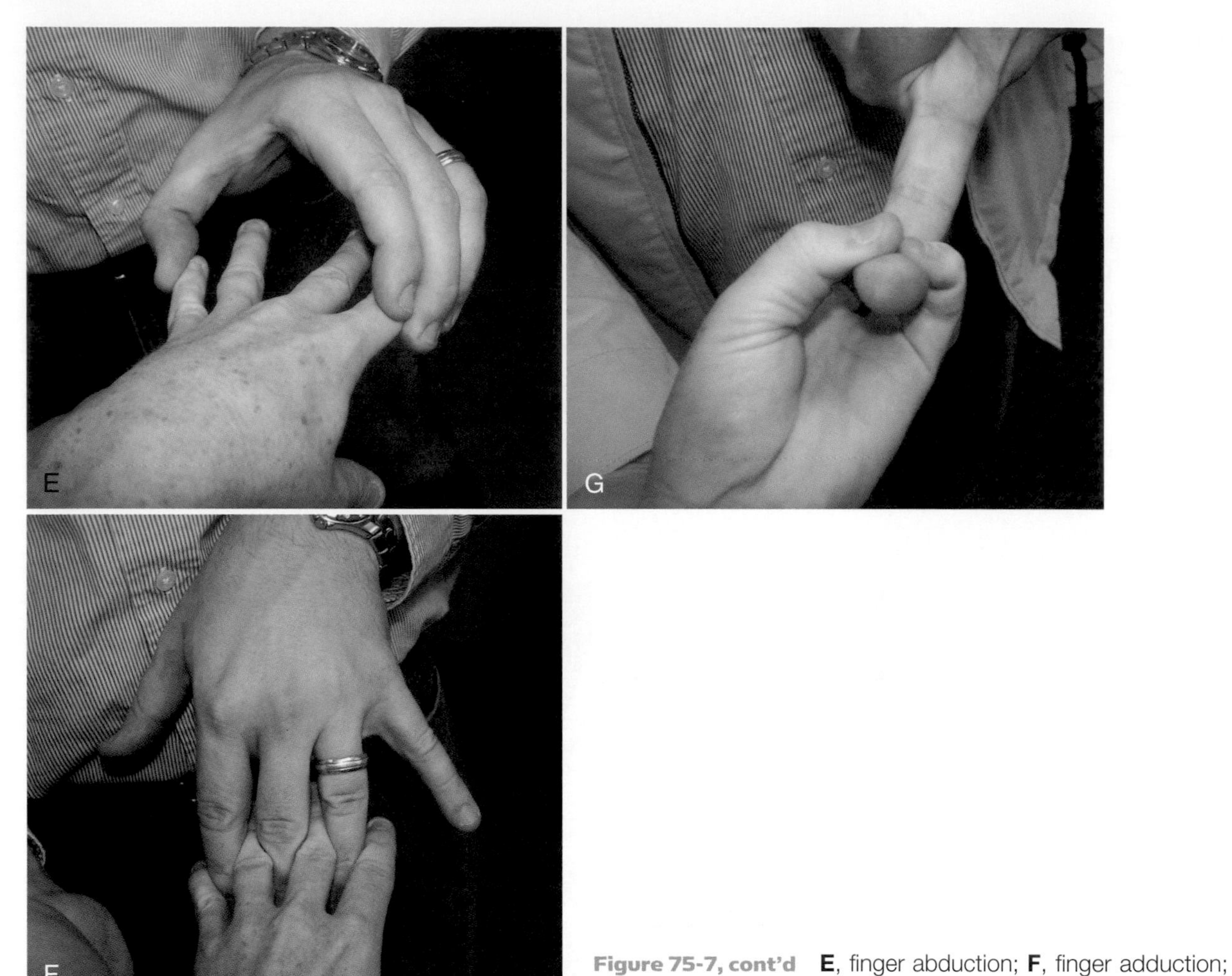

Figure 75-7, cont'd **E**, finger abduction; **F**, finger adduction; **G**, opposition.

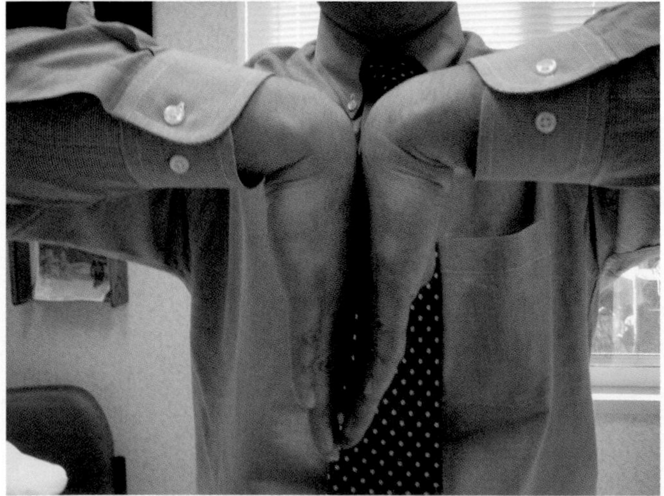

Figure 75-8 Phalen test.

— Positive: reproduction of numbness and paresthesia in the thumb and index finger

- Tinel's sign (Fig. 75-9)
  — Purpose: evaluation for carpal tunnel syndrome
  — How to perform: Tap over the anterior aspect of the wrist.
  — Positive: indicated by reproduction of numbness and paresthesia in the thumb and index finger
- Finkelstein test (Fig. 75-10)
  — Purpose: evaluation for de Quervain's tenosynovitis
  — How to perform: Ask the patient to make a fist, tucking the thumb under the other fingers and then placing the wrist in ulnar deviation.
  — Positive: indicated by reproduction of the pain along the side of the thumb
- Allen test (Fig. 75-11)
  — Purpose: evaluation for a patent radial artery
  — How to perform: With the patient's hand in a fist and elevated, occlude both the ulnar and radial arteries. Ask the patient to open his or her hand, which will appear blanched. Release the pressure on the ulnar artery.
  — Positive: Return of color within 7 seconds indicates a patent radial artery.

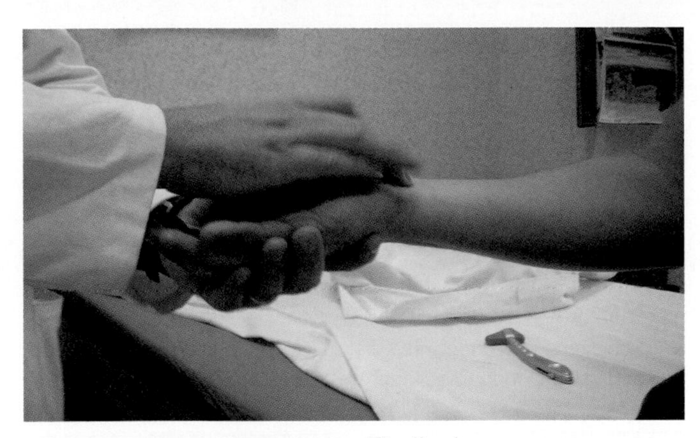

Figure 75-9 Tinel's sign.

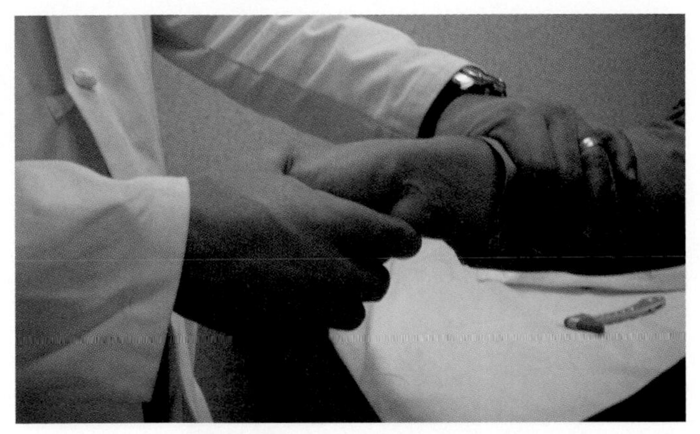

Figure 75-10 Finkelstein test.

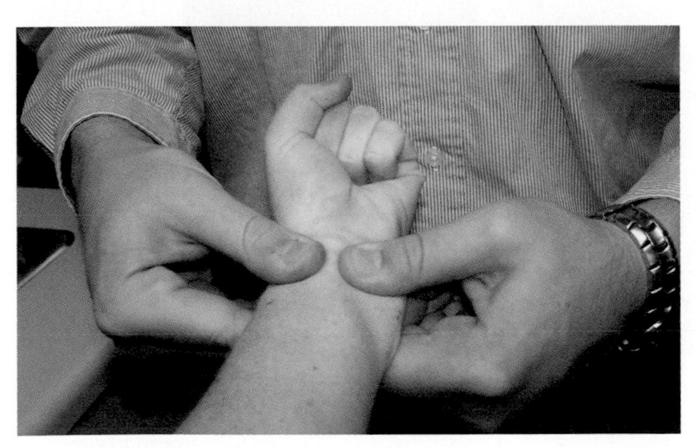

Figure 75-11 Allen test.

- Valgus stress test of the thumb (Fig. 75-12)
  - — Purpose: evaluation for ulnar collateral ligament injury
  - — How to perform: Using one hand to stabilize the thumb proximal to the MCP joint, place the thumb first in 0 degrees of flexion and then 30 degrees of flexion and apply gentle valgus stress to the MCP joint.

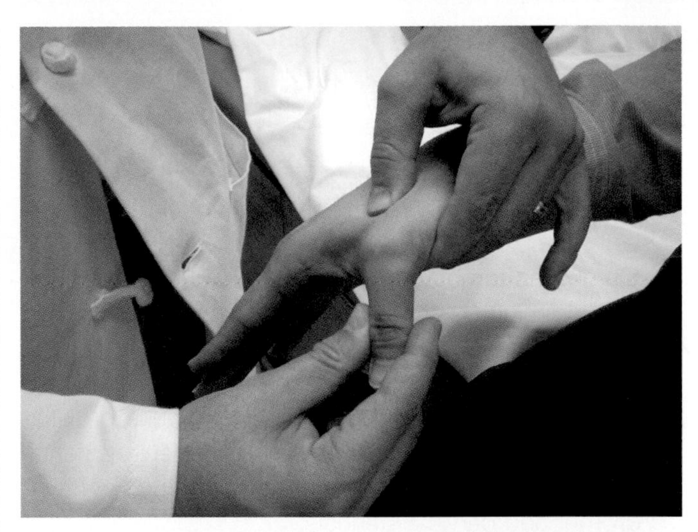

Figure 75-12 Valgus stress test of the thumb.

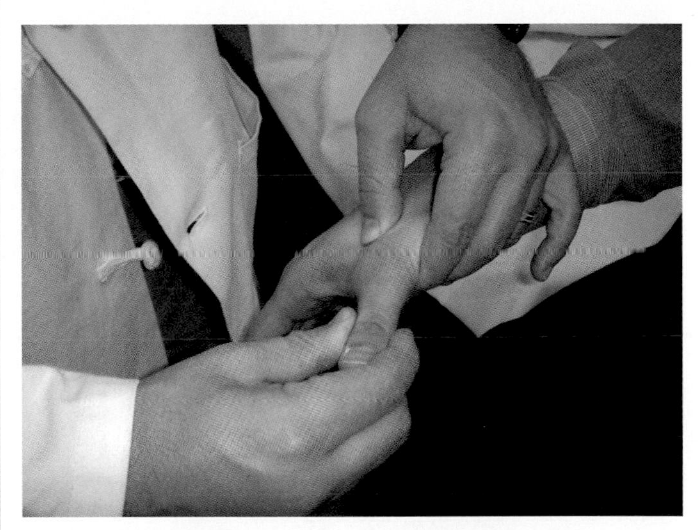

Figure 75-13 Carpometacarpal grind test.

  - — Positive: Opening of the MCP joint indicates rupture of the ulnar collateral ligament of the thumb.
- Carpometacarpal grind test (Fig. 75-13)
  - — Purpose: evaluation for carpometacarpal arthritis
  - — How to perform: Using one hand to stabilize the thumb proximal to the carpometacarpal joint, hold the thumb in the other hand and move it in a circular pattern.
  - — Positive: Reproduction of pain at the carpometacarpal joint is indicative of arthritis there.

Imaging

- Radiography
  - Standard radiographic views of the wrist and hand include anteroposterior, lateral, and oblique views

(Figs. 75-14 and 75-15). Special images are useful when evaluating for certain injuries such as the carpal tunnel view or clenched-fist view (Fig. 75-16).

- Magnetic resonance imaging of the wrist is helpful when evaluating such things as triangular fibrocartilage complex tears.
- Computed tomography is most helpful when evaluating comminuted or severely displaced fractures to aid in preoperative planning.
- Electromyography is a commonly used test in evaluating the wrist and hand because it can help to distinguish various upper extremity nerve entrapments, such as carpal tunnel syndrome, cubital tunnel syndrome, and cervical stenosis.

Suggested Reading

- Green D, Hotchkiss R, Pederson W, Wolfe S (eds): Green's Operative Hand Surgery. Philadelphia: Churchill Livingstone, 2005.
- Hoppenfeld S: Physical Examination of the Spine and Extremities. Norwalk, CT: Appleton & Lange, 1976.
- Loreda RA, Sorge DG, Garcia G: Radiographic evaluation of the wrist: A vanishing art. Semin Roentgenol 2005;40:248–289.
- Reddy RS, Compson J: Examination of the wrist-surface anatomy of the carpal bones. Curr Orthop 2005;19:171–179.
- Schreibman KL, Freeland A, Gilula LA, Yin Y: Imaging of the hand and wrist. Orthop Clin North Am 1997;28:537–582.
- Watson HK, Weinzweig J: Physical examination of the wrist. Hand Clin 1997;13:17–34.
- Young D, Papp S, Giachino A: Physical examination of the wrist. Orthop Clin North Am 2007;38:149–165.

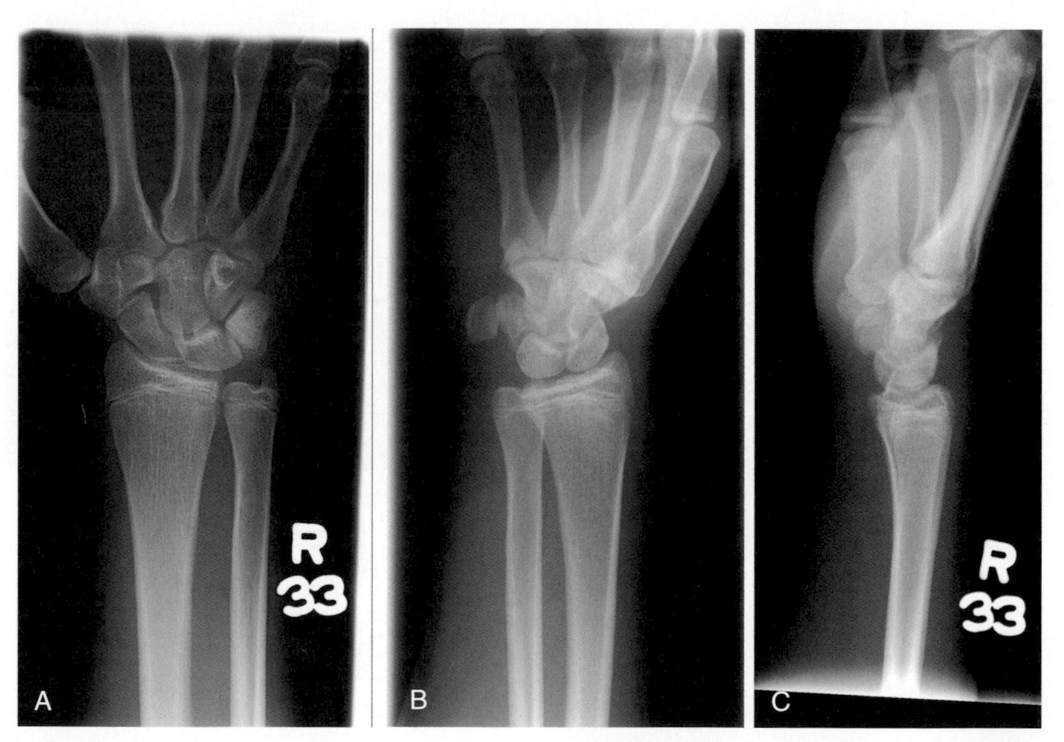

Figure 75-14 Standard radiographic views of the wrist. Anteroposter (**A**), oblique (**B**), and lateral (**C**) views.

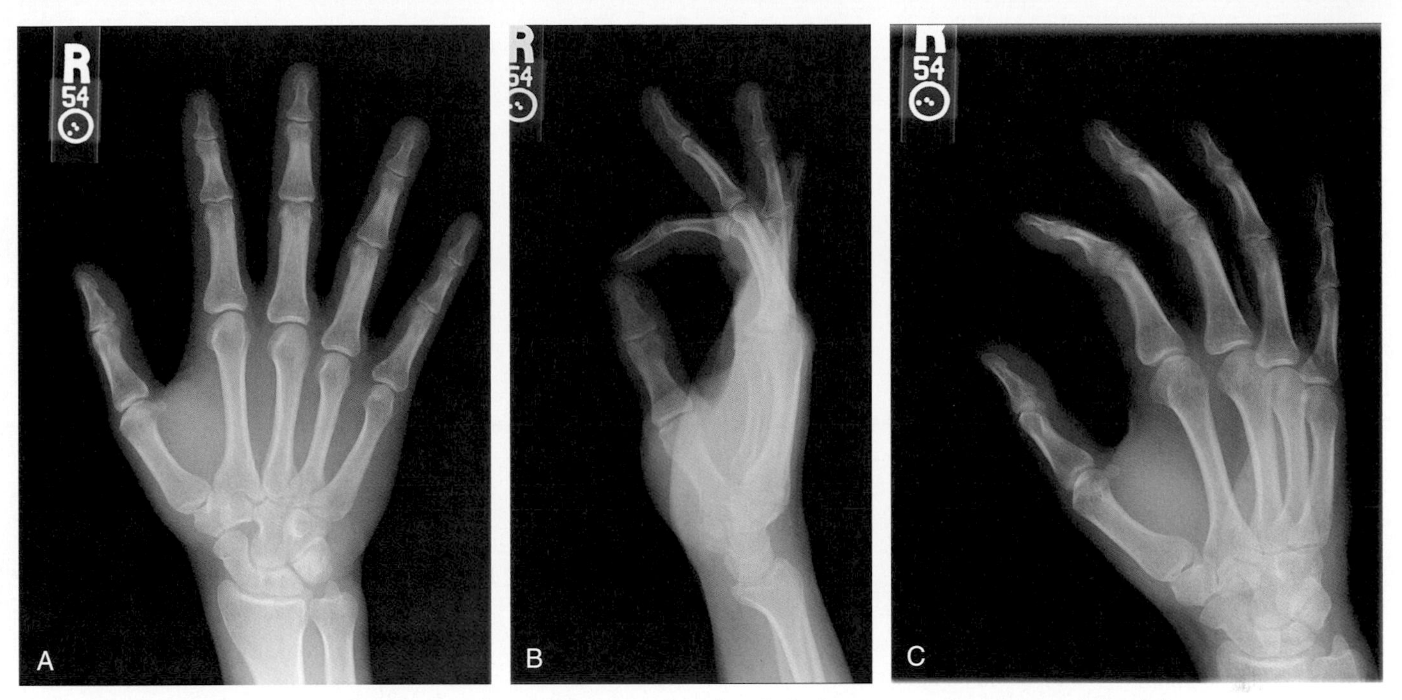

Figure 75-15 Standard radiographic views of the hand. **A**, Anteroposterior; **B**, lateral; **C**, oblique.

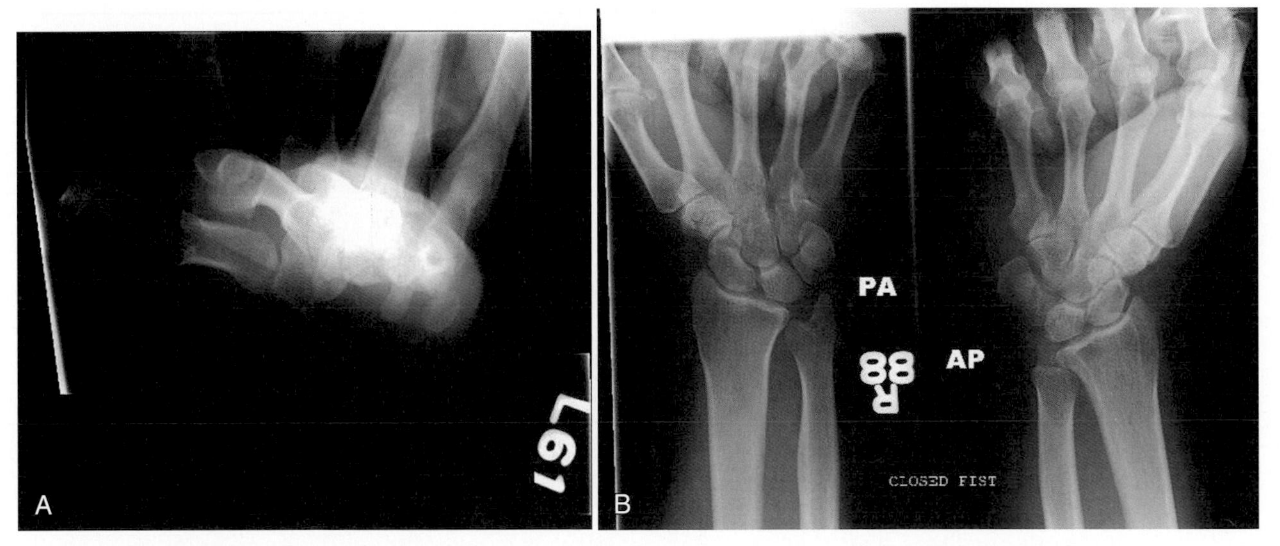

Figure 75-16 Special radiographic views of the wrist. **A**, Carpal tunnel view; **B**, clenched-fist view.

Chapter 76 Scapholunate Ligament Injury

Sara D. Rynders and A. Bobby Chhabra

ICD-9 CODE
842.01 *Carpal Sprain*

Key Concepts

- The scapholunate ligament (SLL) is an interosseous ligament between the scaphoid and lunate that functions as a major stabilizer of the wrist. It is C shaped and strongest at its dorsal attachment with thinner and weaker volar and proximal portions.
- There is a wide spectrum of disorders that can result from injury to the SLL, which are classified based on the type of instability that is present (static versus dynamic) and the acuity of the injury (acute, subacute, and chronic).
- In an uninjured wrist, the lunate is held in a neutral position by the opposing moment arms of the SLL, which has a flexion moment arm, and the lunotriquetral ligament, which has an extension moment arm.
- If the SLL is compromised, the lunate is subject to an unopposed extension force created by the intact lunotriquetral ligament, resulting in an extension deformity of the lunate called dorsal intercalated segment instability (DISI) deformity, which is characteristic of a scapholunate (SL) dissociation.
- Chronic, untreated SL instability will result in a predictable pattern of degenerative changes in the wrist known as scapholunate advanced collapse (SLAC).
- The gold standard of diagnosis is wrist arthroscopy, although magnetic resonance imaging may be helpful in some settings.

History

- The patient may or may not report a history of a wrist sprain, a fall on an outstretched hand, or an injury with an axial load on the wrist.
- The patient may describe a pain or weakness in the wrist with use, especially when the wrist is extended and axially loaded (push-up position).
- There may or may not be a history of edema or a painful "clicking" in the wrist.
- In the late stages of chronic SL instability, patients may report decreased wrist range of motion.

Physical Examination

- Inspection may reveal dorsal wrist edema.
- Palpate the SL interval with the wrist in slight flexion. Identify the soft spot on the dorsum of the wrist just distal to Lister's tubercle. Pain here may indicate an SLL injury (Fig. 76-1).
- Watson's maneuver (Fig. 76-2)
  - The examiner places one hand on the radial aspect of the wrist and with the thumb applies constant pressure over the scaphoid tubercle. The examiner then uses his or her opposite hand to passively move the patient's wrist from ulnar to radial deviation. A positive test result is indicated by a painful "clunk" as the wrist moves from ulnar to radial deviation. This occurs because the pressure over the scaphoid tubercle prevents palmar flexion of the scaphoid, and the proximal pole will subluxate over the dorsal rim of the radius, producing pain.
  - This test must be compared with one done on the uninjured side. Some patients will have a palpable clunk that is not painful and may occur bilaterally. Pain produced during this maneuver is the indication of a positive finding.
- A thorough examination of the wrist should be performed to identify other areas of tenderness and possible injury. A thorough neurovascular examination and examination of the cervical spine, shoulder, and elbow should also be performed.

Imaging

- There are four stages of SL instability.
  - Predynamic instability
    — Partially ruptured or attenuated ligament that allows abnormal movement between the scaphoid and lunate and creates wrist synovitis

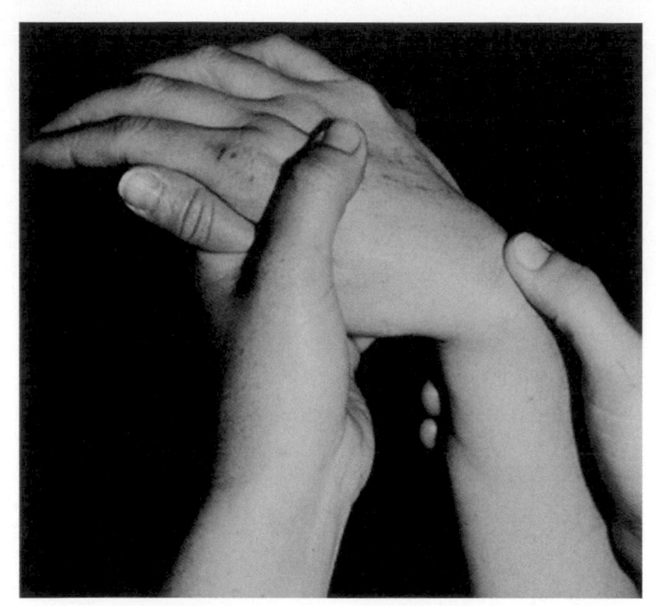

Figure 76-1 Palpation of the scapholunate interval. (From Green D, Hotchkiss R, Pederson W, Wolfe S [eds]: Green's Operative Hand Surgery, Vol. 1, 5th ed. Philadelphia: Churchill Livingstone, 2005, p 492.)

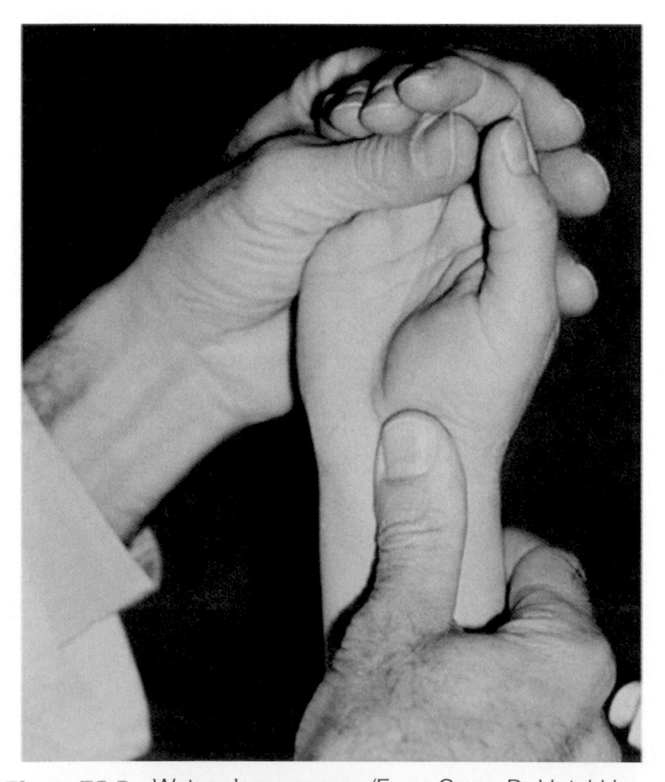

Figure 76-2 Watson's maneuver. (From Green D, Hotchkiss R, Pederson W, Wolfe S [eds]: Green's Operative Hand Surgery, Vol. 1, 5th ed. Philadelphia: Churchill Livingstone, 2005, p 493.)

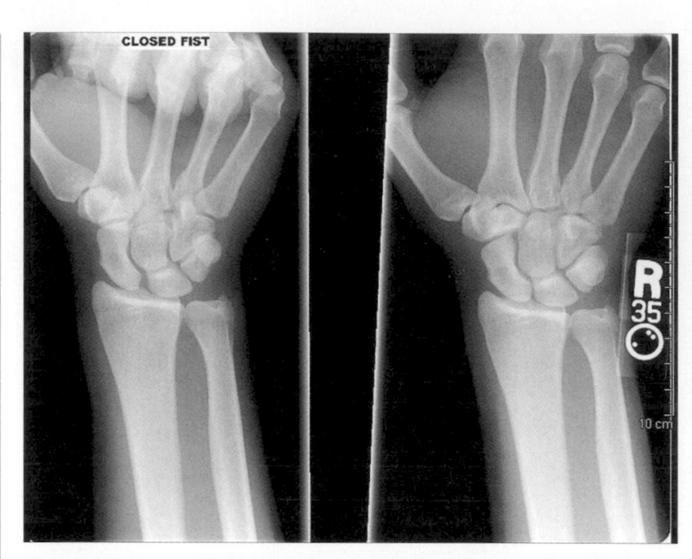

Figure 76-3 *Left,* Stress view ("clinched-fist view") of the wrist shows widening of the scapholunate (SL) interval. *Right,* Normal, non-stress view demonstrating normal SL interval.

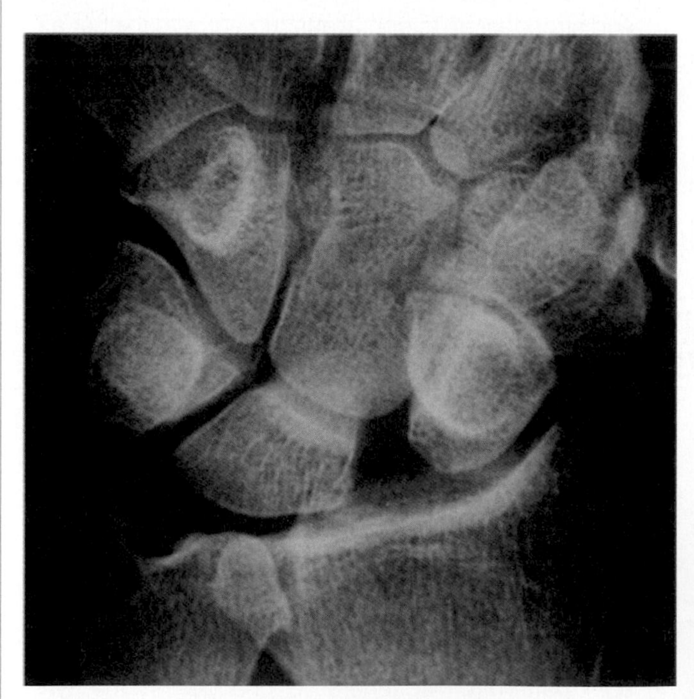

Figure 76-4 Static instability and dorsal intercalated segment instability deformity. (From Green D, Hotchkiss R, Pederson W, Wolfe S [eds]: Green's Operative Hand Surgery, Vol. 1, 5th ed. Philadelphia: Churchill Livingstone, 2005, p 569.)

  - — Radiographs appear normal.
- Dynamic instability (Fig. 76-3)
  - — The palmar or dorsal portions of the SLL are disrupted.
  - — Identified on clenched-fist radiographs as SL interval widening. Nonstress views of the wrist are normal.
- Static instability (Fig. 76-4)

- Injury to the SLL and the secondary stabilizers of the wrist (volar carpal ligaments and dorsal wrist capsule)
- Evidence of SL widening and dorsal intercalated segment instability deformity on nonstress views
- SLAC wrist: Final stage of SL instability; chronic and degenerative arthritis (Fig. 76-5)

- The following should be evaluated on radiographs:
  - Scaphoid ring sign: produced when the SLL has been disrupted and the scaphoid falls into flexion. A distance of less than 7 mm from the ring to the scaphoid proximal pole indicates a rotatory subluxation of the scaphoid (Fig. 76-6).
  - Terry Thomas sign: widening of the SL interval by more than 5 mm (see Fig. 76-6)
    - Must compare with contralateral side
    - If present on nonstress view, a static instability of the wrist is demonstrated
  - Late stages of SLL instability result in a SLAC wrist with the following degenerative changes seen on posteroanterior radiographs (Table 76-1 and Fig. 76-7)
- Lateral view
  - Dorsal intercalated segment instability deformity and increased SL angle (Fig. 76-8)
    - The normal SL angle is 30 to 60 degrees.
    - Dorsal intercalated segment instability deformity creates an angle greater than 70 degrees and is indicative of instability of the SLL.

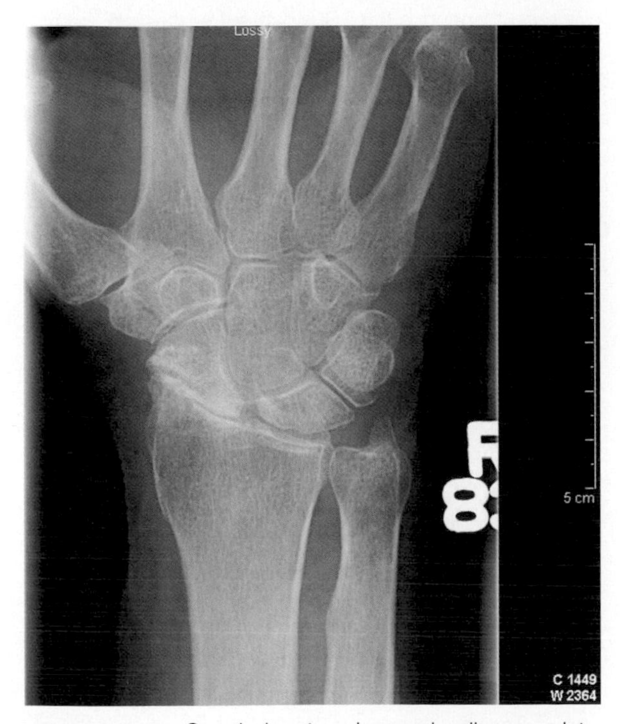

Figure 76-5 Scapholunate advanced collapse wrist.

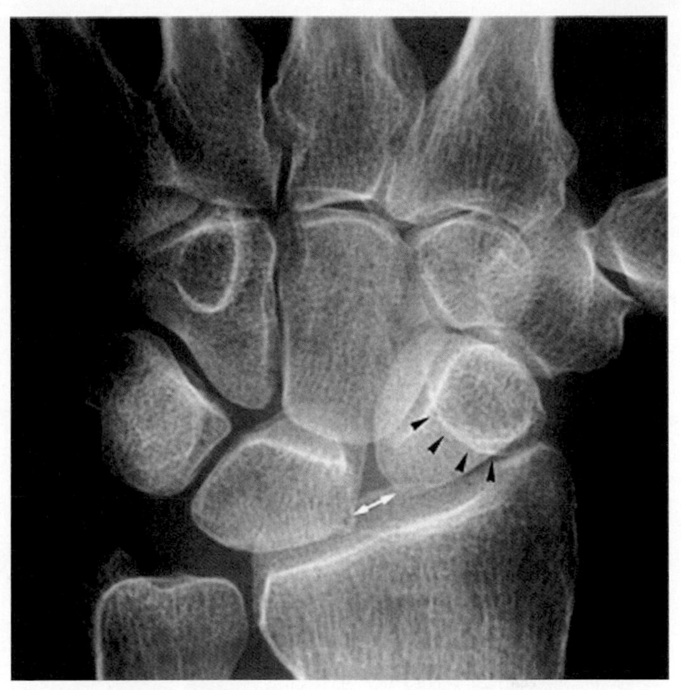

Figure 76-6 Scaphoid ring sign *(black arrowheads)* and Terry Thomas sign *(white arrow)*. (From Green D, Hotchkiss R, Pederson W, Wolfe S [eds]: Green's Operative Hand Surgery, Vol. 1, 5th ed. Philadelphia: Churchill Livingstone, 2005, p 557.)

TABLE 76-1 *Stages of Scapholunate Advanced Collapse Wrist*

Stage	Joint Degeneration
I	Radial styloid-scaphoid articulation; radial styloid beaking
II	Stage I + radioscaphoid joint
III	Stage II + capitolunate joint and proximal migration of capitate
IV	Panarthritis including radiolunate joint

- Posteroanterior clenched-fist view (Fig. 76-9)
  - Increased SL interval by more than 5 mm* indicates a dynamic instability of the SLL.
  - Compare the affected side with the contralateral side.

*There is some controversy surrounding this value. A wide interval may be defined as more than 3 mm if there are correlating physical examination findings and widening of the interval when compared with the uninjured wrist.

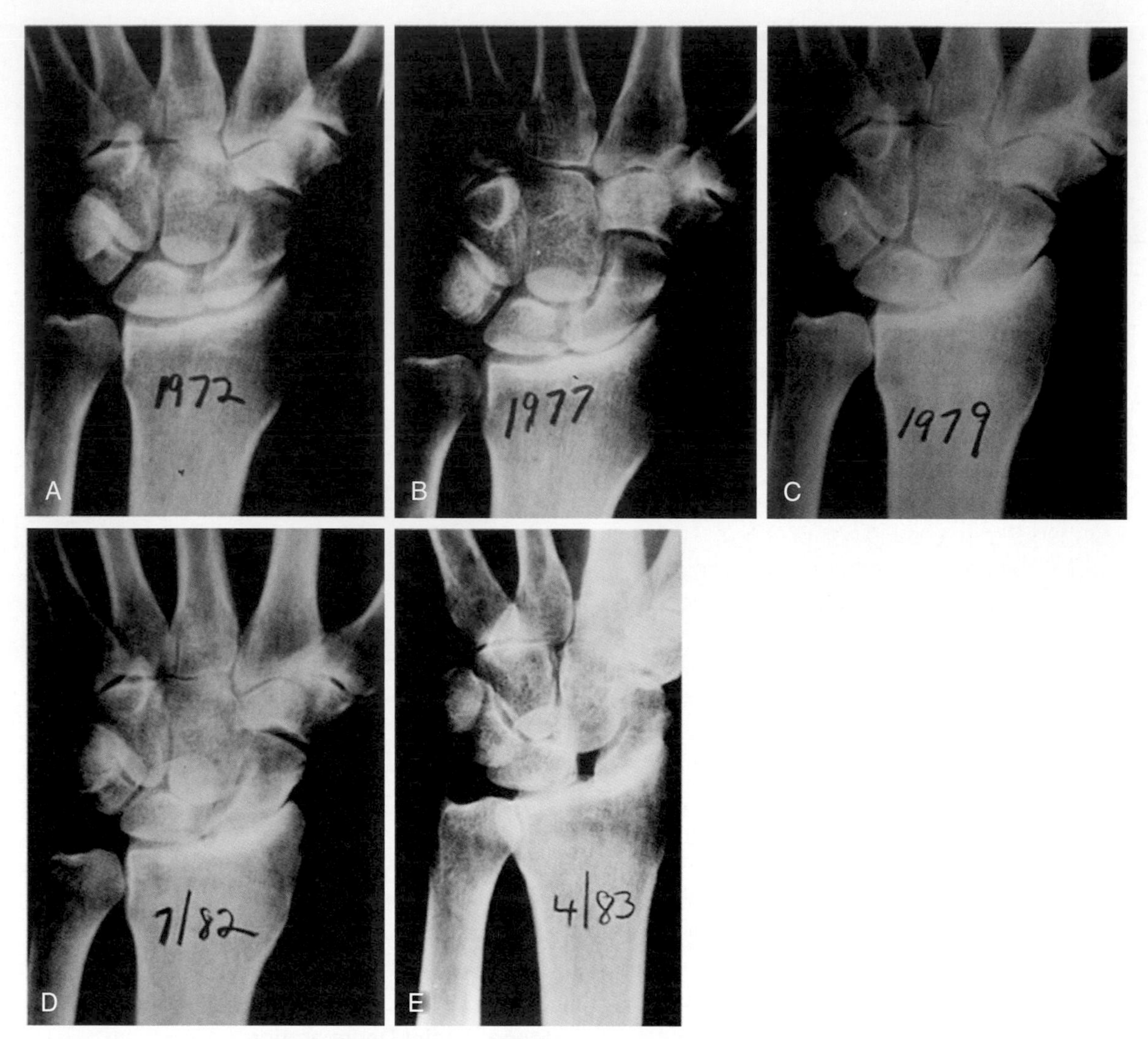

Figure 76-7 Stages of scapholunate (SL) advanced collapse. **A,** No radiographic changes after SL ligament surgery. **B,** Early extension of lunate and narrowing of radioscaphoid joint. **C,** Radioscaphoid arthritis and proximal migration of capitate. **D,** Radiocarpal arthritis and proximal migration of capitate. **E,** Static instability with radiocarpal arthritis, SL interval widening on non-stress view, and proximal migration of capitate. (From Green D, Hotchkiss R, Pederson W, Wolfe S [eds]: Green's Operative Hand Surgery, Vol. 1, 5th ed. Philadelphia: Churchill Livingstone, 2005, p 507.)

Additional Tests

- Magnetic resonance imaging with gadolinium (Fig. 76-10)
- Controversial due to variation in quality of images, radiologist experience, and technique
- High-resolution magnetic resonance imaging may reveal an SLL tear.
- Useful to work through differential diagnosis
- Arthroscopy is the gold standard for diagnosis and treatment.

Differential Diagnosis

- Please see Table 76-2.

Treatment

- At diagnosis
  - Predynamic instability (mild wrist pain and all radiographs are normal, including stress views)
    - — Nonsteroidal anti-inflammatory drugs
    - — Splint or short arm cast immobilization for 4 to 6 weeks
  - Dynamic instability, static instability
    - — Splint immobilization and referral to specialist within 7 to 10 days for an acute injury
  - SLAC wrist
    - — Nonsteroidal anti-inflammatory drugs
    - — Splint or cast immobilization
    - — Avoidance of provocative activity
    - — Radiocarpal injection

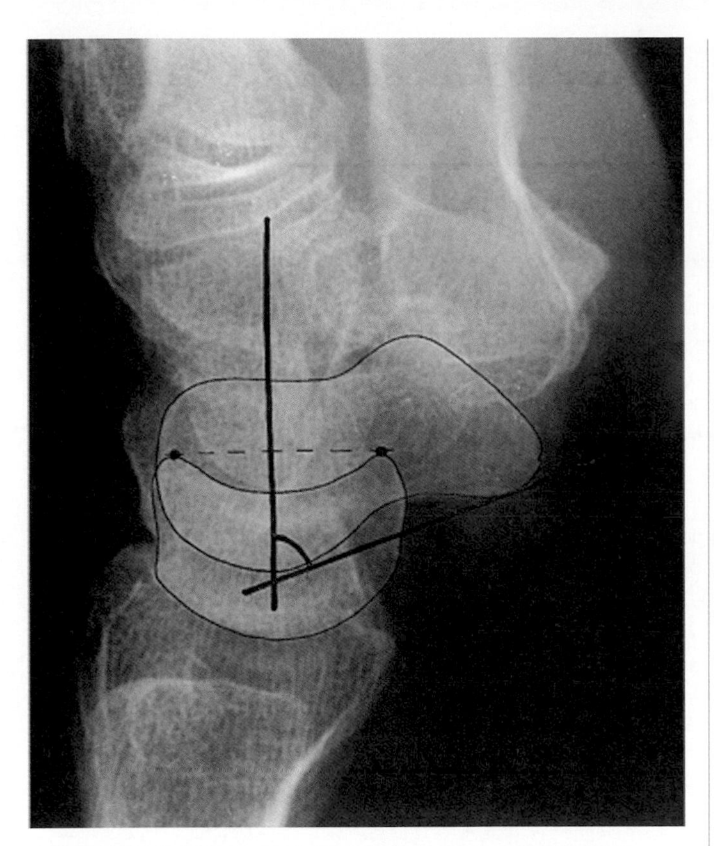

Figure 76-8 Dorsal intercalated segment instability (DISI) deformity and scapholunate (SL) angle. DISI deformity is described as SL angle greater than 70 degrees. (From Green D, Hotchkiss R, Pederson W, Wolfe S [eds]: Green's Operative Hand Surgery, Vol. 1, 5th ed. Philadelphia: Churchill Livingstone, 2005, p 558.)

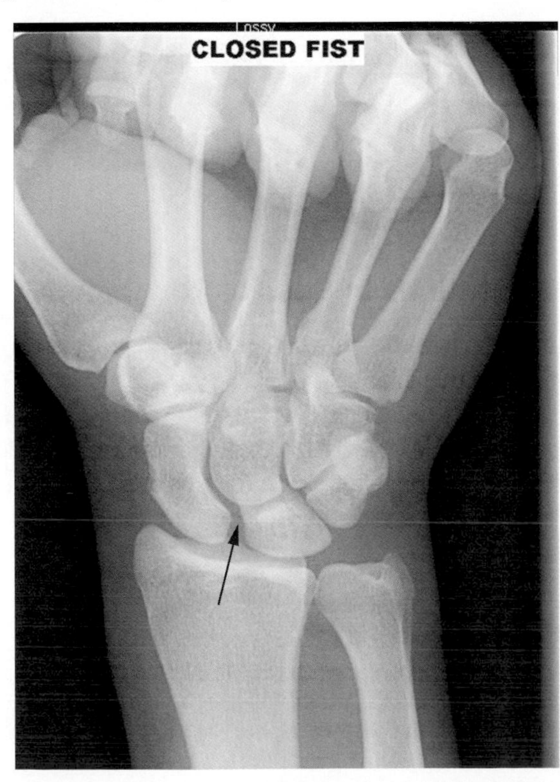

Figure 76-9 Posteroanterior clenched-fist view.

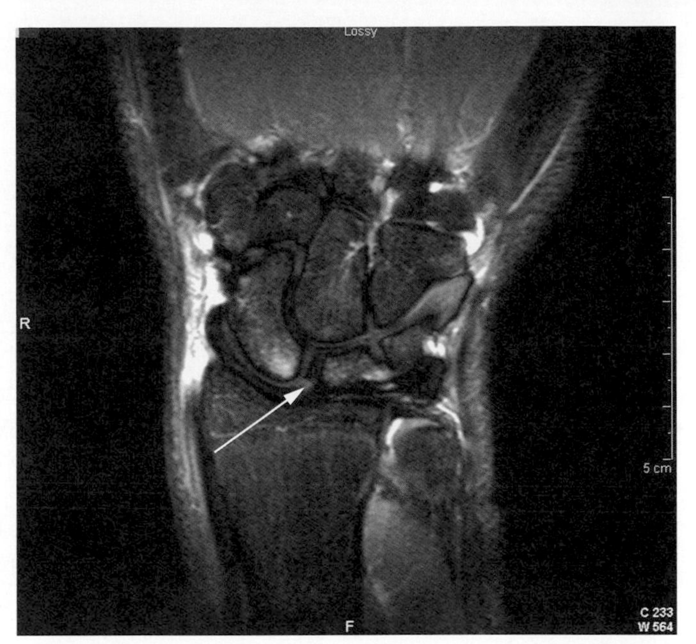

Figure 76-10 Scapholunate ligament tear on MRI (*arrow*).

- Later
  - Predynamic instability
    — Repeat radiographs. If asymptomatic, begin range of motion exercises and gradual return to activity. If symptomatic, refer to a specialist.
  - SLAC wrist: If conservative management fails, refer the patient to a specialist.

When to Refer

- When there are physical examination findings suggestive of an SLL injury or there is evidence of SL interval widening or dorsal intercalated segment instability deformity on plain radiographs (static or dynamic instability)
- If conservative management of a predynamic pattern of instability or SLAC wrist fails
- A patient may require a diagnostic wrist arthroscopy to identify, stage, and repair damage to the SLL.
- Surgical repair options include débridement of the SLL, pinning of the SLL with Kirschner wires, reconstruction with dorsal capsulodesis, tenodesis, or ligament reconstruction.
- Late stages of SLL instability resulting in SLAC wrist may require more involved surgical procedures such as proximal row carpectomy and limited or total wrist fusion.

TABLE 76-2 *Differential Diagnosis*

Condition	Differentiating Features	Chapter Reference
Acute fracture or wrist sprain	History of recent fall or trauma; no evidence of chronic degenerative changes on plain radiographs	96, 79
de Quervain's tenosynovitis	Positive Finkelstein's sign	80
Rheumatoid arthritis	Evidence of erosive arthritis on radiographs; hand and finger deformities such as metacarpophalangeal dislocations; swan neck and boutonnière deformities of fingers	18
Gout	Punch-out lesions on radiographs	18
Calcium pyrophosphate dihydrate deposition or pseudogout	Calcium pyrophosphate dihydrate deposits visible in triangular fibrocartilage complex on plain radiographs	18
Carpal tunnel syndrome	History of numbness, tingling, and pain in the median nerve distribution; pain worse at night; positive provocative maneuvers for carpal tunnel syndrome; normal radiographs; evidence of carpal tunnel syndrome on electromyography/nerve conduction studies	83
Cubital tunnel syndrome or ulnar neuropathy at Guyon's canal	Paresthesias and pain in the ulnar nerve distribution; positive provocative maneuvers for cubital tunnel syndrome at the elbow or in Guyon's canal; normal radiographs; evidence of cubital tunnel syndrome or distal ulnar neuropathy on electromyography/nerve conduction studies	65
Tendonitis of common extensors (extensor carpi ulnaris, extensor radialis carpi brevis, extensor carpi radialis longus, flexor carpi ulnaris, or flexor carpi radialis)	Tenderness to palpation directly over the affected tendon; normal radiographs	81
Triangular fibrocartilage complex injury	Tender to palpation over the triangular fibrocartilage complex; normal radiographs if occurs as isolated injury; magnetic resonance imaging may help to identify triangular fibrocartilage complex tear	79
Ganglion cysts, occult	May have evidence of a palpable, firm, slightly mobile mass; normal radiographs; magnetic resonance imaging can help to identify ganglion cysts	82

Prognosis

- All patients with complete SLL disruptions will develop degenerative changes in the wrist if left untreated.
- Patients whose injuries are recognized early and undergo early ligamentous repair can have an excellent outcome. Injuries that are recognized late or in the presence of degenerative changes are more difficult to treat and often have suboptimal outcomes.

Patient Instructions

- Evaluation by a specialist is important to prevent the development of progressive degenerative changes.

Considerations in Special Populations

- Athletes involved in contact sports are particularly prone to this injury.
- They often present with a remote history of a wrist sprain with a failure to seek treatment, and there should be a high suspicion for a missed SLL injury.
- Referral to a specialist is important to prevent long-term sequelae.

Suggested Reading

- Garcia-Elias M, Geissler W: Carpal instability. In Green D, Hotchkiss R, Pederson W, Wolfe S (eds): Green's Operative Hand Surgery, Vol. 1, 5th ed. Philadelphia: Churchill Livingstone, 2005, pp 535–604.

- Linscheid RL, Dobyns JH, Beaubout JW, et al: Traumatic instability of the wrist: Diagnosis, classification, and pathomechanics. J Bone Joint Surg Am 1972;54A:1612–1632.
- Manuel J, Moran S: The diagnosis and treatment of scapholunate instability. Orthop Clin North Am 2007;38:261–277.
- Walsh J, Berger R, Cooney W: Current status of scapholunate interosseous ligament injuries. J Am Acad Orthop Surg 2002;10:32–42.
- Watson HK, Ballet FL: The SLAC wrist: Scapholunate advanced collapse pattern of degenerative arthritis. J Hand Surg [Am] 1984;5:320–327.
- Watson HK, Winzweig J, Zeppieri J: Physical examination of the wrist. Hand Clin 1997;13:17–34.
- Watson HK, Winzweig J, Zeppieri J: The natural progression of scaphoid instability. Hand Clin 1997;13:39–49.

Chapter 77 Wrist Osteoarthritis

Sara D. Rynders and A. Bobby Chhabra

ICD-9 CODES
715.13 *General Osteoarthritis of Wrist*
716.13 *Traumatic Arthropathy of Wrist*

Key Concepts

- Osteoarthritis (OA) of the wrist typically begins as a local injury and develops into a predictable pattern of degenerative changes.
- The most common cause of wrist OA is chronic scapholunate instability.
- Causes of wrist OA may be primary-degenerative or due to trauma
    - Scapholunate advanced collapse wrist (Fig. 77-1)
    - Scaphoid nonunion advanced collapse wrist (Fig. 77-2)
    - Radiocarpal arthritis (Fig. 77-3)
    - Midcarpal arthritis
    - Distal radioulnar joint arthritis (Fig. 77-4)
    - Pisotriquetral OA
    - Scaphotrapezoid-trapezium (STT) arthritis (or triscaphe arthritis) (Fig. 77-5)
    - Avascular necrosis
        - — Kienböck's disease (avascular necrosis of the lunate) (Fig. 77-6)
        - — Preiser's disease (idiopathic scaphoid avascular necrosis)
- Physical examination is essential to identify and localize the area of tenderness.
- Must obtain radiographs (anteroposterior, lateral, and oblique views) to identify affected joints.
- High suspicion for scapholunate advanced collapse or scaphoid nonunion advanced collapse in a patient who reports a remote history of wrist injury or scaphoid fracture

History

- There may be a history of wrist injury or fracture.
- Wrist pain, morning stiffness, decreased motion, and decreased strength, especially with grip, may be reported.
- Pain is described as an underlying dull ache that becomes sharp with certain movements of the wrist and may fluctuate with activity, weather changes, or temperature changes; patient may rub affected area with other hand while trying to describe symptoms.
- The patient may or may not have an underlying diagnosis of OA in other weight-bearing joints or the hands.
- The patient may describe symptoms of carpal tunnel syndrome due to compression of the median nerve from generalized wrist synovitis.

Physical Examination

- Inspection of the wrist may reveal a normal-appearing wrist or inflammation and nodular changes.
- Palpation is essential to identify the point of maximal tenderness.
- A thorough examination of the wrist should be performed with emphasis on palpating the following sites:
    - Anatomic snuffbox: Tenderness may indicate scaphoid nonunion, scaphoid avascular necrosis, STT OA, radioscaphoid arthritis, or scaphoid fracture.
    - Scaphoid tubercle tenderness may indicate OA involving the scaphoid.
    - Scapholunate interval tenderness may indicate chronic scapholunate ligament injury and scapholunate advanced collapse or scaphoid nonunion advanced collapse wrist, or Kienböck's disease.
    - STT joint, located just proximal to the base of the second metacarpal: pain may indicate STT arthritis (Fig. 77-7)
    - Pisotriquetral joint: pain may indicate pisotriquetral arthritis
    - Diffuse tenderness may represent panarthritis.
- The following tests should be performed.
    - Piano key test: Place one hand on the radius and apply dorsal pressure over the ulnar head. Pain may indicate distal radioulnar joint OA.
    - Perform Watson's maneuver to assess for scapholunate ligament disruption, a precursor to arthritis (see Chapter 76).

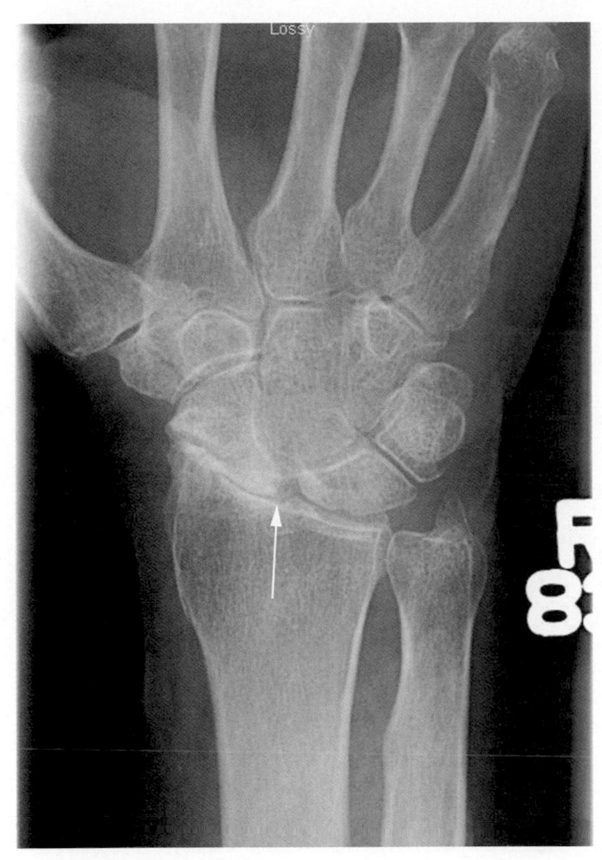

Figure 77-1 Scapholunate advanced collapse (*arrow*).

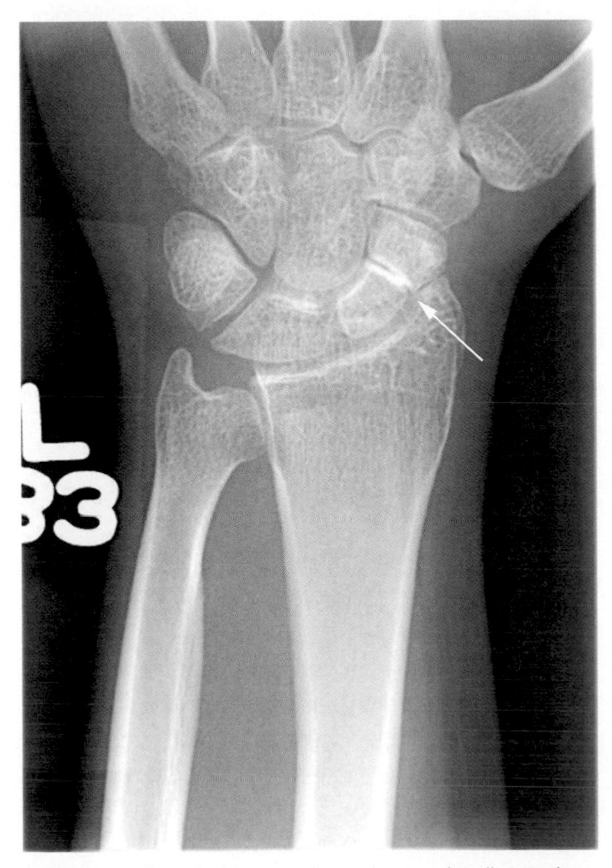

Figure 77-2 Scaphoid nonunion advanced collapse (*arrow*).

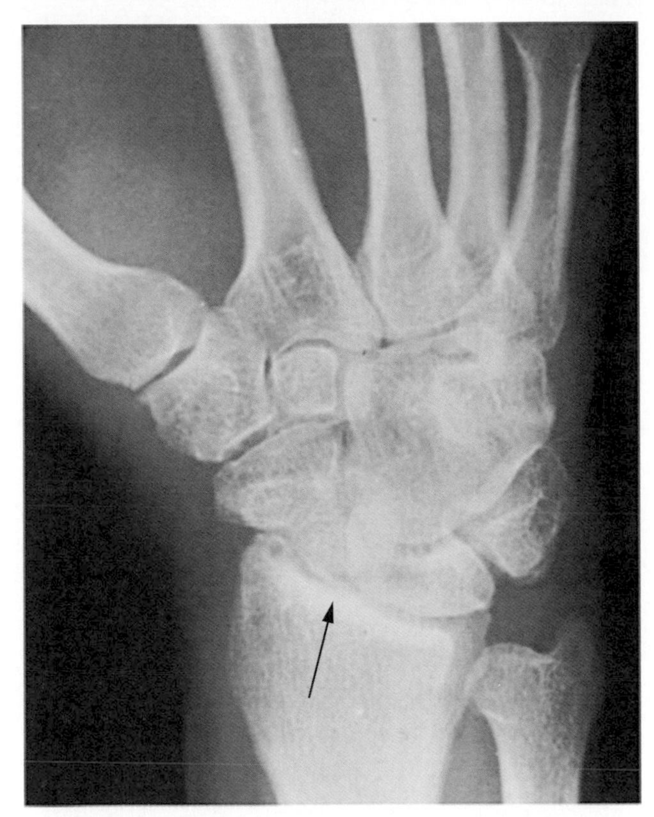

Figure 77-3 Radiocarpal arthritis (*arrow*). (From Green D, Hotchkiss R, Pederson W, Wolfe S [eds]: Green's Operative Hand Surgery, Vol. 1, 5th ed. Philadelphia: Churchill Livingstone, 2005, p 523.)

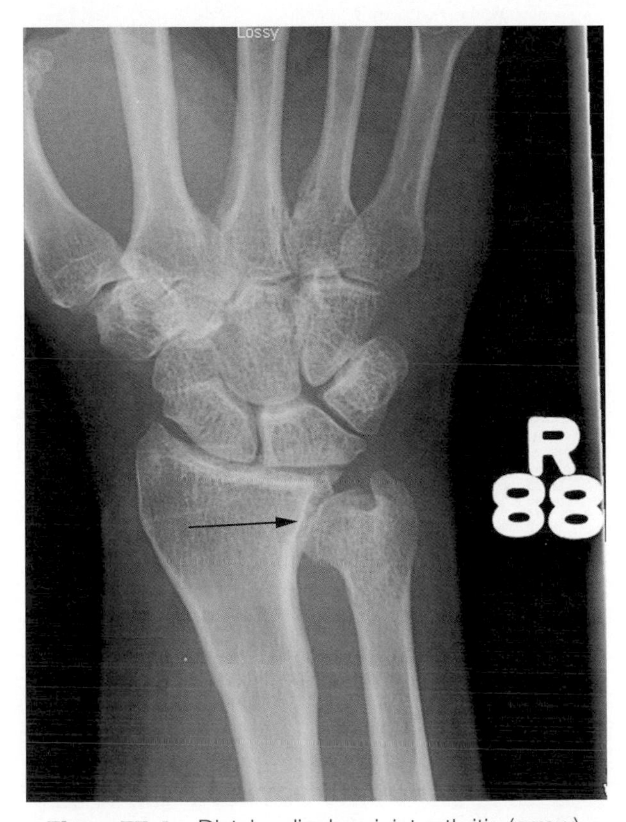

Figure 77-4 Distal radioulnar joint arthritis (*arrow*).

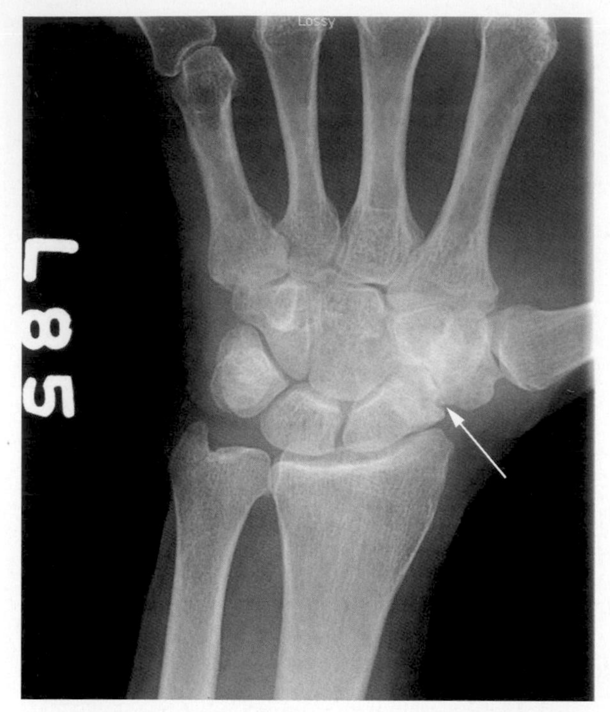

Figure 77-5 Scaphotrapezoid-trapezium arthritis (*arrow*).

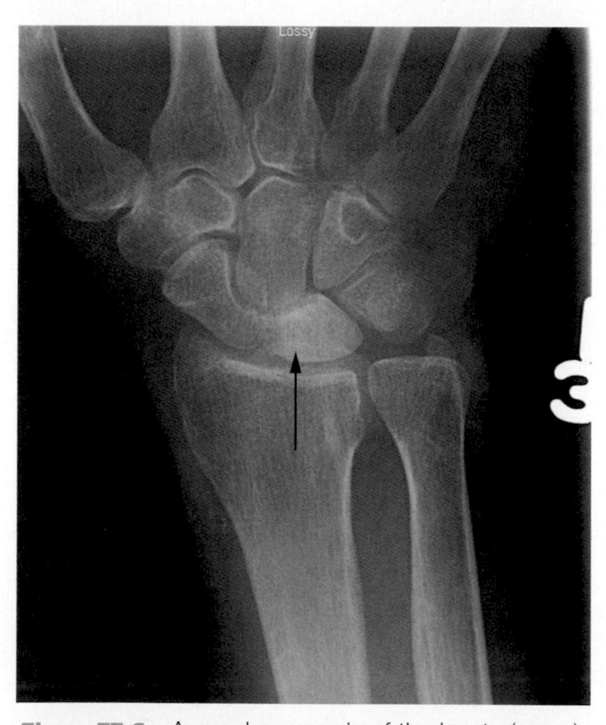

Figure 77-6 Avascular necrosis of the lunate (*arrow*).

- Assess active wrist range of motion. Normal values are listed and any deficiencies or pain should be noted:
  - Flexion: 70 degrees
  - Extension: 80 degrees
  - Radial deviation: 20 degrees
  - Ulnar deviation: 30 degrees

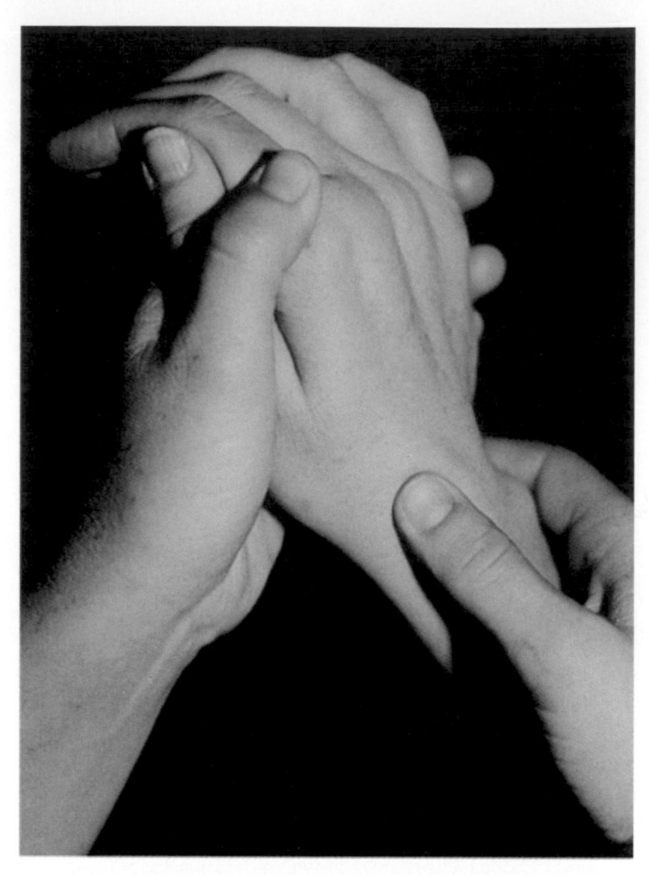

Figure 77-7 Palpation of scaphotrapezoid-trapezium joint. (From Green D, Hotchkiss R, Pederson W, Wolfe S [eds]: Green's Operative Hand Surgery, Vol. 1, 5th ed. Philadelphia: Churchill Livingstone, 2005, p 492.)

- A thorough neurovascular examination of the cervical spine, shoulder, elbow, and wrist should be performed to evaluate for additional pathology.

Imaging

- Obtain anteroposterior, lateral, and oblique views of the wrist as baseline radiographs.
- Staging of specific pathology (Table 77-1; see also Fig. 76-7) as related to SLAC and SNAC wrists
- Additional views:
  - Navicular or scaphoid view to identify scaphoid nonunion or STT arthritis
  - Posteroanterior neutral clenched-fist view to evaluate for scapholunate ligament disruption, which appears as a widening of the scapholunate interval in a clenched fist; may need to obtain contralateral clenched-fist view for comparison (see Chapter 76)
  - Pisiform oblique view to evaluate the pisotriquetral joint

TABLE 77-1 *Stages of Scapholunate Advanced Collapse and Scaphoid Nonunion Advanced Collapse (SNAC) Wrist*

Stage	Joint Degeneration
I	Radial styloid-scaphoid articulation; radial styloid beaking
II	Stage I + radioscaphoid joint (+ scaphocapitate in SNAC)
III	Stage II + capitolunate joint and proximal migration of capitate
IV	Panarthritis including radiolunate joint

Additional Tests

- Computed tomography can evaluate for arthritic changes if none can be identified on plain radiographs.
- Three-phase bone scan to identify area of bone reactivity, which may indicate OA

Differential Diagnosis

- Please see Table 77-2.

Treatment

- At diagnosis
  - Nonsteroidal anti-inflammatory drugs, if tolerated; lifestyle and activity modifications; wrist brace; local modalities such as paraffin baths; and supplements such as glucosamine and chondroitin sulfate may be helpful if not contraindicated.
  - Counseling on the natural history of OA for realistic treatment goals

TABLE 77-2 *Differential Diagnosis*

Condition	Differentiating Features	Chapter Reference
Acute fracture or wrist sprain	History of recent fall or trauma; no evidence of chronic degenerative changes on plain radiographs	79, 96, 97
de Quervain's tenosynovitis	Positive Finkelstein's sign	80
Rheumatoid arthritis	Evidence of erosive arthritis on radiographs; hand and finger deformities such as metacarpophalangeal dislocations; swan neck and boutonnière deformities of fingers	18
Gout	Punch-out lesions on radiographs	18
Calcium pyrophosphate dihydrate deposition or pseudogout	Calcium pyrophosphate dihydrate deposits visible in triangular fibrocartilage complex on plain radiographs	18
Carpal tunnel syndrome	History of numbness, tingling, and pain in the median nerve distribution; pain worse at night; positive provocative maneuvers for carpal tunnel syndrome; normal radiographs; evidence of carpal tunnel syndrome on electromyography/nerve conduction studies	83
Cubital tunnel syndrome or ulnar neuropathy at Guyon's canal	Paresthesias and pain in the ulnar nerve distribution; positive provocative maneuvers for cubital tunnel syndrome at the elbow or in Guyon's canal; normal radiographs; evidence of cubital tunnel syndrome or distal ulnar neuropathy on electromyography/nerve conduction studies	65
Tendonitis of common extensors (extensor carpi ulnaris, extensor radialis carpi brevis, extensor carpi radialis longus, flexor carpi ulnaris, or flexor carpi radialis)	Tenderness to palpation directly over the affected tendon; normal radiographs	81
Triangular fibrocartilage complex injury	Tender to palpation over the triangular fibrocartilage complex; normal radiographs if occurs as isolated injury; magnetic resonance imaging may help to identify triangular fibrocartilage complex tear	79
Ganglion cysts, occult	May have evidence of a palpable, firm, slightly mobile mass; normal radiographs; magnetic resonance imaging can help to identify ganglion cysts	82

- Later (if nonsteroidal anti-inflammatory drugs fail)
    - Fluoroscopically guided corticosteroid injection into affected joint; common injection sites are
        — Radiocarpal joint
        — Distal radioulnar joint
        — STT joint
        — Pisotriquetral joint

When to Refer

- Diagnosis of scaphoid nonunion, scaphoid avascular necrosis, or Kienböck's disease or evidence of acute scapholunate ligament injury because early surgical intervention can prevent progression of arthritis
- When conservative measures fail
- A variety of surgical options are available based on location of arthritis, stage of disease, and patient age and activity level. Options may include proximal row carpectomy, limited versus total wrist arthrodesis, total wrist arthroplasty, and tendon-interposition arthroplasty.

Prognosis

- OA is a chronic progressive disease.
- All patients with a complete scapholunate ligament disruption or an untreated scaphoid nonunion will develop progressive arthritis if left untreated.

Troubleshooting

- Radiocarpal joint injection (see Chapter 105)

Patient Instructions

- OA is a chronic inflammatory condition that does not have a cure, and treatment goals are directed toward limitation of pain.
- Corticosteroid injections take several weeks to become effective.

Considerations in Special Populations

- Young patients who present with wrist pain after traumatic injury should be monitored for occult scaphoid fractures and evidence of scapholunate ligament injury because identification and treatment of these injuries are the key to the prevention of OA.
- Treatment of laborers and young, active patients with wrist arthritis should be geared toward preserving strength and motion for as long as possible.

Suggested Reading

- Cooney WP: Post-traumatic arthritis of the wrist. In Cooney WP, Linscheid RL, Dobyns JH (eds): The Wrist: Diagnosis and Operative Treatment, Vol. 1. St. Louis: Mosby, 1998, pp 588–629.
- Ghazi R: Pisiform ligament complex syndrome and pisotriquetral arthrosis. Hand Clin 2005;21:507–517.
- Hastings H II: Arthrodesis (partial and complete). In Green D, Hotchkiss R, Pederson W, Wolfe S (eds): Green's Operative Hand Surgery, Vol. 1, 5th ed. Philadelphia: Churchill Livingstone, 2005, pp 489–534.
- Parmalee-Peters K, Eathorne S: The wrist: Common injuries and management. Prim Care Clin Office Pract 2005;32:35–70.
- Peterson B, Szabo R: Carpal osteoarthritis. Hand Clin 2006; 22:517–528.
- Weiss K, Rodner C: Osteoarthritis of the wrist. J Hand Surg [Am] 2007;32A:725–746.

Chapter 78 Kienböck's Disease

John B. Thaller

ICD-9 CODES
732.3 *Juvenile Kienböck's Disease*
733.49 *Adult Kienböck's Disease*

Key Concepts

- Kienböck's disease is a condition of avascular necrosis of the lunate.
- The exact etiology of Kienböck's disease remains unknown.
- It is often related to a relative difference in the length of the radius and ulna bones. Specifically it is most common when the ulna is significantly shorter than the ulna.
- Other factors associated with the development of Kienböck's disease include
  - History of trauma
  - Horizontal slope of the distal radius
  - Ligamentous instability of the wrist
- Cadaver studies have demonstrated that a high percentage of lunate bones have only a single blood vessel responsible for nutritional blood flow. This tenuous blood supply is thought to predispose the lunate to avascular necrosis.
- It appears to be more common in men than women and is more common in younger patients.

History

- Signs and symptoms of Kienböck's disease are often vague and insidious in onset.
  - Dorsal or diffuse wrist pain
  - Swelling
  - Stiffness
- A history of trauma may be present in nearly 50% of patients. However, sometimes the trauma is quite minor.

Physical Examination

- Nonspecific examination findings
- Dorsal wrist tenderness over the lunate bone
- Decreased active and passive wrist range of motion
- Dorsal wrist effusion
- Decreased grip strength
- No physical examination finding is specific for Kienböck's disease.

Imaging

- Plain radiographs
  - The Lichtman classification, which is useful for stratification, prognostication, and choosing treatment, is based on plain posteroanterior and lateral radiographs.
    - — Stage I: Plain radiographs may be normal, or there may be a subtle lunate fracture noted. There are no sclerosis and no collapse (Fig. 78-1A).
    - — Stage II: Increased density and sclerosis of the lunate (Fig. 78-2)
    - — Stage IIIa: Lunate collapse with maintained carpal relationships (Fig. 78-3)
    - — Stage IIIb: Lunate collapse with fixed scaphoid rotatory collapse
    - — Stage IV: Extensive pancarpal osteoarthritis
- Magnetic resonance imaging (MRI)
  - In early disease, MRI may be the only radiographic abnormality. If plain radiographs are normal, then MRI may be necessary to establish the correct diagnosis.
  - Decreased signal on T1-weighted images (see Fig. 78-1B)
  - Increased signal on T2-weighted images
  - Fracture or collapse may also be evident on MRI.
- Computed tomography (CT)
  - Often the diagnosis may be confirmed on plain radiographs, but CT is necessary for proper staging of the disease.
  - Figure 78-4 demonstrates a case in which the CT scan significantly altered the staging of the disease and subsequently affected the treatment choice. Plain radiographs appear to be stage I to II, and treatment would be aimed at lunate salvage such as a joint leveling procedure or revascularization of the lunate. However, the CT scan revealed

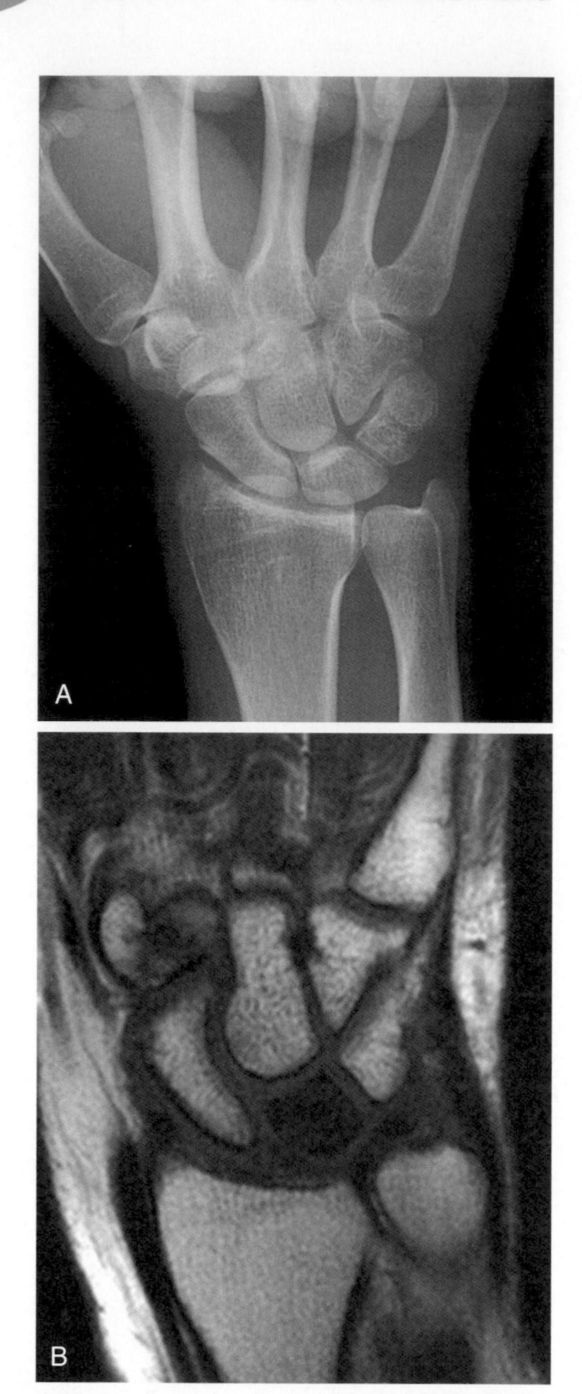

Figure 78-1 **A,** Routine posteroanterior radiograph of a patient with wrist pain with no abnormal radiographic findings. **B,** Coronal magnetic resonance imaging of the same patient with decreased signal on T1, consistent with poor vascularity of the lunate.

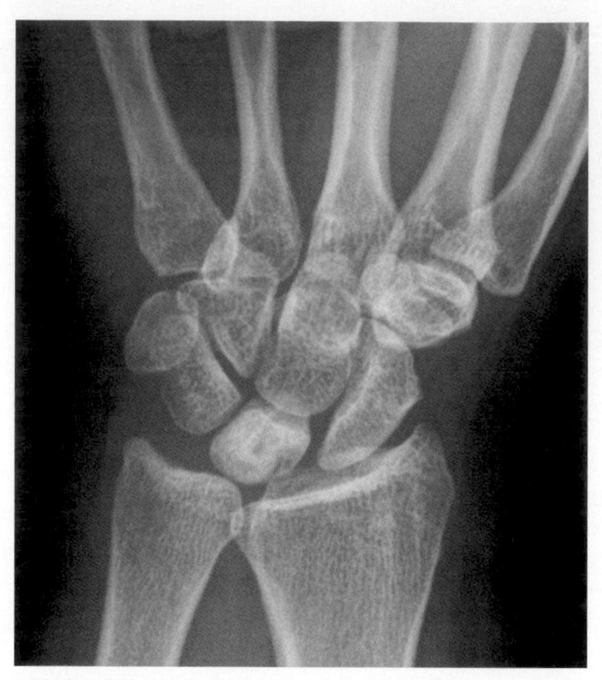

Figure 78-2 Routine posteroanterior radiograph of patient with stage II Kienböck's disease. The lunate shows increased density and sclerosis but no collapse, loss of height, or fracture.

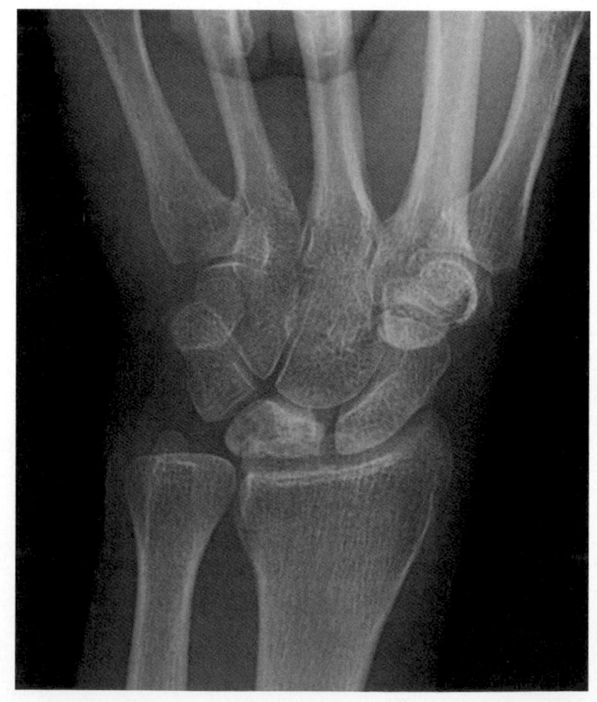

Figure 78-3 Routine posteroanterior radiograph of patient with stage IIIa Kienböck's disease. The lunate shows increased sclerosis as well as collapse and some loss of height more radially than ulnarly.

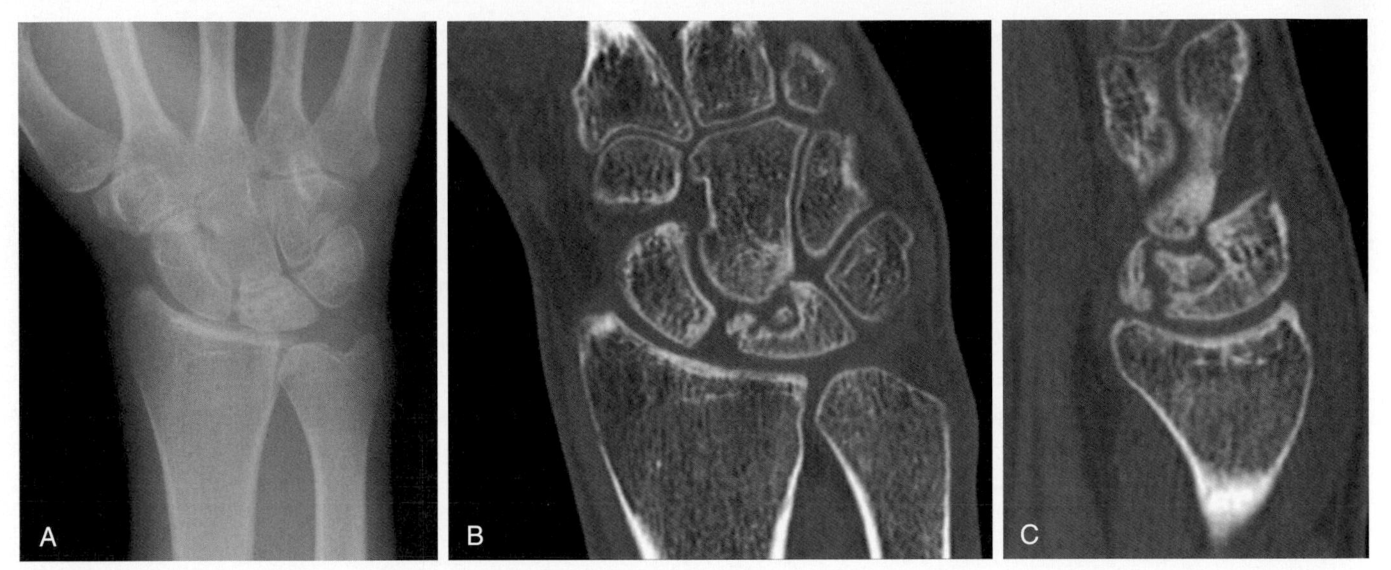

Figure 78-4 **A,** Routine posteroanterior plain radiograph of patient with what appears to be an early stage of Kienböck's disease. Coronal (**B**) and sagittal (**C**) computed tomography scan of the same patient revealing much more advanced collapse and fragmentation than are evident on the plain radiographs. (Photos courtesy of A.Y. Shin, copyright Mayo Foundation.)

TABLE 78-1 *Differential Diagnosis*

Differential Diagnosis	Differentiating Feature
Lunate fracture	A simple lunate fracture may look similar to Kienböck's fragmentation on plain radiographs and computed tomography scans. However, magnetic resonance imaging will be diagnostic in demonstrating avascularity of the lunate in Kienböck's disease.
Wrist sprain	Plain radiography and computed tomography scan may be normal in both conditions, but magnetic resonance imaging will be diagnostic of avascular necrosis, where it should be normal in a wrist sprain.

advanced collapse and fragmentation, which would prevent success with lunate salvage (see Fig. 78-4).

Differential Diagnosis

- Please see Table 78-1.

Treatment

- At diagnosis
  - Initial treatment depends entirely on proper radiographic staging.
  - All patients should have plain radiographs and a CT scan to accurately assess for sclerosis, collapse, and fragmentation.
  - Although MRI may be necessary to establish the early diagnosis of Kienböck's disease, a CT scan is necessary for accurate staging.
  - The role of non-operative treatment in adults with an established diagnosis of Kienböck's disease remains somewhat controversial.
  - In patients with completely normal plain radiographs but a positive MRI, some authors would advocate for a period of immobilization as the initial treatment. Some authors, though, feel that surgical treatment is indicated for all adults with the diagnosis of Kienböck's disease.
- Later
  - Patients with more advanced radiographic disease or patients in whom nonoperative treatment has failed will require surgical intervention.
  - There is no one universally accepted surgical procedure.
  - In patients with an ulnar negative variant, a radial shortening osteotomy has proven successful.
  - In more advanced stages, a vascularized bone graft procedure may be necessary to reintroduce blood supply to the lunate.
  - Patients with Kienböck's stage IIIb and beyond will need a salvage procedure.
  - In these patients, the fragmentation of the lunate and the associated degenerative changes prevent successful reconstruction unless the lunate is

removed or mechanically bypassed with a partial wrist fusion.
- A proximal row carpectomy, partial wrist fusion, or total wrist fusion may often be necessary to provide good pain relief in these advanced cases.

When to Refer

- Any patient with an MRI demonstrating avascular necrosis of the lunate should be referred to a hand surgeon for discussion of treatment options.
- Any patient who initially presents with collapse, fragmentation, or other advanced radiographic changes should also be referred immediately to a hand surgeon.

Prognosis

- Patients who present early and respond to nonoperative treatment can expect an excellent outcome with eventual resolution of symptoms.
- Patients who either present with or progress to further radiographic changes have a much more guarded prognosis.
- Natural history studies seem to demonstrate that the majority of patients will demonstrate progressive radiographic collapse, fragmentation, and arthrosis of the lunate, so the key to a good prognosis remains early recognition and early treatment.

Troubleshooting

- In patients with early disease, the diagnosis may be difficult to make.
- All patients who present with chronic diffuse wrist pain should have plain radiographs.
- If plain radiographs are normal and the patient fails to respond to routine appropriate nonoperative treatment, then MRI is warranted.
- MRI should be diagnostic in the majority of cases.
- CT should then be ordered for accurate staging to evaluate for fracture and fragmentation.

Patient Instructions

- It is often difficult to explain this vexing problem to patients.
- The diagnosis is often difficult to establish, the etiology remains uncertain, and there are multiple treatment options.
- An early frank discussion regarding the diagnosis and the necessity for referral to a hand surgeon will be helpful for the patient.

Considerations in Special Populations

- Younger patients have shown a more favorable outcome after both nonoperative and operative treatments for Kienböck's disease.
- When avascular necrosis without fragmentation is diagnosed in a teenage patient, the initial treatment should always be immobilization.
- Patients being treated non-operatively should be monitored closely. Progression of sclerosis, collapse, or fracture will often indicated that surgical intervention is necessary.

Suggested Reading

- Beckenbaugh RD, Shives TC, Dobyns JH, Linscheid RL: Kienbock's disease: The natural history of Kienbock's disease and consideration of lunate fractures. Clin Orthop Relat Res 1980;149:98–106.
- Gelberman RH, Bauman TD, Menon J, Akeson WH: The vascularity of the lunate bone and Kienböck's disease. J Hand Surg [Am] 1980;5:272–278.
- Iwasaki N, Minami A, Oizumi N, et al: Predictors of clinical results of radial osteotomies for Kienbock's disease. Clin Orthop Relat Res 2003;415:157–162.
- Lichtman DM, Degnan GG: Staging and its use in the determination of treatment modalities for Kienbock's disease. Hand Clin 1993;9:409–416.
- Raven E, Haverkamp D, Marti RK: Outcome of Kienbock's disease 22 years after distal radius shortening osteotomy. Clin Orthop Relat Res 2007;460:137–141.
- Salmon J, Stanley JK, Trail IA: Kienbock's disease: Conservative management versus radial shortening. J Bone Joint Surg Br 2000;82B:820–823.
- Shin A, Bishop A: Vascular anatomy of the distal radius: Implications for vascularized bone grafts. Clin Orthop Relat Res 2001;38:60–67.

Chapter 79 Triangular Fibrocartilage Complex Injuries

Sara D. Rynders and A. Bobby Chhabra

ICD-9 CODE
842.09 *Sprain of Distal Radioulnar Joint*

Key Concepts

- The triangular fibrocartilage complex (TFCC) is located on the ulnar aspect of the wrist and functions as a major stabilizer of the distal radioulnar joint (DRUJ). It is composed of (Fig. 79-1)
  - Fibrocartilage disc
  - Volar and dorsal distal radioulnar ligaments
  - Meniscus homologue
  - Volar ulnocarpal ligaments: ulnolunate and ulnotriquetral ligaments
  - Floor of the extensor carpi ulnaris tendon sheath
- The TFCC carries 18% to 20% of the axial load of the wrist.
  - Any factor that increases the axial load on the ulnar aspect of the wrist puts the TFCC at risk of injury.
- Patients with ulnar positive variance (due to anatomic variation, distal radius malunion, growth arrest, or radial head resection) are at greater risk of developing central TFCC pathology.
- TFCC injuries are classified as (Fig. 79-2)
  - Type 1: traumatic lesions
    - — Type 1A: central TFCC perforation (most common)
    - — Type 1B: base of the ulnar styloid with or without ulnar styloid fracture
    - — Type 1C: carpal detachment (volar ulnolunate ligaments)
    - — Type 1D: radial detachment with or without radial avulsion fracture
  - Type 2: degenerative lesions
    - — Type 2A: thinning of the articular disc
    - — Type 2B: thinning of the articular disc and lunate chondromalacia
    - — Type 2C: central perforation of the TFCC and lunate chondromalacia
    - — Type 2D: central perforation of the TFCC, lunate chondromalacia, and lunotriquetral ligament perforation
    - — Type 2E: central perforation of the TFCC, lunate chondromalacia, lunotriquetral ligament perforation, ulnocarpal arthritis
- Vascular supply
  - The ulnar peripheral TFCC is vascularized, whereas the central aspect of the TFCC is avascular; this principle guides treatment options.
  - Peripheral lesions can usually be repaired as they have a high healing potential; central lesions may be treated conservatively or require arthroscopic débridement because poor vascularity leads to a poor healing potential.
- Posteroanterior neutral view plain radiographs of the wrist must be obtained to assess for ulnar positive variance.
- Arthroscopy remains the gold standard of diagnosis; however, magnetic resonance imaging arthrograms are improving in their diagnostic capabilities.

History

- The patient reports ulnar-sided wrist pain that may increase with power grip or ulnar deviation or may report a "clicking" in the wrist.
- May report a recent or remote history of a fall on an outstretched hand, sudden rotational force, axial loading with distraction, or repetitive loading
- May have a history of distal radius malunion with radial shortening

Physical Examination

- Inspection may reveal a prominent ulnar styloid if the DRUJ is significantly disrupted and there is edema on the ulnar aspect of the wrist.
- Palpate the TFCC on the ulnar aspect of the wrist, distal to the ulnar styloid in the soft spot between the

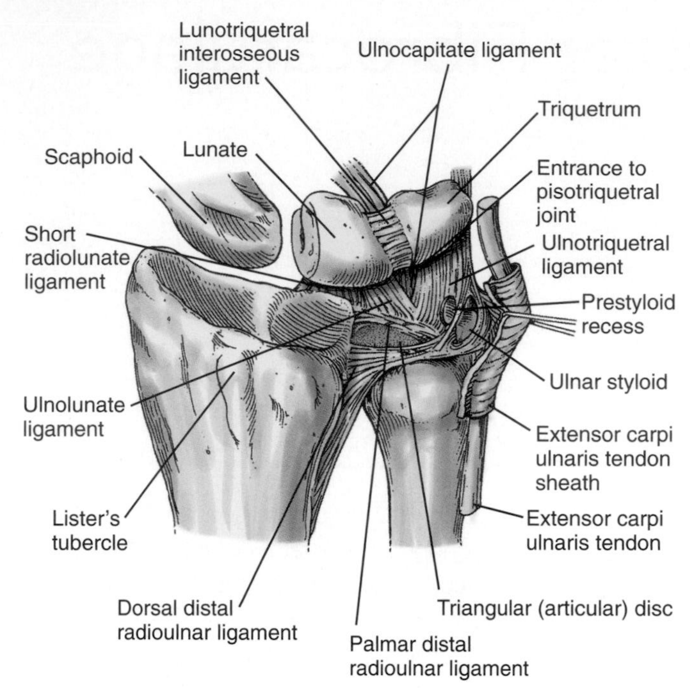

Figure 79-1 Anatomy of the triangular fibrocartilage complex. (Adapted from Cooney WP, Linscheid RL, Dobyns JH [eds]: The Wrist: Diagnosis and Operative Treatment. St Louis: Mosby, 1998.)

extensor carpi ulnaris and flexor carpi ulnaris tendons; tenderness may indicate a peripheral TFCC tear.

- Ulnar grind test:
  - Extend, axially load, and ulnarly deviate the wrist; pain may indicate a TFCC tear.
- Palpate the DRUJ with the wrist in pronation and perform the piano key test.
  - Place one hand on the radius and apply dorsal pressure over the ulnar head.
  - Compare with the opposite side.
  - Increased motion or pain with motion on the injured side can indicate DRUJ instability.
- A thorough examination of all wrist structures should be performed, taking care to isolate the area of tenderness.
- A thorough neurovascular examination of the upper extremity should also be performed.

Imaging

- Posteroanterior neutral and true lateral views of the wrist
  - Posteroanterior neutral position: the arm is abducted to 90 degrees at the shoulder, the elbow is flexed to 90 degrees, and the forearm is in a neutral pronation (Fig. 79-3)

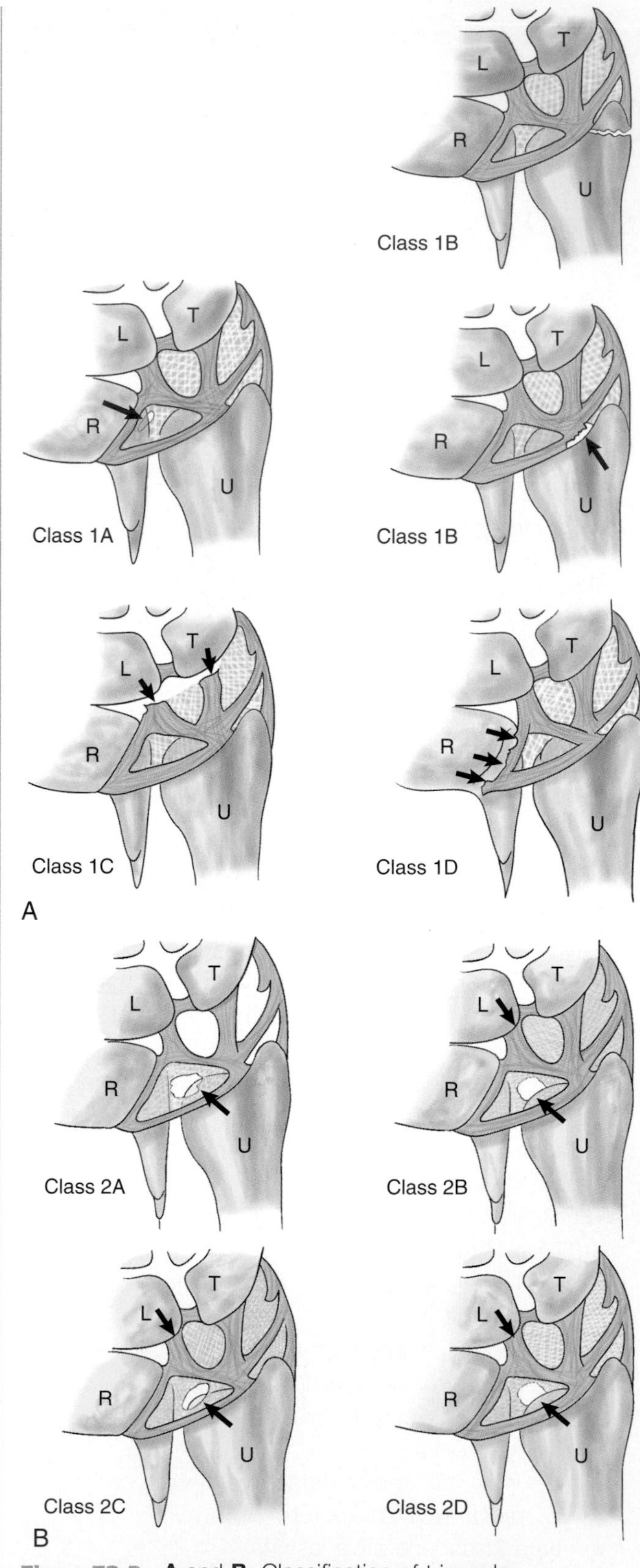

Figure 79-2 **A** and **B,** Classification of triangular fibrocartilage complex injuries. L, lunate; R, radius; T, triquetum; U, ulna. (Adapted from Green D, Hotchkiss R, Pederson W, Wolfe S [eds]: Green's Operative Hand Surgery, Vol. 1, 5th ed. Philadelphia: Churchill Livingstone, 2005.)

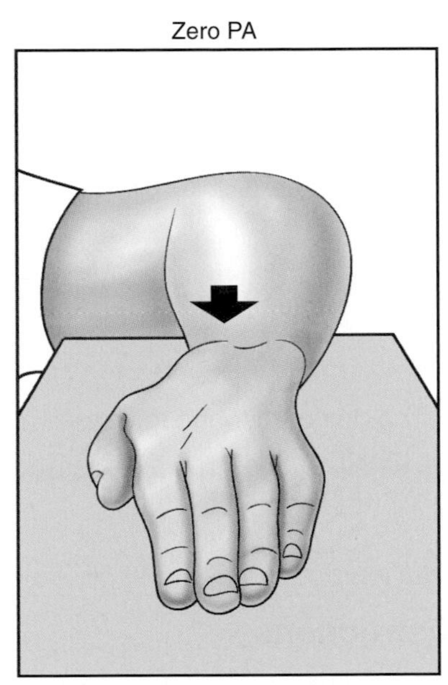

Figure 79-3 Posteroanterior (PA) neutral view. *Arrow* demonstrates the direction of x-ray beam from posterior to anterior. (Adapted from Green D, Hotchkiss R, Pederson W, Wolfe S [eds]: Green's Operative Hand Surgery, Vol. 1, 5th ed. Philadelphia: Churchill Livingstone, 2005.)

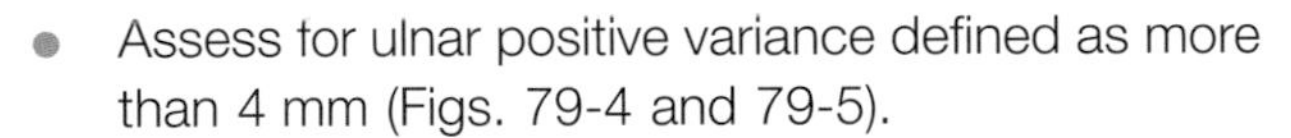

- Assess for ulnar positive variance defined as more than 4 mm (Figs. 79-4 and 79-5).
- Assess for DRUJ widening on a posteroanterior view radiograph and compare with the opposite wrist.
- Assess for DRUJ dislocation on lateral radiographs.
- Radiographs may be normal.

- Additional views
  - Pronated posteroanterior grip view: obtain if a degenerative TFCC lesion is suspected because this view may demonstrate ulnar impaction.

Additional Tests

- Magnetic resonance imaging with gadolinium (Fig. 79-6)
  - Controversial due to variation in quality of images, radiologist experience, and technique
  - High-resolution magnetic resonance imaging may reveal a TFCC tear.
  - Useful to work through the differential diagnosis
- Arthroscopy is the gold standard for diagnosis and treatment.

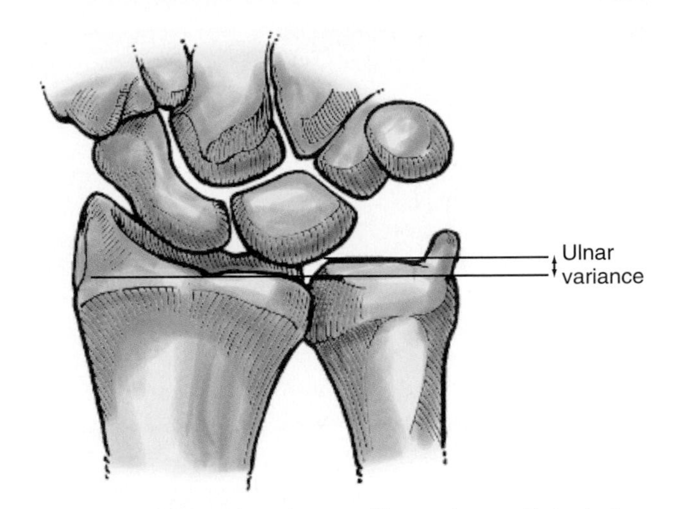

Figure 79-4 Measuring ulnar positive variance. (Adapted from Green D, Hotchkiss R, Pederson W, Wolfe S [eds]: Green's Operative Hand Surgery, Vol. 1, 5th ed. Philadelphia: Churchill Livingstone, 2005.)

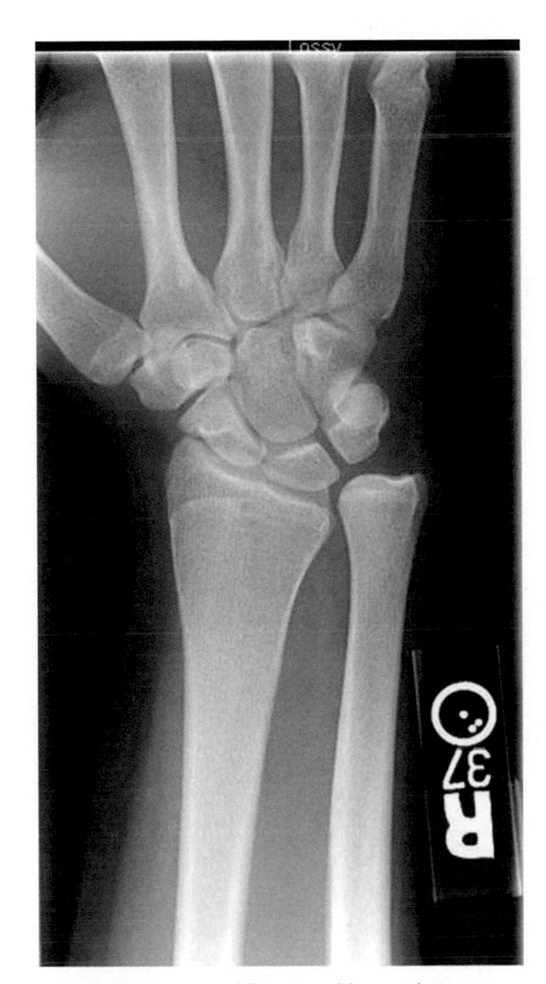

Figure 79-5 Ulnar positive variance.

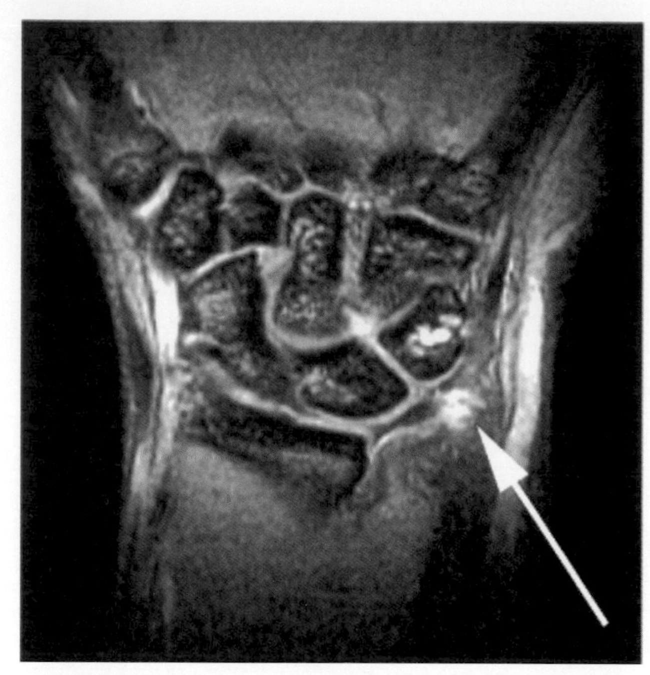

Figure 79-6 Triangular fibrocartilage complex tear *(arrow)* on magnetic resonance imaging.

Differential Diagnosis

- Please see Table 79-1.

Treatment

- At diagnosis
  - If a TFCC tear is suspected in the presence of normal radiographs and no DRUJ instability, immobilize the wrist in a splint for 4 to 6 weeks and initiate nonsteroidal anti-inflammatory drugs for pain relief if tolerated.
- Later
  - Once the patient is pain free, occupational therapy may help facilitate wrist range of motion and guide strengthening after prolonged immobilization.

When to Refer

- Persistent symptoms after 4 to 6 weeks of conservative management
  - Immobilize in a wrist splint and refer to a hand specialist within 7 to 10 days.
- If patient has positive physical examination findings and any of the following, refer immediately
  - Ulnar positive variance
  - Evidence of DRUJ instability
  - Distal radius or ulna fracture
- If surgery is indicated, there are many different options based on the location and type of injury.
- The gold standard of diagnosis is wrist arthroscopy; some injuries may be repaired arthroscopically, whereas others may require ulnar shortening procedures or open repairs.

Prognosis

- Patients who do not respond to conservative management will generally have an excellent outcome with arthroscopic débridement or repair.

Patient Instructions

- If being managed conservatively, the patient should wear a wrist brace at all times except when showering, avoid provocating activities, and avoid heavy lifting.

Considerations in Special Populations

- If a TFCC injury is suspected in a high-level athlete, immobilize the wrist in a splint and perform magnetic resonance imaging. Refer to a hand specialist within 7 days because the patient may require wrist arthroscopy for evaluation and treatment.

Suggested Reading

- Adams BD: Distal radioulnar joint instability. In Green D, Hotchkiss R, Pederson W, Wolfe S (eds): Green's Operative Hand Surgery, Vol. 1, 5th ed. Philadelphia: Churchill Livingstone, 2005, pp 605–644.
- Ahn A, Chang D, Plate A: Triangular fibrocartilage complex tears—a review. Bull Hosp Jt Dis 2006;64(3–4):114–118.
- Cooney WP: Tears of the triangular fibrocartilage of the wrist. In Cooney WP, Linscheid RL, Dobyns JH (eds): The Wrist: Diagnosis and Operative Treatment. St. Louis: Mosby, 1998, pp 710–742.
- Elkowitz SJ, Posner MA: Wrist arthroscopy. Bull Hosp Jt Dis 2006;64(3–4):156–165.
- Palmer AK: Triangular fibrocartilage complex lesions: A classification. J Hand Surg [Am] 1989;14:594–606.
- Palmer AK, Werner FW: The triangular fibrocartilage complex of the wrist—anatomy and function. J Hand Surg [Am] 1981; 6:153–162.
- Parmalee-Peters K, Eathorne S: The wrist: Common injuries and management. Prim Care Clin Office Pract 2005;32:35–70.
- Rettig AC: Athletic injuries of the wrist and hand. Part I: Traumatic injuries of the wrist. Am J Sports Med 2003;31:1028–1048.

TABLE 79-1 *Differential Diagnosis*

Condition	Differentiating Features	Chapter Reference
Extensor carpi ulnar tendonitis	Tenderness to palpation over extensor carpi ulnar tendon sheath; pain with resisted wrist extension	81
Flexor carpi ulnar tendonitis	Tenderness to palpation over flexor carpi ulnar tendon sheath; pain with resisted wrist flexion	81
Pisotriquetral osteoarthritis	Pain over pisotriquetral joint; evidence of pisotriquetral arthritis on radiograph, pisiform oblique view	77
Distal radioulnar joint osteoarthritis	Pain with distal radioulnar joint ballottement; evidence of arthritis at distal radioulnar joint on radiograph	77
Occult ganglion cysts	May have history of wrist mass that increases and decreases in size; visualized on magnetic resonance imaging	82
Cubital tunnel syndrome	Paresthesias in ulnar nerve distribution, worse with elbow flexion or leaning on the elbow; positive provocative maneuvers for cubital tunnel syndrome; electromyography/nerve conduction studies show evidence of cubital tunnel syndrome	65
Ulnar nerve compression at Guyon's canal	Paresthesias in the fourth and fifth digits; tenderness to palpation over Guyon's canal with positive Tinel's sign; electromyography/nerve conduction studies show evidence of ulnar neuropathy at Guyon's canal	65
Hook of hamate fracture	Tenderness over the hook of the hamate; carpal tunnel view shows hook of hamate fracture on radiograph; may require computed tomography scan to diagnose fracture	97
Ulnar artery thrombosis	May or may not have color and temperature changes in the fingers; Allen's test reveals radial artery dominant flow; computed tomography angiography helpful to visualize occult hook of hamate fractures and evidence of thrombosis	21
Essex-Lopresti lesion	History of elbow injury or pain or radial head excision; posteroanterior and lateral views of elbow reveal fracture malunion or resected radial head; must also obtain views of wrist to identify ulnar positive variance	67
Scapholunate ligament disruption	Pain over scapholunate interval; may have a positive Watson's maneuver; posteroanterior clenched-fist radiograph reveals scapholunate widening greater than 5 mm* compared with contralateral side; magnetic resonance imaging shows ligament disruption	76
Lunotriquetral ligament disruption	Positive lunotriquetral shuck test; evidence of volar intercalated segment instability deformity on lateral radiographs; magnetic resonance imaging shows ligament disruption	76
Calcium pyrophosphate dihydrate deposition syndrome or pseudogout	Calcium pyrophosphate dihydrate deposits visible in the triangular fibrocartilage complex on plain radiographs	18

*There is some controversy surrounding this value. A wide interval may be defined as more than 3 mm if there are correlating physical examination findings and widening of the interval compared with the uninjured wrist.

Chapter 80 de Quervain's Tenosynovitis

David Schnur

ICD-9 CODE
727.04 *Radial Styloid Tenosynovitis*

Key Concepts

- Tenosynovitis of the first dorsal compartment of the wrist
  - The abductor pollicis longus and extensor pollicis brevis muscles occupy the first dorsal compartment (Fig. 80-1).
- Fritz de Quervain first described the condition in 1895.
- Attributed to and exacerbated by activities involving thumb abduction with ulnar deviation of the wrist
- Anatomy of the first dorsal compartment can have significant variation
  - The extensor pollicis brevis tendon is absent in 5% to 7% of extremities.
  - The compartment has a longitudinal septum in 24% to 34% of extremities.
  - The abductor pollicis longus muscle often has two or more slips with various insertions.
- Anatomic variation can lead to failure of nonoperative treatment.

History

- Several weeks or months of pain over the radial styloid
- Exacerbated with movement of the thumb
- Can have associated swelling over the radial styloid
- Can have pseudotriggering
- Most common in fourth and fifth decades
- Much more common in women
  - Can occur after childbirth

Physical Examination

- Tenderness on palpation over the first dorsal compartment
  - 1 to 2 cm proximal to the radial styloid
- Finkelstein's test (Fig. 80-2)
  - With the thumb grasped in the palm, ulnar deviation of the wrist causes sharp pain.
- Can have pain with resisted abduction of thumb
- Occasionally associated with a ganglion over the first dorsal compartment

Imaging

- Radiographs
  - Useful to differentiate from carpometacarpal arthritis of the thumb
  - Can rule out radial styloid fracture as the cause of pain
  - Occasionally see localized osteopenia or spurring of the radius
  - Not typically necessary to make the diagnosis
- Magnetic resonance imaging can assist in diagnosis if diagnosis is difficult.

Differential Diagnosis

- Please see Table 80-1.

Treatment

- At diagnosis
  - Splinting or casting can relieve symptoms but is often not curative as a single therapy.
  - Corticosteroid injection should be considered a first-line treatment and can be combined with immobilization.
    - — Occasionally a second injection is necessary.
    - — For details and proper injection technique, refer to Chapter 104.
- Later
  - Surgical release of the first dorsal compartment is typically reserved for patients in whom conservative treatment failed.
    - — A 2-cm transverse incision is made over the first dorsal compartment just proximal to the radial styloid.

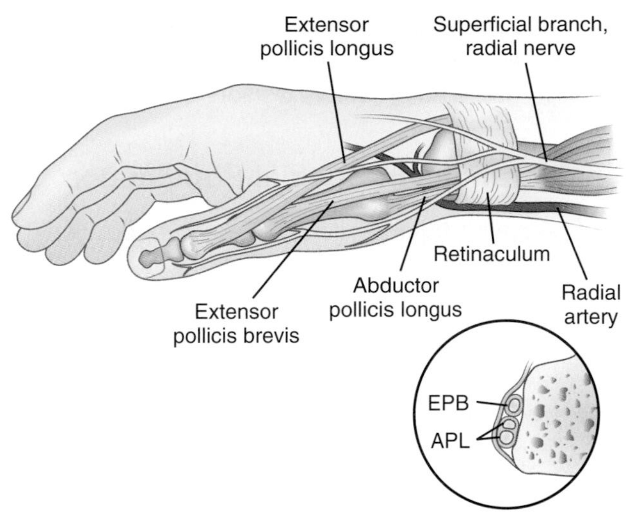

Figure 80-1 Anatomic relationship of the first dorsal compartment. APL, abductor pollicis longus; EPB, extensor pollicis brevis. (Adapted from Green DP, Hotchkiss RN, Pederson WC, Wolfe SW [eds]: Operative Hand Surgery, 5th ed. Philadelphia: Churchill Livingstone, 2005, p 2153, Fig. 60-16. Copyright Elizabeth Martin.)

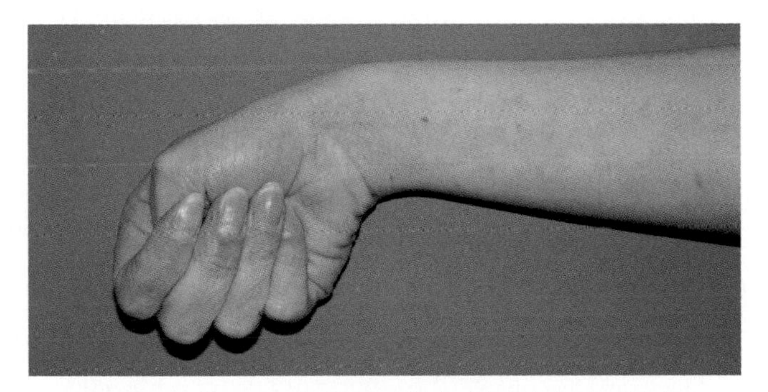

Figure 80-2 Demonstration of Finkelstein's test with the thumb in the palm and the wrist ulnarly deviated.

TABLE 80-1 *Differential Diagnosis*

Diagnosis	Differentiating Features	Chapter Reference
Carpometacarpal arthritis of the thumb	Pain typically more distal, negative Finkelstein's test, positive carpometacarpal grind	84
Radial styloid fracture	History of trauma with positive radiographs, pain over dorsal radial styloid on palpation	96
Radiocarpal arthritis	Pain more dorsal over radiocarpal joint on palpation, radiographs with arthritic changes	77

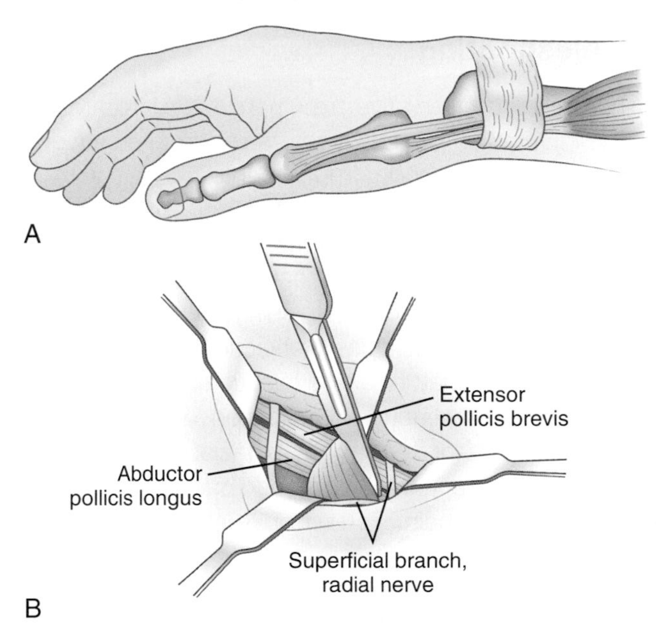

Figure 80-3 Surgical treatment of de Quervain's tenosynovitis. **A,** The first dorsal compartment is approached through a short transverse incision. **B,** The extensor retinaculum is divided longitudinally. (Adapted from Green DP, Hotchkiss RN, Pederson WC, Wolfe SW [eds]: Operative Hand Surgery, 5th ed. Philadelphia: Churchill Livingstone, 2005, p 2153, Fig. 60-17. Copyright Elizabeth Martin.)

— Longitudinal dissection is performed down to the level of the first dorsal compartment with care to protect cutaneous nerves.

— The compartment is released, and care is taken to ensure that intracompartmental septa are divided if present (Fig. 80-3).

When to Refer

- Once the diagnosis is made, timing of the referral is dependent on the comfort of the provider in rendering conservative treatment.
  - If the provider is experienced in corticosteroid injection of the first dorsal compartment, then referral should be made if this therapy fails and operative treatment is necessary.
  - If the provider is not comfortable with giving the injection, then referral should be made at the time of diagnosis.

Prognosis

- Good with conservative measures alone and excellent with surgical intervention

Troubleshooting

- Failure of conservative treatment may indicate anatomic variation or tenosynovitis at the intersection of the first and second compartments.
- The patient should be counseled on the risks of conservative and surgical treatment.
  - Corticosteroid injection can cause hypopigmentation and fat atrophy; this may occur more often than with other types of injections because of the superficial nature of the injection.
  - The most serious complication of surgical intervention is injury to the superficial sensory branch of the radial nerve, which can cause numbness or significant pain. Failure of relief of symptoms is also possible.

Patient Instructions

- Patients should be given details of the disease process.
- Additionally they should be instructed not to lift objects with the hands vertical to the ground using an ulnar to radial deviation motion.
  - This is especially important for mothers of young children with this condition because they tend to lift their children in this fashion.

Considerations in Special Populations

- Conservative treatment in the diabetic population may be less effective.

Suggested Reading

- de Quervain F: On a form of chronic tendovaginitis by Dr. Fritz de Quervain in la Chaux-de-Fonds 1895. Am J Orthop 1997;26:641–644.
- Gundes H, Tosun B: Longitudinal incision in surgical release of de Quervain disease. Tech Hand Up Extrem Surg 2005;9:149–152.
- Kulthanan T, Chareonwat B: Variations in abductor pollicis longus and extensor pollicis brevis tendons in de Quervain syndrome: A surgical and anatomical study. Scand J Plast Reconstr Surg Hand Surg 2007;41:36–38.
- Witt J, Pess G, Gelberman RH: Treatment of de Quervain tenosynovitis. A prospective study of the results of injection of steroids and immobilization in a splint. J Bone Joint Surg Am 1991;73:219–222.
- Wolfe SW: Tenosynovitis. In Green DP, Hotchkiss RN, Pederson WC, Wolfe SW (eds): Operative Hand Surgery, 5th ed. Philadelphia: Churchill Livingstone, 2005, pp 2150–2154.

Chapter 81 Tendinitis of the Wrist

David Schnur

ICD-9 CODE
727.05 *Tenosynovitis, Wrist*

Key Concepts

- Tenosynovitis of the wrist can affect the following tendons (Fig. 81-1)
  - Extensor pollicis longus (EPL)
  - Extensor carpi ulnaris (ECU)
  - Flexor carpi radialis (FCR)
  - Muscle bellies of the abductor pollicis longus and the extensor pollicis brevis (intersection syndrome)
  - Fourth extensor compartment (extensor digitorum communis and extensor indicis proprius)
  - Extensor digiti minimi
- Intersection syndrome describes pain and swelling about the muscle bellies of the abductor pollicis longus and the extensor pollicis brevis at the point in which they cross the radial wrist extensors (Fig. 81-2).
  - Anatomically located 4 cm proximal to the wrist on the dorsoradial aspect
  - Originally thought to occur as a result of friction between the muscle bellies of the abductor pollicis longus and extensor pollicis brevis tendons and the radial wrist extensors; now believed to be entrapment of the second dorsal compartment (extensor carpi radialis longus and extensor carpi radialis brevis)
- EPL tenosynovitis is rare and occurs on the dorsal wrist at Lister's tubercle (the location at which the EPL wraps around and heads for the thumb).
  - If undiagnosed, can lead to tendon rupture
  - Can occur with blunt trauma or fractures of the distal radius
- ECU tenosynovitis is a more common problem and occurs on the dorsoulnar aspect of the wrist.
  - Common cause of ulnar-side wrist pain
  - Can be initiated by a twisting injury of the wrist
  - Can cause dysesthesias along the distribution of the dorsal sensory branch of the ulnar nerve
  - Can cause pain at night
- FCR tendinitis can occur at the point where the tendon crosses the ridge of the trapezium on the volar radial aspect of the wrist.
  - Uncommon
  - Can lead to rupture of the FCR tendon
- Fourth extensor compartment tendinitis most commonly affects the tendons of the ECU to the small and index fingers because of the more acute angle that these tendons take from the compartment to their respective insertions.
  - Uncommon except in rheumatoid arthritis
  - Can occur after a distal radius fracture and has been associated with dorsal hardware on the dorsal distal radius
- Extensor digiti minimi tendinitis is uncommon except in rheumatoid arthritis.

History

- Pain and swelling around the wrist
- Pain with certain motions and activities
- Most commonly worse with activity but can occur at night (especially ECU tendinitis)
- Prolonged pain after blunt trauma or distal radius fracture
- Crepitus with certain conditions may be reported

Physical Examination

- Intersection syndrome
  - Can have swelling and even redness
  - Tenderness to palpation 4 cm proximal to the radial styloid (Fig. 81-3)
  - Pain with wrist extension and radial deviation
  - Occasionally palpable crepitus
- EPL
  - Pain with resisted thumb extension
  - Pain on palpation over Lister's tubercle
  - Swelling at Lister's tubercle
- ECU
  - Pain on palpation of tendon with resisted wrist extension and ulnar deviation

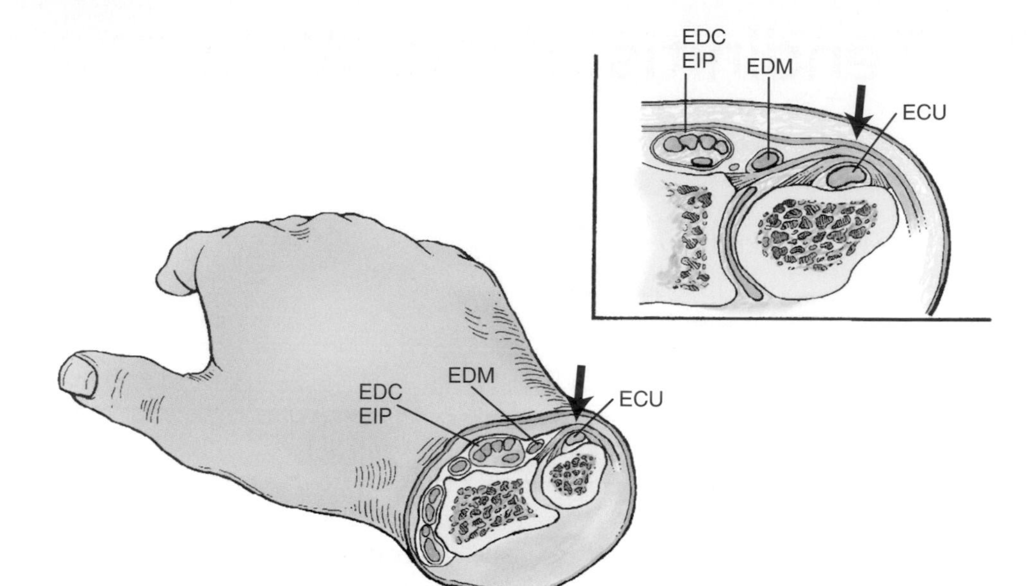

Figure 81-1 Location of the six dorsal compartments of the wrist. Note the contribution of the extensor carpi ulnaris (ECU) tendon sheath to the triangular fibrocartilage complex (*arrow*). EDC, extensor digitorum communis; EDM, extensor digiti minimi; EIP, extensor indicis proprius. (Adapted with permission from Green DP, Hotchkiss RN, Pederson WC, Wolfe SW [eds]: Operative Hand Surgery, 5th ed. Philadelphia: Churchill Livingstone, 2005, p 2151, Fig. 60-13.)

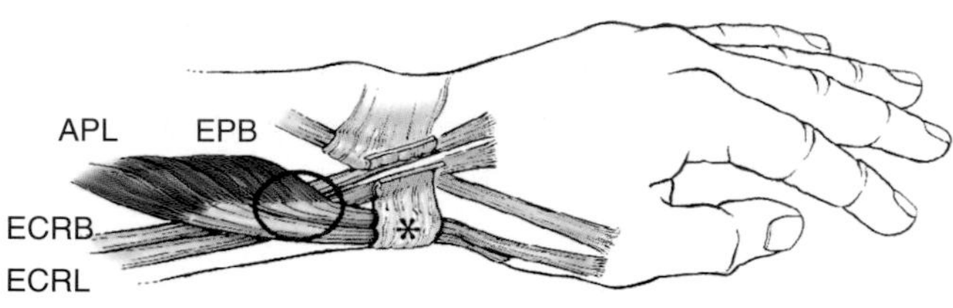

Figure 81-2 Location of the intersection syndrome where the extensor pollicis brevis (EPB) and the abductor pollicis longus (APL) cross the radial wrist extensors (*circled area*). The second dorsal compartment has been released in the manner recommended for the treatment of intersection syndrome. ECRB, extensor carpi radialis brevis; ECRL, extensor carpi radialis longus. (Adapted with permission from Green DP, Hotchkiss RN, Pederson WC, Wolfe SW [eds]: Operative Hand Surgery, 5th ed. Philadelphia: Churchill Livingstone, 2005, p 2155, Fig. 60-19.)

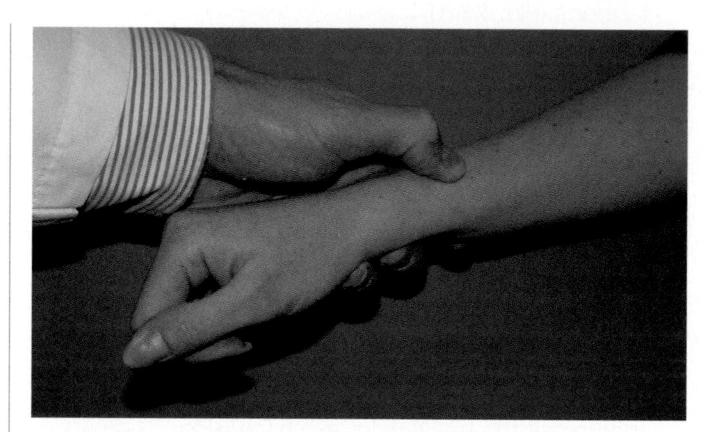

Figure 81-3 Location of pain in patient with intersection syndrome. The extensor pollicis brevis and the abductor pollicis longus cross the radial wrist extensors approximately 4 cm proximal to the radial styloid.

    - Can have palpable crepitus
- FCU
    - Can have swelling over volar wrist
    - Pain on palpation of tendon with resisted wrist flexion
- Fourth dorsal compartment and extensor digiti minimi
    - Swelling and pain on palpation over central dorsal wrist
    - Pain with resisted finger extension

Imaging

- Plain radiographs do not tend to be helpful in the diagnosis except in rare case of calcific tendinitis.
- Magnetic resonance imaging can be used to confirm or assist with diagnosis and will show inflammation around the tendon.

Additional Tests

- Injection of a local anesthetic agent into the respective tendon sheath should give substantial or complete relief of symptoms and can be used for diagnostic purposes.

Differential Diagnosis

- Most other causes of wrist pain are included in the differential diagnosis for tendinitis.
- ECU tendinitis is typically the most difficult diagnosis of the different types of tendinitis.
    - Symptoms may mimic those from both triangular fibrocartilage complex pathology as well as distal radioulnar joint pathology.
- FCR tendinitis can be difficult to diagnose also because its symptoms can mimic those of basal joint arthritis,

scaphoid fractures and nonunions, and volar ganglion cysts.

Treatment

- At diagnosis
  - First-line therapies for the stenotic conditions of the wrist are modification of activity, nonsteroidal anti-inflammatory drugs, and splinting.
  - Immobilization is best accomplished with a well-formed thermoplastic splint with the wrist in approximately 20 degrees of extension.
  - Steroid injection into the tendon sheath can be considered as first-line therapy with immobilization or in cases in which immobilization alone has failed.
- Later
  - Surgical release of the affected tendon should be performed if nonoperative therapy has failed.
  - Intersection syndrome
    - — A longitudinal incision is made over the radial wrist extensors from the level of their insertion and carried proximally approximately 4 cm.
    - — The muscle bellies of the abductor pollicis longus and extensor pollicis brevis are retracted proximally, and the second dorsal compartment is released.
    - — The retinaculum does not need to be reconstructed, and the wrist should be immobilized for 2 weeks.
  - EPL tendinitis
    - — A longitudinal incision is made over Lister's tubercle.
    - — The third dorsal compartment is identified, and the EPL tendon is completely released.
    - — It is translocated to the radial side of the tubercle in a subcutaneous plane.
    - — The compartment is reclosed to prevent the tendon from re-entering the compartment.
    - — After a short period of immobilization (5–7 days), unrestricted activity is allowed.
  - Fourth and fifth compartment tendinitis (extensor digitorum communis, extensor indicis proprius, extensor digiti minimi)
    - — The need for surgical release of these compartments is very rare.
  - ECU tendinitis
    - — A longitudinal incision is made over the ECU tendon.
    - — Care is taken to preserve and protect the dorsal sensory branches of the ulnar nerve.
    - — The entire fibro-osseous canal is released.
    - — Surgical reconstruction of the canal is not necessary.
  - FCR tendinitis
    - — A longitudinal incision is made over the FCR tendon volarly.
    - — Care is taken to protect the palmar cutaneous branch of the median nerve.
    - — The sheath of the tendon is released past the level of the trapezial tubercle.
    - — Any osteophytes on the trapezium should be removed, and any frayed portion of the tendon should be débrided.

When to Refer

- The patient should be referred to a hand specialist if conservative measures have not brought about improvement in 4 to 6 weeks.
- Many of the steroid injections for these conditions are difficult and should be performed only by those with previous experience or by a hand surgeon.

Prognosis

- Good with conservative measures and excellent with operative intervention

Troubleshooting

- With splint immobilization, patients need to wear splint continually
  - Try to assess and ensure patient compliance
- Steroid injections most commonly are not effective because of improper injection location.
  - Lidocaine injection either preceding the steroid or mixed with it will help determine whether the injection is located properly.
- For surgical release, proper diagnosis and adequate tendon release are essential.
  - Continued pain after release may be caused by cutaneous nerve irritation or damage.

Patient Instructions

- Patients need to be educated on the disease process.
- Instruct patients that if splint immobilization is prescribed, it is important to wear the splint full time with the possible exception of bathing and sleeping.
- If a nonsteroidal anti-inflammatory drug is prescribed, then the patient should take it regularly for

the period prescribed and not only as needed for pain.

- If steroid injection is used, then instruct patients that pain may increase for 24 to 48 hours and that effect of the steroid will not be experienced for 5 to 7 days
  - Have patients return in 2 weeks if there is no pain relief.
- When surgery is recommended, then patients should be educated on the risks and benefits of the procedure.

Considerations in Special Populations

- Patients with diabetes should be instructed to monitor their blood sugar level after a steroid injection.
- A steroid injection should be considered first-line therapy in patients who cannot tolerate immobilization.

Suggested Reading

- Brown J, Helms CA: Intersection syndrome of the forearm. Arthritis Rheum 2006;54:2038.
- Costa CR, Morrison WB, Carrino JA: MRI features of intersection syndrome of the forearm. Am J Radiol 2003;181:1245–1249.
- Grundberg AB, Reagan DS: Pathologic anatomy of the forearm: Intersection syndrome. J Hand Surg [Am] 1985;10:299–302.
- Ostric SA, Martin WJ, Derman GH: Intersecting the intersection: A reliable incision for the treatment of de Quervain's and second dorsal compartment tenosynovitis. Plast Reconstr Surg 2007;119:2341–2342.
- Wolfe SW: Tenosynovitis. In Green DP, Hotchkiss RN, Pederson WC, Wolfe SW (eds): Operative Hand Surgery, 5th ed. Philadelphia: Churchill Livingstone, 2005, pp 2137–2158.

Chapter 82 Ganglion Cysts

David Schnur and Jerrod Keith

ICD-9 CODE

727.4 *Ganglion and Cyst of Synovium, Tendon, and Bursa*

Key Concepts

- Most common soft-tissue masses of the hand and wrist, accounting for 50% to 70%
- Most prevalent in women and in second through fourth decades of life
- Not true cysts because they lack an epithelial lining and etiology is not well defined
- Mucin-filled cyst; communicates through a stalk to the adjacent joint capsule, tendon, or tendon sheath
- Aspiration and injection can be curative, but surgical resection reduces the rate of recurrence.
- Dorsal wrist ganglion cysts (60% to 70%)
  - Usually over the dorsal radial aspect of the wrist, between the third and fourth extensor compartments (Fig. 82-1)
  - Arise from the dorsal scapholunate ligament
- Volar wrist ganglion cysts (18% to 20%)
  - Usually occur under the volar wrist crease, just radial to the flexor carpi radialis tendon; these can be quite extensive (Fig. 82-2)
  - Two thirds arise from the radiocarpal joint and one third from the scaphotrapezial joint.
- Volar retinacular cysts (10% to 12%)
  - Arise from the palmar digital sheath in the region of the A1 and A2 pulleys
- Other ganglions
  - Degenerative mucous cysts in the dorsal distal interphalangeal joint of elderly patients
  - Proximal interphalangeal joint
  - Extensor tendons
  - Over first dorsal compartment with de Quervain's disease

History

- Can occur suddenly or develop over several months
- Pain, weakness, and poor cosmetic appearance are the most common reasons for presentation.

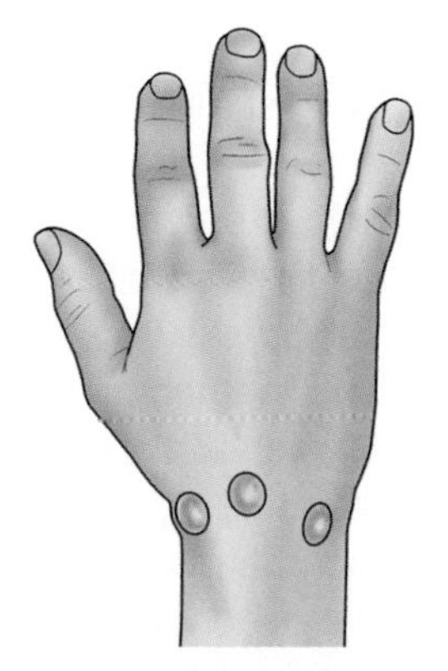

Figure 82-1 Common locations of dorsal wrist ganglion cysts.

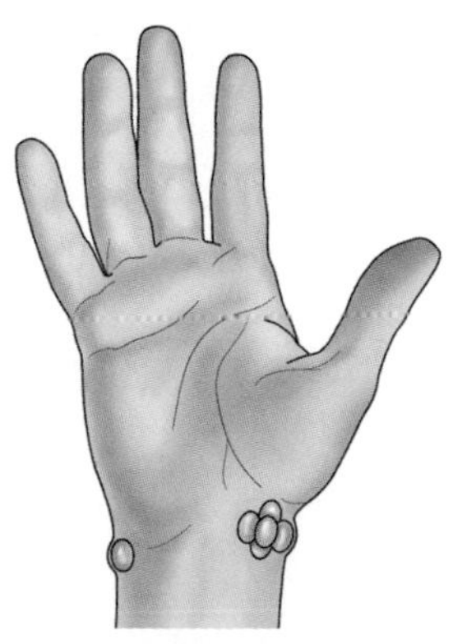

Figure 82-2 Typical locations of volar wrist ganglions.

- At least 10% of patients report antecedent traumatic events.
- Repetitive minor trauma believed to be a factor in development
- Often enlarge with increased activity and subside with rest

Physical Examination

- Thorough examination of the hand and wrist, including provocative maneuvers to rule out carpal instability
- Firm or rubbery, mobile, 1 to 3 cm in size, often nontender
- Smaller cysts may be more painful because they compress the posterior interosseous nerve during emergence through the fourth extensor compartment.
- Carpal tunnel symptoms
  - Compression of the median nerve due to ganglions from the volar carpus within the carpal canal
- Ulnar nerve palsy
  - Compression in Guyon's canal due to ganglions from joints around the hamate
- Longitudinal grooving of the nail may be an early indication of a mucous cyst.
- Heberden's nodes and osteoarthritic changes of the distal interphalangeal joint are often associated with mucous cysts.
- Ganglion cysts remain stationary with flexion and extension, whereas proliferative tenosynovitis does not.
- May transilluminate

Imaging

- Begin with plain radiographs if there is suspicion of an underlying bony abnormality.
  - Intraosseous ganglion cysts appear as radiolucent lesions with well-defined sclerotic borders.
- Ultrasonography and magnetic resonance imaging can be used to diagnose occult ganglion cysts.
  - Ultrasonography shows a well-defined anechoic structure close to a joint with posterior acoustic enhancement.
  - Magnetic resonance imaging shows a homogeneous signal with well-defined margins, which is hyperintense on T2-weighted sequences.

Additional Tests

- Physical examination is usually sufficient.
- Aspiration can be diagnostic and therapeutic.
  - Contents are highly viscous, clear, sticky, jelly-like mucin composed of glucosamine, albumin, globulin, and high concentrations of hyaluronic acid.

Differential Diagnosis

- Dorsal wrist ganglions
  - Giant cell tumor of the tendon sheath, lipoma, a true synovial cyst, tenosynovitis of the extensor tendons, anomalous muscles
- Volar wrist ganglions
  - Similar to dorsal, except anomalous muscles are rare in this area
- Volar retinacular cysts
  - Giant cell tumor of the tendon sheath, epidermoid inclusion cysts, foreign body granuloma, fibroma, lipoma, neurilemoma
- In general, the differential diagnosis includes solid tumors and proliferative tenosynovitis.

Treatment

- Indications for treatment include pain, weakness, and disfigurement.
- Initial conservative management includes supportive splinting, nonsteroidal anti-inflammatory drugs, and aspiration, with or without injection.
  - Injections of steroids or hyaluronidase are often performed.
  - Injection of sclerosing agents is not recommended.
  - At least temporary resolution in as many as 80% of patients with dorsal wrist ganglion cyst aspiration; high rate of recurrence
  - Recurrence rates of volar wrist ganglions after aspiration are much higher.
- Surgical excision should be offered for patients in whom nonoperative treatment fails or who remain symptomatic. Avoid cyst rupture and include the entire stalk.
- Dorsal wrist ganglion excision
  - Transverse incision over the cyst
  - The stalk typically arises from the dorsal aspect of the scapholunate ligament, and the cyst is excised at the base of the stalk along with a portion of the joint capsule (Figs. 82-3 and 82-4).
- Dorsal wrist ganglion can be treated arthroscopically by stalk excision at its origin along the level of the dorsal scapholunate ligament.
- Volar wrist ganglion excision
  - A longitudinal incision curving around the radial aspect of the cyst allows for extension if needed.

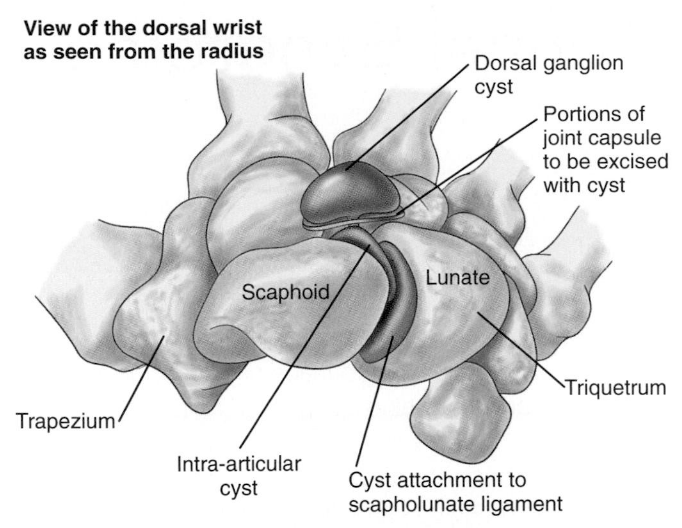

Figure 82-3 Representation of a ganglion cyst with its pedicle attachment to the scapholunate ligament.

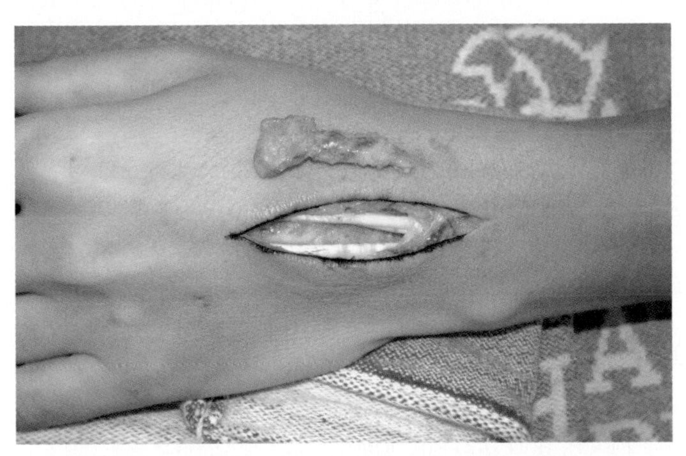

Figure 82-4 Intraoperative view of excised dorsal ganglion cyst and stalk.

    - Often located between the first extensor compartment tendons and the flexor carpi radialis sheath
    - The radial artery is usually intimately involved, and a small portion of the cyst may be left behind.
- Volar retinacular cyst
    - Good success with aspiration and injection; surgery is recommended only after several attempts at conservative management have failed
    - A small window of tendon sheath is excised along with the cyst.
- Degenerative mucous cysts
    - Surgical excision for pain, open wound, or draining

Troubleshooting

- Complete excision of the cyst and stalk at the base reduces the recurrence rate.
- Surgical dissection should be done under magnification to avoid small arterial or nerve branches, as well as to identify the cyst stalk and ligamentous attachments.
- Aspiration of volar wrist ganglions is not often recommended due to the close proximity of the radial artery.
- Allen's test should be performed prior to excision of volar wrist ganglion due to potential radial artery injury.
- Do not close the joint capsule after cyst excision, as it can result in joint stiffness.
- Occult wrist ganglions can be a cause of unexplained wrist pain, and excision is often curative.

Patient Instructions

- Reassure patients that this is not a malignant condition.
- If patients are asymptomatic, treatment can be delayed because the cyst may spontaneously regress.
- Postoperatively the wrist is immobilized in a splint for 7 to 10 days, after which the splint is removed, and the patient should begin wrist motion. Early finger motion is encouraged.

Considerations in Special Populations

- Degenerative mucous cysts usually occur between the fifth and seventh decades of life.

Suggested Reading

- Angelides AC: Ganglions of the hand and wrist. In Green DP, Hotchkiss RN, Pederson WC, Wolfe SW (eds): Green's Operative Hand Surgery, 5th ed. Philadelphia: Churchill Livingstone, 2005.
- Minotti P, Taras J: Ganglion cysts of the wrist. J Am Soc Surg Hand 2002;2:102–107.
- Nahra M, Bucchieri J: Ganglion cysts and other tumor related conditions of the hand and wrist. Hand Clin 2004;20:249–260.
- Nguyen V, Choi J, Davis K: Imaging of wrist masses. Curr Probl Diagn Radiol 2004;33:147–160.
- Young L, Bartell T, Logan S: Ganglions of the hand and wrist. South Med J 1988;81:751–760.

Chapter 83 Carpal Tunnel Syndrome

David Schnur

ICD-9 CODE

354.0 *Carpal Tunnel Syndrome (Median Nerve Entrapment/Partial Thenar Atrophy)*

Key Concepts

- Group of symptoms associated with compression of the median nerve as it passes through the carpal canal
- Most common compression neuropathy of the upper extremity
- Clinical diagnosis but can be confirmed with electrodiagnostic testing
- The volar surface of the carpal canal is the flexor retinaculum, which attaches to the hamate and triquetrum on the ulnar side and the scaphoid and trapezium on the radial side.
- The carpal bones account for the dorsal confines of the canal.
- The median nerve travels through the carpal canal. It gives off the recurrent motor branch at the distal end of the flexor retinaculum. It then divides into the digital nerves and gives sensation to the thumb and index finger and the long and radial sides of the ring finger (Fig. 83-1).
- There may be anatomic variations at the level of the takeoff of the motor branch as well as which fingers are innervated by the nerve.
- Intrinsic muscles innervated by the median nerve include the abductor pollicis brevis muscle, superficial head of the flexor pollicis muscle, opponens pollicis muscle, and lumbrical muscles of the index and long fingers.

History

- Paresthesia in the thumb and index and long fingers and radial aspect of the ring finger
- Pain, typically in the same distribution or in the thenar eminence
- Symptoms often worse at night
- Symptoms may be exacerbated with repetitive motion
- May report weakness and dropping objects

Physical Examination

- Direct compression test
  - The thumb is used to place compression over the median nerve at or just distal to the distal wrist crease for 60 seconds.
  - Paresthesia or replication of symptoms in the median nerve distribution indicates a positive test result.
- Tinel's sign
  - Firm percussion over the median nerve at the level of the carpal canal causing electric shock sensation in the thumb or index, long, or ring finger is considered a positive result.
- Phalen's maneuver
  - Wrist flexed maximally for at least 60 seconds
  - Paresthesia or replication of symptoms indicates a positive result
- Two-point discrimination
  - 5 mm considered normal
- Visual inspection for atrophy of the thenar eminence (Fig. 83-2)
- Strength testing for opposition of the thumb, key pinch, and grip strength

Imaging

- None is necessary unless the diagnosis is in question or there is concern that other pathology may be causing symptoms from secondary compression of the median nerve.

Additional Tests

- Electrodiagnostic studies
  - Electromyography
    - — Evaluates either spontaneous or volitional electrical activity in the muscle
    - — Fibrillation potentials at rest are the earliest signs of muscle denervation.
  - Nerve conduction velocity studies
    - — Can be used to study motor and sensory portions of the nerve

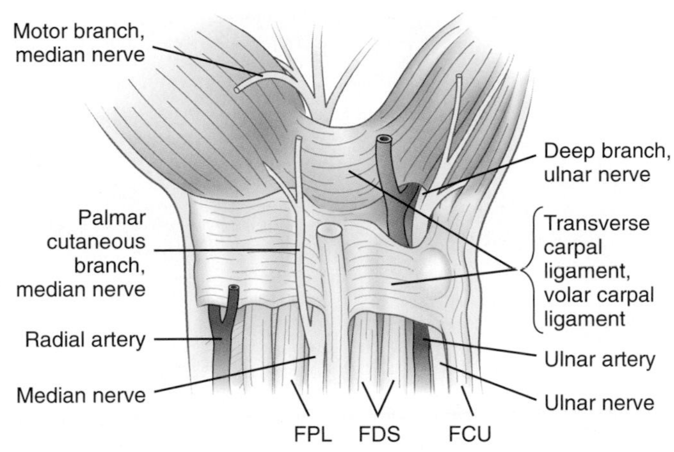

Figure 83-1 Anatomy of the carpal canal. The median nerve gives off the palmar cutaneous branch before entering the canal. The median nerve then travels through the canal and gives off the motor branch. FCU, flexor carpi ulnaris; FDS, flexor digitorum superficialis; FPL, flexor pollicus longus. (Adapted from Green D, Hotchkiss R, Pederson W, Wolfe S [eds]: Green's Operative Hand Surgery, Vol. 1, 5th ed. Philadelphia: Churchill Livingstone, 2005, p 1011, Fig. 28-8. Copyright Elizabeth Martin.)

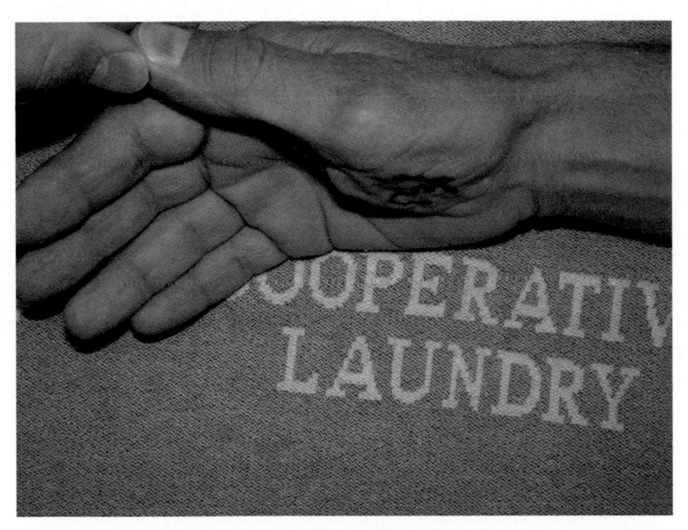

Figure 83-2 Severe atrophy of the thenar musculature.

- — Median motor distal latency considered abnormal if more than 4.5 msec
- — Sensory latencies wrist to digit II more than 3.5 msec or palm to wrist more than 2.2 msec
- — Also compare median and ulnar sensory latencies, with a difference of more than 0.5 msec abnormal with wrist to digit II and a difference of more than 0.3 msec in the palm to wrist

TABLE 83-1 *Differential Diagnosis*

Differential Diagnosis	Differentiating Feature(s)
Proximal median nerve compression	Resisted pronation test replicates symptoms, provocative tests over carpal tunnel negative with pure pronator syndrome
Ulnar nerve compression	Symptoms on ulnar side of the hand, Tinel's sign, and direct compression over cubital tunnel positive

Differential Diagnosis (Table 83-1)

- Median nerve compressions at higher levels can mimic carpal tunnel syndrome (CTS) symptoms or can coexist as a double crush.
  - Compression points of the median nerve proximal to the wrist should always be evaluated when examining patients suspected of having CTS.
- Ulnar nerve compression at the cubital tunnel or through Guyon's canal should be evaluated because it can coexist with or mimic CTS.

Treatment

- At diagnosis
  - First-line treatment of mild to moderate CTS is splinting, oral nonsteroidal anti-inflammatory drugs, and corticosteroid injection.
    - — For splinting, the wrist should be placed in a neutral position (most over-the-counter splints put the wrist in 30 degrees of extension, which can increase pressure in the carpal canal). Because of the nonfunctional position of the wrist in a neutral position, most patients will not tolerate the splint during normal daily activities; therefore, nighttime splinting should be recommended.
    - — Nonsteroidal anti-inflammatory drug use has variable effects on CTS but can be tried as a first-line therapy.
    - — Corticosteroid injection should be considered once the diagnosis of CTS is made. Corticosteroid injection is useful as both a diagnostic tool and a therapeutic modality. Relief from carpal tunnel injection has also been proven to be a good prognostic indicator of relief after surgical intervention. For specifics on steroid injection of the carpal canal, refer to Chapter 106.

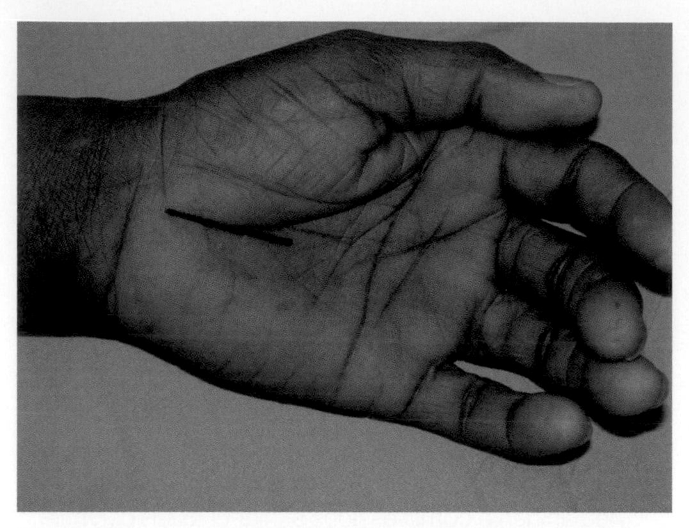

Figure 83-3 Incision placement for release of the carpal tunnel in line with the radial side of the fourth ray.

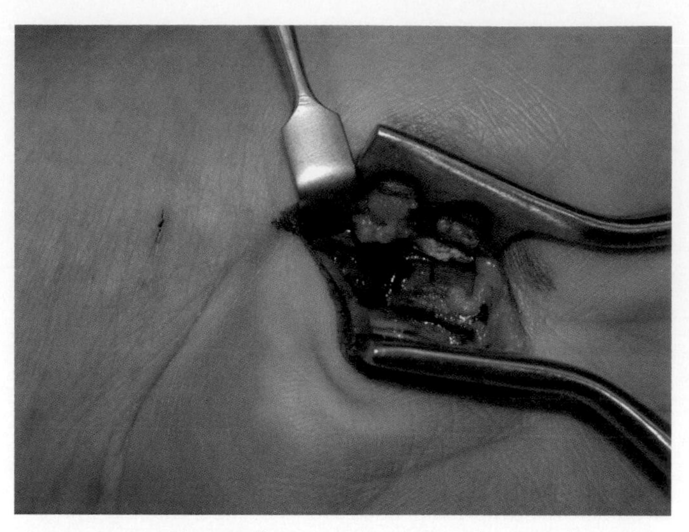

Figure 83-4 The median nerve is seen in the carpal canal. This nerve has significant hyperemia, which is indicative of long-standing compression.

- Later
  - Surgical release of the carpal tunnel should be considered if conservative measures have failed or there is severe disease with significant and worsening of numbness of the fingers rather than just paresthesias.
    - — To release the carpal tunnel, an incision is made in the proximal palm along the radial border of the fourth ray under tourniquet control (Fig. 83-3).
    - — The dissection is performed through the flexor retinaculum to the carpal canal.
    - — The distal end of the retinaculum is identified and divided distally to proximally, taking care to protect the median nerve (Fig. 83-4).
    - — Dissection is performed in the forearm, and the antebrachial fascia is divided.
    - — The tourniquet is released, hemostasis is obtained, and the incision is closed at the level of the skin.
    - — Release of the flexor retinaculum can also be done using endoscopic techniques.

When to Refer

- Referral is dependent on the comfort of the practitioner treating CTS.
- After 1 to 3 months with no improvement of symptoms, splinting and nonsteroidal anti-inflammatory drugs should be augmented with steroid injection or surgery should be considered. At this time, the patient should be referred to a hand specialist. Some hand surgeons appreciate when patients are referred after electrodiagnostic testing, whereas others believe that these tests are not indicated until after failure of carpal tunnel injections. Additionally, patients should be referred if they have a decrease in two-point discrimination or any thenar atrophy.

Prognosis

- The prognosis is excellent.
- Many patients will respond at least temporarily to first-line treatment of CTS.
- Those patients who require surgery will have an excellent chance of significant improvement of symptoms if they are treated in a timely fashion.

Troubleshooting

- If a patient fails treatment with splinting and nonsteroidal anti-inflammatory drugs, compliance may be an issue.
- With failure to decrease or eliminate symptoms after carpal tunnel injection, it is important to assess whether the injection was properly placed. With the addition of local anesthetic to the injection, the patient should be instructed to take note of which, if any, fingers become numb.
- No decrease in pain after surgical intervention is unusual and would call into question the diagnosis of CTS or may indicate that there is another location of compression (double crush).

- Long-standing paresthesia in the fingers may not be improved with surgery, and this should be explained to patients before intervention.

Patient Instructions

- After a diagnosis is made, patients should be educated on the disease process.
- If splinting and nonsteroidal anti-inflammatory drugs are prescribed, it is important to stress to patients that compliance is paramount to improvement.
- With steroid injection, patients are instructed to take note of which, if any, fingers become numb. Patients should also be instructed that symptoms will not improve for 5 to 7 days and that they may increase for 24 to 48 hours.
- Surgical patients should be instructed on the risks of surgery, especially the possibility of permanent nerve damage (a rare complication). They should also be instructed that pain in the palm (pillar pain) can last many months and that in rare cases this pain may be permanent.

Considerations in Special Populations

- When performing steroid injection on diabetic patients, instruct them to monitor and treat elevated blood sugars.
- Pregnant patients have a higher incidence of CTS. These patients can be treated with splinting and a steroid injection. Surgery should only be considered in extreme cases. Although these patients often improve after delivery, those who have significant symptoms should be considered for surgical decompression if further pregnancies are likely.
- Patients with significant loss of two-point discrimination or thenar atrophy and no pain should be considered for surgery to halt progression of their symptoms, although improvement may not be expected.
- Pediatric patients with CTS should have a workup for other pathologic conditions that may cause secondary compression of the median nerve. The diagnosis of lipofibromatous hamartoma of the median nerve should also be entertained. The workup for these patients should include magnetic resonance imaging.

Suggested Reading

- Bland JD: Carpal tunnel syndrome. BMJ 2007;335:343–346.
- Braun RM, Rechnic M, Fowler E: Complications related to carpal tunnel release. Hand Clin 2002;18:347–357.
- Cranford CS, Ho JY, Kalainov DM, Hartigan BJ: Carpal tunnel syndrome. J Am Acad Orthop Surg 2007;15:537–548.
- Gannon C, Muffly M, Rubright RT, Baratz ME: Aberrant nerve in limited open carpal tunnel release. J Hand Surg [Am] 2006;31:1407–1408.
- Green DP: Diagnostic and therapeutic value of carpal tunnel injection. J Hand Surg [Am] 1984;9:850–854.
- Mackinnon SE, Novak CB: Compression neuropathy. In Green D, Hotchkiss R, Pederson W, Wolfe S (eds): Operative Hand Surgery, Vol. 1, 5th ed. Philadelphia: Churchill Livingstone, 2005, pp 999–1046.
- Thoma A, Veltri K, Haines T, Duku E: A systematic review of reviews comparing the effectiveness of endoscopic and open carpal tunnel decompression. Plast Reconstr Surg 2004;113:1184–1191.

Chapter 84 Thumb Basal Joint Arthritis

David Schnur

ICD-9 CODE
715.14 *Osteoarthritis, Localized, Primary (Hand)*

Key Concepts

- Type of osteoarthritis that most commonly affects the trapeziometacarpal (TM) joint of the thumb but can affect all five articulations of the thumb basal joint
- The TM joint is a saddle joint with minimal bony constraints.
- Ligamentous stability is very important for the TM joint.
- The anterior oblique ligament or "beak" ligament is the primary stabilizer of the TM joint.
- Degeneration of the beak ligament results in laxity of the TM joint, which, in turn, results in abnormal translation of the metacarpal on the trapezium, which leads to excessive shear forces on the joint.
- Women have a greater predilection for the disease, with a female-to-male ratio of 10:1.
- Commonly presents in fifth and sixth decades of life
- Because of adduction of the thumb, there may be compensatory hyperextension of the metacarpophalangeal joint and laxity of the volar plate.

History

- Pain at the base of the thumb, particularly during pinch and grasp
- Difficulty turning keys in doors or ignition of car
- Pain and weakness with opening jars
- Occasionally pain less well localized and pain in entire thumb reported
- May report the appearance of the thumb "zigzag"

Physical Examination

- Observation of the thumb may reveal prominence of the base of the thumb metacarpal.
- Hyperextension of the MP joint may be visible with motion or pinch.
- Tenderness at TM joint on palpation
- Grind test
  - Axial load on the thumb combined with circumduction elicits pain and often crepitance in the joint.

Imaging

- Plain radiographs should be adequate to confirm the diagnosis (Fig. 84-1).
- Radiographic staging according to Eaton and Littler
  - Stage 1: normal joint with possible widening
  - Stage 2: joint space narrowing with debris and osteophytes less than 2 mm
  - Stage 3: joint space narrowing with debris and osteophytes greater than 2 mm
  - Stage 4: scaphotrapezial joint space narrowing in addition to TM joint involvement
- Bone scan may be useful if diagnosis is in question (Fig. 84-2).

Additional Tests

- A local anesthetic agent can be injected into the TM joint and should alleviate most of the pain (Fig. 84-3).

Differential Diagnosis

- Please see Table 84-1.

Treatment

- At diagnosis
  - First line treatment for this disease involves nonsteroidal anti-inflammatory drugs, intra-articular steroid injections (see Chapter 107), thenar cone strengthening therapy, and immobilization with a thumb spica splint.
  - These treatments, although not curative, may improve symptoms and delay the need for operative intervention.

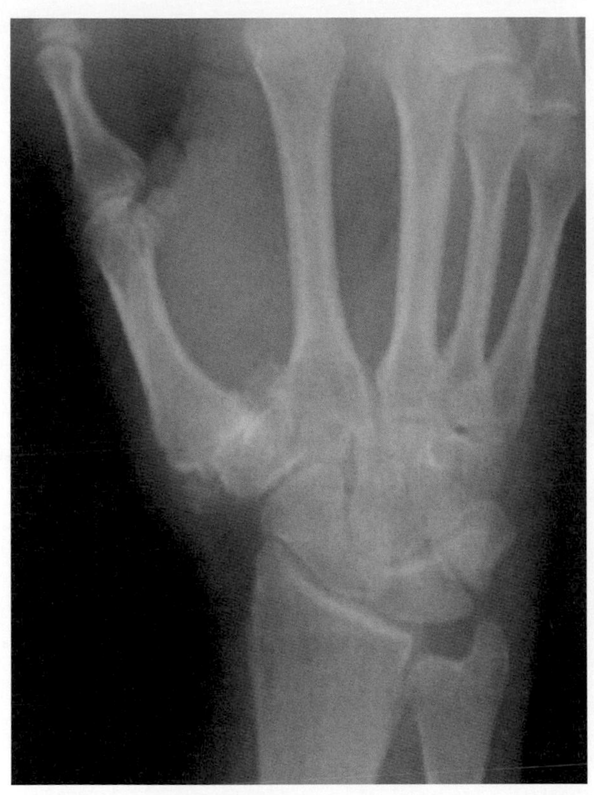

Figure 84-1 Radiographic appearance of basal joint arthritis. Note the narrowing of the joint space and osteophyte formation.

- These therapies may be tried sequentially or may be done in combination.
- Later
  - Once patients have failed nonoperative treatment, surgery should be considered.
  - Many surgical procedures have been described for this disease process; the two most popular procedures for treatment of basilar joint arthritis are TM arthrodesis and trapezium excision with ligament reconstruction and tendon interposition arthroplasty.
  - TM arthrodesis is indicated when the arthropathy is limited to the TM joint and the patient has a high-demand hand (i.e., laborer).
    - — This procedure trades motion for retention of power and strength and long-term durability.
  - Soft-tissue arthroplasties have gained increasing popularity, and of these procedures, the ligament reconstruction and tendon interposition described by Burton and Pellegrini is probably the most common surgery performed.
    - — This involves excision of the trapezium followed by harvest of the flexor carpi radialis tendon (Fig. 84-4).
    - — The tendon is used to reconstruct the beak ligament and then formed into an "anchovy" and used as a soft-tissue spacer between the base of the metacarpal and the scaphoid (Figs. 84-5 and 84-6).
    - — Examination of the scaphotrapezoid joint is essential, and if arthritis is present at this location, it must be addressed simultaneously.

When to Refer

- Referral to a hand specialist for this condition, like many conditions in the hand, depends on the practitioner's comfort with diagnosing TM arthritis and executing nonoperative therapy.
- Certainly once the nonoperative therapies have been instituted and the patient still has significant functional impairment from the disease, the patient should be referred to the hand surgeon for consideration for surgical treatment.

Prognosis

- TM arthritis is a progressive disease and only definitively treated with surgery.
- Nonoperative modalities often alleviate symptoms but only temporarily
- The prognosis for pain relief and good function is excellent after surgical treatment.

Troubleshooting

- The degree of arthritis on radiographs and the severity of symptoms may not correlate.
  - Patients with little change on radiographs may have significant symptoms, and, conversely, patients with severe disease radiographically may have surprisingly mild symptoms.
- Patients who do not respond to nonsteroidal anti-inflammatory drugs, splinting, and therapy should have a corticosteroid injection in the TM joint, if indicated.
- No response or partial response to the steroid injection may indicate scaphotrapezoid trapezium or pantrapezial involvement.
- Continued pain after surgical treatment may indicate unrecognized scaphotrapezoid joint involvement.

Patient Instructions

- Patients should be instructed about the progressive nature of the process once the diagnosis is made.

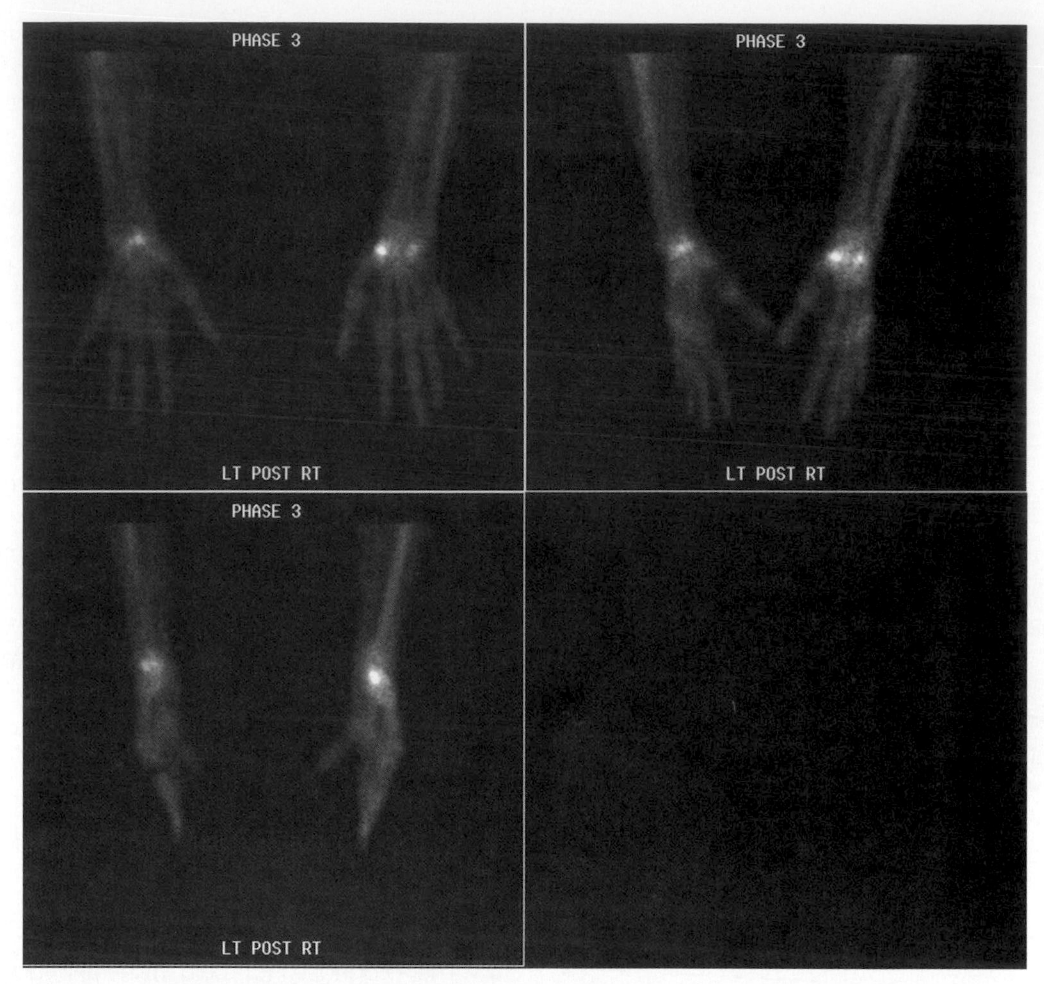

Figure 84-2 Bone scan of patient with basal joint arthritis. Note increased uptake of the trapeziometarpal joint on phase 3. LT, left; RT, right.

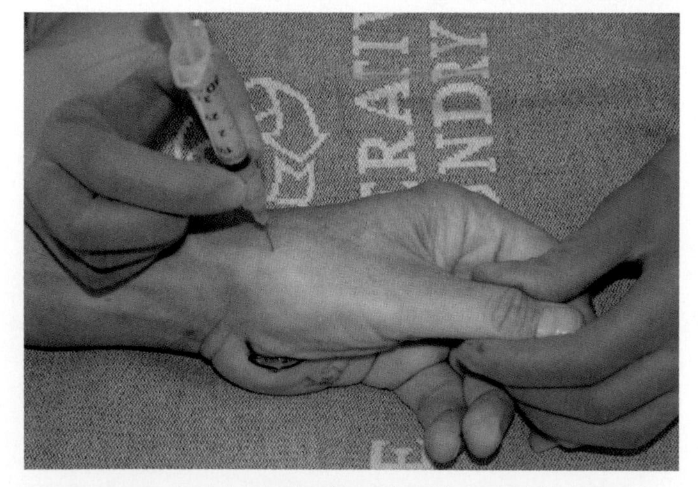

Figure 84-3 Local anesthesia and corticosteroid injected into the trapeziometacarpal joint can help diagnose basal joint arthritis and give relief of symptoms.

TABLE 84-1 *Differential Diagnosis*

Differential Diagnosis	Differentiating Feature	Chapter Reference
de Quervain's tenosynovitis	Pain and tenderness more proximal; positive Finkelstein's test	80
Carpal tunnel syndrome	Often associated with numbness of the fingers; not acutely exacerbated with specific activities	83
Trigger thumb	Pain over A1 pulley and often associated with triggering	86
MCP joint osteoarthritis	Pain at MCP joint and tenderness on palpation of MCP joint; radiographs with arthritic changes at MCP joint	—
Sesamoiditis and subsesamoid arthritis	Pain typically volar over MCP joint	—

MCP, metacarpophalangeal.

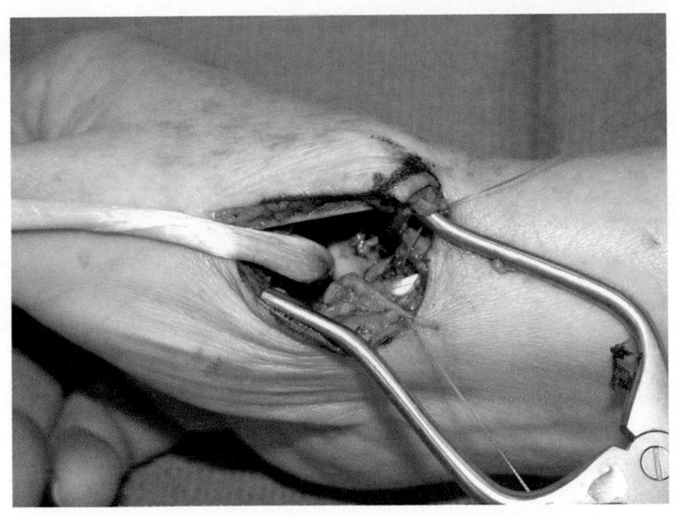

Figure 84-4 Intraoperative appearance after the trapezium has been excised and the flexor carpi radialis tendon has been harvested and kept attached to the base of the index metacarpal.

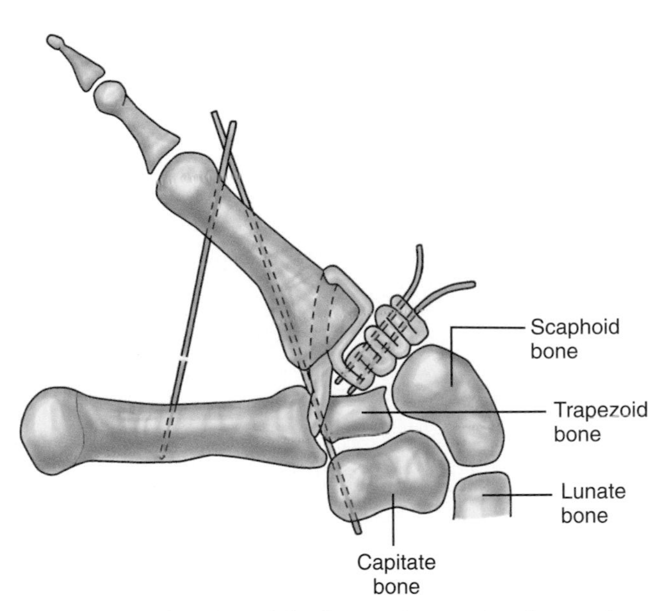

Figure 84-5 Drawing of the ligament reconstruction and tendon interposition once the flexor carpi radialis tendon has been made into an "anchovy" and inserted into the space where the trapezium was before resection. (Adapted with permission from Green DP, Hotchkiss RN, Pederson WC, Wolfe SW [eds]: Operative Hand Surgery, 5th ed. Philadelphia: Churchill Livingstone, 2005.)

- Hand therapists are often an excellent source for patient information and instruction; this is one of the reasons that referral to the therapist for splinting and thenar cone strengthening is helpful.
- For patients undergoing surgery, the entire postoperative course needs to be explained to the patient.

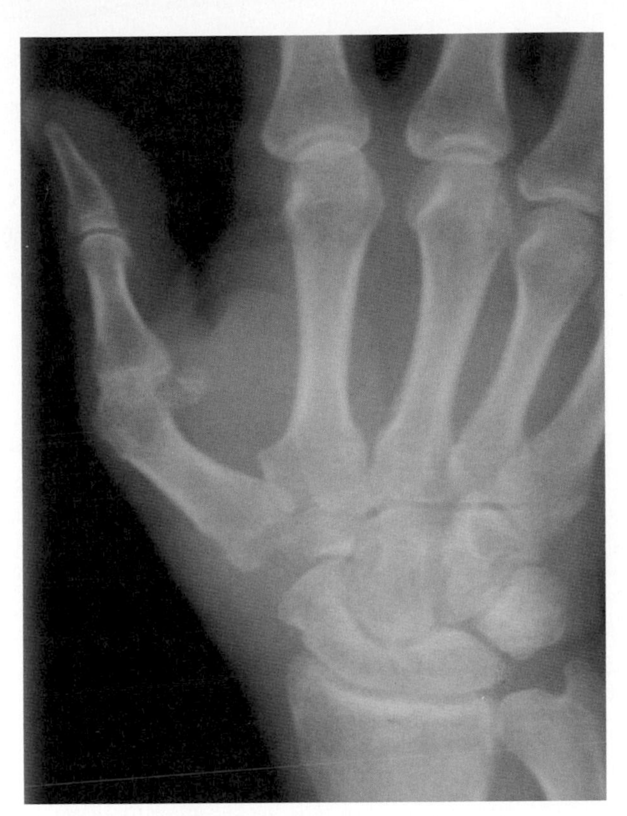

Figure 84-6 Radiographic appearance of the clear space with the flexor carpi radialis "anchovy" between the scaphoid and the base of the thumb metacarpal.

- Additionally, it needs to be stressed to patients undergoing surgery that complete pain relief may not be accomplished until 3 to 6 months postoperatively.
- It also needs to be explained that patients will have some loss of strength compared with the precondition strength.
- Patients typically have loss of strength with basilar joint arthritis and are grateful for the return of power after surgery.

Considerations in Special Populations

- Young patients with high-demand hands should be considered for TM arthrodesis.
- Patients undergoing surgical treatment who have developed more than 30 degrees of hyperextension of the MP joint should have either a capsulodesis or an arthrodesis of this joint.
- Patients with concomitant carpal tunnel syndrome should have carpal tunnel release if the basilar joint arthritis is treated surgically.

Suggested Reading

- Burton R, Pellegrini VD: Surgical management of basal joint arthritis of the thumb: Part II. Ligament reconstruction with tendon interposition arthroplasty. J Hand Surg [Am] 1986;11: 325–332.

- Damen A, van der Lei B, Robinson PH: Carpometacarpal arthritis of the thumb. J Hand Surg [Am] 1996;21:807–812.
- Luria S, Waitayawinya T, Nemechek N, et al: Biomechanical analysis of trapeziectomy, ligament reconstruction with tendon interposition, and tie-in trapezium implant arthroplasty for thumb carpometacarpal arthritis: A cadaver study. J Hand Surg [Am] 2007;32:697–706.
- Tomaino MM, King J, Leit M: Thumb basal joint arthritis. In Green DP, Hotchkiss RN, Pederson WC, Wolfe SW (eds): Operative Hand Surgery, 5th ed. Philadelphia: Churchill Livingstone, 2005, pp 461–485.

Chapter 85 Ulnar Collateral Ligament Injuries of the Thumb (Gamekeeper's Thumb, Skier's Thumb)

Jack Ingari and Gary Blum

ICD-9 CODE

842.12 *Sprain Metacarpophalangeal Joint*

Key Concepts

- Common injury among ball-handling athletes and skiers, resulting from acute valgus and hyperextension force to thumb metacarpophalangeal (MCP) joint (skier's thumb)
- Instability can also be chronic, typically resulting from inadequate treatment of an acute tear or treatment of an unrecognized Stener lesion (gamekeeper's thumb).
- Stener lesion: Interposition of the adductor aponeurosis at the time of a complete tear, which will prevent adequate healing
- May be associated with a fracture, most commonly an avulsion fracture at the base of the proximal phalanx

History

- Acute injury
  - Typically results from a fall on an outstretched hand with the thumb abducted, causing a sudden abduction (valgus) force to the thumb MCP joint and injury to the ulnar collateral ligament (Fig. 85-1)
  - Patients will present with a painful, swollen thumb MCP joint.
- Chronic injury
  - Attenuation over time due to occupational use (classic gamekeeper's thumb) is less common.
  - Presentation more than 6 weeks after injury
  - Patients present with pain, swelling, weakness, and instability, typically with activities requiring pinch.

Physical Examination

- Swelling, ecchymosis, and localized tenderness to the ulnar aspect of the MCP joint
- May be able to diagnose a Stener lesion by palpation of a mass just proximal to the MCP joint
- Important to distinguish between partial and complete ruptures of the ulnar collateral ligament
  - Complete rupture: With radial stress, more than 30 degrees of laxity in full extension and slight flexion, as well as more than 15 degrees of laxity compared with the contralateral thumb (Fig. 85-2)
  - A more practical measure may be the presence or absence of an endpoint; complete tears will present with a joint that can be opened completely with radial stress without resistance.
- Guarding secondary to pain and muscle spasm may limit complete examination, and therefore stress testing should be done under some form of anesthesia.
  - Intra-articular injection of local anesthetic
  - Local infiltration of the ligament
  - Median and radial nerve blocks at the wrist
- Always compare with the uninjured contralateral thumb

Imaging

- Radiographs
  - Posterolateral, lateral, and oblique views of the thumb
  - Acutely, looking for fracture (avulsion or intra-articular) and joint subluxation
  - Chronically, also looking for the presence of arthritic changes

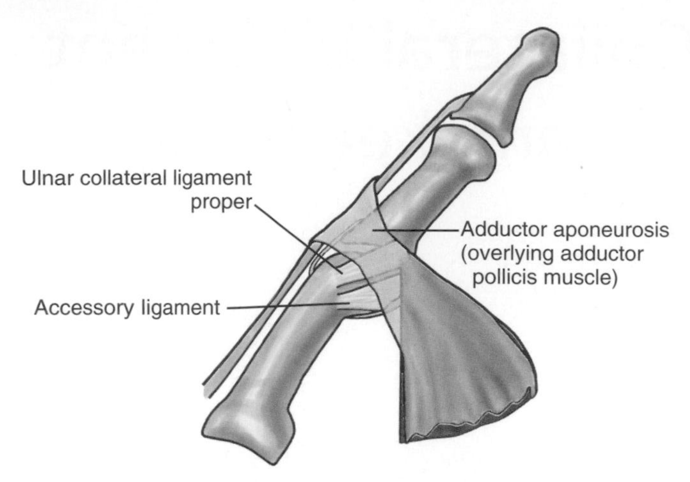

Figure 85-1 Ulnar collateral ligament.

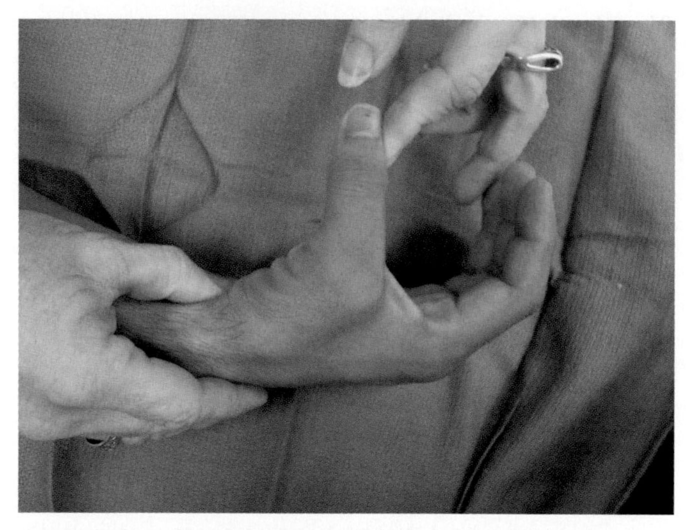

Figure 85-2 Complete rupture of ulner collateral ligament with angulation of greater than 30 degrees found on radial stress exam.

- Obtain radiographs before clinical stress examination to avoid potential displacement of nondisplaced fractures
- Ultrasonography
  - Noninvasive
  - Relatively inexpensive
  - Sensitivity and specificity high (75% to 95%) for Stener and non-Stener lesions, but may decrease if the procedure is delayed
- Magnetic resonance imaging
  - May be more accurate than ultrasonography, especially when magnetic resonance arthrography is performed
  - Interpretation dependent on quality of equipment
  - Experienced radiologist important
  - Higher cost
- Stress radiographs can be considered when
  - There is no fracture.
  - Distinction between complete and partial injury cannot by made on clinical examination.

Differential Diagnosis

- Generalized laxity: Compare with contralateral side and examine multiple joints
- Proximal phalanx fracture: May or may not occur in conjunction with injury to the ulnar collateral ligament

Treatment

- At diagnosis
  - Acute, partial tears
    - — General agreement that these injuries can be treated nonoperatively using a thumb spica cast for 3 to 4 weeks
    - — May consider a thermoplastic thumb spica splint in compliant patients
  - Acute, complete tears
    - — Theoretically, complete tears without a Stener lesion can be treated with cast immobilization.
    - — The most predictable result is likely with operative exploration and repair, which can be done with a variety of techniques (Fig. 85-3); dependent on location of tear
    - — Associated fractures are also indications for operative management.
      - — Displaced intra-articular fractures involving more than 25% of the base of the proximal phalanx
      - — Avulsion fracture with greater than 5 mm of displacement
  - Chronic, partial tears
    - — Consider intra-articular corticosteroid injection followed by cast or splint immobilization and nonsteroidal anti-inflammatory drugs for 3 weeks
  - Chronic, complete tears
    - — Can be treated like partial tears as a temporizing measure or in sedentary patients
    - — Most patients are candidates for operative exploration and repair versus ligament reconstruction, particularly those desiring to return to athletic endeavors.
    - — MCP fusion may be required in cases of advanced joint degeneration.
- Later
  - Acute, partial tears
    - — Four weeks of cast immobilization in a thumb spica cast or splint can be followed by range

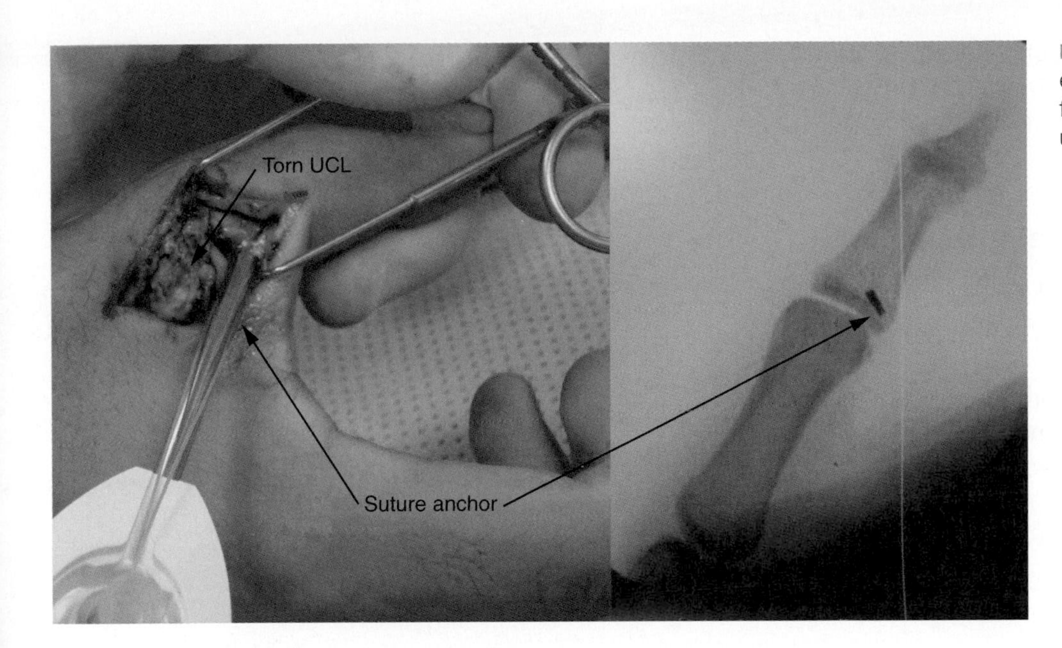

Figure 85-3 Operative exploration and repair techniques for acute, complete tears. UCL, ulnar collateral ligament.

of motion therapy and return to activities as comfort allows.

- Acute, complete tears
  - — Surgically repaired tears will also be immobilized for 4 weeks in a thumb spica cast.
  - — This is followed by use of a removable splint for 2 to 3 weeks, during which time range of motion exercises of the thumb MCP joint are initiated.
  - — Full, unrestricted activity can be allowed at 12 weeks, assuming return of near-normal range of motion and strength.
  - — Athletes returning to contact sports should protect the thumb with splinting or tape for an additional 4 weeks.
- Chronic tears
  - — After ligament reconstruction, the initial cast is left on for 6 weeks rather than 4, and unrestricted activity is delayed for 16 to 18 weeks.

When to Refer

- All acute, complete tears, with and without fractures
- All chronic tears
- Cases in which differentiating between partial and complete tears is deemed difficult

Prognosis

- Operative treatment
  - Complete tears
    - — When treated operatively within 3 weeks, can expect more than 90% good to excellent results
    - — Pain and stiffness are typically minimal.
    - — Return to athletic activities as high as 95%
    - — Traction injury to the crossing branches of the sensory branch of the radial nerve is the most common complication.
  - Chronic tears
    - — Overall satisfaction is very high.
    - — Consistent restoration of thumb stability
    - — Mild, occasional pain may be seen in as many as 33% of patients
    - — Restoration of motion usually 80% to 90% of contralateral side

Troubleshooting

- Although physical examination alone is usually sufficient to make the diagnosis, do not hesitate to refer when distinguishing between partial and complete tears is difficult.
- Absence of an endpoint may be the most clinically relevant indicator of a complete tear.
- All patients with pain to the ulnar side of the thumb MCP joint and a typical history should have a radiograph first.

Patient Instructions

- Early treatment of acute partial (nonoperative) and complete (operative) tears is best.

- Counsel patients that although results of acute repairs and chronic reconstructions are favorable, optimal results require as long as a 4-month commitment to rehabilitation.

Considerations in Special Populations

- Acute injuries to the thumb MCP joint ulnar collateral ligament are typically seen in the younger, athletic population.
- Older, sedentary patients with chronic instability can typically be treated symptomatically; should osteoarthritis develop, there are favorable results with MCP fusion.

Suggested Reading

- Campbell CS: Gamekeeper's thumb. J Bone Joint Surg Br 1995;37B:148–149.
- Green DP, Rowland SA: Fractures and dislocations of the hand. In Rockwood CA Jr, Green DP, Bucholz RW (eds): Fractures in Adults, 4th ed. Philadelphia: Lippincott, 1996, pp 707–716.
- Heyman P: Injuries to the ulnar collateral ligament of the thumb metacarpophalangeal joint. J Am Acad Orthop Surg 1997; 5:224–229.
- Richard JR: Gamekeeper's thumb: Ulnar collateral ligament injury. Am Fam Physician 1996;53:1775–1780.
- Stener B: Displacement of the ruptured ulnar collateral ligament of the metacarpophalangeal joint of the thumb: A clinical and anatomical study. J Bone Joint Surg Br 1962;44B:869–879.

Chapter 86 Trigger Finger

Megan M. Wood and Jack Ingari

ICD-9 CODES
727.03 *Trigger Finger, Acquired*
756.89 *Trigger Finger, Congenital*

Key Concepts

- Stenosing tenosynovitis, commonly known as trigger finger
- Mechanical symptoms of locking, catching, or popping when inflamed flexor tendons pass through a narrowed and restricted A1 pulley in the hand
- Normal gliding of flexor digitorum superficialis and flexor digitorum profundus tendons is disrupted, leading to increased resistance as tendons pull through the A1 pulley. Tendon entrapment creates a cycle of further inflammation and constriction at the pulley and ultimately worsening of symptoms (Fig. 86-1).
- The A1 pulley becomes grossly thickened with the histologic response of an increase in collagen and hyperplasia. Microscopic examination reveals fibrocartilaginous metaplasia of the inner layer of the surface of the pulley.
- The digits affected in order of prevalence: thumb, middle, ring, index, small
- Lifetime incidence of 2% after the age of 30 years; 10% incidence with diabetes
- Affects women two to six times more than men
- Peak incidence at 55 to 60 years of age
- Idiopathic trigger finger most common
- Systemic risk factors include
  - Diabetes
  - Rheumatoid arthritis
  - Collagen vascular disorders
  - Dupuytren's disease
  - Gout
  - Renal disease
- Local trauma as risk factor
  - Activities with power grip cause shearing at the edges of the A1 pulley.
  - Recent surgery

History

- Grade I: pretriggering
  - Early symptoms consist of generalized dull ache and pain in the area of the A1 pulley located over the metacarpal head in the palm of the hand; there may not be reproducible catching.
  - Pain can be referred to the entire digit of the affected hand; patients may incorrectly localize pain to the proximal interphalangeal joint of the affected finger.
  - Feelings of morning stiffness and swelling of finger also reported
- Grade II: active
  - Later symptoms of reproducible locking or catching during flexion and extension of fingers; the patient can actively extend the digit.
- Grade III: passive
  - With increasing severity, the involved digit becomes locked and passive extension is necessary to unlock the digit.
- Grade IV: contracture
  - Most severe trigger fingers still have reproducible catching but also have a fixed flexion contracture at the proximal interphalangeal joint.
  - In extreme cases, the patient may present with a permanently locked finger.

Physical Examination

- Tenderness over the A1 pulley; in palmar flexion, a crease over the metacarpal head
- Palpable nodule in the flexor digitorum superficialis tendon moves with flexion
- Popping sensation over the A1 pulley with flexion or extension of the digit
- Triggering may not be reproducible by the examiner, but the patient is usually able to reproduce the offending click with maximal active flexion (Fig. 86-2).

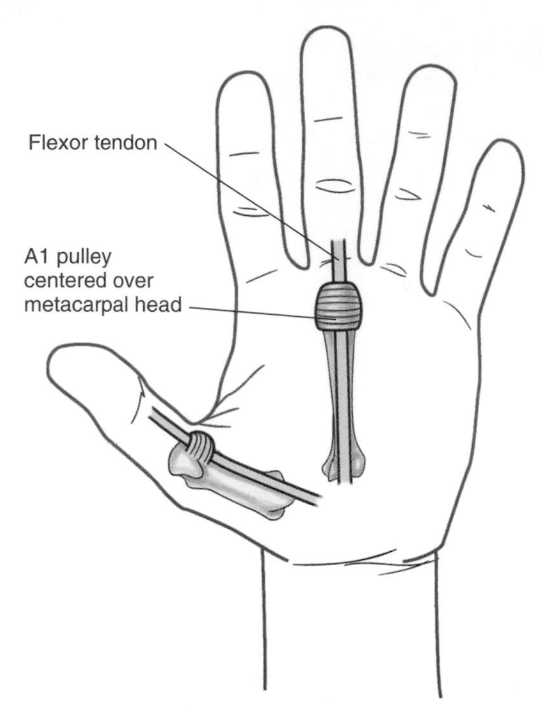

Figure 86-1 Flexor tendon with the pulley system.

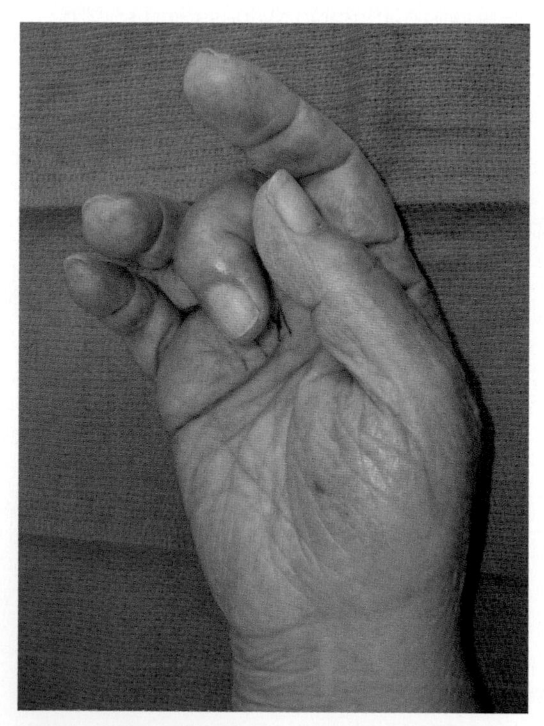

Figure 86-2 Example of locked trigger finger.

Imaging

- No imaging is necessary.
- The diagnosis of trigger finger is overtly clinical, based on history and examination.
- Plain radiographs are obtained only if suspicion of other pathology exists.

TABLE 86-1 *Differential Diagnosis*

Condition	Differentiating Feature
Dupuytren's disease (see Chapter 92)	Nodular cords do not move with tendons with flexion and extension
Metacarpophalangeal joint locking	Locked metacarpophalangeal joint but proximal and distal phalangeal joints flex normally; often associated with collateral ligament impingement on metacarpal head osteophyte; rarely caused by abnormal sesamoids

Differential Diagnosis

- Please see Table 86-1.

Treatment

- At diagnosis
  - Patients with symptoms of pretriggering without reproducible locking can be treated with nonsteroidal anti-inflammatory drugs, splinting in extension, or stretching (Fig. 86-3).
- Later
  - Patients with palpable mechanical symptoms of triggering should be treated with corticosteroid injection as the first-line treatment (see Chapter 108 for technique); a series of up to three injections may be given.

When to Refer

- Patients in whom conservative measures, including steroid injections, have failed or those who have a locked finger should be referred to a hand surgeon for evaluation of operative treatment.
- Only actively triggering fingers should be considered for operative intervention.
- Surgical treatment includes either a day surgery procedure with release of the A1 pulley, or some experienced hand surgeons may perform an office-based procedure of percutaneous release of the A1 pulley.

Prognosis

- As many as 80% of patients have resolution of symptoms after one steroid injection.
- After three injections, the success rate may increase to 97%.
- Surgical treatment will relieve mechanical symptoms with few complications.

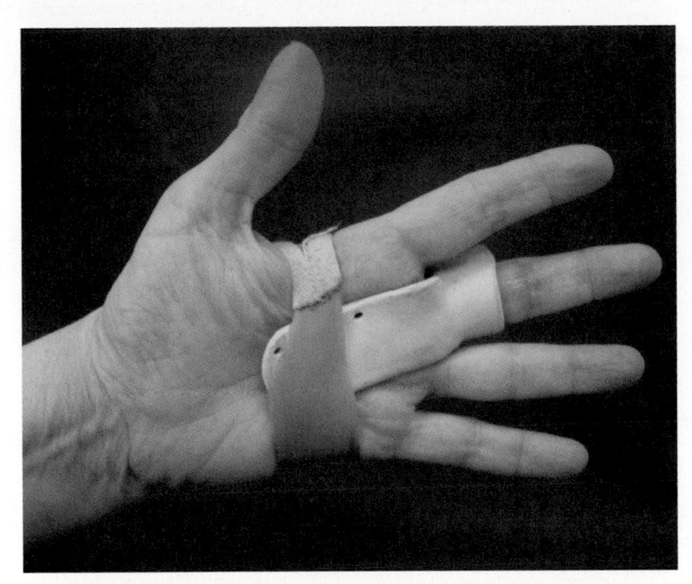

Figure 86-3 Example of splinting for trigger finger.

- Patients may complain of prolonged soreness after surgical release, but mechanical symptoms resolve immediately after surgical treatment.

Troubleshooting

- Multiple steroid injections can theoretically cause rupture of tendons despite only one report in the literature. However, most series of steroid injections are limited to three.
- Diabetics should be counseled that they may have a transient increase in blood sugar levels after corticosteroid injection.
- Steroid injections are proven to be more effective in nondiabetic patients compared with those with diabetes, and patients without diabetes are significantly less likely to require surgical release than diabetics.

Patient Instructions

- Steroid injection may cause a painful postinjection flare that can be treated with a few days of oral anti-inflammatory medication.
- Patients with previous trigger fingers are at increased risk of developing triggering in other digits.
- Active use of fingers is encouraged after injection and surgical release.
- Formal hand therapy is rarely needed to improve hand function.

Considerations in Special Populations

- Although diabetic patients are less likely to respond as well as patients with idiopathic trigger finger, steroid injection should still be initially attempted.

Pediatric Triggering

- True trigger finger is rare in children.
- Most commonly, children have "congenital trigger thumb," although this is not truly a congenital condition because it does not occur at birth. It develops later and more properly is a "developmental trigger thumb."
- Develops at approximately 2 years of age
- Mechanical symptoms may be noted, but at presentation the thumb is locked in fixed flexion at the interphalangeal joint.
- A nodule or Notta's node is commonly palpated at the A1 pulley.
- Flexor tendon thickening is seen without constriction or hyperplasia of the A1 pulley in congenital trigger thumb.

Treatment

- Nonoperative treatment such as splinting is rarely effective.
- Children do not tolerate injections.
- Surgical treatment of release of the A1 pulley is most effective to resolve symptoms of locked thumb.
- Nodule dissipates with time.

Suggested Reading

- Baumgarten KM, Gerlach D, Boyer MI: Corticosteroid injection in diabetic patients with trigger finger. J Bone Joint Surg Am 2007;89A:2604–2611.
- Eastwood DM, Gupta KJ, Johnson DP: Percutaneous release of the trigger finger: An office procedure. J Hand Surg [Am] 1992;17A:114–117.
- Marks MR, Gunther SF: Efficacy of cortisone injection in treatment of trigger fingers and thumbs. J Hand Surg [Am] 1989;14A: 722–727.
- Newport ML, Lane LB, Stuchin SA: Treatment of trigger finger by steroid injection. J Hand Surg [Am] 1990;15A:748–750.
- Saldana MJ: Trigger digits: Diagnosis and treatment. J Am Acad Orthop Surg 2001;9:246–252.
- Turowski GA, Zdankiewicz TD, Thompson JG: Results of surgical treatment of trigger finger. J Hand Surg [Am] 1997;22A:145–149.

Chapter 87 Flexor Tendon Injuries

Robert C. Chadderdon and Jonathan E. Isaacs

ICD-9 CODES

882.2 *Open Wound of Hand with Tendon Involvement*

883.2 *Open Wound of Finger with Tendon Involvement*

842.10 *Finger Sprain (Traumatic Injury to Ligament or Tendon)*

727.64 *Rupture of Flexor Tendons of Hand and Wrist, Nontraumatic*

Key Concepts

- Flexor tendons are commonly injured structures. Injuries usually result in a significant functional deficit if they are not properly treated.
- Timely surgical treatment is based on anatomic location of injury.
- Specific treatment recommendations vary tremendously based on the anatomic locations (zones) of ruptures/lacerations and the time from injury.
- Injuries can involve the flexor digitorum superficialis (FDS), flexor digitorum profundus (FDP), or both; a physical examination can help determine this.
- Frequent association with adjacent nerve/vessel injuries, most of which require surgical repair
- Surgical treatment for complete lacerations and ruptures is usually necessary.
- Postoperative peritendinous adhesions are a major concern and can result in poor tendon gliding, stiffness, and functional disability.
- Appropriate rehabilitation is critical (balance between decreasing adhesion formation while protecting the repair).

Anatomy

- There are two flexor tendons to each digit extending from the FDS muscle bellies and the FDP muscle belly, and one flexor tendon to the thumb extending from the flexor pollicis longus muscle belly.
- The FDS and FDP muscle bellies are in the volar forearm and the tendons, which form in the distal forearm, go through the carpal tunnel, and continue to insert on the base of the proximal phalanges and distal phalanges, respectively.
- The flexor pollicis longus tendon also traverses the carpal tunnel and inserts on the base of the distal phalanx of the thumb.
- The FDS is superficial (volar) to the FDP until approximately the metacarpophalangeal (MCP) joint, where it splits (Camper's chiasma); the FDP tendon continues through the chiasm to become the more superficial tendon, and the two slips of the FDS insert on the palmar surface at the base of the middle phalanx (Fig. 87-1).

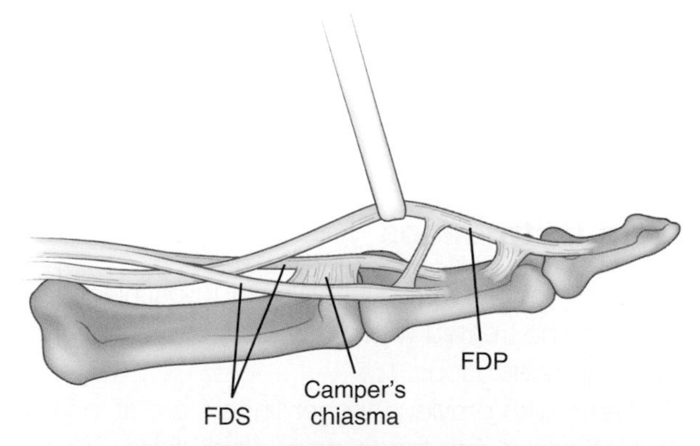

Figure 87-1 The flexor digitorum superficialis (FDS) is volar to the flexor digitorum profundus (FDP) until approximately the metacarpophalangeal joint, where it splits. The FDP tendon continues through the chiasm to become the more superficial tendon, and the two slips of the FDS insert on the palmar surface at the base of the middle phalanx. (Adapted from Green DP, Hotchkiss RN, Pederson WC, Wolfe SW [eds]: Green's Operative Hand Surgery, 5th ed. New York: Churchill Livingstone, 2005, Fig. 7-3. Copyright Elizabeth Martin.)

- Just proximal to the MCP joint, the FDS and FDP are enclosed by a common flexor tendon sheath (Fig. 87-2).
  - The sheath contains synovial fluid and facilitates gliding and nutritional supply of tendons.
  - The sheath is composed of several annular and cruciate pulleys that stabilize the tendons and act as a mechanical fulcrum for flexion.
- Flexor tendons are divided into five anatomic zones (Fig. 87-3).
  - Zone I: the portion of the FDP distal to the insertion of the FDS
  - Zone II ("no man's land"): from the decussation to the insertion of the FDS
  - Zone III: origin of the lumbricals (the intrinsic hand muscles), just proximal to the splitting of the FDS
  - Zone IV: carpal tunnel
  - Zone V: proximal to the carpal tunnel
- The FDS flexes the proximal interphalangeal (PIP) joint and secondarily the MCP and wrist joints.
- The FDP flexes the distal interphalangeal (DIP) joint and secondarily the PIP, MCP, and wrist joints.
- The lumbricals originate in the palm from the tendons of the FDP and insert distally and dorsally to the extensor mechanism at the level of the proximal phalanx.

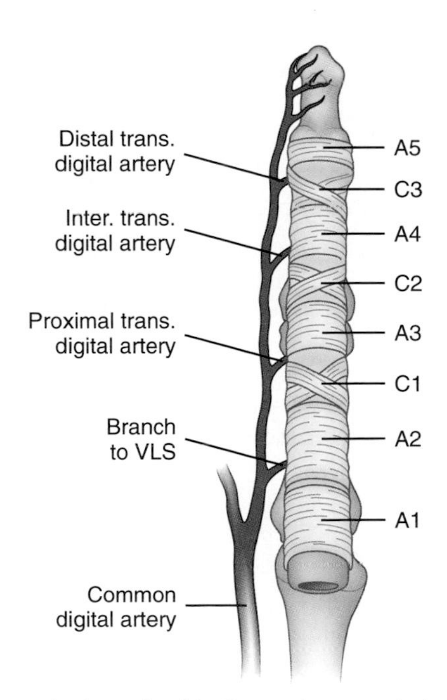

Figure 87-2 Just proximal to the metacarpophalangeal joint, the flexor digitorum superficialis and flexor digitorum profundus become enclosed by a common flexor tendon sheath, which is composed of several annular and cruciate pulleys. VLS, vinculum longum. (Adapted from Green DP, Hotchkiss RN, Pederson WC, Wolfe SW [eds]: Green's Operative Hand Surgery, 5th ed. New York: Churchill Livingstone, 2005, Fig. 7-4. Copyright Elizabeth Martin.)

  - Four lumbricals, one to each digit except the thumb
  - The action of the lumbrical is simultaneous flexion of the MCP joint and extension of the PIP and DIP joints.
  - Intrinsic and extrinsic muscles must function together for normal finger motion.
- The blood supply to the tendons is a combination of diffusion (via synovial fluid bathing the tendon) and perfusion (via vincula, which are interval soft-tissue attachments between the phalanges and the dorsal surface of the FDP and FDS).
- The digital neurovascular bundles lie just radial and ulnar to the flexor tendons and are thus susceptible to concurrent injury with lacerations/punctures; the nerve lies just volar to the artery and vein.

History

- Usually the result of an acute event, usually a laceration/puncture
- Obvious loss of finger flexion (PIP, DIP, or both, depending on level of injury)
- Lacerations frequently will involve injury to adjacent neurovascular structures, and the patient may report numbness distal to the injury.
- Inquire about the position of the hand at the time of injury: if the fingers were flexed, the level of tendon injury will be distal to the skin wound; if the fingers

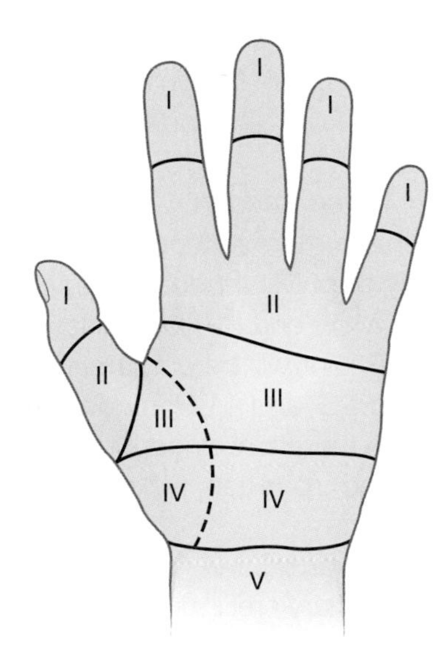

Figure 87-3 Flexor tendons are divided into five anatomic zones (I to V) that can be demarcated by superficial landmarks. Knowledge of these zones is useful in describing the injury. (Adapted from Green DP, Hotchkiss RN, Pederson WC, Wolfe SW [eds]: Green's Operative Hand Surgery, 5th ed. New York: Churchill Livingstone, 2005, Fig. 7-2. Copyright Elizabeth Martin.)

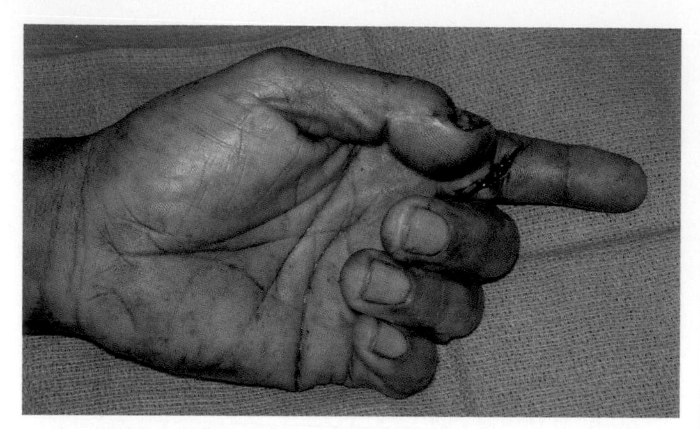

Figure 87-4 Example of a tendon laceration. Note the loss of the normal cascade and the patient's inability to flex the injured finger.

were extended, the tendon injury is approximately at the level of the wound.

- Patients present with the inability to flex the involved finger(s) (Fig. 87-4).
- Ruptures typically occur in the setting of chronic attrition, as may be seen in patients with rheumatoid arthritis or in association with retained plates or screws previously used to fix a wrist or hand fracture.

Physical Examination

- Observation
  - Lacerations/punctures: Do not probe or try to retrieve lacerated flexor tendons.
  - Posture of hand and fingers: With the hand in a resting position, the fingers are normally held in a flexed posture, with flexion increasing in a cascading fashion from the index finger to the small finger.
    - — The injured tendon will cause its finger to assume a more extended posture.
    - — If only the FDP tendon is injured, then flexion of the MCP and PIP joints may be normal and the DIP joint will be abnormally extended.
    - — If the FDS and FDP tendons are both disrupted, the entire finger will fall into a resting extended position, clearly disrupting the arcade.
- Neurovascular examination
  - Assess capillary refill in the affected digit(s): sluggish or absent refill may indicate a devascularized digit, which requires emergent surgical intervention.
  - Assess sensation to light touch on both the ulnar and radial sides of the digit(s): sensation that is absent or altered compared with noninjured fingers indicates likely damage to the neurovascular bundle; this can alert the surgeon that microvascular repair may be necessary.

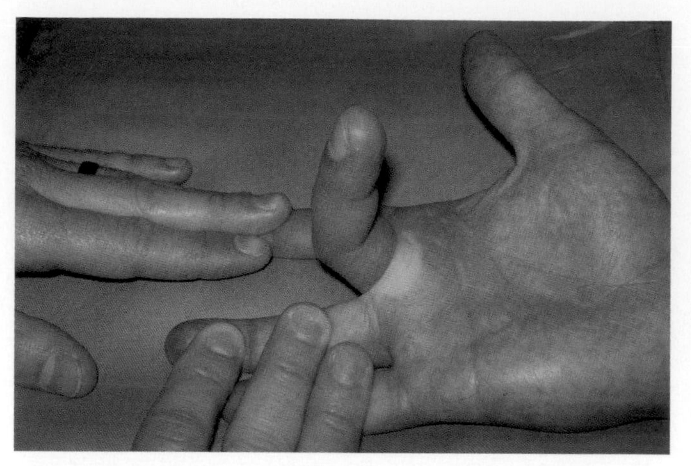

Figure 87-5 To test the integrity of the flexor digitorum superficialis, keep all other fingers extended, including the distal interphalangeal joints, and ask the patient to flex the affected finger. If the tendon is intact, the finger will flex at the proximal interphalangeal and metacarpophalangeal joints.

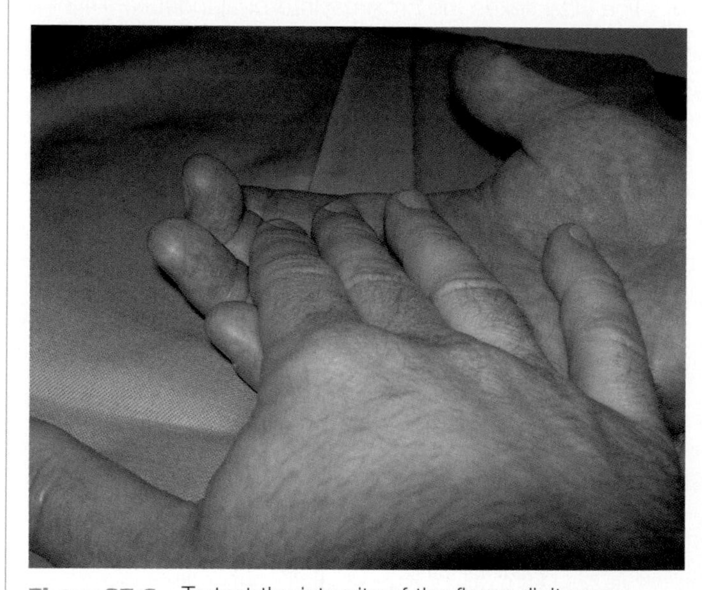

Figure 87-6 To test the integrity of the flexor digitorum profundus, isolate the distal interphalangeal joint by holding the metacarpophalangeal and proximal interphalangeal joints extended, and ask the patient to flex the finger.

- Check the integrity of the tendons
  - Independently examine the FDP and FDS tendons.
    - — FDS: Keep all other fingers extended, including the DIP joints, and ask the patient to flex the affected finger; if the tendon is intact, it will flex at the PIP and MCP joints (Fig. 87-5).
    - — FDP: Isolate the DIP joint by holding the MCP and PIP joints extended and ask the patient to flex the finger (Fig. 87-6).

- Alternative techniques
  - — Passively extend the patient's wrist, and the tenodesis effect should cause all fingers with intact tendons to flex accordingly.
  - — Squeeze the volar forearm musculature, which should cause all digits to flex slightly; if a tendon has been transected, it will not respond.
- With partial transections, a normal arcade may be present, and the patient may still have intact function.
  - — Pain with flexion against resistance may indicate partial injury.
  - — Clicking or catching may occur during motion.

Imaging

- The mechanism of injury may have also caused injury to the phalanges or joint surfaces that plain radiographs of the hand/finger can delineate.
- Other modalities are typically not indicated in a primary injury.
- Magnetic resonance imaging or ultrasonography can be used to differentiate between post-repair tendon adhesions and re-rupture.

Treatment

- At diagnosis
  - If the injury is caused by a laceration/puncture, administer intravenous antibiotics and assess the need for a tetanus update.
  - Irrigate the wound, apply a clean dressing, and apply a splint (dorsal splint with the wrist in neutral flexion and the MCP joints in 60 to 70 degrees of flexion).
  - Consult with a hand surgeon, who may ask to close the skin wound with sutures before applying a dressing or splint.
  - Chronic ruptures from attrition (i.e., rheumatoid arthritis) can be splinted for comfort.
- Later
  - Complete disruption of a flexor tendon will typically require surgical repair, as will many partial tendon injuries.
    - — This may be accompanied by microsurgical repair of the digital neurovascular structures.
  - Surgical options are based on the level of injury, degree of contamination, soft-tissue damage, and time from injury.

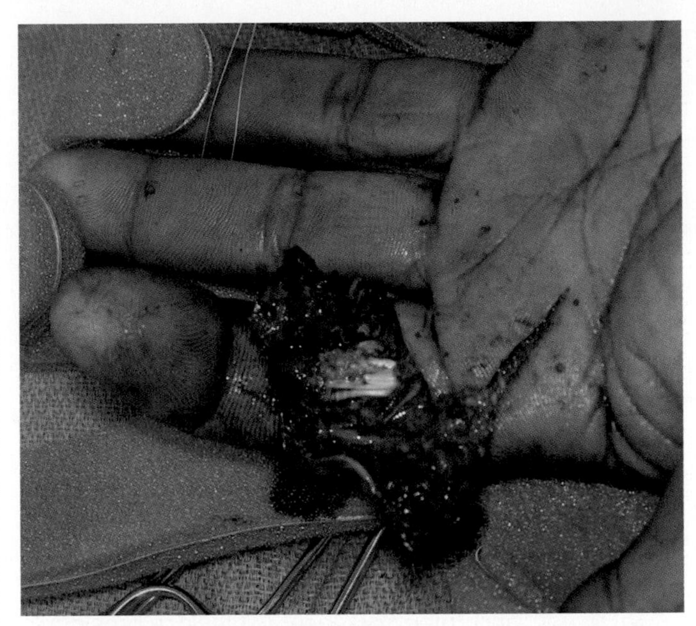

Figure 87-7 Intraoperative view of an acute zone II flexor digitorum profundus and flexor digitorum superficialis tendon repair. Note the tight sheath above and below the repair, which is one reason why adhesions and loss of motion are so problematic.

Surgical Repair

Acute Repair

- In clean wounds, primary end-to-end repair can usually be performed within 1 to 2 weeks of injury.
  - Zone I: similar to repair of avulsion injuries (Jersey finger) (see Chapter 90)
  - Zone II: FDP tendon typically repaired end-to-end with four deep core sutures and a running epitenon suture
    - — FDS tendons usually repaired separately with simple suture techniques, change to FDP tendon typically repaired end to end with a four-strand core suture technique and a running epitenon suture; FDS tendons usually repaired separately with simple suture techniques (Fig. 87-7)
    - — Repair of pulleys/tendon sheath is done as necessary.
  - Zones III to V: FDS and FDP are repaired independently with core sutures with or without running epitenon suture
    - — Repair or excision of a damaged lumbrical in zone III depending on injury

Delayed/Staged Repair

- In delayed presentations (more than 3–4 weeks), cases of re-rupture, excessive scarring of repair, dirty wounds, and some acute zone II injuries, staged repair is indicated.

- Stage I: the FDS and/or FDP is excised, and a prosthetic (i.e., silicone) rod is placed.
  - — Pulley system is reconstructed as needed at this time
  - — Stays in approximately 3 months; range of motion preserved with therapy
- Stage II: the prosthetic graft is removed, and the tendon graft is placed within the sheath and sutured to the proximal and distal stumps.

Basics of Rehabilitation

- Multiple protocols have been described for different injuries.
- Initial postoperative immobilization with the MCP joints in flexion and interphalangeal joints in extension to avoid contractures
- Regular follow-up with a hand therapist is imperative to optimal outcome.
- In general, motion is started within a few days to decrease tendon adhesions and improve excursion/motion.
  - Initially, passive flexion (or carefully controlled/protected active flexion) and active extension are performed within the confines of a dorsal extension block splint.
- Gradual supervised progression over 3 to 4 months of increased extension, active flexion, and active flexion against resistance until full activity is allowed

When to Refer

- If the examiner is confident that the patient has a complete or partial tendon injury, with or without concomitant neurovascular injury, he or she should refer the patient to a surgeon for repair.
  - Surgery preferably occurs within 1 to 2 weeks of an injury and ideally within 24 hours.
  - Repairs after 2 weeks are complicated by retraction of tendons and scarring, and the chance of a poor outcome is greater.

Prognosis

- Variable
- Dependent on anatomic location(s) of injury, time until surgery, coexisting injuries, quality of repair, and patient compliance with postoperative rehabilitation
- Appropriate rehabilitation with a hand therapist is critical to achieving an optimal outcome.
- The most common complication is postoperative tendon adhesions, which can lead to a decreased range of motion and stiffness.
- Another complication is re-rupture of the repaired tendon (most commonly 1–2 weeks postoperatively), often requiring two-stage repair as described previously.

Considerations in Special Populations

- Children do not require the same postoperative protocols; they are unable to comply with the complex instructions. However, this population does quite well with 4 weeks of immobilization and then unrestricted activity.

Suggested Reading

- Beredjiklian PK: Biologic aspects of flexor tendon laceration and repair. J Bone Joint Surg Am 2003;85A:539–550.
- Boyer M, Taras JS, Kaufman RA: Flexor tendon injury. In Green DP, Hotchkiss RN, Pederson WC, Wolfe SW (eds): Green's Operative Hand Surgery, 5th ed. New York: Churchill Livingstone, 2005, pp 219–276.
- Boyer MI, Strickland JW, Engles D, et al: Flexor tendon repair and rehabilitation: State of the art in 2002. Instr Course Lect 2003;52:137–161.
- Freilich AM, Chhabra AB: Secondary flexor tendon reconstruction, a review. J Hand Surg [Am] 2007;32A:1436–1442.
- Newmeyer WL, Manske PR: No man's land revisited: The primary flexor tendon repair controversy. J Hand Surg [Am] 2004;29A:1–5.
- Tang JB, Zhang Y, Cao Y, Xie RG: Core suture purchase affects strength of tendon repairs. J Hand Surg [Am] 2005;30A:1262–1266.

Chapter 88 Boutonniere Deformity

Jack Ingari and Daniel T. Fletcher, Jr.

ICD-9 CODE

736.21 *Central Slip Extensor Tendon Injury (Boutonniere)*

Key Concepts

- Also known as *buttonhole deformity*
- Deformity of the finger involving flexion of the proximal interphalangeal (PIP) joint and hyperextension of the distal interphalangeal (DIP) joint (Fig. 88-1)
- Caused by disruption or attenuation of the central slip of the extensor expansion (Fig. 88-2)
- Traumatic, infectious, or inflammatory etiology
- The balance of the finger extensor mechanism is altered, which over time leads to fixed volar subluxation of the lateral bands and focus of extension force exclusively on the distal joint. This causes loss of active PIP joint extension and hyperextension of the DIP joint, respectively.
- If left untreated, fixed flexion occurs at the PIP joint secondary to volar plate and oblique retinacular ligament contracture.

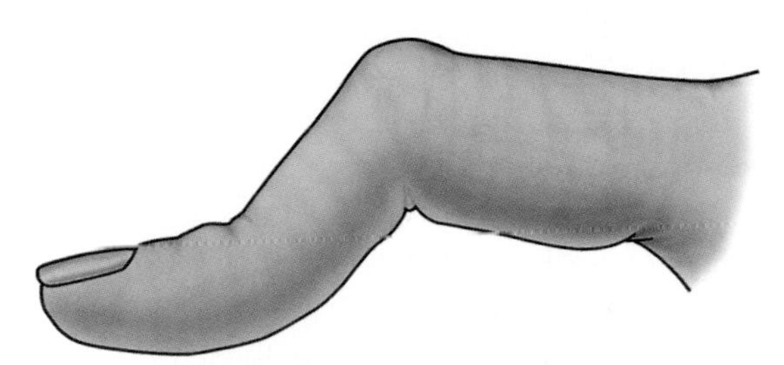

Figure 88-1 Extensor tenotomy for supple boutonniere deformity. The deformity is characteristic of the chronic boutonniere deformity. (Adapted from Green DP, Hotchkiss RN, Pederson WC, Wolfe SW [eds]: Green's Operative Hand Surgery, 5th ed. Philadelphia: Churchill Livingstone, 2005, Fig. 6-22A.)

History

- Closed Injury
- Forced flexion of an actively extended PIP joint ("jammed" finger)
- Crush injury
- Volar dislocation of the PIP joint
- Open injury
- Laceration over the PIP joint
- Open wound at the level of the PIP joint with tendon necrosis
- Burns
- Infection
- Subcutaneous infection
- Intra-articular infection of the PIP joint
- Inflammatory
- Rheumatoid and other inflammatory arthritides
- Gout

Physical Examination

- Acute
    - The examiner must have a high index of suspicion because the deformity may evolve over the course of 1 week after the initial injury.

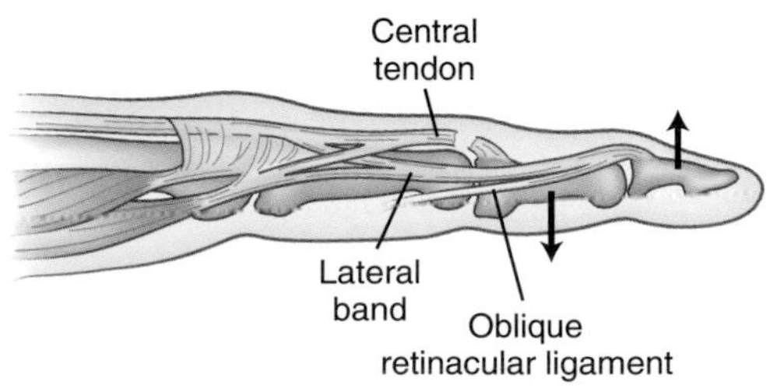

Figure 88-2 Pathomechanics of the boutonniere deformity. Attenuation of the central slip results in unopposed flexion at the proximal interphalangeal joint. (Adapted from Green DP, Hotchkiss RN, Pederson WC, Wolfe SW [eds]: Green's Operative Hand Surgery, 5th ed. Philadelphia: Churchill Livingstone, 2005, Fig. 6-21A.)

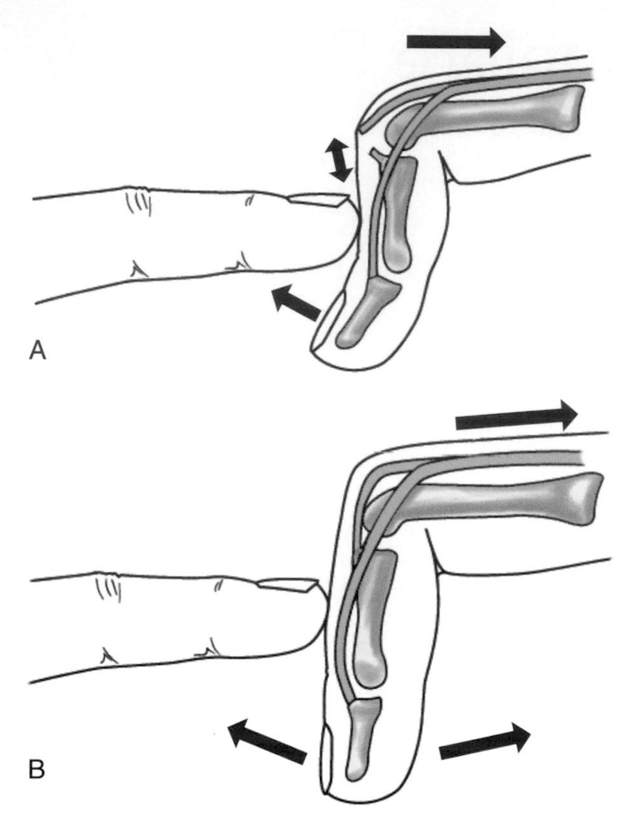

Figure 88-3 Elson test. **A**, With a disrupted central slip, attempted active extension of the proximal interphalangeal joint against resistance allows proximal movement of the origin of the lateral bands holding the distal joint in extension. **B**, With an intact central slip, attempted active extension of the proximal interphalangeal joint against resistance affects the middle phalanx but leaves the distal joint flail.

- PIP joint effusion
- Localized tenderness over the dorsal aspect of the PIP joint at the insertion of the central tendon
- Elson test (Fig. 88-3)
  — A positive test result is demonstrated when the patient bends the PIP joint 90 degrees over the edge of a table and, with resisted middle phalanx extension the DIP joint, goes into rigid extension (all the forces are distributed to the terminal tendon through the intact lateral bands).
  — A negative test result is demonstrated when the DIP joint remains floppy with this maneuver.
- Chronic
  - Assess the PIP and DIP joints for flexibility and evidence of arthritis.

Imaging

- Radiographs of acute and chronic injuries are imperative in determining the mode of treatment.

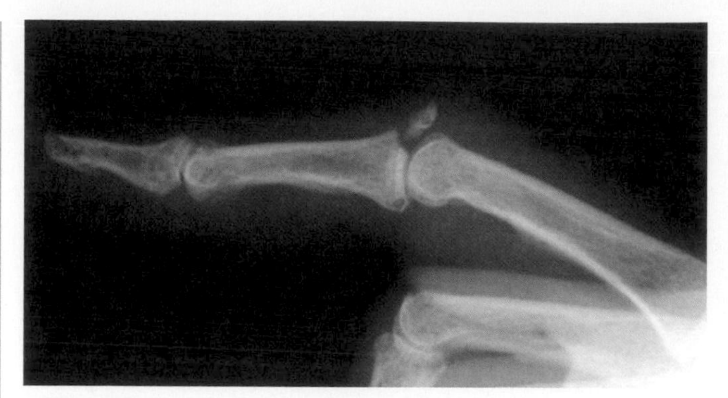

Figure 88-4 An avulsed bone fragment at the insertion of the central slip. (From Green DP, Hotchkiss RN, Pederson WC, Wolfe SW [eds]: Green's Operative Hand Surgery, 5th ed. Philadelphia: Churchill Livingstone, 2005, Fig. 6-17B.)

- Standard views of the affected digit should include anteroposterior, lateral, and oblique views.
- Acute: Fractures and volar subluxations are often seen (Fig. 88-4).
- Chronic: Arthritic changes may be present from infection or inflammatory arthritis.

Differential Diagnosis

- Pseudo-boutonniere deformity
  - Flexion contracture of the PIP joint but without restriction if DIP joint mobility
  - Extensor mechanism is unaffected
  - Caused by PIP joint hyperextension injury that results in fibrosis of the volar ligamentous complex
  - Radiographs often demonstrate avulsion fractures of the PIP volar plate and calcification about the volar mechanism of the proximal phalanx.

Treatment

- Depends on the chronicity of the injury and the flexibility of the digit
- Acute injuries (0–2 weeks)
  - Lacerations require exploration and anatomic reapproximation of the central slip.
  - Closed injuries not involving a fracture require 6 weeks of immobilization of the PIP joint in extension, leaving the DIP joint free (Fig. 88-5).
  - Flexion of the DIP joint draws the extensor mechanism distally and facilitates dorsal translation of the lateral bands.
  - Closed injuries involving a fracture or dislocation require reduction followed by an assessment of joint stability.

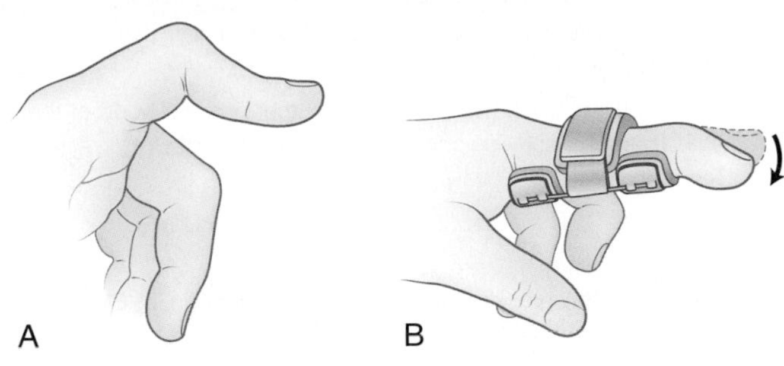

Figure 88-5 **A**, Schematic representation of a boutonniere deformity. **B**, A Bunnell splint is applied to maintain extension at the proximal interphalangeal (PIP) joint. The strap over the PIP joint is progressively tightened until the PIP joint is fully extended. The patient is encouraged to actively and passively flex the distal interphalangeal joint. The splint is worn until the patient can maintain active extension of the PIP joint. (Adapted from Green DP, Hotchkiss RN, Pederson WC, Wolfe SW [eds]: Green's Operative Hand Surgery, 5th ed. Philadelphia: Churchill Livingstone, 2005, Fig. 6-16A and B. Copyright Elizabeth Martin.)

  - If the reduction is adequate and the joint is stable, immobilize the PIP joint with the DIP joint free for 6 weeks.
  - If the reduction cannot be obtained or the joint is unstable, open reduction and internal fixation are required.
- Subacute injuries (2–8 weeks)
  - Treat supple PIP joints like acute closed injuries without fractures, except leave the splint on for 8 weeks.
  - Stiff PIP joints require treatment to regain full mobility.
  - Dynamic or progressive static splints can be used.
  - If full motion is restored, leave the splint on for an additional 8 weeks.
  - If motion cannot be restored, treat the injury like a chronic stiff boutonniere determity (see the following).
- Chronic injuries (>8 weeks)
  - Probably will not be amenable to splint therapy
  - The status of the PIP and DIP joints determines the treatment protocol in these long-standing injuries.
  - Flexible PIP joints require operative rebalancing of the extensor mechanism through anatomic repair, reconstruction using local tissue, or tendon grafting.
  - Treatment of stiff PIP joints requires staged treatment.
  - The first priority is to re-establish joint motion through splinting or surgery.
  - Once full motion is established, an extensor tendon reconstruction is typically required.
  - Arthritic PIP joints require arthroplasty or fusion depending on whether the extensor mechanism is intact or disrupted, respectively.

When to Refer

- Open injuries
- Fractures or irreducible dislocations requiring open reduction and internal fixation
- Residual deformity after failure of splinting program
- Flexion contracture unresponsive to conservative treatment

Troubleshooting

- Early diagnosis is essential for successful treatment.
- The examiner must have a high index of suspicion of central slip injury during the acute phase because a boutonniere deformity may be delayed.
- In a stiff deformity, full extension must be obtained either through splinting or surgical release before definitive treatment can be performed.
- It is important to differentiate between boutonniere and pseudo-boutonniere deformities because surgery for either condition when the other is actually the problem will have poor results.
- The most common complication encountered in treating acute closed deformities is incomplete correction.
- Full flexion of the PIP and DIP joints with an extension lag of 20 degrees or less produces a finger with few functional limitations.

Patient Instructions

- The splint for acute injury must be worn full time for a minimum of 6 weeks.
- An additional 6 weeks of night splinting follows for protection.
- Concomitant active and passive flexion of the DIP joint must be done during splint wear.

Considerations in Special Populations

- Rheumatoid arthritis patients can be treated with a similar algorithm.
- It is important to address the wrist pathology before surgical treatment of boutonniere deformity in these patients.

- Severe rheumatoid boutonniere deformities often require joint fusion.

Suggested Reading

- Baratz ME, Schmidt CC, Hughes TB: Extensor tendon injuries. In Green DP, Hotchkiss RN, Pederson WC, Wolfe SW (eds): Green's Operative Hand Surgery, 5th ed. Philadelphia: Churchill Livingstone, 2005, pp 199–205.
- Coons MS, Green SG: Boutonniere deformity. Hand Clin 1995;11:387–402.
- Elson RA: Rupture of the central slip of the extensor hood of the finger, a test for early diagnosis. J Bone Joint Surg Br 1986;68B:229–231.
- Massengill JB: The boutonniere deformity. Hand Clin 1992;8:787–801.
- Souter WA: The problem of boutonniere deformity. Clin Orthop Relat Res 1974;104:116–133.

Chapter 89 Mallet Finger

Steven L. Henry and Jack Ingari

ICD-9 CODE
736.1 *Mallet Finger*

Key Concepts

- A mallet finger (also known as *drop finger* or *baseball finger*) is a finger that droops at the tip due to an injury to the terminal extensor mechanism.
- The terminal extensor mechanism is composed of a broad, flat terminal tendon that spans the distal interphalangeal (DIP) joint to insert at the dorsal base of the distal phalanx (Fig. 89-1).
- An isolated injury to the terminal extensor mechanism will cause an extensor lag (i.e., loss of active extension) at the DIP joint.
- Specific injuries to the terminal extensor mechanism include
    - Rupture of the terminal tendon
    - Laceration of the terminal tendon
    - Fracture of the distal phalanx at the terminal tendon's insertion

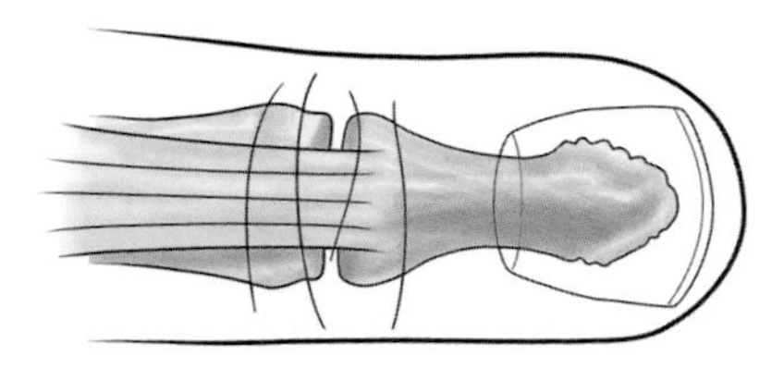

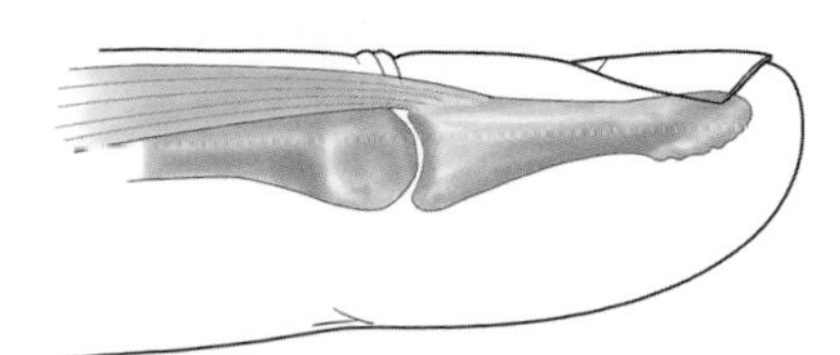

Figure 89-1 The thin, flat terminal tendon (*blue*) inserts at the dorsal lip of the base of the distal phalanx, just distal to the distal interphalangeal joint. Note that the tendon is immediately subcutaneous, the joint is immediately deep to the tendon, and the nail bed begins just distal to the tendon insertion.

- As the more proximal joints are typically uninjured, the finger acquires the classic mallet posture, a drooping tip on an otherwise normal digit (Fig. 89-2).
- When the terminal tendon is disrupted, forces on the extensor mechanism are no longer transmitted across the DIP joint, but rather are concentrated at the proximal interphalangeal (PIP) joint.
    - Thus, in addition to an extensor lag at the DIP joint (i.e., a mallet deformity), a terminal tendon injury can also produce a hyperextension deformity at the PIP joint.
    - This condition, called a compensatory swan neck deformity (Fig. 89-3), is particularly common in patients with naturally hyperextensible PIP joints.
- Over time, mallet and swan neck deformities can become fixed; for this reason, it is desirable that treatment for a mallet finger be initiated reasonably promptly.

History

- The typical chief symptom is an inability to extend the DIP joint.
- Many patients present with a history of a sports-related injury (e.g., jammed finger) or a traumatic event such as a knife accident.
    - These patients will likely have significant pain at the site of injury.
- Often, however, the trauma is surprisingly minor; examples include inadvertently banging a fingertip against a desk drawer and catching a fingertip on the edge of a pocket.
    - These patients may have little or no pain.
    - Such scenarios are typical in older patients and are probably indicative of an attritional tendon rupture from arthritic changes at the DIP joint.

Physical Examination

- Often there is edema and erythema over the dorsal DIP joint region.

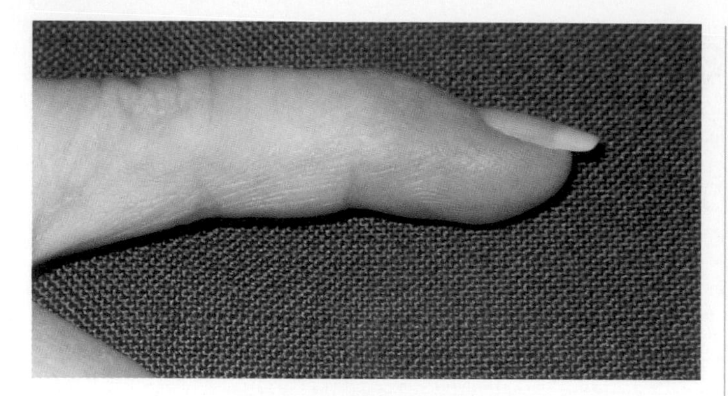

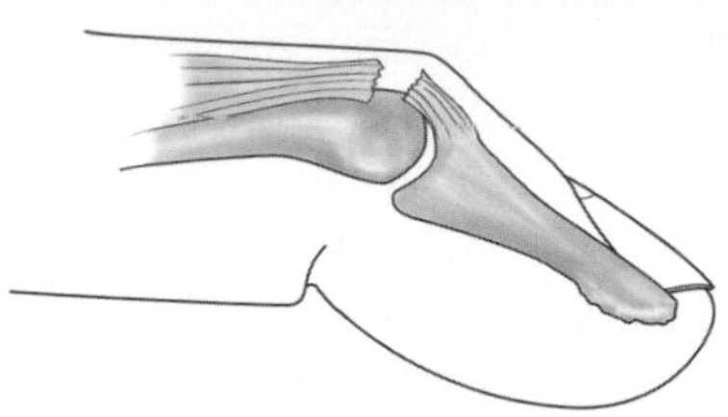

Figure 89-2 The mallet posture is due to discontinuity of the extensor mechanism across the distal interphalangeal joint. In this case, the discontinuity was due to closed rupture of the terminal tendon. Lacerations/abrasions of the tendon and fractures of the distal phalanx at the tendon's insertion can also create the mallet posture.

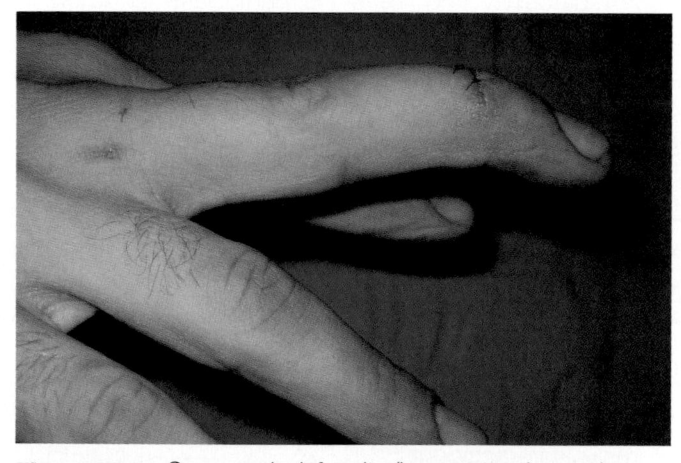

Figure 89-3 Swan neck deformity (hyperextension at the proximal interphalangeal joint and flexion at the distal interphalangeal joint) can be seen with mallet injuries, especially in people with naturally hyperextensible proximal interphalangeal joints.

- There may be a laceration or abrasion over the dorsal middle phalanx or DIP joint regions.
- Usually (but not always) there is mild to moderate tenderness at the site of injury.
- An extensor lag at the DIP joint is usually immediately evident, but occasionally the lag takes time to develop.
  - This presentation is more typical of attritional ruptures, in which a few wispy fibers of tendon or scar tissue remain in continuity.

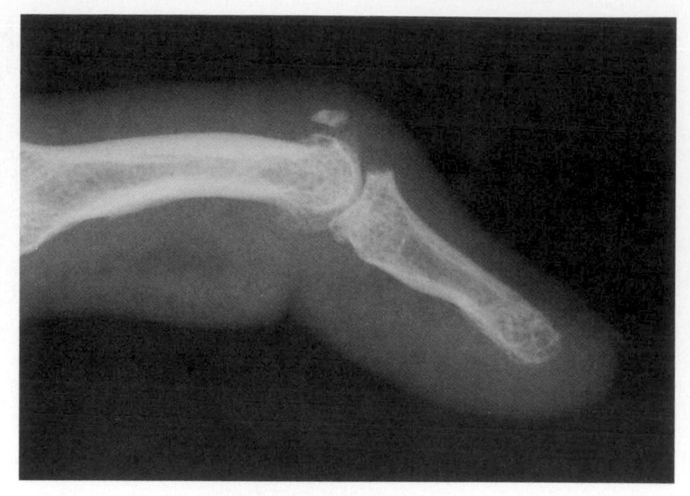

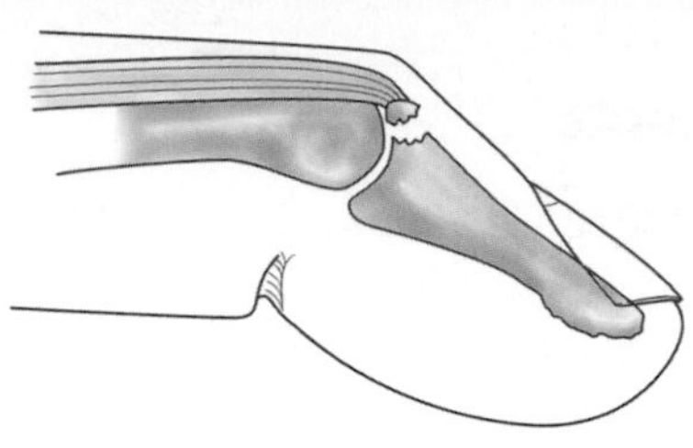

Figure 89-4 Many mallet injuries involve fractures of the distal phalanx. In most cases, the fragment is small and represents an avulsion of the tendon insertion. The distal phalanx remains properly located at the distal interphalangeal joint. These injuries usually heal well with splinting.

  - In these early cases, a lag will become evident if the patient is asked to make a tight fist (stretching the remaining fibers) and then extend the fingers.
- Flexor function is typically not affected.
- Passive extension is usually intact, unless the injury is chronic, in which case a fixed flexion contracture may develop.
- Hyperextension may be present at the PIP joint (i.e., compensatory swan neck deformity).

Imaging

- Radiographs should be obtained for all mallet fingers.
  - Order three views (posteroanterior, lateral, and oblique) of the individual digit.
  - It is important to get a true lateral view, which is most likely to reveal dorsal fractures.
  - Attempts to image all digits simultaneously rarely result in true lateral views.
  - Many mallet injuries involve a small fracture of the dorsal lip of the distal phalanx, where the tendon insertion is avulsed along with a small piece of bone (Fig. 89-4).

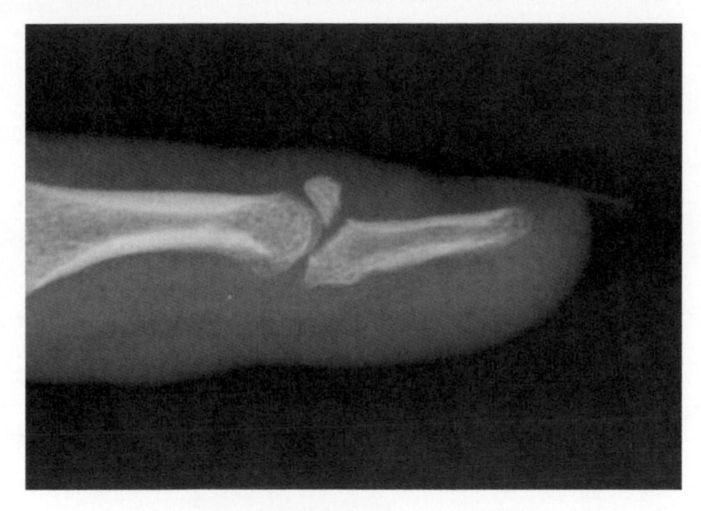

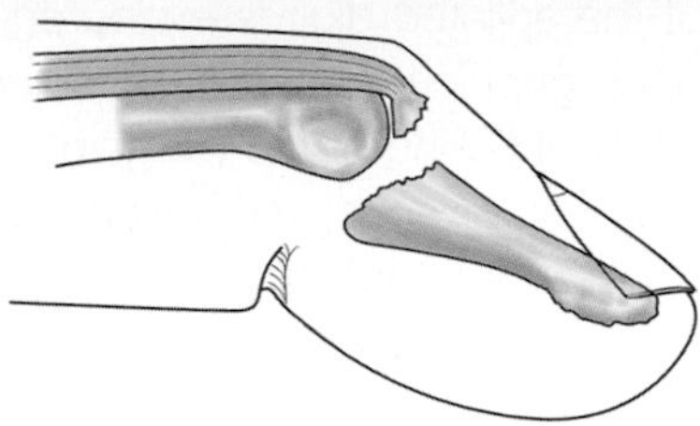

Figure 89-5 Distal phalanx fractures that encompass a large portion of the articular surface may lead to incongruity of the distal interphalangeal joint and volar subluxation of the distal phalanx. These cases may require surgery.

- If the fracture fragment is large (i.e., >30% of the articular surface), volar subluxation of the distal phalanx can occur (Fig. 89-5).
- Additional imaging tests, such as computed tomography or magnetic resonance imaging, are usually not indicated.

Differential Diagnosis

- An isolated extensor lag at the DIP joint is virtually pathognomonic for an injury of the terminal extensor tendon or its bony insertion.
- Some patients with arthritis can develop primary hyperextension at the PIP joint with secondary drooping of the distal phalanx; this is called a primary swan neck deformity.
  - The feature distinguishing a primary swan neck deformity from a compensatory one is the presence of (typically long-standing) pain and swelling at the PIP joint before the development of the deformity.
- A fixed flexion contracture of the DIP joint can be seen with both long-standing mallet injuries and unrelated disorders of the joint or flexor mechanism; the distinction is usually evident from the history.
- Rarely an exostosis (bony growth) of the dorsal DIP joint region can create the appearance of a mallet deformity; such a pseudo-mallet can be distinguished with radiographs.

Treatment

- Relatively few mallet injuries require surgical intervention; the exceptions are
  - Lacerations or abrasions of the terminal tendon
  - Fractures involving more than 30% of the articular surface or volar subluxation of the distal phalanx
  - Otherwise nonoperative injuries in patients who cannot perform their work duties while wearing a splint
- The remainder (and majority) of mallet injuries, including those involving tendon ruptures or small avulsion fractures, can be treated with splinting of the DIP joint in slight hyperextension.
  - Even chronic mallet fingers can often be improved significantly with a course of splinting.
  - Only the DIP joint needs to be splinted; in fact, it is desirable to leave the PIP joint free, not only to prevent stiffness, but also because flexion at this joint relieves tension on the terminal extensor tendon.
- The standard splinting protocol calls for full-time splinting for 6 weeks (counted from the date splinting was initiated, not the date of injury) followed by splinting only at night for 2 weeks.
  - Should the DIP joint be flexed at any time during the full-time splinting period, the 6-week time frame starts over.
  - If during the 2-week nighttime splinting period, the extensor lag begins to return, the patient resumes full-time splinting for another 2 weeks, again followed by 2 weeks of nighttime splinting.
- Types of splints
  - Aluminum-foam splint (Fig. 89-6)
    - — This is preferably placed dorsally to facilitate continued use of the digit.
    - — A slight bend is created in the aluminum to maintain the DIP joint in approximately 5 degrees of hyperextension.
      - — *More aggressive hyperextension can cause ischemia of the skin dorsal to the DIP joint and must therefore be avoided.*
  - Stack splint (Fig. 89-7)
    - — This is a prefabricated plastic splint designed specifically for mallet fingers.

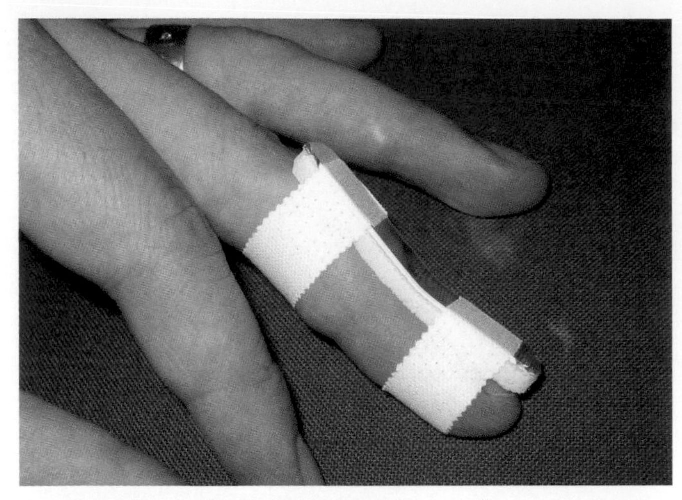

Figure 89-6 A piece of aluminum-foam splint material can be fashioned into an effective mallet splint. The material should be cut to a length that spans the middle and distal phalanges and leaves the proximal interphalangeal joint free. A small bend in the aluminum keeps the distal interphalangeal joint in mild (5 degrees) of hyperextension.

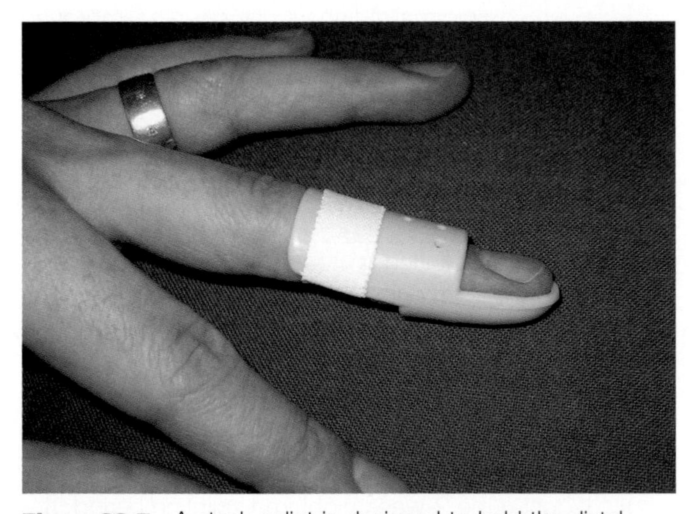

Figure 89-7 A stack splint is designed to hold the distal interphalangeal joint in extension while permitting full motion at the proximal interphalangeal joint. These splints come in multiple sizes and should be selected to provide a snug but comfortable fit.

- It is available in various sizes and should be selected to provide a snug but comfortable fit.
- It may be necessary to use a larger size initially to accommodate wound dressings or edema and then downsize as the finger heals.
- Occasionally these splints do not provide the proper degree of hyperextension at the DIP joint; a trick is to apply moleskin to the inside of the splint on the surface in contact with the volar fingertip to push the joint into the desired 5 degrees of hyperextension.

- Customized thermoplastic splint constructed by an occupational therapist
- The patient should be given the following instructions:
  - During the period of full-time splinting, the splint should be removed only to cleanse the finger and splint.
  - To avoid inadvertent flexion of the DIP joint, the splint should be worn in the shower; afterward, the splint may be removed to wash and dry the finger and splint, taking great care not to flex the DIP joint. The splint is then immediately replaced.
  - Use of the splinted digit is encouraged, although strenuous gripping should be avoided to prevent unintentional flexing of the DIP joint.
- With this splinting protocol, the majority of patients will achieve a satisfactory outcome, although a slight (and usually inconsequential) residual extensor lag is common, as is a persistent prominence over the dorsal DIP joint region.
- Some hand surgeons recommend operative repair of mallet injuries in an effort to obviate a residual extensor lag, which in some cases is significant enough to create a functional and/or cosmetic impairment.
  - Outcomes for operative repair are usually good as well, although stiffness preventing full flexion, rather than an extensor lag, is a risk; the argument hinges on whether it is better to lose terminal extension or terminal flexion and whether the patient wishes to avoid surgery.
- Lacerations of the terminal tendon should be repaired at the time of skin closure.
  - These repairs can often be achieved in the clinic or emergency department settings, assuming the wound is clean and fresh.
  - The repair technique is a matter of personal preference, but an acceptable method would be to place figure-of-eight or horizontal mattress stitches using a permanent (e.g., Ethibond) or long-lasting absorbable (e.g., Vicryl) suture, size 3-0 or 4-0 (Fig. 89-8).
  - Very distal lacerations, where the tendon is extremely thin, can be very difficult or impossible to repair directly, and simultaneous approximation of the skin and tendon in a single layer (tenodermodesis) is an effective alternative (Fig. 89-9).
  - In these cases, a nonabsorbable monofilament suture (nylon or Prolene, size 3-0 or 4-0), as would be used for skin closure, is preferred.

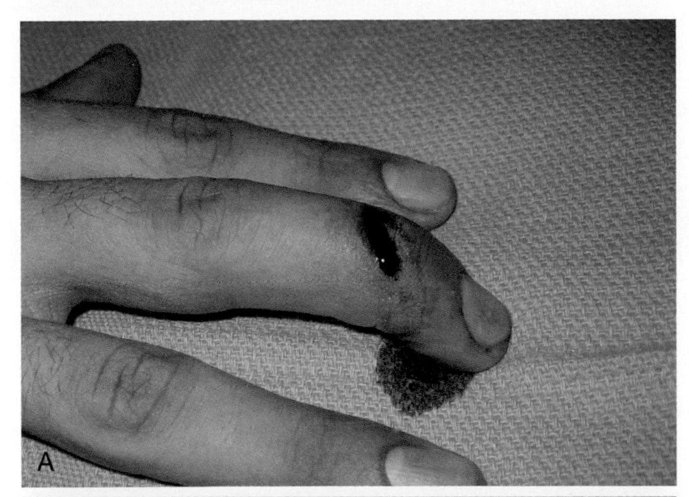

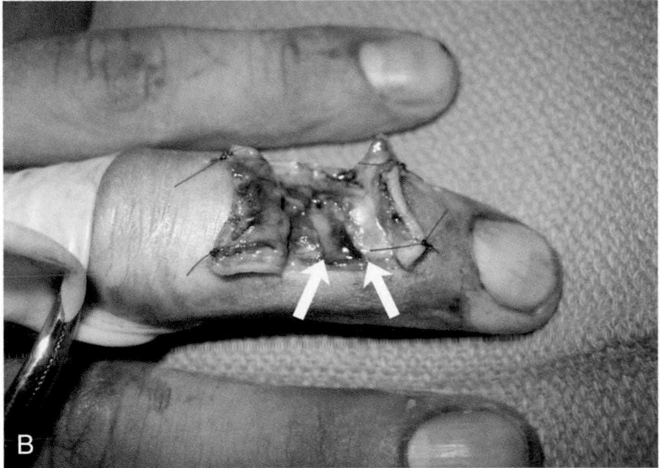

Figure 89-8 Tendon lacerations can be repaired at the time of skin repair. **A,** In this case, an oblique laceration was present across the dorsum of the middle phalanx. **B**, Flaps of dorsal skin have been created proximally and distally to facilitate exposure of the tendon edges (*arrows*). A 1-inch Penrose drain has been wrapped around the digit proximally as a tourniquet. The tendon will be repaired with multiple figure-of-eight stitches using 3-0 Vicryl.

- All terminal tendon repairs should be protected postoperatively with the splinting protocol described previously.

When to Refer

- Abrasion injuries in which there is a segmental loss of tendon substance, as might be seen with a power tool or motorcycle accident
- Distal phalanx fractures that encompass more than one third of the articular surface, which may lead to volar subluxation of the distal phalanx and/or post-traumatic arthritis of the DIP joint
    - Although many hand surgeons contend that even these injuries can be treated with splinting alone, many others believe that operative reduction and fixation with a pin or screw is necessary.

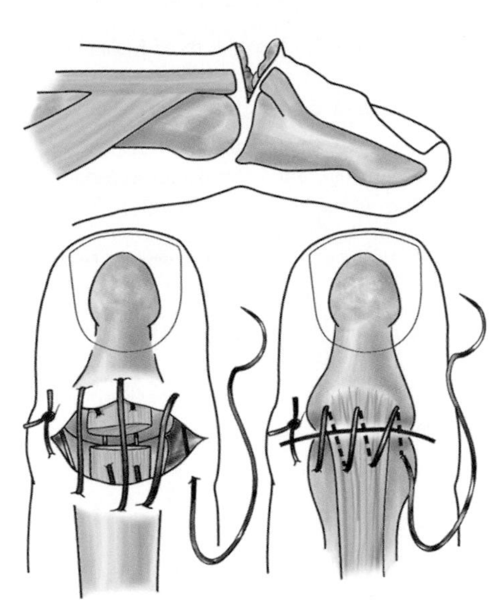

Figure 89-9 Lacerations of the terminal tendon very near its insertion where the tendon is extremely thin can be repaired with a single suture that simultaneously approximates the skin and tendon.

- Those who could otherwise be treated nonoperatively but who cannot wear a splint at work (such as surgical personnel or food preparers) can be treated with a pin across the DIP joint.
- Those in whom a prolonged course of splinting failed
- Those with a fixed DIP and/or PIP deformity
- Children in whom treatment can be difficult due to poor compliance with splinting

Suggested Reading

- Baratz ME, Schmidt CC, Hughes TB: Extensor tendon injuries. In Green DP, Hotchkiss RN, Pederson WC, Wolfe SW (eds): Green's Operative Hand Surgery, 5th ed. Philadelphia: Churchill Livingstone, 2005, pp 199–205.
- Garberman SF, Diao W, Peimer CA: Mallet finger: Results of early versus delayed closed treatment. J Hand Surg [Am] 1994; 19A:850–852.
- Handoll HH, Vaghela MV: Interventions for treating mallet finger injuries. Cochrane Database Syst Rev 2004;3:CD004574.
- Kalainov DM, Hoepfner PE, Hartigan BJ, et al: Nonsurgical treatment of closed mallet finger fractures. J Hand Surg [Am] 2005;30A:580–586.
- Katzman BM, Klein DM, Mesa J, et al: Immobilization of the mallet finger: Effects on the extensor tendon. J Hand Surg [Br] 1999;24B:80–84.
- Kronlage SC, Faust D: Open reduction and screw fixation of mallet fractures. J Hand Surg [Br] 2004;29B:135–138.
- Nakamura K, Nanjyo B: Reassessment of surgery for mallet finger. Plast Reconstr Surg 1994;93:141–149.

- Okafor B, Mbubaegbu C, Munshi I, et al: Mallet deformity of the finger: Five-year follow-up of conservative treatment. J Bone Joint Surg Br 1997;79B:544–547.
- Rayan GM, Mullins PT: Skin necrosis complicating mallet finger splinting and vascularity of the distal interphalangeal joint overlying skin. J Hand Surg [Am] 1987;12A:548–552.
- Takami H, Takahashi S, Ando M: Operative treatment of mallet finger due to intra-articular fracture of the distal phalanx. Arch Orthop Trauma Surg 2000;120:9–13.

Chapter 90 Jersey Finger (Flexor Digitorum Profundus Avulsion)

Jack Ingari

ICD-9 CODE
727.64 *Flexor Digitorum Profundus Tendon Rupture*

Key Concepts

- Flexor tendon ruptures from insertion onto the distal phalanx of a digit from a forceful extension on a flexed digit, typically in an athlete grabbing a jersey (Fig. 90-1)
- Occurs most commonly in the ring finger (~75%)
- Can occur with or without fracture
- If seen early, operative repair is indicated.
- If missed and patient asymptomatic, no treatment needed
- If missed and a tender palmar mass develops, the tendon stump can be excised
- If missed and the distal interphalangeal (DIP) joint is unstable, it can be fused
- Early referral of suspected jersey finger leads to the best results.

History

- The player feels a "pop" in the finger after grabbing another player's jersey.
- Ring finger involved 75% of the time
- Unable to flex at DIP after injury
- May describe finger was "jammed" or twisted
- The mechanism is forced extension on the tip of the clenched, flexed digit.
- Often missed acutely and presents late with inability to flex at the DIP joint

Physical Examination

- The resting posture of the hand is disrupted with the injured finger held extended (Fig. 90-2).
- Tender at the insertion of the flexor tendon at the base of the distal phalanx
- Also tender at the location of the tendon stump
- The tendon retracts into the palm (type I), to the A2 pulley (type II), or to the A4 pulley (type III).
- Unable to actively flex the distal phalanx against resistance

Imaging

- Plain radiographs of the involved digit will reveal fractures, if present.
- Magnetic resonance imaging can reveal the level of tendon retraction.
    - Magnetic resonance imaging not needed to make diagnosis
    - May be useful if the level of tendon is uncertain

Differential Diagnosis

- Phalangeal fractures can cause pain and mimic flexor digitorum profundus avulsion.
    - The patient is unable to flex the DIP joint due to pain.
    - Radiographs help make the diagnosis of fracture.
    - Fracture can accompany tendon rupture.

Treatment

- Tendon retraction and time from injury are key
    - Type I: The tendon is retracted into the palm, and surgical repair is needed within 7 to 10 days due to a compromised blood supply to the tendon.
    - Type II: The tendon retracts to the A2 pulley and can be repaired up to 3 months later because the tendon blood supply is largely intact.
    - Type III: The tendon retracts to the A4 pulley with a bone fragment; the bone fragment should be surgically fixed within 2 weeks.
- Early referral to an orthopaedic hand surgeon for surgical repair is the best option (Fig. 90-3).

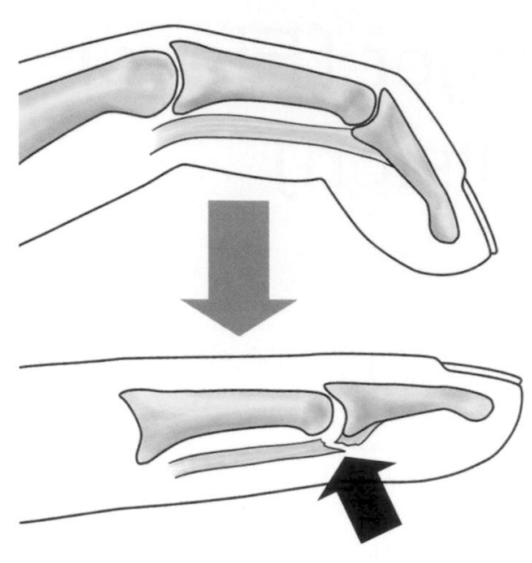

Figure 90-1 When a flexed digit is "jerked" into extension, rupture of the flexor digitorum profundus tendon (jersey finger) can occur.

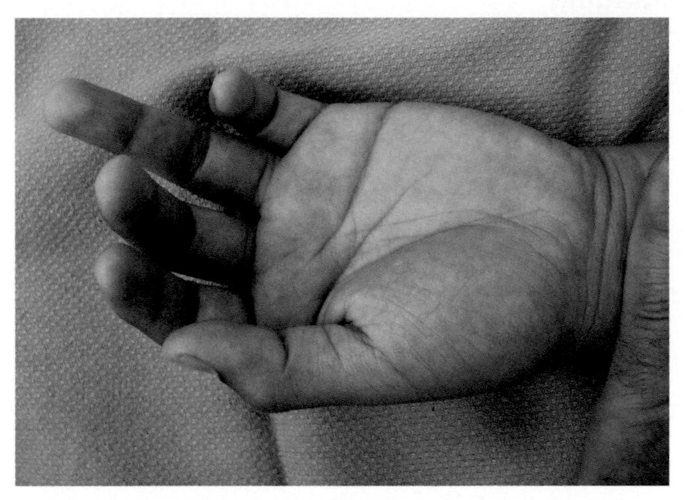

Figure 90-2 Loss of normal flexion posture with ring finger (injured) held in extension.

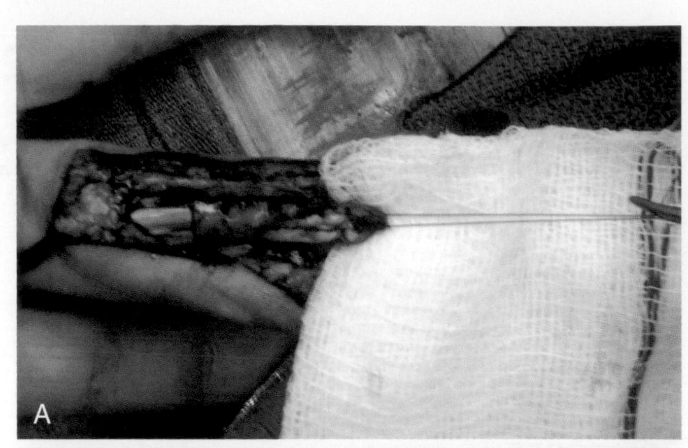

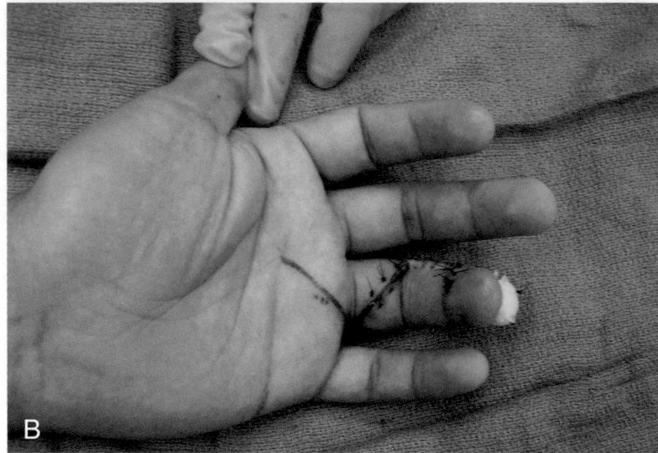

Figure 90-3 **A**, Intraoperative photograph of ruptured flexor tendon before final repair. **B**, Resting, flexed posture of ring finger restored after surgical repair of flexor digitorum profundus avulsion (jersey finger).

Patient Instructions

- To restore active DIP flexion, early surgical repair is needed.
- If missed or left untreated, a painful mass (tendon stump) in the palm or a "floppy" DIP joint can develop.
- If a painful palmar mass develops late, it can be excised.
- If a late, unstable DIP joint is bothersome, fusion can help.

Suggested Reading

- Leddy JP: Avulsions of the flexor digitorum profundus. Hand Clin 1985;1:77–83.
- Murphy BA, Mass DP: Zone I flexor tendon injuries. Hand Clin 2005;21:167–171.
- Pannunzio ME: Rugger jersey finger. Am J Orthop 2004;33:596.
- Peterson JJ, Bancroft LW: Injuries of the fingers and thumb in the athlete. Clin Sports Med 2006:25:527–542, vii–viii.
- Tuttle HG, Olvey SP, Stern PJ: Tendon avulsion injuries of the distal phalanx. Clin Orthop Relat Res 2006;445:157–168.

Chapter 91 Nail Bed Injuries

Michael Feldman and Jonathan E. Isaacs

ICD-9 Codes

816.2 *Fracture of One or More Phalanges of Hand (Distal Phalanx or Phalanges)*
883 *Open Wounds of Finger(s)*
886 *Traumatic Amputation of Other Finger (2) (Complete) (Partial)*
915 *Superficial Injury of Finger(s)*
923.3 *Contusion of Upper Limb (Finger)*
959.9 *Injury to Finger, Other and Unspecified*

Key Concepts

- The goal of treatment of nail bed injuries is to restore anatomy, which will allow return of function and maximize cosmetic result.
- Anatomy and physiology (Fig. 91-1)
  - The germinal matrix, sterile matrix, and dorsal nail bed make up the nail bed.
    - — Germinal matrix: specialized cells that generate the majority of the nail plate; located proximal to the lunula
    - — Sterile matrix: contributes to the nail bed; located distal to the germinal matrix, acts to promote nail plate adherence to the nail bed
    - — Dorsal nail bed: gives the nail plate its hard shiny coat
- Nail plate: the "nail"
- Lunula: curved white portion of the proximal nail plate; overlies the distal portion of the germinal matrix
- Eponychium: thin layer of skin that extends over the dorsal nail bed and nail plate, forms the nail fold
- Perionychium: the folds of skin alongside of the nail plate
- Hyponychium: the area between the distal nail plate and skin of the fingertip that acts as a barrier to infection
- Nerve supply to perionychium via dorsal branches of the volar digital nerves
  - Arterial supply to the nail via two dorsal branches of the volar digital arteries
  - Four primary functions of the fingernail
    - — Protection of the fingertip
    - — Improved tactile sensation (counterforce)
    - — Regulation of peripheral circulation
    - — Assist in picking up objects
- The nail plate grows an average of 0.1 mm/day or 100 days for complete growth, but distal growth is halted for 3 weeks as the proximal nail thickens.

History

- Determine the mechanism of injury.
  - Usually the result of crush or pinching type mechanism
- Determine when the injury occurred.
- Record comorbidities that may interfere with wound healing.
  - Advise against smoking or use of nicotine products.

Physical Examination

- Look for an obvious (open) or more subtle (closed) injury in which the patient has pain/swelling and hematoma under an intact and adherent nail plate.
- If the injury involves more than just the nail bed, assess for tissue viability and loss of sensation.
- May or may not involve the bone (radiograph necessary)

Treatment

Closed Nail Bed Injuries

- Can treat symptomatically or can remove nail plate and fix nail bed
  - If large nail bed defect not repaired, then theoretical concern that abnormal nail regrowth (thick ridge) may result, although several studies suggest that there is no difference in repaired versus unrepaired groups
    - — Historically, a subungual hematoma involving more than 50% of the nail plate indicates significant underlying nail bed laceration
    - — Displaced fracture under nail bed compatible with significant underlying nail bed laceration, although this usually results in loss of nail adherence (open injury)

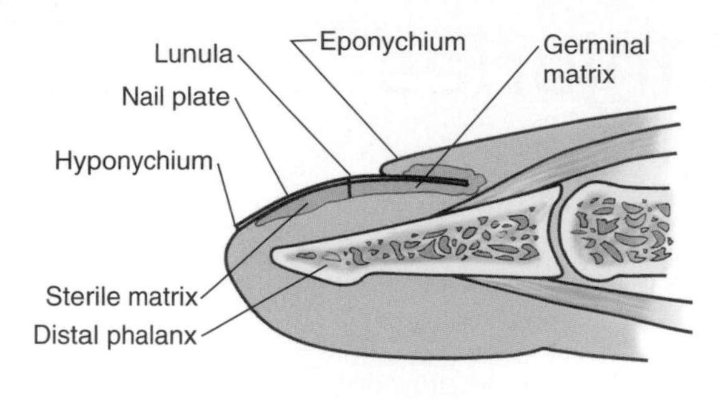

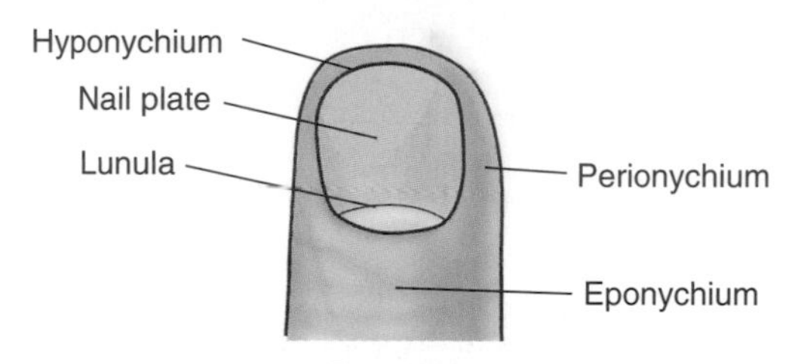

Figure 91-1 Fingertip anatomy.

- Pressure from hematoma under nail plate often very painful
    - If no repair is planned, then trephination (creation of hematoma drainage hole) with an electrocautery device, the heated tip of a paper clip, or a large-bore needle may alleviate discomfort.
        - — Heat dissipated by underlying blood
        - — Large-bore needle spun like a drill tip until it has gone through the nail plate (be careful not to damage the underlying nail bed)

Open Nail Bed Injuries

- Nail partially or completely avulsed from nail bed
- If underlying fracture, treat as open fracture with irrigation/débridement and antibiotics.
- Usually repair of soft tissue is enough to align bone fragments.
- A displaced distal shaft fracture may require pinning (with Kirschner wire or percutaneously placed 20-gauge needle "drilled" across tip of finger by hand).
- Injuries are often intimidating, but after hemostasis is obtained and adequate irrigation performed, the "pieces" will often come together quite nicely.
- Steps to repair
    - Digital block
    - Copious irrigation, usually with saline
    - Prep and drape hand (sterile procedure)
    - Tourniquet control is obtained with a finger Tournicot or a sterile Penrose drain wrapped around the base of the finger.
    - Remove any partially avulsed or remaining nail plate with a hemostat or by separating its connection with the nail bed using a Freer elevator (be careful not to avulse more of the nail bed).
    - Repair the skin surrounding the nail bed with 5-0 nylon sutures first.
    - Meticulously reapproximate the wound edges of the nail bed with a 6-0 spatulated chromic suture under loupe magnification.
    - Place a new "nail plate" to act as a spacer under the nail fold and to splint the nail bed.
        - — If the nail plate is mostly intact, it can be cleaned and replaced.
        - — Other options include
            - — A silicone sheet
            - — A piece of the foil packaging from the suture
            - — Dry Nu Gauze or Xeroform with the petroleum scraped off (this will absorb some of the blood, and once this dries and hardens it will actually make a protective "nail plate")
    - The spacer is held in place with a 5-0 nylon suture that should be removed in 1 to 2 weeks (Fig. 91-2).
    - The wound is dressed with nonadherent gauze (Xeroform or Adaptec) followed by a 2 × 2 gauze patch and a protective aluminum splint held in place with Coban that only covers the distal finger.

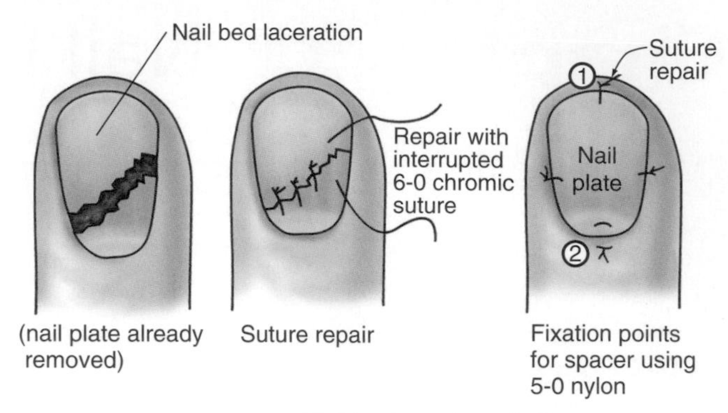

Figure 91-2 Nail bed repair technique.

- Any injury that involves the germinal matrix (extends proximal to the eponychial fold) will require appropriate exposure of the injured area. In these situations, the fold must be incised and raised as a skin flap that is based proximally. Accurate repair and exposure of the germinal matrix is essential to a good outcome. The edges of the releasing incisions are repaired with simple interrupted 5-0 nylon sutures afterward (Fig. 91-3).
- Treatment of more extensive injury may require referral to a hand specialist.

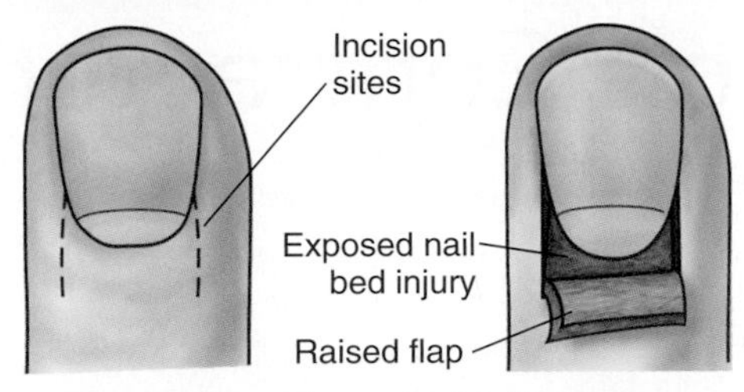

Figure 91-3 Eponychial fold exposure.

- In cases of severe crush injury or partial tip amputation with an avulsed nail bed, the nail bed may be reconstructed with a nail bed graft.
- Loss of more than 50% of supporting bone (partial amputation) is an indication for nail ablation, which requires the excision of the germinal matrix.

Prognosis

- The final functional and cosmetic outcome depends on the amount of nail bed that remains intact, the severity of the injury (worse with crush injuries), and the patient's comorbidities.
- The patient may, on average, expect full nail growth in approximately 2 to 5 months. There is normally a lag in nail growth after this type of injury. The new nail may have temporary divots or stripes that will usually improve with time.

Considerations in Special Populations

- Pediatric nail bed injuries typically require the involvement of a hand surgeon.
- They are more likely to need conscious sedation or a trip to the operating room for repair.
- Consider a more restrictive dressing (such as a cast) to prevent disruption or contamination of the repair.

Patient Instructions

- Strict hand elevation to decrease swelling and pain
- Leave the dressing intact until return appointment to minimize disruption to the repair.
- Avoid getting the repaired site dirty or wet; avoid using the injured extremity until cleared to do so by the physician.

Suggested Reading

- Brown R, Zook E, Russell R: Fingertip reconstruction with flaps and nail bed grafts. J Hand Surg [Am] 1999;24A:345–351.
- Hatoko M, Iioka H, Tanka A, et al: Hard-palate and mucosal graft in the management of severe pincer-nail deformity. Plast Reconstr Surg 2003;112:835–839.
- Ogo K: Does the nail bed really regenerate? Plast Reconstr Surg 1987;80:445–447.
- Richards A, Crick A, Cole R: A novel method of securing the nail following nail bed repair. Plast Reconstr Surg 1999;103: 1983–1985.
- Roser S, Gellman H: Comparison of nail bed repair versus nail trephination for subungual hematomas in children. J Hand Surg [Am] 1999;24A:1166–1170.
- Trumble TE (ed): Principles of Hand Surgery and Therapy. Philadelphia: Saunders, 2000, pp 192–194.

Chapter 92 Dupuytren's Contracture

Khurram Pervaiz and Jonathan E. Isaacs

ICD-9 CODE
728.6 *Contracture of Palmer Fascia*

Key Concepts

- Slowly progressive fibroproliferative disease of the palmar fascia (Fig. 92-1)
- Results in characteristic cord and nodule formation in the palm and fingers
- Usually painless but can result in digital flexion contractures, which may inhibit function
- The only current treatment (not cure) is surgical.
- Demographics
  - More prevalent in persons of Northern European descent
  - Five percent to 15% of men in the United States older than 50 are affected.
  - More common in males (80%)
  - Males often have an earlier onset and more aggressive disease progression.
  - Bilateral involvement 65% of the time
- Etiology
  - Multifaceted and not completely understood although possible theories include
    - Genetic predisposition: positive family history in 27% to 68% of patients
    - Immunologic or benign neoplastic changes in the palmar fascia
    - Trauma
    - The palmar subdermal fat pads undergo age-related thinning in the populations most prone to Dupuytren's contracture. This may expose the underlying fascia to repetitive traumatic shear and compression forces that may trigger an excessive reparative process in the palmar fascia leading to Dupuytren-type changes.
- Associated conditions
  - Diabetes mellitus
  - Alcoholism
  - Human immunodeficiency virus infection
  - Epilepsy (antiseizure medication)
  - Trauma
  - Manual labor
  - Cigarette smoking
  - Previous myocardial infarction

History

- Insidious onset and progression
- Painless cord and nodule-like thickenings in the palm that may extend into the digits are usually noticed first.
- Nodules are occasionally tender.
- Flexion contractures of the involved fingers progress with time and cord formation.
- In nondiabetic patients, the ring and little fingers are most commonly affected and the thumb and index finger are least involved.
- Diabetic patients usually have more predominant involvement of the radial side of the hand.

Physical Examination (Fig. 92-2)

- Firm palpable nodules in the distal palm and fingers that are rarely tender to palpation
- Palpable painless cords extending from the midpalm toward and into the fingers
- Palmar skin in the diseased area blanches on active finger extension.
- Grooves or pits in the palmar skin denoting adherence to the underlying diseased fascia
- Tender knuckle pads over the dorsal aspect of the proximal interphalangeal joints may be seen in more aggressive disease.
- Metacarpophalangeal or proximal interphalangeal joint flexion contractures with possible compensatory distal interphalangeal joint hyperextension contracture; alternatively, the distal interphalangeal joints may not be involved or are rarely part of flexion contracture.

Stages of Dupuytren's Contracture

- Proliferative
  - The most biologically active stage characterized by the development of nodules composed of fibroblasts and type III collagen

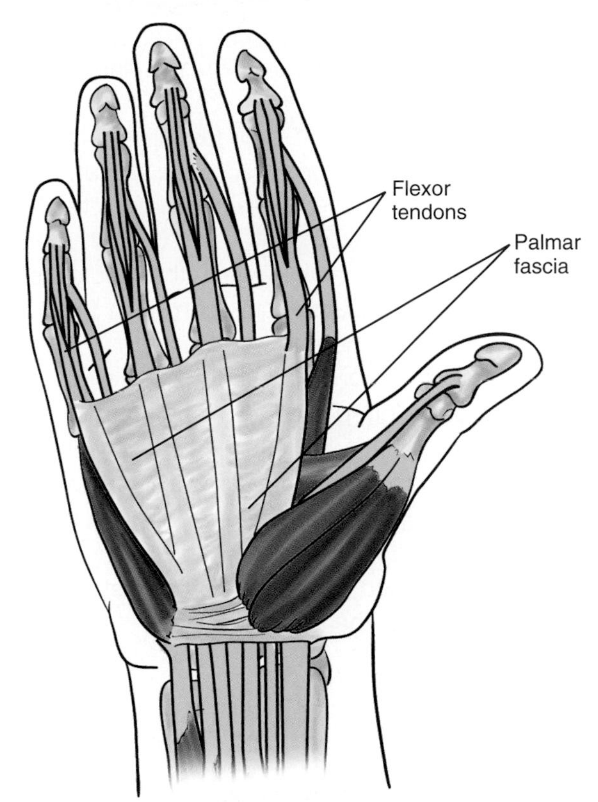

Figure 92-1 Gross anatomic depiction of palmar fascia.

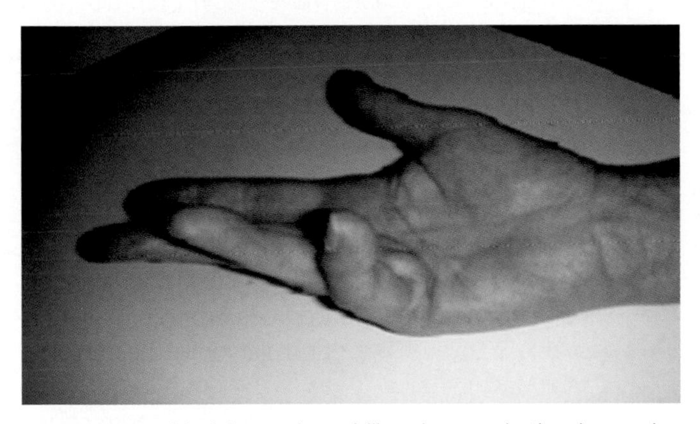

Figure 92-2 Nodule- and cord-like changes in the ring and little fingers resulting in characteristic flexion contractures of the involved digits. (Courtesy of Bobby Chhabra, MD.)

- Involutional: Cords and skin pits develop as normal palmar fibroblasts transform into myofibroblasts. These cells deposit collagen, which thickens the cords and has contractile components that draw the tissue tightly together and pull the fingers down.
- Residual: The most biologically quiescent phase is characterized by nodular regression but also metacarpophalangeal joint and proximal interphalangeal joint contractures. Tendon-like cords are visible underlying the palmar skin and contain densely packed inelastic, longitudinally oriented, predominantly type I collagen fibers. At this stage, relatively few cells remain.

Surgical Anatomy of the Diseased Palmar Fascia

- A normal anatomic structure, the central aponeurosis, is the core of Dupuytren's disease activity.
- It is a triangular fascial layer with its apex proximal.
- Its fibers are oriented longitudinally, transversely, and vertically.
- The longitudinal fibers fan out as pretendinous bands toward the digits, and each bifurcates distally.
- Each bifurcation has three layers: A superficial layer inserts into the dermis; a middle layer continues to the digit as the spiral band; and a deep layer passes almost vertically and dorsally.
- Transverse fibers make up the natatory ligament located in the distal part of the palm and the transverse ligament of the palmar aponeurosis.
- In Dupuytren's disease, as these normal fascial structures (referred to as bands) become thickened and contracted, they are referred to as cords (Fig. 92-3).

Types of Cords and Their Relationship to Neurovascular Anatomy

- Cords are diseased and transformed bands of tissue.

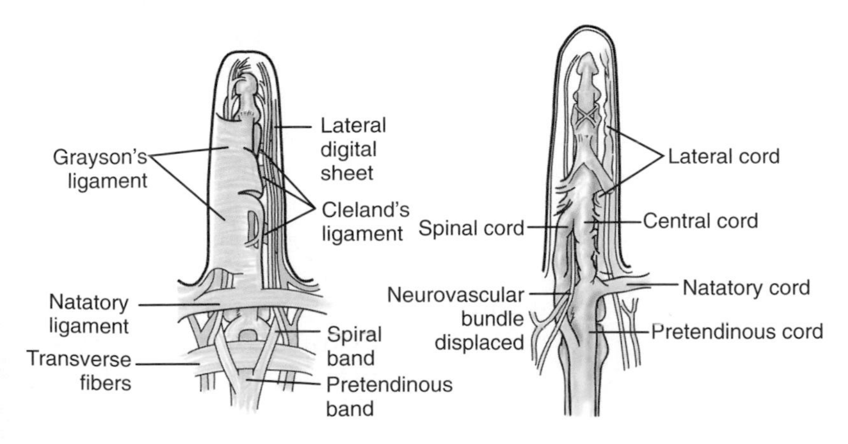

Figure 92-3 Normal palmar and digital fascial structures become nodular and contractile, resulting in characteristic finger contractures and palpable cords.

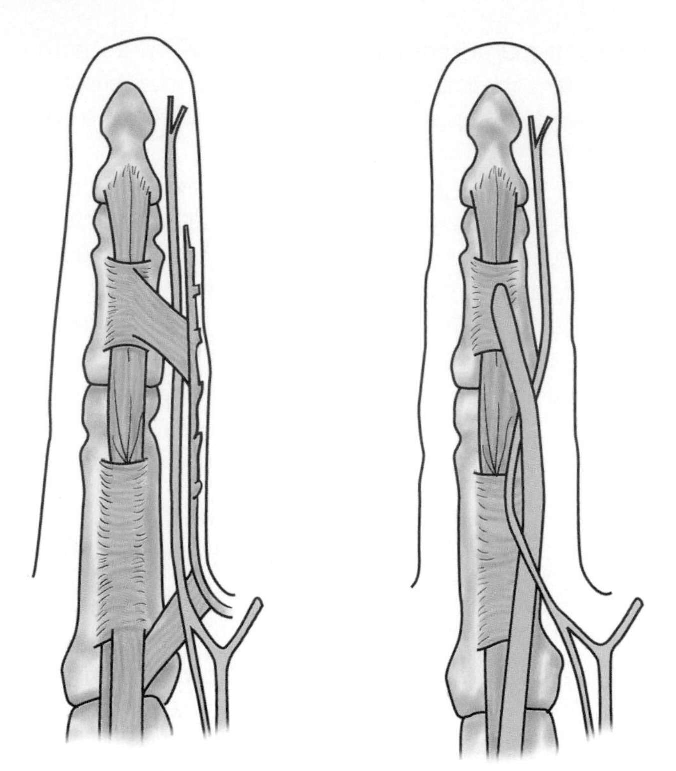

Figure 92-4 The spiral cord wraps around the digital neurovascular bundle and pulls it superficial and midline. This puts the bundle at risk during surgical dissection.

- Central cord
  - This is a direct extension of the pretendinous band in the palm that remains directly subcutaneous.
  - It lies between the neurovascular bundles.
  - Over the proximal phalanx, the cord is intimately attached to the skin but not to the tendon sheath.
  - If it extends distally, it attaches to the tendon sheath and periosteum of the middle phalanx, usually on one or the other side, but a symmetrical attachment is seen occasionally.
- Spiral cord (Fig. 92-4)
  - The spiral cord arises from the pretendinous fibers of the palmar fascia.
  - It runs behind the neurovascular bundles just distal to the metacarpophalangeal joint and joins the lateral digital sheet.
  - From there, it extends in front of the neurovascular bundle and inserts on the flexor sheath of the middle phalanx.
  - The spiral cord thus winds around the neurovascular bundle (hence, its name).
  - It usually causes severe proximal interphalangeal joint contracture.
  - The distorted anatomy of the neurovascular bundle, which displaces medially and centrally, renders it at risk of injury during surgery.

- Lateral cord
  - This is an involvement of the lateral digital sheet.
  - The natatory ligament is almost always involved.
  - This cord attaches primarily to the skin and generally does not cause severe proximal interphalangeal joint contracture.
  - The cord does not disturb the neurovascular bundle except that its bulk can push the bundle toward the midline.
  - A distal extension of the lateral cord can rarely cause distal interphalangeal joint contracture.
- Adductor cord
  - In the little finger, a cord coming off the abductor digiti minimi muscle is often found on the ulnar border of the finger.
  - This may lead to contracture of the distal interphalangeal joint of the little finger.

Treatment

- Nonsurgical
  - There is no consistently successful nonsurgical treatment option.
  - Collagenase injections have shown promise, but are still in preclinical trials.
- Surgical
  - The goal of surgical treatment is to excise or incise the diseased fascia.
  - This treatment does not cure the disease, but is meant to delay progression and restore function by at least partially relieving contractures.
  - Surgery is indicated with metacarpophalangeal joint contracture of 30 degrees or more (patient is unable to place the hand flat onto the tabletop [table test]).
  - Treated metacarpophalangeal joint contractures usually do not recur.
  - Proximal interphalangeal joint contractures, particularly those of long duration, are more difficult to treat, so surgery is indicated as soon as proximal interphalangeal joint contractures are observed and become functionally inhibitive.
- Procedures
  - Fasciotomy involves incising (cutting) the involved fascia.
    - It may provide short-term relief with less surgical morbidity, but is associated with a very high recurrence rate.
    - It is reserved for elderly or debilitated patients who are unable to tolerate a more lengthy procedure.

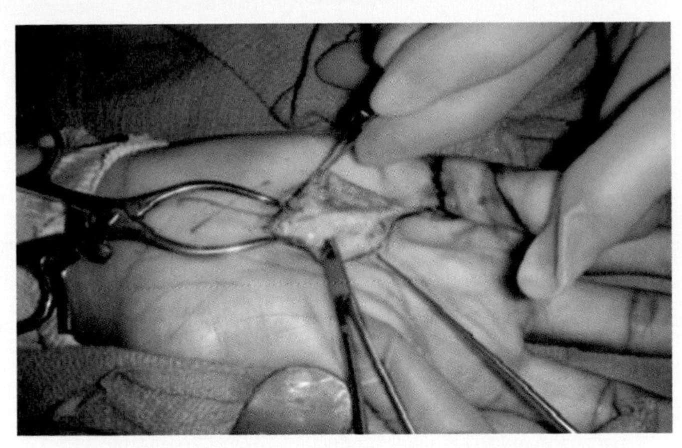

Figure 92-5 Intraoperative view of the diseased palmar fascia being excised. (Courtesy of Bobby Chhabra, MD.)

- Needle fasciotomy involves release of Dupuytren's cords using a blade or the bevel of a needle through the skin in a percutaneous fashion, affording short-term relief; the recurrence rate is 50% at 3 to 5 years in some studies.
  - Dermofasciectomy involves removing the diseased fascia and the overlying skin. The wound is either left open to heal secondarily (open palm technique) or resurfaced with a full thickness skin graft. Recurrence rates are quite low, but because of the radical nature of this procedure, it is usually reserved for patients with recurrent or severe disease.
  - Regional fasciectomy, the most widely used surgical procedure, involves excising only grossly involved fascia (Fig. 92-5).
    - This approach has proved successful in correcting metacarpophalangeal joint contractures and some proximal interphalangeal joint contractures and carries an acceptably low morbidity rate.
  - Dynamic external fixators may be used as an adjuvant to surgical release in a patient with severe contractures.
  - Amputation of an absolutely nonfunctional digit that has failed to respond to previously mentioned therapies remains an option.
- Postoperative
  - Rehabilitation is a gradual process of increased activity and decreased splinting to achieve optimal restoration of movement.
    - Frequent visits to the occupational therapist help to restore preoperative flexion and to maintain extension gained at the time of surgery.

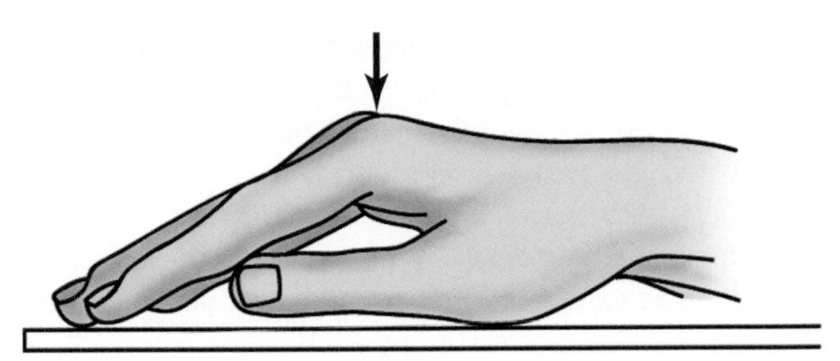

Figure 92-6 The table test. When the patient can no longer place his or her hand flat on a tabletop, it is time to refer the patient.

    - Patient motivation and severity of disease dictate the intensity and duration of therapy.
  - Final results are realized in approximately 6 weeks.
  - The patient can expect to return to normal activities in 2 to 3 months.

Complications

- The incidence of complications is 20%.
- The most common complications are postoperative joint stiffness and loss of preoperative flexion.
- Other complications include hematoma, skin loss, infection, nerve injury, vascular injury, prolonged edema, and reflex sympathetic dystrophy.

Prognosis

- The long-term overall recurrence rate is approximately 50% and can be in the same area of the hand or in a new area.
- Metacarpophalangeal joint contractures are readily corrected with surgery (80% to 96%) and usually do not recur.
- Proximal interphalangeal joint contractures are usually not completely corrected (20% to 56% are corrected) and occasionally may be exacerbated by surgery (25%).

When to Refer

- Observation is the mainstay of early treatment, and referral is not necessary until surgery is indicated by the inability to place the hand flat on a table (table test) (Fig. 92-6).

Considerations in Special Populations

- A subset of patients have a more aggressive and rapidly progressive form of the disease referred to as

Dupuytren's diathesis. These patients are characterized by onset before age 40, a positive family history, and bilateral involvement. The knuckle pads may be involved as well as other body parts (Ledderhose disease [fibrosis in the feet] and Peyronie's disease [fibrosis in the penis]). These patients have a poor prognosis with limited response to surgical treatment and a high rate of recurrence.

Suggested Reading

- Adamietz B, Keilholz L, Grunert J, Sauer R: Radiotherapy of early stage Dupuytren disease. Long-term results after a median follow-up period of 10 years [in German]. Strahlenther Onkol 2001;177:604–610.
- Badalamente MA, Hurst LC: Efficacy and safety of injectable mixed collagenase subtypes in the treatment of Dupuytren's contracture. J Hand Surg [Am] 2007;32A:767–774.
- Cordova A, Tripoli M, Corradino B, et al: Dupuytren's contracture: An update of biomolecular aspects and therapeutic perspectives. J Hand Surg [Br] 2005;30B:557–562.
- Hindocha S, John S, Stanley JK, et al: The heritability of Dupuytren's disease: Familial aggregation and its clinical significance. J Hand Surg [Am] 2006;31A:204–210.
- Ketchum LD, Donahue TK: The injection of nodules of Dupuytren's disease with triamcinolone acetonide. J Hand Surg [Am] 2000;25A:1157–1162.
- Loos B, Puschkin V, Horch RE: 50 years experience with Dupuytren's contracture in the Erlangen University Hospital—a retrospective analysis of 2919 operated hands from 1956 to 2006. BMC Musculoskelet Disord 2007;8:60.
- Rayan GM: Clinical presentation and types of Dupuytren's disease. Hand Clin 1999;15:87–96, vii.
- Rayan GM: Dupuytren's disease: Anatomy, pathology, presentation, and treatment. Instr Course Lect 2007;56: 101–111.
- Reilly RM, Stern PJ, Goldfarb CA: A retrospective review of the management of Dupuytren's nodules. J Hand Surg [Am] 2005;30A:1014–1018.
- Seegenschmiedt MH, Olschewski T, Guntrum F: Radiotherapy optimization in early-stage Dupuytren's contracture: First results of a randomized clinical study. Int J Radiat Oncol Biol Phys 2001;49:785–798.
- Shaw RB Jr, Chong AK, Zhang A, et al: Dupuytren's disease: History, diagnosis, and treatment. Plast Reconstr Surg 2007; 120:44e–54e.
- Smith AC: Diagnosis and indications for surgical treatment. Hand Clin 1991;7:635–643.

Chapter 93 Hand Tumors

Dan A. Zlotolow

ICD-9 CODES

170.5	*Chondrosarcoma*
171.2	*Epithelioid Sarcoma*
172.6	*Melanoma*
213.4	*Giant Cell Tumor of Bone*
213.5	*Osteochondroma*
213.5	*Enchondroma*
214.1	*Lipoma*
228.01	*Glomus Tumor*
228.01	*Hemangioma*
715.14	*Carpometacarpal Boss*
727.02	*Giant Cell Tumor of the Tendon Sheath*
727.05	*Tenosynovitis*
727.42	*Retinacular Cyst*
782.2	*Epidermal Inclusion Cyst*

Key Concepts

- Most tumors in the hand are benign.
- Painful or fast-growing tumors need an urgent workup.
- Intraosseous tumors are common and can lead to fracture with minor trauma.
- Expansile bone lesions, even if benign, can be aggressive.
- A dark streak in the fingernail of a light-skinned person is a subungual melanoma until proven otherwise.
- Most malignancies in the hand involve the skin.
- Solid tumors do not transilluminate.
- The diagnosis needs to be certain before the problem is treated with "observation."

History

- The growth rate of the tumor is important for identifying aggressive lesions.
- Previous trauma can cause deformity that can mimic a tumor.
- Minor injury resulting in a fracture is suspicious for an enchondroma.
- Inflammatory arthropathies with boggy synovitis or tenosynovitis can mimic periarticular or peritendinous tumors.
- History of tophaceous gout
- Northern European (Viking) ancestry, antiseizure medications, smoking, and alcohol abuse history consistent with Dupuytren's disease

Physical Examination

- Overlying skin changes (lesions involving the skin are of concern for malignancy)
- Coloration (hemangiomas have a blue tint)
- Pulse/bruit (vascular malformations and aneurysms)
- Consistency (giant cell tumors of the tendon sheath and tenosynovitis are boggy, lipomas are firm in one direction and fluctuant in the other, cysts and bony masses are firm)
- Transillumination with a penlight (only positive in clear fluid-filled masses such as ganglia and early tenosynovitis)
- Adherence to underlying tissues (mobile discrete masses tend to be benign)
- Glomus tumors demonstrate pinpoint tenderness, are most common under the nail, have a slight bluish tint, and cause pain with exposure to ice-cold water (Fig. 93-1).
- Tinel's sign (tapping over the mass creates shooting pain in the nerve distribution) indicates a neural tumor or neuroma.
- Look for signs of infection (blanching erythema, induration, warmth, fluctuance).

Imaging

- Enchondromas often present as incidental findings on radiographs (Fig. 93-2).
- Look for scalloping/expansion of the bone cortex (indicates an aggressive lesion).
- Expansile lesions of bone (enchondroma, aneurysmal bone cyst, giant cell tumor of bone, chondrosarcoma)
- Periarticular masses can be evaluated with radiographs, which typically demonstrate degenerative changes in a joint with large osteophytes in patients with osteoarthritis or joint erosions with a soft-tissue mass in patients with inflammatory arthropathies.

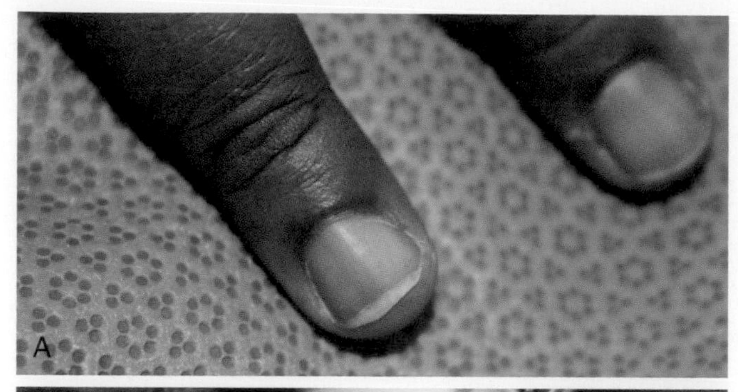

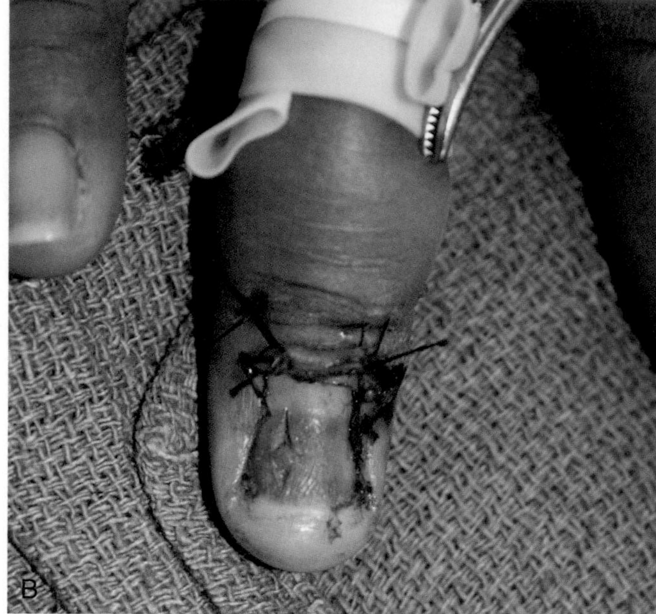

Figure 93-1 Glomus tumors are most common under the nail plate and classically present with a slight bluish tint, cold sensitivity, and severe point tenderness. Note the subtle appearance clinically (**A**) and the typical tumor size intraoperatively (**B**).

- Magnetic resonance imaging with or without contrast medium may demonstrate lesion if large enough; useful for glomus tumors, hemangiomas, tenosynovitis, and lipomas
- Angiography to identify aneurysms, hemangiomas, and arteriovenous malformations

Additional Tests

- White blood cell count, platelet count, erythrocyte sedimentation rate, and C-reactive protein to differentiate a tumor from an infection
- Uric acid levels and joint aspiration to rule out gout
- Rheumatoid panel to evaluate for rheumatoid arthritis

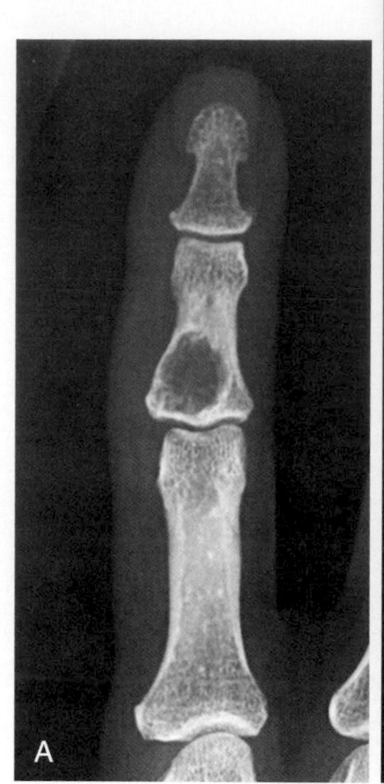

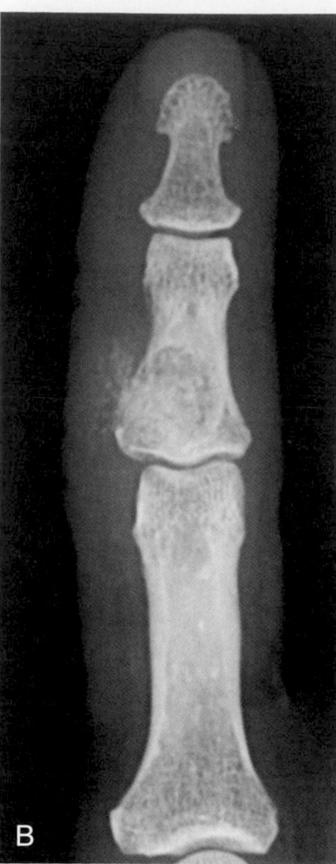

Figure 93-2 Enchondromas are either incidental findings on radiographs or present with pain (impending fracture) (**A**) or a pathologic fracture. Although these lesions meet many radiographic and histologic criteria for malignant lesions, they are overwhelmingly benign. Simple curettage and bone grafting are usually curative (**B**).

Differential Diagnosis

- Please see Table 93-1.

Treatment

- At diagnosis
  - If lesion is stable in size, does not cause pain, and is mobile, patient reassurance is indicated
- Later
  - Regular periods of observation, initially every 3 to 6 months, are warranted, with eventual yearly checkups if the mass does not change.

When to Refer

- Any lesion involving the skin requires a referral to a dermatologist and/or a hand surgeon to rule out a malignancy.
- Any patient with a lesion that changes in character or size, causes pain, is rigidly fixed to underlying tissues,

TABLE 93-1 *Differential Diagnosis*

Differential Diagnosis	Differentiating Feature	Chapter Reference
Chondrosarcoma	Firm mass, stippled calcification on radiograph, cartilage on magnetic resonance imaging	93
Epithelioid sarcoma	Can be confused with Dupuytren's nodule; look for ulcerations	93
Melanoma	Pigmented skin lesion	93
Giant cell tumor of bone	Expansile epiphyseal lesion	93
Osteochondroma	Epiphyseal or metaphyseal lesion of cartilage and bone growing away from the physis	93
Enchondroma (see Fig. 93-2)	Expansile cartilaginous mass	93
Lipoma	Firm in one direction, fluctuant in the other	93
Glomus tumor (see Fig. 93-1)	Pinpoint tenderness, bluish, cold intolerance	93
Hemangioma	Bluish tint	93
Carpometacarpal boss (Fig. 93-3)	Firm mass over carpometacarpal joints	93
Giant cell tumor of the tendon sheath	Boggy, dark on all magnetic resonance imaging sequences, high hemosiderin content	93
Dupuytren's nodule (Fig. 93-4)	Firm nonulcerating cord in palm or digit along fascial tracks	92
Tenosynovitis (Fig. 93-5)	Boggy, moves with the tendons, can transilluminate	81
Retinacular cyst	Firm, transilluminable mass over tendon sheath	81
Epidermal inclusion cyst	Pattern of enlarging and shrinking, filled with keratin	93
Traumatic nail bed deformity	Ridging or split of the nail associated with an injury to the nail bed	91
Neuroma	Positive Tinel's sign over tumor	93
Arthritis	Pain with joint motion, osteophytes, and loss of joint space on radiograph	77
Gout	Uric acid crystal deposits, multiarticular, tophi	18

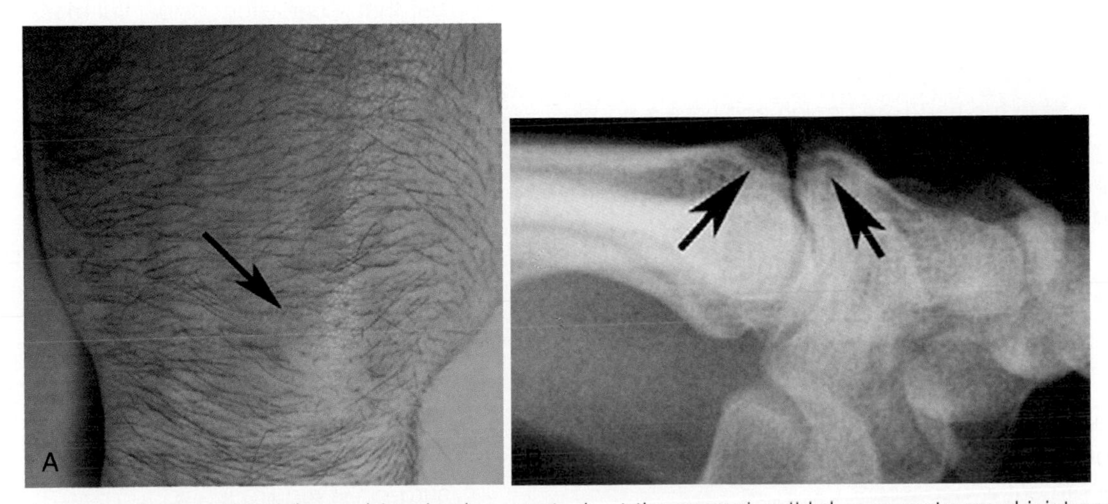

Figure 93-3 A carpometacarpal boss (*arrows*) is a benign exostosis at the second or third carpometacarpal joint and is often confused with a dorsal wrist ganglion. The differentiating features are its more distal location (**A**) and its more firm and immobile character on palpation. Radiographs will show the typical "volcano" appearance of the carpometacarpal joint (**B**). (From Park MJ, Namdari S, Weiss APC: The carpal boss: Review of diagnosis and treatment. J Hand Surg [Am] 2008;33A:446–449.)

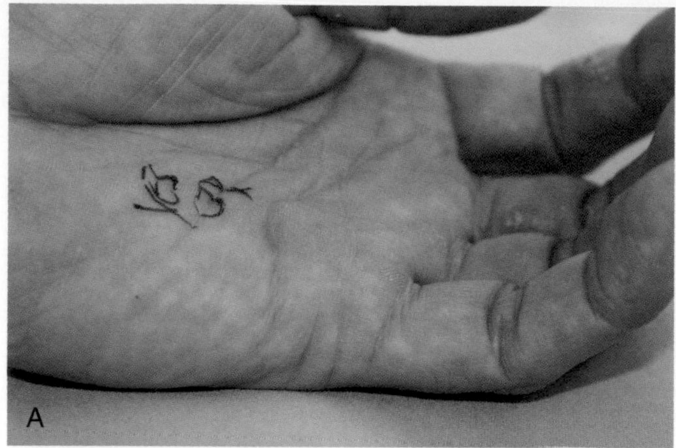

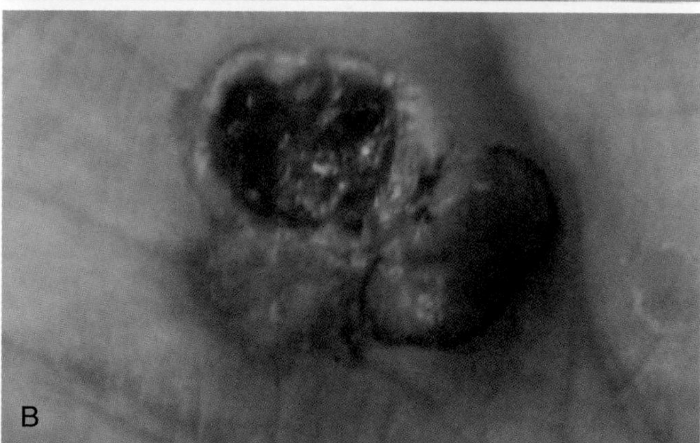

Figure 93-4 A Dupuytren's nodule is often mistaken for a soft-tissue tumor (**A**). Be aware that epithelioid sarcomas can present with a similar appearance, although ulcerations and pain are differentiating factors (**B**). (**B,** From Pai KK, Pai SB, Sripathi H, et al: Epithelioid sarcoma: A diagnostic challenge. Indian J Dermatol Venereol Leprol 2006;72:446–448.)

or does not transilluminate should be referred to a hand surgeon.

Prognosis

- Most masses in the hand are benign and have a good prognosis.
- Even malignant lesions, if caught early, can typically be cured with wide excision.

Patient Instructions

- Enchondroma
  - If the tumor is an incidental radiographic finding, explain to the patient that these benign tumors can be found in up to 30% of the population and that no treatment is necessary.
  - If the tumor is painful or associated with fracture, refer the patient to a hand surgeon urgently with reassurance that the prognosis is good.

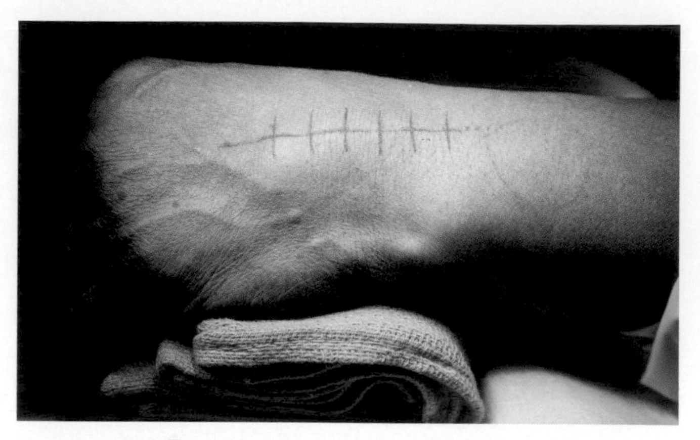

Figure 93-5 Extensor tenosynovitis has an appearance similar to that of dorsal wrist ganglia. However, tenosynovitis is marked by proximal termination at the extensor retinaculum, motion with extensor tendon motion, and a softer consistency on palpation.

- Retinacular cyst
  - If the cyst is small or painless, explain that the mass is a marker of a minor injury to the flexor sheath of the finger and that the mass may disappear on its own.
  - If the cyst is large or painful, refer the patient to a hand surgeon for aspiration or excision.
- Epidermal inclusion cyst
  - A benign mass composed of incarcerated skin keratin that may be self-limited or exhibit periodic episodes of worsening, then resolving, pain
  - It can be removed if symptomatic, and recurrence is rare.
- Extensor tenosynovitis
  - If the mass is painless or recent, reassure the patient that the mass will likely go away on its own, but that a persistent or painful mass can damage the extensor tendons and lead to delayed tendon rupture.
  - If the mass is painful or long-standing, refer the patient to a hand surgeon urgently to excise the mass before tendon rupture occurs.
- Hemangioma
  - If the lesion is painless, reassure the patient.
  - If the lesion is painful, refer the patient to a hand surgeon for excision.
- Chondrosarcoma
  - Most lesions are low grade and rarely metastasize.
  - An urgent referral to an oncologist and a hand surgeon is required.
- Giant cell tumor of the tendon sheath
  - Can degrade the tendon and should be removed if painful

- Giant cell tumor
  - Can be aggressive benign lesion and should be evaluated by an oncologist
  - Often requires a wide excision to effect a cure
- Osteochondroma
  - Benign lesions that can cause tendon or local tissue irritation
  - Can be removed if symptomatic, but malignant transformation uncommon in solitary lesion
- Melanoma
  - Inform the patient of the need for an urgent dermatologic evaluation.
- Epithelioid sarcoma
  - Despite its benign appearance, it can be a very aggressive malignancy.
  - Requires wide excision and lymph node biopsy
- Lipoma
  - Benign tumor that can be observed or removed if unsightly
- Carpometacarpal boss
  - An osteophyte at the carpometacarpal joint that can be removed if painful
- Glomus tumor
  - Removal is effective in relieving pain
  - Recurrence is rare, but a second primary tumor may develop.

Considerations in Special Populations

- Gout
  - Tophaceous gout can cause large and sometimes ulcerating lesions filled with a white uric acid paste that is the consistency of toothpaste.
- Rheumatoid arthritis
  - Rheumatoid nodules can be firm and mimic soft-tissue tumors.
  - Periarticular synovitis can cause large, painful soft-tissue masses.
  - Tenosynovitis can be particularly aggressive and result in early tendon rupture.
- Osteoarthritis
  - Osteophytes can resemble firm, immobile tumors near joints.
  - Associated synovial cysts can develop as part of a degenerative process.
  - Radiographic evaluation to differentiate from other tumors

Suggested Reading

- Bos GD, Pritchard DJ, Reiman HM, et al: Epithelioid sarcoma. An analysis of fifty-one cases. J Bone Joint Surg Am 1988;70A: 862–870.
- Buecker PJ, Villafuerte JE, Hornicek FJ, et al: Improved survival for sarcomas of the wrist and hand. J Hand Surg [Am] 2006;31A:452–455.
- Harness NG, Mankin HJ: Giant-cell tumor of the distal forearm. J Hand Surg [Am] 2004;29A:188–193.
- Jewusiak EM, Spence KF, Sell KW: Solitary benign enchondroma of the long bones of the hand: Results of curettage and packing with freeze-dried cancellous bone allograft. J Bone Joint Surg Am 1971;53A:1587–1590.
- McDermott EM, Weiss APC: Glomus tumors. J Hand Surg [Am] 2006;31A:1397–1400.
- O'Connor MI, Bancroft LW: Benign and malignant cartilage tumors of the hand. Hand Clin 2004;20:317–323.
- Park MJ, Namdari S, Weiss APC: The carpal boss: Review of diagnosis and treatment. J Hand Surg [Am] 2008;33A:446–449.
- Rizzo M, Beckenbaugh RD: Treatment of mucous cysts of the fingers: Review of 134 cases with minimum 2-year follow-up evaluation. J Hand Surg 2003;28(3):519–524.
- Simon M, Finn H: Diagnostic strategy for bone and soft tissue tumors. J Bone Joint Surg Am 1993;75A:622–631.

Chapter 94 Hand Infections

Robert P. Waugh and Dan A. Zlotolow

ICD-9 CODES

680.4	*Carbuncle and Furuncle, Hand (Finger, Thumb, Wrist)*
681.01	*Felon (Pulp Abscess or Whitlow Excluding Herpetic Whitlow)*
681.02	*Onychia and Paronychia of Finger*
727.05	*Other Tenosynovitis of Hand and Wrist*

Key Concepts

- Acute infections of the hand can present as surgical emergencies.
- Common hand infections include those of the skin (cellulitis, soft-tissue abscesses), the nail (paronychia), or the finger tip pulp (felon).
- More serious but less common infections include those of the flexor tendon sheath (pyogenic flexor tenosynovitis) and necrotizing fasciitis.
- It is important and sometimes difficult to distinguish between inflammatory and infectious processes.
- Infections are influenced substantially by host factors contributing to immunocompromise, including diabetes, human immunodeficiency virus, alcoholism, malnutrition, and steroid use.
- Treatment of pyogenic infection is directed toward identifying the pathogen (holding antibiotics until a culture is taken), as well as decompressing and draining any infected fluid collections.
- More serious hand infections require emergent referral to a hand surgeon for definitive management; these include necrotizing fasciitis, pyogenic flexor tenosynovitis, deep space abscesses, and joint infections.
- Never culture an open wound because this will only grow the patient's colonizing skin flora. A true culture can only be obtained from a wound that you have created after the skin has been prepped.
- Persistent infections should be evaluated for osteomyelitis.

History

- Pertinent parts of the patient's medical history include identifying any risk factors for immunocompromise as well as the tetanus immunization status.
- Patients may be able to recall the precipitating factors leading to infection, which can be of help in planning operative management and directing antibiotic treatment (e.g., dog bites versus IV drug injections versus rusty nails).
- Patients with gout or other inflammatory arthritides may present similarly to those with infection and will usually improve with nonsteroidal anti-inflammatory drugs.
  - They should be monitored closely for the first 24 to 48 hours for improvement to ensure that the diagnosis is correct.
- Injuries in patients who present with a "fight bite" laceration on their metacarpophalangeal joint are very likely to be intra-articular given the proximity of the joint capsule to the skin in a clenched fist.
  - These innocuous looking wounds require surgical exploration (Fig. 94-1).

Physical Examination

- Infections present with erythema, pain, and tenderness in the affected area.
  - The examiner should evaluate the area for fluctuance or induration to distinguish cellulitis from an underlying abscess.
- Paronychia, the most common hand infection, presents with erythema and tenderness along the nail fold and can progress to an abscess in this space (Fig. 94-2A).
- The anatomy of a fingertip infection (felon) (Fig. 94-3) may obscure the diagnosis because these deep infections can present with pain and moderate swelling only, without evidence of underlying pus.
  - Felons require incision and decompression (see Fig. 94-2B).
- Watch for Kanavel's four cardinal signs of pyogenic flexor tenosynovitis; all four must be present to make the diagnosis (this is a surgical emergency!):
  - Fusiform swelling of the entire digit
  - Extreme tenderness along the course of the flexor tendon
  - Exquisite pain on passive extension of the finger
  - A resting position of the finger in a semiflexed position

- Deep space infections present with swelling of the entire hand, usually more pronounced dorsally. In addition, wide thumb abduction, semiflexed fingers, and isolated swelling of the hypothenar area suggest fluid collection in these spaces.

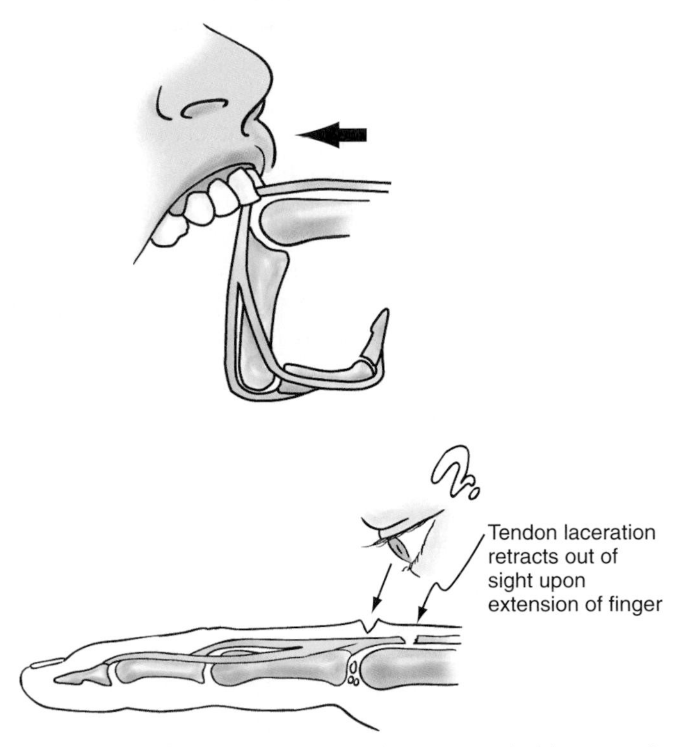

Figure 94-1 A punch to the mouth accompanied by a small laceration near the metacarpophalangeal joint should raise suspicion of a fight bite. This injury is characterized by its benign appearance and severe sequelae, which can include tendon rupture, septic arthritis, and osteomyelitis. (Adapted from Carter PR: Common Hand Injuries and Infections. A Practical Approach to Early Management. Philadelphia: WB Saunders, 1983, p 206.)

Imaging

- Plain radiographs are an important part of the evaluation of hand infections. It is vital to identify foreign objects such as hypodermic needles or tooth fragments as well as gas collections in the wound. Plain radiographs can also reveal underlying fractures and osteomyelitis.

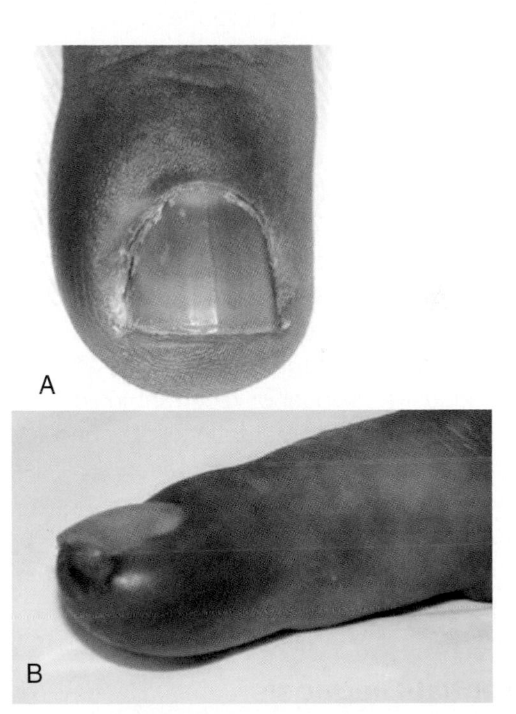

Figure 94-2 Clinical appearance of a paronychia (**A**) and a felon (**B**). (Part A from Rigopoulos D, Larios G, Gregoriou S, Alevios A: Acute and chronic paronychia. Am Fam Physician 2008;77:341; part B from Clark D: Common acute hand infections. Am Fam Physician 2003;68:2170.)

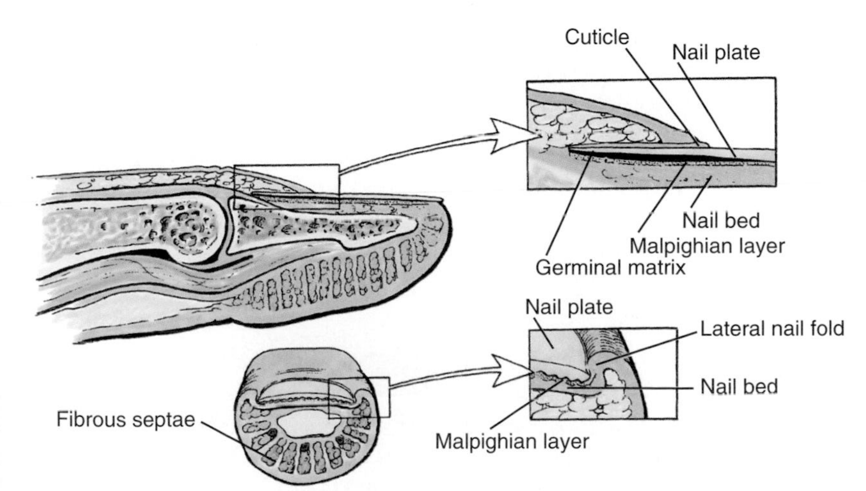

Figure 94-3 Anatomy of the fingertip. Note the fibrous septae in the fingertip pulp that must be transected to decompress a felon. The nail is a modified hair that grows at the rate of 1 mm per week. Infections deep to the eponychium and the lateral nail fold (paronychia) can be drained by elevating the eponychial fold bluntly and the lateral fold sharply with a blade pointing away from the center of the nail. (Adapted from Carter PR: Common Hand Injuries and Infections. A Practical Approach to Early Management. Philadelphia: WB Saunders, 1983, p 37.)

- Although a good history and physical examination usually obviate the need for advanced imaging studies, computed tomography can be helpful in identifying deep fluid collections in some cases.
- Magnetic resonance imaging should be performed if radiographs do not show evidence of osteomyelitis, but the suspicion remains high.

Additional Tests

- Laboratory tests should include
  - Complete blood count with manual differentiation
  - C-reactive protein
  - Erythrocyte sedimentation rate
  - The white blood cell count (WBC) may be normal, especially in long-standing infections.
  - C-reactive protein and erythrocyte sedimentation rate are nonspecific infection markers that help to establish a baseline value that the clinician can follow over time. Infection markers that do not decrease or begin to increase after treatment suggest a residual or recurrent infection.
  - Erythrocyte sedimentation rate and C-reactive protein will also be increased in inflammatory conditions.
  - A random glucose level may reveal previously undiagnosed diabetes, a condition that predisposes one to infection and complicates healing.

Differential Diagnosis

- Please see Table 94-1.

TABLE 94-1 *Differential Diagnosis*

Condition	Differentiating Feature
Local abscess	Demarcated fluctuance or induration
Deep space abscess	Swelling of the entire hand, especially dorsally
"Fight bite"	History of fistfight, small laceration over the metacarpophalangeal joint
Septic arthritis	Exquisite pain with passive or active motion of the joint
Pyogenic flexor tenosynovitis	Positive Kanavel's signs
Felon	Swelling and tenderness distal to the distal interphalangeal joint
Paronychia	Erythema and occasionally pus at the nail fold
Gout	History of gout, improvement with nonsteroidal anti-inflammatory drugs

Treatment

- In the office or emergency department
  - Acute paronychia
    - — Drain by using a blade pointing away from the center of the nail and opening the lateral nail fold and bluntly elevating the eponychial fold from the nail plate to evacuate the exudate. Obtain a sample for culture. Pack the nail fold open (Fig. 94-4).
    - — After drainage, the patient should soak the finger two to three times per day in a hot diluted povidone-iodine solution and change the wet-to-dry dressings also two to three times daily. Once-daily dry dressings are appropriate after 3 or 4 days when the incision has stopped draining.
    - — Place the patient on 7 to 10 days of oral antibiotics.
  - Felons
    - — Under digital block, carry the incision down the side of the finger away from the thumb except for the small finger, where the incision should be made facing the thumb. Begin your incision 0.5 cm distal to the distal interphalangeal crease and stop just as the finger starts to curve toward the fingertip (Fig. 94-5A).
    - — Open the incision bluntly; the palmar aspect of the distal phalanx is the roof of the incision deeply. Spread down into the pulp to break up the septae containing the infection (see Fig. 94-5B). Culture and then irrigate the wound.
    - — Pack the wound open with iodoform gauze and have the patient change the dressing two to three times daily for 3 to 4 days and then convert to once-daily dry dressings.
    - — Place the patient on 7 to 10 days of oral antibiotics.
    - — Have the patient follow up in approximately 5 days for a wound check.

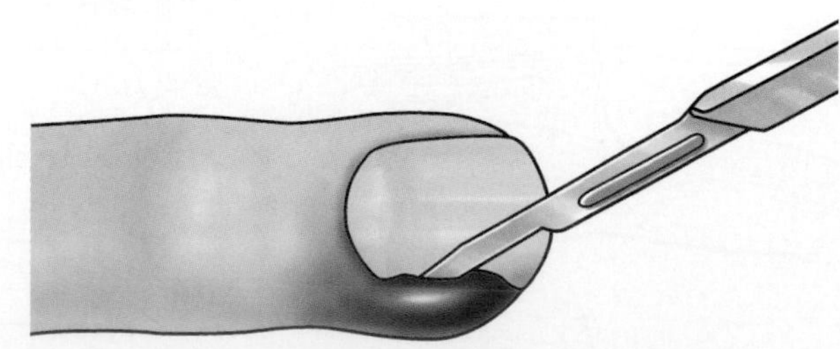

Figure 94-4 Incision for paronychia involving the lateral nail fold. (Adapted from Rockwell P: Acute and chronic paronychia. Am Fam Physician 2001;63:1115.)

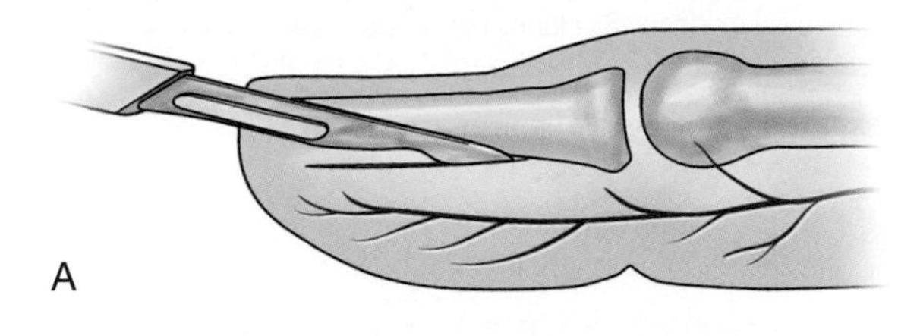

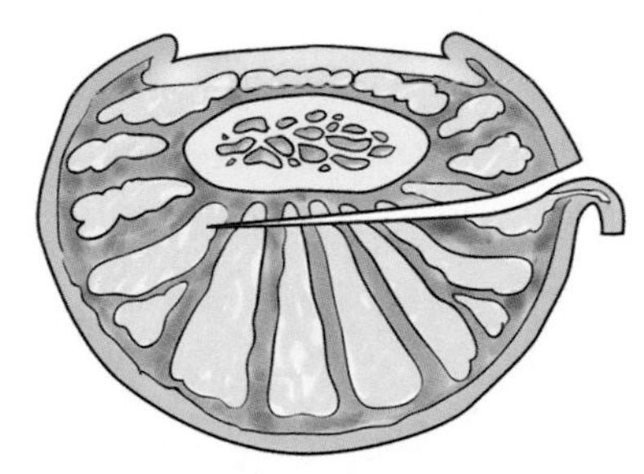

Figure 94-5 Incision for a felon. Note that the incision is just lateral to the nail fold and away from the digital nerve (**A**). The dissection should proceed just under the phalanx to open all the septae of the pulp (**B**). (Adapted from Clark D: Common acute hand infections. Am Fam Physician 2003;68:2171.)

- Local abscesses
  - Treat these abscesses in a fashion similar to that for abscesses elsewhere in the body.
  - Carry the incision across the abscess through the skin sharply and expose the abscess space bluntly. Use an adequate incision to expose the entire abscess. Evacuate all infected contents and irrigate the wound. Do not attempt to drain volar hand abscesses in the office.
  - Pack the wound open with iodoform gauze and have the patient change the dressing two to three times daily for 3 to 4 days and then convert to once-daily dry dressings.
  - Place the patient on 7 to 10 days of oral antibiotics.
  - Have the patient follow up in approximately 5 days for a wound check.

When to Refer?

- Patients who exhibit Kanavel's signs, show evidence of deep space infections, or have puncture wounds that enter joints are likely to require surgical exploration, débridement, and irrigation. These patients should be referred to a hand surgeon that day. Refrain from administering antibiotics unless the patient is septic because this will make it difficult to identify an organism at the time of surgery.

Prognosis

- Most patients with hand infections do well once the infection is controlled. However, inadequately treated infections can lead to serious consequences. The swelling and edema of an untreated infection causes increased tissue pressure and can result in tissue necrosis. Likewise, untreated pyogenic flexor tenosynovitis can lead to tendon rupture.

Troubleshooting

- The most common complication of a treated hand infection is recurrence. This is usually due to incomplete débridement or failure to allow the wound to stay open after evacuation of the abscess cavity. The tendency of inexperienced clinicians is to make the incision too small and be too timid in packing the wound.
- Recurrent exposure to the cause of the infection is also common (e.g., IV drug abusers, certain manual laborers, frequently manicured women). Counsel patients on the risk factors for hand infections to reduce recurrent infection.

Patient Instructions

- Patients should be meticulous about dressing changes. If they are not able to change their dressings by themselves or with the help of someone else, they may need home nursing assistance or in some cases inpatient admission.
- Be sure to instruct patients to complete their entire antibiotic regimen.
- Patients should keep their hand dry when showering and should absolutely avoid submerging it if bathing.

Considerations in Special Populations

- Be aware that patients with diabetes or those on long-term steroid treatment are likely to take longer to heal. Aggressive management of underlying medical problems as well as proper nutrition will optimize their recovery.

Suggested Reading

- Boles D, Schmidt C: Pyogenic flexor tenosynovitis. Hand Clin 1998;14:567–578.
- Boyes J (ed): Infections. In Bunnell's Surgery of the Hand. Philadelphia: JB Lippincott, 1970, pp 613–642.

- Brook I: Paronychia: A mixed infection. J Hand Surg [Br] 1993;18:358–359.
- Connor R, Kimbrough R, Dabezies E: Hand infections in patients with diabetes mellitus. Orthopedics 2001;24:1057–1060.
- Glass K: Factors related to the resolution of treated hand infections. J Hand Surg [Am] 1982;7:388–394.
- Gonzalez M, Garst J, Nourbash P, et al: Abscesses of the upper extremity from drug abuse by injection. J Hand Surg [Am] 1993;18:868–870.
- Hausman M, Lisser S: Hand infections. Orthop Clin North Am 1992;23:171–185.
- Jebsen P: Infections of the fingertip: Paronychias and felons. Hand Clin 1998;5:547–555.
- Patzakis M, Wilkins J, Bassett R: Surgical findings in clenched-fist injuries. Clin Orthop Relat Res 1987;220:237–240.
- Zook E: Infection of the nail apparatus: Paronychia. In Krull EA, Zook EG, Baran R (eds): Nail Surgery: A Text and Atlas. Philadelphia: Lippincott Williams & Wilkins, 2001, pp 195–200.

Chapter 95 Hand Dislocations

Dan A. Zlotolow and R. Bryan Butler

ICD-9 CODES
833.01 *Dislocation Radioulnar Joint, Distal*
833.02 *Dislocation Radiocarpal Joint*
833.03 *Dislocation Midcarpal Joint*
833.04 *Dislocation Carpometacarpal Joint*
834.01 *Dislocation Metacarpophalangeal Joint*

Key Concepts

- A dislocation is a complete disruption of joint congruity.
- A subluxation implies that at least a portion of the articulating surfaces are still in contact.
- The progression of joint injury begins with a mild sprain with no joint laxity through ligament disruption, joint subluxation, and finally dislocation.
- Closed reduction is most often accomplished with traction, slight exaggeration of deformity, and correction of deformity.
- Soft-tissue interposition can block closed reductions in some dislocations.
- Be aware of associated fractures.
- Open dislocations are a surgical emergency.
- Dislocations are often missed, even by experienced practitioners.

History

- The mechanism of injury is very helpful for identifying associated injuries.
- Assess whether the dislocation is recurrent (has happened before) or chronic (has occurred in the past but was never reduced).
- Determine the energy that went into causing the dislocation.

Physical Examination

- High-energy injuries warrant a thorough secondary survey including the lower limbs, spine, and both upper limbs.
- Look for open wounds that may indicate an open dislocation (assume it is open until proven otherwise).
- Evaluate the compartments of the forearm and hand to make sure they are soft.
- Identify associated neurovascular compromise by checking sensation to light touch and capillary refill.
- Check for generalized ligamentous laxity.

Imaging

- Plain radiographs are essential for diagnosis.
- A good radiographic series usually obviates the need for advanced imaging studies and includes true anteroposterior and true lateral views.
- Computed tomography can be helpful if bony detail is obscured, as for carpometacarpal dislocations (Fig. 95-1) or distal radioulnar joint dislocations (Fig. 95-2).
- Magnetic resonance imaging is rarely needed and may be used to determine associated injuries preoperatively.

Additional Tests

- No additional tests are routinely necessary.

Differential Diagnosis

- Please see Table 95-1.

Treatment

- Radiocarpal or midcarpal dislocations (Fig. 95-3)
    - These are difficult reductions to accomplish and will likely require an orthopaedic consultation at the time of injury.
    - Traction, volar pressure on the lunate, and wrist flexion are typically effective.
- Distal radioulnar joint dislocations
    - Depending on the direction of the dislocation, these will reduce in either pronation or supination
    - Use a sugar tong splint to hold the wrist and the forearm in the position of reduction.
- Carpometacarpal dislocations
    - Closed reduction requires traction and direct pressure over the dislocated metacarpal joint.

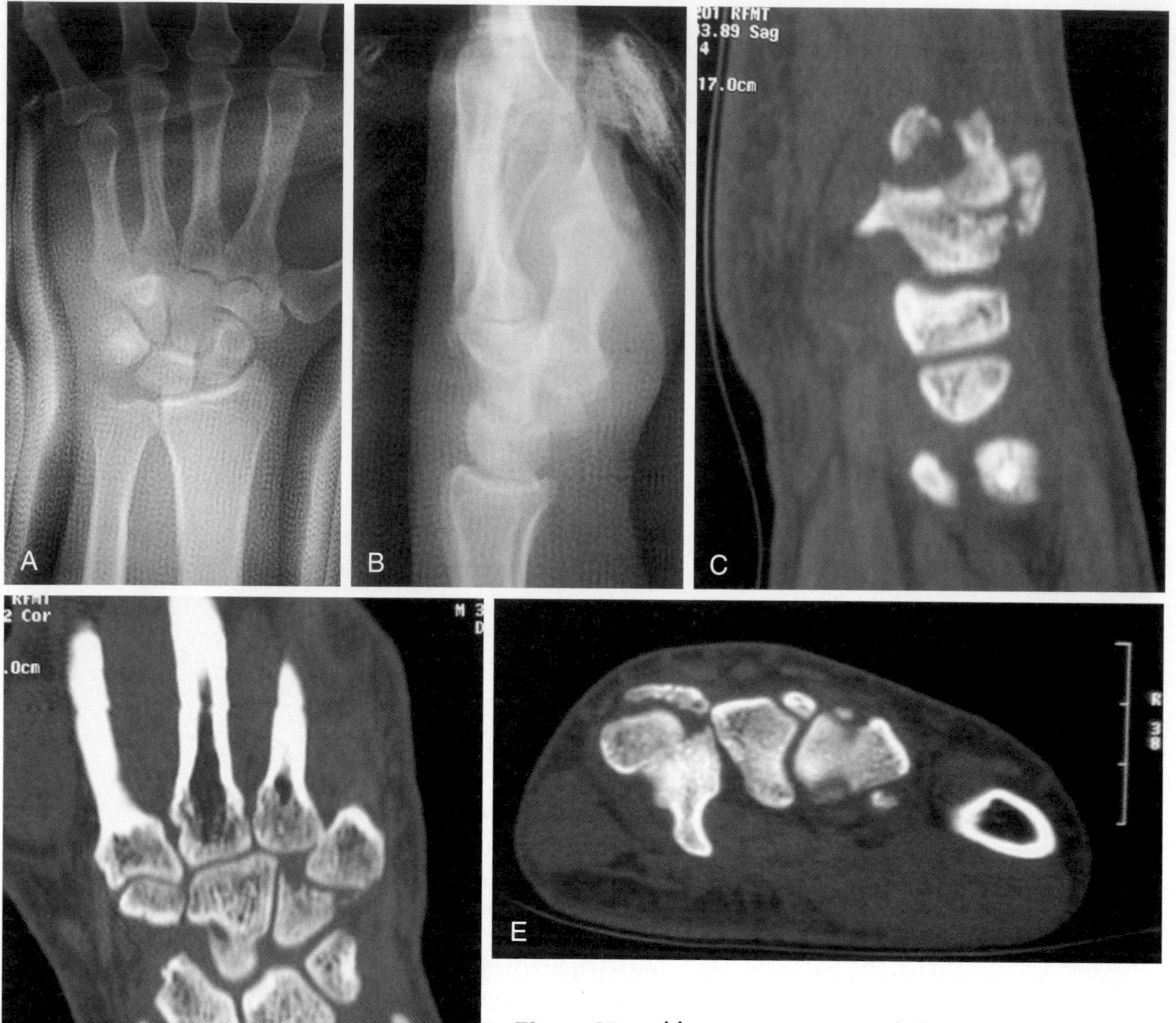

Figure 95-1 Many carpometacarpal dislocations are missed on initial radiographs. A high index of suspicion and computed tomography scanning may be necessary to make the diagnosis. Note the subtle findings on the anteroposterior (**A**) and lateral (**B**) radiographs compared with the computed tomography scan (**C** to **E**). Computed tomography in this case shows impaction of the fifth metacarpal base into the body of the hamate.

   - These are inherently unstable injuries and difficult to assess on plain radiographs.
   - Postreduction computed tomography scans are necessary to assess the quality of the reduction.
   - Place in an ulnar gutter or clamshell splint with the wrist in neutral position, the metacarpophalangeal joints in flexion, and the interphalangeal joints free.
- Metacarpophalangeal dislocations
   - Soft-tissue interposition can prevent closed reduction.
   - Reduce by using traction, exaggeration of deformity, and translation.
   - Place in an ulnar gutter or clamshell splint with the wrist in extension, the metacarpophalangeal joints in flexion, and the proximal interphalangeal joints in extension.
- Interphalangeal dislocations
   - Soft-tissue interposition can prevent closed reduction
   - Reduce by using traction, exaggeration of deformity, and translation
- Dorsal dislocation (Fig. 95-4)
   - If the joint is stable in full extension, buddy tape to adjoining finger
   - If the joint tends to redislocate, place in an extension block splint to allow a stable range of motion.
   - Always place finger splints on the dorsum of the finger.

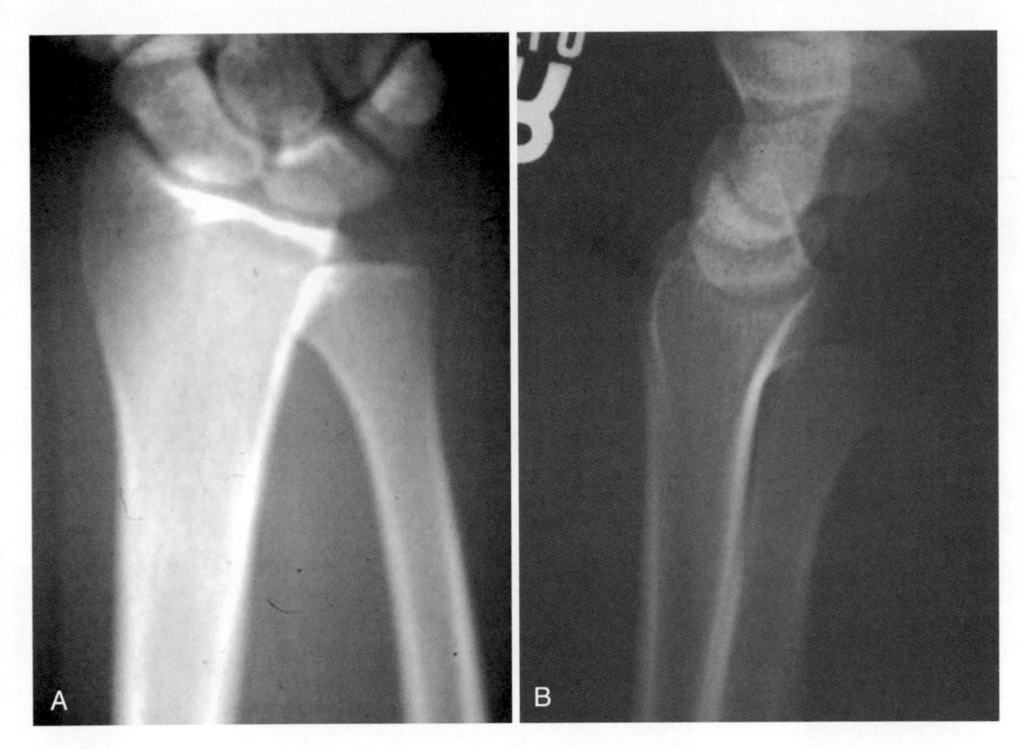

Figure 95-2 **A**, Distal radioulnar joint dislocation. **B,** A true lateral radiograph, identified by overlap of the distal pole of the scaphoid with the pisiform, is necessary to make the diagnosis. (From Szabo B: Distal radioulnar joint instability. J Bone Joint Surg Am 2006;88A:884–894.)

- Volar dislocation
  - More rare; splint the proximal interphalangeal joint in extension

When to Refer

- Any open dislocation
- Any suspicion of compartment syndrome
- Irreducible dislocations
- High-energy mechanism

Prognosis

- Most patients will have some residual loss of motion at the dislocated joint, even if optimal treatment is provided.

TABLE 95-1 *Differential Diagnosis*

Differential Diagnosis	Differentiating Feature	Chapter Reference
Sprain, grade I	No joint laxity with stress testing	79
Sprain, grade II	Laxity present, but ligament is intact with firm endpoint	79
Sprain, grade III	Complete ligament injury with no endpoint on stress testing	79
Subluxation	Joint not concentrically reduced, but articular surfaces remain in contact	79

- Outcome is principally dependent on patient compliance with their therapy protocol and on their propensity for scarring.

Troubleshooting

- Appropriate reduction maneuvers can avoid catastrophes such as soft-tissue interposition, neurovascular injury, and iatrogenic fracture.
- A well-made splint can make the difference between a good outcome and a recurrently dislocated or ankylosed/arthritic joint.

Patient Instructions

- Ice and elevation are critical to limit swelling.
- For radiocarpal or intercarpal dislocations, patients should be referred to a hand surgeon within a couple of days for definitive management as long as a closed reduction was achieved.

Considerations in Special Populations

- Children with unossified epiphyses may have complete Salter I fractures that can mimic dislocations.
- Patients with ligamentous laxity have a propensity for dislocation and should be counseled about their condition.

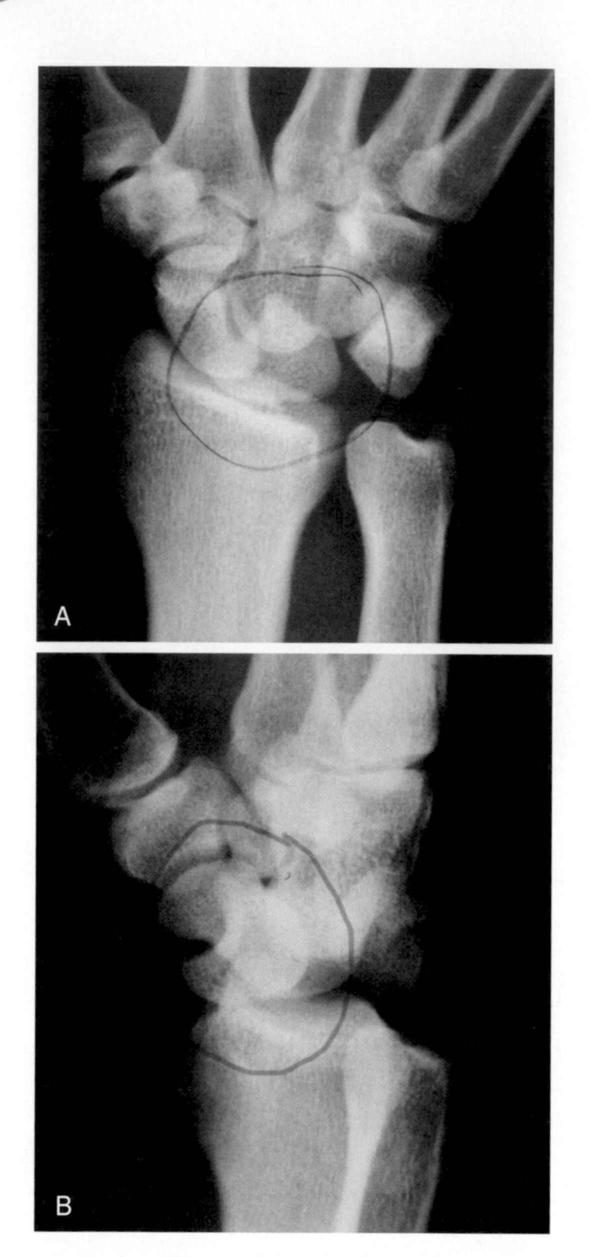

Figure 95-3 A perilunate dislocation is a high-energy injury with a fair long-term prognosis. Although the radiographic findings are well understood, this injury is underdiagnosed, resulting in complete loss of wrist function for the patient and legal entanglements for the physician. Note the triangular appearance of the lunate on the anteroposterior view (**A**), as well as the "empty cup" appearance of the lunate on the lateral view (**B**).

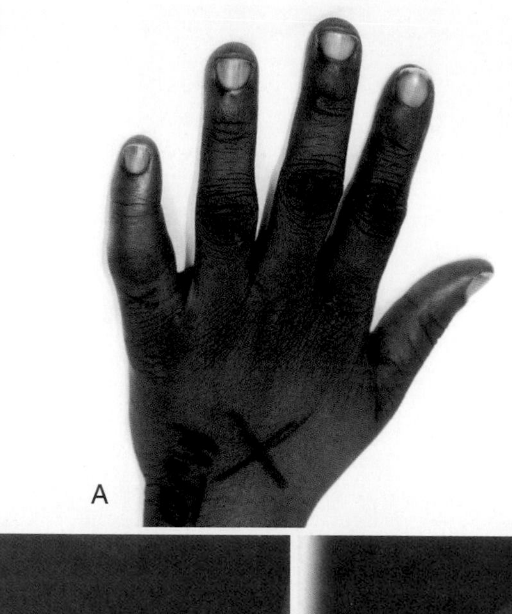

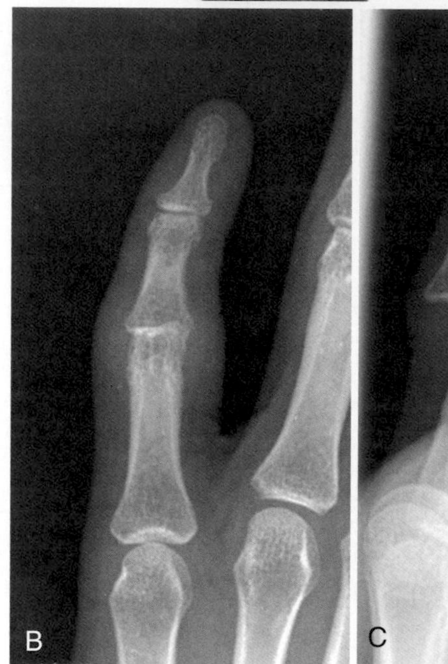

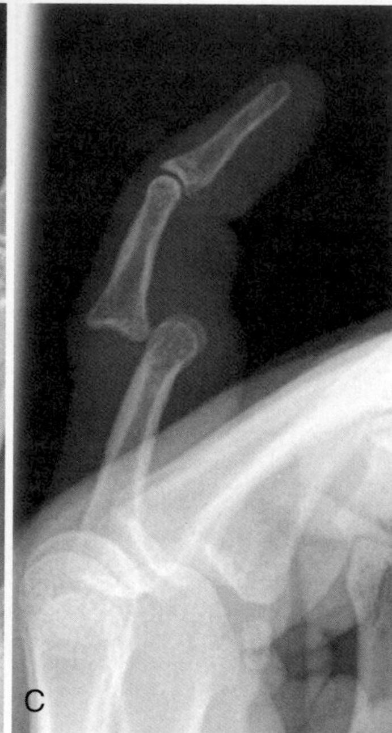

Figure 95-4 **A,** Proximal interphalangeal dislocations can have a benign clinical appearance. **B,** An anteroposterior radiograph will often not demonstrate the dislocation. **C,** A good lateral radiograph is crucial.

Suggested Reading

- Adkinson JW, Chapman MW: Treatment of acute lunate and perilunate dislocations. Clin Orthop Relat Res 1982;164:199–207.
- Betz RR, Browne EZ, Perry GB, Resnick EJ: The complex volar metacarpophalangeal joint dislocation. A case report and review of the literature. J Bone Joint Surg Am 1982;64A:1374–1375.
- Bowers WH: The proximal interphalangeal joint volar plate. II. A clinical study of hyperextension injury. J Hand Surg [Am] 1981;6A:77–81.
- Deshmukh NV, Sonanis SV, Stothard J: Neglected volar dislocations of the interphalangeal joint. Hand Surg 2004; 9:71–75.
- Dobyns JH, McElfresh EC: Extension block splinting. Hand Clin 1994;10:229–237.
- Mueller JJ: Carpometacarpal dislocations: Report of five cases and review of the literature. J Hand Surg [Am] 1986;11A: 184–188.

Chapter 96 Distal Radius Fracture

Trevor Starnes and A. Bobby Chhabra

ICD-9 CODES
813.4 *Distal Radius Fracture, Closed*
813.5 *Distal Radius Fracture, Open*

Key Concepts

- The most common fracture of the upper extremity
- Bimodal age distribution
  - Adolescent: high energy; fall from a height, motor vehicle accident, athletics
  - Elderly: low energy; fall from standing position
  - Osteoporosis is a critical risk factor.
- Mechanism: fall on outstretched hand
- Fracture on tension side (volar) and comminution on compression side (dorsal)
- Axial load in forearm is split 80% radius and 20% ulna

History

- Important to obtain the following information
  - Age
  - Hand dominance
  - Mechanism of injury: high versus low energy
  - Comorbidities
  - Activity level
  - Occupation

Physical Examination

- Skin and soft-tissue swelling
- Painful and limited range of motion of wrist
- Deformity and angulation
  - Dorsal displacement: Colles' fracture (90% of distal radius fractures)
  - Volar displacement: Smith's fracture
- Neurovascular status, especially median nerve
  - Carpal tunnel compression symptoms present in 13% to 23% of injuries
- Palpate the anatomic snuffbox for tenderness, which may suggest a scaphoid fracture.
- Examine finger and thumb motion to confirm tendon continuity.
- Always examine the ipsilateral hand, elbow, and shoulder for associated injuries.

Imaging

- Posteroanterior and lateral radiographs
  - Normal values
    - — Radial inclination: 22 degrees (range, 13–30 degrees) (Fig. 96-1)
    - — Radial length: 11 to 12 mm (range, 8–18 mm) (Fig. 96-2)
    - — Volar tilt: 11 degrees (range, 1–21 degrees) (see Fig. 96-1)
  - Evaluate the distal radioulnar joint.
  - Evaluate for associated carpal injuries.
  - Evaluate for associated ulnar fracture.
- Navicular or scaphoid view
  - Evaluate the scaphoid for fracture.
- Elbow anteroposterior and lateral views with any associated pain
  - Evaluate for associated injury.
  - Monteggia's fractures: proximal ulnar fracture with radial head dislocation
  - Galeazzi's fractures: radial diaphysis fracture at the junction of the middle and distal thirds with associated disruption of distal radioulnar joint

Differential Diagnosis

- Please see Table 96-1.
- Description of fracture
  - Open versus closed
  - Intra-articular versus extra-articular
  - Comminution: dorsal versus volar
  - Loss of radial height: radial shortening
  - Displacement and angulation
  - Look for an associated distal ulnar fracture.

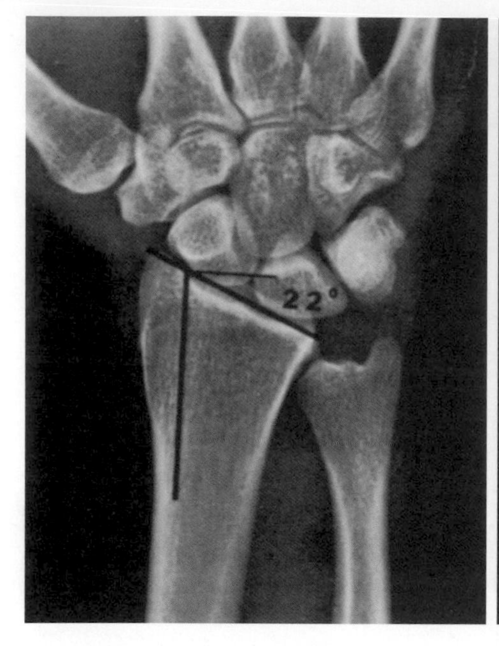

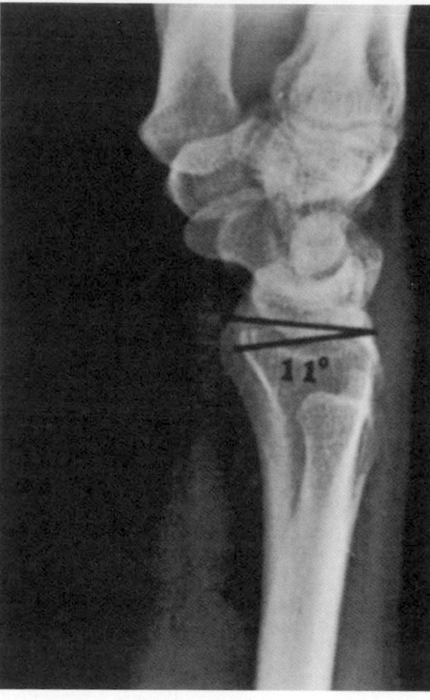

Figure 96-1 The anteroposterior radiograph on the *left* illustrates normal radial inclination of approximately 22 degrees. The lateral radiograph on the *right* illustrates normal volar tilt of the distal articular surface of approximately 11 degrees. (From Green DP, Hotchkiss RN, Pederson WC, Wolfe SW [eds]: Green's Operative Hand Surgery, 5th ed. Philadelphia: Churchill Livingstone, 2005, Fig. 16-7.)

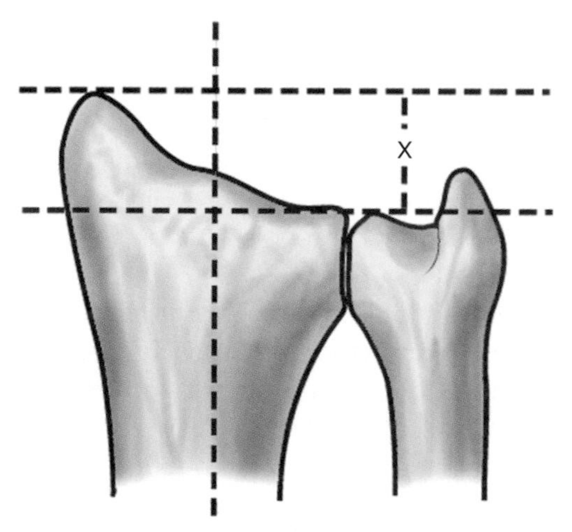

Figure 96-2 Radial length is the distance from the tip of the radial styloid to the ulnar articular surface on an anteroposterior radiograph (X). Radial length averages 11 to 12 mm, with a range of 8 to 18 mm.

TABLE 96-1 *Differential Diagnosis*

Fracture Eponym	Differentiating Features
Colles' fracture	Dorsal comminution, dorsal displacement, dorsal angulation (apex volar), radial shortening, silver fork deformity (Fig. 96-3)
Smith's fracture	Volar displacement, volar angulation (apex dorsal), unstable fracture, garden spade deformity (Fig. 96-4)
Barton's fracture	Dorsal rim displacement of distal radius, unstable articular fracture-subluxation with carpus displacement (see Fig. 96-4)
Volar Barton's fracture	Volar rim displacement of distal radius, unstable articular fracture-subluxation with carpus displacement (see Fig. 96-4)
Chauffeur's fracture	Radial styloid fracture with carpus displaced ulnarly (Fig. 96-5)
Die-punch fracture	Depression of lunate fossa with proximal migration of lunate (see Fig. 96-5)

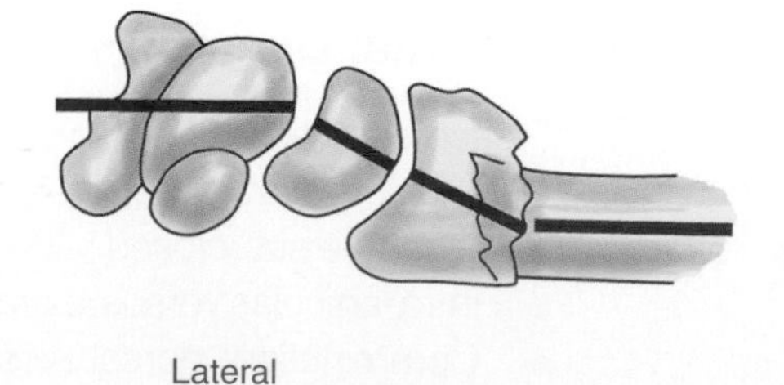

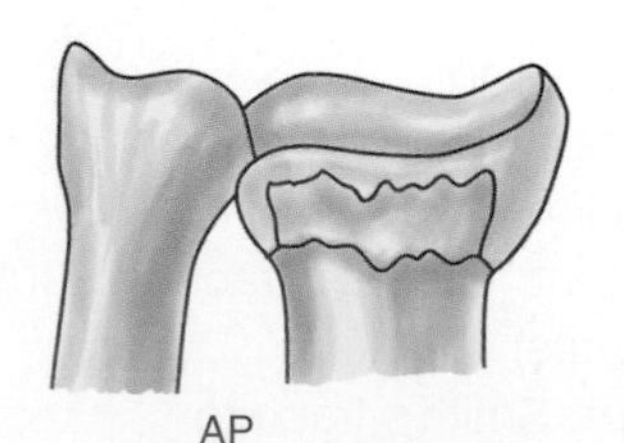

Figure 96-3 Representation of the typical deformity seen in a Colles' fracture. Dorsal comminution and displacement with shortening of the radius relative to the ulna are present. AP, anteroposterior. (Adapted from Green DP, Hotchkiss RN, Pederson WC, Wolfe SW [eds]: Green's Operative Hand Surgery, 5th ed. Philadelphia: Churchill Livingstone, 2005, Fig. 16-8.)

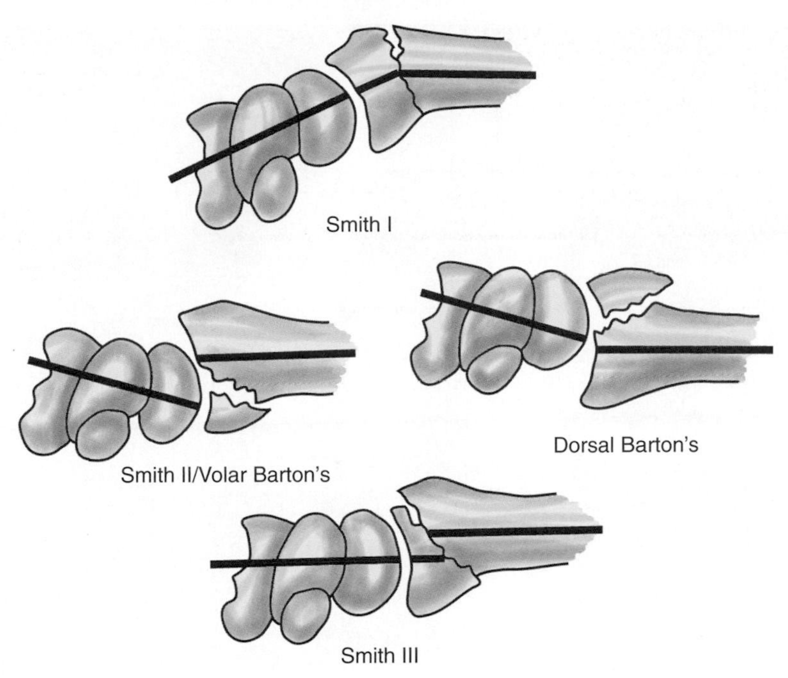

Figure 96-4 Thomas' classification of Smith's fractures. Type I Smith's fracture: extra-articular fracture with palmar angulation and displacement of the distal fragment. Type II Smith's fracture: intra-articular fracture with volar and proximal displacement of the distal fragment along with the carpus. Type III Smith's fracture: extra-articular fracture with volar displacement of the distal fragment and carpus. (In type III, the fracture line is more oblique than in a type I fracture.) A type II Smith's fracture is essentially a volar Barton's fracture. A dorsal Barton's fracture, illustrated for comparison, shows the dorsal and proximal displacement of the carpus and distal fragment on the radial shaft. (Adapted from Green DP, Hotchkiss RN, Pederson WC, Wolfe SW [eds]: Green's Operative Hand Surgery, 5th ed. Philadelphia: Churchill Livingstone, 2005, Fig. 16-9.)

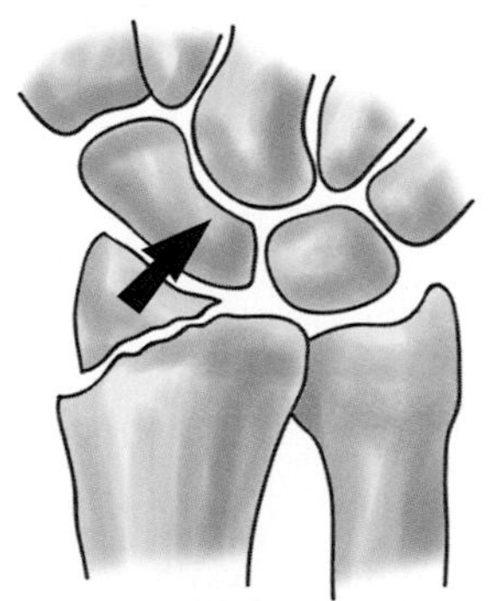

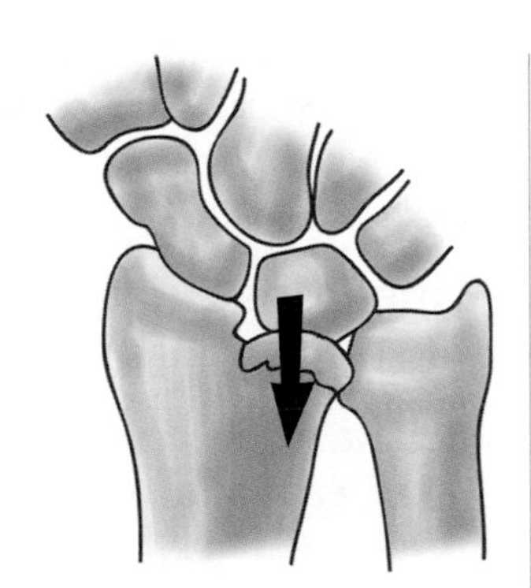

Figure 96-5 A chauffeur's fracture is illustrated with the carpus displaced ulnarly by the radial styloid fracture. A lunate load (die-punch) fracture is shown with a depression of the lunate fossa of the radius that allows proximal migration of the lunate and/or proximal carpal row. *Arrows* represent deforming forces and displacement. (Adapted from Green DP, Hotchkiss RN, Pederson WC, Wolfe SW [eds]: Green's Operative Hand Surgery, 5th ed. Philadelphia: Churchill Livingstone, 2005, Fig. 16-10.)

Treatment

- Initial treatment
  - Radiographs to define injury
  - Nondisplaced fracture (Fig. 96-6)
    - — Sugar tong splint
    - — Referral to orthopaedist to be seen in 5 to 7 days
  - Displaced fracture (Fig. 96-7)
    - — Closed reduction and splinting (see Chapter 101)
    - — Hematoma block
    - — Finger traps and traction
    - — Sugar tong splint (Fig. 96-8)
    - — Referral to orthopaedist to be seen in 3 to 5 days
  - Acceptable reduction (Fig. 96-9)
    - — Radial shortening less than 2 mm
    - — Neutral tilt
    - — Articular step-off less than 1 mm

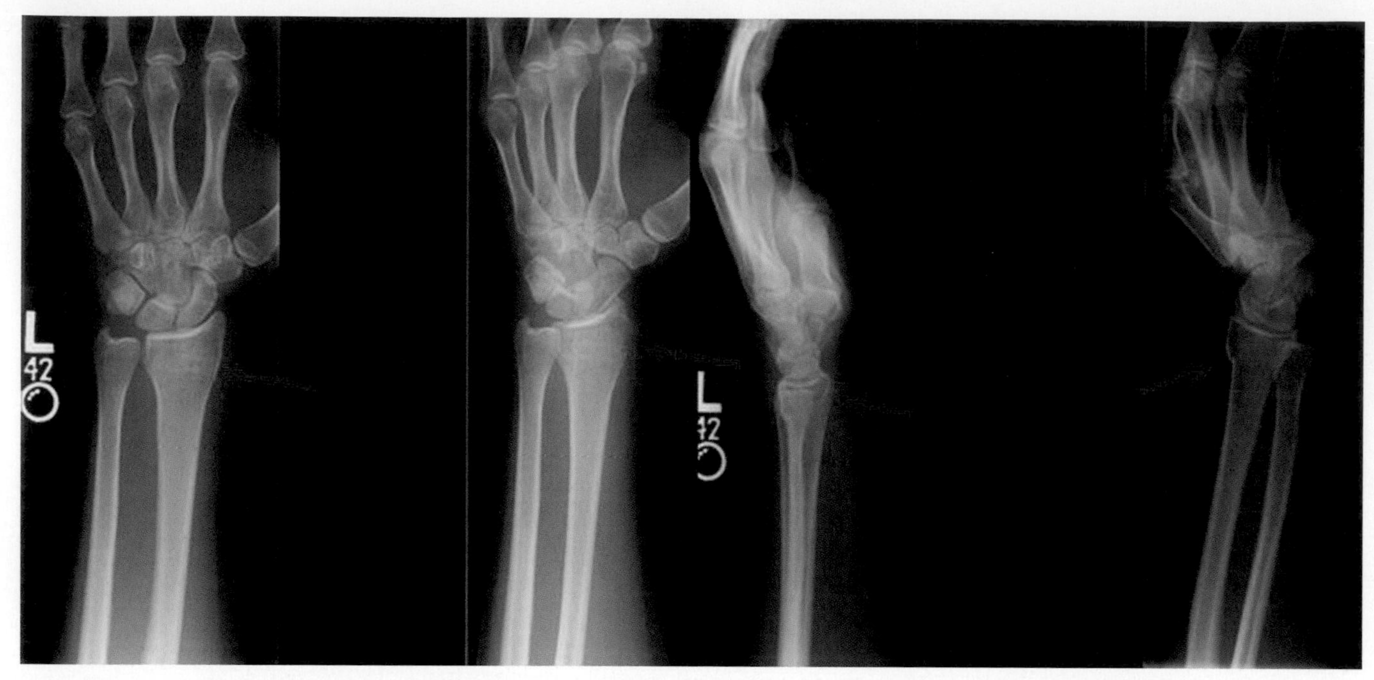

Figure 96-6 Nondisplaced distal radius fracture (*arrow*). Treat in splint followed by cast. (From left to right, Posteroanterior, oblique, lateral, and oblique views of the left wrist are shown.)

When to Refer

- Refer to orthopaedist for all distal radius fractures
  - Nonoperative
    - — Nondisplaced fractures
    - — Stable fracture patterns with acceptable reduction
    - — Elderly (older than 65 years) or low-demand patients with comorbidities with reasonable reduction
  - Operative
    - — Open fractures
    - — Unstable fracture patterns: comminution or intra-articular
    - — Associated neurovascular or tendon injuries
    - — Unacceptable reduction
    - — Young active patient
- Complications
  - Post-traumatic arthritis
  - Malunion
  - Nonunion
  - Median neuropathy
  - Finger and wrist stiffness
  - Tendon ruptures: extensor pollicis longus tendon
  - Chronic regional pain syndrome or reflex sympathetic dystrophy

Patient Instructions

- Keep the splint clean and dry.
- Elevate the arm above the heart for 48 hours to decrease swelling and pain.
- Take pain medications as prescribed.
- Follow up with orthopaedist as instructed

Considerations in Special Populations

- Pediatric patients
  - Salter-Harris classification (Fig. 96-10)
  - Only one reduction attempt should be made to prevent further damage to the physis.
  - High potential for remodeling
  - Referral to orthopaedist for all displaced and physeal fractures

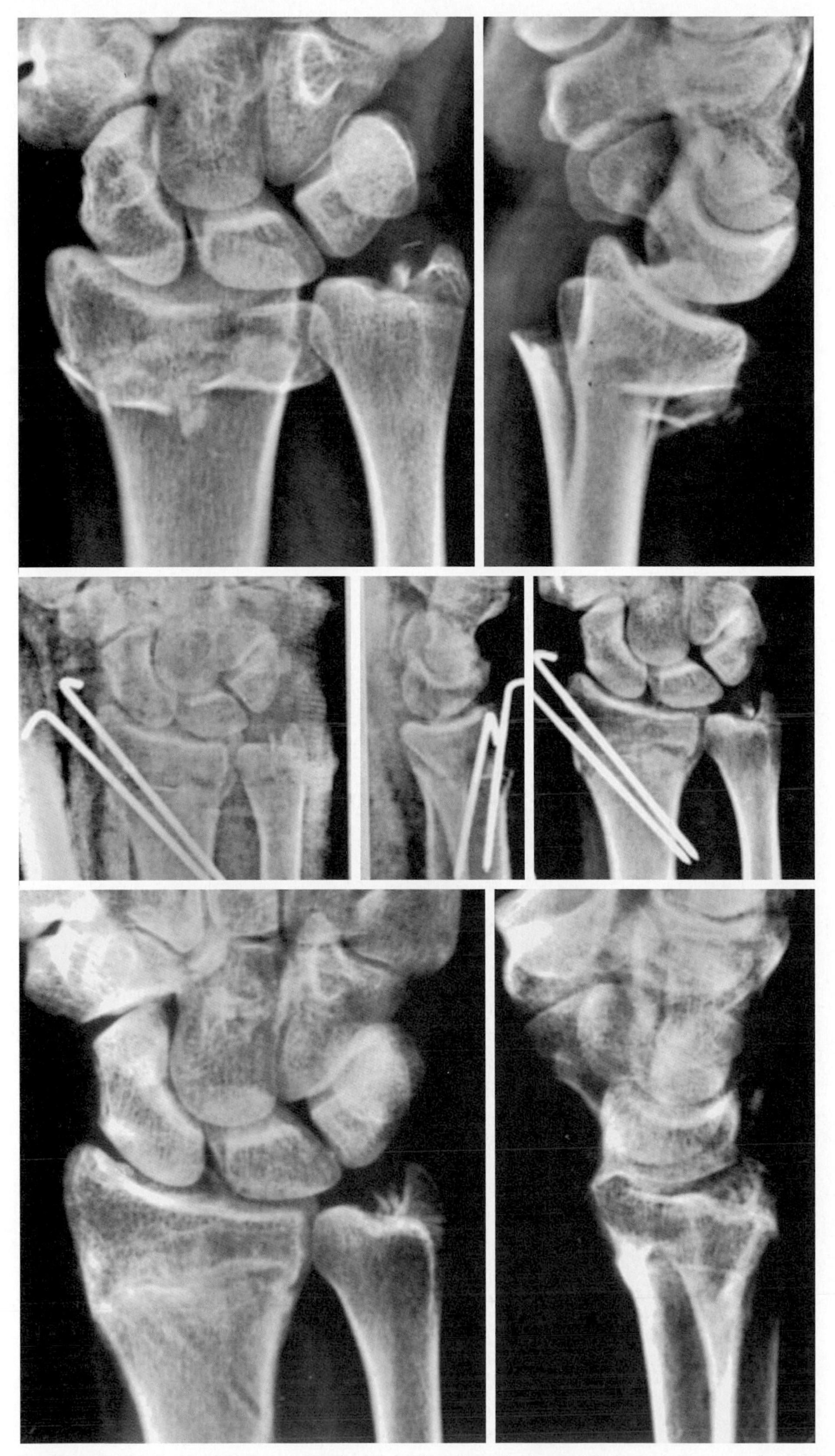

Figure 96-7 Unstable dorsally displaced fracture associated with a dorsal die-punch fragment treated by closed manipulation, intrafocal pinning, and cast fixation for 5 weeks. Follow-up radiographs at 6 months reveal an anatomic result. (From Green DP, Hotchkiss RN, Pederson WC, Wolfe SW [eds]: Green's Operative Hand Surgery, 5th ed. Philadelphia: Churchill Livingstone, 2005, Fig. 16-26.)

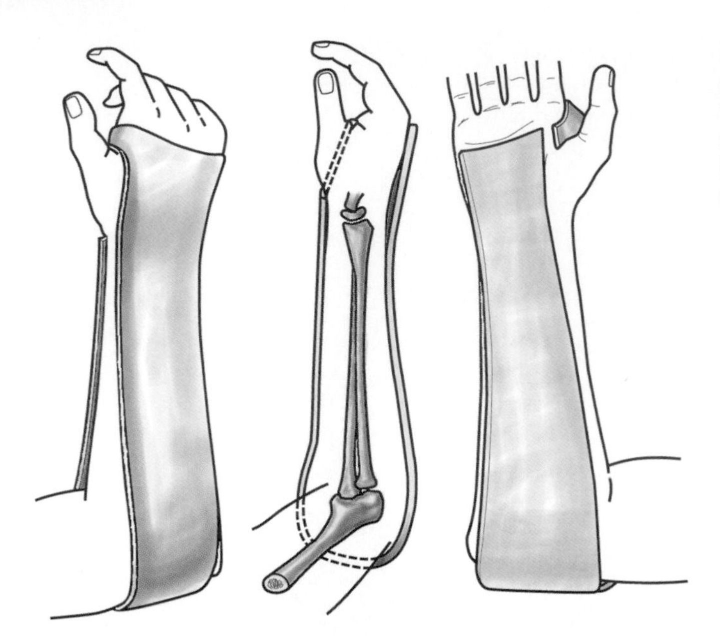

Figure 96-8 Sugar tong splint for a distal radius fracture. This splint controls forearm rotation while allowing for some elbow flexion. The palmar crease should be free to allow full metacarpophalangeal flexion. (From Green DP, Hotchkiss RN, Pederson WC, Wolfe SW [eds]: Green's Operative Hand Surgery, 5th ed. Philadelphia: Churchill Livingstone, 2005, Fig. 16-23.)

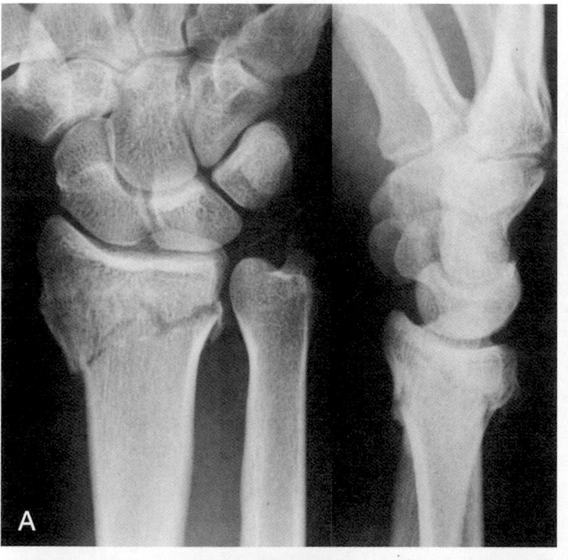

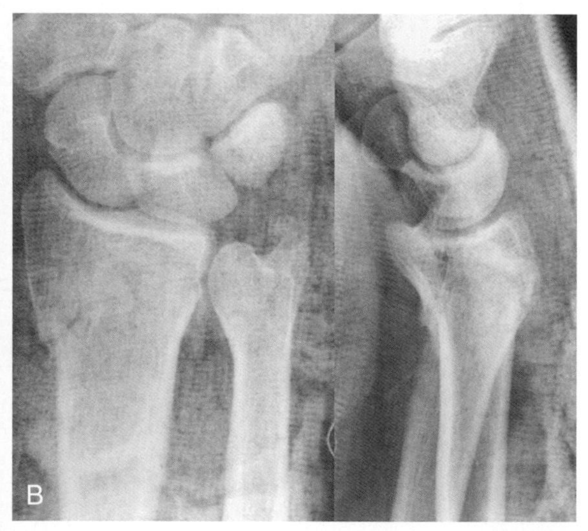

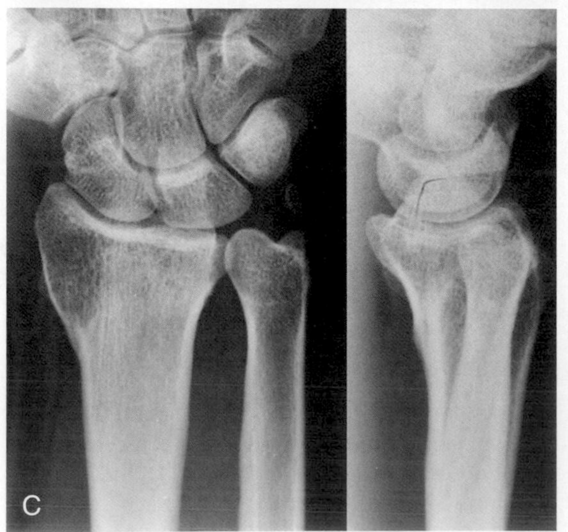

Figure 96-9 **A,** Typical radiographic appearance of a Colles' fracture in a young adult. **B,** The fracture was manually reduced and held in slight flexion, ulnar deviation, and slight pronation in a sugar tong splint for 3 weeks, followed by a short-arm cast for another 3 weeks. **C,** Follow-up radiographs at 1 year reveal loss of 2 mm of length but maintenance of normal volar and ulnar tilt. Notice the asymptomatic nonunion of the tip of the ulnar styloid. (From Green DP, Hotchkiss RN, Pederson WC, Wolfe SW [eds]: Green's Operative Hand Surgery, 5th ed. Philadelphia: Churchill Livingstone, 2005, Fig. 16-22.)

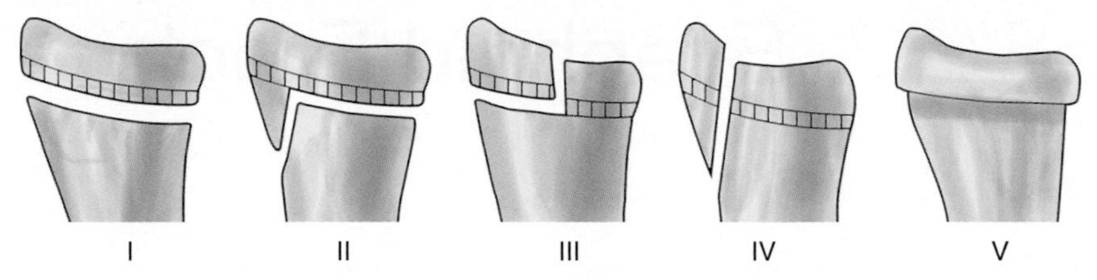

Figure 96-10 Salter-Harris classification of distal radial epiphyseal fractures in children. Type V is a crush injury. (Adapted from Green DP, Hotchkiss RN, Pederson WC, Wolfe SW [eds]: Green's Operative Hand Surgery, 5th ed. Philadelphia: Churchill Livingstone, 2005, Fig. 16-63.)

Suggested Reading

- Fernandez DL, Palmer AK: Fractures of the distal radius. In Green DP, Hotchkiss RN, Pederson WC, Wolfe SW (eds): Green's Operative Hand Surgery, 5th ed. Philadelphia: Churchill Livingstone, 2005, pp 929–985.
- Jiuliano JA, Jupiter J: Distal radius fractures. In Trumble TE, Budoff JE, Cornwall R (eds): Hand, Elbow, and Shoulder: Core Knowledge in Orthopaedics. Philadelphia: Mosby, 2006, pp 84–101.
- Koval KJ, Zuckerman JD: Handbook of Fractures, 3rd ed. Philadelphia: Lippincott Williams & Wilkins, 2006, pp 226–236.
- Ruch D: Fractures of the distal radius and ulna. In Bucholz RW, Heckman JD, Court-Brown C (eds): Rockwood and Green's Fractures in Adults, 6th ed. Philadelphia: Lippincott Williams & Wilkins, 2006, pp 909–988.

Chapter 97 Scaphoid Fracture

Trevor Starnes and A. Bobby Chhabra

ICD-9 CODE
814.1 *Scaphoid Fracture of the Wrist*

Key Concepts

- Most common carpal bone fracture
- Mechanism: fall on outstretched hand
- Eighty percent of scaphoid covered with articular cartilage
- Vascular supply (Fig. 97-1)
  - Branches off radial artery
  - Enters dorsally and distally and courses proximally
  - Fractures through waist and proximal third render the proximal fragment at risk of avascular necrosis
- The scaphoid links the proximal and distal carpal rows.
- Carpal bones are connected by capsular and interosseous ligaments.

History

- It is mportant to obtain the following information:
  - History of sprain with persistent pain and swelling
  - Age
  - Hand dominance
  - Mechanism of injury
  - Comorbidities
  - Activity level
  - Occupation

Physical Examination

- Skin and soft-tissue swelling
- Painful and limited range of motion of wrist
  - Tenderness to deep palpation in anatomic snuffbox
  - Between extensor pollicis longus and extensor pollicis brevis muscles
  - Scaphoid shift test
    - Pain with dorsal to volar shifting of scaphoid
    - Watson test
    - Pain and dorsal scaphoid subluxation as wrist moves from ulnar to radial deviation with compression of scaphoid tuberosity
- Deformity and angulation
- Neurovascular status
- Examine finger and thumb motion to confirm tendon continuity.
- Always examine ipsilateral hand, elbow, and shoulder for associated injuries.

Imaging

- Posteroanterior view with hand in a fist and lateral view radiographs (Fig. 97-2)
  - Evaluate distal radius, ulna, and all carpal bones.
  - Evaluate lateral radiograph for perilunate dislocation (Fig. 97-3).
  - Evaluate distal radioulnar joint
- Scaphoid view
  - Evaluate scaphoid for fracture.
  - Ulnar deviation of wrist assists in fracture definition (Fig. 97-4).
- Scaphoid radial oblique view, supinated posteroanterior view
- Fracture description
  - Pattern (Fig. 97-5)
    - Horizontal oblique
    - Transverse
    - Vertical oblique
  - Stability
    - Stable, nondisplaced fracture with no step-off
    - Unstable
      - Displacement more than 1 mm
      - Scapholunate angle more than 60 degrees (Fig. 97-6)
      - Lunatocapitate angle more than 15 degrees (see Fig. 97-6)
  - Location (Fig. 97-7)
    - Tuberosity
    - Distal third

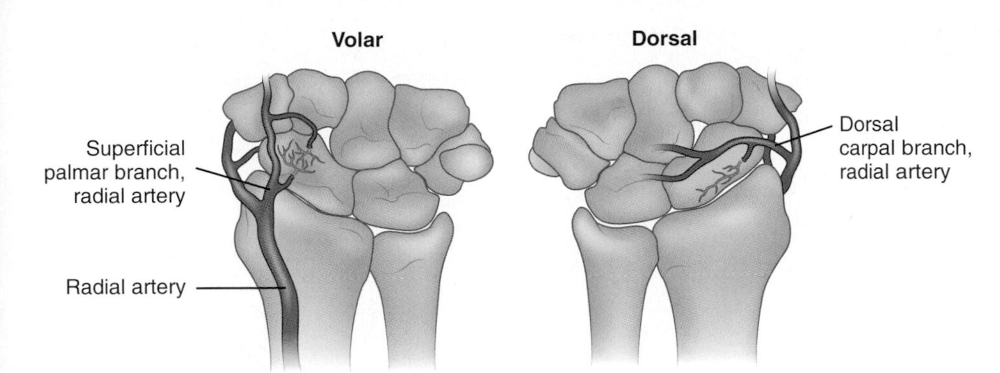

Figure 97-1 Schematic representation of the blood supply of the scaphoid. (Adapted from Green DP, Hotchkiss RN, Pederson WC, Wolfe SW [eds]: Green's Operative Hand Surgery, 5th ed. Philadelphia: Churchill Livingstone, 2005, Fig. 17-4. Copyright Elizabeth Martin.)

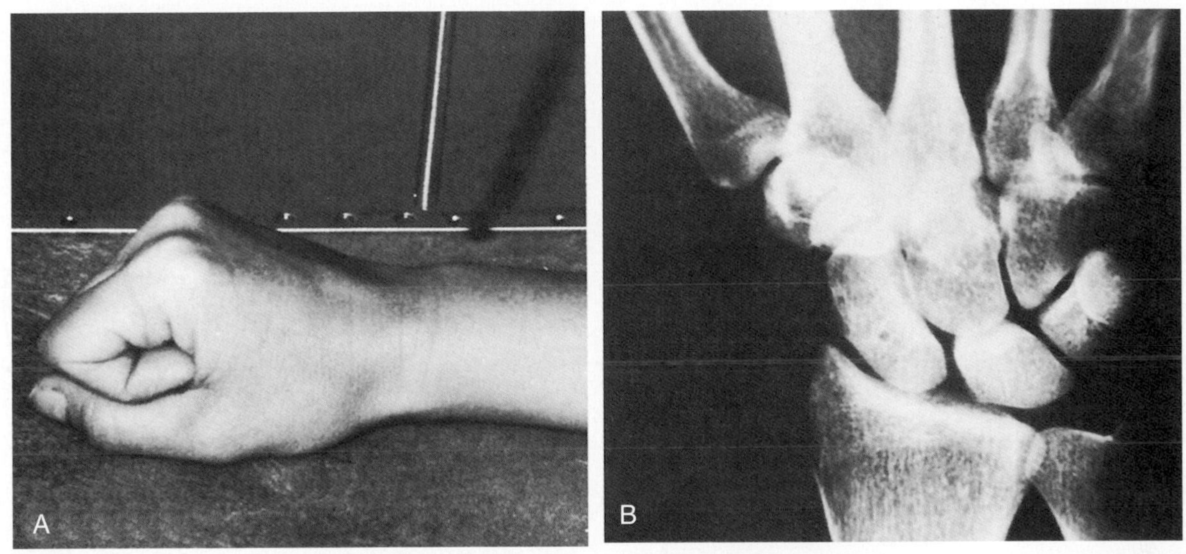

Figure 97-2 **A,** Positioning for a posteroanterior radiograph obtained with the fingers flexed into a fist. **B,** Slight dorsiflexion is produced to place the longitudinal axis of the scaphoid in a plane more nearly parallel to that of the film. (From Green DP, Hotchkiss RN, Pederson WC, Wolfe SW [eds]: Green's Operative Hand Surgery, 5th ed. Philadelphia: Churchill Livingstone, 2005, Fig. 17-5.)

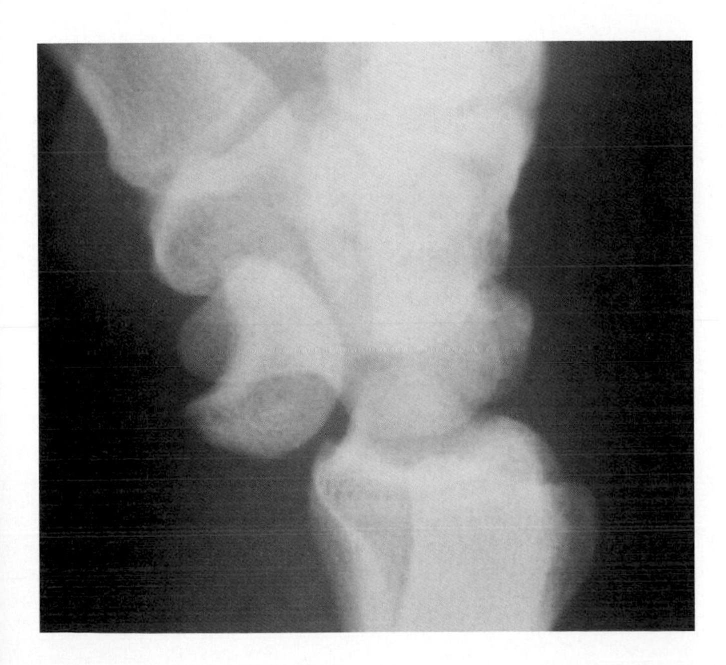

Figure 97-3 On a lateral radiograph, the lunate is displaced volarly while the capitate is articulating with the radius. (From Fractures and dislocation of the carpus. In Trumble TE [ed]: Principles of Hand Surgery and Therapy. Philadelphia: WB Saunders, 2000, Fig. 10-44.)

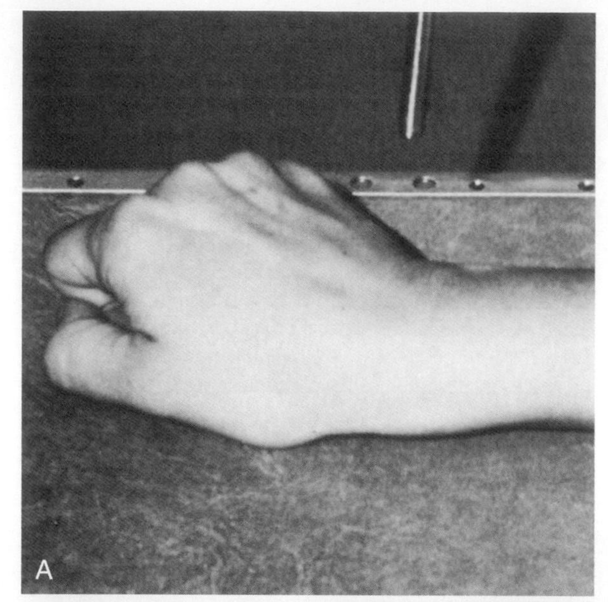

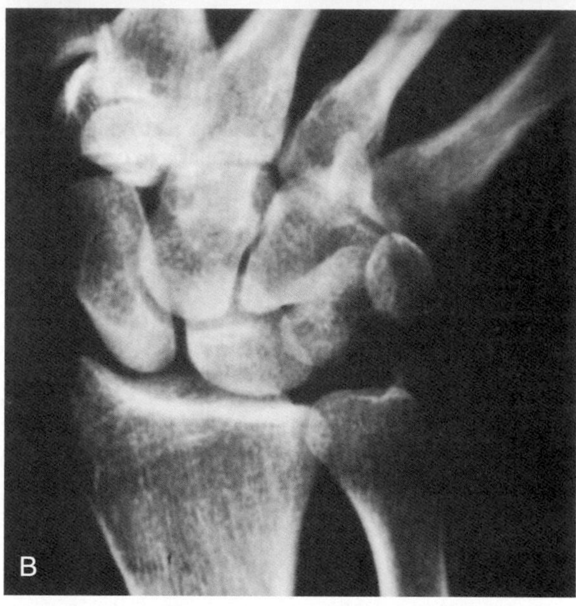

Figure 97-4 A better profile of the entire scaphoid is obtained in the posteroanterior view with the fingers flexed into a fist (**A**) and the wrist in ulnar deviation (**B**). (From Green DP, Hotchkiss RN, Pederson WC, Wolfe SW [eds]: Green's Operative Hand Surgery, 5th ed. Philadelphia: Churchill Livingstone, 2005, Fig. 17-6.)

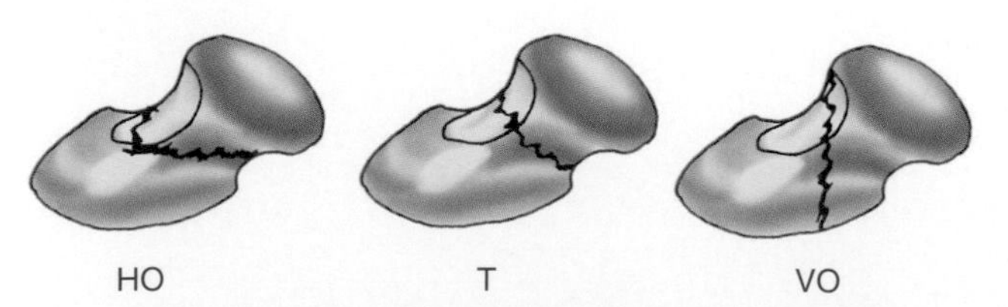

Figure 97-5 Classification of fractures of the scaphoid (Russe). HO, horizontal oblique; T, transverse; VO, vertical oblique. (Adapted from Taleisnik J: The Wrist. New York, Churchill Livingstone, 1985.© 1985, Elizabeth Roselius.)

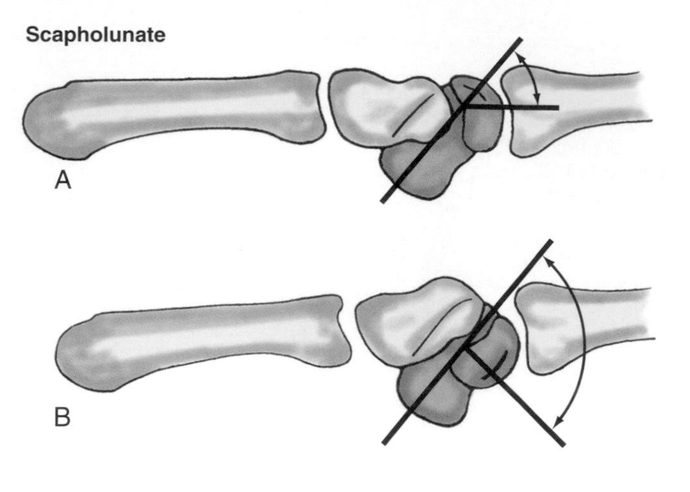

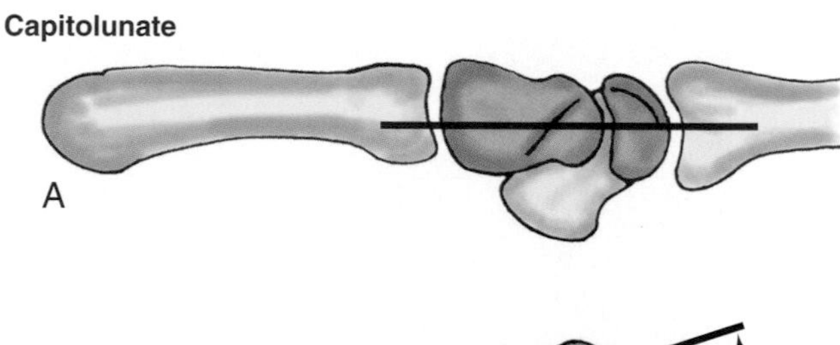

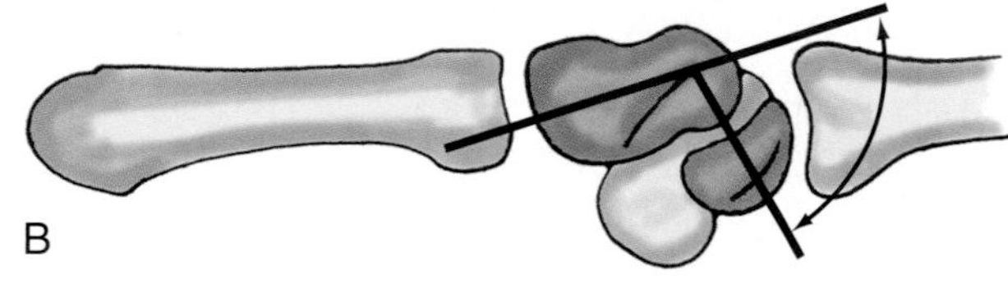

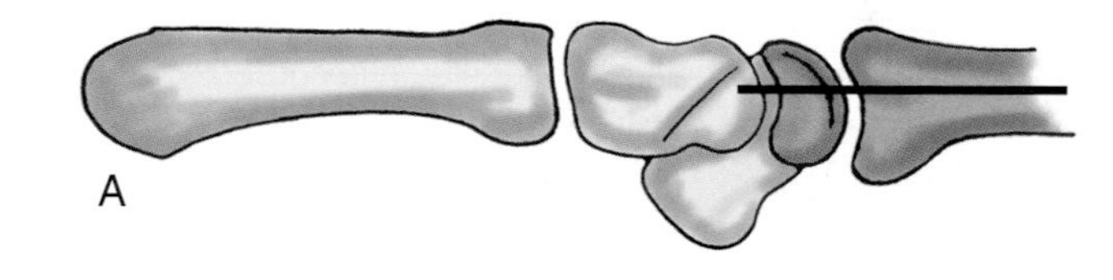

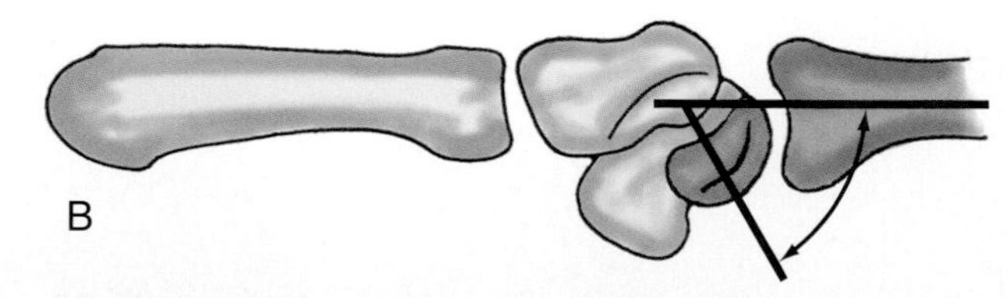

Figure 97-6 The carpal bone angles are of considerable aid in identifying carpal instability patterns. In each illustration the normal angle (**A**) is shown in comparison with the abnormal angle (**B**) seen when there is dorsal intercalary segmental carpal instability. The scapholunate angle, when greater than 80 degrees, is definitive evidence of either a scapholunate dissociation or a palmarly displaced scaphoid fracture. The capitolunate angle should theoretically be 0 degrees with the wrist in neutral, but the normal range probably extends to as much as 15 degrees. The radiolunate angle is abnormal if it exceeds 15 degrees. (Adapted from Green DP, Hotchkiss RN, Pederson WC [eds]: Green's Operative Hand Surgery, 4th ed. New York: Churchill Livingstone, 1999, Fig. 28-13.)

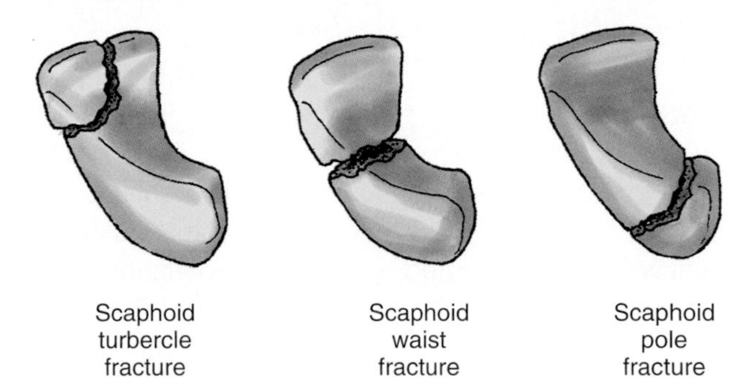

Figure 97-7 Scaphoid fractures can be simply described as involving the distal pole or tubercle, waist, or proximal pole. (Adapted from Knoll VE, Trumble TE: Scaphoid fractures and nonunions. In Trumble TE, Cornwall R, Budoff J [eds]: Core Knowledge in Orthopaedics: Hand, Elbow, and Shoulder. Philadelphia: Mosby, 2005, Fig. 8-8.)

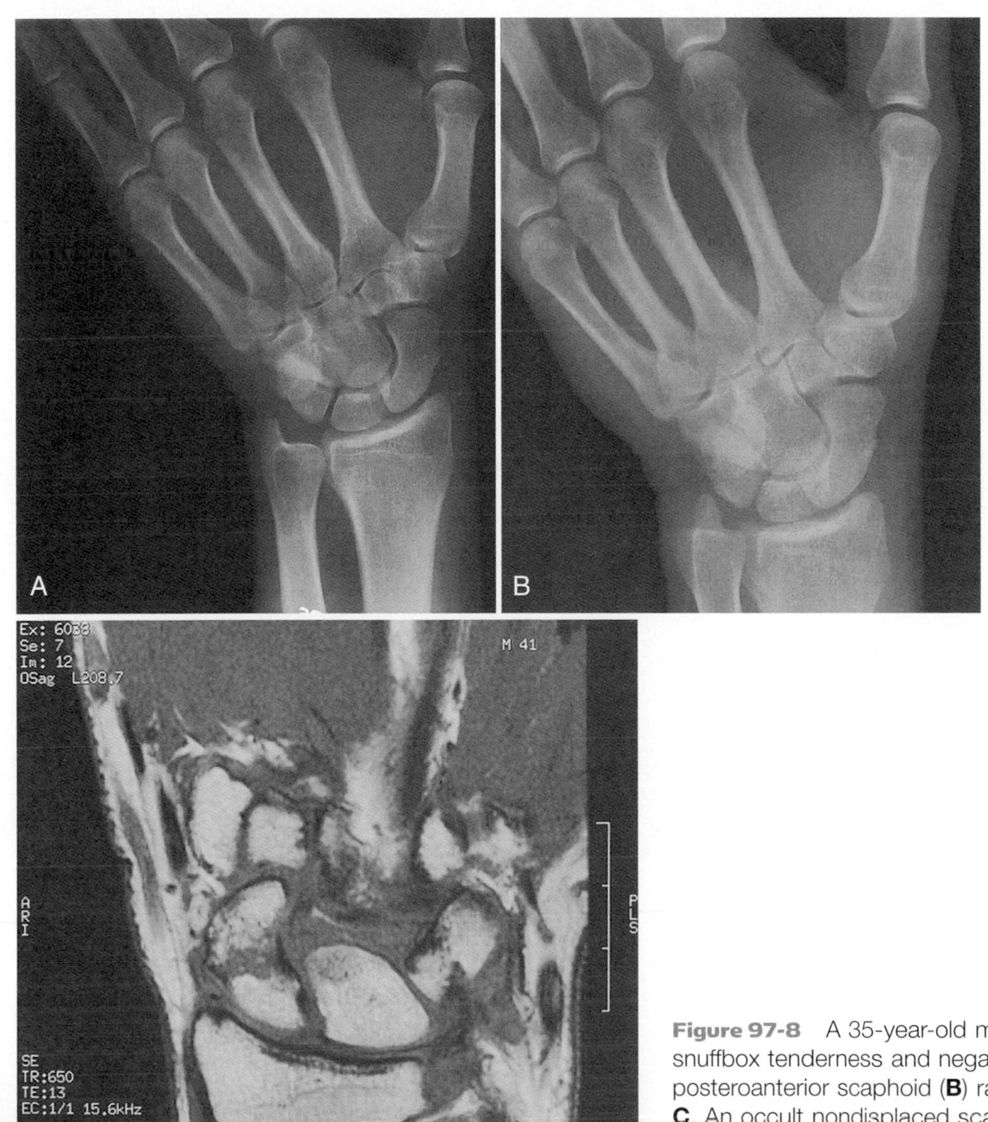

Figure 97-8 A 35-year-old man presented with persistent snuffbox tenderness and negative posteroanterior (**A**) and posteroanterior scaphoid (**B**) radiographs at 1 week post-injury. **C**, An occult nondisplaced scaphoid fracture was detected with magnetic resonance imaging. (From Green DP, Hotchkiss RN, Pederson WC, Wolfe SW [eds]: Green's Operative Hand Surgery, 5th ed. Philadelphia: Churchill Livingstone, 2005, Fig. 17-10.)

- Middle third or waist (most common)
- Proximal third

- MRI, bone scan, computed tomography (CT)
  - Initial radiographs nondiagnostic in 25% of cases
  - Studies to be used to evaluate for occult scaphoid fracture (Fig. 97-8)
- Elbow anteroposterior and lateral with any associated pain
  - Evaluate for associated injury.
  - Monteggia's fractures: proximal ulnar fracture with radial head dislocation
  - Galeazzi's fractures: radial diaphysis fracture at the junction of the middle and distal thirds with associated disruption of the distal radioulnar joint

Treatment

- At diagnosis
  - Radiographs to define injury
  - Thumb spica splint for all suspected and defined injuries
  - Injury with positive examination but normal radiographs
    - Immobilize for 12 to 14 days
    - Repeat radiographs if still symptomatic
    - If negative, consider MRI, CT, or bone scan, with MRI being the most diagnostic (see Fig. 97-8)
  - If acute diagnosis necessary (athlete), consider MRI immediately to detect occult fractures
- Nonoperative
  - Stable, nondisplaced fractures
    - Short arm thumb spica cast with wrist in neutral position for 6 to 8 weeks
    - Then short arm spica cast for an additional 4 to 6 weeks until radiographic evidence of union
    - Follow up every 3 months for 1 year to confirm union.
  - Nonoperative union rates, based on blood supply
    - Distal third: 100% union
    - Middle third: 80% to 90% union
    - Proximal third: 60% to 70% union
  - Expected time to union
    - Tuberosity: 6 weeks
    - Distal third: 6 to 8 weeks
    - Middle third: 8 to 12 weeks
    - Proximal third: 12 to 24 weeks
- Operative
  - Unstable fractures with displacement
  - Proximal pole fractures
  - Nonunion after attempting nonoperative treatment
  - Fractures associated with other injuries (perilunate dislocation)
  - Open reduction with internal fixation
    - Compression screw (Fig. 97-9)
    - Open versus percutaneous techniques
    - With or without bone graft
    - Union rate of 93% to 97%
    - Begin aggressive range of motion when radiographic union evident

Complications

- Delayed union, nonunion, and malunion are seen more often with proximal fractures.
- May require delayed open reduction and internal fixation with bone graft
- Osteonecrosis is more common with proximal pole fractures.
- Early wrist osteoarthritis is seen with untreated nonunion or malunion.

When to Refer

- All scaphoid fractures should be referred to an orthopaedic surgeon or hand specialist.
- Delay in diagnosis and treatment results in a high rate of nonunion and poor functional outcome.

Patient Instructions

- Keep the splint clean and dry.
- Elevate the arm above the heart for 48 hours to decrease swelling and pain.
- Take pain medications as prescribed.
- Follow up with an orthopaedist as instructed.
- Good results with cast immobilization for tuberosity and distal third fractures
- Surgery is commonly performed for middle and proximal third fractures to enhance union rates.
- Increased risk of osteonecrosis with proximal third fractures; early surgery is recommended to enhance healing rates (even in nondisplaced fractures)

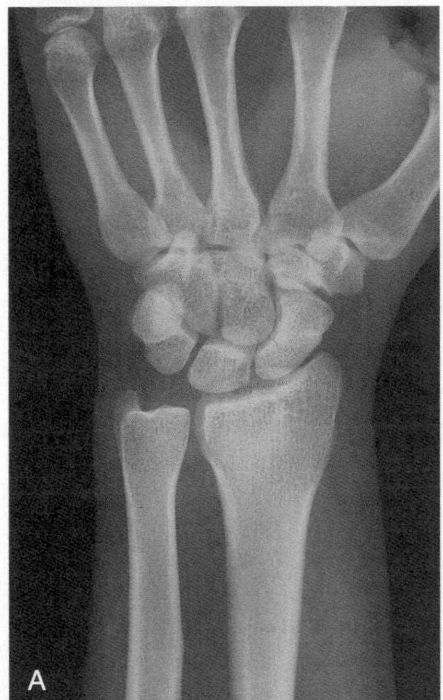

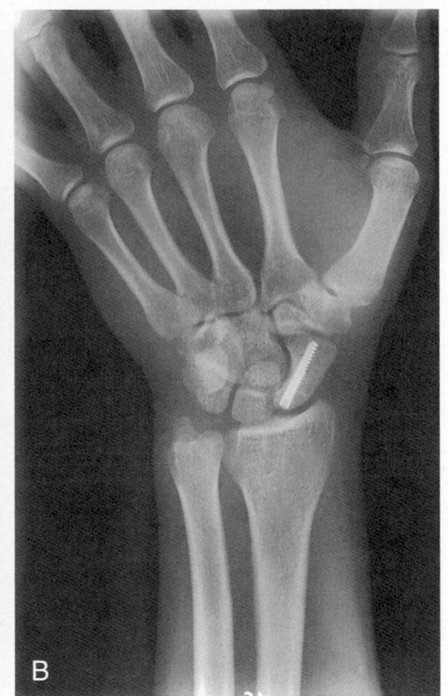

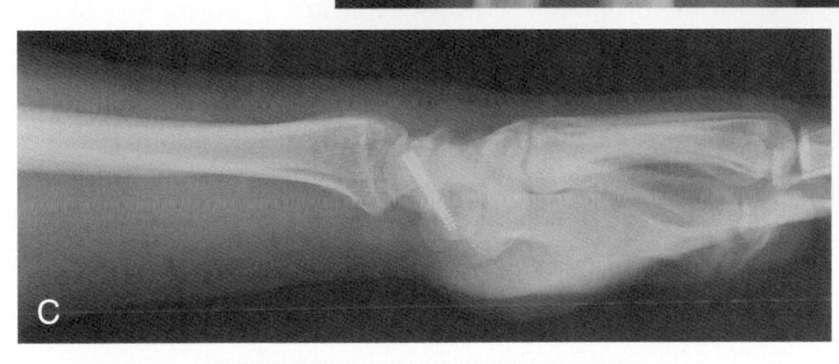

Figure 97-9 **A**, A 24-year-old football player suffered a nondisplaced scaphoid fracture in mid-season. Posteroanterior scaphoid (**B**) and lateral (**C**) radiographs showing a compression screw placed percutaneously. The patient returned to practice at 6 weeks. (From Green DP, Hotchkiss RN, Pederson WC, Wolfe SW [eds]: Green's Operative Hand Surgery, 5th ed. Philadelphia: Churchill Livingstone, 2005, Fig. 17-14.)

Suggested Reading

- Amadio PC, Moran SL: Fractures of the carpal bones. In Green DP, Hotchkiss RN, Pederson WC, Wolfe SW (eds): Green's Operative Hand Surgery, 5th ed. Philadelphia: Churchill Livingstone, 2005, pp 711–768.
- Gaebler C: Fractures and dislocations of the carpus. In Bucholz RW, Heckman JD, Court-Brown C (eds): Rockwood and Green's Fractures in Adults, 6th ed. Philadelphia: Lippincott Williams & Wilkins, 2006, pp 857–908.
- Knoll VD, Trumble TE: Scaphoid fractures and nonunions. In Trumble TE, Budoff JE, Cornwall R (eds): Hand, Elbow, and Shoulder: Core Knowledge in Orthopaedics. Philadelphia: Mosby, 2006, pp 116–131.
- Koval KJ, Zuckerman JD: Handbook of Fractures, 3rd ed. Philadelphia: Lippincott Williams & Wilkins, 2006, pp 237–256.

Chapter 98 Thumb Fractures

Sara D. Rynders and A. Bobby Chhabra

ICD-9 CODE
815.01 *Thumb Metacarpal Base Fracture, Closed*

Key Concepts

- Injuries to the thumb commonly result from a fall, an industrial accident, or an athletic injury.
- The most common thumb fracture is Bennett's fracture.
- Thumb metacarpal fractures are prone to displacement due to the deforming forces created by tendon attachments (Fig. 98-1).
- The key to an optimal outcome is a good reduction; all intra-articular fractures should be reduced with less than 1 mm step-off.

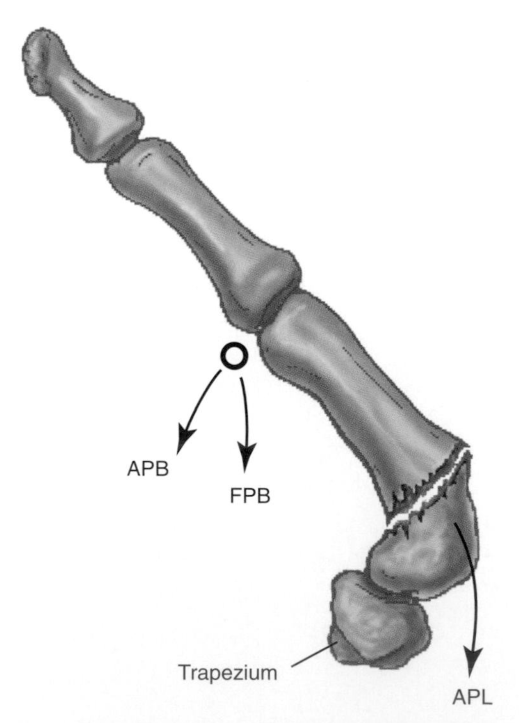

Figure 98-1 Thumb anatomy. Extensor tendon attachments. AP, anteroposterior; APB, abductor pollicis brevis; APL, abductor pollicis longus; FPB, flexor pollicis brevis.

- Improperly treated Bennett's or Rolando's fractures can result in traumatic arthritis of the thumb carpometacarpal joint and cause severe impairment of thumb function.

Types of Fractures

- Bennett's fracture (Fig. 98-2)
  - Intra-articular oblique fracture through the ulnar-volar metacarpal base; ulnar fracture fragment (Bennett fragment) varies in size and remains attached to the trapezium by the anterior oblique ligament.
  - There is subsequent proximal and radial subluxation of the remainder of the metacarpal base from

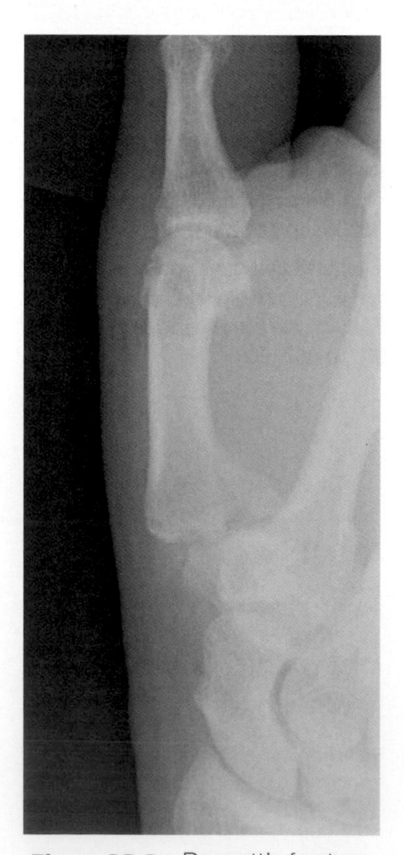

Figure 98-2 Bennett's fracture.

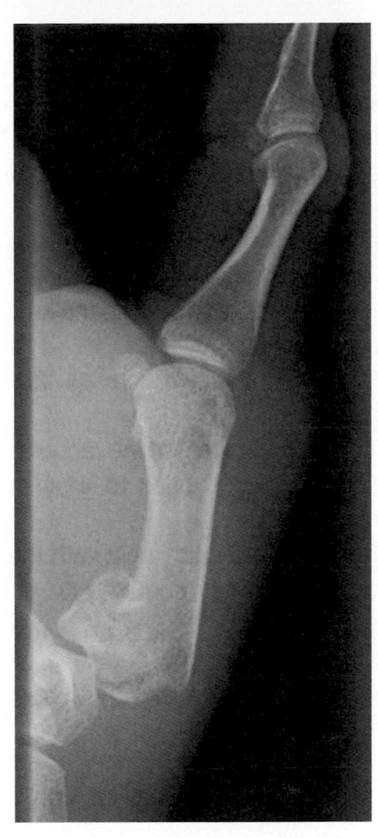

Figure 98-3 Rolando's fracture.

the carpometacarpal joint due to the pull of the abductor pollicis longus tendon, which inserts on the radial side of the metacarpal base.
  - All require surgical fixation.
- Rolando's fracture (Fig. 98-3)
  - Intra-articular Y- or T-shaped fracture with both a radial fragment and an ulnar fragment
  - Also includes comminuted intra-articular base fractures
  - All require surgical fixation.
- Extra-articular metacarpal shaft fractures (Fig. 98-4)
  - Uncommon and usually located transversely or obliquely just above the metacarpal base
  - This fracture has a tendency to dorsally angulate due to the forces of the various tendon attachments on the thumb. As much as 20 degrees of angulation may be accepted because the multiplanar motion of the thumb carpometacarpal joint is able to compensate.

History

- Patient may report a history of a fall or an injury to the thumb or a hyperflexion, hyperextension, or hyperabduction type of mechanism.

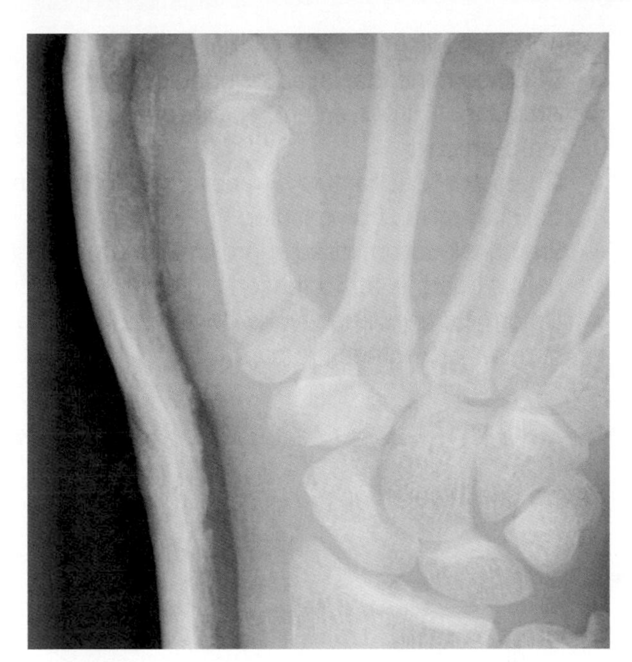

Figure 98-4 Extra-articular metacarpal fracture.

- Patient may report pain, edema, and loss of thumb range of motion.

Physical Examination

- Inspection may reveal edema or a deformity of the thumb or its metacarpal. Identify any open injuries.
- The fracture site will be exquisitely tender to palpation, and crepitus or gross instability may be present.
- Assess the patient's active range of motion in all planes and check for rotational deformity.
- Assess ligamentous stability by applying varus and valgus stress to all joints (this should be performed only after radiographs have confirmed no evidence of a ligament avulsion fracture).
- Sensation should be checked over the radial and ulnar borders of the thumb and any deficits should be noted.
- Capillary refill should be tested; normal is less than 2 seconds.
- Always assess for secondary injuries with a thorough wrist and hand examination. Be sure to palpate the anatomic snuffbox to assess for scaphoid tenderness, which may indicate a scaphoid fracture.

Imaging

- Anteroposterior, lateral, and oblique views of the thumb should be obtained, and the thumb carpometacarpal joint should be included in the views.

- Note the following
  - Displacement: displaced or nondisplaced
  - Articular involvement: intra-articular or extra-articular
  - Character of fracture: transverse, longitudinal, oblique, spiral, comminuted
  - Fracture location: distal or proximal phalanx, metacarpal head, shaft, or base
  - Deformity: angulation (volar/dorsal, radially/ulnarly, number of degrees), rotation

Differential Diagnosis

- Please see Table 98-1.

Treatment

- Bennett's fracture
  - Fracture is considered unstable
  - Place patient in a thumb spica splint and refer to a hand specialist to be seen within 7 days of injury.
  - Surgery is necessary for these fractures.

TABLE 98-1 *Differential Diagnosis*

Condition	Differentiating Feature
Thumb carpometacarpal osteoarthritis (see Chapter 84)	No history of injury; tenderness to palpation at the thumb carpometacarpal joint; positive carpometacarpal grind test; radiographs: arthritis changes evident at thumb carpometacarpal joint
de Quervain's tenosynovitis (see Chapter 80)	Tenderness to palpation over first extensor compartment; positive Finkelstein's sign; negative radiographs
Trigger finger (see Chapter 80)	Tenderness to palpation over thumb A1 pulley; palpable tender nodule or evidence of triggering at A1 pulley; negative radiographs
Ulnar collateral or radial collateral ligament sprain (see Chapter 85)	Tenderness to palpation over ulnar collateral or radial collateral ligament at thumb metacarpophalangeal joint; laxity of metacarpophalangeal joint with varus or valgus stress in flexion or extension; radiographs may reveal a small avulsion fracture
Scaphoid fracture (see Chapter 97)	Tenderness to palpation at anatomic snuffbox; scaphoid tubercle tenderness; radiographs may reveal a scaphoid fracture

- Rolando's fracture
  - Fracture is considered unstable
  - Place in a thumb spica splint and refer to a hand specialist to be seen within 7 days of injury.
  - Surgery is necessary for these fractures.
- Extra-articular base fractures
  - At diagnosis
    - — Closed reduction under a local block should be attempted to minimize the amount of dorsal angulation.
    - — May accept as much as 20 degrees of angulation
    - — A thumb spica splint should be applied and worn for 1 week to allow the edema to subside.
    - — Then a thumb spica cast with the interphalangeal joint free should be applied for 3 weeks.
    - — Repeat radiographs once the cast has been applied to ensure that the fracture has maintained alignment.
  - Later
    - — After 3 weeks of cast immobilization, repeat radiographs. If the fracture shows evidence of healing, transition the patient into a removable thumb spica splint and begin range of motion therapy.

When to Refer

- More than 20 degrees of angulation
- More than 2 mm of shortening
- Rotation
- Open fracture

Prognosis

- All intra-articular fractures are at risk of developing traumatic arthritis. This risk is minimized by adequate articular reduction with a step-off of less than 1 mm.

Patient Instructions

- Patients may require a referral to a hand therapist to restore thumb range of motion after cast immobilization or surgery.
- If a fracture requires surgical treatment, there are several options that the surgeon may recommend including closed reduction and percutaneous pinning, open reduction and internal fixation, or external fixation.

Considerations in Special Populations

- Athletes are prone to thumb injuries and should be referred to a hand specialist for early intervention and return to play.
- Manual laborers are also prone to thumb injuries. If adequate fracture reduction is not obtained, there may be a significant impact on their ability to perform their job duties.

Suggested Reading

- Calandruccio JH, Jobe MT: Fractures, dislocations, and ligamentous injuries. In Canale ST, Beaty JH (eds): Campbell's Operative Orthopaedics, Vol. 4, 11th ed. Philadelphia: Mosby, 2008, pp 3921–3940.
- Henry M: Fractures and dislocations of the hand. In Bucholz RW, Heckman JD (eds): Rockwood and Green's Fractures in Adults, Vol. 1, 5th ed. Philadelphia: Lippincott Williams & Wilkins, 2001, pp 726–732.
- Laub DR Jr, Priano SV: Hand, fracture and dislocations: Thumb. E-medicine. Available at: www.emedicine.com/plastic/topic513.htm. Accessed March 12, 2009.
- Rettig AC: Athletic injuries of the wrist and hand: Part II: Overuse injuries of the wrist and traumatic injuries to the hand. Am J Sports Med 2004;2:262.
- Soyer AD: Fractures of the base of the first metacarpal: Current treatment options. J Am Acad Orthop Surg 1999;7:403–412.
- Stern PJ: Fractures of the metacarpals and phalanges. In Green DP, Hotchkiss RN, Pederson WC, Wolfe SW (eds): Green's Operative Hand Surgery, Vol. 1, 5th ed. Philadelphia: Churchill Livingstone, 2005, pp 330–339.

Chapter 99 Metacarpal Fractures

Trevor Starnes and A. Bobby Chhabra

ICD-9 CODES
815.0 *Fracture of Metacarpal Bone(s), Closed*
815.1 *Fracture of Metacarpal Bone(s), Open*
815.02 *Base of the Metacarpal Bone(s)*
815.03 *Shaft of the Metacarpal Bone(s)*
815.04 *Neck of the Metacarpal Bone(s)*

Key Concepts

- Along with phalangeal fractures, most common fracture in upper extremity
- "Hand fractures can be complicated by deformity from no treatment, stiffness from overtreatment, and both deformity and stiffness from poor treatment." (Swanson)
- Twenty-seven percent of finger fractures are treated inappropriately in the emergency department.
  - Inaccurate reduction
  - Inappropriate splinting

History

- Important to obtain the following information
  - Age
  - Hand dominance
  - Mechanism of injury
  - Comorbidities
  - Occupation

Physical Examination

- Skin and soft-tissue swelling
- Painful and limited range of motion
- Neurovascular status
  - Capillary refill less than 2 seconds
  - Two-point discrimination
- Rotational and angulation deformity
  - Grip to evaluate rotation (Fig. 99-1)
- Always examine the ipsilateral hand, elbow, and shoulder for associated injuries.
- "Fight bite:" curved laceration over metacarpophalangeal joint = open fracture or open joint and should be thoroughly irrigated (Fig. 99-2)

Imaging

- Posteroanterior, lateral, and oblique radiographs of the affected digit
- Description of fracture
  - Open versus closed
  - Bone involved and location within bone
  - Displacement and angulation
  - Comminution
  - Intra-articular versus extra-articular

Differential Diagnosis

- Metacarpal head fracture (Fig. 99-3)
  - Axial loading or direct trauma
  - Often intra-articular
- Metacarpal neck fracture (Fig. 99-4)
  - Boxer's fracture
  - Often involves ring and small fingers
- Metacarpal shaft fracture (Fig. 99-5)
  - Transverse: often apex dorsal angulation
  - Oblique or spiral: rotational malalignment
  - Comminuted: shortening
- Metacarpal base fracture (Fig. 99-6)
  - Rare injuries in index and long fingers
  - Intra-articular fracture of ring or small finger
    - — Reverse Bennett's fracture: fracture dislocation of small finger metacarpal: hamate joint
- Metacarpophalangeal joint dislocations (Fig. 99-7)
  - Dorsal dislocation
    - — More common
    - — Usually involve thumb and index finger
    - — Simple (reducible) or complex (irreducible)
  - Volar dislocation
    - — Less common
    - — Usually complex (irreducible)

Treatment

- Metacarpal head
  - Radiographs to define injury
  - Closed reduction and splinting
    - — Require anatomic reduction to establish joint congruity

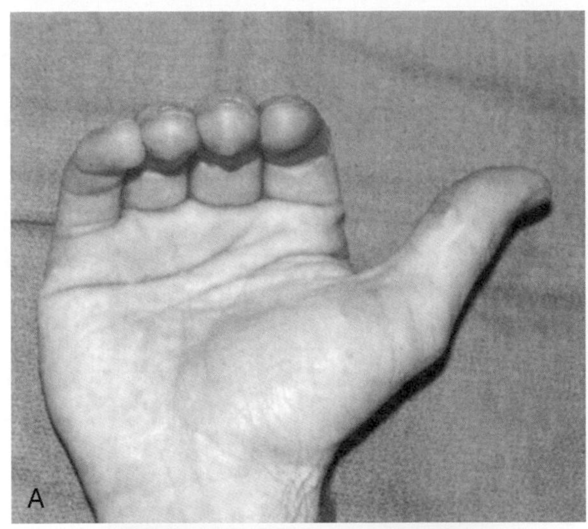

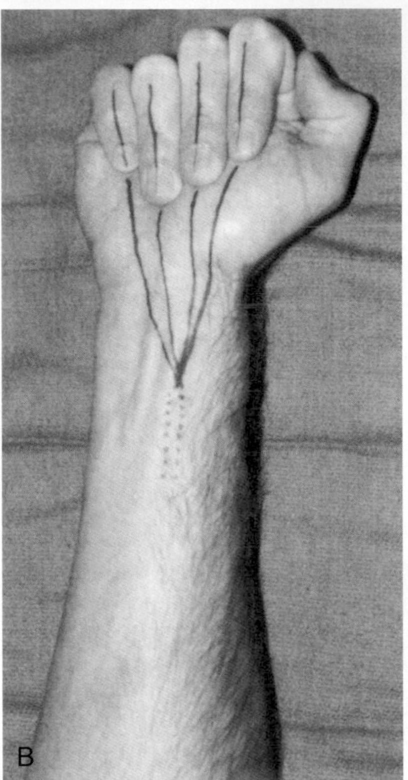

Figure 99-1 **A**, Evaluation of rotational discrepancy in the digits has been described to include nail plate alignment, which is rather inaccurate. **B**, Viewing axially along the segment of the ray in question to evaluate the parallelism of the next digital segment is most accurate. When the digits are flexed, both metacarpophalangeal and proximal interphalangeal joints align to converge at a point overlying the flexor carpi radialis tendon above the level of the wrist. (From Bucholz RW, Heckman JD, Court-Brown C [eds]: Rockwood and Green's Fractures in Adults, 6th ed. Philadelphia: Lippincott Williams & Wilkins, 2006, Fig. 24-2.)

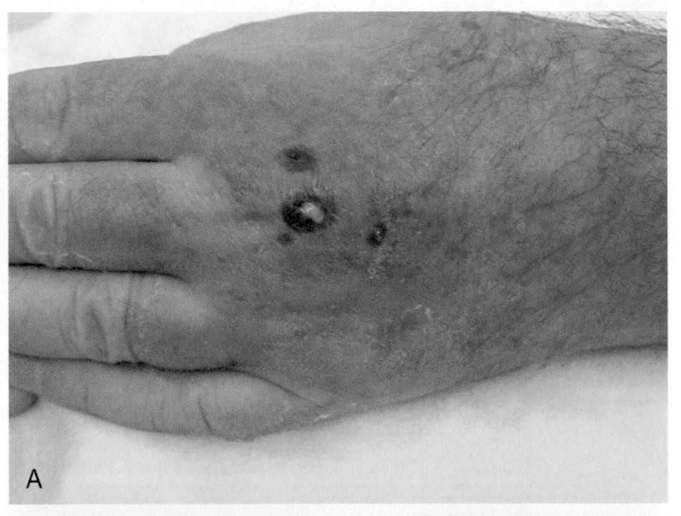

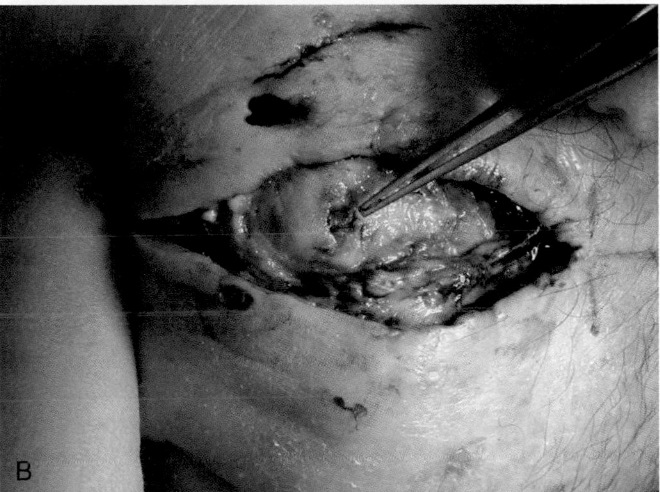

Figure 99-2 **A**, Fight bite with laceration over metacarpophalangeal joint. **B**, Open irrigation and débridement demonstrate tooth indentation in bone.

    - Splint in intrinsic plus position (Fig. 99-8)
    - Early range of motion
  - Operative indications
    - Unstable fractures or if more than 1 mm step-off
    - Fight bite: open fracture with high incidence of infection; treat with antibiotics to cover human mouth organisms
    - Open reduction and internal fixation versus closed reduction and percutaneous pinning
- Metacarpal neck
  - Radiographs to define injury
    - Often volar comminution with dorsal angulation
  - Closed reduction and splinting in intrinsic plus position: Jahss maneuver (Fig. 99-9)
  - Acceptable reduction

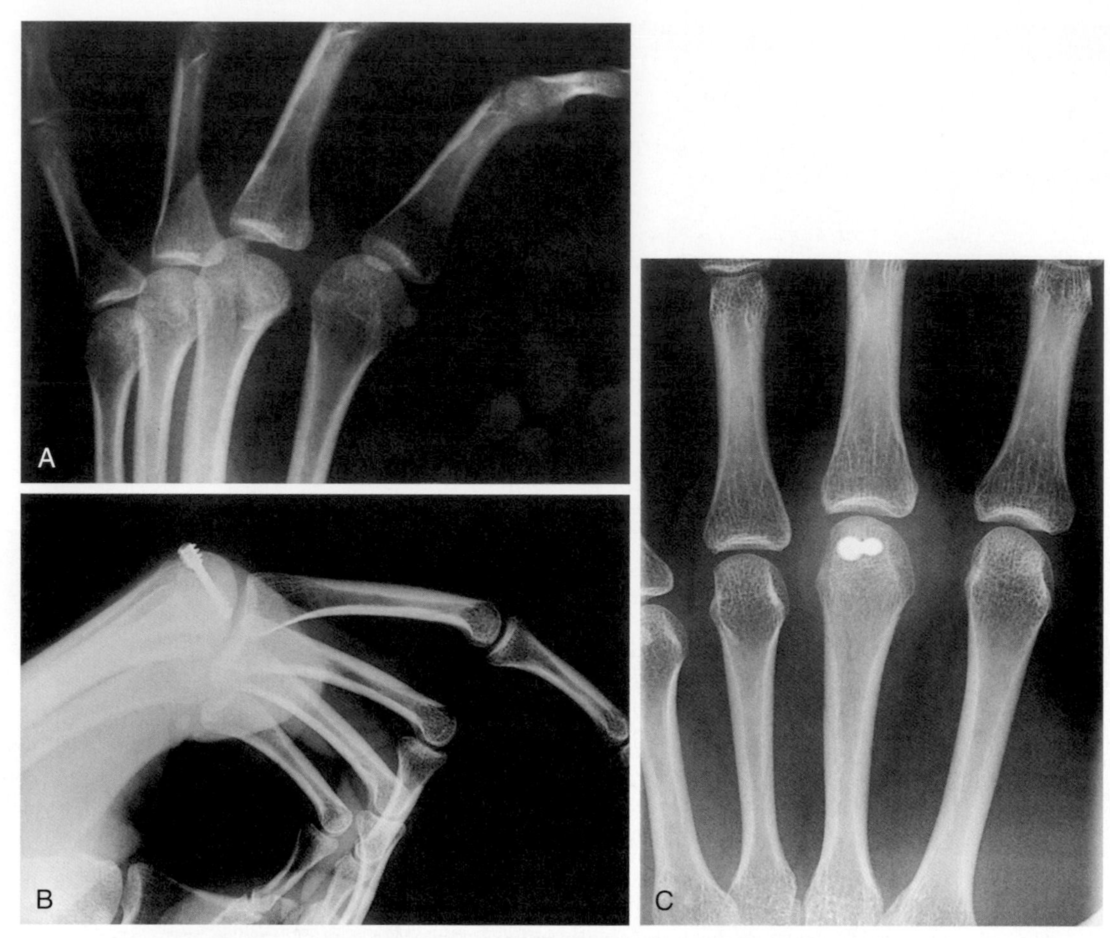

Figure 99-3 **A**, Displaced intra-articular sagittal slice fracture of the middle finger metacarpal head. Postoperative posteroanterior (**B**) and lateral (**C**) views show anatomic reduction and fixation with a Herbert screw. Full metacarpophalangeal mobility was restored. (From Green DP, Hotchkiss RN, Pederson WC, Wolfe SW [eds]: Green's Operative Hand Surgery, 5th ed. Philadelphia: Churchill Livingstone, 2005, Fig. 8-2.)

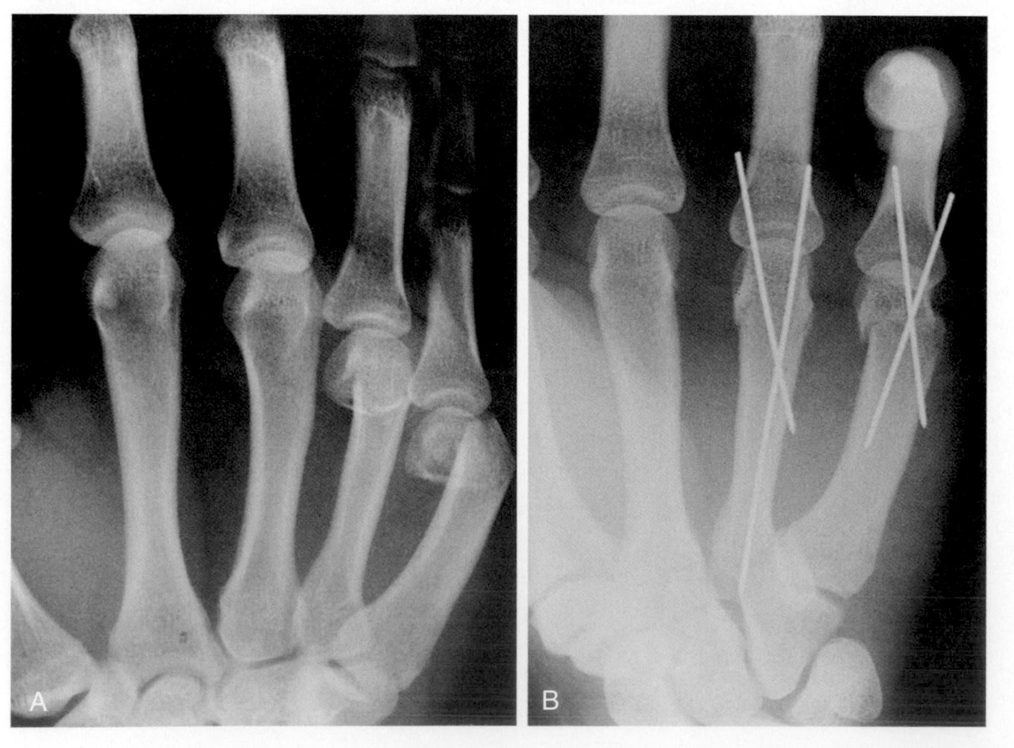

Figure 99-4 **A**, Severely displaced neck fractures of the ring and small finger metacarpals. **B**, Closed reduction using the Jahss maneuver and percutaneous crossed pins. (From Green DP, Hotchkiss RN, Pederson WC, Wolfe SW [eds]: Green's Operative Hand Surgery, 5th ed. Philadelphia: Churchill Livingstone, 2005, Fig. 8-6.)

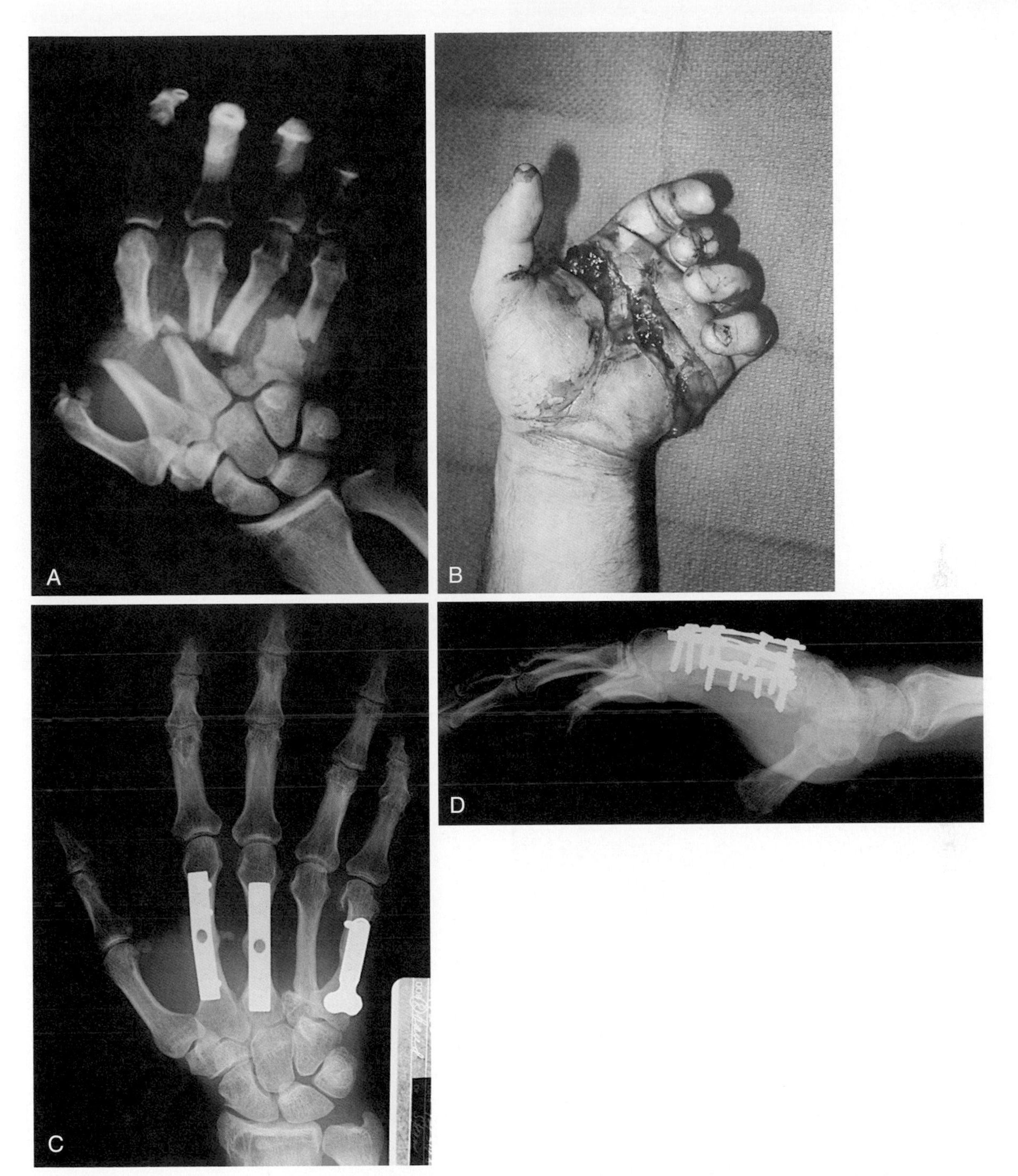

Figure 99-5 Plate fixation for metacarpal shaft fractures. **A**, Shaft fractures of all four metacarpals. **B**, The fractures were open and revascularization was required. **C**, Anteroposterior radiograph showing healed fractures. Plate fixation provided a stable framework for microvascular repairs. **D**, Lateral view. (From Green DP, Hotchkiss RN, Pederson WC, Wolfe SW [eds]: Green's Operative Hand Surgery, 5th ed. Philadelphia: Churchill Livingstone, 2005, Fig. 8-14.)

  - — Index and long fingers: less than 15 degrees of angulation
  - — Ring and small fingers: less than 45 degrees of angulation
- Unstable fractures require open reduction and internal fixation versus closed reduction and percutaneous pinning.

- Metacarpal shaft
  - Radiographs to define injury
  - Closed reduction and splinting in intrinsic plus position
  - Operative indications
    - — Open fractures
    - — Multiple metacarpal fractures

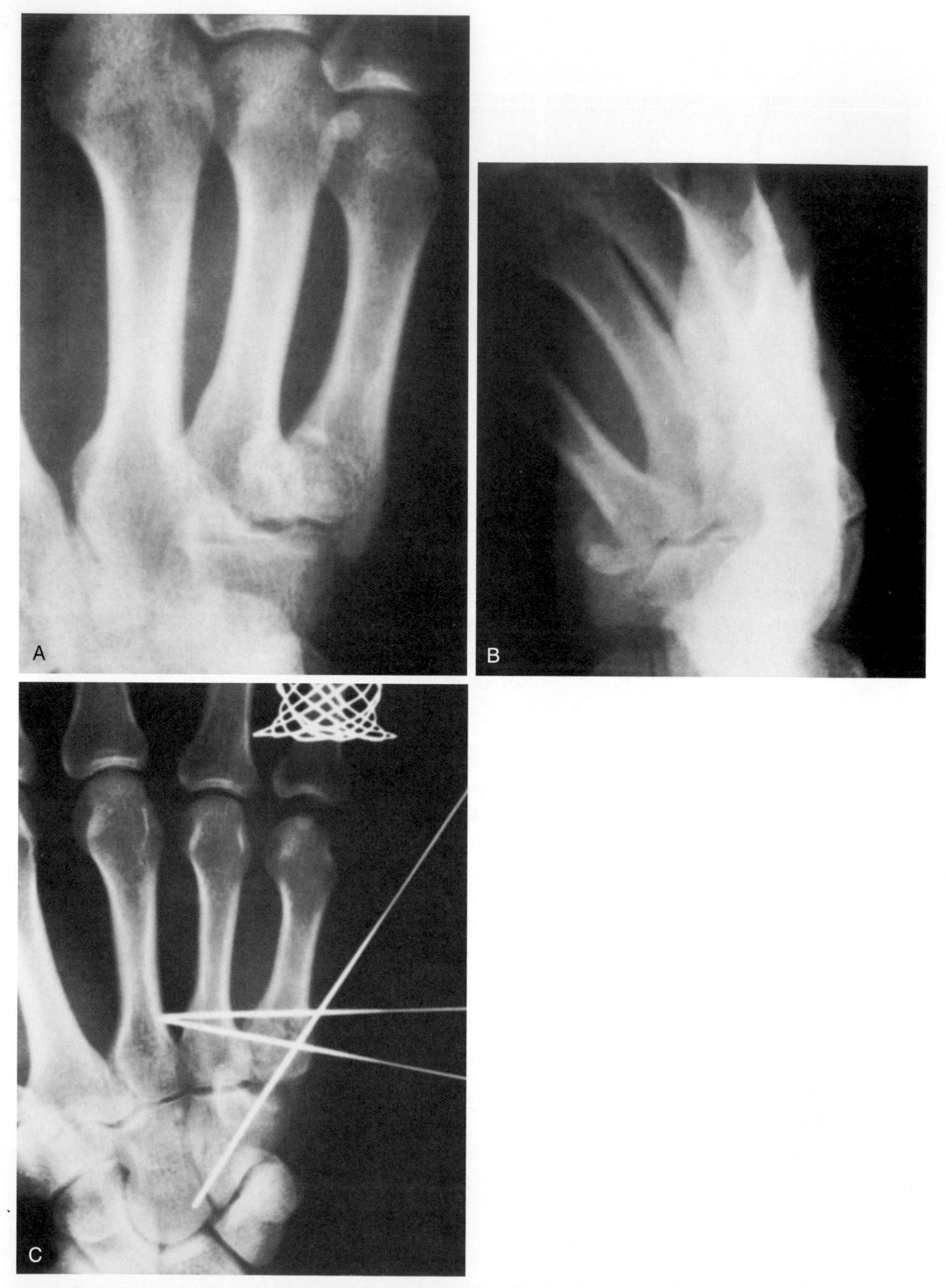

Figure 99-6 **A**, An intra-articular fracture of the base of the fifth metacarpal with proximal and dorsal subluxation of the carpometacarpal joint. **B**, An oblique view taken with the hand pronated 30 degrees from its fully supinated position shows the extent of the intra-articular injury. **C**, Reduction was obtained by longitudinal traction and lateral pressure on the displaced bone. Firm fixation with a transarticular pin as well as transfixation pins into the adjacent metacarpal allowed early motion. (From Green DP, Hotchkiss RN, Pederson WC, Wolfe SW [eds]: Green's Operative Hand Surgery, 5th ed. Philadelphia: Churchill Livingstone, 2005, Fig. 8-18.)

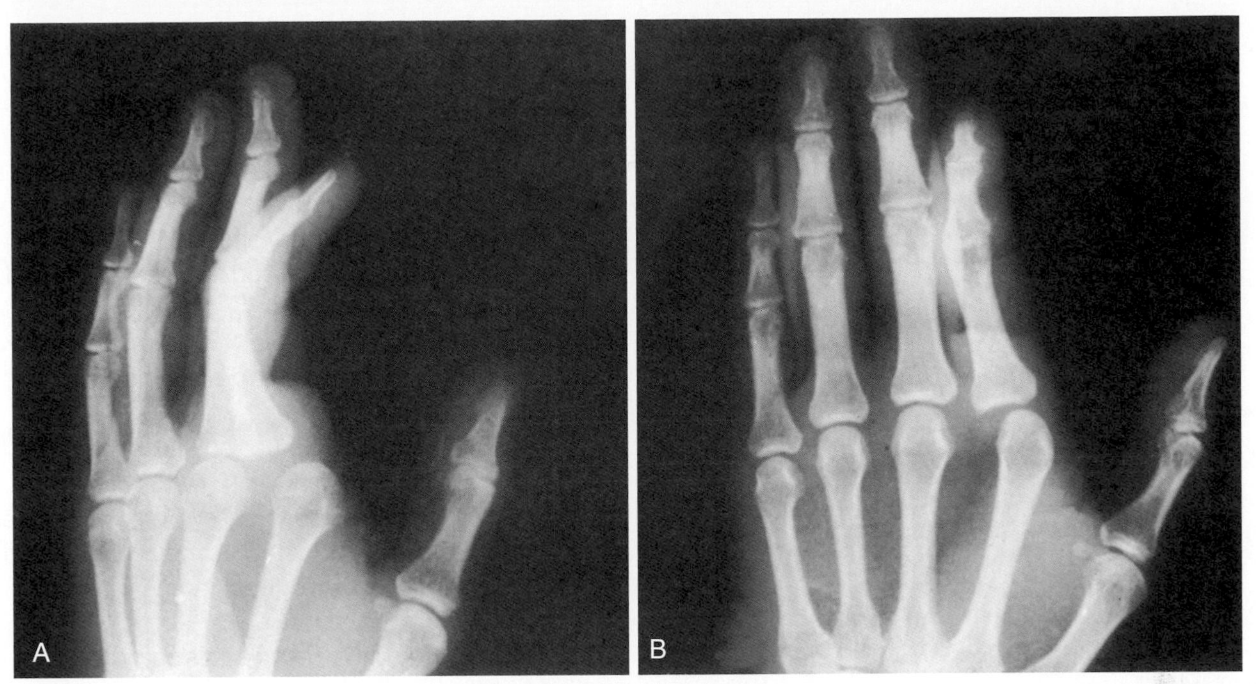

Figure 99-7 Radiographs of a dorsal irreducible (complex) dislocation. **A,** An oblique view shows the dorsal dislocation and widened joint space caused by interposition of the volar plate. **B**, The ulnar shift of the proximal phalanx suggests rupture of the radial collateral ligament. (From Green DP, Hotchkiss RN, Pederson WC, Wolfe SW [eds]: Green's Operative Hand Surgery, 5th ed. Philadelphia: Churchill Livingstone, 2005, Fig. 9-13.)

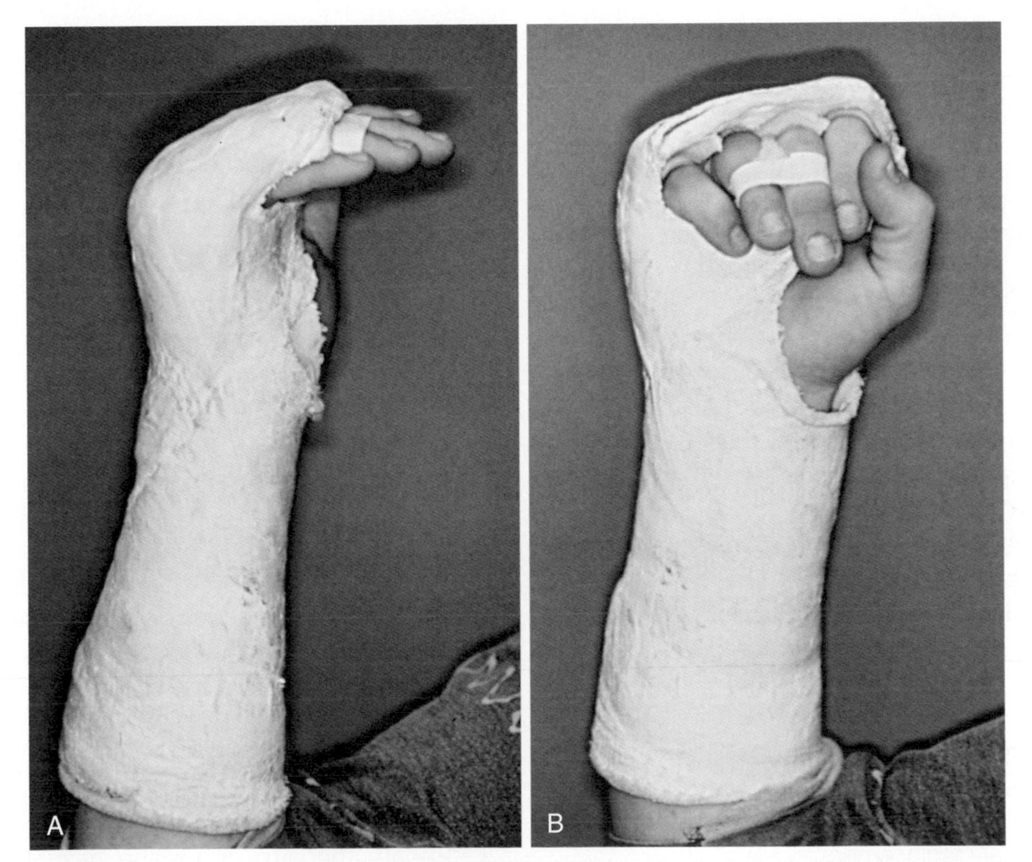

Figure 99-8 Clam-digger cast for a metacarpal shaft fracture. The wrist is extended 30 degrees, the metacarpophalangeal joints are flexed 80 to 90 degrees, and the interphalangeal joints are extended. Active range of motion is encouraged, and supplemental buddy taping can help control rotation. (From Green DP, Hotchkiss RN, Pederson WC, Wolfe SW [eds]: Green's Operative Hand Surgery, 5th ed. Philadelphia: Churchill Livingstone, 2005, Fig. 8-9.)

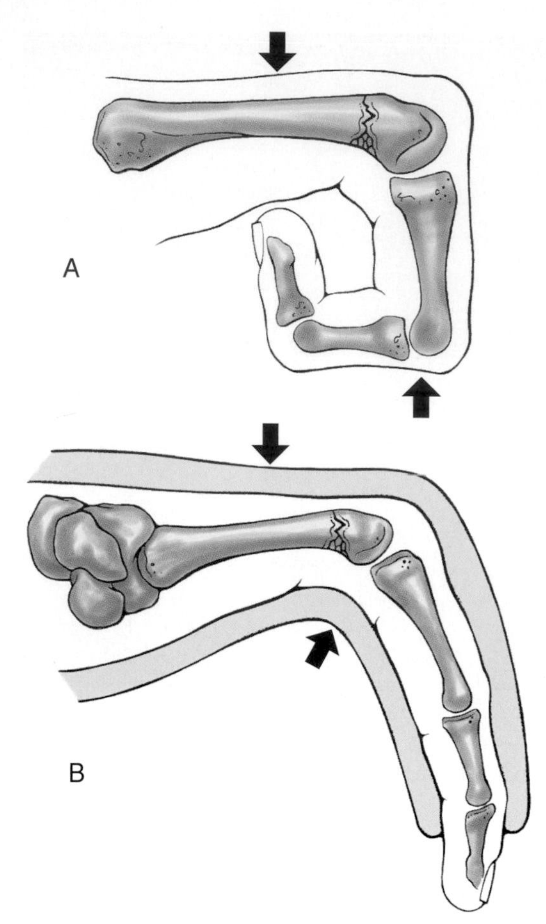

Figure 99-9 **A**, The Jahss maneuver for reduction of a metacarpal neck fracture. *Arrows* indicate the direction of pressure application for fracture reduction. **B**, After reduction, the fingers are held in an intrinsic-plus (safe) position in an ulnar gutter splint with molding as indicated by *arrows*. (Adapted from Green DP, Hotchkiss RN, Pederson WC, Wolfe SW [eds]: Green's Operative Hand Surgery, 5th ed. Philadelphia: Churchill Livingstone, 2005, Fig. 8-5.)

- — Associated neurovascular or tendon injuries
- — Failure of attempted closed reduction
- — Rotational deformity more than 10 degrees
- — Dorsal angulation more than 10 degrees for index and long fingers
- — Dorsal angulation more than 20 degrees for ring and small fingers
- Open reduction and internal fixation with plate and screws or closed reduction and percutaneous pinning
- Metacarpal base
  - Radiographs to define injury
  - Closed reduction and splinting
    - — Base of the index, long, and ring fingers; minimal displacement
    - — Associated with ligament avulsion
    - — Early range of motion
  - Reverse Bennett's fracture
    - — Metacarpal displaced by pull of extensor carpi ulnaris and flexor carpi ulnaris muscles
    - — Radiograph of hand in 30 degrees of pronation
    - — Often requires open reduction and internal fixation or closed reduction and percutaneous pinning to restore articular surface
    - — A fracture diagnosed late can be treated conservatively with the option for fusion of the carpometacarpal joint if pain continues.
- Metacarpophalangeal joint dislocations
  - Dorsal dislocation
    - — Reducible when phalanx is still in contact with metacarpal head
    - — Dorsal pressure to base of proximal phalanx to maintain contact with metacarpal head and prevent volar plate entrapment
    - — Traction is contraindicated.
    - — Irreducible or complex dislocations occur when the volar plate is interposed in the metacarpophalangeal joint.
    - — Complex dislocations require open reduction.
    - — After reduction, place into a splint in the intrinsic plus position
  - Volar dislocation
    - — Often complex and irreducible by closed means
    - — Require open reduction
    - — After reduction, place into a splint in intrinsic plus position
- Complications
  - Stiffness
  - Posttraumatic arthritis
  - Malunion: may cause weakness of grip or pain
  - Malrotation: may result in scissoring and overlap of digits
  - Nonunion
  - Tendon adhesions

When to Refer

- All metacarpal fractures or joint dislocations should be referred to an orthopaedist or hand specialist for evaluation and definitive treatment.

Patient Instructions

- Keep splint clean and dry.
- Elevate the arm above the heart for 48 hours to decrease swelling and pain.
- Take pain medications as prescribed.
- Follow-up with the orthopaedist as instructed

Suggested Reading

- Glickel SZ, Barron OA, Catalano LW: Dislocations and ligament injuries in the digits. In Green DP, Hotchkiss RN, Pederson WC, Wolfe SW (eds): Green's Operative Hand Surgery, 5th ed. Philadelphia: Churchill Livingstone, 2005, pp 343–388.
- Henry MH: Fractures and dislocations of the hand. In Bucholz RW, Heckman JD, Court-Brown C (eds): Rockwood and Green's Fractures in Adults, 6th ed. Philadelphia: Lippincott Williams & Wilkins, 2006, pp 771–855.
- Koval KJ, Zuckerman JD: Handbook of Fractures, 3rd ed. Philadelphia: Lippincott Williams & Wilkins, 2006, pp 257–274.
- Markiewitz AD: Fractures and dislocations involving the metacarpal bone. In Trumble TE, Budoff JE, Cornwall R (eds): Hand, Elbow, and Shoulder: Core Knowledge in Orthopaedics. Philadelphia: Mosby, 2006, pp 38–55.
- Stern PJ: Fractures of the metacarpals and phalanges. In Green DP, Hotchkiss RN, Pederson WC, Wolfe SW (eds): Green's Operative Hand Surgery, 5th ed. Philadelphia: Churchill Livingstone, 2005, pp 277–341.
- Swanson AB: Fractures involving the digits of the hand. Orthop Clin North Am 1970;1:261–274.

Chapter 100 Phalangeal Fractures

Trevor Starnes and A. Bobby Chhabra

ICD-9 CODES

816.0 *Fracture of Phalanx or Phalanges, Unspecified*
816.1 *Fracture of Middle or Proximal Phalanx or Phalanges*
816.2 *Fracture of Distal Phalanx or Phalanges*
816.3 *Fracture of Phalanges, Multiple Sites*

Key Concepts

- Most common fracture in upper extremity
- The primary goal is to maintain joint motion and congruity.
- "Hand fractures can be complicated by deformity from no treatment, stiffness from overtreatment, and both deformity and stiffness from poor treatment." (A.B. Swanson)
- Twenty-seven percent of finger fractures are treated inappropriately in the emergency department.
  - Inaccurate reduction
  - Inappropriate splinting
- The proximal interphalangeal (PIP) joint is the most unforgiving joint in the hand.
- Prolonged mobilization has a deleterious effect on the overall outcome.

History

- Important to obtain the following information
  - Age
  - Hand dominance
  - Mechanism of injury
  - Comorbidities
  - Occupation

Physical Examination

- Skin and soft-tissue swelling
- Nail bed injuries
- Painful and limited range of motion
  - Examine each joint for congruent range of motion.
- Neurovascular status
  - Capillary refill less than 2 seconds
  - Two-point discrimination
- Rotational and angulation deformity
  - Grip to evaluate rotation (see Fig. 99-1)
- Check tenodesis effect
  - Wrist flexion results in finger extension.
  - Wrist extension results in finger flexion.
  - Abnormality of the normal cascade of fingers suggests injury.
  - Possible tendon injury on fracture fragment
- Complete examination may require injection of a local anesthetic agent.
  - Check the nerve status before administering a local anesthetic agent.
- Always examine the ipsilateral hand, elbow, and shoulder for associated injuries.

Imaging

- Posteroanterior, lateral, and oblique radiographs of affected digit
- Description of fracture
  - Open versus closed
  - Bone involved and location within bone
  - Displacement and angulation
  - Comminution
  - Intra-articular versus extra-articular

Differential Diagnosis

- Proximal phalanx fracture
  - Intra-articular
    - — Condyle fractures
      - — Unicondylar (Fig. 100-1)
      - — Bicondylar (Fig. 100-2)

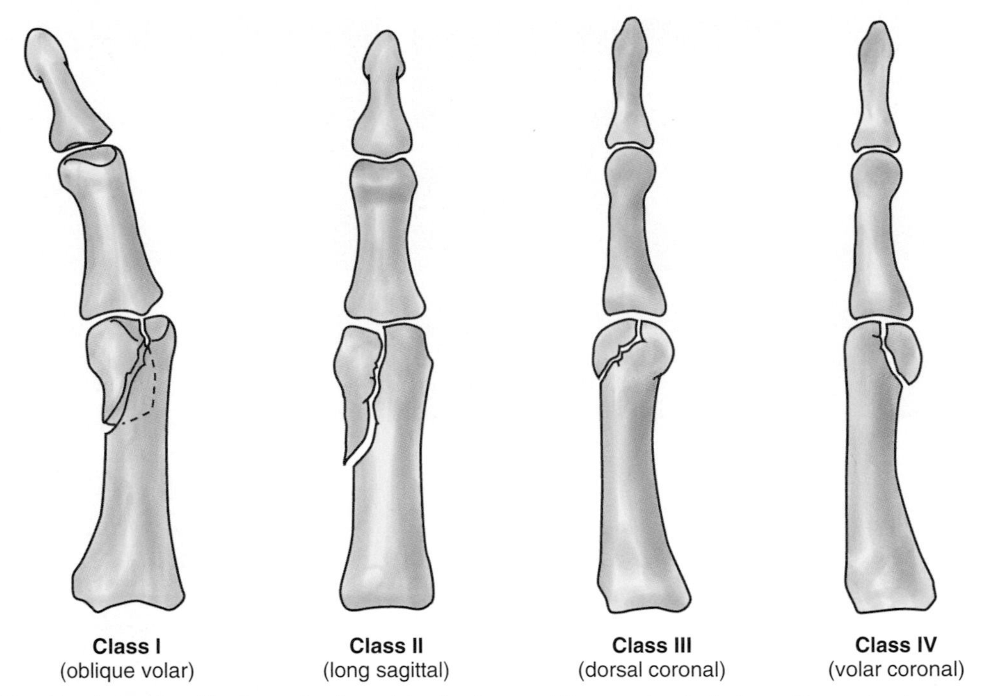

Figure 100-1 Weiss-Hastings classification of unicondylar fractures of the proximal phalanx. These fractures are nearly all unstable and nearly always require operative fixation. (Adapted from Weiss APC, Hastings HH: Distal unicondylar fractures of the proximal phalanx. J Hand Surg [Am] 1993;18A:594–599.)

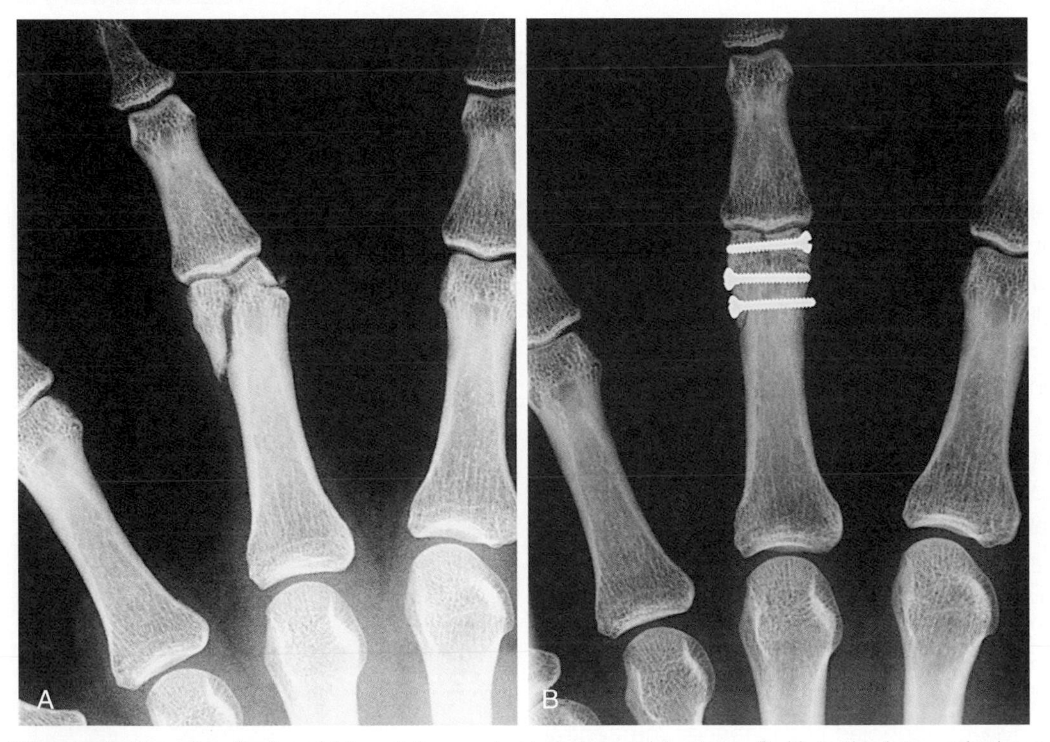

Figure 100-2 Open reduction of a displaced bicondylar proximal phalangeal fracture. **A**, Note the intra-articular component and angular deformity. **B**, Anatomic reduction with three lag screws. (Courtesy of T.R. Kiefhaber, MD. From Green DP, Hotchkiss RN, Pederson WC, Wolfe SW [eds]: Green's Operative Hand Surgery, 5th ed. Philadelphia: Churchill Livingstone, 2005.)

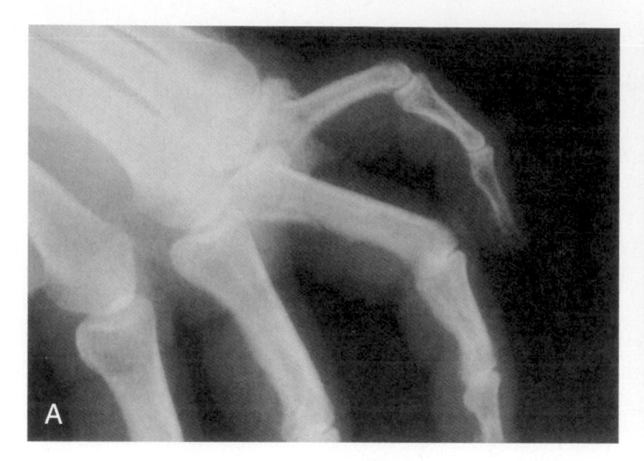

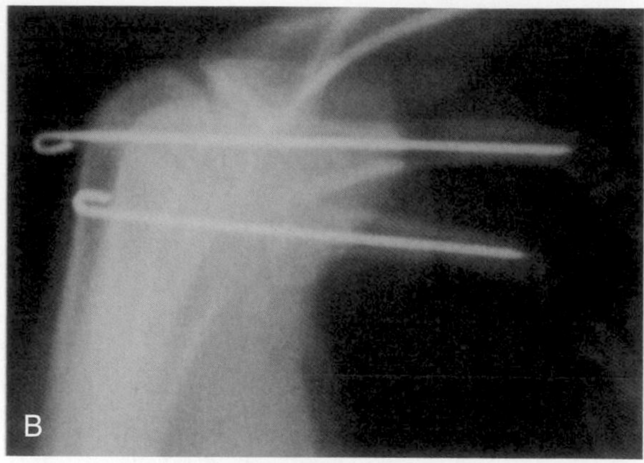

C

Figure 100-3 Transverse fractures at the base of P1 (**A**) have inherent soft tissue stability once reduced and can be stabilized by a single wire per fracture (passing through the metacarpal head) (**B**). **C**, This is best demonstrated on an oblique view. (From Bucholz RW, Court-Brown C, Tornetta P, et al [eds]: Rockwood and Green's Fractures in Adults, 6th ed. Philadelphia: Lippincott, Williams & Wilkins, 2006, Fig. 24-53.)

- Extra-articular
  — Transverse: stable fracture pattern (Fig. 100-3)
  — Oblique: unstable (Fig. 100-4)
  — Spiral: unstable (Fig. 100-5)
  — Comminuted: unstable (Fig. 100-6)
- PIP joint dislocation
  - Dorsal dislocation (Fig. 100-7)
    — Hyperextension of the PIP joint
    — Evaluate for associated fracture
    — Pilon fracture of the middle phalanx
  - Volar dislocation (Fig. 100-8)
    — Less common
    — Can disrupt extensor mechanism (central slip)
  - Volar rotary subluxation (Fig. 100-9)
    — Condyle buttonholes in the tear of the central tendon
- Middle phalanx fracture
  - Intra-articular
    — Condyle fractures
      — Unicondylar
      — Bicondylar

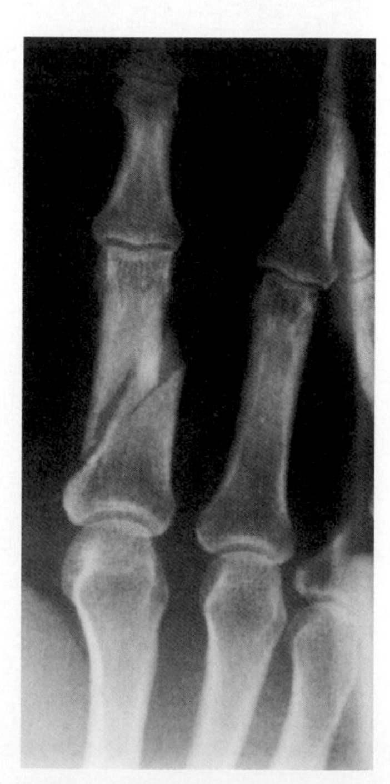

Figure 100-4 Fracture patterns appearing in P1 include oblique fractures of the shaft. (From Bucholz RW, Heckman JD, Court-Brown C, et al [eds]: Rockwood and Green's Fractures in Adults, 6th ed. Philadelphia: Lippincott Williams & Wilkins, 2006.)

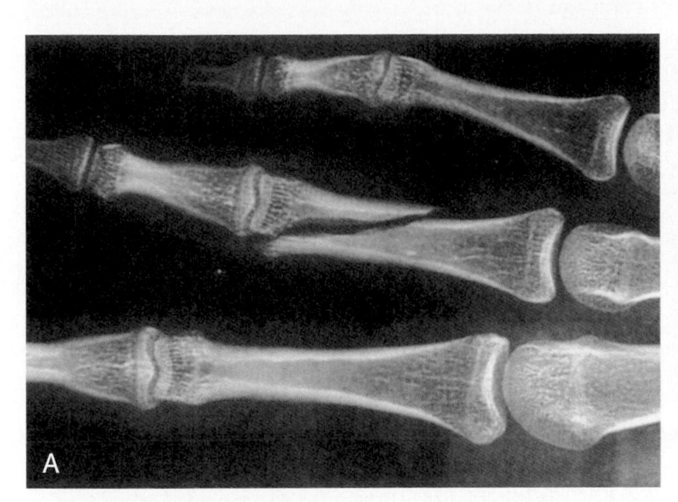

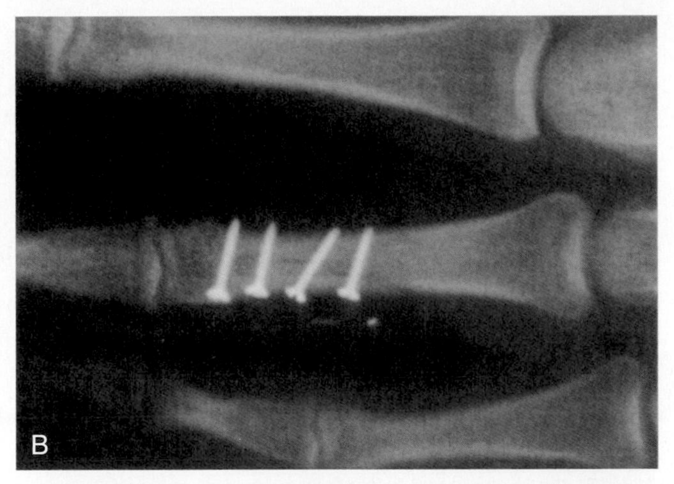

Figure 100-5 Long oblique fractures of the shaft (**A**) with shortening can achieve an exact reduction and stability sufficient to withstand early motion using lag screw fixation only (**B**). (From Bucholz RW, Heckman JD, Court-Brown C, et al [eds]: Rockwood and Green's Fractures in Adults, 6th ed. Philadelphia: Lippincott Williams & Wilkins, 2006.)

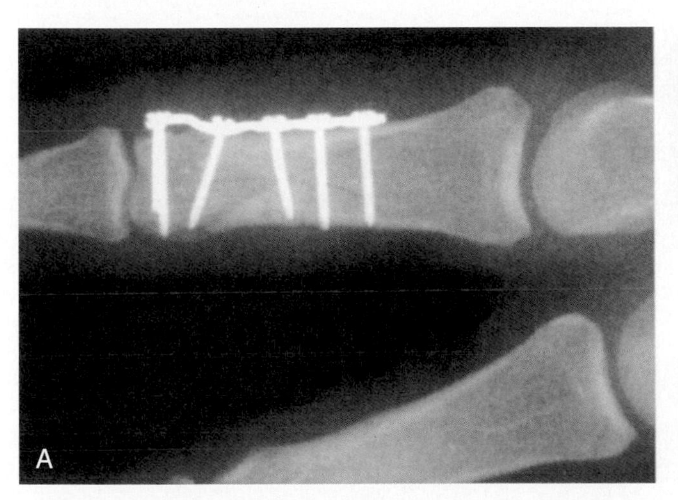

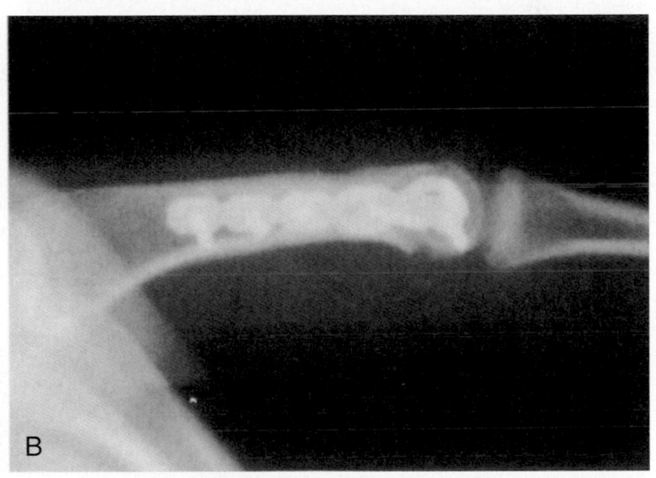

Figure 100-6 Comminuted fractures involving the head and shaft of P1 (**A**) can be stabilized for early motion with a condylar blade plate (**B**) placed laterally in the mid-axial plane. (From Bucholz RW, Heckman JD, Court-Brown C, et al [eds]: Rockwood and Green's Fractures in Adults, 6th ed. Philadelphia: Lippincott Williams & Wilkins, 2006.)

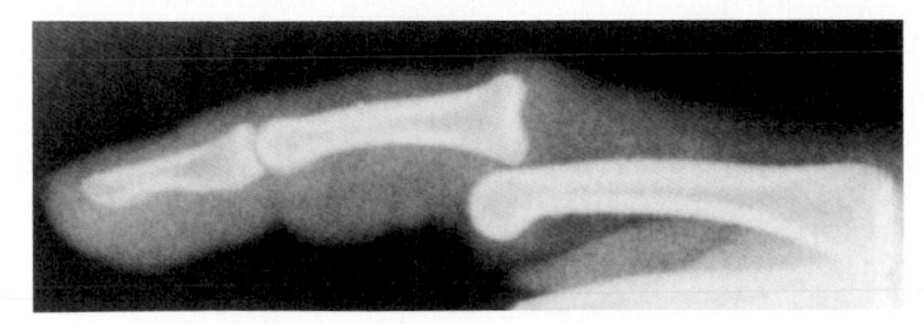

Figure 100-7 Dorsal dislocation, a common variant of a proximal interphalangeal joint dislocation. (From Bucholz RW, Heckman JD, Court-Brown C, et al [eds]: Rockwood and Green's Fractures in Adults, 6th ed. Philadelphia: Lippincott Williams & Wilkins, 2006.)

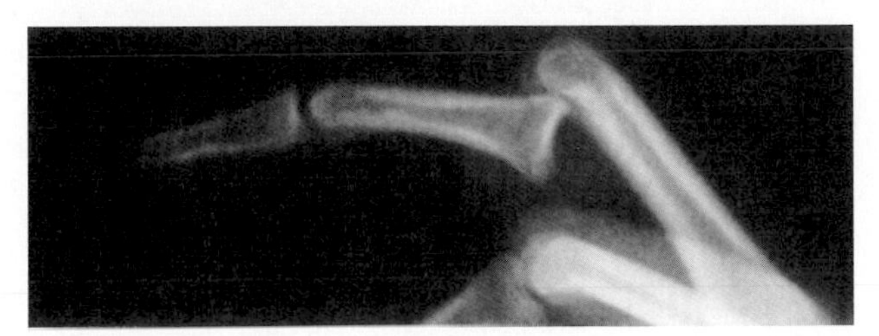

Figure 100-8 Pure volar dislocation with a central slip disruption, a less common variant of a proximal interphalangeal joint dislocation. (From Bucholz RW, Heckman JD, Court-Brown C, et al [eds]: Rockwood and Green's Fractures in Adults, 6th ed. Philadelphia: Lippincott Williams & Wilkins, 2006.)

- Extra-articular
  - — Transverse: stable fracture pattern
  - — Oblique: unstable
  - — Spiral: unstable
  - — Comminuted: unstable
- Distal interphalangeal (DIP) joint dislocation (Fig. 100-10)
  - Injury due to hyperextension, hyperflexion, or impaction

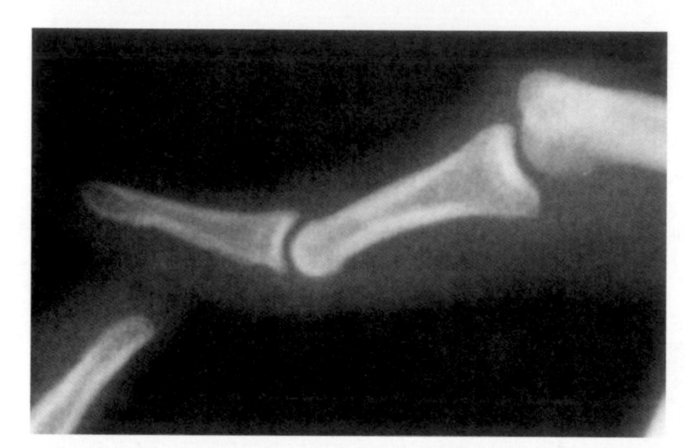

Figure 100-9 Volar rotatory subluxation, a rare variant of proximal interphalangeal joint dislocation (note that P2 is seen as a true lateral view, whereas P1 is seen in oblique profile). (From Bucholz RW, Heckman JD, Court-Brown C, et al [eds]: Rockwood and Green's Fractures in Adults, 6th ed. Philadelphia: Lippincott Williams & Wilkins, 2006.)

  - Most often dorsal or lateral
  - Hinge joint with strong collateral ligaments
- Distal phalanx fractures (Fig. 100-11)
  - Most common hand fracture
  - Thumb and middle finger most common
  - Tuft fracture (see Fig. 100-11C)
    - — Crush injury
    - — Often seen with a nail matrix injury or laceration = open fracture
    - — Painful subungual hematoma
  - Shaft fracture
    - — Transverse (see Fig. 100-11B)
    - — Longitudinal (see Fig. 100-11A)
- Intra-articular fracture (see Fig. 100-11G)
  - — Bony mallet: avulsion of extensor tendon from the distal phalanx (see Fig. 100-11D)
  - — Flexor digitorum profundus avulsion from the distal phalanx (see Fig. 100-11F)

Treatment

- Early motion after adequate initial healing is key to prevent stiffness.
- Splint the injured joint only and avoid crossing surrounding joints.
- If there is associated tendon or neurovascular injury requiring surgery, then also stabilize the bone injury at the same operative intervention.

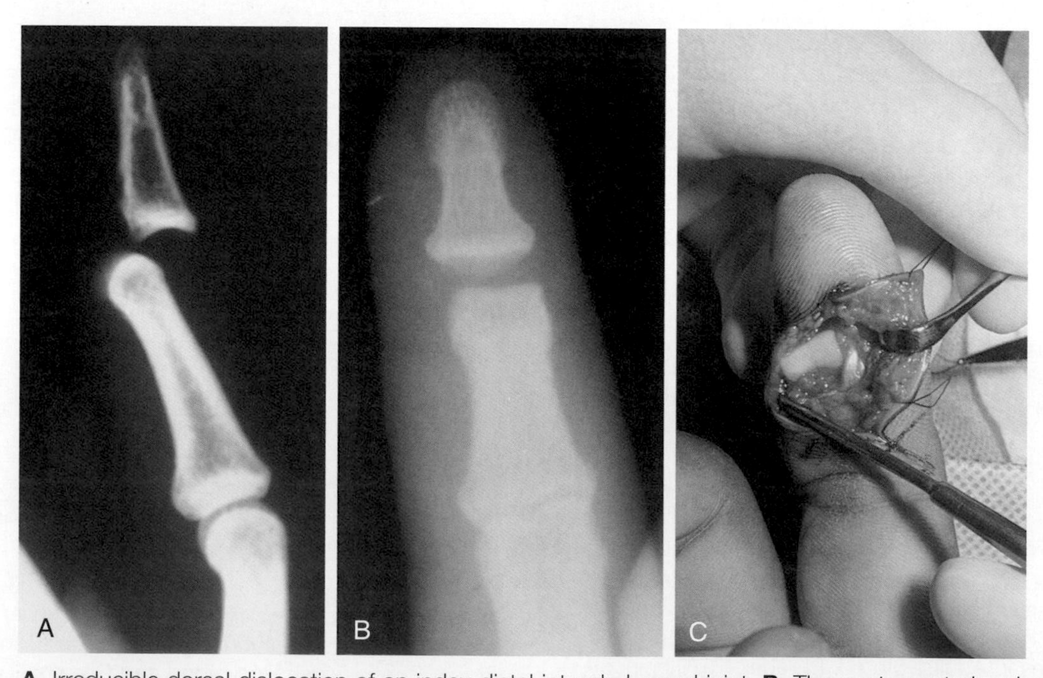

Figure 100-10 **A,** Irreducible dorsal dislocation of an index distal interphalangeal joint. **B,** The posteroanterior view shows a wide gap between the middle and distal phalanges suggestive of soft-tissue interposition. This appearance is typical of an irreducible dislocation in which the interposed soft tissue prevents reduction of the joint. These injuries are commonly open, and, at exploration (**C**), the head of the middle phalanx was seen ulnar to the displaced flexor tendon. The volar plate was interposed between the base of the distal phalanx and the head of the middle phalanx. (From Green DP, Hotchkiss RN, Pederson WC, Wolfe SW [eds]: Green's Operative Hand Surgery, 5th ed. Philadelphia: Churchill Livingstone, 2005.)

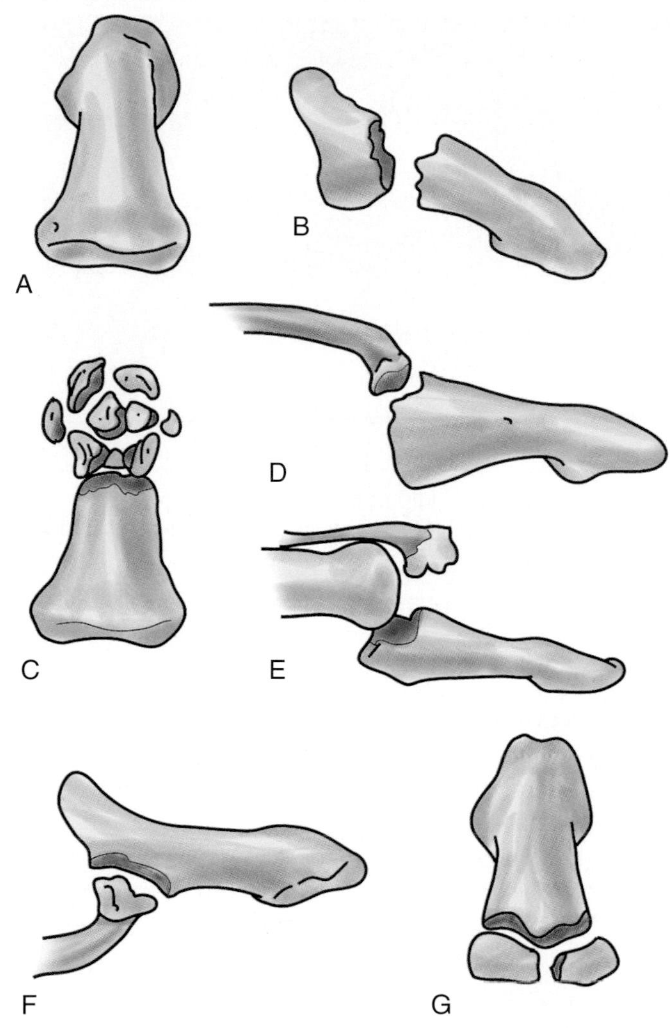

Figure 100-11 Fracture patterns seen in the distal phalanx include the longitudinal shaft (**A**), transverse shaft (**B**), tuft (**C**), dorsal base avulsion (**D**), dorsal base shear (**E**), volar base (**F**), and complete articular (**G**). (From Bucholz RW, Heckman JD, Court-Brown C, et al [eds]: Rockwood and Green's Fractures in Adults, 6th ed. Philadelphia: Lippincott Williams & Wilkins, 2006.)

- Proximal phalanx
  - Extra-articular fractures
    - — Stable (transverse) and nondisplaced
      - — Closed reduction with axial traction
      - — Buddy taping for 3 to 4 weeks
      - — Monitor closely for displacement.
    - — Unstable (spiral, oblique, comminuted)
      - — Closed reduction and splinting in intrinsic plus position
      - — Often require closed reduction and percutaneous pinning or open reduction and internal fixation (see Figs. 100-3, 100-5, and 100-6)
      - — Refer to a hand specialist.
  - Intra-articular fractures
    - — Unstable or displaced
    - — Condylar fractures
    - — Closed reduction to align fracture fragments via axial traction
    - — Splint in intrinsic plus position with radial or ulnar gutter splints
    - — Nonoperative
      - — Closed minimally displaced fractures with acceptable alignment
      - — Monitor closely for displacement.
    - — Operative (see Fig. 100-2)
      - — Open fractures
      - — Significant shortening or malrotation
      - — Articular step-off
      - — Failed closed treatment: displaced extra-articular fractures
- PIP joint dislocation
  - Dorsal dislocation with no fracture
    - — Longitudinal traction for reduction and buddy taping for several weeks until pain has resolved
    - — Early motion is encouraged if the dislocation is stable after reduction.
  - Dorsal dislocation with fracture
    - — The goal is a congruous articular surface and early motion.
    - — Extension block splinting (Fig. 100-12) or open reduction and internal fixation
    - — Refer to a hand specialist.
  - Volar dislocation with no fracture
    - — Extensor mechanism (central slip) injury
    - — Longitudinal traction for reduction
    - — Extension splinting of proximal interphalangeal joint for 6 weeks to prevent boutonniere deformity
    - — Refer to a hand specialist.
  - Volar dislocation with fracture
    - — Dorsal bony avulsion may require open reduction and internal fixation.
    - — Refer to a hand specialist.
  - Volar rotary subluxation
    - — Difficult closed reduction often requires open reduction.
    - — Refer to a hand specialist.
- Middle phalanx
  - Extra-articular fractures
    - — Stable (transverse) and nondisplaced
      - — Closed reduction with axial traction
      - — Buddy taping for 3 to 4 weeks
      - — Monitor closely for displacement.

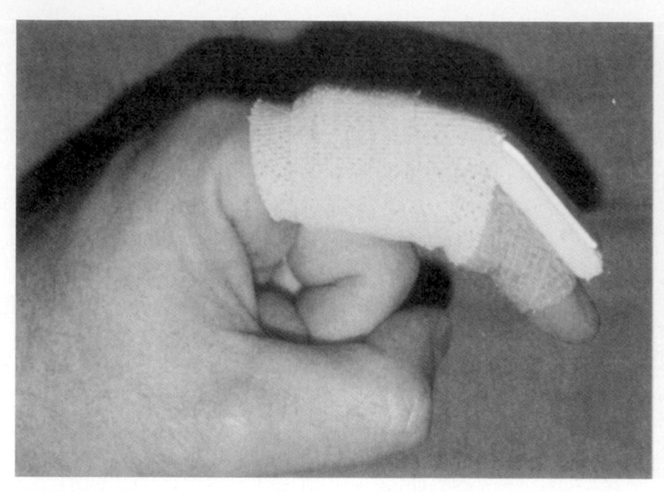
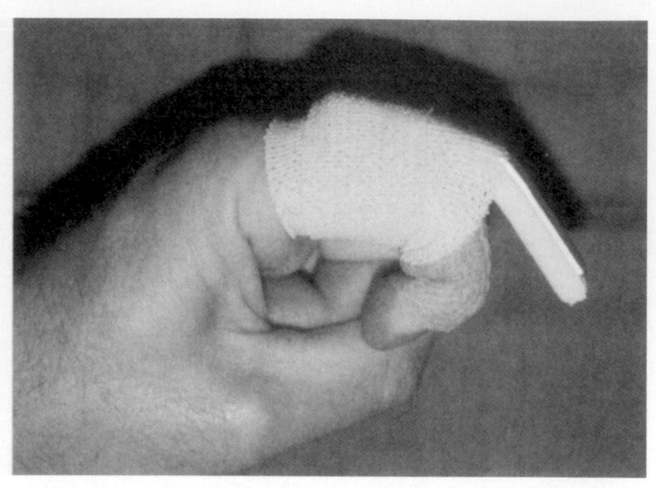

Figure 100-12 Extension block splinting requires that the dorsal surface of the proximal interphalangeal joint and proximal phalanx not be capable of pulling away from the splint. (From Bucholz RW, Heckman JD, Court-Brown C, et al [eds]: Rockwood and Green's Fractures in Adults, 6th ed. Philadelphia: Lippincott Williams & Wilkins, 2006.)

- — Unstable (spiral, oblique, comminuted)
  - — Closed reduction and splinting in intrinsic plus position
  - — Often require closed reduction and percutaneous pinning or open reduction and internal fixation
  - — Refer to a hand specialist.
- Intra-articular fractures
  - — Unstable or displaced
  - — Closed reduction to align fracture fragments via axial traction
  - — Splint in intrinsic plus position with radial or ulnar gutter splints
  - — Nonoperative
    - — Closed minimally displaced fractures with acceptable alignment
  - — Operative
    - — Open fractures
    - — Significant shortening
    - — Articular step-off
    - — Failed closed treatment: displaced extra-articular fractures
- DIP joint dislocation
  - Reduce closed injuries with traction.
  - Open injuries are due to a minimal soft-tissue envelope 60% of the time.
    - — Thorough irrigation, antibiotics, and reduction
    - — Nail bed injuries require repair with absorbable suture.
  - Splint DIP joint in flexion for 2 to 3 weeks
  - Volar dislocation immobilized in DIP joint extension splint for 6 to 8 weeks
- Distal phalanx
  - Tuft fracture
    - — Decompression of subungual hematoma with needle
    - — Nail bed repair: repair all nail matrix lacerations with absorbable suture after thorough irrigation and antibiotics (see Chapter 91)
    - — Immobilize with aluminum foam splint
  - Shaft fracture
    - — Transverse
      - — Nondisplaced: aluminum foam splint including DIP joint for 3 to 4 weeks
      - — Displaced: closed reduction and percutaneous pinning (often requires nail bed repair); refer to a hand specialist
  - Intra-articular fracture
    - — Bony mallet
      - — DIP joint extension splint for 6 to 8 weeks (see Chapter 89)
      - — Refer to a hand specialist.
    - — Flexor digitorum profundus avulsion
      - — Flexor tendon repair (see Chapter 87)
      - — Refer to a hand specialist.
- Complications
  - Stiffness
  - Hyperesthesia, cold intolerance, or numbness
  - Post-traumatic arthritis
  - Malunion: may cause weakness of grip or pain
  - Malrotation: may result in scissoring and overlap of digits
  - Nonunion

When to Refer

- All phalangeal fractures and complicated interphalangeal dislocations should be referred to an orthopaedist or a hand specialist for evaluation.

Patient Instructions

- Keep the splint clean and dry.
- Elevate the arm above the heart for 48 hours to decrease swelling and pain.
- Take pain medications as prescribed.
- Follow up with an orthopaedist as instructed.
- Early motion and therapy are very important after adequate initial healing.

Suggested Reading

- Glickel SZ, Barron OA, Catalano LW: Dislocations and ligament injuries in the digits. In Green DP, Hotchkiss RN, Pederson WC, Wolfe SW (eds): Green's Operative Hand Surgery, 5th ed. Philadelphia: Churchill Livingstone, 2005, pp 343–388.
- Henry MH: Fractures and dislocations of the hand. In Bucholz RW, Heckman JD, Court-Brown C (eds): Rockwood and Green's Fractures in Adults, 6th ed. Philadelphia: Lippincott Williams & Wilkins, 2006, pp 771–855.
- Koval KJ, Zuckerman JD: Handbook of Fractures, 3rd ed. Philadelphia: Lippincott Williams & Wilkins, 2006, pp 257–274.
- Slade JF, Magit DP: Phalangeal fractures and dislocations. In Trumble TE, Budoff JE, Cornwall R (eds): Hand, Elbow, and Shoulder: Core Knowledge in Orthopaedics. Philadelphia: Mosby, 2006, pp 22–37.
- Stern PJ: Fractures of the metacarpals and phalanges. In Green DP, Hotchkiss RN, Pederson WC, Wolfe SW (eds): Green's Operative Hand Surgery, 5th ed. Philadelphia: Churchill Livingstone, 2005, pp 277–341.
- Swanson AB: Fractures involving the digits of the hand. Orthop Clin North Am 1970;1:261–274.

Chapter 101 Distal Radius Fracture Reduction

Trevor Starnes and A. Bobby Chhabra

CPT CODES

25600 *Closed Treatment of Distal Radial Fracture (e.g., Colles' or Smith's Type) or Epiphyseal Separation, Includes Closed Treatment of Fracture of Ulnar Styloid, When Performed; without Manipulation*

25605 *Closed Treatment of Distal Radial Fracture (e.g., Colles' or Smith's Type) or Epiphyseal Separation, Includes Closed Treatment of Fracture of Ulnar Styloid, When Performed; with Manipulation*

Equipment

- Lidocaine for hematoma block
- Finger traps and an IV pole for traction
- Countertraction weight
- Soft roll padding
- Sugar tong splinting material (plaster or fiberglass)
- Ace bandage

Contraindications

- Nondisplaced fractures may worsen alignment.
- Stable fracture patterns with acceptable reduction
  - Radial shortening less than 2 mm
  - Neutral tilt
  - Articular step-off less than 1 mm
- Elderly (older than 65 years old) or low-demand patients with comorbidities with reasonable alignment and may not tolerate reduction

Technique and Tips

- Complete full physical examination before reduction
  - Skin and soft-tissue swelling
  - Painful and limited range of motion of wrist
  - Deformity and angulation
    - — Dorsal displacement: Colles' fracture (90% of distal radius fractures)
    - — Volar displacement: Smith's fracture
  - Neurovascular status, especially median nerve
    - — Carpal tunnel compression symptoms are present in 13% to 23% of injuries.
  - Palpate anatomic snuffbox for tenderness that may suggest scaphoid fracture
  - Examine finger and thumb motion to confirm tendon continuity.
  - Always examine the ipsilateral hand, elbow, and shoulder for associated injuries.
- Provide adequate anesthesia
- Hematoma block (Fig. 101-1)
    - — 10 mL of 1% lidocaine without epinephrine
    - — Prepare skin with povidone-iodine and alcohol.
    - — Inject at the level of the fracture on the dorsal wrist in the middle of the radius.
    - — Draw back after the needle is placed; you should see blood to confirm proper placement.
    - — Inject 10 mL of lidocaine.
  - May provide fast-acting IV pain medication such as fentanyl
  - Conscious IV sedation may be required in children and some adults.
- Place the thumb and index and middle fingers in finger traps, making sure that the fit is tight (Fig. 101-2).
  - Using only these digits provides the ulnar deviation often needed to aid in reduction.
  - Protect the skin, especially in the elderly, with tape.
- Hang the upper extremity in finger traps from an IV pole (see Fig. 101-2).
  - Patient placed supine on bed
  - Shoulder at 90 degrees abduction and neutral external rotation
  - The elbow should be at 90 degrees of flexion.
  - Hang 5 to 15 pounds of countertraction from the distal humerus.
  - Confirm patient comfort once positioned
  - Allow the countertraction weight to work using ligamentotaxis for approximately 5 minutes.

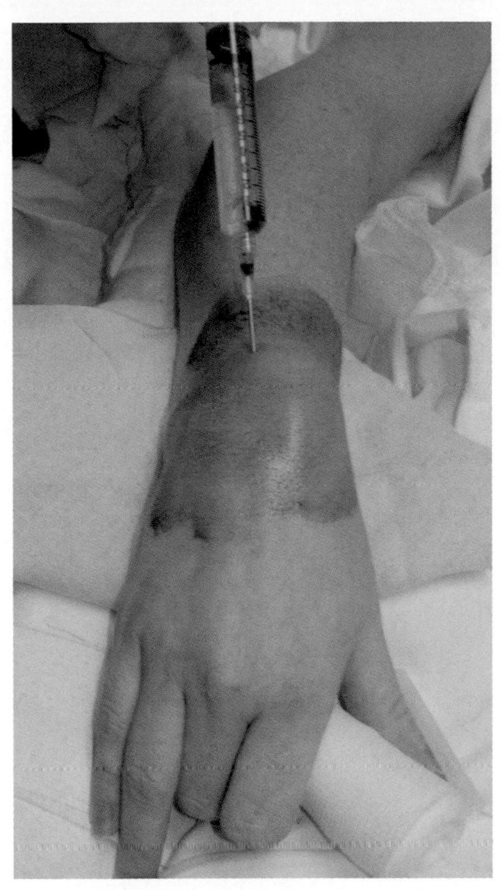

Figure 101-1 Hematoma block: 10 mL of 1% lidocaine without epinephrine injected at the level of the fracture on the dorsal wrist in the middle of the radius. Draw back after the needle is placed; you should see blood to confirm proper placement.

- Closed manipulation of dorsally displaced fractures (Fig. 101-3)
  - Longitudinal traction to release the fracture fragments
  - Reproduce the fracture mechanism by hyperextending the wrist.
  - Pull longitudinal traction while flexing the wrist and placing direct pressure on the dorsal fracture fragment with your thumb.
  - Be careful not to tear fragile skin in the elderly.
  - Palpate the distal radius dorsally to confirm improvement in dorsal displacement.
  - May use fluoroscopy at this point to confirm reduction
  - Sometimes takes several attempts to completely unlock fragments and obtain adequate reduction
- Splint placement
  - Wrap the arm including the distal humerus, elbow, forearm, wrist, and proximal hand to the metacarpophalangeal joints with a soft roll.

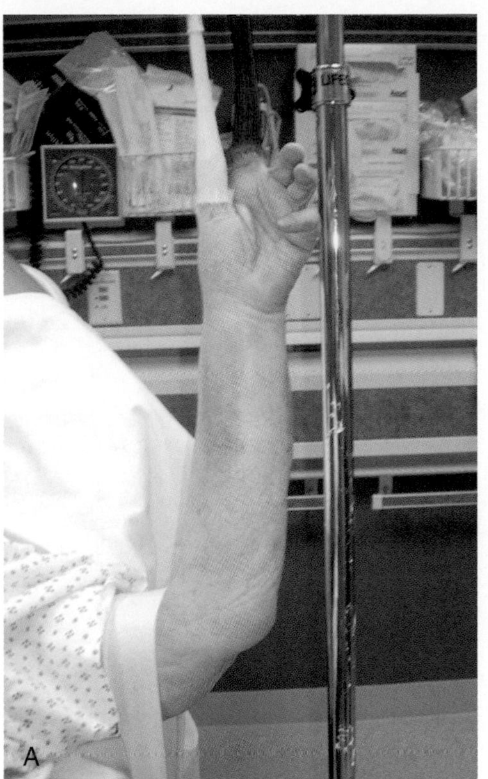

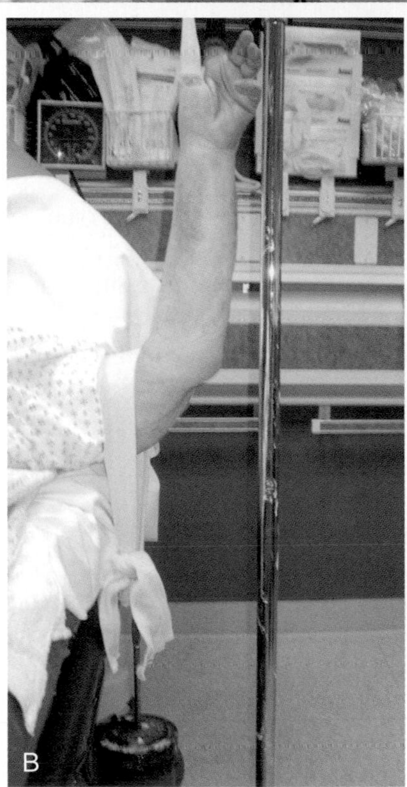

Figure 101-2 **A**, The upper extremity is hung in finger traps from an IV pole. **B**, Five to 15 pounds of countertraction is hung from the distal humerus. Confirm patient comfort once the patient is positioned. Allow the countertraction weight to work using ligamentotaxis for approximately 5 minutes.

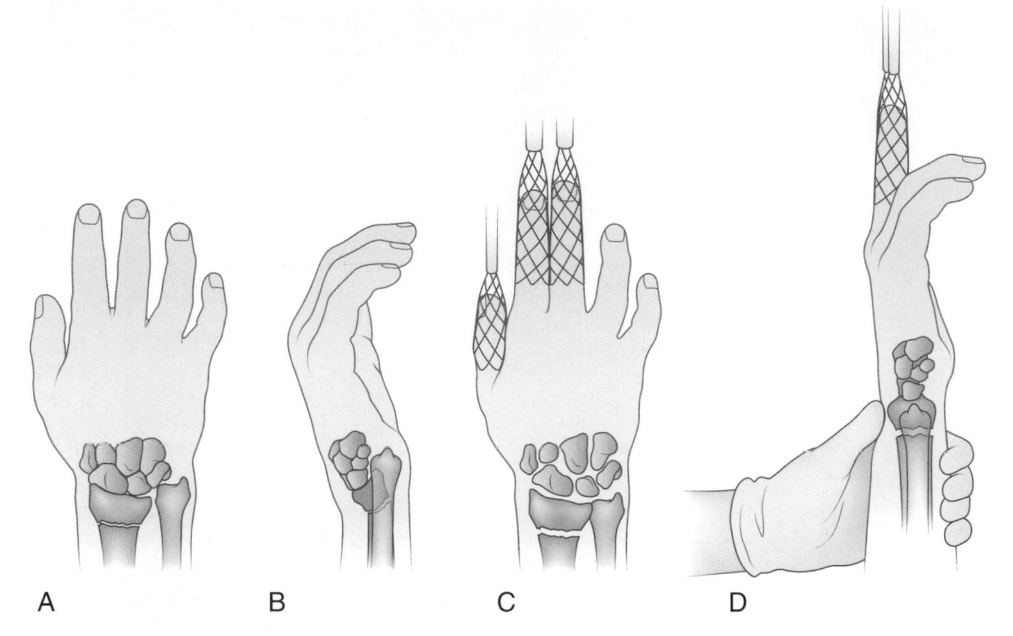

Figure 101-3 Posteroanterior (**A**) and lateral (**B**) views of distal radius (Colles') fracture. Posteroanterior (**C**) and lateral (**D**) views of our recommended reduction of this fracture. After suspending the arm from finger traps and allowing for fracture disimpaction, pressure is applied with the thumb over the distal fragment. (Adapted from Green DP, Hotchkiss RN, Pederson WC, Wolfe SW [eds]: Green's Operative Hand Surgery, 5th ed. Philadelphia: Churchill Livingstone, 2005, Fig. 16-21. Copyright Elizabeth Martin.)

  - May take the thumb out of the finger trap at this point to place the soft roll around the thumb in the first web space
  - Leave the index finger in the trap to make placement of the splint easier while the arm is hanging.
  - Confirm that padding is adequate, especially at the bony prominences at the elbow.
- Place a sugar tong splint using plaster or fiberglass around the elbow and on the dorsal and volar surfaces of the forearm with the forearm in a neutral position (Fig. 101-4).
  - Dorsally: Stop the splint at the metacarpophalangeal joints to allow finger motion.
  - Volarly: Stop at the proximal palmar skin crease to allow metacarpophalangeal flexion to 90 degrees.
- Wrap the splinting material with an Ace bandage.
- Three-point molding of the splint (Fig. 101-5)
  - Place one hand dorsally distal to the fracture.
  - Place the second hand volarly proximal to the fracture.
  - The third point is at the elbow dorsally.
- Try to obtain a dorsal buttress to prevent collapse.
  - Avoid excessive wrist flexion as it can cause median nerve compression symptoms.
  - Place in slight ulnar deviation and neutral forearm rotation
- Postreduction examination
  - Always obtain postreduction radiographs after the splint has been placed.

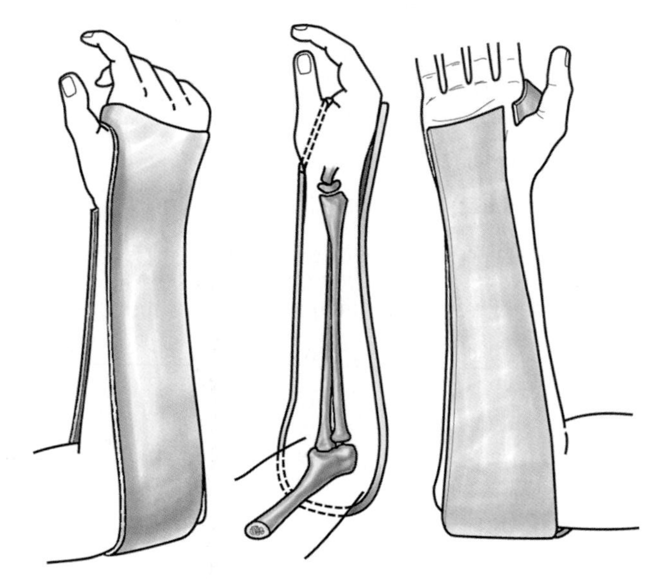

Figure 101-4 Sugar tong splint for a distal radius fracture. This splint controls forearm rotation while allowing for some elbow flexion. The palmar crease should be free to allow full metacarpophalangeal flexion. (Adapted from Green DP, Hotchkiss RN, Pederson WC, Wolfe SW [eds]: Green's Operative Hand Surgery, 5th ed. Philadelphia: Churchill Livingstone, 2005, Fig. 16-23.)

  - Always perform a complete postreduction examination including sensation, motor, and vascular examination.
- Refer to an orthopaedist for all distal radius fractures
  - New radiographs to be obtained within 1 week to confirm maintenance of reduction

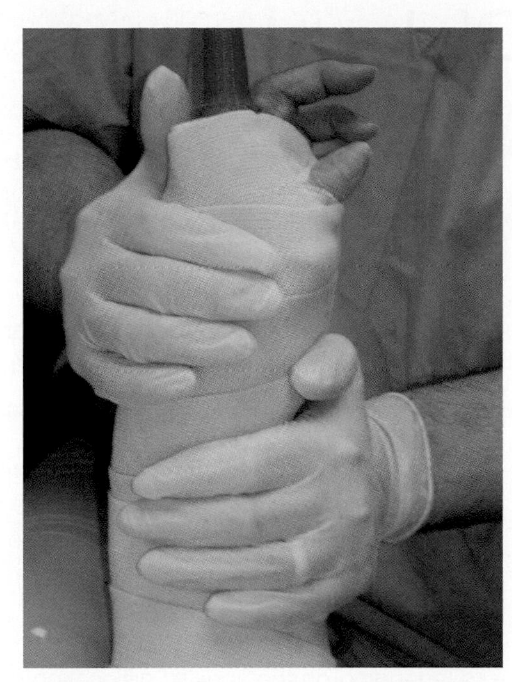

Figure 101-5 Three-point molding of the splint. Place one hand dorsally distal to the fracture and the other hand volarly proximal to the fracture. Your knee can be used as the third point at the elbow dorsally.

- May tighten the splint by rewrapping the bandage as swelling decreases
- If definitive nonoperative therapy, orthopaedist will change the splint to a cast when the swelling has decreased

Considerations in Special Populations

- Pediatrics
  - Often requires IV conscious sedation
  - Only one reduction attempt should be made to prevent further damage to the physis
  - High potential for remodeling
  - Refer to an orthopaedist for all displaced and physeal fractures

Troubleshooting

- Inadequate reduction may be secondary to inadequate pain control and anesthesia.
- Provide adequate pain control to allow for adequate traction.

Patient Instructions

- Keep the splint clean and dry.
- Elevate the arm above the heart for 48 hours to decrease swelling and pain.
- Take pain medications as prescribed.
- Follow up with an orthopaedist as instructed.

Suggested Reading

- Fernandez DL, Palmer AK: Fractures of the distal radius. In Green DP, Hotchkiss RN, Pederson WC, Wolfe SW (eds): Green's Operative Hand Surgery, 5th ed. Philadelphia: Churchill Livingstone, 2005, pp 929–985.
- Jiuliano JA, Jupiter J: Distal radius fractures. In Trumble TE, Budoff JE, Cornwall R (eds): Core Knowledge in Orthopaedics: Hand, Elbow, and Shoulder. Philadelphia: Mosby, 2006, pp 84–101.
- Koval KJ, Zuckerman JD: Handbook of Fractures, 3rd ed. Philadelphia: Lippincott Williams & Wilkins, 2006, pp 226–236.
- Ruch D: Fractures of the distal radius and ulna. In Bucholz RW, Heckman JD, Court-Brown C (eds): Rockwood and Green's Fractures in Adults, 6th ed. Philadelphia: Lippincott Williams & Wilkins, 2006, pp 909–988.

Chapter 102 Finger Dislocations

Robert Neff, Nathan Richardson, and Jonathan E. Isaacs

ICD-9 CODES
834.00 *Dislocation Finger, Unspecified*
834.01 *Metacarpophalangeal Dislocation*
834.02 *Interphalangeal Joint Dislocation*
834.10 *Open Dislocation, Unspecified*
834.11 *Open Metacarpophalangeal Dislocation*
834.12 *Open Interphalangeal Joint Dislocation*

Key Concepts

- The proximal interphalangeal (PIP) joint is a commonly dislocated joint due to a relative lack of protection and a long lever arm.
- Dislocations of the distal interphalangeal (DIP) and metacarpophalangeal (MCP) joints are less common.
- DIP joint dislocations are often open injuries due to the thin, adherent soft-tissue envelope.
- MCP joint dislocations are more likely to require an open reduction.
- Dislocations are described by the direction of displacement of the distal aspect of the digit: dorsal, volar, and lateral. Dorsal dislocation is the most common injury pattern.
- Treatment depends on the degree of ligament and bony injury and the presence or absence of residual instability.
- The method of reduction must be performed accurately so as not to exacerbate the injury.

Anatomy

- The MCP, DIP, and PIP joints share a similar anatomy in the basic form of a three-sided box. The floor is formed by the volar plate and the sides by collateral ligaments (Fig. 102-1).
  - Volar plate
    — A stout volar capsule thickening that inserts into the periosteum; it is more firmly attached proximally to the joint and is suspended by insertions of the collateral ligaments
    — Its primary function is to resist hyperextension.
    — Often avulsed in dislocations, the volar plate can block reduction if it becomes interposed within the joint.
  - Collateral ligaments
    — Stout lateral capsular thickenings that originate on the dorsolateral aspect of the more proximal bone; run obliquely to insert on the volar-lateral 40% of the distal articular rim
    — Primary restraints to radial and ulnar deviation
    — Depending on the specific dislocation mechanism, the collateral ligaments are often disrupted. This disruption can occur partially or in whole and can affect joint stability.
- Extensor mechanism
  - Two components: The central mechanism inserts just distal to the PIP joint (central slip) and again just distal to the DIP joint (terminal tendon).
  - The lateral band extends from the intrinsic muscles of the hand and inserts into the extensor hood.
  - This anatomy is important because both the central slip and terminal tendon are vulnerable to avulsion injury during volar dislocations.
  - Dislocations of MCP and PIP joints can become trapped between the lateral band and the central mechanism.

History

- Finger dislocations are generally referred after spontaneous reduction or reduction by the patient, trainer, or parent.
- Often describe a mechanism of jamming, hyperextension, or twisting
- May describe chronic instability, pain, or swelling

Physical Examination

- Swelling and ecchymosis are common. Unreduced dislocations are usually obvious, although they may be obscured by swelling. Open dislocations are not uncommon and skin integrity should be carefully assessed.

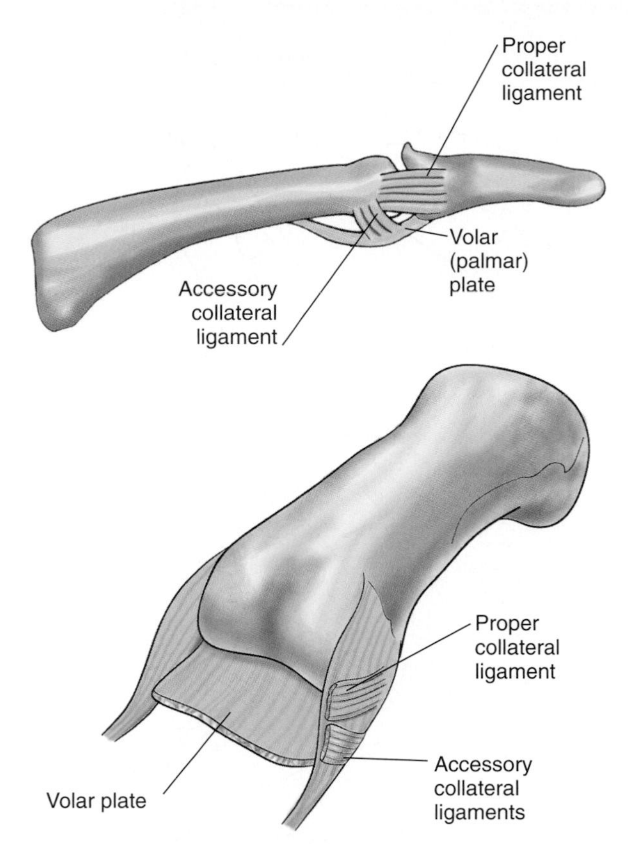

Figure 102-1 The metacarpophalangeal, proximal interphalangeal, and distal interphalangeal joints share a basic three-sided box architecture. The volar plate forms the floor and resists hyperextension, whereas stout collateral ligaments protect from lateral forces.

- A focused neurovascular examination includes sensory testing and capillary refill documented before reduction or digital block.
- Palpate to localize points of tenderness to identify ligament, volar plate, bone, and tendon injuries both before and after reduction.
- Check range of motion and stability postreduction. Redislocation or subluxation during active range of motion indicates gross instability.
- Next, evaluate stability with gentle lateral stress and hyperextension; this may indicate subtle instability.
- Isolate the injured joint and test for active flexion and extension to identify associated tendon injuries.

Imaging

- Anteroposterior and lateral views of the affected joint pre- and postreduction to guide and confirm reduction and to evaluate for associated bony injury (perform before testing for instability)
- Fluoroscopic stress views are often helpful to evaluate stability.
- Other imaging modalities (such as magnetic resonance imaging) are not usually necessary or helpful.

Classification

- In general, dislocations are described according to the location of the distal component relative to the proximal component. Associated bone and soft-tissue injuries further stratify dislocations and help not only to communicate adequately the injury severity but also to help guide treatment strategy and predict outcome.
    - Dorsal, volar, lateral
    - Associated with or without fracture
    - Stable versus unstable
    - Reducible (simple) versus irreducible (complex)
    - Chronic or acute

Treatment

- Digital block or proper anesthesia is mandatory for reduction and stability testing.
- Complex (i.e., irreducible) dislocations require surgical exploration.
- Open injuries need appropriate irrigation/débridement and antibiotic treatment.
- Avoid prolonged immobilization; simple/stable injuries are generally conducive to brief periods of immobilization followed by protected range of motion.

DIP (and Thumb Interphalangeal) Joint Dislocations

- Reduction maneuver: slow, steady traction of the distal phalanx accompanied by direct pressure over the deformity
- Treatment depends on stability and associated tendon injury
    - If grossly unstable, the DIP joint needs operative fixation. If instability is subtle, splint the joint in 20 degrees of flexion for 2 weeks and then reevaluate it. A stable joint can be treated symptomatically with temporary splinting (1–2 weeks) followed by early mobilization when tolerated.
    - Loss of active extension, with or without a small dorsal bone fragment, requires prolonged (6 weeks) splinting in full extension. This represents an extensor tendon avulsion or tear (Fig. 102-2).
    - Avoid splinting across the PIP joint, which can cause stiffness, and hyperextension of the DIP, which can cause maceration of the dorsal skin.
- Small fractures should be treated the same as a sprain (with treatment based on stability as previously described).

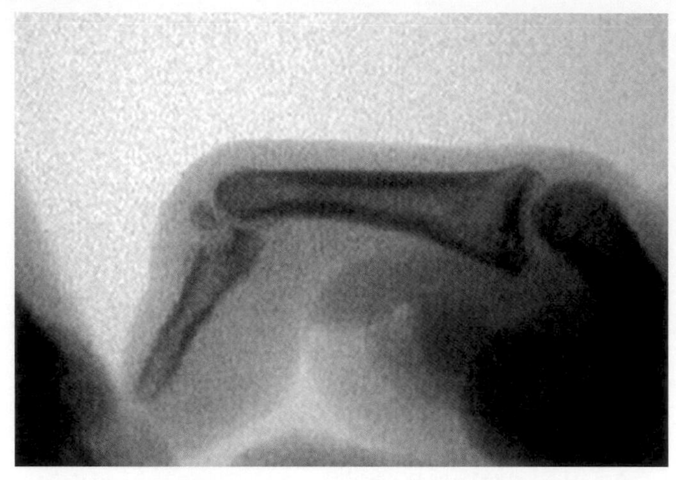

Figure 102-2 Distal interphalangeal bony mallet injury. Postreduction radiographs and active strength testing reveal associated injuries, such as this fracture involving the articular surface and insertion of the extensor tendon. This injury pattern necessitates referral to a hand surgeon for possible surgical stabilization (versus prolonged extension splinting). (From Green DP, Hotchkiss RN, Pederson WC, Wolfe SW [eds]: Green's Operative Hand Surgery, 5th ed. Philadelphia: Churchill Livingstone, 2005.)

- Significant fractures (>40% of the joint surface) should be splinted and the patient referred to a hand specialist for possible fixation.

PIP Joint Dislocations

- Dorsal
  - Most dorsal dislocations are reduced with gentle distal traction while applying volarly directed pressure over the PIP joint (Fig. 102-3).
  - Treatment depends on stability
    - — If grossly unstable, the collateral ligaments need operative fixation.
    - — If instability is subtle, splint in 20 degrees of flexion for 3 weeks and then re-evaluate the joint.
    - — A stable joint can be treated symptomatically with temporary splinting (1–2 weeks) followed by early mobilization (buddy taping) when tolerated.
  - In cases of fracture-dislocation, treatment may depend on the size of the articular fracture fragment.
    - — Small fragments (<10% or volar lip avulsions) can be treated the same as dislocations based on the joint stability.
    - — Large fragments (>40% of the joint surface) are typically grossly unstable. These should be splinted for comfort and promptly referred to a specialist for surgical fixation. Surgical options will include open reduction with internal fixation, dynamic external fixation, and volar plate advancement.
    - — Intermediate fragments (10% to 40%) can often be stable after reduction when kept in slight flexion (Fig. 102-4). These can be treated by extension block splinting in 30 degrees of flexion, followed by weekly reduction of the splint by 10 degrees until full extension is achieved. Maintenance of reduction must be verified weekly (Fig. 102-5). This can be difficult to judge and referral to a specialist would be appropriate.

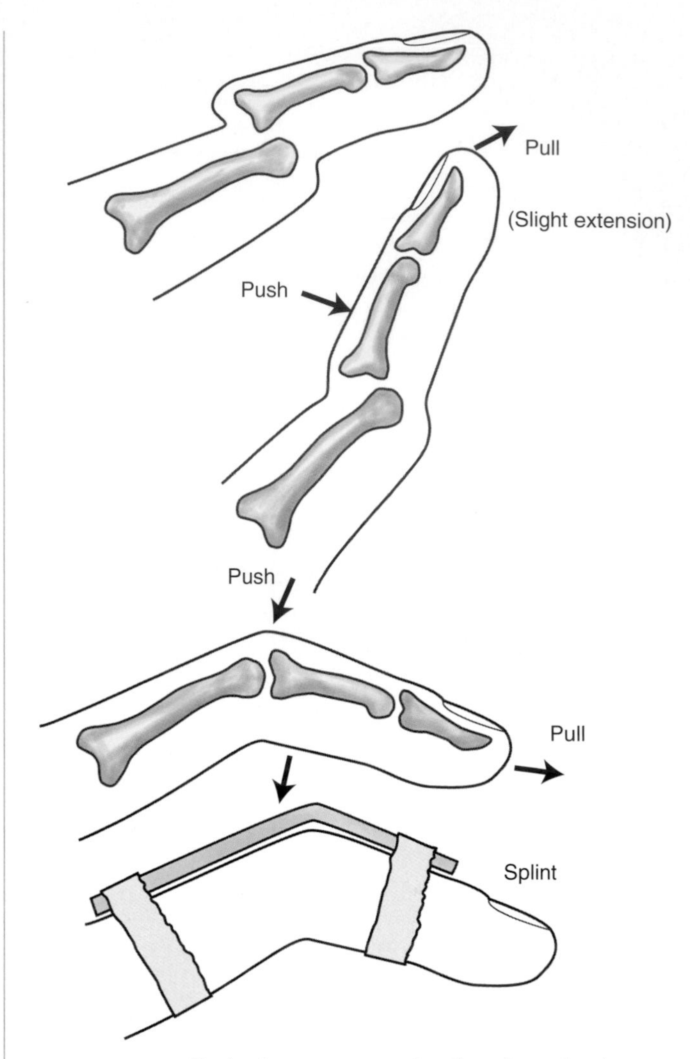

Figure 102-3 Reduction maneuver for dorsal proximal interphalangeal dislocation. Gentle traction and slight exaggeration of deformity, followed by volar pressure to slide the joint back into place.

- Volar
  - Rare and often unstable; easy to reduce but difficult to maintain; these injuries are often open
  - Always involve a central slip tear that results in a boutonnière deformity if not recognized and

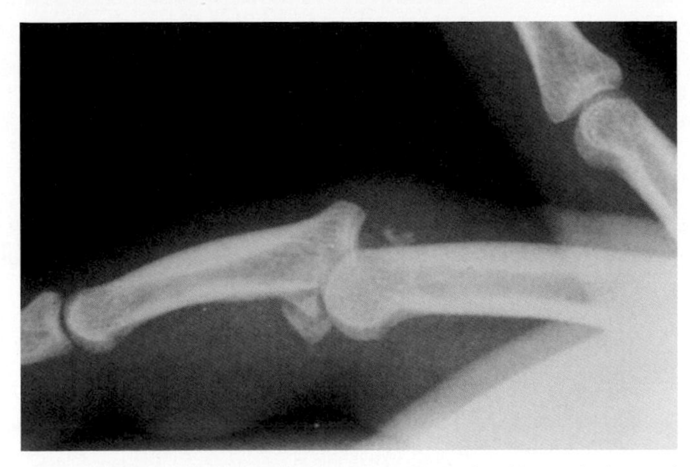

Figure 102-4 Fracture/dislocation of proximal interphalangeal joint involving approximately 40% of the volar articular surface of the middle phalanx. Fractures/dislocations involving less than 40% of the articular surface are amenable to extension block splinting. (From Green DP, Hotchkiss RN, Pederson WC, Wolfe SW [eds]: Green's Operative Hand Surgery, 5th ed. Philadelphia: Churchill Livingstone, 2005.)

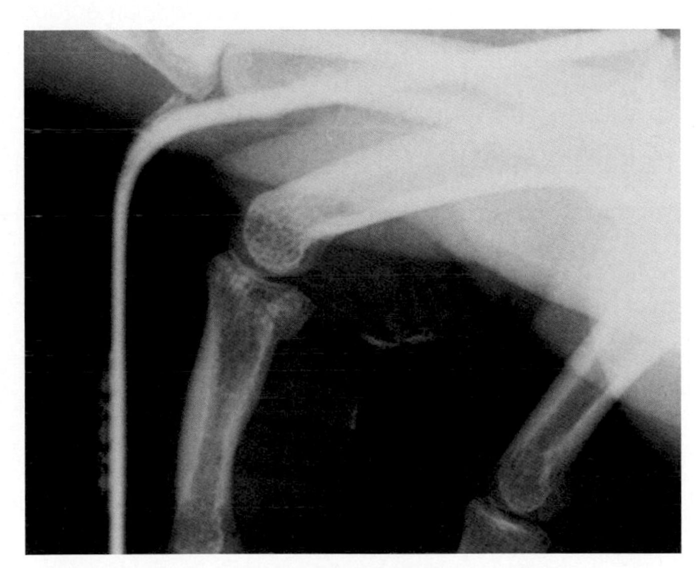

Figure 102-5 Extension block splinting of proximal interphalangeal (PIP) joint. Extension block splinting, as with this stable fracture dislocation, allows active flexion at the PIP joint. The splint is extended at weekly intervals. (From Green DP, Hotchkiss RN, Pederson WC, Wolfe SW [eds]: Green's Operative Hand Surgery, 5th ed. Philadelphia: Churchill Livingstone, 2005.)

treated; this requires supervised therapy and the patient should be referred to a hand surgeon

- A variant of volar dislocations, rotational subluxation poses a reduction dilemma. This pattern can be recognized on a lateral radiograph: the proximal phalanx will appear in profile as a true lateral and the middle phalanx as an oblique view (not a true lateral). The head of the proximal phalanx is incarcerated between the lateral band and extensor mechanism. Traction alone may result in a "Chinese finger trap" effect, in which increased longitudinal traction acts to tension the soft tissue and form a tightening noose around the proximal phalanx neck that blocks reduction.
- To avoid this pitfall, reduction is attempted by gentle flexion of the PIP and MCP joints (to relax the lateral bands) followed by axial and rotational force to finesse the proximal phalanx to anatomic position. Exaggeration of the deformity often aids in the reduction. If it is unsuccessful, open reduction will be required.
- Splinting
  - Stable volar dislocations of the PIP joint should be placed in full extension of the PIP joint only (the same treatment as for an isolated boutonnière deformity); this will approximate the central slip to allow healing.
  - Motion of both the MCP and DIP joints is encouraged to avoid stiffness and actually aids in healing of the extensor tendon.
  - Splinting should be continued for 6 weeks.

Lateral Dislocations

- Often spontaneously or easily reduced; they may be stable with buddy taping of simple splinting (in slight flexion)
- Generally involve partial or complete disruption of the collateral ligaments
- Blocks to reduction can include an interposed collateral ligament, extensor tendon entrapment, and buttonholing through the dorsal apparatus; these typically require operative exploration.
- Most can be treated by conservative means, including buddy taping and active range of motion to prevent stiffness. Joints grossly unstable to lateral stress (>20 degrees of joint angulation) should be referred to a hand specialist.

MCP Finger and Thumb Dislocations

- Dorsal
  - Dislocation may be simple (base of the proximal phalanx stays in contact with the head of the metacarpal) or complex (base of the proximal phalanx is bayoneted and dorsal to the head of the metacarpal). Simple dislocations usually present with the dislocated finger appearing to point straight in the air away from the joint. Complex dislocations are characterized by puckering of the palmar skin, shortening of the digit, and extensive swelling at the MCP joint.

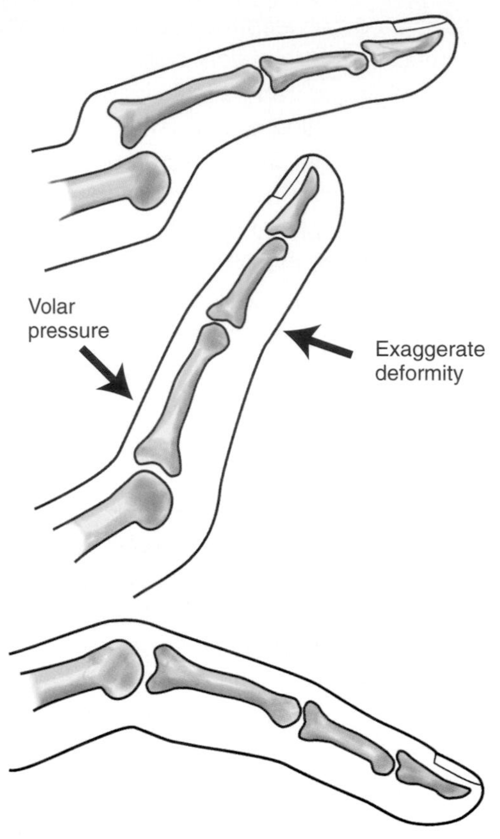

Figure 102-6 Reduction maneuver for dorsal metacarpophalangeal joint dislocation. The examiner grasps the injured hand with fingers on the patient's palm and thumb on the dorsal surface of the base of the proximal phalanx. Avoid axial traction. A volar-directed force is then applied with the examiner's thumbs to slide the joint back into place.

- Reduction for simple dislocations must be done in the following manner (to avoid converting to a complex dislocation).
  — The examiner grasps the injured hand with his or her fingers on the patient's palm.
  — The examiner's thumbs are placed on the dorsal surface of the base of the proximal phalanx; the wrist is flexed to relax the flexor tendons.
  — A volar-directed force is then applied with the examiner's thumbs, and the joint should slide back into place.
  — Avoid axial traction to prevent interposition of the volar plate into the MCP joint (Fig. 102-6).
- Complex dislocations are irreducible due to entrapment of the volar plate and generally require open treatment and should be referred to a hand surgeon.
- Splinting
  — Extension block splint, with fingers flexed enough to ensure a stable reduction
  — Encourage patients to fully flex the fingers.
  — Each week the extension block is reduced 10 degrees until full extension is achieved.
  — Buddy taping alone is not adequate for initial treatment.

Troubleshooting

- Attempts at reduction are generally always recommended; however, certain injuries render the joint irreducible under closed means. Prompt referral to a specialist is indicated.
- Meticulous pre- and postreduction examination of perfusion, sensation, and skin integrity is mandatory.
- Proper digital or regional anesthesia will often yield superior results in both the reduction maneuver and accurate stability testing.
- Associated significant bony or unstable ligamentous injuries warrant referral to a hand surgeon.
- Chronically unstable joints generally will not respond to prolonged immobilization and require ligamentous reconstruction.
- Overtreatment (prolonged splinting) often results in stiffness and flexion contractures (of the PIP joints) and extension contractures (of the MCP joints).
- Prolonged swelling and discomfort for several months even in a stable joint are not uncommon.

Suggested Reading

- Carter PR: Common Hand Injuries and Infections: A Practical Approach to Early Treatment. Philadelphia: WB Saunders, 1983, pp 107–122.
- Daniels JM II, Zook EG, Lynch JM: Hand and wrist injuries: Part II. Emergent evaluation. Am Fam Physician 2004; 69:1949–1956.
- Doyle JR: Orthopaedic Essentials Series: Hand and Wrist. Philadelphia: Lippincott Williams & Wilkins, 2006, pp 144–157.
- Freiberg A, Pollard BA, Macdonald MR, Duncan MJ: Management of proximal interphalangeal joint injuries. Hand Clin 2006;22:235–242.
- Glickel SZ, Barron OA, Eaton RG: Dislocations and ligament injuries in the digits. In Green DP, Hotchkiss RN, Pederson WC, Wolfe SW [eds]: Green's Operative Hand Surgery, 5th ed. Philadelphia: Churchill Livingstone, 2005, pp 343–388.
- Graham TJ, Mullen DJ: Athletic injuries of the adult hand. In DeLee JC, Drez D Jr, Miller MD (eds): DeLee and Drez's Orthopaedic Sports Medicine, 2nd ed. Philadelphia: WB Saunders, 2002, pp 1381–1430.
- Seiler JG III: Essentials of Hand Surgery. American Society for Surgery of the Hand. Philadelphia: Lippincott Williams & Wilkins, 2002, pp 343–387.
- Trumble TE: Principles of Hand Surgery and Therapy. Philadelphia: WB Saunders, 2000, pp 41–89.

Chapter 103 Aspiration of Ganglion Cyst

David Schnur

CPT CODE

20612 *Aspiration and/or Injection of Ganglion Cyst Any Location*

Equipment

- Syringe (3–5 mL)
- 18-Gauge needle (to draw up medicine)
- 27-Gauge needle (⅝ inch)
- Local anesthetic (1% to 2% lidocaine plain)
- Corticosteroid (optional)
- Sterile prep solution (alcohol or povidone-iodine)
- Hemostat (if using injectable agent)
- Ethyl chloride, optional but suggested
- Sterile gauze and adhesive bandage

Indication

- Diagnosed ganglion cyst with pain or loss of function
- Mass with suspected diagnosis of a ganglion cyst

Contraindications

- Ganglion cyst of the volar wrist
- Volar retinacular ganglion less than 3 or 4 mm

Instructions/Technique

- Verbal consent is obtained and the correct side is verified.
- Have the patient wash the wrist with soap and water for 1 to 2 minutes.
- Place the patient in a semirecumbent or recumbent position.
- Place 1 mL of a local anesthetic agent in the syringe.
- Prep the area with alcohol or povidone-iodine.
- Use ethyl chloride for patient comfort (recommended).
- Using a 27-gauge needle, inject the skin overlying the ganglion.
- Use an 18-gauge needle to aspirate the ganglion (Fig. 103-1).
- Fluid in the ganglion is clear or clear yellow and viscous (Fig. 103-2).
- If injecting a corticosteroid, use a hemostat to remove the syringe and leave the needle in the cyst.
- Fill the syringe with the corticosteroid using an 18-gauge needle.
- Reattach the syringe and inject the agent into the cyst.
- Massage the area of the cyst in an attempt to express any additional fluid (not recommended if corticosteroid is injected into the cyst because corticosteroids expressed into subcutaneous tissue may cause fat atrophy or hypopigmentation).
- Apply an adhesive bandage.
- With successful aspiration, immediate reduction in the size of the cyst or disappearance of the cyst should be observed and symptoms improved or resolved.

Considerations in Special Populations

- Diabetic patients may experience an increase in blood sugar level if corticosteroids are injected and should be instructed to check it and treat themselves appropriately.

Troubleshooting

- Unsuccessful aspiration of a mass may indicate that it is a solid mass.

Patient Instructions

- Aspiration should improve symptoms.
- Patients should be instructed about the possibility or probability of recurrence of the cyst.
- After one or two recurrences, patients should be considered for surgery if symptomatic.

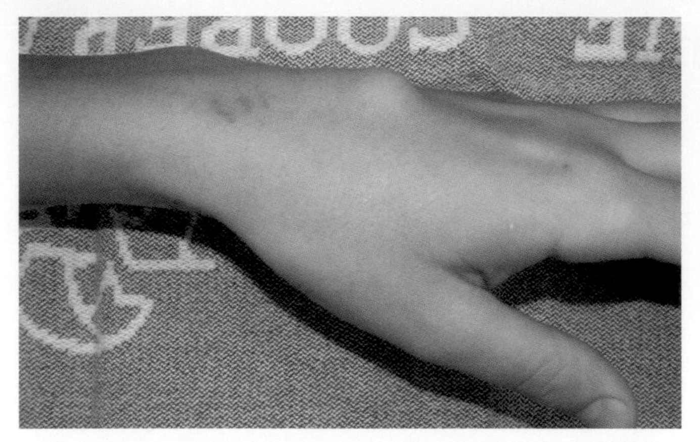

Figure 103-1 Typical appearance of a dorsal wrist ganglion. The needle is inserted directly into the ganglion, aiming slightly proximally until clear or clear yellow viscous fluid is aspirated.

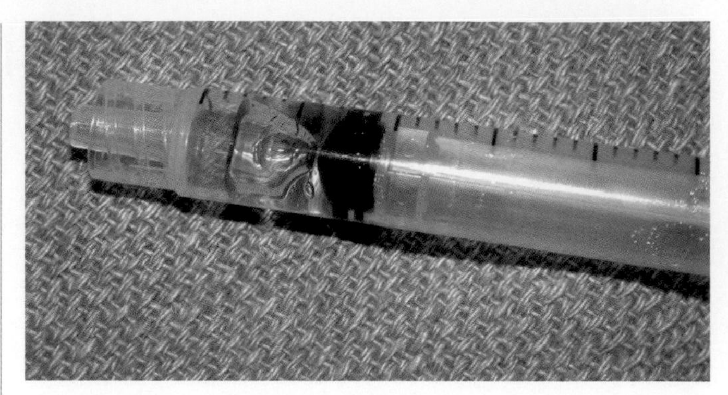

Figure 103-2 Appearance of viscous cyst fluid in the syringe after aspiration.

Chapter 104 de Quervain's/First Dorsal Compartment Injection

David Schnur

CPT CODE

20550 *Injection; Single Tendon Sheath, or Ligament, Aponeurosis*

Equipment

- Injection syringe (3–5 mL)
- 18-Gauge needle (to draw up medicine)
- 25-Gauge needle
- Local anesthetic (1% to 2% lidocaine plain)
- Injectable agent (corticosteroid of choice)
- Sterile prep solution (alcohol or povidone-iodine)
- Hemostat
- Ethyl chloride, optional but suggested
- Sterile gauze and adhesive bandage

Indications

- Tenosynovitis of the first dorsal compartment
- Pain consistent with de Quervain's tenosynovitis
- Loss of function of the thumb

Contraindications

- Fat atrophy or hypopigmentation with previous injection
- Multiple injections (more than three) without effect
- Brittle diabetics may experience an increase in the blood sugar level with injections.
- Allergy to commercial corticosteroid preparations

Instructions/Technique

- Verbal consent is obtained and the correct side is verified.
- Have the patient wash the wrist with soap and water for 1 to 2 minutes.
- Place the patient in a semirecumbent or recumbent position.
- Place 1 to 2 mL of a local anesthetic in the syringe.
- Identify the location of the first dorsal compartment while the patient abducts the thumb and mark it (Fig. 104-1).
- Prep the area with alcohol or povidone-iodine.
- Use ethyl chloride for patient comfort (recommended).
- Insert a 25-gauge needle with local anesthetic in the first dorsal compartment with the needle aimed slightly distally to proximally, entering the compartment just proximal to the radial styloid (Fig. 104-2).
- Inject approximately 1 mL of a local anesthetic agent into the compartment.
- May encounter resistance with injection that suddenly gives way as local anesthetic passes through the compartment
- Having the patient abduct the thumb at this point may confirm the correct location (the syringe will move with the thumb).
- Using a hemostat, remove the syringe and leave the needle in the first dorsal compartment.
- Fill the syringe with corticosteroid using an 18-gauge needle.
- Reattach the syringe and inject the steroid into the compartment.
- Remove the needle quickly to minimize steroid infiltration into subcutaneous tissue.
- Apply an adhesive bandage.
- If the local anesthetic agent is injected into the correct location, Finkelstein's test should elicit significantly less pain.

Considerations in Special Populations

- Diabetic patients may experience an increase in the blood sugar level and should be instructed to check it and treat themselves appropriately.

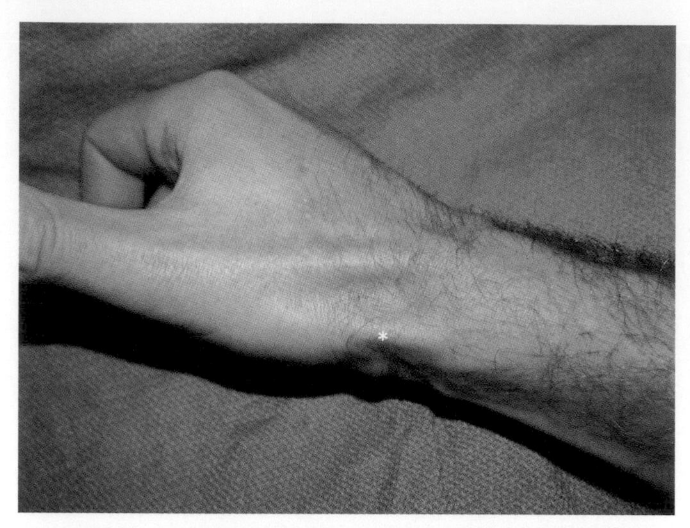

Figure 104-1 With the thumb extended and abducted from the hand, the tendons of the first dorsal compartment can be identified *(asterisk).* Mark this location with a pen to the compartment when the thumb is relaxed.

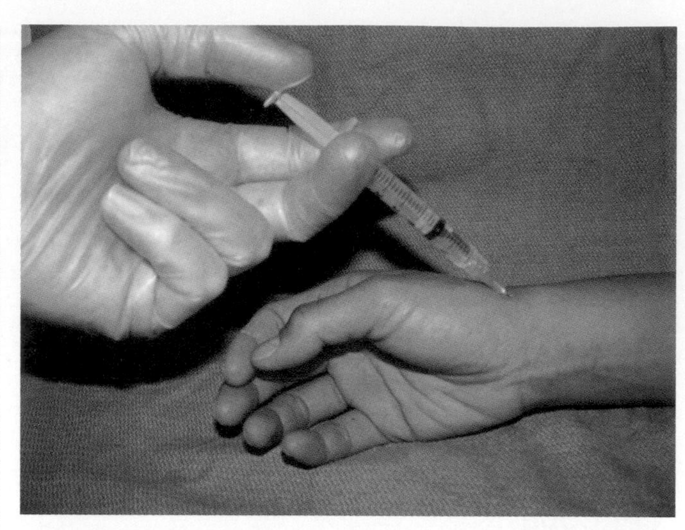

Figure 104-2 The first dorsal compartment is injected just proximal to the tip of the radial styloid with the needle aimed slightly proximally.

Troubleshooting

- If the local anesthetic does not inject or is very difficult to inject, gently reposition the needle because it may be in the tendon.
- Minimize volumes of injection because the corticosteroid will pass into the subcutaneous tissue proximal to the compartment and may cause fat atrophy or hypopigmentation.
- Be sure to warn dark-skinned individuals about the possibility of hypopigmentation.
- Failure or partial relief of symptoms may indicate a septum within the compartment separating tendons.

Patient Instructions

- Explain to the patient that it will take several days to experience the effects of the corticosteroid.
- Occasionally patients will have increased pain in the 24 hours after the injection; consider giving a prescription for pain medication.
- Splinting is optional after injection but may aid in the short-term relief of symptoms.
- Tell the patient to return after 2 weeks for a second injection if symptoms persist.

Chapter 105 Radiocarpal Joint Injection

Dan A. Zlotolow

CPT CODE

20605 *Intermediate Joint or Bursa Injection*

Make sure to include a modifier 25 if also billing for the office visit under the same diagnosis code. One cannot bill for the office visit if the purpose of the visit is for the injection.

Radiocarpal Joint Injection

- Wrist injection/aspiration
- Triangular fibrocartilage complex injection

Equipment (Fig. 105-1)

- Two 3-mL syringes
- Two large-bore needles
- One ⅝-inch 25-gauge needle
- 2% lidocaine without epinephrine
- 0.5% bupivacaine without epinephrine
- 40 mg/mL triamcinolone acetonide (or other corticosteroid of your choice)
- Alcohol wipes or povidone-iodine prep sticks
- Ethyl chloride spray
- 2 × 2-inch gauze
- Small self-adhesive bandage

Indications

- Aspiration
  - Suspected joint infection
  - Gouty arthritis
- Injection
  - Osteoarthritis
  - Rheumatoid arthritis
  - Posttraumatic joint stiffness
  - Wrist pain that has failed splinting and activity modification

Contraindications

- Aspiration
  - Overlying cellulitis
- Injection
  - Suspected septic arthritis
  - Overlying skin compromise

Instructions/Technique

- Load one syringe with 1.5 mL of 2% lidocaine and 1.5 mL of 0.5% bupivacaine using the large-bore needle, and then change to the 25-gauge needle.
- Load the other syringe with 0.5 mL of 2% lidocaine and 1 mL of triamcinolone acetonide using the other large-bore needle.
- Obtain verbal or written consent for the procedure (if mandated by your facility).
- Identify the correct site and side for the injection/aspiration.
- Mark the soft spot 1 cm distal to Lister's tubercle for a radiocarpal injection.
- Mark the soft spot just distal to the distal radioulnar joint for a triangular fibrocartilage complex injection (Fig. 105-2).
- Prep the skin with an antiseptic solution (Fig. 105-3).
- Use a short burst of ethyl chloride to numb the skin
- Inject a small wheel of local anesthetic from the first syringe, slowly infiltrating the area with local anesthetic until the joint is reached (Fig. 105-4).
- Keeping light thumb pressure on the plunger at all times facilitates identification of joint penetration (the resistance should ease after a slight pop is felt).
- While maintaining the needle in the joint, switch syringes and inject the contents of the second syringe into the joint (Fig. 105-5).

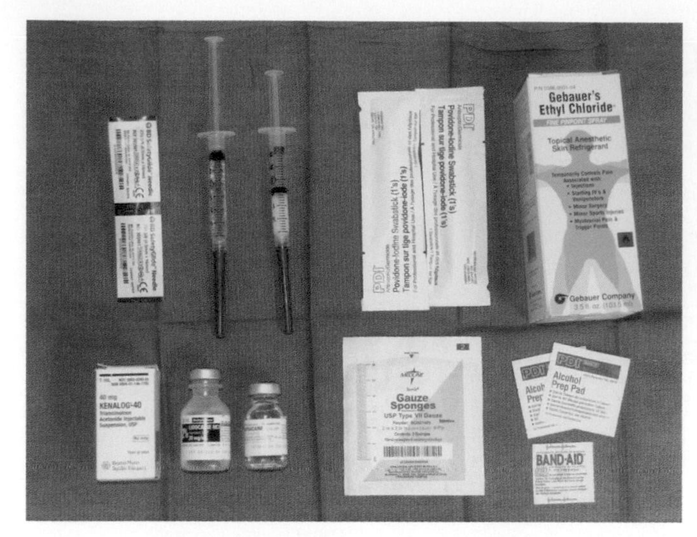

Figure 105-1 Recommended supplies.

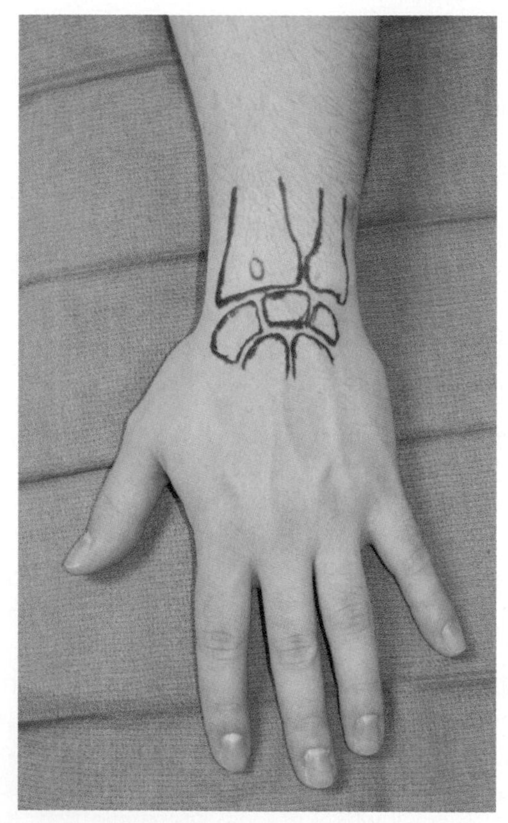

Figure 105-2 Identify the landmarks for the injection sites.

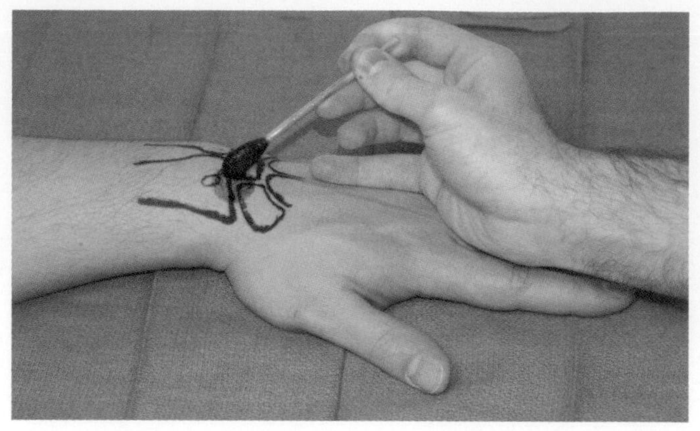

Figure 105-3 Use an antiseptic solution to prep the skin.

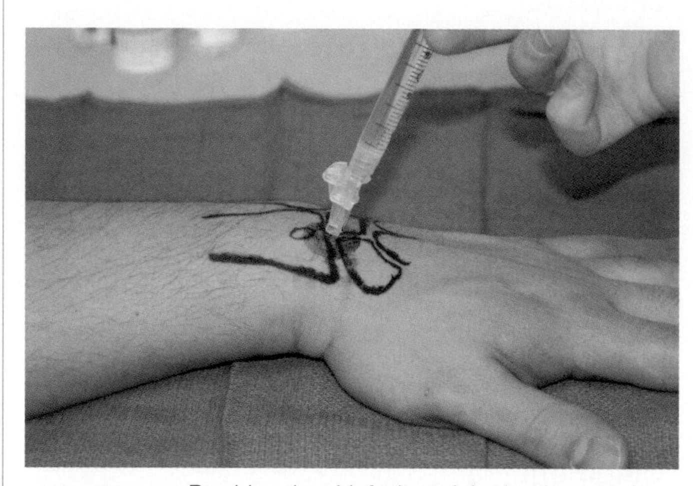

Figure 105-4 Provide a local infusion of the bupivacaine/lidocaine mix as you search for the joint (note that the thumb is always on the plunger to aid with proprioception).

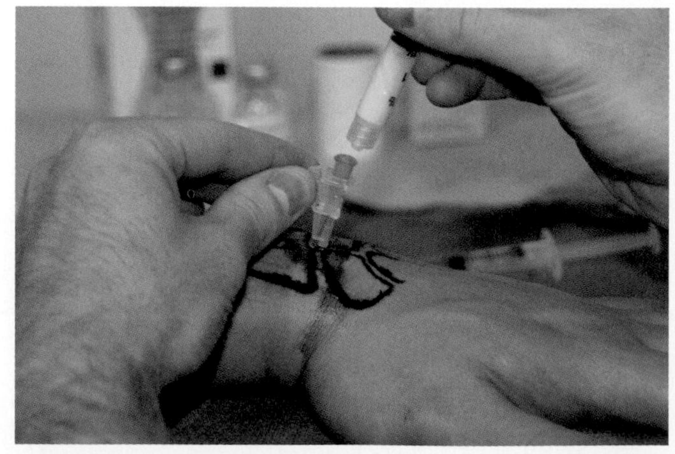

Figure 105-5 While keeping the needle in the joint, switch syringes.

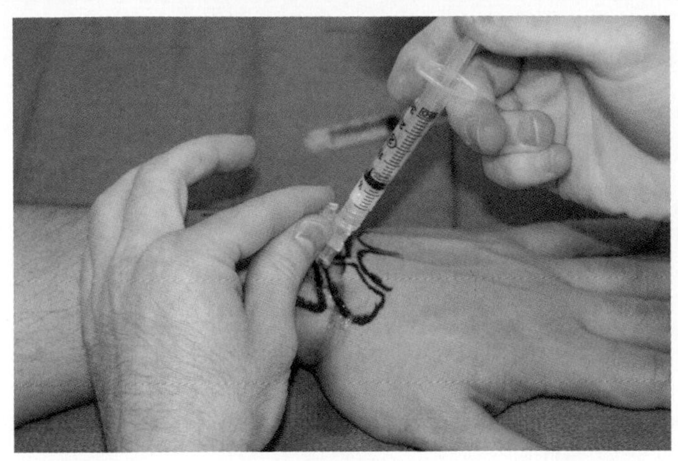

Figure 105-6 Inject the triamcinolone acetonide into the joint.

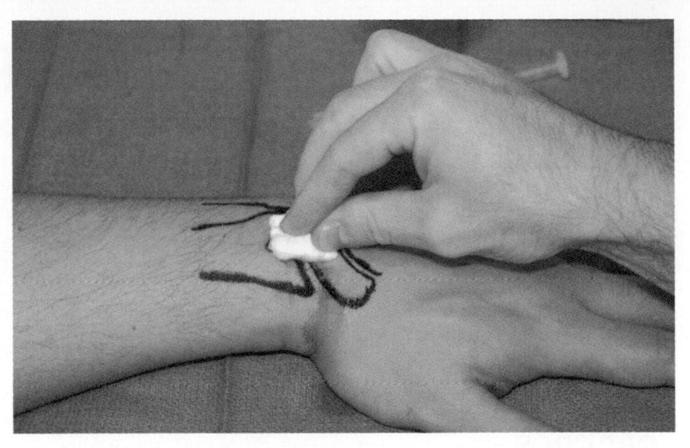

Figure 105-7 Apply a bandage and hold pressure to prevent bleeding.

- If resistance is experienced, move the needle slightly in or out until the injectate goes in easily (Fig. 105-6).
- Remove the needle and apply pressure with the gauze bandage (Fig. 105-7).
- Place a sterile self-adhesive bandage over the injection site.

Considerations in Special Populations

- Patients with diabetes should be cautioned that corticosteroid injections may increase their blood sugar levels.
- Patients with hypertrophic osteoarthritis may have tight joint spaces, which makes injection difficult.

Troubleshooting

- If the joint is difficult to enter, walk along the bone with the needle until the needle "falls" into the joint.

Patient Instructions

- Instruct patients to ice the wrist in the evening and to take whatever medication they take for a headache before going to bed.
- Increasing levels of pain, an enlarging effusion, or fever should merit an urgent visit back to the physician's office or emergency department for evaluation of septic arthritis.
- The effects of the triamcinolone actonide may not be noticed until up to 2 weeks after the injection.

Chapter 106 Carpal Tunnel Injection

David Schnur

CPT CODE

20526 *Injection, Therapeutic (e.g., Local Anesthetic, Corticosteroid), Carpal Tunnel*

Equipment

- Injection syringe (3–5 mL)
- 18-Gauge needle (to draw up medicine)
- 25-Gauge needle (1.5 inches)
- Local anesthetic (1% to 2% lidocaine plain)
- Injectable agent (corticosteroid of choice)
- Sterile prep solution (alcohol or povidone-iodine) (Fig. 106-1)
- Hemostat
- Ethyl chloride, optional but suggested
- Sterile gauze and adhesive bandage

Indications

- Diagnosed carpal tunnel syndrome
- Suspected carpal tunnel syndrome based on history and physical examination
- Pain
- Subjective numbness in the thumb and index and long fingers

Contraindications

- Marked increase in two-point discrimination or severe carpal tunnel syndrome based on electromyography/nerve conduction velocity (surgery should be considered as initial treatment)
- Anticoagulation with significant increase in prothrombin time or partial thromboplastin time
- Fat atrophy or hypopigmentation with previous injection
- Multiple injections (more than three) without effect
- Brittle diabetics may experience an increase in the blood sugar level with injections.
- Allergy to commercial corticosteroid preparations

Instructions/Technique

- Verbal consent is obtained and the correct side is verified.
- Have the patient wash the wrist with soap and water for 1 to 2 minutes.
- Place the patient in a semirecumbent or recumbent position.
- Place 1 to 2 mL of a local anesthetic agent in a syringe.
- Prep the area with alcohol or povidone-iodine.
- Use ethyl chloride for patient comfort (recommended).
- Insert the 25-gauge needle with local anesthetic into the carpal canal.
  - The needle should be inserted into the skin at the level of the proximal wrist crease and aimed toward the metacarpophalangeal joints of the fingers.
  - The thumb or index finger is used to locate the hook of the hamate.
  - The needle is inserted just ulnar to the palmaris longus tendon and aimed just radial to the hook of the hamate (Figs. 106-2 and 106-3).
  - Once the needle is inserted to the level of the hub, the patient is asked to wiggle the fingers slightly.
  - If the needle is in the correct position, the syringe will move with the fingers.
  - If at any time during the insertion of the needle the patient experiences shooting pain or shock into the fingers, the needle should be pulled out and reinserted.
- Inject approximately 1 mL of local anesthetic into the carpal canal.
- Using a hemostat, remove the syringe and leave the needle in the carpal canal.
- Fill the syringe with a corticosteroid using an 18-gauge needle.
- Reattach the syringe and inject the corticosteroid into the carpal canal.

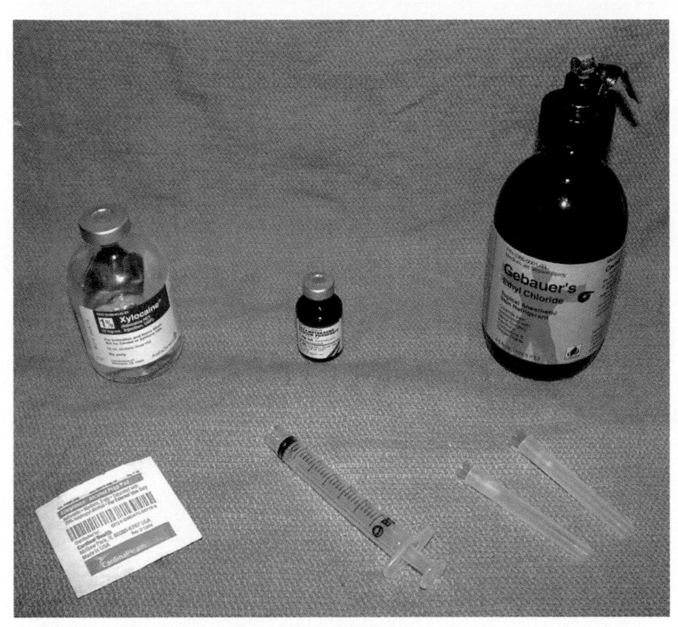

Figure 106-1 Set-up for carpal tunnel injection: local anesthetic agent, corticosteroid, ethyl chloride, alcohol swab, needles, and a syringe.

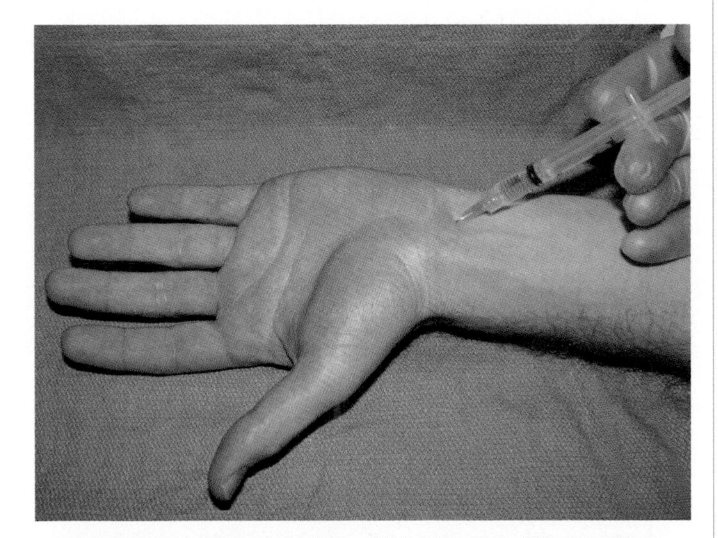

Figure 106-2 Demonstration of injection into the carpal canal. The needle is inserted just proximal to the wrist crease, directed distally, and inserted at an angle of approximately 30 degrees.

- Remove the needle quickly to minimize steroid infiltration into the subcutaneous tissue.
- Apply an adhesive bandage.
- Have the patient flex and extend the fingers multiple times.
- Numbness in the thumb or index, long, or radial ring finger indicates correct placement of the corticosteroid.

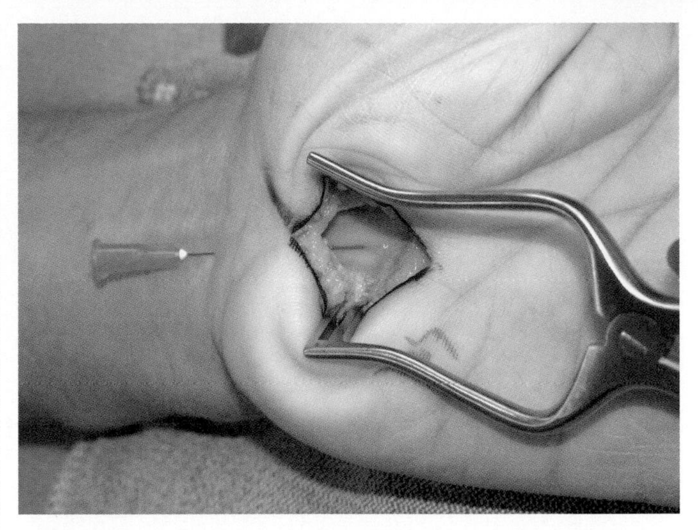

Figure 106-3 With the needle in the proper position for injection, the end of the needle is seen in the carpal canal.

- Absence of numbness is not predictive of the location of the corticosteroid.
- Relief of symptoms strongly supports the diagnosis of carpal tunnel syndrome.
- Relief of symptoms has been shown to be predictive of relief of symptoms with surgical release.

Considerations in Special Populations

- Diabetic patients may experience an increase in the blood sugar level and should be instructed to check it and treat themselves appropriately.

Troubleshooting

- If the local anesthetic does not inject or is very difficult to inject, then gently reposition the needle because it may be in the tendon.
- Be sure to warn dark-skinned individuals about the possibility of hypopigmentation.
- Water-soluble corticosteroids have a lower chance of nerve damage if they are accidentally injected into a nerve.
- If the patient has a sensation of electrical shock in the fingers or the needle does not move when the fingers are wiggled, then pull the needle tip out into the subcutaneous tissue and redirect it.

Patient Instructions

- Explain to the patient that it will take several days to experience the effects of the corticosteroid.

- Occasionally patients will have increased pain in the 24 hours after the injection; consider giving a prescription for pain medication.
- Splinting is optional after injection but may aid in the short-term relief of symptoms.
- Tell the patient to return after 2 weeks for a second injection if symptoms persist.
- Successful injection should relieve symptoms for at least 6 weeks but can give considerably longer relief.

Chapter 107 Carpometacarpal Injection

David Schnur

CPT CODE

20605 *Arthrocentesis, Aspiration, and/or Injection Intermediate Joint or Bursa*

Equipment

- Injection syringe (3–5 mL)
- 18-Gauge needle (to draw up medicine)
- 25-Gauge needle (⅝ inches)
- Local anesthetic agent (1 to 2% lidocaine plain)
- Injectable agent (corticosteroid of choice)
- Sterile prep solution (alcohol or povidone-iodine)
- Hemostat
- Ethyl chloride, optional but suggested
- Sterile gauze and adhesive bandage

Indications

- Diagnosed carpometacarpal (CMC) arthritis
- Suspected CMC arthritis based on history, physical examination, and radiographs
- Pain
- Loss of function of the thumb
- Failed conservative treatment (splinting and therapy)

Contraindications

- Anticoagulation with significant increase in prothrombin time or partial thromboplastin time
- Fat atrophy or hypopigmentation with previous injection
- Multiple injections (more than three) without effect
- Brittle diabetics may experience an increase in the blood sugar level with injections.
- Allergy to commercial corticosteroid preparations

Instructions/Technique

- Verbal consent is obtained and the correct side is verified.
- Have the patient wash the wrist with soap and water for 1 to 2 minutes.
- Place the patient in a semirecumbent or recumbent position.
- Place 0.5 mL of local anesthetic agent in a syringe.
- Identify the location of the CMC joint and mark it (just proximal to the prominence of the base of the thumb metacarpal) (Fig. 107-1).
- Prep the area with alcohol or povidone-iodine.
- Use ethyl chloride for patient comfort (recommended).
- Place traction on the thumb to open the joint space.
- Insert a 25-gauge needle with the local anesthetic into the CMC joint (Fig. 107-2).
- Inject approximately 0.5 mL of local anesthetic into the joint.
- May encounter resistance with small joints; can put less than 0.5 mL into the joint
- Using a hemostat, remove the syringe and leave the needle in the CMC joint.
- Fill the syringe with the corticosteroid using an 18-gauge needle (typically 1 mL of corticosteroid).
- Reattach the syringe and inject the corticosteroid into the joint.
- May not be able to get the full 1 mL of anesthetic into the joint
- Remove the needle quickly to minimize corticosteroid infiltration into subcutaneous tissue.
- Apply an adhesive bandage.
- If the local anesthetic is injected into the correct location, a grind test should elicit significantly less pain.

Considerations in Special Populations

- Diabetic patients may experience an increase in the blood sugar level and should be instructed to check it and treat themselves appropriately.

Troubleshooting

- If the local anesthetic does not inject or is very difficult to inject, then gently reposition the needle by “walking” the needle either proximally or distally as needed.

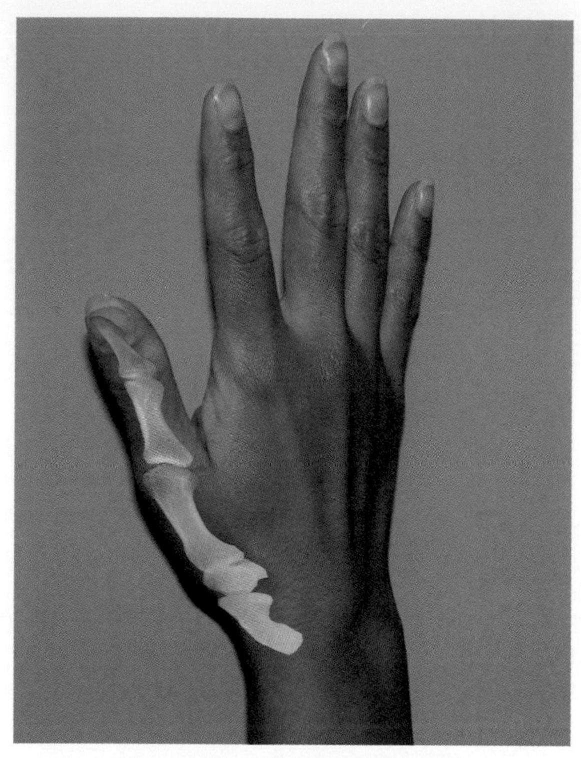

Figure 107-1 Topographic relationship of the carpometacarpal joint to the thumb.

- Most joints will be slightly difficult to inject because of the small volume, but occasionally a very arthritic joint will easily accept larger volumes.
- Be sure to warn dark-skinned individuals about the possibility of hypopigmentation.
- Significant resistance to injection may not be encountered with patients with advanced disease; this can be due to the loss of integrity of the CMC joint.

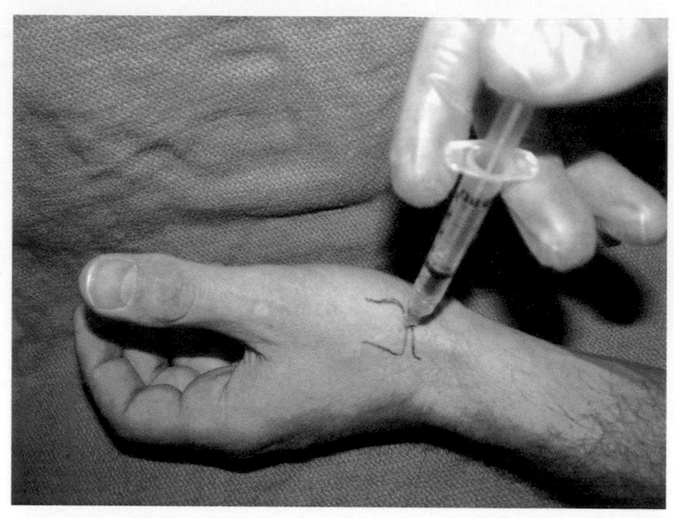

Figure 107-2 Needle inserted in the carpometacarpal joint of the thumb.

Patient Instructions

- Explain to the patient that it will take several days to experience the effects of the corticosteroid.
- Occasionally patients will have increased pain in the 24 hours after the injection; consider giving a prescription for pain medication.
- Splinting is optional after injection but may aid in the short-term relief of symptoms.
- Tell the patient to return after 2 weeks for a second injection if symptoms persist.

Chapter 108 Trigger Finger Injection

Jack Ingari

CPT CODE

20550 *Injection, Tendon Sheath, Ligament, Trigger Points, or Ganglion Cyst*

Key Points

- As many as 90% to 95% of trigger fingers may resolve after one to three corticosteroid injections, which is a very good nonoperative option.

Equipment (Fig. 108-1)

- 5 mL-syringe
- 18-Gauge needle
- 25-Gauge, ⅝-inch needle
- Alcohol prep pads
- Adhesive bandage
- Rubber surgical gloves (optional but recommended)
- 1% lidocaine, without epinephrine
- Corticosteroid (dexamethasone 8 mg/mL is author's preference; triamcinolone acetonide and betamethasone are acceptable alternatives)

Contraindications

- Known or suspected suppurative flexor tenosynovitis is a contraindication for corticosteroid injection.

Technique

- Place the patient's involved hand, palm facing up (supinated), on examination table or other flat surface.
- Prepare the syringe by using the 18-gauge needle to mix 1 mL of 1% lidocaine without epinephrine and 1 mL of corticosteroid (e.g., 1 mL of 8 mg/mL dexamethasone).
- Use alcohol prep pads to cleanse the top of each medication bottle before aspiration of the medication into the syringe.
- Discard the 18-gauge needle and place a 25-gauge, ⅝-inch needle on the syringe.
- Use a sterile alcohol prep to cleanse the involved digit in the area of the proposed injection.
- Inject the mixture of lidocaine and corticosteroid into the area of the A1 pulley (Fig. 108-2).
- Penetrate the dermis (Fig. 108-3).
- The injection is efficacious whether it is in the tendon sheath or superficial to it.
- Place a bandage over the injection site.

Considerations in Special Populations

- Diabetics may experience a transient increase in serum glucose levels (75% higher than the preinjection level at postinjection day 1), lasting as long 5 days.
- The efficacy of the injection is lessened in diabetics; resolution of triggering is still possible in approximately 50% of cases.

Troubleshooting

- If unable to inject, the needle may be embedded in the tendon; withdraw or advance it slightly and continue to exert gentle pressure on the syringe plunger until fluid flows easily.
- If unsure of the correct depth, any depth deep to dermis is acceptable, typically 3 to 5 mm deep from the skin surface
- If after one injection, symptoms are not relieved after 1 to 2 weeks, a second injection has been shown to be helpful in as many as 85% to 90% of patients.
- If symptomatic triggering persists or recurs after three injections, refer for consideration of surgical management.
- Avoid neurovascular bundles by staying in the midline of the digit.

Patient Instructions

- Counsel patients that injection may cause painful throbbing at the injection site (steroid flare) on the night of the injection, and pain medication (a nonsteroidal anti-inflammatory drug or narcotic) can be used on the night of injection if needed.

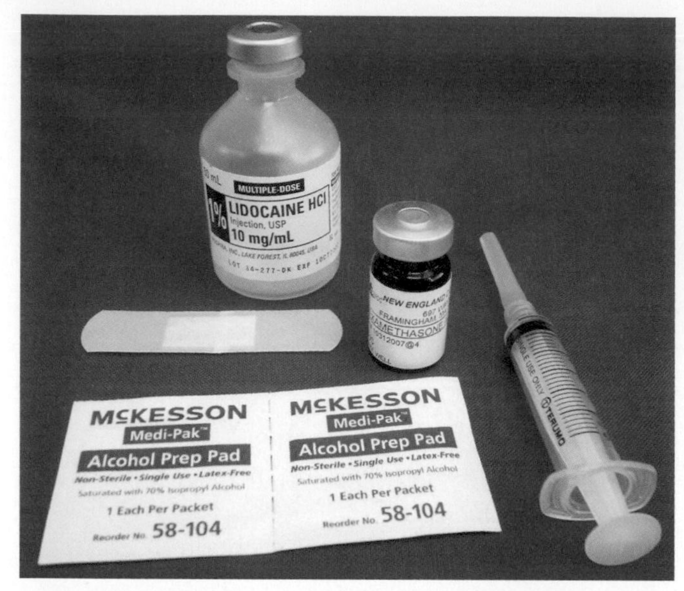

Figure 108-1 Equipment required for a trigger finger injection.

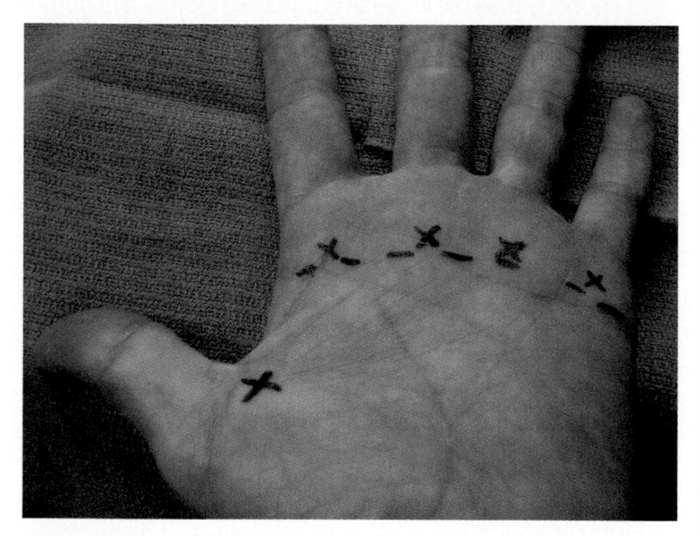

Figure 108-2 A line drawn from the proximal palmar crease radially to the distal palmar crease ulnarly provides a good landmark for trigger finger injections. X marks the spot for needle penetration of the skin.

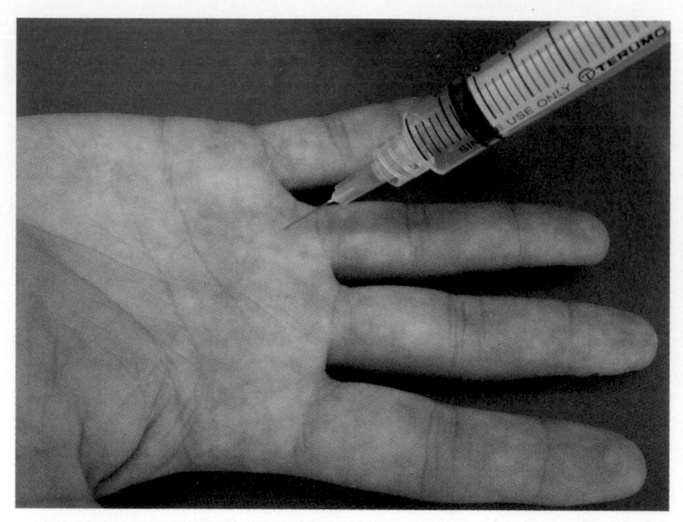

Figure 108-3 A 25-gauge needle is inserted through the skin in the area of the A1 pulley.

- Counsel patients regarding anesthesia in the digit, which lasts as long as 2 hours after injection, due to lidocaine.
- The bandage can be removed 1 to 2 hours after injection.
- The corticosteroid may take several days to provide symptom relief.
- If symptoms are not relieved after 1 to 2 weeks, the patient should return for consideration of a second injection.
- Follow-up as needed if symptoms recur

Chapter 109 Digital Blocks

Daniel Luppens and Jonathan E. Isaacs

CPT Codes

- Do not list a separate CPT code for digital block.
- Code for the procedure that is being performed.
- Digital block is always included in this code.

Equipment

- Use a 10-mL syringe and 1.5-inch 25-gauge needle.
- Local anesthetic agent as recommended in the following

Indications/Contraindications

- Digital block provides significant digital anesthesia with minimal morbidity.
- This is an effective technique any time that part or all of a digit requires anesthesia to allow a patient to tolerate an examination or procedures.
- Avoid blocking fingers with a tenuous vascular supply.
- A definitive neurovascular examination should be performed before blocking a digit.

Instructions/Technique

- Digital nerve block is possible because of predictable nerve anatomy
  - Two digital nerves run parallel to the flexor tendon sheath.
  - Each sends a main branch to the dorsal skin from approximately the proximal interphalangeal joint distally.
  - The proximal dorsal skin of the digits receives innervation from separate cutaneous nerve fibers (Fig. 109-1).
- Quantity given: Use small amounts to decrease injection discomfort and pressure on surrounding soft tissues and vessels.
- Choose the appropriate anesthetic agent depending on the clinical situation.
  - Alkalization of a local anesthetic agent may reduce pain on infiltration and speed onset. Use 1 mL of 8.4% bicarbonate for every 10 mL of lidocaine (a lower concentration of sodium bicarbonate should be used with bupivacaine to avoid precipitate).
    - — However, studies do not consistently show improvement in pain ratings or speed of onset with buffering.
    - — Slow injection was more effective at reducing pain on injection than buffering in one large study.
  - Lidocaine provides 1 to 3 hours of anesthesia.
  - Ropivacaine and bupivacaine provide 10 to 15 hours of anesthesia, with even longer durations reported in some studies.
- Onset is 1 to 3 minutes with lidocaine and 3 to 5 minutes with ropivacaine or bupivacaine.
- Allow at least 10 minutes to elapse from the time of injection regardless of the anesthetic agent for more reliable and complete anesthesia.
- Approach
  - Dorsal (Fig. 109-2)
    - — Insert the needle at the base of the digit dorsally just proximal to the web and advance it until the needle can be seen (or felt) tenting the skin of the palm just proximal to the web.
    - — Inject while withdrawing the needle.
    - — Before removing the needle completely, redirect it across the extensor surface of the finger and make a skin wheal (for dorsal nerve fibers).
    - — Remove the needle and inject again on the other side of the finger.
    - — Two to 3 mL of the local anesthetic should be injected on each side of the finger.
    - — Avoid inadvertent ring block by using small amounts of anesthetic.
  - Volar (Fig. 109-3)
    - — Inject 2 to 3 mL of local anesthetic agent subcutaneously near the distal palmar crease.
    - — Aim a few millimeters radially and then ulnar to the midline to inject anesthetic around both digital nerves.
    - — A more direct approach to the digital nerve but can be more painful

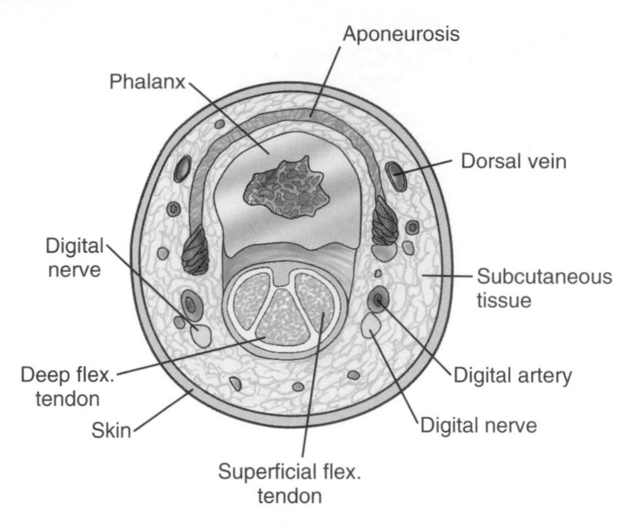

Figure 109-1 Digital nerve anatomy. flex, flexor.

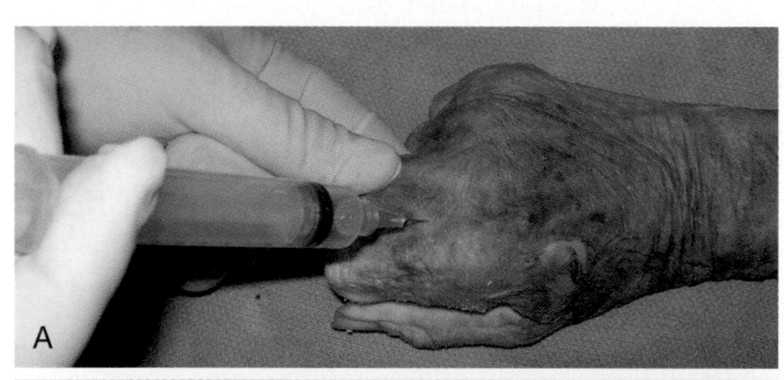

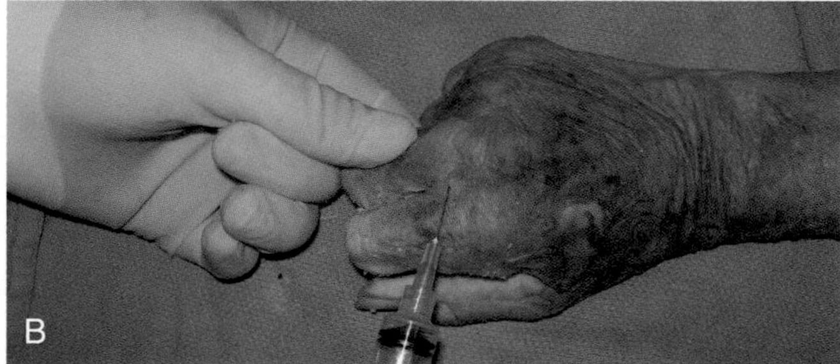

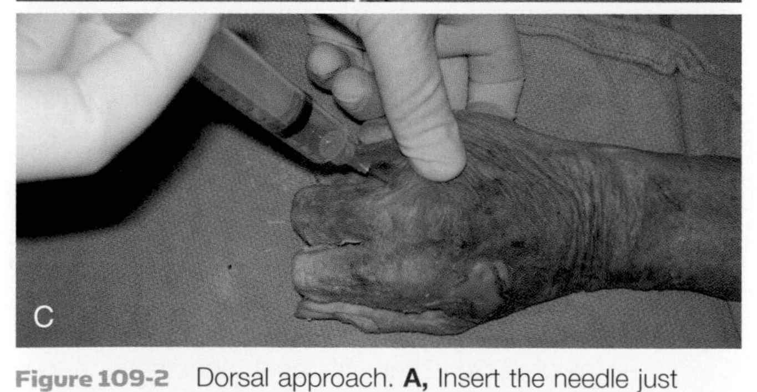

Figure 109-2 Dorsal approach. **A,** Insert the needle just lateral to the base of the proximal phalanx and advance in a slight proximal direction to, but not through, the palmar skin. Inject 2–3 mL while slowing withdrawing the needle. **B,** Redirect the needle within the subcutaneous tissue across the dorsal aspect of the base of the finger. Inject 1–2 mL while slowing withdrawing the needle. **C,** Reposition the needle to the contralateral side of the digit. Advance and inject as described in part A.

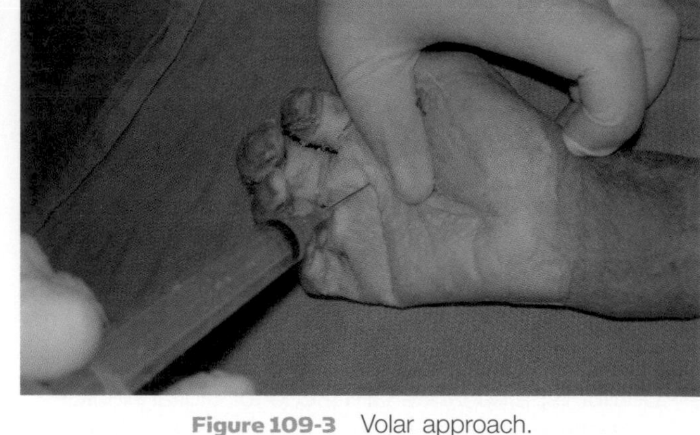

Figure 109-3 Volar approach.

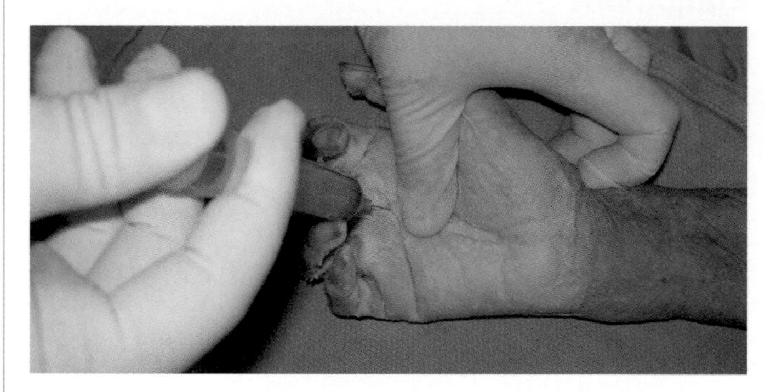

Figure 109-4 Flexor tendon sheath technique.

  - May require dorsal supplement for procedures involving the dorsum of the finger.
- Flexor tendon sheath technique (Fig. 109-4)
  - Inject approximately 2 mL of anesthetic agent into the flexor tendon sheath at the distal palmar crease.
  - Insert the needle through skin, tendon sheath, and tendon down to bone.
  - Apply gentle pressure to the syringe plunger as the needle is withdrawn 1 to 2 mm.
  - As the needle tip enters the potential space of the flexor tendon sheath, resistance will suddenly decrease and the anesthetic agent will be injected into the sheath.
  - Because the digital nerves run along the sides of the sheath, the anesthetic slowly leaks out of the sheath onto both digital nerves.
  - The time of onset and effectiveness of anesthesia are comparable to those of the subcutaneous technique (dorsal), but this technique may be more painful.

Considerations in Special Populations

- Digital blocks can be used on most patients as long as doses are weight appropriate.

Troubleshooting

- Inadequate anesthesia may indicate that the injection did not properly infiltrate adjacent to the digital nerves. Make sure adequate time is given for the block to set up before resorting to repeat injection.
- Anesthetic toxicity must be considered with repeat injections or injection of multiple digits. Maximum recommended doses are as follows: lidocaine, 8 to 11 mg/kg; bupivacaine, 2.5 to 3.5 mg/kg; ropivacaine, 2.5 to 3.5 mg/kg.
- Ischemic injury after digital block is very rare (<1%), but has been reported sporadically in the literature.
    - Addition of epinephrine does not seem to increase complications in current studies.

Patient Instructions

- Patients should be warned not to expect sensation to return to their finger for at least several hours.

Suggested Reading

- Braun H, Harris ML: Operations on extremities. In Braun H, Harris ML (eds): Local Anesthesia: Its Scientific Basis and Practical Use, 2nd ed. New York: Lea & Febiger, 1924, pp 366–367.
- Chiu DTW: Transthecal digital nerve block. J Hand Surg 1990;15:471–473.
- Cummings AJ, William TB, Lynne EM: Modified transthecal digital block versus traditional digital block for anesthesia of the finger. J Hand Surg 2004:29:44–48.
- Keramidas EG, Rodopoulou SG, Tsoutsos D: Comparison of transthecal digital block and traditional digital block of the finger. Plast Reconstr Surg 2004;114:1131–1134.
- Wilhelmi BJ, Blackwell SJ, Miller JH, et al. Do not use epinephrine in digital blocks: Myth or truth? Plast Reconstr Surg 2001;107:393–396.

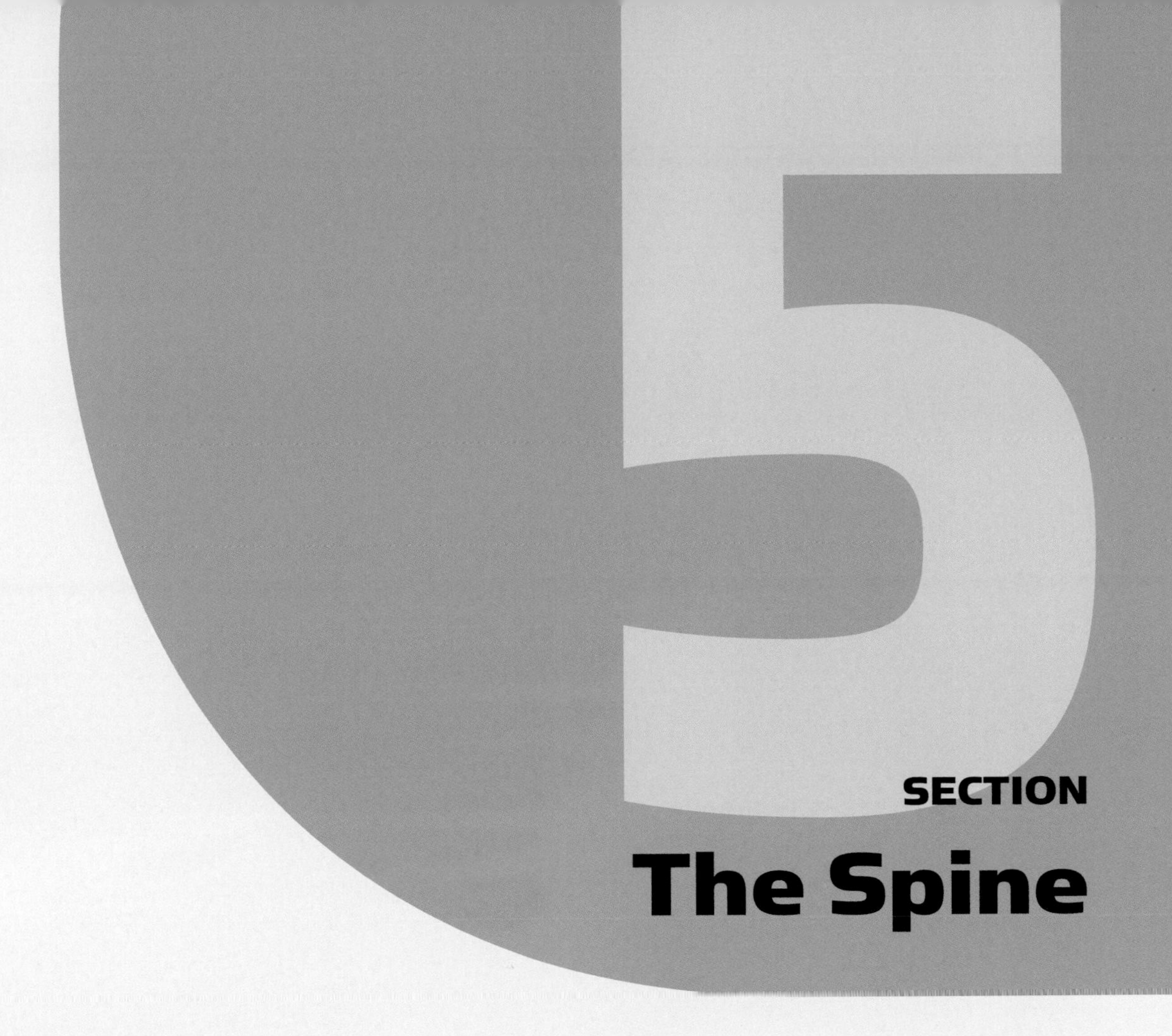

SECTION

The Spine

Chapter 110 Overview of the Spine

Uma Srikumaran and A. Jay Khanna

Anatomy

Spinal Column

- The spinal column is made up of 33 vertebrae: 7 cervical, 12 thoracic, 5 lumbar, 5 sacral, and 4 coccygeal vertebrae.
- Although each vertebra has a distinctive shape based on its location in the spine, with a few exceptions, they share a common structure.
- In general, a single vertebra is made up of the vertebral body, bilateral pedicles, bilateral superior and inferior facets, bilateral lamina, bilateral transverse processes, and the spinous process (Fig. 110-1).
- The intervertebral disc lies between two vertebral bodies and is made up of the annulus fibrosus and the nucleus pulposus (see Fig. 110-1).
- It is important to evaluate the overall alignment of the spine in both the sagittal and coronal planes (Fig. 110-2).
  - Coronal plane alignment is evaluated with anteroposterior standing radiographs, and sagittal plane alignment is evaluated with lateral standing radiographs.
- The normal range of cervical lordosis is approximately 30 to 50 degrees, normal thoracic kyphosis ranges from 20 to 50 degrees, and normal lumbar lordosis ranges from 30 to 80 degrees.

Ligaments

- Several important ligaments connect the vertebrae and provide strength and stability, including the anterior and posterior longitudinal ligaments, which attach to the anterior and posterior aspects of the vertebral body.
- The ligamentum flavum connects the lamina, and the interspinous and supraspinous ligaments connect the spinous processes (Fig. 110-3).

Muscles

- The spine is further stabilized by the musculature of the back and neck (Figs. 110-4 and 110-5).

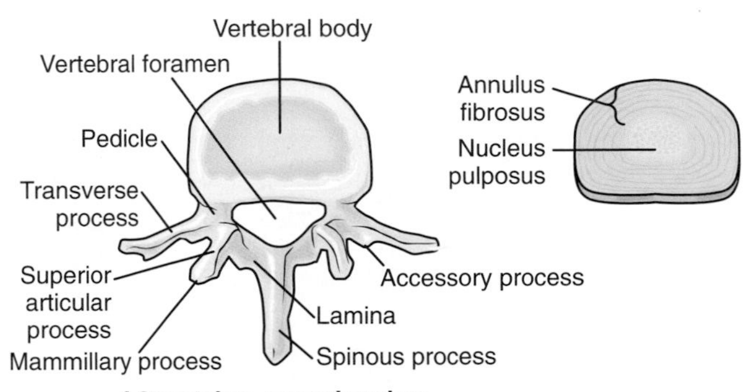

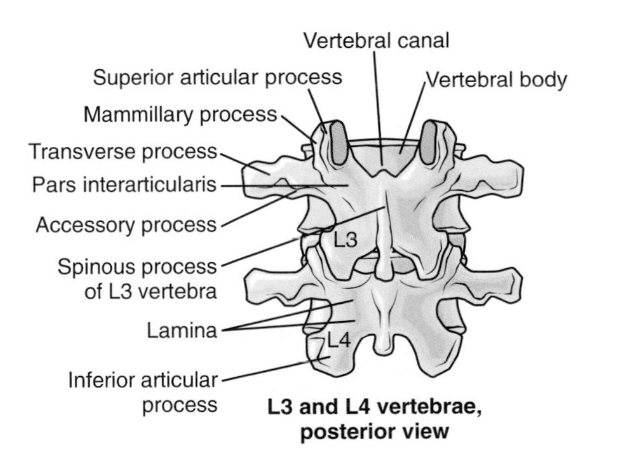

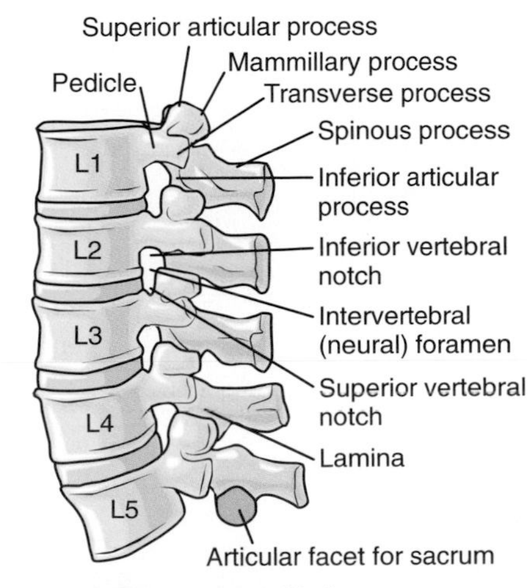

Figure 110-1 The bony anatomy of the lumbar vertebrae and the intervertebral disc.

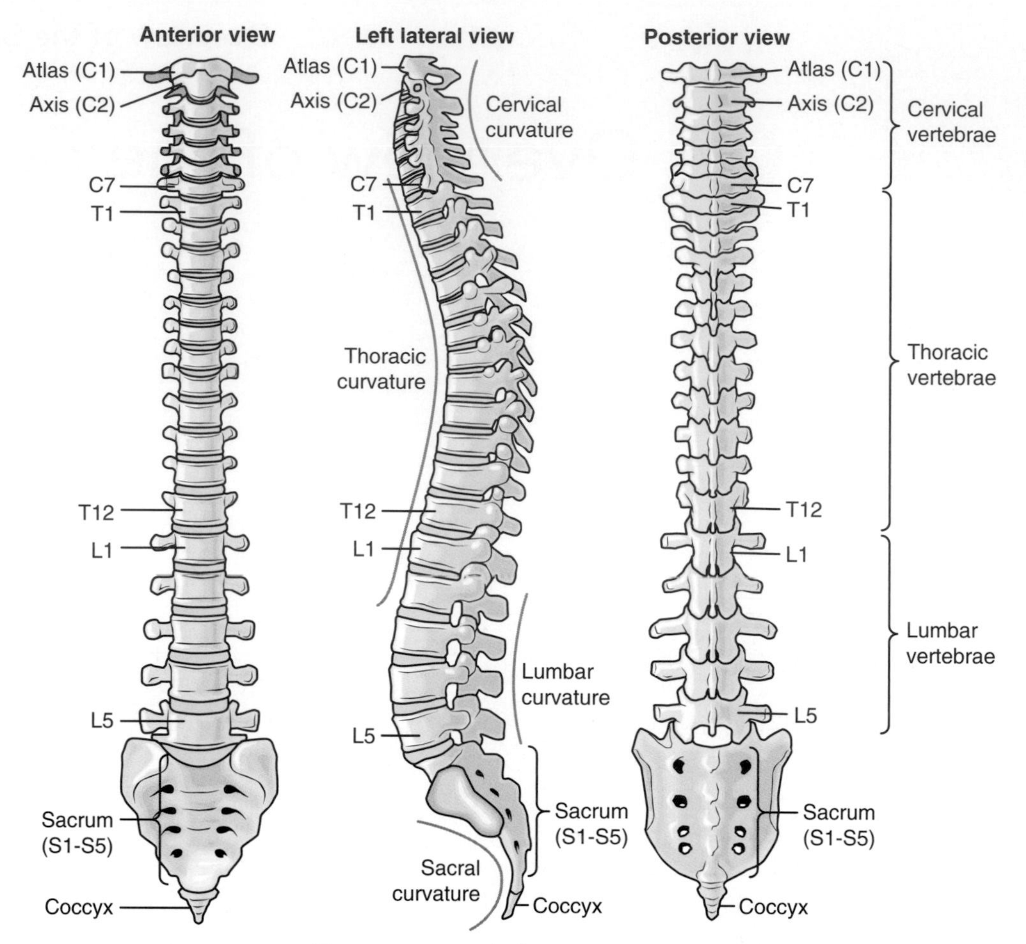

Figure 110-2 The anatomy and alignment of the vertebral column.

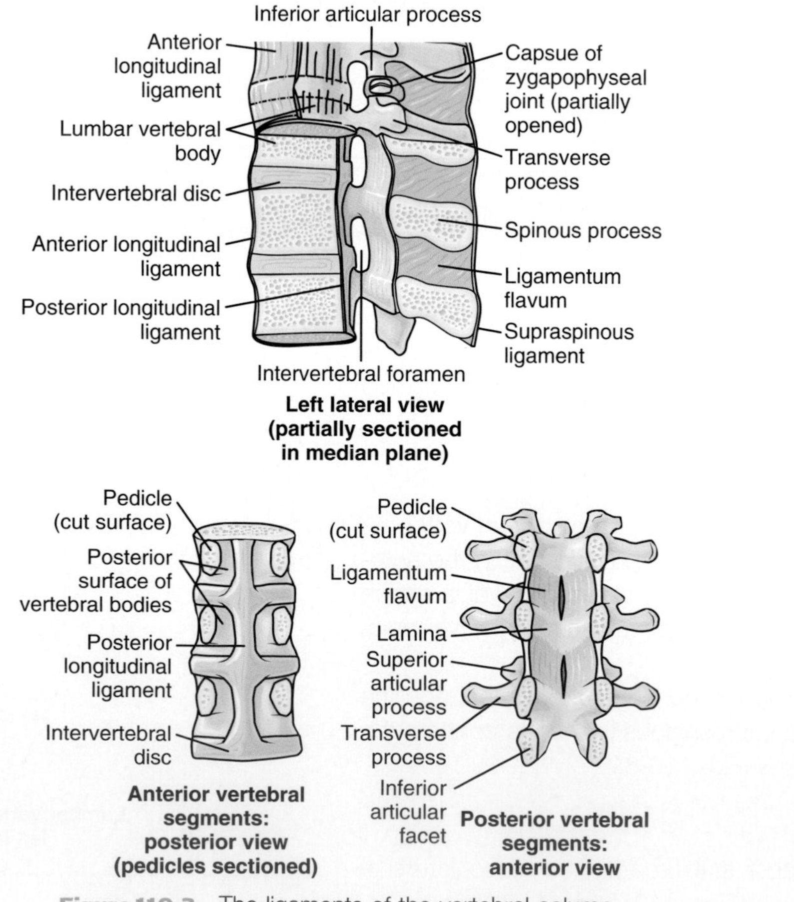

Figure 110-3 The ligaments of the vertebral column.

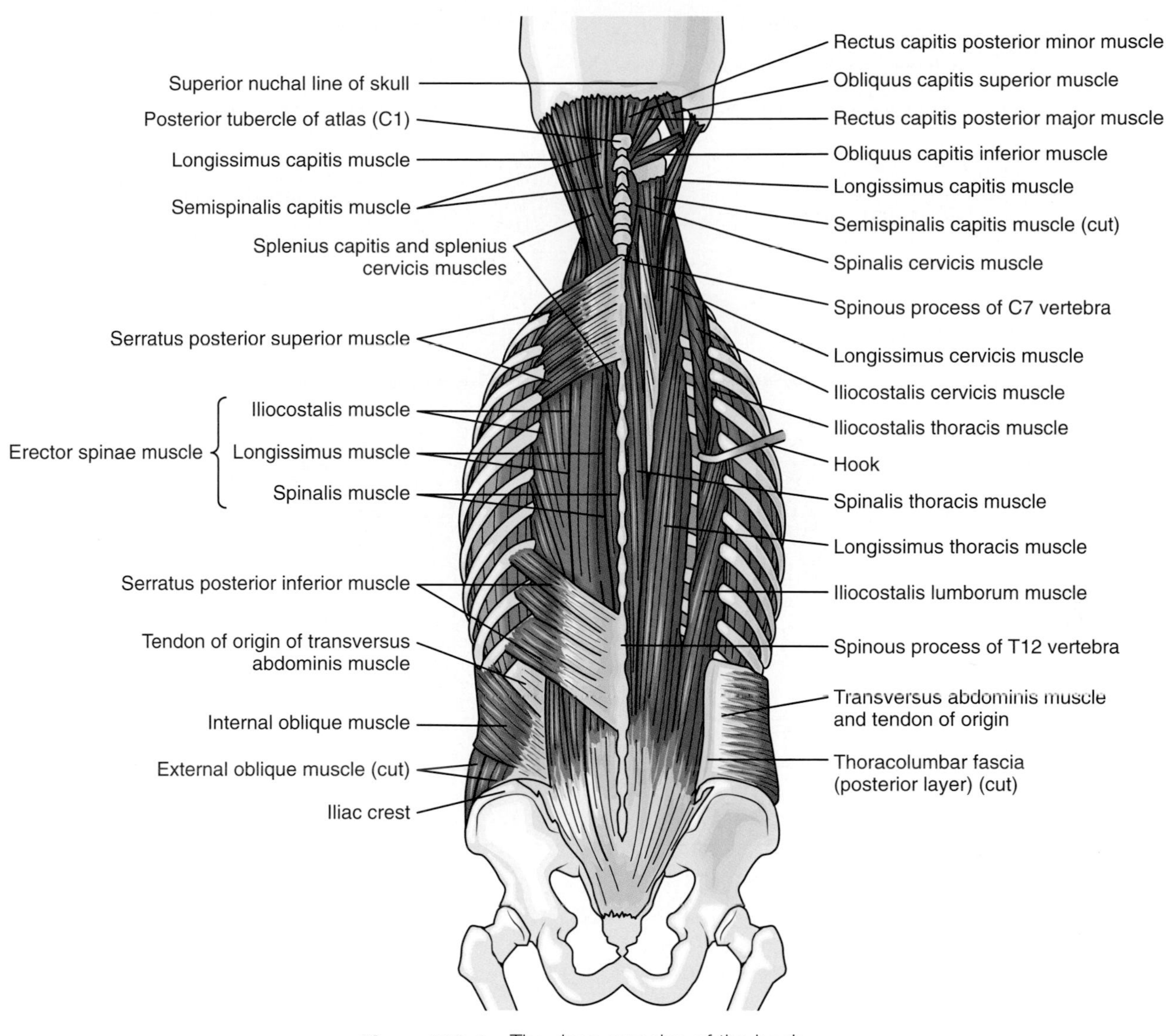

Figure 110-4 The deep muscles of the back.

- At the deepest level, the iliocostalis, longissimus, and spinalis muscles comprise the erector spinae muscle and lie between the transverse and spinous processes of adjacent segments.
  - Superficial to this layer are the rhomboids, serratus posterior, trapezius, and latissimus dorsi muscle groups.

Spinal Cord

- The spinal cord lies within the bony canal created by the vertebral column.
- Thirty-one pairs of nerve roots exit this column through the intervertebral foramina: 8 cervical, 12 thoracic, 5 lumbar, 5 sacral, and 1 coccygeal nerve roots (Fig. 110-6).

Patient Evaluation

History

- As with any patient, a comprehensive history and physical examination are essential components of the diagnosis and decision-making process.
- The complete history begins with the chief complaint and details of the patient's symptoms.
  - Important details include the duration of symptoms or pain, exacerbating and alleviating factors, the anatomic distribution of symptoms, the onset of symptoms, and the quality and severity of the pain.
- For the spine patient, specific attention should be given to the precise distribution of the symptoms in an

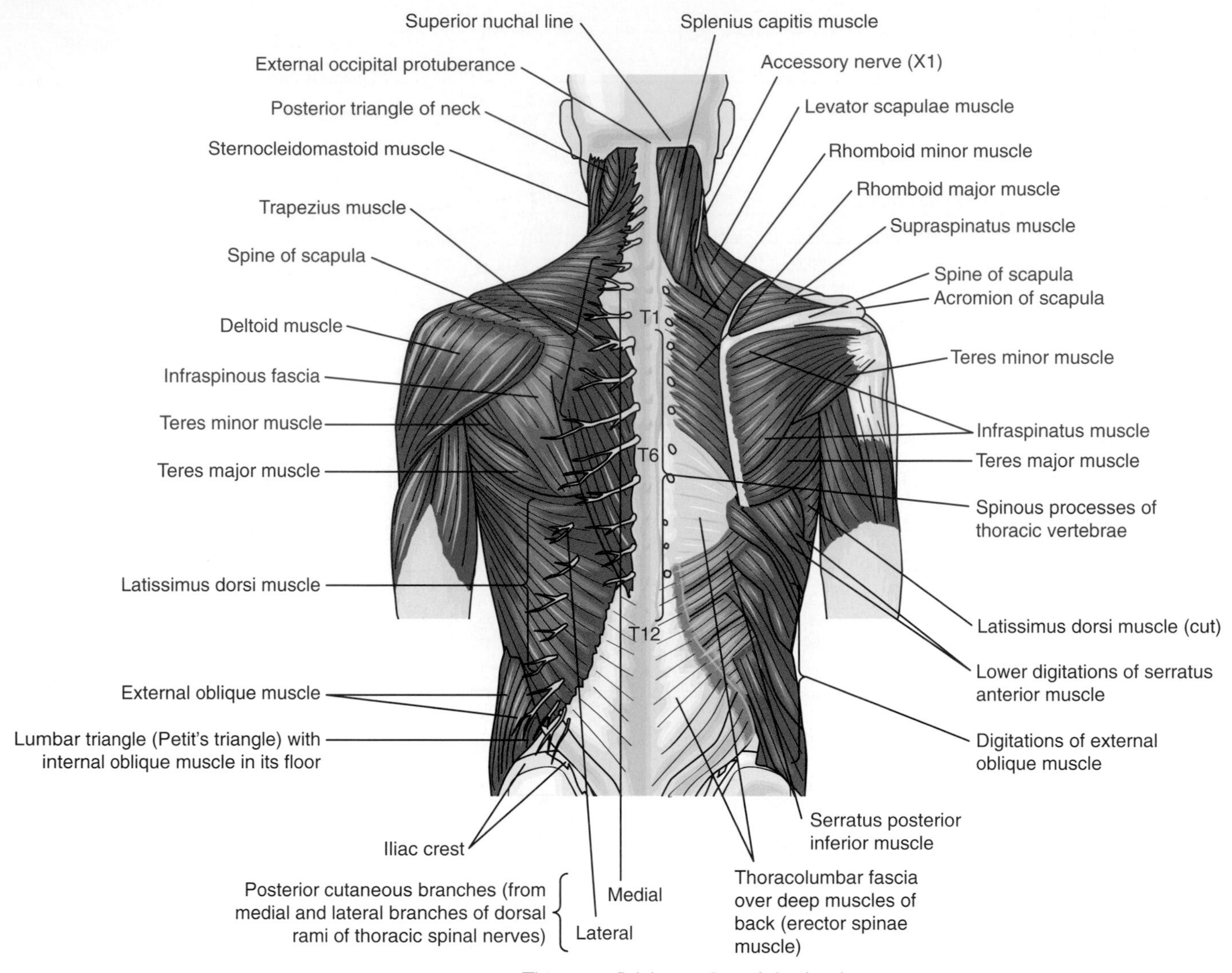

Figure 110-5 The superficial muscles of the back.

effort to determine whether the symptoms fit into a particular dermatome or neural pattern.

- A detailed history regarding the neurologic deficits should be documented.
  - For patients with a traumatic injury or a history of trauma, the clinician should note the mechanism of injury.
  - A thorough description of previous evaluations and treatments, especially spine surgery, is also important.
  - Finally, an occupational history should be obtained.
- It is important to use the history along with the physical examination to differentiate patients with myelopathy (dysfunction from spinal cord compression) and those with radiculopathy (dysfunction of nerve roots).
  - Patients with radiculopathy often present with pain in a specific distribution in the upper or lower extremity, weakness and atrophy of particular muscle groups, and decreased muscle tone.
  - Patients with myelopathy will present with the opposite spectrum of findings, including generalized weakness and no dermatomal pain. Patients with myelopathy also have a more nonspecific history, reporting frequent falls, gait and balance instability, paresthesias in a bilateral pattern, and difficulty with fine motor control, including buttoning a shirt, handwriting, or turning a doorknob.
- Attention should be given to determining the effect of various actions on the patient's symptoms.
  - Patients with neurogenic claudication often have improvement of their symptoms with leaning forward (e.g., on a grocery cart).
  - Patients with discogenic pain often have improvement in and worsening of symptoms with exten-

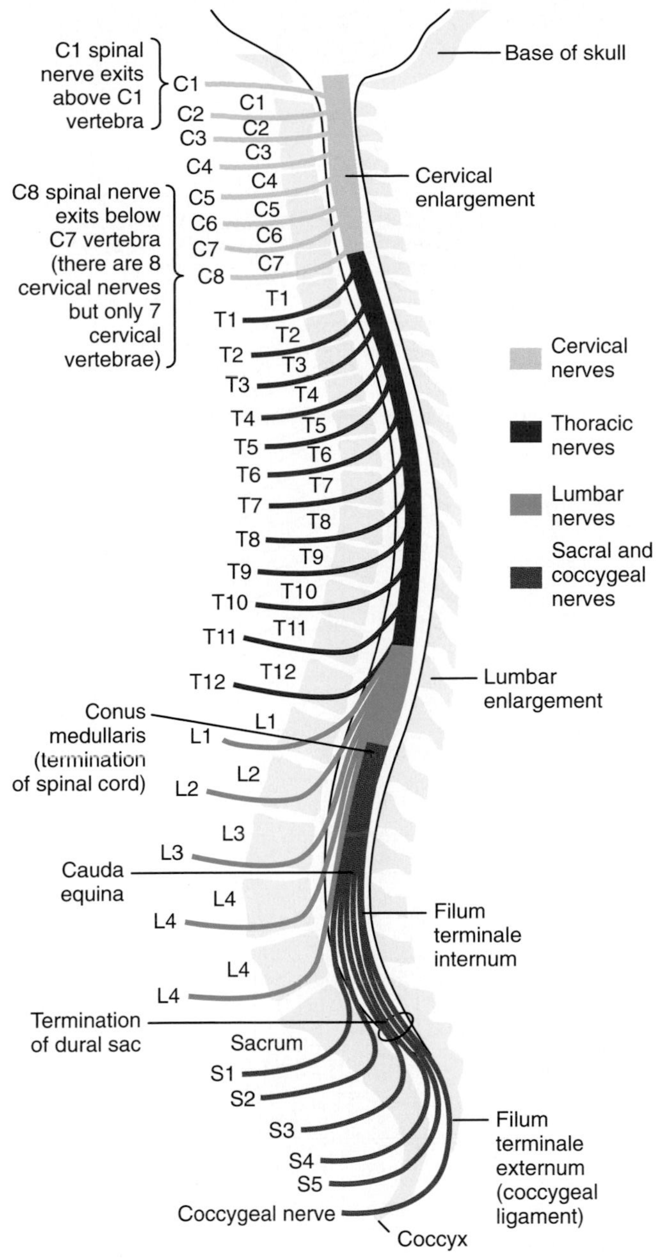

Figure 110-6 The spinal cord and segmental nerves.

sion and flexion, respectively, of the lumbar or cervical spine.

- Finally, it is important to ascertain the presence of any "red flags" that may suggest systemic illnesses and the need for more immediate imaging and aggressive evaluation.
  - These findings include fevers, chills, night sweats, unexpected weight loss, loss of appetite, and night pain.
  - Cauda equina syndrome, characterized by perineal or saddle paresthesia, lower extremity motor and sensory deficits, and bowel or bladder difficulties, also requires immediate imaging and evaluation for surgical intervention.

Physical Examination

- A thorough and complete physical examination is crucial so that findings can be correlated with the patient's symptoms and imaging studies to make diagnostic determinations and guide therapeutic interventions.
- The physical examination is divided into the following areas: inspection and palpation, range-of-motion evaluation, and neurologic examination.

Inspection and Palpation

- Inspection begins with a general evaluation of appearance, weight, posture, and gait.
- Determination of any deformity, such as scoliosis and excessive kyphosis/lordosis, is important.
- Evaluation of the skin involves looking for signs of infection or of underlying disease, such as café au lait marks and patches of hair.
- Palpation should include evaluation of the bony architecture and the paraspinal musculature; the extremities should be examined for associated or concurrent abnormalities.
- Careful palpation can reveal points of bony tenderness, areas of soft-tissue pain, or areas of swelling.

Range-of-Motion Evaluation

- Active range of motion is assessed for all areas of the spine.
- Flexion, extension, rotation, and lateral bending can all be evaluated.
- Attention to positions that cause or alleviate symptoms can provide insight into the source of the abnormality.
  - However, in the emergency setting, as with a patient who has a history of trauma, range-of-motion evaluation may not be appropriate, and spinal precautions should be followed during the entire examination.

Neurologic Examination

- The neurologic examination includes evaluation of sensation, motor function, and reflexes.
  - The sensory examination should be documented with regard to the distribution of dermatomes (Fig. 110-7).
  - Motor function is graded on a 0- to 5-point scale by testing motor groups that correlate with particular neurologic levels (Fig. 110-8 and Table 110-1).
    - — 5: Full motion against gravity with maximum resistance

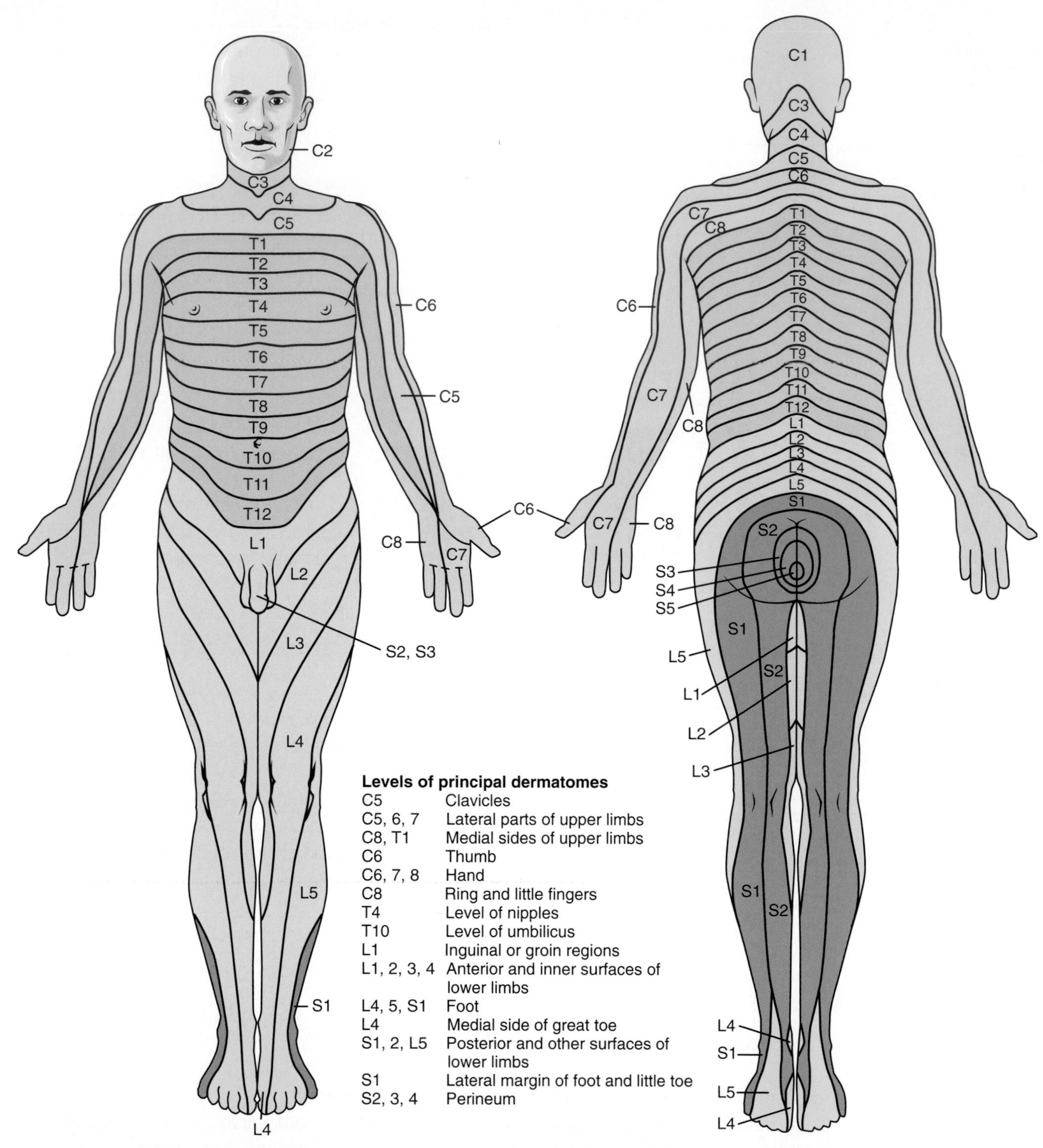

Figure 110-7 Schematic demarcation of dermatomes. There is actually considerable overlap between any two adjacent dermatomes.

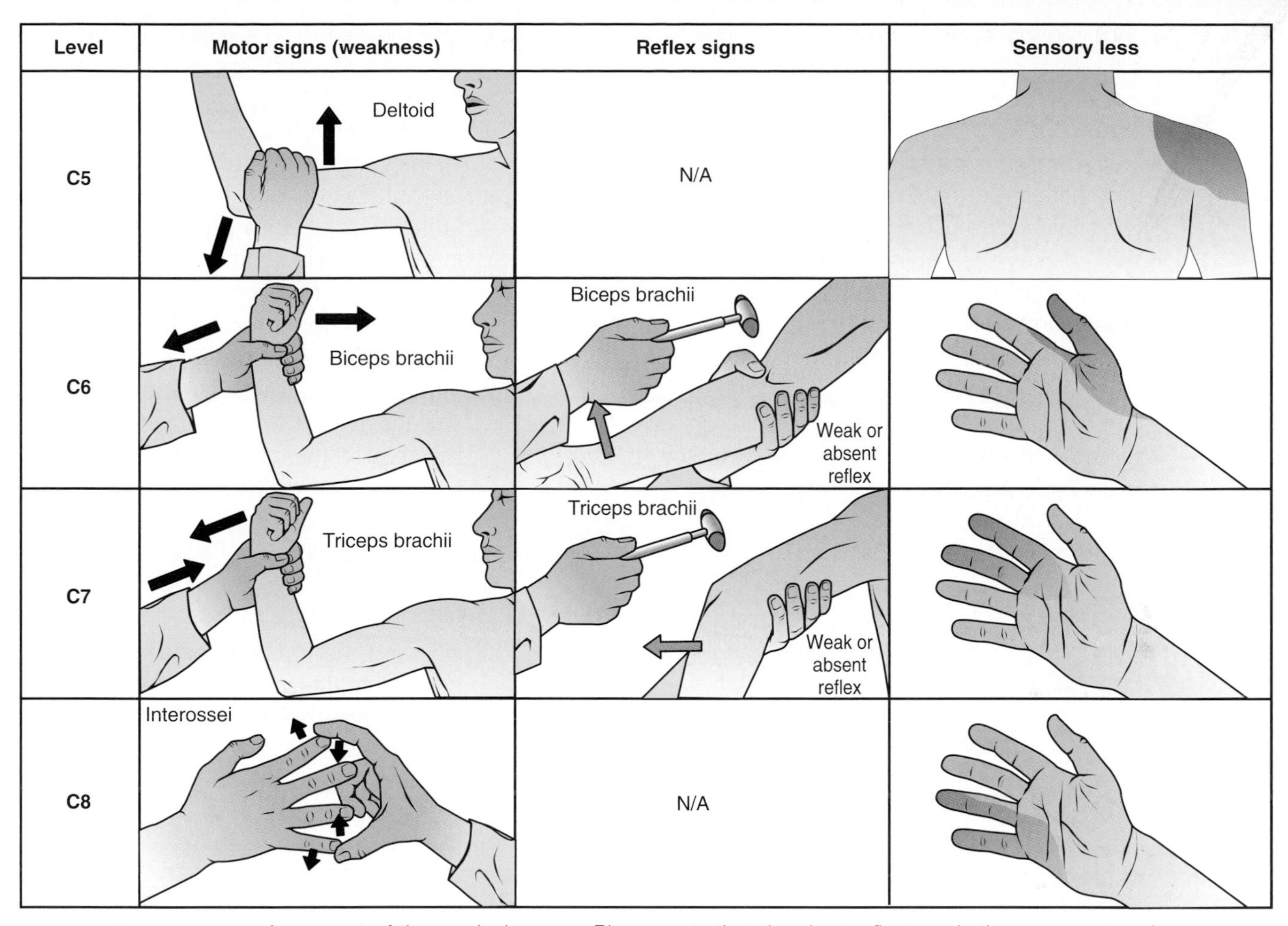

Figure 110-8 Assessent of the cervical nerves. Please note that the chart reflects only the upper extremity.

TABLE 110-1 *Motor Function: Evaluation of Nerve Roots*

Neurologic Level	Sensation	Motor	Reflex
C5	Lateral shoulder/arm	Deltoid (shoulder abduction)	Biceps tendon
C6	Radial forearm	Biceps/wrist extensors (elbow flexion, wrist extension)	Brachioradialis tendon
C7	Middle finger	Triceps/wrist flexors/finger extensors (elbow extension, wrist flexion, finger extension)	Triceps tendon
C8	Ulnar forearm	Interossei/finger flexors (finger abduction/adduction, finger flexion)	None
T1	Medial arm	Interossei (finger abduction/adduction)	None
T12, L1, L2, L3	Anterior thigh	Iliopsoas (hip flexion)	None
L2, L3, L4	Anterior thigh	Quadriceps/adductors (knee extension, leg adduction)	None
L4	Medial lower leg and foot	Tibialis anterior (foot dorsiflexion/inversion)	Patellar tendon
L5	Dorsum of foot and lateral lower leg	Extensor hallucis longus (great-toe dorsiflexion)	None
S1	Lateral/plantar aspect of foot	Peroneus longus/brevis (foot plantar flexion/eversion)	Achilles tendon
S2, S3, S4	Perianal	Bladder, intrinsic foot muscles	None

— 4: Full motion against gravity with moderate resistance
— 3: Full motion against gravity with no resistance
— 2: Full motion in gravity-eliminated position
— 1: No motion, but muscle contraction noted
— 0: No motion or muscle contraction

- Abnormal reflexes should also be elicited.
  — Clonus: evaluates for upper motor neuron injury (Fig. 110-9)
    — Abruptly dorsiflex the ankle and count the beats of ankle motion.
    — Positive: more than four beats of flexion
  — Babinski's sign: evaluates for upper motor neuron injury (Fig. 110-10)

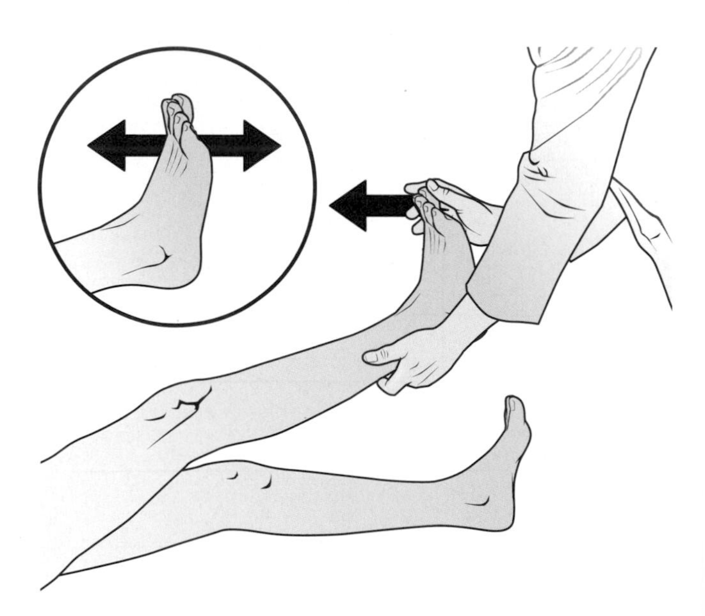

Figure 110-9 Evaluation of clonus.

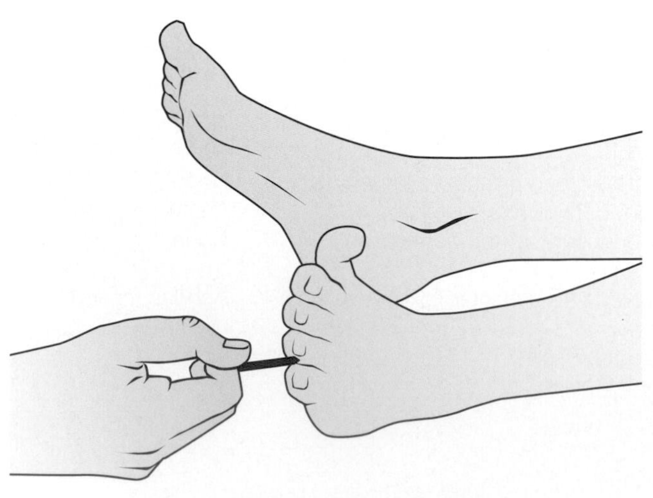

Figure 110-10 Babinski's sign.

    — Use the handle of a reflex hammer to rub along the plantar aspect of the foot from the heel to the toes.
    — Positive: great-toe extension
  — Hoffmann's sign: evaluates for cervical myelopathy (Fig. 110-11)
    — Flick the distal phalanx of the middle finger in a palmar direction.
    — Positive: the fingers and thumb flex; additional tests performed to aid in diagnosis
  — Spurling's maneuver: distinguishes shoulder pain from radicular pain (Fig. 110-12)
    — Ask the patient to rotate and laterally flex the head to the affected side.
    — Positive: maneuver exacerbates the patient's radicular pain
  — Adson's test: evaluates for thoracic outlet syndrome/cervical rib (Fig. 110-13)
    — Feel for the radial pulse on the affected side and then abduct, extend, and externally rotate the arm. Ask the patient to take a deep breath and turn the head to the affected side.
    — Positive: diminished radial pulse with maneuver
  — Straight leg raise: evaluates for sciatica (Fig. 110-14)
    — With the patient supine, raise the leg on the affected side.
    — Positive: The maneuver produces or exacerbates radicular symptoms.
  — Waddell sign: identifies nonorganic symptoms, unlikely to improve with intervention
    — Gentle rolling of the skin over the back produces radicular symptoms.
    — Twisting the torso with motion through the knees produces back pain.

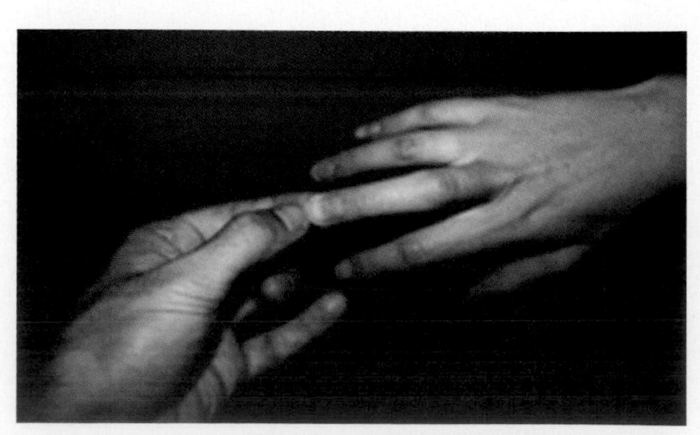

Figure 110-11 Hoffmann's sign.

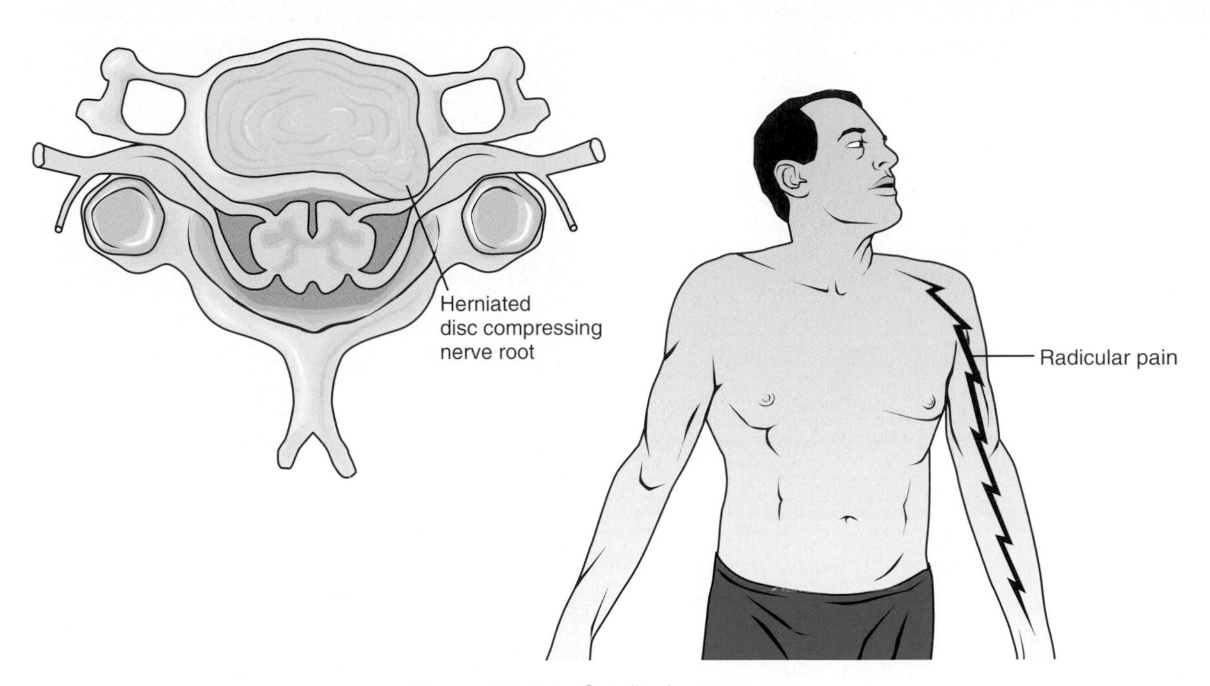

Figure 110-12 Spurling's maneuver.

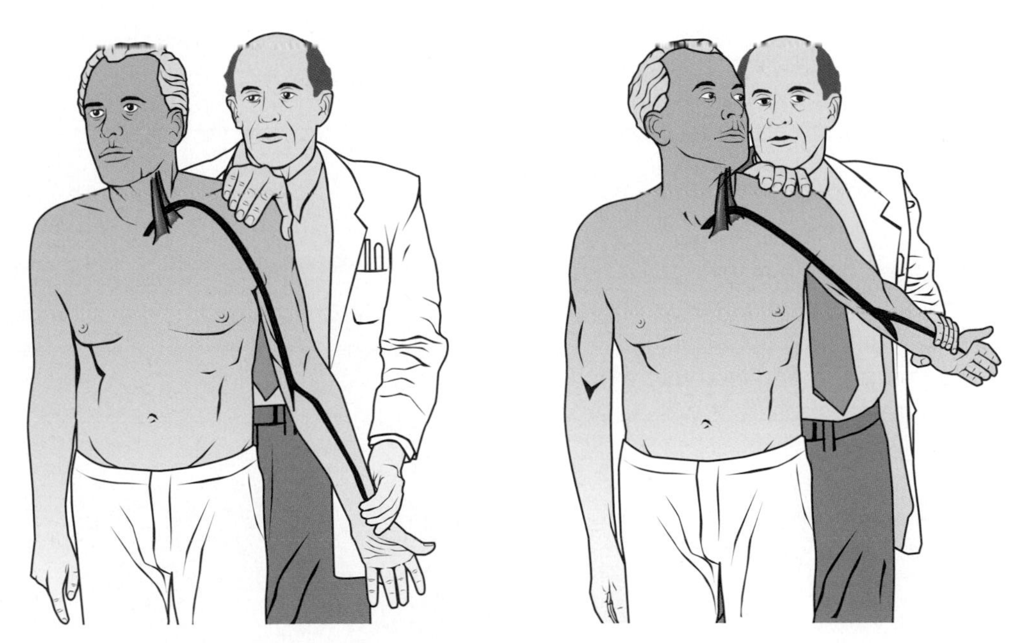

Figure 110-13 Adson's test.

— Slight axial compression to the head produces pain.
— Supine and seated straight leg raise tests produce different responses.
— Positive: Three or more positive responses indicate a likely nonorganic abnormality.

- During the physical examination, it is important to look for clues that would help further differentiate radiculopathic and myelopathic pain.
  - Such findings include weakness, diminished reflexes, decreased muscle tone, and a dermatomal distribution of pain for radicular pathology.

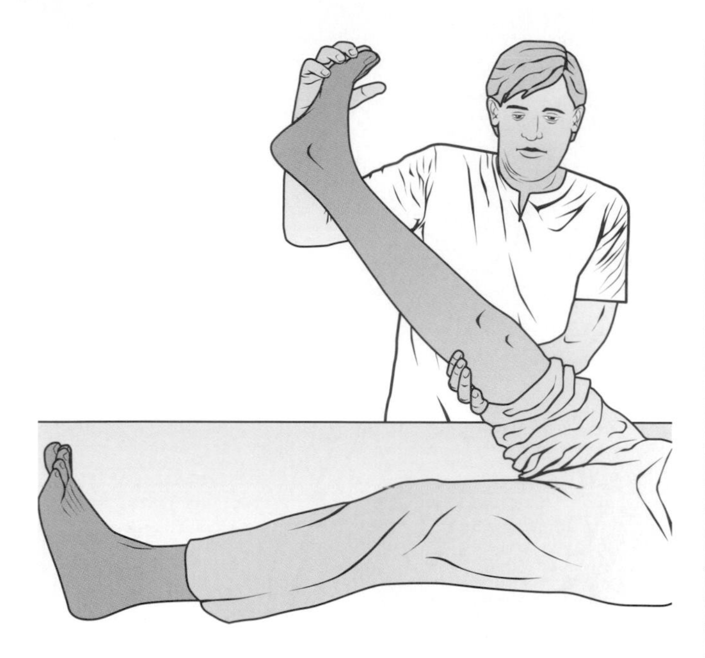

Figure 110-14 Straight leg raise.

- Myelopathic findings include increased muscle tone, hyperreflexia, decreased balance, gait abnormalities, and the presence of upper motor neuron signs.

Imaging

- Imaging the spine based on the results of the history and physical examination is an important part of the diagnostic and therapeutic protocol algorithm.
- There are multiple imaging modalities with which to evaluate spinal abnormalities, each of which has different strengths and weaknesses.
- An understanding of spinal anatomy, normal variations, and the incidence of degenerative changes is critical for the appropriate interpretation of imaging studies.
- In addition, reviewing the radiologist's reports and discussing the findings with the radiologist can be a valuable practice.
- Conventional radiography (Fig. 110-15)
    - This modality is often the initial imaging modality of choice because of its ease of acquisition and cost-effectiveness.
    - Anteroposterior, lateral, and oblique views of the spinal area of interest are customary.
    - Dynamic view radiographs, such as flexion and extension, are often obtained to evaluate for instability.

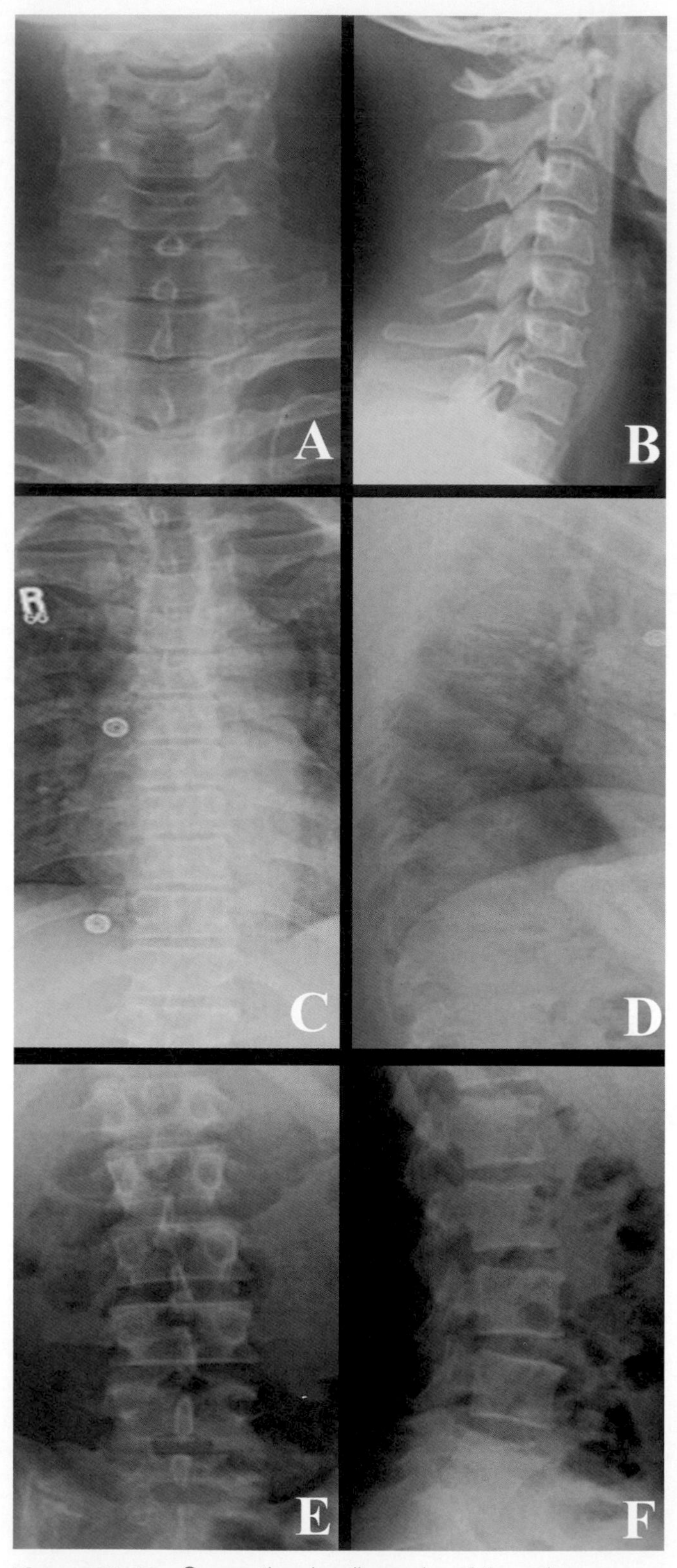

Figure 110-15 Conventional radiographs of the spine. **A**, Anteroposterior cervical spine; **B**, lateral cervical spine; **C**, anteroposterior thoracic spine; **D**, lateral thoracic spine; **E**, anteroposterior lumbar spine; **F**, lateral lumbar spine.

- Computed tomography
  - This cross-sectional imaging modality is well suited in the trauma setting for evaluation of fractures.
  - Computed tomography can also accurately assess the amount of bony destruction from a variety of pathologic processes and assist in preoperative planning.
- Magnetic resonance imaging
  - Magnetic resonance imaging provides high levels of anatomic resolution with respect to both bone and soft tissue.
  - It is commonly used for the evaluation of the degenerative spine, ligamentous injuries, and infectious or neoplastic processes.
  - Most clinicians consider magnetic resonance imaging to be the advanced imaging modality of choice for evaluation of the spine.
- Nuclear scintigraphy (bone scan)
  - Often used to evaluate for metastatic disease, stress fractures, and infection

Suggested Reading

- Bono CM, Garfin SR, Tornetta P, Einhorn TA (eds): Spine. Philadelphia: Lippincott Williams & Wilkins, 2004.
- Emery SE: Cervical spondylotic myelopathy: Diagnosis and treatment. J Am Acad Orthop Surg 2001;9:376–388.
- Fayad LM, Fishman EK: Computed tomography of musculoskeletal pathology. Orthopedics 2006;29:1076–1082.
- Hoppenfeld S (ed): Physical Examination of the Spine and Extremities. East Norwalk, CT: Appleton-Century-Crofts, 1976.
- Khanna AJ, Carbone JJ, Kebaish KM, et al: Magnetic resonance imaging of the cervical spine: Current techniques and spectrum of disease. J Bone Joint Surg Am 2002;84A:70–80.
- Khanna AJ, Shindle MK, Wasserman BA: Imaging of the spine. In McLain RF, Markman M, Bukowski RM, et al (eds): Cancer in the Spine: Comprehensive Care. Totowa, NJ: Humana Press, 2006, pp 73–81.
- Rhee JM, Yoon T, Riew KD: Cervical radiculopathy. J Am Acad Orthop Surg 2007;15:486–494.
- Scoliosis Research Society: White paper on sagittal alignment. Available at: www.srs.org/professionals/resources/sagittal_plane_white_paper.pdf. Accessed February 3, 2009.
- Waddell G, McCulloch JA, Kummel E, et al: Nonorganic physical signs in low-back pain. Spine 1980;5:117–125.

Chapter 111 Whiplash (Cervical Strain)

George S. Gluck and Sameer Mathur

ICD-9 CODE
847.0 *Cervical Sprain/Strain*

Key Concepts

- Whiplash has been used to describe both the injury and the resulting neck pain.
- The syndrome can include neck pain with decreased range of motion, occipital neuralgia, upper back pain, shoulder girdle pain, headache, dizziness, tinnitus, memory loss, visual disturbances, temporomandibular joint pain, dysphagia, hoarseness, and depression.
- More than 50% of patients are improved by 3 months and 75% by 12 months.
- Persistent pain after 6 months is classified as chronic whiplash.
- Prognostic factors for worse outcomes include psychosocial factors, litigation, female gender, radiating pain, and high initial intensity of pain.
- Common sources of neck pain after whiplash injury include the facets, nerve roots, cervical disks, and other supporting soft-tissue structures.
- Cervical radiographs are obtained when a cervical spine fracture, instability, or neurologic deficits (paresthesias, numbness, weakness) are suspected.
- Magnetic resonance imaging is not warranted in the acute or subacute setting after whiplash injury without neurologic abnormalities detected on examination.
- Initial treatment should consist of patient education, reassurance, symptomatic treatment, and discontinuing any cervical orthosis as soon as possible.
- Surgery for axial neck pain is controversial and is indicated in a small subset of patients.

History

- Acceleration-deceleration injury: rear end collision or block/tackle delivered during contact sports (e.g., football, ice hockey)
- Headache and neck pain at rest or with motion
- May have numbness, tingling, or weakness in the extremities
- May report loss of consciousness or amnesia of the event
- Inquire about duration and intensity of symptoms, employment status, psychiatric illness, and desire to pursue legal recourse.

Physical Examination

- Observation
  - Neck stiffness
- Palpation
  - Midline and paraspinal cervical tenderness/muscle spasm
- Range of motion
  - Cervical flexion/extension, rotation, and lateral bending
  - Assess after fracture and instability have been ruled out.
- Special tests
  - Complete neurologic examination, including upper and lower extremity sensation, strength, and reflexes.

Imaging

- Radiographs: Anteroposterior, lateral, and open-mouth views are necessary in the setting of trauma with pain or neurologic deficit.
  - All seven cervical vertebrae must be visualized; obtain swimmer's view, if necessary (Fig. 111-1).
  - Soft-tissue swelling with anterior displacement of the pharyngeal air shadow may signify disruption of the intervertebral disc or anterior longitudinal ligament.
- Abnormal swelling in adults includes more than 10 mm at C1, more than 4 mm at C3-C4, and more than 15 mm at C5-C7.

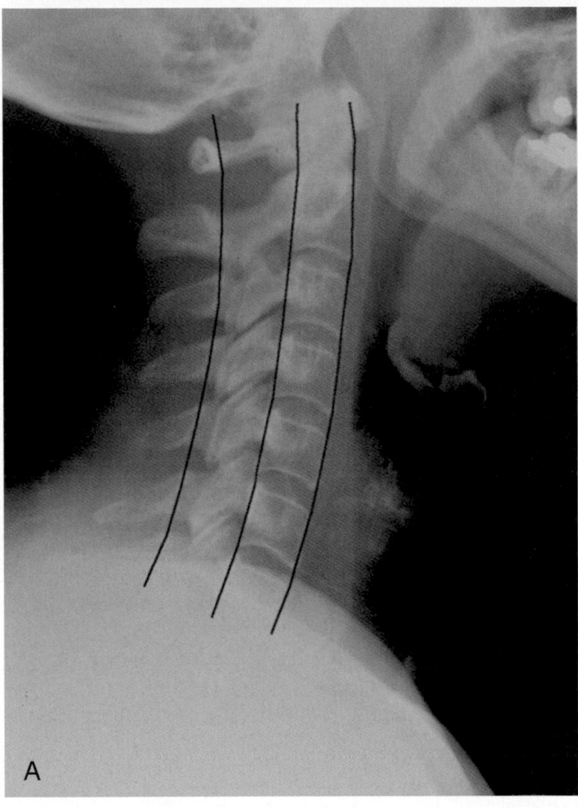

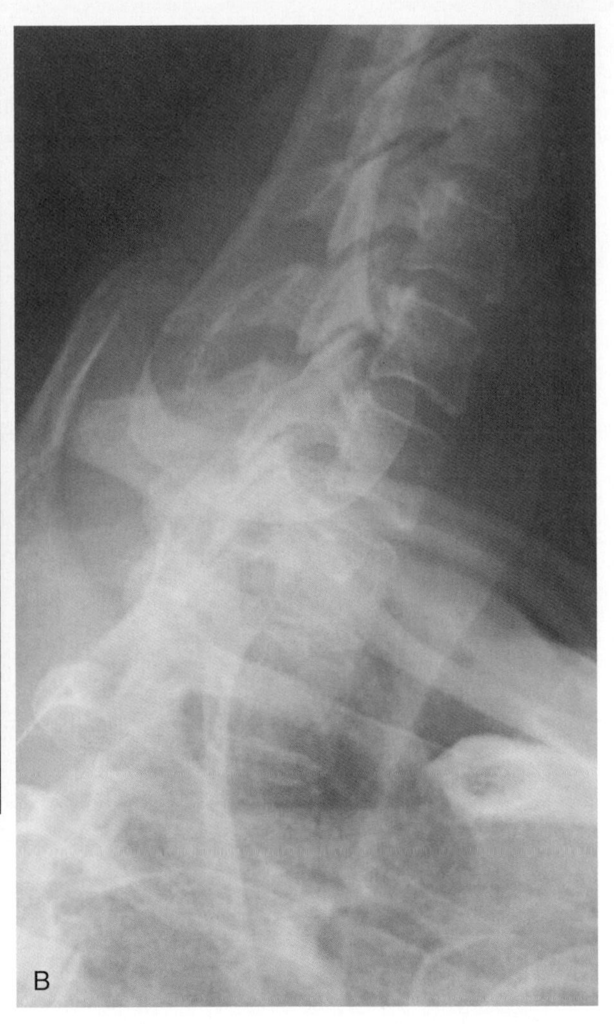

Figure 111-1 Cervical spine radiographs. **A**, Lateral view. **B**, Swimmer's view.

- Signs of instability include translation of more than 3.5 mm, angular displacement of more than 11 degrees, an atlas-dens interval of more than mm (5 mm in children), and asymmetry or widening of more than 2 mm on an odontoid view.
  - Flexion-extension views are best performed in a delayed fashion when acute spasm has subsided in the awake and alert patient without neurologic deficit to confirm ligamentous stability.
- Computed tomography
  - May be obtained to rule out fractures; more sensitive than radiographs
- Magnetic resonance imaging
  - Performed if ligamentous injury is suspected or neurologic deficits are present
  - Should not be used as a screening tool; high rate of false positives
  - May be used to identify the cause of persistent arm pain or other signs of nerve root compression

Differential Diagnosis

- Cervical disc herniation
- Cervical stenosis
- Cervical spine tumor or infection
- Dislocation or subluxation of the spine ("jumped facet")
- Spinal fracture
- Ligamentous injury/instability
- Exacerbation of degenerative or inflammatory arthritis (degenerative disc disease, facet arthritis)

Treatment

- At diagnosis
  - Patients may return to full activity as tolerated and discontinue cervical orthoses once they are clinically or radiographically cleared to do so.
  - Refrain from contact sports until full range of motion returns.

- Clinical follow-up for symptom assessment
- Medications: pain medications (limit narcotic use to acute setting if indicated), muscle relaxants, and tricyclic antidepressants or anticonvulsants (e.g., gabapentin, pregabalin) for chronic neuropathic pain
- Physical therapy: range of motion/stretching/strengthening, home cervical traction, body mechanics and ergonomics, and overcoming fear-based avoidance of activity
- Percutaneous radiofrequency neurotomy may relieve chronic pain after whiplash injury.

- Later
  - Surgery to address disc herniation, instability, or canal/foraminal stenosis may be necessary for persistent radicular pain, numbness, or weakness (Fig. 111-2).

When to Refer

- Patients with numbness, weakness, radicular extremity pain, or pain refractory to initial treatment should undergo cervical spine magnetic resonance imaging, and referral to a spine surgeon should be considered.

Prognosis

- The natural history is good with full recovery in 56% of patients at 3 months, 70% at 6 months, and 76% at 12 months. At 24 months, as many as 18% of patients remain symptomatic.

Troubleshooting

- Patients should be counseled on the warning signs of worsening weakness, numbness, or bowel/bladder incontinence.
- Should neurologic symptoms or pain persist, further workup and invasive treatment may be indicated.

Patient Instructions

- Educate patients on the prognosis and the importance of returning to full activity and employment.

Considerations in Special Populations

- Patients with previous cervical spine surgery and hardware placement need to have their implants evaluated for position change or damage.

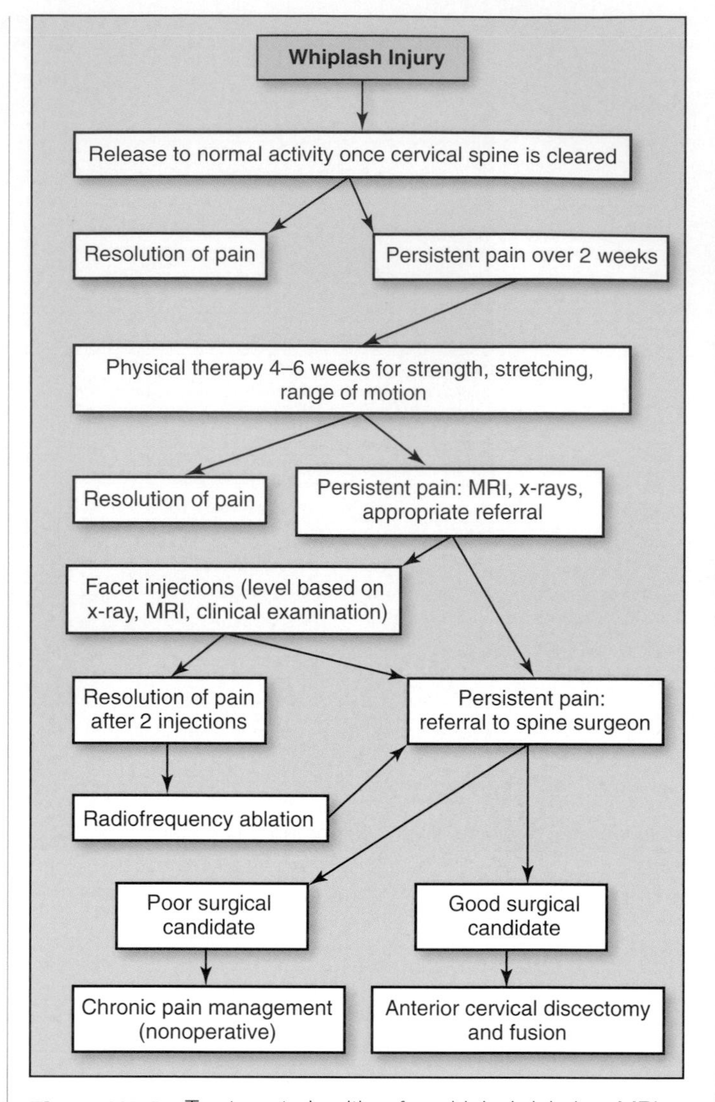

Figure 111-2 Treatment algorithm for whiplash injuries. MRI, magnetic resonance imaging.

- Litigant patients appear to do as well as nonlitigant patients when undergoing radiofrequency neurotomy for chronic neck pain or headache.
- Patients with rheumatoid arthritis are at increased risk of ligamentous cervical spine injury from trauma.

Suggested Reading

- Cusick JF, Pintar FA, Yoganandan N: Whiplash syndrome. Spine 2001;26:1252–1258.
- Gun RT, Osti OL, O'Riordan A, et al: Risk factors for prolonged disability after whiplash injury: A prospective study. Spine 2005;30:386–391.
- Hartling L, Brison RJ, Ardern C, et al: Prognostic value of the Quebec classification of whiplash-associated disorders. Spine 2001;26:36–41.
- Lord S, Barnsley L, Wallis BJ, et al: Chronic cervical zygapophyseal joint pain after whiplash: A placebo-controlled prevalence study. Spine 1996;21:1737–1744.

- Lord SM, Barnsley L, Wallis BJ, et al: Percutaneous radiofrequency neurotomy for chronic cervical zygapophyseal joint pain. N Engl J Med 1996;335:1721–1726.
- Olson VL: Whiplash-associated chronic headache treated with home cervical traction. Phys Ther 1997;77:417–424.
- Panjabi MM, Shigeki I, Pearson AM, et al: Injury mechanisms of the cervical intervertebral disc during simulated whiplash. Spine 2004;29:1217–1225.
- Pierre C, Cassidy JD, Carroll L, et al: A systematic review of the prognosis of acute whiplash and a new conceptual framework to synthesize the literature. Spine 2001;26:E445–E458.
- Rosenfeld M, Gunnarsson R, Borenstein P: Early intervention in whiplash-associated disorders: A comparison of two treatment protocols. Spine 2000;25:1782–1787.
- Sapir DA, Gorup JM: Radiofrequency medial branch neurotomy in litigant and nonlitigant patients with cervical whiplash: A prospective study. Spine 2001;26:E268–E273.

Chapter 112 Cervical Disc Disease

R. Todd Allen and Howard An

ICD-9 CODES

722.4	*Degenerative Disc Disease, Cervical*
724.9	*Foraminal Encroachment (Compression) of Nerve Root, Cervical*
723.4	*Cervical Radiculitis, Radicular Syndrome of Upper Extremity, Brachial Neuritis*
722.0	*Cervical Disc Disorder without Myelopathy*
722.71	*Cervical Disc Disorder with Myelopathy*

Key Concepts

- Degenerative changes in the cervical spine are universal in the elderly, making clinical correlation critically important in the diagnosis of cervical disc disorders.
- Intervertebral disc (IVD) protrusions are more common in males aged 30 to 50 years.
- IVDs are composed of an outer annulus fibrosus and an inner gelatinous nucleus pulposus.
- Cervical IVDs are present between the second through seventh vertebrae; are thicker anteriorly, contributing to normal (31–40 degrees) cervical lordosis; and have oblique posterior clefts that articulate with uncinate processes of the vertebrae above and below (joints of Luschka) (Fig. 112-1).
- Cervical disc disease is a normal wear-and-tear process of the aging spine due to genetic and environmental factors (see Fig. 112-1).
- IVD space narrowing, protrusion/herniation, local kyphosis, facet arthrosis, and osteophytes can lead to nerve root and/or cord compression, instability, and/or kyphosis.
- Factors accelerating cervical disc degeneration include smoking, poor posture, trauma, mechanical effects (occupational, diving, lifting, vibration), autoimmune processes, and atherosclerosis (or processes disrupting the blood supply).

History

- Rule out nonmechanical pain (pain at rest, night pain, constant throbbing pain) that may suggest infection, neoplasm, or pathologic fracture.
- Distinguish between axial neck pain, radiculopathy, myelopathy, or a combination of these disorders.
    - Axial neck pain: typically low grade with stiffness, worse with neck extension, often referred to pericervical, suboccipital, or periscapular areas
    - Radiculopathy: pain or paresthesia in a dermatomal distribution, muscle group weakness follows worsening nerve root dysfunction
    - Myelopathy: altered/unsteady gait and hand involvement (fine motor skill difficulty); late findings include weakness, bowel/bladder dysfunction
- Lower nerve root typically involved (e.g., C6 root in C5-C6 disc herniation)

Physical Examination (Figs. 112-2 and 112-3)

- Observation
    - Elevation of one shoulder (relieving nerve root pressure)
    - Muscle tone, atrophy, myelopathy of the hand
    - Slow, unsteady gait, postural changes, cervical lordosis loss
- Palpation
    - Tender pericervical musculature with or without spasm
    - Inconsistent bony tenderness
- Range of motion
    - Decreased extension worsens uncinate and facet joint pain.
    - Decreased flexion worsens muscular pain.
- Special tests
    - Complete neurologic examination
    - Radiculopathy: nerve root dysfunction leads to pain, weakness, atrophy, hyporeflexia
        - — Spurling's sign: symptoms exacerbated by neck extension and rotation/lateral bending toward the symptomatic side; ameliorated by neck flexion and deviation to the opposite side
        - — Shoulder abduction relief sign: abducting shoulder relieves pain from nerve root compression
    - Myelopathy: hyperreflexia, positive Babinski's sign, clonus, weakness
        - — Hoffmann's sign: Flicking the terminal phalanx of the third or fourth finger produces

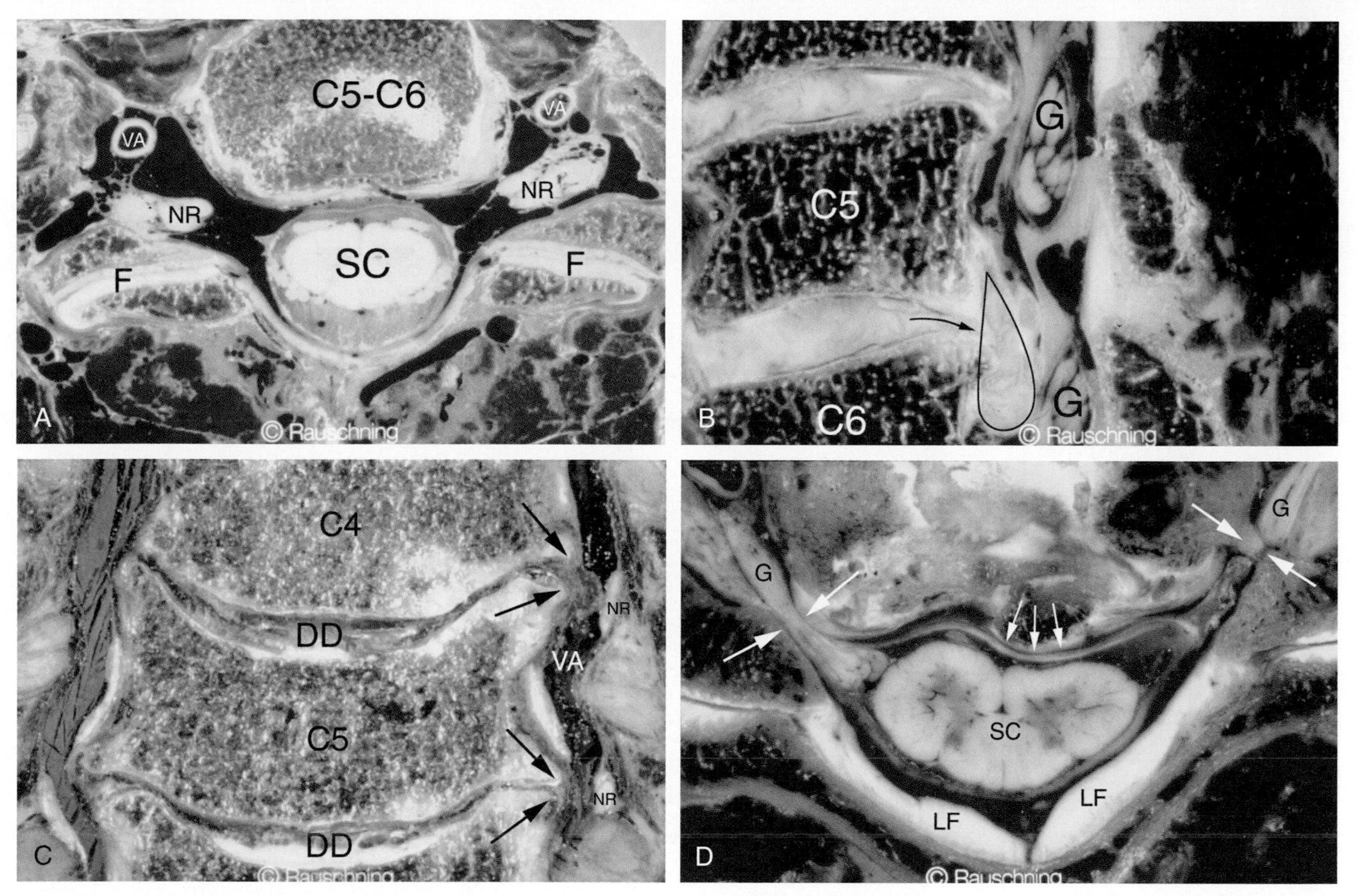

Figure 112-1 Normal (**A**) and degenerative (**B** to **D**) cervical spine anatomy. **A**, Axial cross section showing a normal C5-C6 level and the relationship of nerve roots (NR), facets (F), spinal cord (SC), and vertebral artery (VA). **B**, Parasagittal section showing a teardrop-shaped disc extrusion (herniation), compressing the ganglion (G) of the C6 nerve root. **C**, Coronal section showing severe disc degeneration (DD; cervical spondylosis), collapse, and uncinate process osteophytes (*arrows*). **D**, Axial section showing late-stage cervical disc disease, with osteophytes centrally (*small arrows*) and peripherally compressing the ganglia (*large arrows*), as well as thickened ligamentum flava (LF). (From Gallego J, Schnuerer AP, Manuel C: Basic Anatomy and Pathology of the Spine. Memphis: Medtronic Sofamor Danek, 2001; photographs by Wolfgang Rauschning, MD, PhD.)

rapid flexion of the terminal phalanx of the thumb.
- — Myelopathic hand: intrinsic wasting, positive finger "escape" sign (failure of adduction and/or extension ability of ulnar digits of hand, leading to drift outward or "escape")
- — Grip release test: slowed ability to grip and release
- — Lhermitte's sign: electric shock sensation with neck flexion

Imaging (Fig. 112-4)

- Clinical correlation is poor after the age of 40 years; many patients with cervical disc disease and IVD herniations remain asymptomatic.
- Radiographs
  - Anteroposterior and lateral views: narrowed IVD space, facet arthrosis, osteophytes, spinal canal narrowing (lateral view only)
  - Oblique view: foraminal narrowing
  - Flexion/extension lateral view: more than 3.5 mm translation or 11 degrees of angulation consistent with instability
- Computed tomography
  - Better evaluates ossification of posterior longitudinal ligament, foraminal stenosis, and extent of bony cord compression
  - Cervical canal midsagittal diameter less than 10 mm indicates absolute stenosis; 10 to 13 mm is relative stenosis.
  - Foraminal stenosis: 45-degree oblique reconstruction images

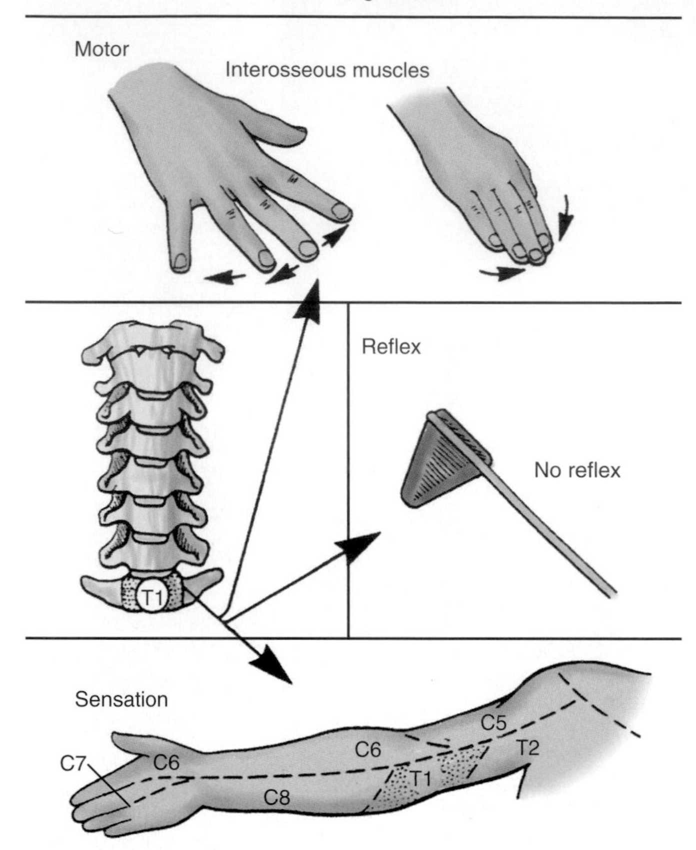

Figure 112-2 Upper extremity neurologic evaluation of the T1 level. (Adapted with permission from Klein JD, Garfin SR: History and physical examination. In Weinstein JN, Rydevik B, Sonntag VKG [eds]: Essentials of the Spine. New York: Raven Press, 1995, pp 71–95.)

- Magnetic resonance imaging (MRI)
  - Imaging test of choice for cervical, thoracic, and lumbar disc disease
  - Best for spinal cord lesions (syringomyelia, tumors, infection)

Additional Tests

- Computed tomography myelography: useful if patient unable to undergo MRI and in patients with complex deformities or previous surgery with metal implants
- Electromyography: adjunctive test to help rule out other etiologies of nerve root dysfunction (brachial neuritis, peripheral nerve compression)

Differential Diagnosis

- Trauma: cervical sprain, traumatic neuritis (brachial plexus traction), post-traumatic instability
- Tumor: superior sulcus tumor (C8 radiculopathy, Horner syndrome), cord tumor, metastatic disease, primary bone tumor
- Inflammatory condition: rheumatoid arthritis, seronegative arthropathies
- Infection: discitis, osteomyelitis, soft-tissue abscess
- Shoulder disorder: rotator cuff tear, impingement syndrome, instability
- Neurologic disorder: demyelinating disease, anterior horn cell disease
- Other: thoracic outlet syndrome, reflex sympathetic dystrophy, angina pectoris, peripheral nerve entrapments (carpal tunnel, ulnar tunnel syndromes; may coexist as double crush syndrome), temporomandibular disorders, medications

Treatment

- At diagnosis
  - Nonoperative treatment measures for cervical disc disease and radiculopathy may be divided into three phases.
    - Acute painful phase (1–2 weeks): nonsteroidal anti-inflammatory drugs, oral steroids if more severe, short-term analgesics, ice/heat, activity and posture modifications, soft collar or home traction may be helpful
    - Intermediate healing phase (2–4 weeks): stretching/motion first priority, then isometric exercises, physical therapy modalities if not improving
    - Rehabilitation phase (>4 weeks): cardiovascular and strengthening exercises, workplace modifications (ergonomics)
- Later
  - Without worsening or progressive neurologic dysfunction, nonoperative modalities for a minimum of 6 to 12 weeks should generally be explored before surgery is considered.
  - Surgical indications include spinal cord or nerve root impingement with neurologic dysfunction (radiculopathy, weakness, myelopathy) failing to resolve with nonoperative measures.
  - Surgical options include posterior foraminotomy (radiculopathy with or without weakness due to foraminal nerve root impingement with no neck pain); anterior cervical discectomy and fusion (for radiculopathy with or without weakness, often with neck pain, cervical disc disease with herniation, osteophytes, and anterior pathology); and cervical disc replacement (promising early results in patients with less bony cervical disc disease and low/moderate demands).

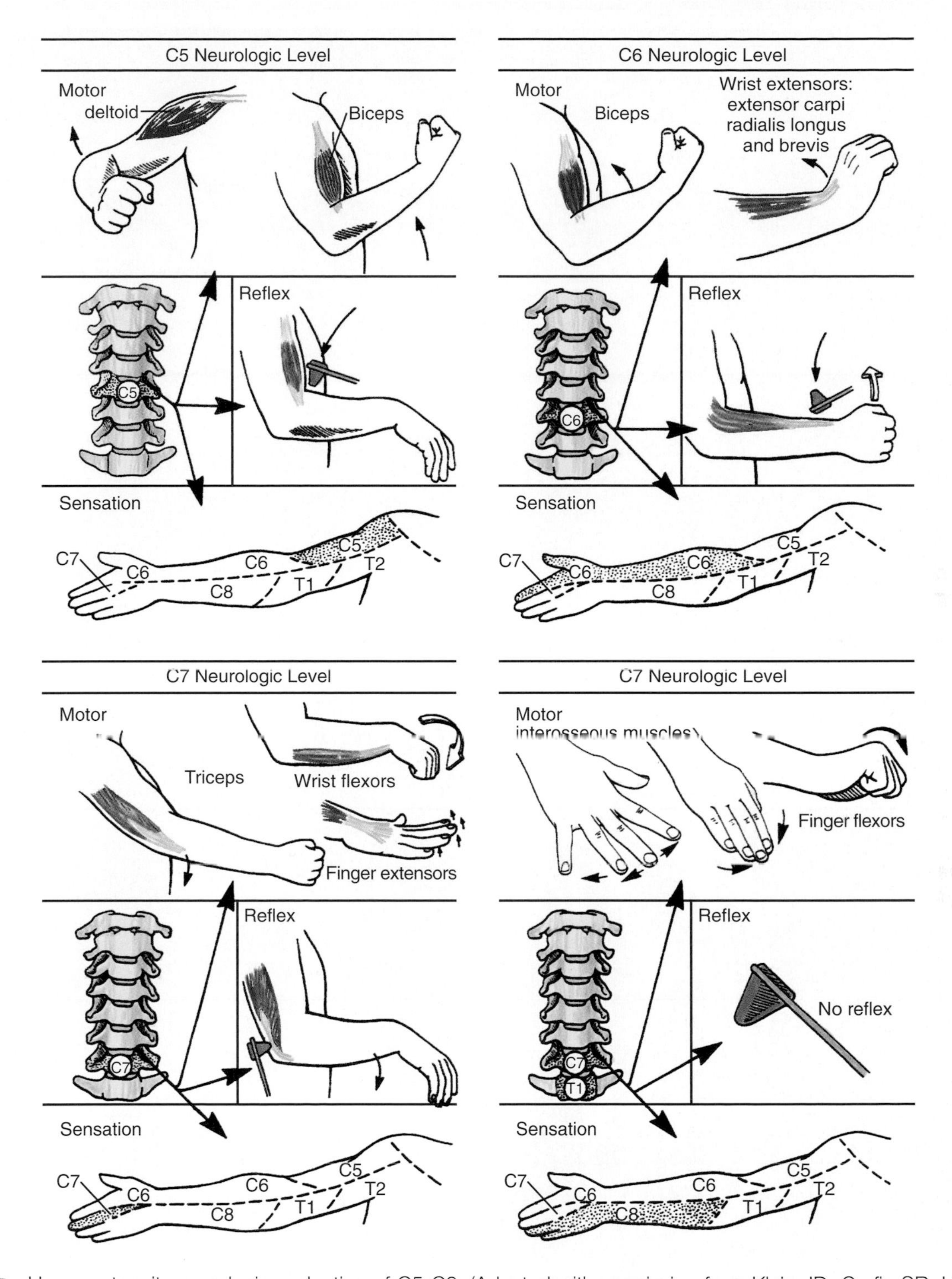

Figure 112-3 Upper extremity neurologic evaluation of C5-C8. (Adapted with permission from Klein JD, Garfin SR: History and physical examination. In Weinstein JN, Rydevik B, Sonntag VKG [eds]: Essentials of the Spine. New York: Raven Press, 1995, pp 71–95.)

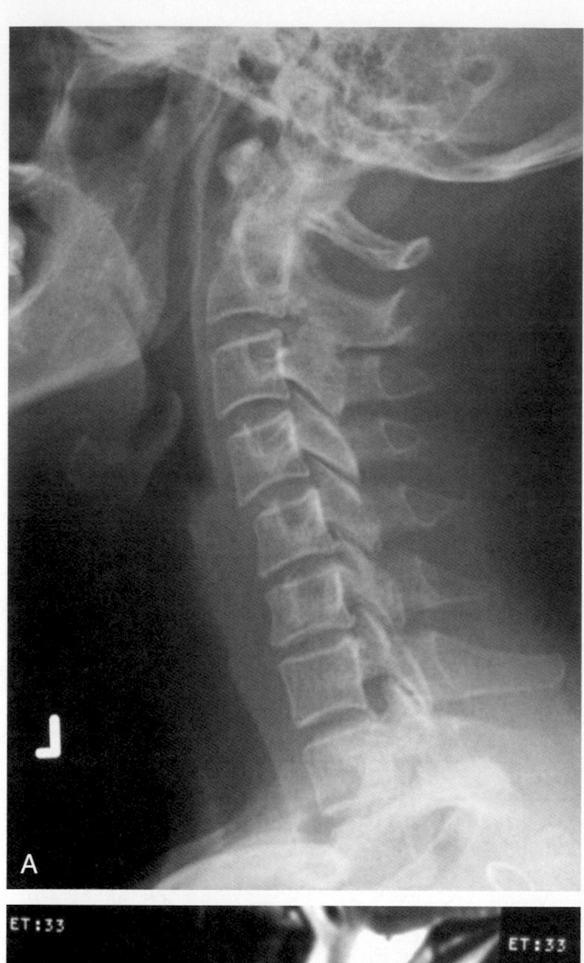

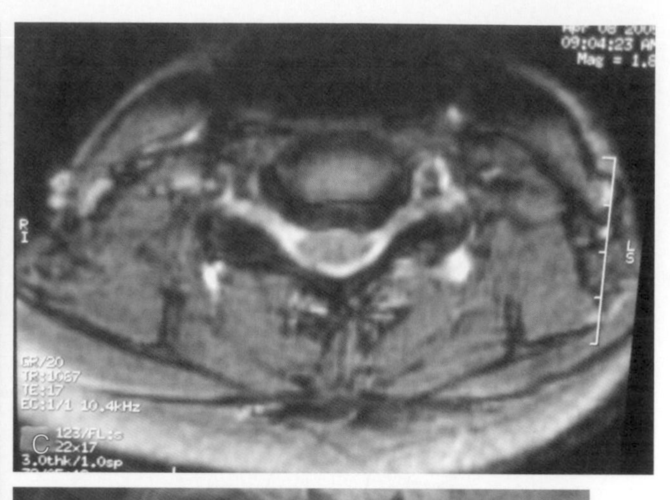

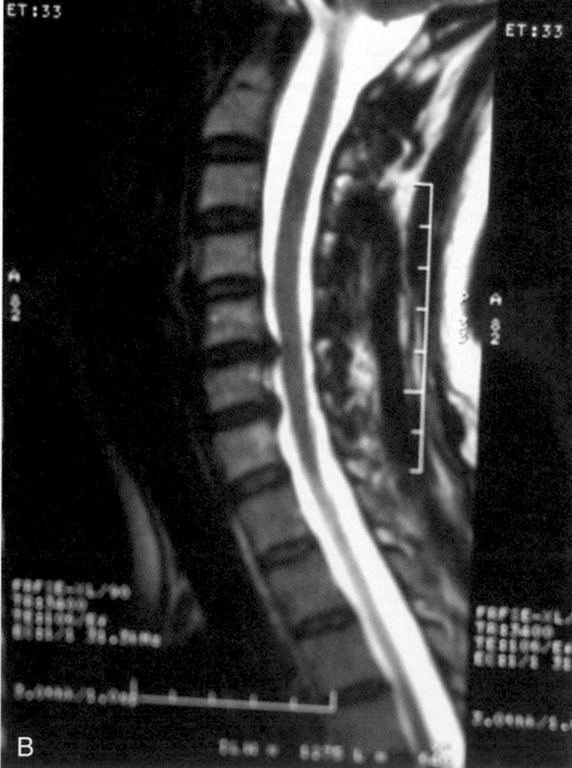

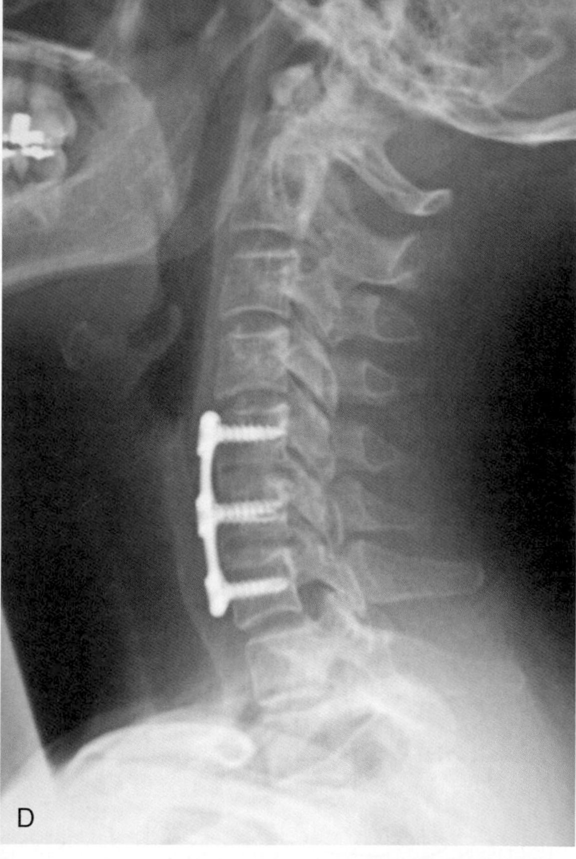

Figure 112-4 **A**, Lateral cervical spine radiograph in a patient with C6 and C7 radiculopathy due to cervical disc disease, most pronounced at C5-C6 and C6-C7, with disc space narrowing and loss of lordosis. **B**, Sagittal cervical spine magnetic resonance imaging showing disc herniations at C5-C6 and C6-C7. **C**, Axial magnetic resonance imaging showing C5-C6 disc herniation. **D**, Postoperative lateral radiograph showing two-level anterior discectomies and fusion of C5-C6 and C6-C7 with structural iliac crest allograft and supplemental plate fixation.

When to Refer

- Patients with signs of cervical myelopathy, progressive nerve root or cord compression, or neurologic dysfunction should be referred.
- Red flags requiring more aggressive evaluation include symptoms unrelieved by rest, night pain, constant aching, and insidious pain that becomes rapidly progressive/intense or fails to resolve for a prolonged period (consider infection, tumor, osteopenic/pathologic fractures).
- Acutely progressive symptoms, including loss of ambulation and bowel/bladder dysfunction, warrant immediate referral or emergency care.

Prognosis

- Axial neck pain typically resolves or improves with nonoperative treatment, and 70% to 80% of patients with radiculopathy can be successfully treated with 2 to 3 months of nonoperative modalities.
- Surgical outcomes for radiculopathy are good for pain relief and good to fair for some recovery of motor and sensory function.
- Surgical results are less predictable for axial neck and referred pain.

Troubleshooting

- Close, serial follow-up is needed in cases of nerve root or spinal cord dysfunction.
- A comprehensive history and examination are critical, helping to rule out other etiologies in the differential diagnosis if examination and imaging studies do not correlate with patient symptoms.

Patient Instructions

- Counsel patients about what to expect with nonoperative treatment and to aggressively adhere to physical therapy recommendations, continuing these at home.
- Counsel patients about when to return if they are failing to improve or worsening and include counseling about the risks and benefits of surgery.

Considerations in Special Populations

- Patients with inflammatory arthritides or ligamentous laxity (rheumatoid arthritis, ankylosing spondylitis, diffuse idiopathic skeletal hyperostosis [DISH]) should be carefully evaluated for recent mild trauma, instability, and neurologic status. Any signs of trauma or neurologic dysfunction in these patients may indicate instability or fracture, necessitating hard collar placement in the office and immediate referral.
- Chronic pain can lead to deconditioning. Extensive physical therapy, conditioning, and pain management referrals should be considered before orthopaedic referral for operative treatment in the absence of ongoing neurologic dysfunction.

Suggested Reading

- An HS, Singh K (eds): Synopsis of Spine Surgery, 2nd ed. New York: Thieme, 2007.
- Boden SD, McCowin PR, Davis DO, et al: Abnormal magnetic resonance scans of the cervical spine in asymptomatic subjects. A prospective investigation. J Bone Joint Surg Am 1990;72A:1178–1184.
- Dwyer A, Aprill C, Bogduk N: Cervical zygapophyseal joint pain patterns. A study in normal volunteers. Spine 1990;15:453–457.
- Emery SE: Cervical spondylotic myelopathy: Diagnosis and treatment. J Am Acad Orthop Surg 2001;9:376–388.
- Gore DR, Sepic SB, Gardner GM, et al: Neck pain: A long term follow-up of 205 patients. Spine 1987;12:1–5.
- Grauer JN, Beiner JM, Albert TJ: Cervical disk disease. In Vacarro AR (ed): Orthopaedic Knowledge Update 8: Home Study Syllabus. Rosemont, IL: American Academy of Orthopaedic Surgeons, 2005, pp 527–534.
- Haak M: History and physical examination. In Spivak J, Connolly P (eds): Orthopaedic Knowledge Update Spine 3. Rosemont, IL: American Academy of Orthopaedic Surgeons, 2006, pp 43–56.
- Rao R, Bagaria V: Pathophysiology of degenerative disk disease and related symptoms. In Spivak J, Connolly P (eds): Orthopaedic Knowledge Update Spine 3. Rosemont, IL: American Academy of Orthopaedic Surgeons, 2006, pp 35–42.
- Rhee JM, Yoon T, Riew KD: Cervical radiculopathy. J Am Acad Orthop Surg 2007;15:486–494.
- Sampath P, Bendebba M, Davis JD, et al: Outcome of patients treated for cervical myelopathy: A prospective, multicenter study with independent clinical review. Spine 2000;25:670–676.

Chapter 113 Cervical Spondylosis

Tony Y. Tannoury and Jared Toman

ICD-9 CODE
722.4 *Degeneration of Cervical Intervertebral Disc*

Key Concepts

- Spondylosis is an aging process defined as osteophytosis secondary to degenerative disc disease (DDD).
- Fifty percent of individuals older than 40 years of age and 95% of individuals older than 60 years of age have some degree of disc degeneration.
- Genetics and repetitive motion jobs/sports play an important role in the development of DDD.
- A defining characteristic of the process is desiccation of the intervertebral disc, which affects disc height and compliance.
- Pathoanatomic features include marginal osteophytosis, ligamentous ossification, facet joint arthrosis, and stenosis of the spinal canal and foramen (Fig. 113-1).
- Cervical spondylosis may present with varying degrees of axial neck pain, radiculopathy, and/or myelopathy.

History

- Axial neck pain
  - Discogenic pain located in the posterior neck, aggravated by extension and rotation of the head (myofascial pain exacerbated with flexion)
  - Associated morning symptoms, weight loss, polyarticular involvement, or nonmechanical neck pain raise suspicion of inflammatory arthritis or neoplasm.
  - Neck or shoulder girdle pain can be referred from the thorax or abdomen.
- Cervical radiculopathy (nerve root compression)
  - Arm pain (99% of affected patients), sensory deficits (85%), neck pain (80%), motor deficits (68%), and shoulder pain (52%)
  - Upper cervical radiculopathies present as suboccipital pain with referral to the back of the ear, and lower cervical radiculopathies manifest along specific dermatomes in the upper extremity (Fig. 113-2).
  - Radiculopathy due to spondylosis is more frequent in patients older than 55 years of age. In patients younger than 55 years, symptoms are more likely due to herniated nucleus pulposus (soft disc disease).
- Cervical myelopathy (spinal cord compression)
  - Loss of fine motor skills and hand coordination
  - Myelopathy hand: loss of dexterity and sensation, wasting of the intrinsic hand muscles, slowed finger movement, and positive finger escape sign
  - May report awkward gait or difficulty with balance

Physical Examination

- Observation
  - Often nonspecific
  - Observe gait
- Palpation
  - May have paracervical tenderness
- Range of motion
  - Assess flexion/extension, rotation, lateral bending
- Special tests
  - Detailed motor and sensory assessment
  - Spurling's maneuver to reproduce radiculopathic symptoms (Fig. 113-3)
  - Long tract upper motor neuron signs (hyperreflexia, clonus) or pathologic reflexes may be present in myelopathy.
  - Late myelopathic findings are associated with a poorer prognosis for recovery and include fasciculations, atrophy, and loss of sphincter function.

Imaging

- Radiographs: anteroposterior and lateral views of the cervical spine
  - Degenerative changes, such as disc space narrowing, facet and uncovertebral joint osteophytes, and endplate sclerosis, are extremely common in

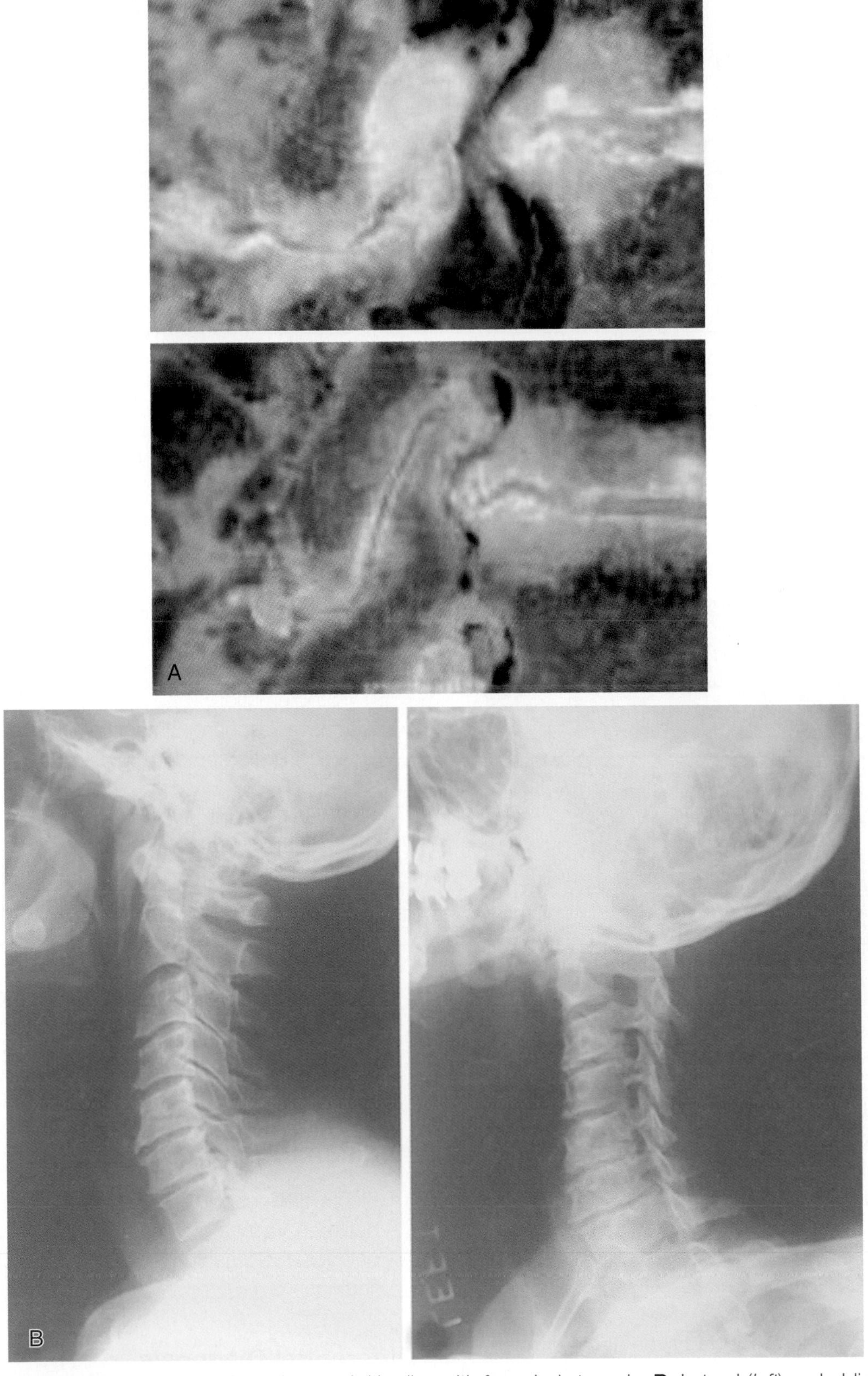

Figure 113-1 **A**, Pathoanatomic section through an arthritic disc with foraminal stenosis. **B**, Lateral (*left*) and oblique (*right*) radiographs evaluating the neural foramina.

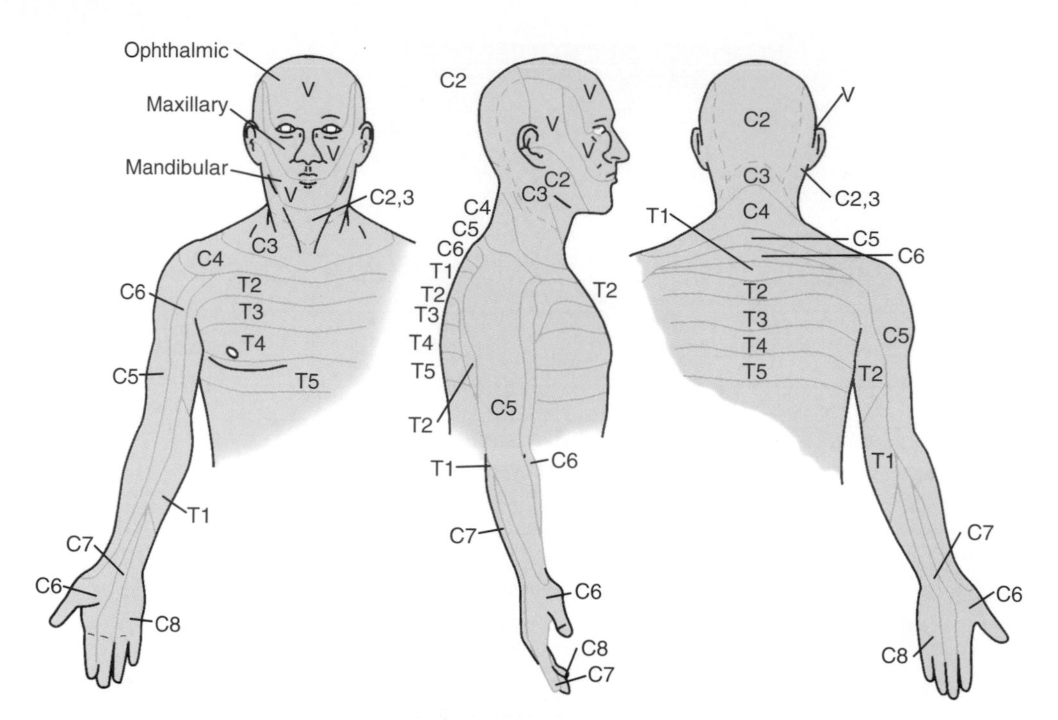

Figure 113-2 Dermatomal distribution of different spinal levels.

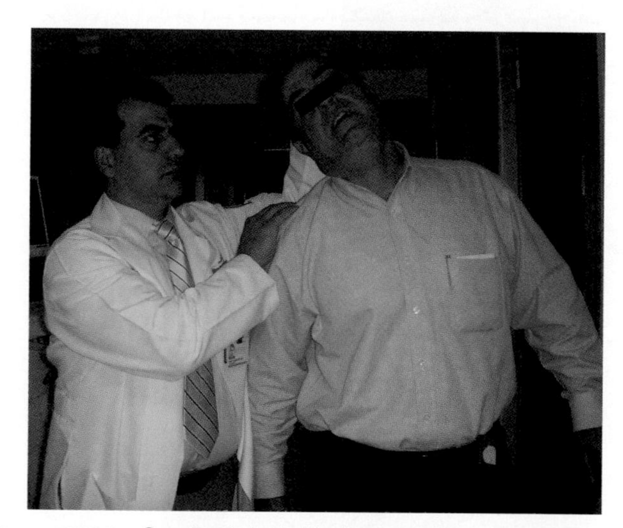

Figure 113-3 Spurling's test. Neck extension and lateral bending narrows the foramen and reproduces radiculopathy.

the adult population older than 55 years of age and may not be diagnostic of spondylosis.
  - Spondylotic bars, however, are more suggestive of the disease.
  - Lateral flexion-extension views (in atraumatic patients) are used to measure cervical range of motion and identify ankylosed segments.
- Computed tomography
  - Preferred imaging modality for definition of bony detail: vertebral artery foramina, spinal canal, neural foramina, facet and uncovertebral joints
  - Can help quantify the impact of compressive osteophytes and ossification of the posterior longitudinal ligament
  - Computed tomography myelography: largely replaced by magnetic resonance imaging; useful in postsurgical patients in whom metal artifact is problematic.
- Magnetic resonance imaging
  - Diagnostic standard for evaluation of the cervical spine
  - May be too sensitive and subject to overinterpretation
  - In myelopathy, signal changes on T2-weighted images represent intramedullary cord pathology such as edema, ischemia, inflammation, and gliosis (Fig. 113-4).
  - High signal intensity on T2-weighted images and low signal on T1-weighted images suggest a more severe lesion, such as necrosis and myelomalacia, indicative of late-stage disease.

Additional Tests

- Electrodiagnostic studies may help differentiate between various causes of neuropathy in the setting of equivocal imaging studies or clinical examination findings.

Differential Diagnosis

- Axial neck pain: inflammatory arthritis, tumor, shoulder condition, thorax or abdominal condition
- Cervical radiculopathy: peripheral compressive neuropathy, diabetic neuropathy

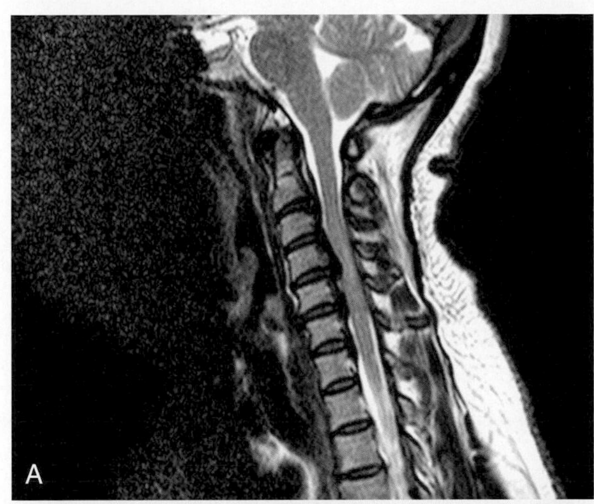

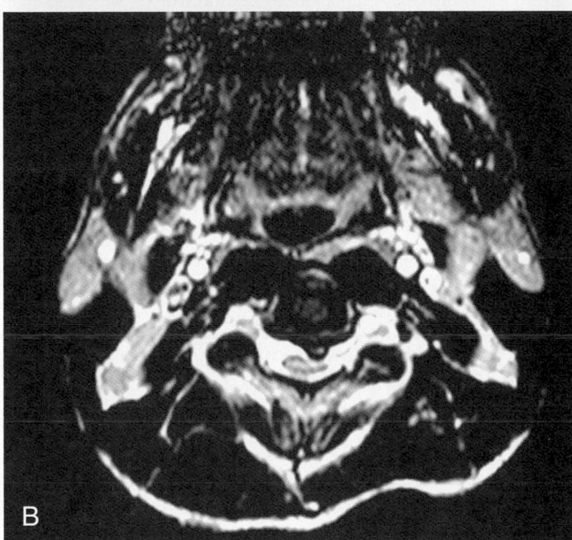

Figure 113-4 **A**, Sagittal T2-weighted magnetic resonance imaging of the cervical spine indicating multiple-level disc herniations causing spinal cord compression. Myelomalacia (spinal cord signal) is present behind the C4 vertebra. **B**, Axial T2-weighted magnetic resonance image indicating the disc herniation and indentation of the spinal cord.

- Cervical myelopathy: amyotrophic lateral sclerosis, intracranial process, myelitis, demyelinating condition, intraspinal tumor, syringomyelia, Chiari malformation

Treatment

- At diagnosis
  - The course of cervical spondylosis is extremely variable.
  - Periods of symptomatic remission and quiescence can be interspersed with exacerbations or a stepwise chronic deterioration; therefore, in the absence of severe myelopathic symptoms, conservative management should be instituted first.
    - — Avoid activities that provoke neck pain; use of a soft collar with mild neck flexion may alleviate acute pain and spasm.
    - — Nonsteroidal anti-inflammatory agents, corticosteroids, muscle relaxants, and antidepressants to relieve neck pain and flares of established radiculopathy
    - — Opioid analgesics may be used in the acute setting, but are a suboptimal choice for long-term management owing to their high potential for abuse and tolerance.
    - — Physical therapy may be effective in addressing painful symptoms.
- Later
  - The decision to proceed with surgery should be based on symptoms and clinical examination, not abnormal imaging studies.
  - Imaging should help in planning an operative intervention or confirming the root diagnosis.
  - Surgical approaches are based on the extent of disease and sagittal contour of the spine.
    - — Anterior cervical discectomy/corpectomy and fusion is most commonly performed and offers direct spinal cord decompression, with success rates greater than 90% for spondylosis.
    - — Posterior decompression (laminectomy) with or without fusion is contraindicated in the setting of cervical kyphosis.
    - — Fusion is indicated in the setting of instability and axial neck pain.
    - — Foraminotomy may be performed open or using a minimally invasive technique.
    - — Laminoplasty is indicated for multilevel involvement (e.g., ossification of the posterior longitudinal ligament).
    - — Cervical disc replacement may be another option (long-term data are lacking).
    - — Combined anterior/posterior procedures: If more than a two-level corpectomy is necessary, supplementing it with posterior instrumented fusion is recommended because of the unacceptably high rate of mechanical failure and graft dislodgement.

When to Refer

- Indications for referral include failure of conservative management, neurologic symptoms associated with weakness or nonresponsive to conservative management, and myelopathic symptoms.

Prognosis

- Success rates for nonoperative management of symptoms stemming from cervical spondylosis are highly variable.
- Treatment of isolated neck pain is typically most successful, with 70% to 80% of patients responding favorably. For cervical radiculopathy, as many as 60% of patients have complete or partial long-term relief.
- Medical management is rarely as successful in the treatment of cervical myelopathy; its natural progression is a stepwise increase in severity of symptoms over time.

Troubleshooting

- When a mismatch exists between the patient's symptoms and the diagnostic examinations, consider re-evaluation of clinical and diagnostic tests, nerve conduction/velocity tests, and referral to a hand/upper extremity specialist or neurologist.

Patient Instructions

- Instruct patients that it may take several weeks before physical therapy helps.
- Patients should seek re-evaluation in the case of new red flags indicating diseases that would require immediate attention, such as myelopathy (generalized weakness, loss of balance or dexterity, loss of bowel/bladder function), malignancy (constitutional symptoms, unintentional weight loss, loss of appetite, fatigue), and systemic diseases.

Suggested Reading

- Albert TJ, Murrell SE: Surgical management of cervical radiculopathy. J Am Acad Orthop Surg 1999;7:368–376.
- Connell MD, Wiesel SW: Natural history and pathogenesis of cervical disk disease. Orthop Clin North Am 1992;23:369–380.
- Edwards CC 2nd, Heller JG, Murakami H: Corpectomy versus laminoplasty for multilevel cervical myelopathy: An independent matched-cohort analysis. Spine 2002;27:1168–1175.
- Emery SE: Cervical spondylotic myelopathy: Diagnosis and treatment. J Am Acad Orthop Surg 2001;9:376–388.
- Garfin SR: Cervical degenerative disorders: Etiology, presentation, and imaging studies. Instr Course Lect 2000;49:335–338.
- Henderson CM, Hennessy RG, Shuey HM Jr, et al: Posterior-lateral foraminotomy as an exclusive operative technique for cervical radiculopathy: A review of 846 consecutively operated cases. Neurosurgery 1983;13:504–512.
- Ono K, Ebara S, Fuji T, et al: Myelopathy hand. New clinical signs of cervical cord damage. J Bone Joint Surg Br 1987;69B:215–219.
- Roa RD, Currier BL, Albert TJ, et al: Degenerative cervical spondylosis: Clinical syndromes, pathogenesis and management. J Bone Joint Surg Am 2007;89A:1360–1378.
- Shafaie FF, Wippold FJ 2nd, Gado M, et al: Comparison of computed tomography myelography and magnetic resonance imaging in the evaluation of cervical spondylotic myelopathy and radiculopathy. Spine 1999;24:1781–1785.
- Shedid D, Benzel EC: Cervical spondylosis anatomy: Pathophysiology and biomechanics. Neurosurgery 2007;60(Suppl):7–13.

Chapter 114 Cervical Spinal Stenosis

S. Tim Yoon and Brett A. Freedman

ICD-9 CODES

721.1 *Cervical Spondylosis with Myelopathy*
722.70 *Intervertebral Disc Disorder with Myelopathy, Unspecified Region*
722.71 *Intervertebral Disc Disorder with Myelopathy, Cervical Region*
723.0 *Spinal Stenosis of Cervical Region*

Key Concepts

- Cervical spondylotic myelopathy is the most common cause of spinal cord dysfunction (paresis/paralysis) in patients older than 55 years of age.
- Cervical spinal stenosis is a multifactorial phenomenon, with acquired and congenital etiologies, that results in a reduced anteroposterior (AP) canal diameter.
- Cervical spondylotic myelopathy likely represents a combination of compressive and ischemic insults. Long tract signs tend to occur first (biceps hyperreflexia), and hypertonia and pathologic reflexes follow.
- Myelopathy can occur without significant axial neck pain or radiculopathy.
- Myelopathy is usually progressive, and surgical intervention to decompress the spinal cord should be considered when there are functional deficits. Surgery ceases progression of myelopathy and leads to neurologic improvement in as many as 75% of cases.
- Ultimately, the diagnosis of myelopathy is a clinical one, based on the history and examination findings in the presence of cord compression on imaging studies.

History

- Typical symptom onset at age 50 to 60 years; younger in congenital stenosis
- Natural history patterns: no progression, stepwise progression (most common; 75%), slow steady decline, and rapid progression (least common)
- Hand clumsiness; decreased dexterity with buttons, coins, and handwriting
- Altered gait: problems with balance, new need for walking aid
- Generalized weakness, easily fatigued, and decreased walking tolerance
- Neck pain can be present, but tends not to be a prominent component.
- Inquire about duration of symptoms, previous treatments and results, bowel/bladder/erectile function, medical history (previous neck trauma or surgery, history of cancer), smoking, and occupation.
- Evaluate shoulder symptoms with a shoulder examination.

Physical Examination

- Observation
  - Previous scars, altered cervical spine alignment (loss of lordosis)
  - Wide-based, shuffling gait; inability to walk heel to toe
  - Ability to stand on toes: check plantarflexion strength and balance
- Palpation
  - Identify masses, tender points, deformity, and paraspinal spasm
- Special tests
  - Complete motor, sensory, and reflex examination
  - Rectal examination: Record tone, sensation, wink (reflexive anal contraction when skin contacted), or bulbocavernosus reflex (pinch glans/clitoris or tug on Foley catheter to elicit reflexive anal sphincter contraction).
  - Myelopathy signs: Hoffmann's, hyperreflexia (absent in 30%), abnormal reflexes (inverted radial reflex), clonus, Babinski's, dysdiadochokinesia (alternating clapping, grip release test), Lhermitte's (flexing/extending neck shoots electric pain down spine)

- Postvoid residual: sterile catheter placed after patient attempts to fully void, should be less than 100 mL; also check urinanalysis
- Nurick score for myelopathy (as many as 75% of patients improve one grade with surgery)
  — 0: Signs/symptoms of radiculopathy, but no myelopathy
  — 1: Myelopathy signs, but no difficulty walking
  — 2: Myelopathy, slight difficulty walking, does not restrict employment
  — 3: Myelopathy, difficulty walking, no full-time job, still independent
  — 4: Myelopathy, assisted ambulation only
  — 5: Myelopathy, wheelchair only

Imaging

- Because spondylosis is present in more than 70% of normal elderly patients, imaging studies alone cannot diagnose cervical spondylotic myelopathy.
- Radiographs: anteroposterior, lateral, and flexion/extension lateral views
  - Spondylosis: disc height loss, osteophytes, retrolisthesis (typically C3-C4 or C4-C5), lost cervical lordosis, signs of fractures or other pathology
  - Spinal canal AP diameter: normal, more than 17 mm on lateral view; cord compression (from spinal stenosis) occurs with canal diameter of less than 13 mm
  - Torg ratio: AP canal diameter/AP vertebral body length; commonly used to describe the congenital component of cervical spinal stenosis; normal is more than 1; a Torg ratio of less than 0.8 indicates cervical stenosis
  - Flexion/extension views demonstrate dynamic stenosis and intervertebral instability. Listhesis of more than 2 to 3.5 mm decreases canal dimensions.
- Computed tomography
  - Best for defining bony anatomy and quality. Computed tomography myelography is useful for patients intolerant of magnetic resonance imaging or those with previous metallic implants.
  - The AP canal dimension is most useful for cervical stenosis. Additionally, a cross-sectional area of less than 30 to 50 mm^2 has been correlated with poor outcomes.
  - Look for osteophytes, facet alignment (trauma), facet hypertrophy, and extraosseous calcifications including chronic disc protrusions or ossification of the posterior longitudinal ligament (Fig. 114-1).

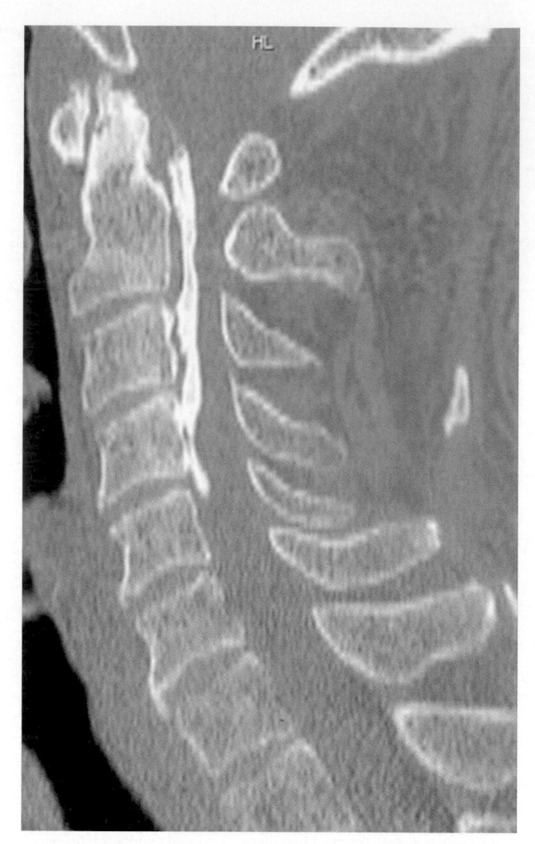

Figure 114-1 Mid-sagittal reconstructed image from a noncontrast computed tomography scan demonstrating advanced ossification of the posterior longitudinal ligament from C2 to C4 causing severe cervical stenosis.

- Magnetic resonance imaging
  - Best for visualizing soft-tissue structures compressing the spinal cord; can demonstrate cord signal changes, a relative prognosticator of poor outcome; can identify ligamentous injuries
  - Myelomalacia (softening of the cord) results from repeated ischemic and hemorrhagic insults to the spinal cord, seen on T2-weighted images as a white grainy signal within the normally gray cord.
  - With progressive stenosis, the T2-weighted cerebrospinal fluid signal is reduced and the cord becomes deformed, usually in the AP direction (bean shaped).
  - Myelopathic signs/symptoms are usually present when the AP diameter of the cord is reduced to 30% of its normal value.

Additional Tests

- Electromyography may distinguish peripheral neuropathy from radicular and myelopathic conditions.
- Advanced brain imaging studies may rule out a central cause of symptoms.

Differential Diagnosis

- Peripheral neuropathy (compressive, metabolic, or diabetes related)
- Cerebral vascular accident
- Progressive intrinsic neurologic or muscular disorders: multiple sclerosis, metabolic myopathy, Parkinson's disease, amyotrophic lateral sclerosis (Lou Gehrig's disease)
- Syringomyelia, Arnold-Chiari malformation, hydrocephalus
- Primary or metastatic intramedullary spinal cord tumor
- Infection: epidural abscess, vertebral osteomyelitis, spondylodiscitis

Treatment

- At diagnosis
  - Acute myelopathy (spinal cord injury) requires immediate attention.
  - On the field, the player's helmet and shoulder pads should be left on, the face mask removed if airway access is needed, and cervical immobilization instituted.
- Later
  - Cervical spondylotic myelopathy is typically progressive. Thus, in symptomatic patients, surgery is the preferred treatment.
  - Most patients have congenital narrowing of their canal that becomes critical with acquired changes with aging or acutely after trauma.
  - Because there are no reliable predictors of progression, watchful waiting can be tried in patients with mild symptoms or those with such poor general health that there is a high risk of severe complications.
  - Collars or exercises can be used, but their efficacy is unproven.
  - Corticosteroids can be useful as a temporizing measure in patients with new cord compression and progressive myelopathy.
  - Surgical options are based on the etiology and level of stenosis.
  - Posterior approaches: laminectomy with or without posterior spinal fusion or laminoplasty (Fig. 114-2); more commonly considered for multilevel (more than three levels) stenosis; severe fixed kyphosis is a contraindication to a posterior-only approach
  - Anterior approaches: anterior cervical discectomy and fusion or corpectomy and fusion (Figs. 114-3 and 114-4); allows direct decompression of the spinal cord; transient dysphagia is common, but typically resolves within 6 months
  - Combined approaches: reserved for complex cases

When to Refer

- Cervical stenosis without signs or symptoms of myelopathy is usually not a surgical disease.
  - However, when myelopathy is present, prompt referral is warranted.
  - If myelopathy is progressing, urgent referral is indicated.

Prognosis

- The natural history of cervical spondylotic myelopathy is progressive neurologic deterioration in the majority of patients.
- With surgical treatment, progression of myelopathy is prevented and the majority of patients have some improvement in neurologic function.
- Cord signal changes on magnetic resonance imaging, an AP canal diameter less than 10 to 13 mm, and the preoperative nonambulatory status (high Nurick grade) predict a poor outcome.

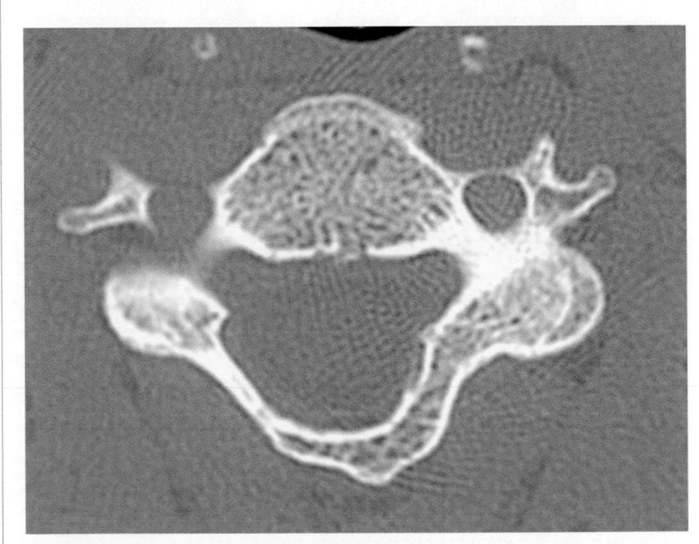

Figure 114-2 Axial computed tomography image 12 months after an open-door laminoplasty in which a cortical allograft was used to maintain "the door" open. The hinge is healed on the left, and the bone graft on the right has incorporated and remodeled.

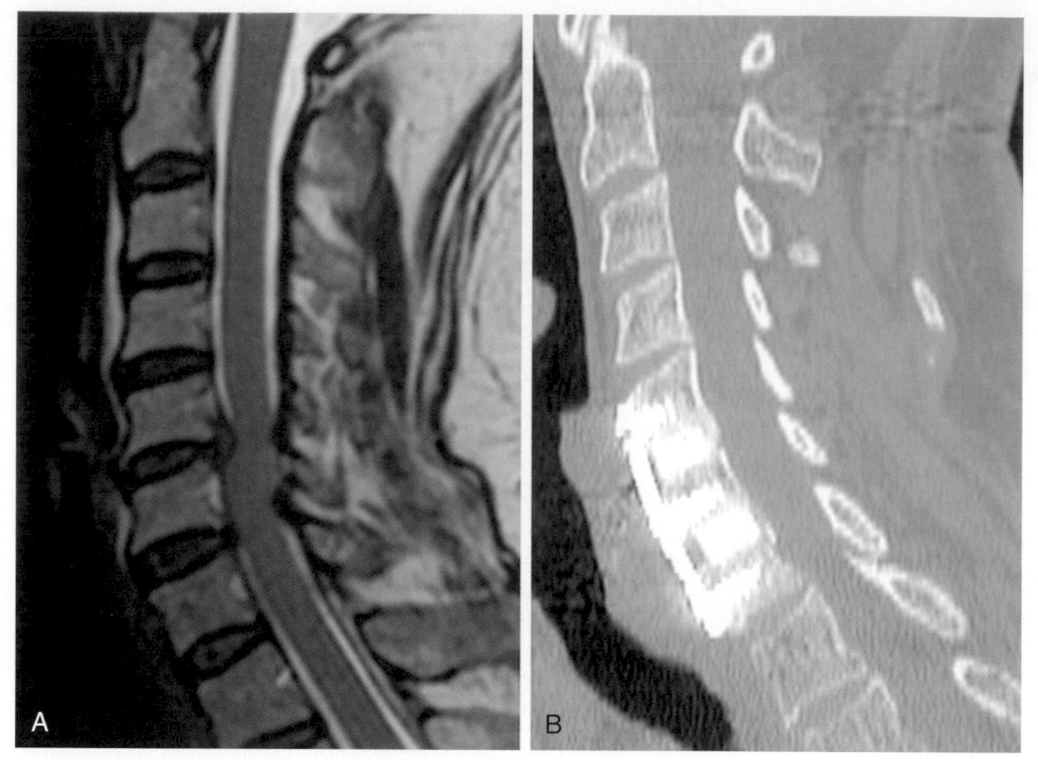

Figure 114-3 T2-weighted sagittal magnetic resonance images demonstrating cord compression at the C5-C6 and C6-C7 levels from disc herniations. **A,** Additionally, there is posterior compression from ligamentum flavum infolding. **B,** Healed two-level anterior cervical discectomy and fusion with cortical allograft and anterior cervical plate fixation.

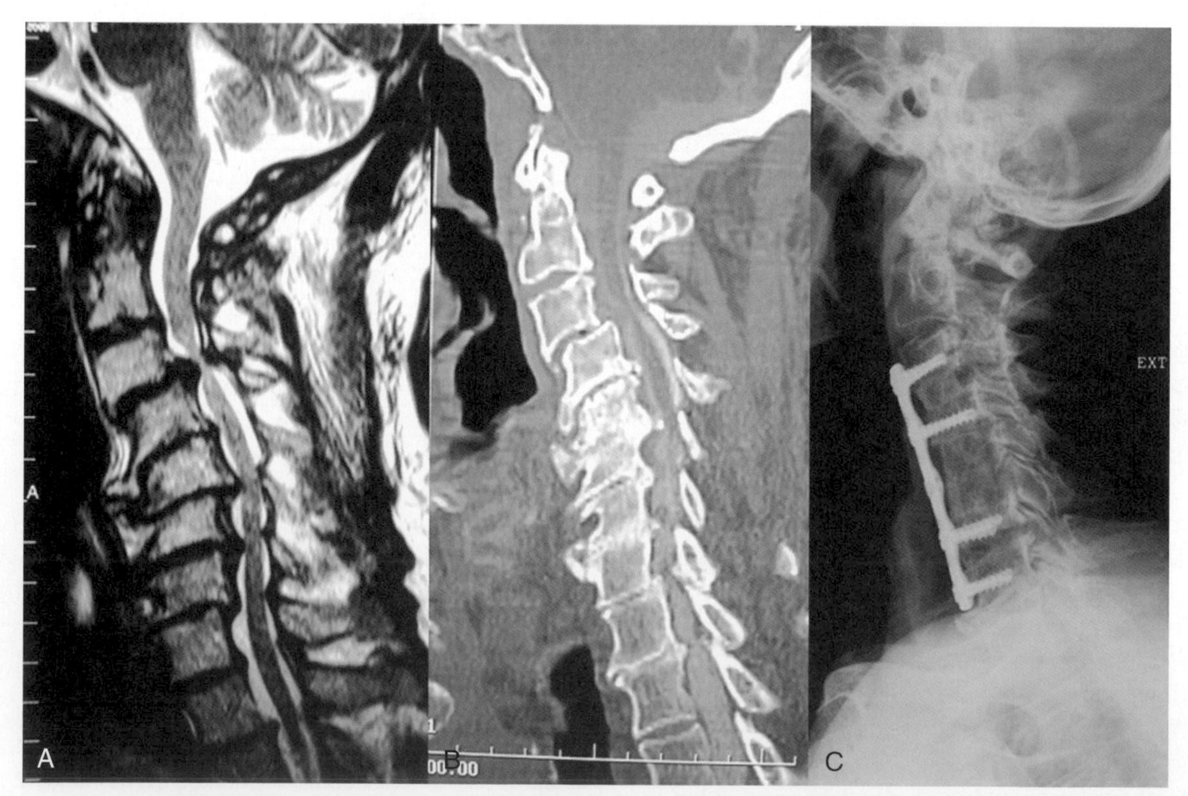

Figure 114-4 Severe multi-level cervical spondylotic myelopathy. Note the classic imaging findings of cervical myelopathy seen on T2-weighted sagittal magnetic resonance image (**A**) and sagittal reconstruction of the computed tomography myelogram (**B**). **C,** This complex compressive pathology was treated with a hybrid anterior technique (C3-C4 and C6-C7 anterior cervical discectomy and fusion and C5 corpectomy with strut allograft).

Troubleshooting

- Establish realistic expectations. The main goal of surgery in patients with myelopathy is to halt progression of the disease.
- Document the neurologic examination immediately preoperatively and postoperatively. Serial examination should be performed during the in-patient stay.
- Rule out other causes; 14% of patients with poor outcomes after surgery for cervical spondylotic myelopathy were later determined to have alternative or additional diagnoses such as myopathy, Parkinson's disease, and cerebellar ataxia.
- Poor neurologic recovery or worsening should prompt repeat imaging.

Patient Instructions

- If a nonoperative approach is tried, the surgeon must clearly instruct the patient to observe for and report any evidence of a progressive neurologic deficit. This warning should include the obvious (muscle weakness, sensory deficits) as well as the not so obvious (changes in bowel/bladder/erectile function, altered gait and balance, reduced hand dexterity).

Considerations in Special Populations

- Football players
    - Cervical cord neurapraxia is a condition associated with cervical canal stenosis.
    - Spear tackling (axial load and hyperflexion) may result in acute, transient (typically 10–15 minutes) burning sensations in the upper extremities, with or without motor deficits.
    - Cervical cord neurapraxia does not predict future permanent neurologic deficit; however, the recurrence rate is 56%.
    - Return to play requires careful discussion. Return is contraindicated in patients with a Torg ratio of less than 0.8, loss of cervical lordosis, or evidence of cord damage on magnetic resonance imaging.
- Ossification of the posterior longitudinal ligament is often a multilevel disease, and progressive enlargement is expected. Thus, it is important to establish the specific diagnosis (computed tomography) and plan surgery that addresses the global nature of the disorder (laminoplasty).
- Patients with Klippel-Feil syndrome frequently have congenitally narrowed spinal canals.

Suggested Reading

- Bohlman HH, Emery SE: The pathophysiology of cervical spondylosis and myelopathy. Spine 1988;13:843–846.
- Clarke E, Robinson PK: Cervical myelopathy: A complication of cervical spondylosis. Brain 1956;79:483–510.
- Emery SE: Cervical spondylotic myelopathy: Diagnosis and treatment. J Am Acad Orthop Surg 2001;9:376–388.
- Hilibrand AS, Carlson GD, Palumbo MA, et al: Radiculopathy and myelopathy at segments adjacent to the site of a previous anterior cervical arthrodesis. J Bone Joint Surg Am 1999; 81A:519–528.
- Nurick S: The natural history and the results of surgical treatment of the spinal cord disorder associated with cervical spondylosis. Brain 1972;95:101–108.
- Torg JS, Naranja RJ Jr, Pavlov H, et al: The relationship of developmental narrowing of the cervical spinal canal to reversible and irreversible injury of the cervical spinal cord in football players. J Bone Joint Surg Am 1996;78A:1308–1314.

Chapter 115 Spinal Cord Injury

Matthew G. Zmurko and D. Greg Anderson

ICD-9 CODES

806.0 *Fracture of Vertebral Column with Spinal Cord Injury, Cervical*
806.2 *Fracture of Vertebral Column with Spinal Cord Injury, Thoracic*
806.4 *Fracture of Vertebral Column with Spinal Cord Injury, Lumbar*
806.6 *Fracture of Vertebral Column with Spinal Cord Injury, Sacrum, and Coccyx*

Key Concepts

- Approximately 11,000 spinal cord injuries occur each year in North America, the majority in young, active individuals as a result of trauma.
  - Motor vehicle accidents are the most common cause, followed by diving, sporting events, falls, and acts of violence.
- No effective means of treatment exists to repair the neural injury and restore spinal cord function below the level of injury.
- After an acute traumatic spinal cord injury, two mechanisms of damage occur:
  - Primary injury: acute contusion of the cord, which occurs at the time of injury as a result of a spinal column fracture, dislocation, or acute cord compression
  - Secondary injury: begins over the hours and days after the acute injury and involves an inflammatory cascade and secondary pathologic changes that worsen the primary insult to the cord
- Using a pharmacologic means of blocking a secondary injury (e.g., high-dose steroid protocol) is an area of research and debate.

History

- Mechanism of injury, including thorough history regarding traumatic event
- Associated injuries
  - Bowel injury in seatbelt mechanism
  - Facial injuries in cervical hyperextension mechanism
- Search for noncontiguous fractures (image the entire spinal axis).

Physical Examination

- Observation
  - Airway, breathing, and circulation
  - Paradoxical diaphragmatic breathing pattern
  - Neurogenic shock; results from loss of sympathetic tone with hemodynamic instability including bradycardia and hypotension
- Palpation
  - Log roll patient to examine spine from occiput to sacrum during secondary examination
  - Tenderness, swelling, deformity
  - Reproducible, focal spinous process tenderness is a sensitive indication of spinal column injury.
  - Palpable gaps between spinous processes indicative of distraction injury
- Special tests
  - Complete neurologic examination
  - Sacral sparing (perianal sensation intact) represents an incomplete spinal cord lesion with a better prognosis.
  - Bulbocavernosus reflex: anal contraction on squeezing the glans penis or pulling on the Foley urinary catheter; return of the bulbocavernosus reflex (or a window of 48 hours) signals the end of spinal shock
  - American Spinal Injury Association Impairment Scale (Table 115-1): standard for assessing and classifying spinal cord injury; the level of neurologic function is defined as the most caudal level with at least grade III motor function

Imaging

- Radiographs: anteroposterior, lateral, and odontoid views of the cervical spine
  - Occiput to T1: if unable to visualize C7-T1, other techniques are employed (e.g., swimmer's view, oblique view, computed tomography)
  - Eighty-five percent of all traumatic injuries are visualized on the lateral radiograph.

TABLE 115-1 *American Spinal Injury Association Impairment Scale*

A	Complete	No motor or sensory function preserved in the sacral segments S4-S5
B	Incomplete	Sensory but no motor function preserved below the neurologic level; includes the sacral segments S4-S5
C	Incomplete	Motor function preserved below the neurologic level; more than half of the key muscles below the neurologic level have a muscle grade < 3
D	Incomplete	Motor function preserved below the neurologic level; at least half of the key muscles below the neurologic level have a muscle grade ≥ 3
E	Normal	Sensory and motor functions are normal.

- Soft-tissue swelling in the retropharyngeal space (>7 mm at C2) may suggest spinal column injury.
- If a cervical spinal fracture is found, the entire spine needs to be imaged because there is a 10% chance of noncontiguous spinal injuries.
- Computed tomography
  - Most sensitive imaging modality in diagnosing fractures of the cervical spine
- Magnetic resonance imaging
  - Not as sensitive in identifying cervical spine fractures as radiographs and computed tomography
  - Gold standard in soft-tissue assessment, including the spinal cord
  - Required before open or closed reduction if patient is not awake and alert

Differential Diagnosis

- Complete spinal cord injury: no motor or sensory function below level of injury
- Incomplete spinal cord injury: Below the level of injury, the spinal cord acts as an upper motor neuron injury, whereas at the level of injury, the cord produces lower motor neuron findings.
  - Brown-Séquard syndrome (best prognosis): penetrating trauma or unilateral facet dislocation and/or fracture; results in ipsilateral muscle paralysis and loss of proprioception/vibratory sense with contralateral loss of pain and temperature sensation below the level of injury
  - Central cord syndrome (second best prognosis): hyperextension injury, typically in older individuals with spinal stenosis; upper extremities (especially hands) weaker than the lower extremities
  - Anterior cord syndrome (poorest prognosis): flexion-compression injury; results in minimal distal motor function; injury to the spinothalamic tracts leads to loss of sensitivity to pain and temperature
  - Posterior cord syndrome (very rare): isolated injury to the dorsal columns; results in loss of proprioception, vibration sense, and deep pressure

Treatment

- At diagnosis
  - The goal for cervical fractures and dislocations is to achieve an anatomic, pain-free, and mobile spine without neurologic deficit. Trauma protocols should be instituted at the initial presentation, including spine immobilization.
  - Neurogenic shock requires aggressive hemodynamic monitoring to maintain appropriate cardiac output and a mean blood pressure of 85 to 90 mmHg.
    - The goal is to maintain cord perfusion to minimize secondary damage.
    - Best treated with vasopressors and atropine
  - Medical therapies are directed at limiting the effect of secondary injuries that follow the initial insult to the spinal cord.
    - Methylprednisolone: 30 mg/kg IV bolus and 5.4 mg/kg/hr for 23 hours for patients with spinal cord injury less than 8 hours to treatment
- Later
  - There is little question about the benefits of spinal cord decompression.
  - The surgical approach is typically dictated by the injury pattern.

When to Refer

- All patients with spinal cord injuries require referral.

Prognosis

- Greater functional recovery occurs when there is more initial sparing of motor and sensory function distal to the level of injury. The root return phenomenon has been observed after decompression of the spinal cord in patients with complete cervical neurologic injuries.

Considerations in Special Populations

- In elderly patients with preexisting stenosis, hyperextension injuries may result in central cord syndrome.

Suggested Reading

- Aebi M, Mohler J, Zach GA, et al: Indications, surgical technique, and results of 100 surgically treated fractures and fracture-dislocations of the cervical spine. Clin Orthop Relat Res 1986;203:244–257.
- Bracken MB: Treatment of acute spinal cord injury with methylprednisolone: Results of a multicenter, randomized clinical trial. J Neurotrauma 1991;8:S47–S50.
- Bracken MB, Shepard MJ, Collins WF, et al: A randomized, controlled trial of methylprednisolone or naloxone in the treatment of acute spinal cord injury. N Engl J Med 1990;322:1404–1411.
- Bracken MB, Shepard MJ, Holford TR, et al: Administration of methylprednisolone for 24 or 48 hours or tirilazad mesylate for 48 hours in the treatment of acute spinal cord injury. Results of the third national acute spinal cord injury randomized controlled trial. JAMA 1997;277:1597–1604.
- Bracken MB, Shepard MJ, Holford TR, et al: Methylprednisolone or tirilazad mesylate administration after acute spinal cord injury: 1 year follow up. Results of the third national acute spinal cord injury randomized controlled trial. J Neurosurg 1998;89:699–706.
- Fehlings MG, Tator CH: An evidence-based review of decompressive surgery in acute spinal cord injury: Rationale, indications, and timing based on experimental and clinical studies. J Neurosurg 1999;91:1–11.
- Hurlbert RJ: Strategies of medical intervention in the management of acute spinal cord injury. Spine 2006;31:S16–S21.
- Levi L, Wolf A, Rigamonti D: Anterior decompression in cervical spine trauma: Does the timing of surgery affect the outcome? Neurosurgery 1991;29:216–222.
- Tsutsumi S, Ueta T, Shiba K, et al. Effects of the second national acute spinal cord injury study of high-dose methylprednisolone therapy on acute cervical spinal cord injury—results in spinal injuries center. Spine 2006;31:2992–2996.
- Vaccaro AR, Daugherty RJ, Sheehan TP, et al: Neurologic outcome of early versus late surgery for cervical spinal cord injury. Spine 1997;22:2609–2613.

Chapter 116 Burners/Stingers (Brachial Plexopathy)

Sanjitpal S. Gill and Michael A. Townsend

ICD-9 CODE
953.4 *Injury to Nerve Roots and Spinal Plexus, Brachial Plexus*

Key Concepts

- Burners and stingers are injuries to the brachial plexus resulting from traction, compression, or direct trauma.
- The brachial plexus is composed of cervical nerve roots C5 through T1.
- C5-C6 most commonly affected (Fig. 116-1)
  - Deltoid, biceps, rotator cuff (supraspinatus, infraspinatus) muscles
- Reversible, unilateral upper extremity pain, radiculopathy, and weakness
- One of the most common cervical spine injuries in athletes
- Most common in collision and contact sports; as many as 65% of college football players report stingers during their 4-year career.
- Symptoms typically resolve within minutes of the injury.
- Limited evidence-based guidelines make return to activity decisions difficult, especially after recurrent episodes.

History

- Posttraumatic syndrome
  - Traction: sudden shoulder depression with lateral head deviation
  - Compression: extension, ipsilateral compression, rotation to affected side
- Root injury in narrowed foramen; more common in mature athletes
  - Direct trauma: direct blow or compression from shoulder pad and superior medial scapula (Erb's point)
- Unilateral burning or tingling sensation in the entire arm
- Transient inability to actively use the arm (dead arm syndrome)
- Neurologic symptoms rarely follow a strict dermatomal pattern.
- If symptoms are bilateral, the concern is for cervical spine injury or transient quadriparesis.

Physical Examination

- Observation
  - Splinting of the affected arm (Fig. 116-2)
  - Shoulder depression
- Palpation
  - Rule out tenderness over the spinous processes and clavicle.
  - May have positive Tinel's sign at Erb's point
- Range of motion
  - Always perform active motion first.
- Special tests
  - Spurling's test: Cervical extension, lateral flexion to the side of the injury, and gentle axial compression reproduce radicular symptoms (Fig. 116-3).
- Testing for compression through stenotic foramen
  - Thorough neurologic examination

Imaging

- Radiographs
  - Anteroposterior view: coronal alignment
  - Lateral view: may have loss of cervical lordosis from spasm
  - Oblique views: to evaluate cervical foramina
  - Flexion/extension views: instability, less useful in acute setting
  - Torg ratio: ratio of sagittal spinal canal width to sagittal vertebral body width; measures degree of congenital spinal stenosis

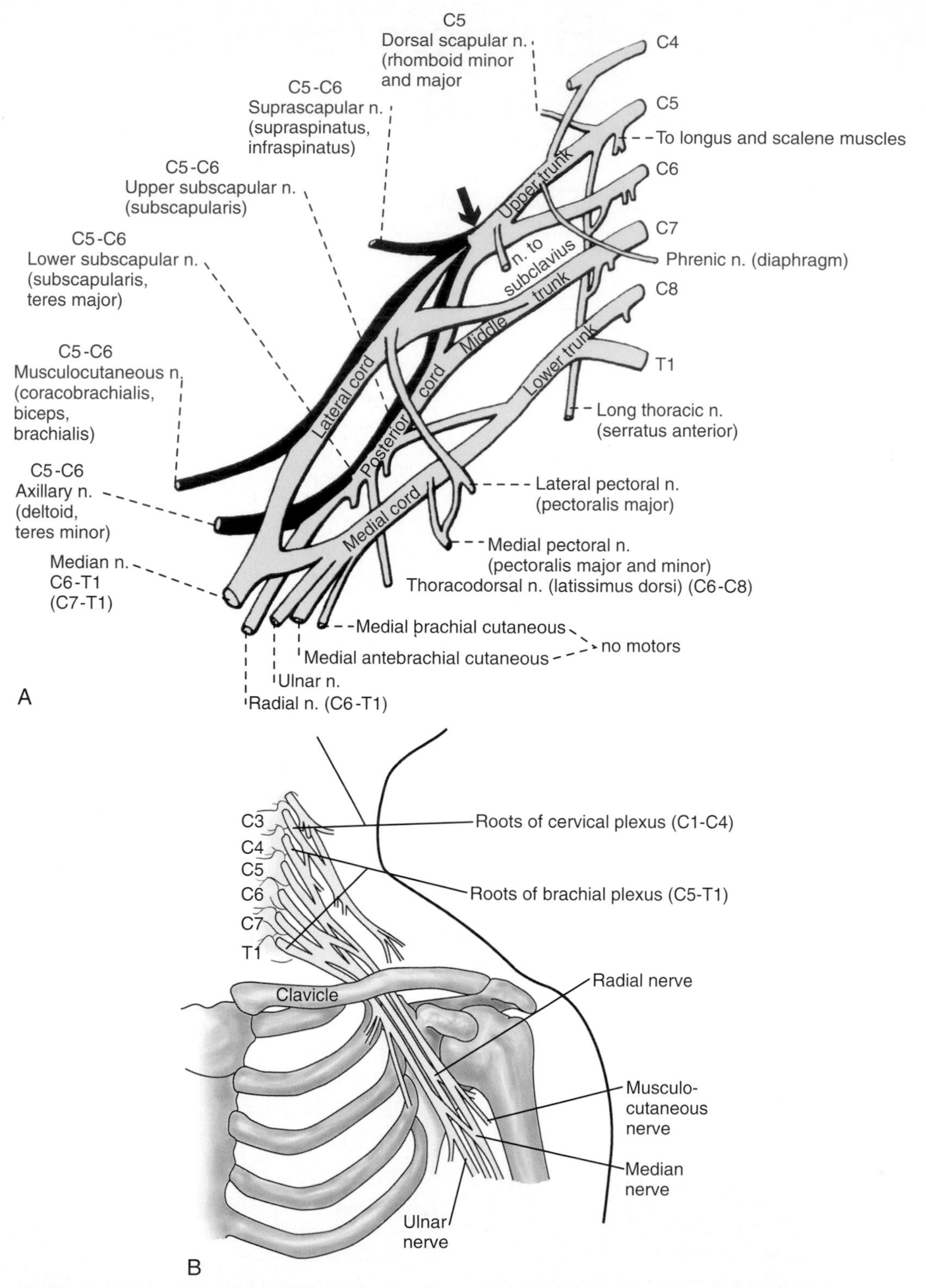

Figure 116-1 **A**, Stingers and burners commonly affect the upper trunk of the brachial plexus creating weakness of the deltoid, biceps, and rotator cuff muscles. **B**, The relationship of the brachial plexus to the surrounding anatomic structures including the clavicle and chest wall. (Part A adapted from DeLee JC, Drez D Jr, Miller MD [eds]: DeLee & Drez's Orthopaedic Sports Medicine, Vol. 1, 2nd ed. Philadelphia: WB Saunders, 2003, p 797; Part B copyright William B. Westwood, 1997)

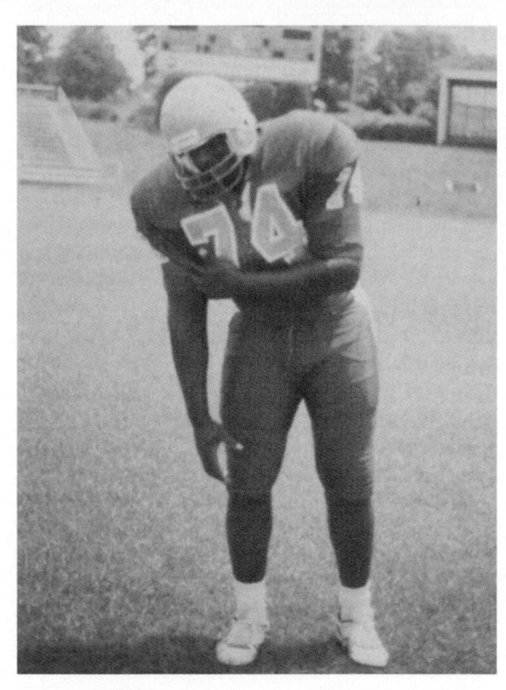

Figure 116-2 Common clinical presentation of an athlete with a stinger that has to support the weight of the arm while leaving the field due to pain or muscle weakness. (From Pritchard JC: Football and Other Contact Sports Injuries: Diagnosis and Treatment. In Buschbacher RM, Braddom RL [eds]: Sports Medicine and Rehabilitation: A Sport Specific Approach. Philadelphia: Hanley and Belfus, 1994, p 172.)

- A ratio of less than 0.8 suggests an increased risk of recurrence.
- Magnetic resonance imaging
    - To evaluate suspected spinal cord or nerve root injury, herniated cervical disc, foraminal stenosis, canal stenosis, spinal cord edema

Additional Tests

- Electromyography
    - Most useful 2 to 4 weeks after injury if persistent symptoms
    - After clinical return of normal strength, as many as 80% of patients show electromyographic abnormalities that may persist for more than 5 years.

Differential Diagnosis

- Cervical spine injury
- Cervical cord neurapraxia (transient quadriparesis)
- Clavicle fracture
- Herniated cervical disc
- Rotator cuff injury

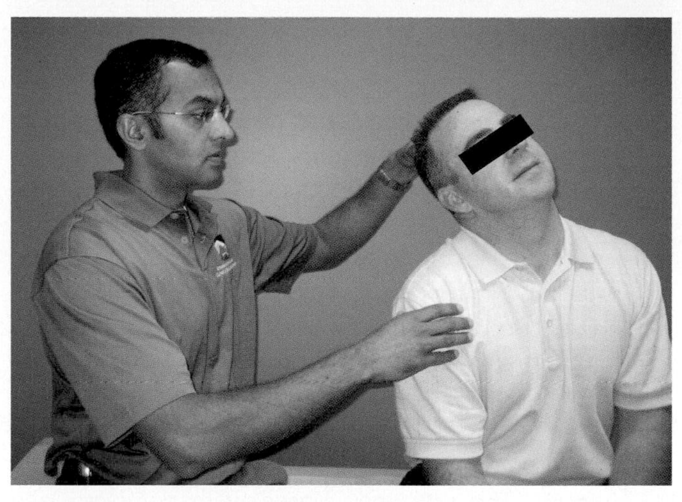

Figure 116-3 Spurling's test is used to re-create foraminal stenosis by ipsilateral extension and rotation.

- Stress fracture of first rib
- Thoracic outlet syndrome
- Parsonage-Turner syndrome

Treatment

- At diagnosis
    - If applicable, remove from competition until complete resolution of symptoms and cervical spine injury excluded
    - Treatment is largely supportive; a sling may help rest the affected extremity until symptoms improve.
- Later
    - Rehabilitation program to restore strength and motion of cervical spine and upper extremity
    - Athletes should not be allowed to return to competition without a full, pain-free cervical range of motion. This is paramount in preventing more serious spinal cord injury.
    - The use of neck rolls, a neck-shoulder-cervical orthosis (cowboy collar), and/or pads at the base of the neck in football players can help minimize recurrence.

When to Refer

- If cervical spine injury is suspected (axial neck pain), immobilization and full radiographic evaluation are warranted.
- Specialist referral if symptoms last longer than 1 week and there are positive findings suggestive of nerve root injury, bilateral symptoms, or recurrent symptoms

Prognosis

- It varies depending on severity.
  - Grade 1: neurapraxia. All nerve structures remain intact (most common). Complete resolution of symptoms typically occurs in minutes, but may take as long as 6 weeks.
  - Grade 2: axonotmesis. There are axonal disruption and wallerian degeneration distal to the injury site. Recovery is complete, but it may take months. An intact epineurium allows axonal regrowth at a rate of approximately 1 mm/day.
  - Grade 3: neurotmesis. Complete disruption of axons, endoneurium, perineurium, and epineurium. The prognosis varies, with complete loss common.

Troubleshooting

- Red flags include bilateral symptoms, lower extremity involvement, painful range of motion, axial tenderness, persistent burning, neurologic deficit, and altered consciousness.
- Immobilize and perform a complete clinical/radiographic evaluation.

Patient Instructions

- Patients should continue sling use until pain resolves. Monitor for elbow stiffness.
- Instruct athletes to report all instances of recurrence.
- Patients may resume activity when full, pain-free range of motion and full upper extremity strength return.

Suggested Reading

- Feinberg JH: Burners and stingers. Phys Med Rehabil Clin N Am 2000;11:771–784.
- Hoppenfeld S: Physical examination of the cervical spine. In Hoppenfeld S (ed): Physical Examination of the Spine and Extremities. Norwalk, CT: Appleton-Century-Crofts, 1976, pp 105–132.
- Kasow DB, Curl WW: “Stingers” in adolescent athletes. Instr Course Lect 2006;55:711–716.
- Kelley JD: Brachial plexus injuries: Evaluating and treating “burners.” J Musculoskel Med 1997;14:70–80.
- Olson DE, McBroom SA, Nelson BD, et al: Unilateral cervical nerve injuries: Brachial plexopathies. Curr Sports Med Rep 2007;6:43–49.
- Safran MR: Nerve injury about the shoulder. Part 2: Long thoracic nerve, spinal accessory nerve, burners/stingers, thoracic outlet syndrome. Am J Sports Med 2004;32:1063–1076.
- Weinberg J, Rokito S, Silber JS: Etiology, treatment, and prevention of athletic “stingers.” Clin Sports Med 2003;22:493–500.

Chapter 117 Thoracolumbar Strain

James Beazell

ICD-9 CODES
724.2 *Lumbago*
847.2 *Lumbar Strain*

Key Concepts

- Low back pain (LBP) affects more than 90% of the adult population at some point in their lifetime.
- A biopsychosocial approach has been proposed based on patient presentation and attitudes regarding work and activity.
- Nonspecific LBP is a heterogeneous condition and includes a number of different clinical entities.
- Previous research suggested a wait-and-see approach for acute LBP.
- A treatment-based classification system has been proposed for acute LBP, based on response to specific treatment interventions.
- Manipulation may be successful in alleviating pain in patients with recent onset of LBP and no lower extremity symptoms.
- Patients with impaired motor control and movement abnormalities benefit from core stabilization exercises.

History

- Localized LBP
- Inquire about onset and duration of pain, previous episodes of LBP, history of trauma, presence of lower extremity symptoms, history of depression, and occupational concerns.
- Red flags requiring special attention should be identified (Table 117-1).
- Multiple episodes of LBP, often due to minor incidents, may indicate clinical instability.

Physical Examination

- Observation
  - Postural assessment
- Palpation
  - Tenderness of paraspinal musculature, sacroiliac joints, and pubic symphysis
- Range of motion
  - Often decreased secondary to pain
  - Evaluate hip and knee range of motion
  - Evaluate for aberrant motions (e.g., Gower's sign: using hands to walk up thighs to return from forward bending in standing)
- Special tests
  - Neurologic examination
  - Prone instability test: Assess segmental stiffness and pain in a resting state and during active contraction. The test is considered positive if pain is provoked in the resting state and eliminated during active muscle contraction (Fig. 117-1).
  - Nerve tension tests: straight leg raise (sciatic nerve), prone knee bend (femoral nerve)
  - Crossed straight leg raise (straight leg raise in uninvolved leg reproduces symptoms in involved leg); useful in detecting disc herniation
  - Provocative tests for sacroiliac dysfunction: posterior pelvic pain provocation (Fig. 117-2), iliac compression and gapping, Gaenslen's test, and sacral thrust

Imaging

- Radiographs: anteroposterior and lateral views
  - Obtain if symptoms not resolving despite conservative treatment or if objective neurologic findings present
  - Avoid the nocebo effect by overemphasizing degenerative changes.
  - Magnetic resonance imaging: typically not necessary unless diagnosis in question

Differential Diagnosis

- Facet syndrome: pain relieved by recumbency, diagnostic block
- Spinal stenosis: pain relieved with flexion

TABLE 117-1 *Red Flags for Low Back Pain*

Fractures	Cauda Equina Syndrome	Cancer	Ankylosing Spondylitis	Spinal Infection
Fracture due to major trauma, e.g., motor vehicle accident, fall	Saddle numbness; bladder dysfunction of recent onset; progressive neurologic deficit in the lower extremity	Age older than 50 yr; history of cancer; unexplained weight loss; no relief with bed rest	Male; morning stiffness; age younger than 35 yr at onset; no relief with lying down; relief with exercise or movement; chest expansion restricted	Recent fever; recent bacterial infection; IV drug abuse; immunosuppression

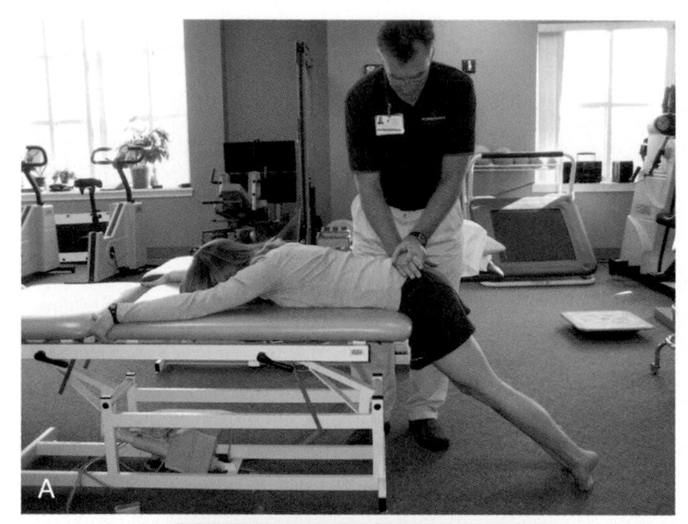

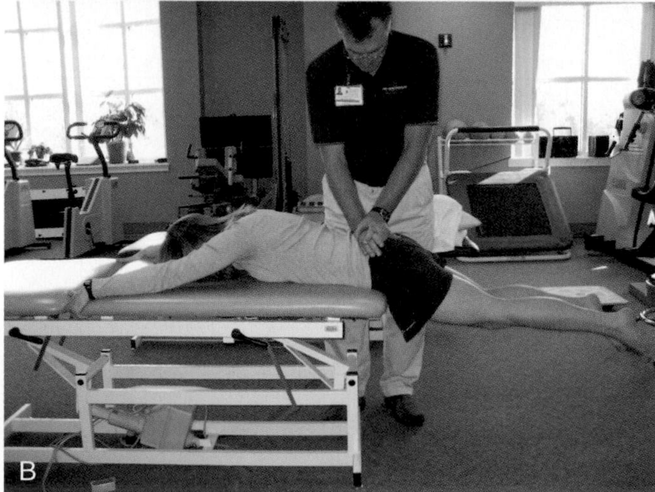

Figure 117-1 Prone instability test. **A**, Starting position with lower extremities in contact with the floor. Posteroanterior glide is performed at each lumbar segment. **B**, If a painful lumbar segment is identified, the test is repeated at that segment in conjunction with active lumbar and hip extension to lift the legs from the ground.

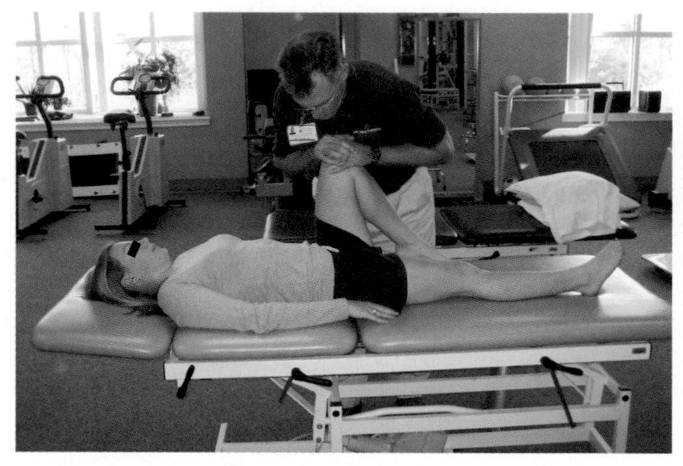

Figure 117-2 Posterior pelvic pain provocation test.

- Spondylolysis/listhesis: pain with or without instability with extension, radiographs
- Sacroiliac dysfunction: provocative tests

Treatment

- At diagnosis
    - Symptomatic treatments should be instituted. Early referral for physical therapy may help to determine the appropriate classification and direct treatment (Fig. 117-3). Recent onset and lack of pain below the knee indicate a high likelihood of a positive response to lumbosacral manipulation.
    - Treatment-based classification system
        - Specific exercise category: initial treatment to include repeated movements that centralize symptoms (e.g., repeated extension causes leg symptoms to decrease or centralize into low back)
        - Manipulation category: initial treatment with lumbosacral manipulation or specific segmental manipulation

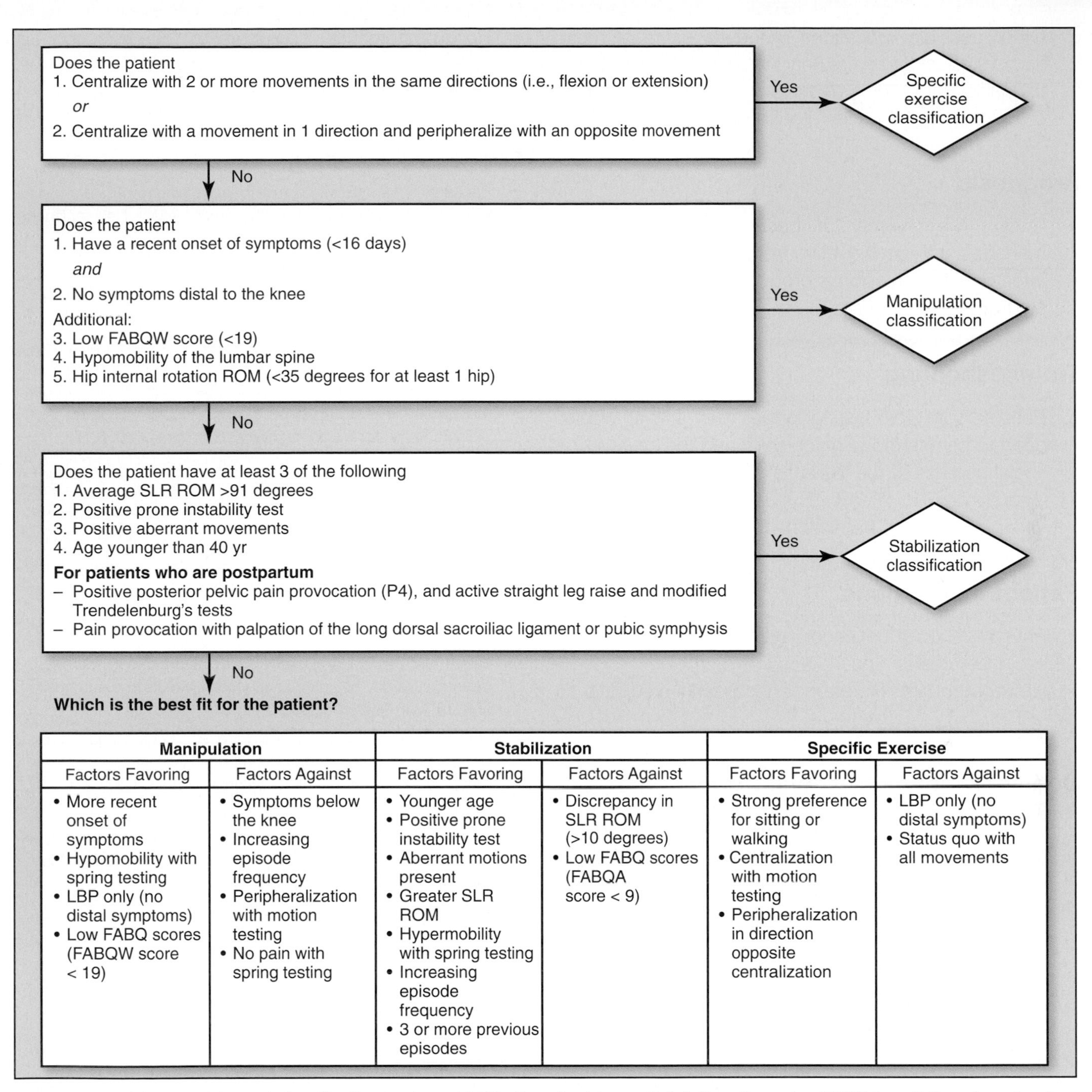

Manipulation		Stabilization		Specific Exercise	
Factors Favoring	Factors Against	Factors Favoring	Factors Against	Factors Favoring	Factors Against
• More recent onset of symptoms • Hypomobility with spring testing • LBP only (no distal symptoms) • Low FABQ scores (FABQW score < 19)	• Symptoms below the knee • Increasing episode frequency • Peripheralization with motion testing • No pain with spring testing	• Younger age • Positive prone instability test • Aberrant motions present • Greater SLR ROM • Hypermobility with spring testing • Increasing episode frequency • 3 or more previous episodes	• Discrepancy in SLR ROM (>10 degrees) • Low FABQ scores (FABQA score < 9)	• Strong preference for sitting or walking • Centralization with motion testing • Peripheralization in direction opposite centralization	• LBP only (no distal symptoms) • Status quo with all movements

Figure 117-3 Treatment-based classification system. FABQ, Fear-Avoidance Belief Questionnaire; FABQA, activity subscale of FABQ; FABQW, work subscale of FABQ; LBP, low back pain; ROM, range of motion; SLR, straight leg raise. (Adapted from Fritz JM, Cleland JA, Childs JD: Subgrouping patients with low back pain: Evolution of a classification approach to physical therapy. J Orthop Sports Phys Ther 2007;37:290–302.)

    — Stabilization category: core stabilization exercises with initial emphasis on the transversus abdominis, multifidus, and pelvic floor muscles, and the diaphragm

- Later
  - Progression of stabilization exercises
  - Specific exercise feedback can restore the normal neuromuscular feedforward function of the transversus abdominis muscle.
  - Local versus global activation of the transversus abdominis, pelvic floor, and multifidus muscles, and the diaphragm should be the basic goal of the exercise program.

When to Refer

- Patients with red flags, neurologic findings, or persistent symptoms despite an appropriate trial of conservative management should be referred.

- Other possible indications include a score of more than 19 out of 24 on the Fear Avoidance Beliefs Questionnaire (FABQ) or a depression score of more than 3 out of 6 on the patient health questionnaire.

Prognosis

- Good: The majority of patients are successfully managed with conservative treatments.
- A history of depression is prognostic for a slow recovery from back pain.

Troubleshooting

- Patients with pain lasting longer than 4 to 6 weeks need to be referred to a specialist and the biopsychosocial aspects of the patient's case considered.
- One percent to 2% of LBP is due to radiculopathy secondary to disc herniation.

Patient Instructions

- Patients should be encouraged to stay active and avoid bed rest.
- Radiographic results are not necessarily predictive of LBP.

Considerations in Special Populations

- Low back pain is commonly reported in the athletic population and may be present in as many as 20% of sports injuries.
- Poor posture may contribute to LBP in school-age children.

Suggested Reading

- Benedetti F, Lanotte M, Lopiano L, et al: When words are painful: Unraveling the mechanisms of the nocebo effect. Neuroscience 2007;147:260–271.
- Childs JD, Fritz JM, Flynn TW, et al: A clinical prediction rule to identify patients with low back pain most likely to benefit from spinal manipulation: A validation study. Ann Intern Med 2004;141:920–928.
- Cleland JA, Fritz JM, Brennan GP: Predictive validity of initial fear avoidance beliefs in patients with low back pain receiving physical therapy: Is the FABQ a useful screening tool for identifying patients at risk for a poor recovery? Eur Spine J 2008;17:70–79.
- Fritz JM, Childs JD, Flynn TW: Pragmatic application of a clinical prediction rule in primary care to identify patients with low back pain with a good prognosis following a brief spinal manipulation intervention. BMC Fam Pract 2005;6:29.
- Fritz JM, Cleland JA, Childs JD: Subgrouping patients with low back pain: Evolution of a classification approach to physical therapy. J Orthop Sports Phys Ther 2007;37:290–302.
- Laslett M, Aprill CN, McDonald B, et al: Diagnosis of sacroiliac joint pain: Validity of individual provocation tests and composites of tests. Man Ther 2005;10:207–218.
- Mens JM, Vleeming A, Snijders CJ, et al: Validity of the active straight leg raise test for measuring disease severity in patients with posterior pelvic pain after pregnancy. Spine 2002;27:196–200.
- Tsao H, Hodges PW: Immediate changes in feedforward postural adjustments following voluntary motor training. Exp Brain Res 2007;181:537–546.

Chapter 118 Thoracolumbar Disc Disease

R. Todd Allen and Frank M. Phillips

ICD-9 CODES

722.51	*Degeneration of Thoracic Disc(s)*
722 52	*Degeneration of Lumbar Disc(s)*
724.9	*Foraminal Encroachment (Compression) of Nerve Root, Thoracic or Lumbar*
724.4	*Thoracic or Lumbosacral Neuritis or Radiculitis*
722.11	*Thoracic Disc Disorder without Myelopathy*
722.72	*Thoracic Disc Disorder with Myelopathy*
722.10	*Lumbar Disc Disorder without Myelopathy*
722.73	*Lumbar Disc Disorder with Myelopathy*

Key Concepts

- Intervertebral discs consist of an outer annulus fibrosus (AF) and an inner nucleus pulposus (NP) (Fig. 118-1).
- Disc degeneration begins with decreased NP water and proteoglycan content, impairing its load-bearing ability. As degeneration progresses, type II collagen replaces type I and tears/fissures develop in the AF. Vertebral endplates calcify, impairing nutrient diffusion to the intervertebral disc (see Fig. 118-1).
- With degeneration, disc bulging or herniation may occur, facet joints may become arthritic and hypertrophy, vertebral body osteophytes develop, and the ligamentum flavum thickens. The result is spinal canal narrowing (stenosis), which can result in neural compression (central, lateral recess, or foraminal).
- Intervertebral disc degeneration is an inevitable consequence of aging and is frequently asymptomatic. Correlation of symptoms with the physical examination and imaging findings is a critical part of patient evaluation.
- Thoracic disc herniation: most cases are asymptomatic; usually occurring in the third through sixth decades
  - Of all symptomatic intervertebral disc herniations, less than 4% occur in the thoracic spine, most commonly in the caudal third.
  - Thoracic spinal kyphosis increases susceptibility to injury from herniation.
- Lumbar herniated NP (HNP); most common at L4-L5, then L5-S1
  - Mean age at onset: younger than 35 years, unusual at younger than 20 or older than 60 years
  - Rare in children; slippage of entire disc and endplate (slipped vertebral apophyses) may mimic a herniated disc
  - Herniation types
    - — Protrusion (NP contained within annulus)
    - — Extrusion (NP through annulus with or without posterior longitudinal ligament tear)
    - — Sequestered (complete displacement of NP, often with free disc fragment)
- Cauda equina syndrome: may be caused by a very large HNP (especially midline), leading to perineal sensation loss, severe pain, leg weakness, and loss of voluntary bowel/bladder control; this is a surgical emergency

History

- Red flags
  - Pain at rest, night pain, or constant aching/throbbing pain may indicate infection, neoplasm, or pathologic/osteopenic fracture.
  - Cauda equina syndrome
- Degenerative disc disease: usually asymptomatic; may present with axial low back pain
  - Lumbar back pain is mechanical (increased with spinal loading) and exacerbated by lumbar flexion and sitting (increases intradiscal pressure).
- Thoracic herniated disc: highly variable presentation; onset typically insidious
  - Axial thoracic pain; Valsalva maneuver typically worsens pain
  - Radicular pain radiates around the chest wall in a dermatomal pattern.
  - Dermatomal sensory changes (paresthesias, dysesthesias)

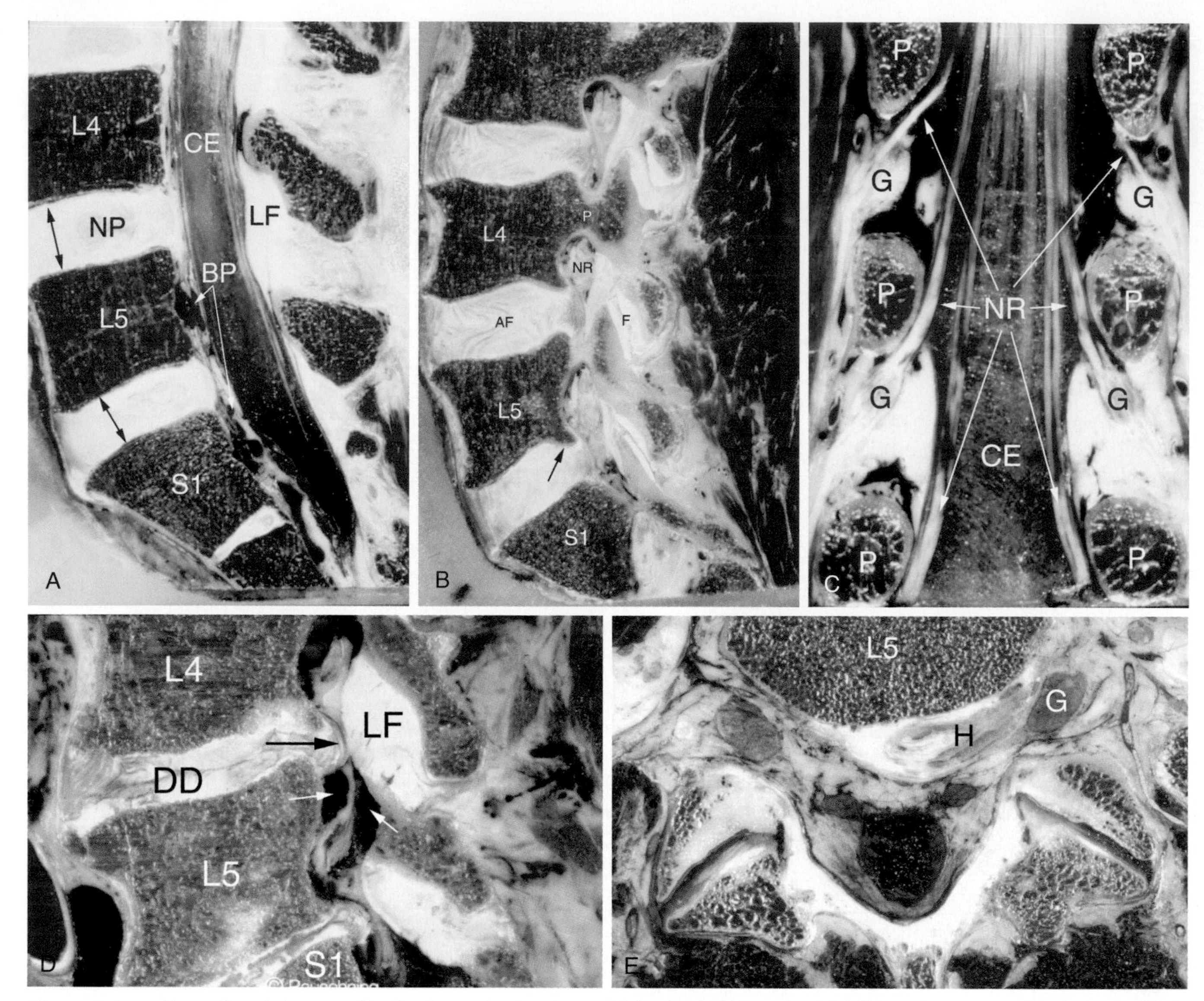

Figure 118-1 Normal and degenerative lumbar spine anatomy. Midsagittal (**A**), parasagittal (**B**), and coronal (**C**) views of a normal lumbar spine. Note maintained disc heights, nerve roots (NR) exiting below the pedicles and out the neural foramen. The coronal section shows the cauda equina (CE) and the location of nerve root ganglia (G) in relation to the pedicle. **D**, Sagittal view of a degenerative lumbar segment. Note the narrowed degenerative disc (DD), posterior disc bulge, ligamentum flavum (LF) hypertrophy, and narrowed intervertebral foramen for the exiting nerve root. **E**, Axial view of a herniated disc. AF, annulus fibrosus; NP, nucleus pulposus; P. (Used with permission from Gallego J, Schnuerer AP, Manuel C: Basic Anatomy and Pathology of the Spine. Medtronic Sofamor Danek, USA, Inc., Memphis, TN, 2001; photographs by Wolfgang Rauschning, MD, PhD.)

- Spinal cord compression may lead to myelopathy with lower extremity hyperreflexia, spasticity/clonus, unsteady gait, numbness, variable weakness, and/or more severe findings of bowel/bladder dysfunction.
- Lumbar herniated disc
  - Classically presents with sciatica or radiating leg pain (with or without paresthesia, dysesthesia) in a dermatomal distribution
    - — Usually worse with coughing or sneezing (increased intraspinal pressure) and with sitting or lumbar flexion (nerve root stretch)
    - — Leg pain frequently greater than back pain
  - May lead to dermatomal sensory, motor, or reflex loss
  - Classic posterolateral herniations impinge on the traversing nerve root (e.g., L5 root with L4-L5 posterolateral herniation).
  - Central herniations: axial pain with or without unilateral (or even bilateral) radiculopathy; if large enough, watch for cauda equina syndrome
  - Far lateral or foraminal herniation; more common in older patients; impinges on exiting nerve root (e.g., L3 root at L3-L4 disc space)

Physical Examination

- Observation
  - Spinal alignment in coronal (scoliosis) and sagittal (kyphosis) planes
  - Muscle atrophy
  - Gait
- Palpation
  - Paraspinal muscle spasm/tenderness
  - Sciatic notch tenderness (in radiculopathy)
  - Step-off may indicate spondylolisthesis.
- Range of motion
  - Usually decreased secondary to pain
  - Low back pain in extension suggests posterior element pathology (facet arthritis); low back pain with flexion (loads intervertebral disc) suggests discogenic pain; leg pain with lumbar flexion (increased nerve tension) suggests radiculopathy.
  - With a posterolateral HNP, ipsilateral lateral bending may exaggerate the radiculopathy as the root is stretched over the herniated disc. In axillary herniated discs, lateral bending away from the symptomatic side will stretch the root.
  - A painful dysrhythmic range of motion may indicate mechanical instability.
  - Special tests (Table 118-1)
  - Complete motor/sensory/reflex examination (Fig. 118-2)
  - Waddell's nonorganic tests: assess for malingering or secondary gain
    - — Nonanatomic superficial tenderness; stimulation tests (axial loading and rotation); flip test (straight leg raise positive while supine, but negative while sitting); nonanatomic weakness and sensory findings; overreaction.

TABLE 118-1 *Common Provocative Tests for Radiculopathy*

Test	Outcome
SLR, sitting and supine	Reproduction/aggravation of radicular pain in exact dermatomal pattern of involved root with elevation of involved leg (sciatic nerve involvement should produce pain distal to knee)
Contralateral SLR	SLR of nonpainful limb causes tension of involved root but from opposite side, causing radiculopathy; may suggest sequestered or extruded large disc fragment
Bowstring sign	Pressure over popliteal fossa aggravates SLR radicular pain
Lasègue's sign	Ankle dorsiflexion aggravates SLR radiculopathy
Femoral nerve stretch test	While patient is prone, examiner extends hip/leg (with or without flexed knee) to stretch femoral nerve roots L2-L4; painful if irritated

SLR, straight leg raise.

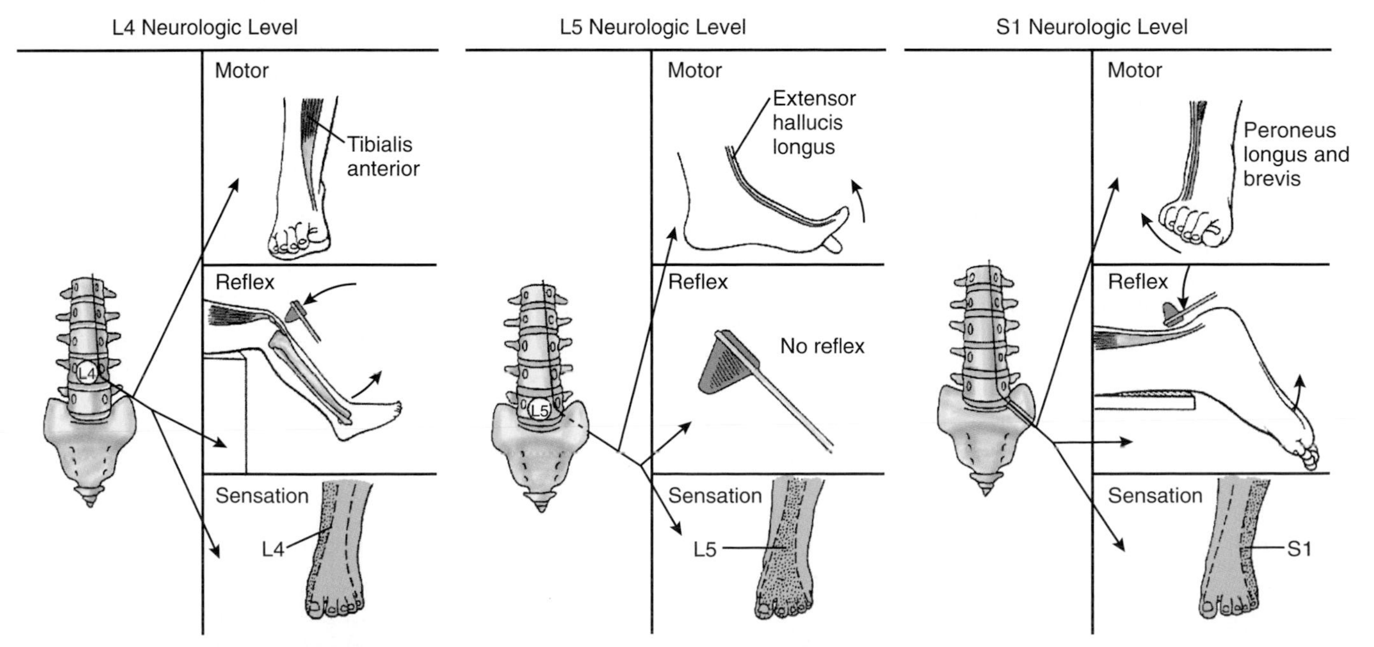

Figure 118-2 Neurologic evaluation of the lower extremity, L4-S1 levels. (Adapted with permission from Klein JD, Garfin SR: History and physical examination. In Weinstein JN, Rydevik B, Sonntag VKG [eds]: Essentials of the Spine. New York: Raven Press, 1995, pp 71–95.)

Imaging

- Eighty percent of individuals older than 55 years of age have radiographic degenerative changes; most are asymptomatic, making correlation with the history/examination most important.
- Radiographs: anteroposterior, lateral, and oblique views
  - Degenerative findings: disc space narrowing, vertebral endplate sclerosis, osteophytes, facet arthrosis/hypertrophy
  - Deformity/instability: coronal (anteroposterior) and sagittal (lateral) plane spinal alignment
    — Assess for scoliosis, kyphosis, pelvic obliquity
  - Spondylolysis/spondylolisthesis detection
  - May detect tumors (pedicle destruction) or fractures
- Magnetic resonance imaging (Fig. 118-3)
  - Imaging study of choice, but high incidence of abnormalities in asymptomatic patients
  - Best screening tool for neural compression/spine lesions/tumors/infection
  - Gadolinium increases accuracy of complex pathology (tumor, infection).
- Computed tomography myelography
  - More than 80% sensitivity for a herniated disc or stenosis but invasive (with myelography); radiation dose relatively high
  - Useful if magnetic resonance imaging contraindicated or in patients with complex problems (e.g., previous surgery with metal implants, complex deformities)

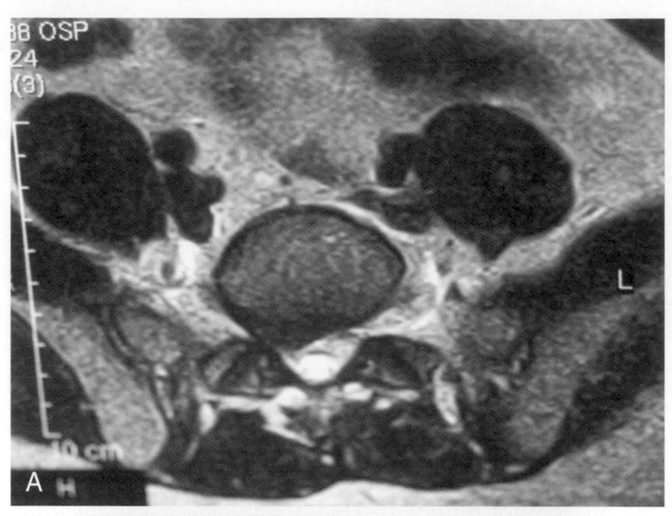

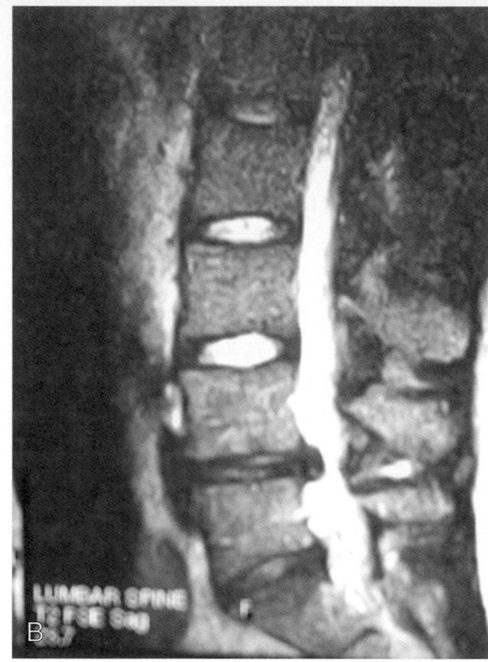

Figure 118-3 **A**, Axial magnetic resonance image of a herniated disc at L4-L5. **B**, Sagittal magnetic resonance image of L4-L5 and L5-S1 disc degeneration. Note the loss of disc height, decreased signal intensity, and disc herniation at L4-L5, causing pain and L5 radiculopathy in this patient.

Additional Tests

- Discography: reproduces concordant pain with intradiscal injection; may be useful in surgical workup of axial back pain
- Electromyography may help to rule out nonspinal etiologies of neural dysfunction.

Differential Diagnosis

- Trauma: sprain/strain, traction neuritis, compression fractures, rib fractures
- Neoplasm: metastatic disease, primary bone/cord tumors
- Infection: discitis, osteomyelitis, soft-tissue/epidural abscess, tuberculosis
- Inflammatory conditions: rheumatoid arthritis, seronegative spondyloarthropathies (ankylosing spondylitis, Reiter syndrome)
- Neurologic conditions
  - Demyelinating disease, anterior horn cell disease, intraspinal cyst
- Visceral conditions
  - Abdominal/renal problems, inflammatory bowel disease
- Other
  - Cardiac disorders, pulmonary disorders, herpes zoster, polymyalgia rheumatica, myofascial syndrome, diffuse idiopathic skeletal hyperostosis, scoliosis or kyphotic deformities, osteomalacia/osteoporosis, Paget's disease, psychogenic disorders

Treatment

- At diagnosis
  - Nonoperative treatment in the acute phase includes nonsteroidal anti-inflammatory drugs, short-term analgesics, ice/heat, and activity modifications with gradual mobilization. Physical therapy with core strengthening, lumbar strengthening/stabilization, and a cardiovascular program can be beneficial (prevents deconditioning).
  - Epidural steroid injections for radiculopathy (not axial back pain)
  - Unproven methods, such as prolonged bed rest (>24 hours) and long-term use of muscle relaxants or braces, may lead to deconditioning, longer recovery times, and delays in return to work and function.
- Later
  - Surgical indications include severe radicular pain unresponsive to a comprehensive nonoperative program (at least 6–12 weeks), spinal cord dysfunction/myelopathy (thoracic HNP), and progressive or profound motor deficit/cauda equina syndrome (lumbar HNP) that requires emergent surgical intervention.
  - Surgical procedures
    — HNP with radiculopathy: discectomy (removal of offending disc fragment); more than 90% success rate
    — Degenerative disc disease with axial low back pain: fusion, disc replacement; results inconsistent

When to Refer

- Patients with progressive or profound neurologic symptoms, signs of myelopathy, or HNP and pain (without neurologic findings) in whom a reasonable course of nonsurgical care fails
- The presence of any red flags requires more aggressive evaluation and emergent referral.

Prognosis

- Asymptomatic HNPs generally have a benign clinical course and can be managed nonoperatively. Recovery in a patient with symptomatic lumbar HNPs causing radiculopathy is approximately 50% in 1 month, with 75% recovery by 1 year. For low back pain, 50% to 60% of patients recover in 1 week and 95% recover in 3 months.
- Surgical success for HNP is enhanced if radicular pain is associated with positive tension signs and imaging studies correlate with the clinical picture.
  - Results in more rapid improvement of sciatica than nonsurgical care, but differences become less pronounced over time
  - Surgical results unaffected by period of observation

Troubleshooting

- Close, serial follow-up is essential.
- A comprehensive history and examination are critical to an accurate diagnosis.
- Consider referral if the diagnosis is uncertain.
- Acute soft-tissue injury (strain/sprain) usually improves over days to weeks.
- Degenerative changes with an acute flare-up (axial and/or radicular pain) may take weeks to months to resolve.

Patient Instructions

- Counsel patients on expectations with nonoperative treatment, when to return if failing to improve or worsening, and risks/benefits/anticipated outcomes of surgery.
- Patients with low back pain should be instructed to stay in shape, quit smoking (risk factor for disc degeneration), maintain their ideal weight, and learn proper techniquesof sitting, standing, lifting, and pushing/pulling.

Suggested Reading

- An HS, Singh K (eds): Synopsis of Spine Surgery, 2nd ed. New York: Thieme, 2007.
- Andersson GB: Epidemiological features of chronic low-back pain. Lancet 1999;354:581–585.
- Buttermann GR: Treatment of lumbar disc herniation: Epidural steroid injection compared with discectomy: A prospective, randomized controlled study. J Bone Joint Surg Am 2004; 86A:670–679.
- Grauer JN, Beiner JM, Albert TJ: Lumbar disc disease. In Vacarro AR (ed): Orthopaedic Knowledge Update 8: Home Study Syllabus. Rosemont, IL: American Academy of Orthopaedic Surgeons, 2005, pp 539–552.
- Grauer JN, Beiner JM, Albert TJ: Thoracic disc disease. In Vacarro AR (ed): Orthopaedic Knowledge Update 8: Home Study Syllabus. Rosemont, IL: American Academy of Orthopaedic Surgeons, 2005, pp 535–538.
- Haak M: History and physical examination. In Spivak J, Connolly P (eds): Orthopaedic Knowledge Update Spine 3. Rosemont, IL: American Academy of Orthopaedic Surgeons, 2006, pp 43–56.

- Rao R, Bagaria V: Pathophysiology of degenerative disk disease and related symptoms. In Spivak J, Connolly P (eds): Orthopaedic Knowledge Update Spine 3. Rosemont, IL: American Academy of Orthopaedic Surgeons, 2006, pp 35–42.
- Vanichkachorn JS, Vaccaro AR: Thoracic disk disease: Diagnosis and treatment. J Am Acad Orthop Surg 2000;8:159–169.
- Videman T, Battie MC, Gibbons LE, et al: Associations between back pain history and lumbar MRI findings. Spine 2003;28:582–588.

Chapter 119 Cauda Equina Syndrome

Clinton W. Howard and Rex Marco

ICD-9 CODE
344.6 *Cauda Equina Syndrome*

Key Concepts

- The spinal cord in adults usually terminates at L1.
- The continuing nerve roots are termed the cauda equina (horse's tail).
- The cauda equina is a connection between the central nervous system and the peripheral nervous system.
- Cauda equina syndrome is a spectrum of clinical findings that imply significant compression of the cauda equina nerve roots.
- Symptoms and signs include low back pain, unilateral or bilateral sciatica, lower extremity motor weakness, sensory disturbance in the saddle/perineal area, and loss of bowel/bladder/sexual function.
- Common etiologies include lumbar spinal stenosis, herniated nucleus pulposus, spinal trauma, neoplasm, infection, spina bifida, and tethered cord.
- Treatment is dependent on etiology.
- If not addressed, it can progress to permanent neurologic deficits.

History

- Etiology predicts the presentation of symptoms.
- If secondary to a chronic process (stenosis), gradual onset of symptoms; if secondary to acute process (herniated nucleus pulposus), acute onset of symptoms
- Symptoms are usually unilateral with severe radicular pain.
- Loss of bowel/bladder control and sexual function

Physical Examination

- Observation
  - Nonspecific
- Palpation
  - Sensation decreased, saddle anesthesia
- Range of motion
  - Muscle tone typically decreased; however, if injury is higher at the conus medullaris, may be spastic
- Special tests
  - Decreased muscle strength: Assess muscle function to determine the level of injury.
  - Decreased lower extremity reflexes
  - Bulbocavernosus usually absent or diminished; can help define completeness of injury
  - Anal sphincter tone usually diminished or absent

Imaging

- Radiographs: anteroposterior and lateral views of the lumbar and thoracolumbar spine
  - Evaluate for spondylosis (may suggest stenosis), spondylolisthesis, lytic or blastic lesions, fractures
  - Flexion-extension views; may demonstrate segmental instability and spondylolisthesis
- Magnetic resonance imaging with contrast is the test of choice; evaluates for intradural neoplasm, discogenic causes, and stenosis (Fig. 119-1)
- Computed tomography myelography can show intra- or extradural pathology.

Differential Diagnosis

- Amyotrophic lateral sclerosis: weakness, atrophy, fasciculations
- Diabetic neuropathy: numbness, impotence, dysesthesia, muscle weakness
- Human immunodeficiency virus myelopathy: urinary hesitancy, clumsiness
- Spinal cord infarction
  - Acute onset, often heralded by sudden and severe back pain that may radiate caudad
  - Associated with bilateral weakness, paresthesias, and sensory loss
  - Loss of sphincter control with hesitancy and inability to void or defecate becomes evident within a few hours.
- Syringomyelia: cyst in the central spinal cord can cause myelopathy and urinary incontinence

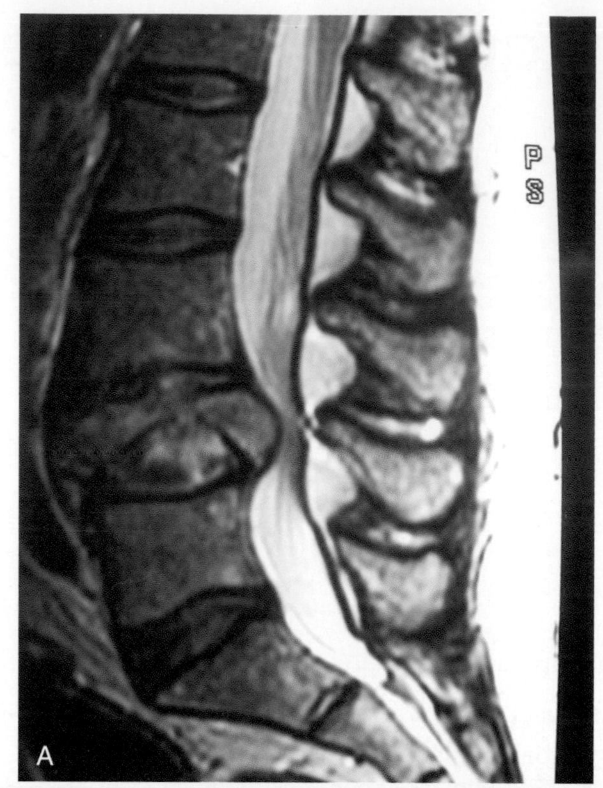

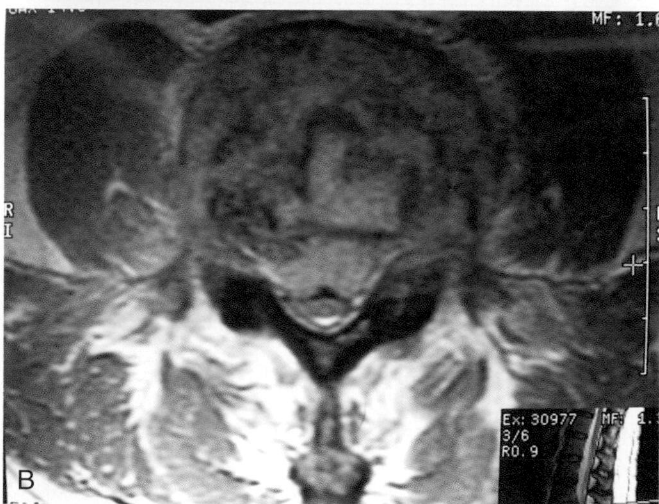

Figure 119-1 T2-weighted sagittal (**A**) and axial (**B**) magnetic resonance imaging of the lumbar spine showing anterior encroachment and compression on the cauda equina from metastatic breast cancer.

Treatment

- Based on etiology
  - Traumatic fracture: methylprednisolone, 30 mg/kg initial dose, then 5.4 mg/kg × 23 hours if symptom onset is less than 3 hours or continue 48 hours if onset is more than 3 hours and less than 8 hours
  - Surgical decompression of cauda equina
  - Herniated disc: discectomy
  - Neoplasm: If etiology is unknown, consider biopsy. Surgical decompression should be considered.
  - Stenosis: Consider corticosteroids. Consider laminectomy and decompression.

When to Refer

- Urgent referral should occur when symptoms of cauda equina syndrome are present.
- If not addressed in timely fashion, may result in permanent neurologic deficits
- Imaging helps in diagnosis and dictates treatment.

Prognosis

- Timing of decompression has significant effect on outcome.
- Those patients decompressed less than 24 hours from the onset of symptoms, compared with more than 24 hours, have increased return of bladder function.
- However, if there are circumstances in which decompression cannot be performed immediately, there is some benefit to decompression even 48 hours after symptom onset.

Patient Instructions

- Patients should seek medical assistance if they are having any symptoms consistent with cauda equina syndrome.

Suggested Reading

- Ahn UM, Ahn NU, Buchowksi MS, et al: Cauda equina syndrome secondary to lumbar disc herniation: A meta-analysis of surgical outcomes. Spine 2000;25:1515–1522.
- Dinning TAR, Schaeffer HR: Discogenic compression of the cauda equina: A surgical emergency. Aust N Z J Surg 1993;63:927–934.
- Gleave JR, Macfarlane R: Cauda equina syndrome: What is the relationship between timing of surgery and outcome? Br J Neurosurg 2002;16:325–328.
- Kennedy JG, Soffe KE, McGrath A, et al: Predictors of outcome in cauda equina syndrome. Eur Spine J 1999;8:317–322.
- Kostuik JP: Controversies in cauda equina syndrome and lumbar disk herniation. Curr Opin Orthopaed 1993;4:125–128.
- Kostuik JP, Harrington I, Alexander D, et al: Cauda equina syndrome and lumbar disc herniation. J Bone Joint Surg Am 1986;68A:386–391.
- O'Laoire SA, Crockard HA, Thomas DG: Prognosis for sphincter recovery after operation for cauda equina compression owing to lumbar disc prolapse. Br Med J 1981;282:1852–1854.

Chapter 120 Thoracolumbar Stenosis

Jeffrey C. Wang and Joseph S. Kim

ICD-9 CODES
724.01 *Spinal Stenosis, Thoracic Region*
724.02 *Spinal Stenosis, Lumbar Region*

LUMBAR STENOSIS

Key Concepts

- Spinal stenosis is narrowing of the spinal canal or neuroforamen resulting in compression of the lumbar thecal sac in central stenosis and/or spinal nerve roots in lateral stenosis.
  - Lateral stenosis is narrowing of the lateral recess of the canal and/or neuroforamen.
  - Central stenosis is narrowing of the central spinal canal.
- Classified as either congenital/developmental or acquired/degenerative
- The most common type is degenerative, with an incidence of 1.7% to 8%.
- Neural compression manifests as constellation of symptoms: low back pain, neurogenic claudication, and/or lower extremity radicular pain
- Symptoms typically develop during the fifth to sixth decades secondary to osteoarthritic changes in the lumbar spine, which lead to pathologic compression of the thecal sac and/or nerve roots (Figs. 120-1 and 120-2).

History

- Long history of low back pain with recent onset of referred pain to the buttocks and/or lower extremities
- Radicular leg pain in a strict dermatomal distribution is relatively uncommon, unless there is concomitant lateral stenosis or disc herniation compressing a specific nerve root.
- Neurogenic claudication (lower extremity pain, paresthesia, and/or weakness with walking/standing) is pathognomonic for lumbar spinal stenosis.
  - Usually bilateral, but not necessarily symmetrical
- Symptoms are rapidly relieved by sitting down or leaning forward, for example, holding onto a shopping cart when walking (shopping cart sign).
- Flexion of the lumbar spine increases the space available for the neural elements and decreases the degree of compression.
- Night pain is uncommon.

Physical Examination

- Despite severe symptoms, patients have few findings on physical examination.
- Observation
  - Characteristic forward stooped posture
  - Decreased lumbar lordosis
- Range of motion: deceased, especially extension
- Special tests
  - Complete neurologic examination, usually normal, despite subjective reports of weakness and paresthesia
    - — When motor weakness is present, it is mild and typically affects the L5 and S1 nerve roots.
    - — Focal deficits more common with lateral stenosis
    - — Deep tendon reflexes may be diminished.
  - Pathologic upper motor neuron reflexes (Babinski's sign, clonus) are uncommon in lumbar stenosis.
    - — Their presence warrants an evaluation for concurrent cervical or thoracic stenosis with cord compression.
  - Nerve tension signs (straight leg raise) usually negative, even in patients with radicular pain

Imaging

- Imaging studies used to confirm the clinical diagnosis and plan operative treatment, if indicated
- Radiographs
  - Upright anteroposterior, lateral, flexion/extension views
  - Obtained in patients having symptoms for less than 6 weeks to exclude pathologic conditions such as tumor, infection, and fracture

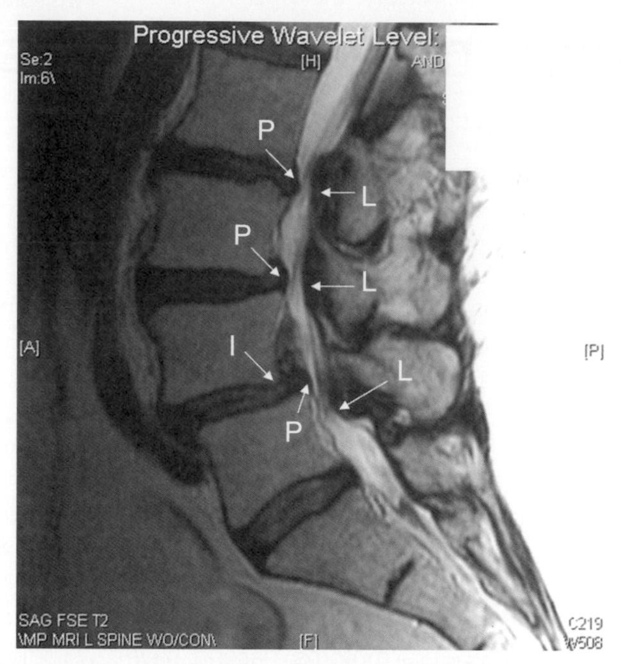

Figure 120-1 Sagittal T2-weighted magnetic resonance image of an elderly patient with three-level degenerative lumbar stenosis at L2–3, L3–4, and L4–5, as well as degenerative spondylolisthesis (I) at L4–5. Disc protrusions (P) and thickened ligamentum flavum infolding (L) contribute to marked narrowing of the thecal sac.

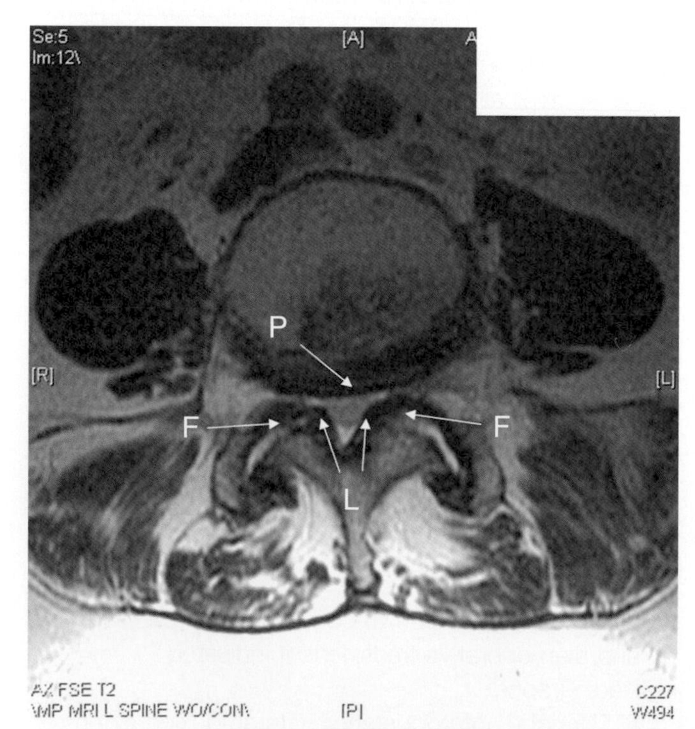

Figure 120-2 Axial T2-weighted magnetic resonance image of the same patient at the level of L4–5. Significant compression of the thecal sac occurs secondary to disc protrusion (P), hypertrophic deformity of the osteoarthritic facet joints (F), and thickened ligamentum flavum infolding (L).

- Dynamic flexion and extension radiographs needed to identify associated instability (e.g., spondylolisthesis)
- Degenerative changes such as intervertebral disc space narrowing, facet osteoarthrosis, osteophyte formation, and endplate sclerosis are ubiquitous in the adult population and are not diagnostic.

- Magnetic resonance imaging
  - Also a confirmatory, not diagnostic, modality; 21% of asymptomatic individuals aged 60 to 80 years have evidence of lumbar stenosis on magnetic resonance imaging
  - Indications include severe symptoms, neurologic deficits, failure of conservative measures, and surgical planning.
- Computed tomography–myelography
  - Useful in patients with contraindications to magnetic resonance imaging (e.g., pacemaker, aneurysm clip, severe claustrophobia)

Additional Tests

- Electrodiagnostic studies are rarely useful.
- Approximately 80% of patients with lumbar stenosis have positive findings of radiculopathy. The presence of these findings supports the diagnosis, but their absence does not rule it out.

Differential Diagnosis

- Peripheral vascular disease: vascular claudication, leg pain not relieved by leaning forward
- Hip/knee osteoarthritis: decreased/painful range of motion
- Peripheral neuropathy: dysesthesias in stocking/glove distribution

Treatment

- At diagnosis
  - Start with a brief period of rest to avoid painful activities, short-term use of a lumbar corset, acetaminophen/nonsteroidal anti-inflammatory drugs, and judicious use of mild narcotics.
  - Follow with a course of physical therapy to promote core muscle strengthening, conditioning, weight loss, and flexibility.
- Later
  - Lumbar epidural steroid injections are reserved for patients in whom medical treatments and physical therapy fail.

- Injections are generally more effective for radicular leg pain than for low back pain.

When to Refer

- Patients with persistent symptoms despite a course of conservative measures for 6 to 12 weeks or objective neurologic deficits (relatively uncommon) should be referred to a spine surgeon.
  - Surgical options include lumbar decompression with or without fusion, depending on the presence or absence of lumbar instability.
- Unless there is progressive neurologic deficit or bowel/bladder dysfunction, the decision for surgical intervention is left to the patient.
- Delayed surgery does not seem to worsen surgical outcomes.

Prognosis

- Fifty percent of patients improve with conservative measures, 20% have no change in their level of symptoms, and 30% have progressive worsening and require surgical treatment.
- Surgical outcomes are generally favorable for patients with severe to moderate symptoms with relatively low rates of complications.

Patient Instructions

- Initial treatment is conservative with nonsteroidal anti-inflammatory drugs, physical therapy, and injections.
- Surgical treatment is generally considered once these conservative measures have failed.
- The ultimate decision for surgical intervention and its timing are entirely up to the patient and guided by the level of symptoms.

THORACIC STENOSIS

Key Concepts

- Less common than stenosis of the cervical or lumbar spine
- Usually results from acquired degenerative changes in the setting of a congenitally narrowed thoracic canal
- The lower thoracic spine is most frequently affected.
- Because the spinal cord ends at L1 or L2, thoracic stenosis can compress both the spinal cord and its accompanying nerve roots.
- Clinical presentation is highly variable with a wide spectrum of neurologic dysfunction
- Patients may report axial back pain with radiating pain to the chest wall, sensory abnormalities, and/or weakness of the lower extremities.
- Pathologic upper motor neuron reflexes and hyperreflexia may be present in the setting of significant cord compression.
- Concomitant symptoms and signs of cervical or lumbar stenosis are commonly present and complicate the clinical presentation.
- Advanced imaging is critical to the diagnosis. Magnetic resonance imaging and computed tomography–myelography are both effective modalities for assessing neural element compression.
- Conservative treatment with short-term bracing, pharmacologic measures, and physical therapy is reasonable in the absence of myelopathy or major neurologic deficits.
- Surgical decompression is indicated when there is debilitating neurologic dysfunction and/or myelopathy.

Suggested Reading

- Amundsen T, Weber H, Nordal NJ, et al: Lumbar spinal stenosis: Conservative or surgical management? A prospective 10 year study. Spine 2000;25:1424–1436.
- Palumbo MA, Hilibrand AS, Hart R, et al: Surgical treatment of thoracic spinal stenosis: Two to nine year follow-up. Spine 2001;26:558–566.
- Sengupta D, Herkowitz HN: Lumbar spinal stenosis treatment strategies and indications for surgery. Orthop Clin North Am 2003;34:281–295.
- Spivak JM: Degenerative lumbar spinal stenosis: Current concepts review. J Bone Joint Surg Am 1998;80A:1053–1066.
- Weinstein JN, Lurie JD, Tosteson TD, et al: Surgical versus nonsurgical treatment for lumbar degenerative spondylolisthesis. N Engl J Med 2007;356:2257–2270.

Chapter 121 Spondylolysis and Spondylolisthesis

Christopher J. DeWald

ICD-9 CODES
756.12 *Spondylolisthesis*
756.13 *Congenital Spondylolisthesis*
738.4 *Degenerative Spondylolisthesis*

Key Concepts

Spondylolysis

- Stress fracture of the posterior elements of the spine through the pars interarticularis (junction between superior/inferior facets) (Fig. 121-1)
- Inferior facet of cranial vertebrae repetitively impacts the adjacent vertebrae at the pars interarticularis.
- Stress fracture most commonly occurs during adolescence.
- Genetic factors (6% prevalence in white males versus 1% in African-American females) and environmental factors (e.g., gymnastics, football, soccer) play a role.

Spondylolisthesis

- Slippage of one vertebra on another, graded by percentage of slippage: I, less than 25%; II, 25% to 50%; III, 50% to 75%; IV, 75% to 100%; V, more than 100%
- Lytic spondylolisthesis occurs most commonly in the lower lumbar spine (85% at L5 and 10% at L4).
- Classic classification of Wiltse (Box 121-1) and functional classification of Marchetti and Bartolozzi (Box 121-2)
- Pediatric: risk of severe progression in high dysplastic developmental types
- Adolescent to young adult: continuum of spondylolysis to low-grade isthmic/lytic spondylolisthesis resulting from progressive disc degeneration at the spondylolytic level (L5-S1 most common)
- Older adult: degenerative spondylolisthesis developing from disc degeneration without previous spondylolysis resulting in spinal stenosis with neurogenic claudication (L4-L5 most common)

History

- Patients with either spondylolysis or spondylolisthesis may be asymptomatic or have mild to moderate low back pain.
- Spondylolysis typically occurs during adolescence and is the most common identifiable cause of back pain in children.
- The most common presenting symptom in lytic spondylolisthesis is the development of unilateral leg (radicular) pain at the level of the lysis or stenosis.
- Degenerative spondylolisthesis results in neurogenic claudication in older patients (older than 50 years); pain or heaviness in legs with standing/walking, improved with bending/sitting

Physical Examination

- Observation
  - Typically normal
  - Phalen-Dickson gait and posture in children with progressive high-grade spondylolisthesis and radicular pain (Fig. 121-2)
  - Accentuated lumbar lordosis in high-grade spondylolisthesis
  - Prominence of the spinous process of the lytic lamina in the lower lumbar spine
- Palpation
  - Typically nontender
  - Step-off of the lytic vertebra's spinous process to the cephalad spinous process
- Range of motion
  - Normal in most cases
  - Extension limited due to pain in adolescents with spondylolysis
  - Tight hamstring muscles noted in adolescents with spondylolisthesis
  - Extension significantly limited in adults with degenerative spondylolisthesis

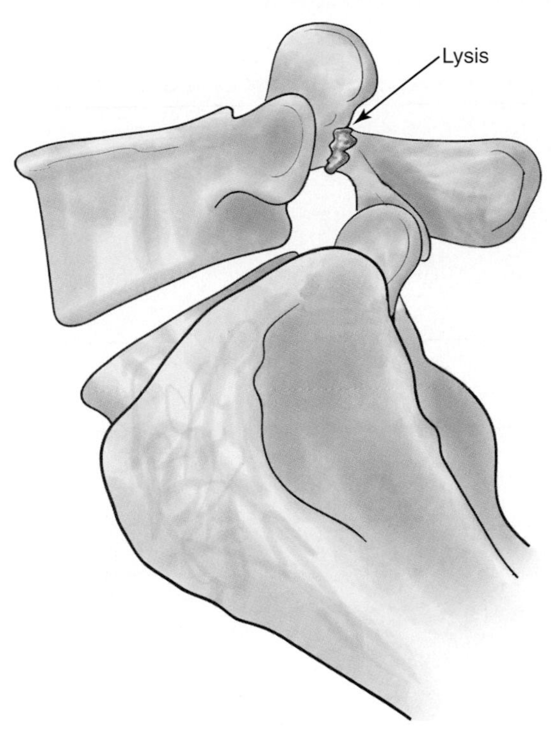

Figure 121-1 Diagram of vertebral body with lysis of the pars interarticularis.

BOX 121-1 *Wiltse Classification*

Dysplastic: congenital abnormalities of the upper sacrum or the arch of L5 permitting slippage to occur
Isthmic: defect in the pars interarticularis
  Lytic: fatigue fracture of the pars
  Elongated but intact pars
  Acute fracture
Degenerative: long-standing intersegmental instability
Traumatic: fractures in areas of the bony hook other than the pars
Pathologic: destruction of the posterior elements from generalized or localized bone pathology

BOX 121-2 *Marchetti-Bartolozzi Classification*

Developmental
High dysplastic with lysis or elongation
Low dysplastic with lysis or elongation

Acquired
Traumatic, due to acute or stress fracture
Postsurgical, caused by direct or indirect surgery
Pathologic, due to local or systemic pathology
Degenerative, found in primary or secondary degenerative conditions

- Special tests
  - Neurologic examination
    — Typically normal
    — Achilles reflexes may be diminished, and, rarely, decreased motor strength can occur in degenerative spondylolisthesis with long-standing severe stenosis.

Imaging

- Radiographs
  - Supine anteroposterior, lateral, and oblique lumbosacral views
    — To evaluate for the presence of spondylolysis (Fig. 121-3) and/or spondylolisthesis (Figs. 121-4 and 121-5).
    — To determine the degree of bony dysplasia (trapezoidal L5, rounded sacral endplate, spina bifida of posterior elements, sacral verticalization, elongated pars)
  - Standing lateral lumbosacral view
    — Required to determine grade of spondylolisthesis
    — Measures the true severity and instability (compared with supine view) of slippage in known spondylolisthesis
- Computed tomography
  - Best study (sagittal reconstruction) to confirm presence of spondylolysis (see Fig. 121-3) and determine presence or absence of healing
  - Not necessary in most cases of spondylolisthesis because slip is evident on plain radiographs
  - May assist in defining bony details of dysplastic spondylolisthesis
- Bone scan
  - Solely used to determine acuity in adolescent spondylolysis; "hot" scan suggests acute fracture or stress reaction
  - Single-photon emission computed tomography images are required to determine the location of uptake at the pars (see Fig. 121-3).
  - A "cold" scan does not rule out the presence of a spondylolysis.
- Magnetic resonance imaging
  - Not particularly helpful in the diagnosis or treatment of spondylolysis; best method to rule out other etiologies of back pain in adolescents (e.g., disc herniation)
  - Best additional study for spondylolisthesis, particularly with developmental high-grade types
  - Determines severity of spinal stenosis in degenerative spondylolisthesis (see Fig. 121-5)

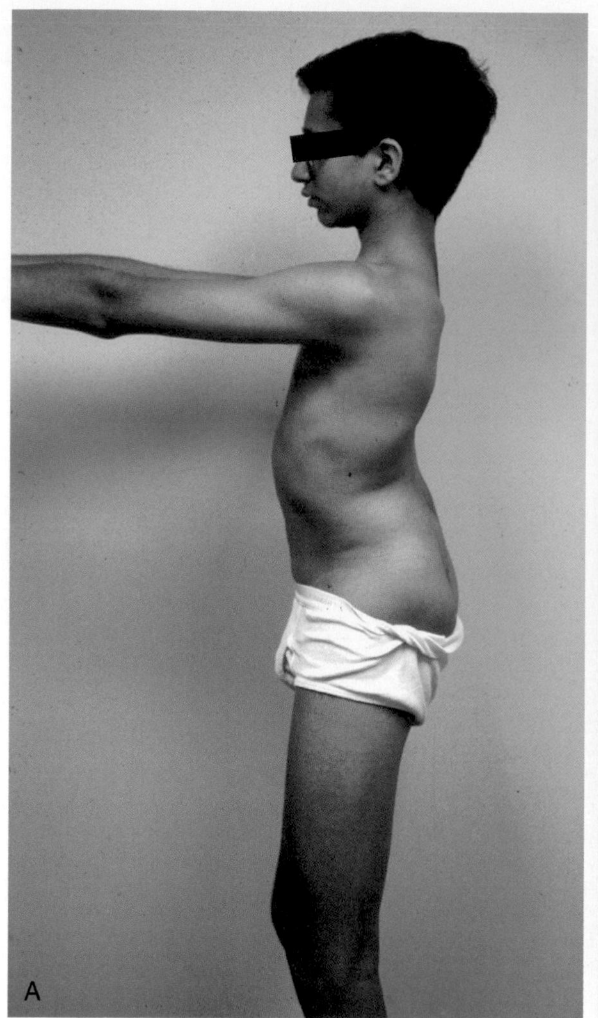

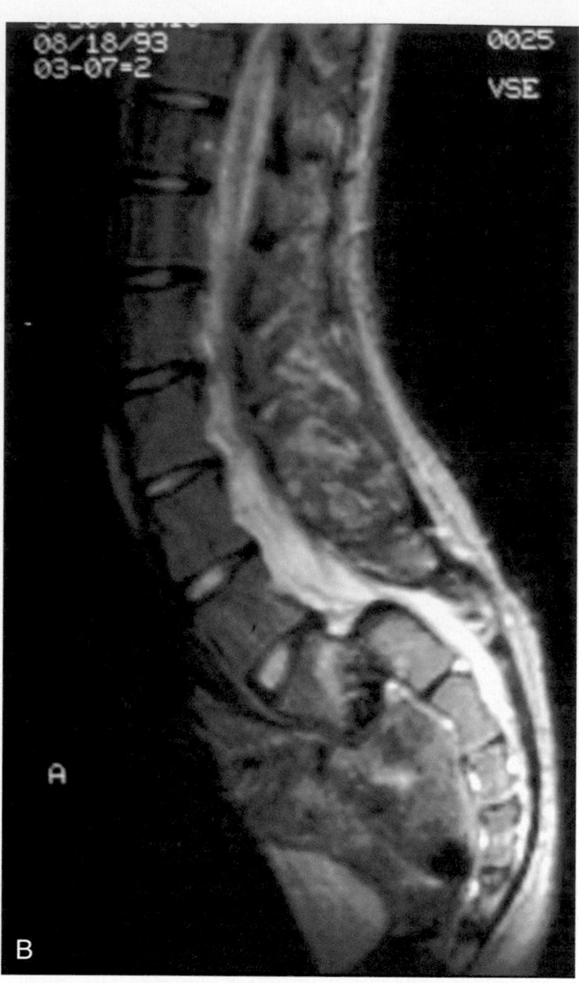

Figure 121-2 **A**, Phalen-Dixon sign in an adolescent with high-grade spondylolisthesis. **B**, Magnetic resonance image of developmental high-grade spondylolisthesis.

Differential Diagnosis

- Disc herniation
- Bony tumor: osteoid osteoma
- Infection: discitis, osteomyelitis
- Mechanical back pain
- Low back strain

Treatment

Spondylolysis

- At diagnosis
  - Treatment is based on symptoms.
  - Stop the specific activity or sport, start nonsteroidal anti-inflammatory drugs if needed, and consider physical therapy.
  - If the patient significantly symptomatic or a bone scan reveals uptake (hot) at the pars, a hypolordotic lumbosacral orthosis is used for 3 months.
- Later
  - If pain persists, surgical options include L5-S1 posterior spinal fusion (younger patients) and repair of the pars (adolescents, midlumbar lysis).

When to Refer

- Significant back pain lasting more than 1 to 2 weeks should be referred for further evaluation.
- Referral is not necessary for asymptomatic patients with radiographic spondylolysis, without listhesis/slippage.

Prognosis

- Good
  - The majority of patients respond well to bracing, whether or not the spondylolysis heals.
  - If pain resolves, patients may return to sports. The results of surgical intervention are also successful if patients do not improve with activity modification, bracing, and physical therapy.

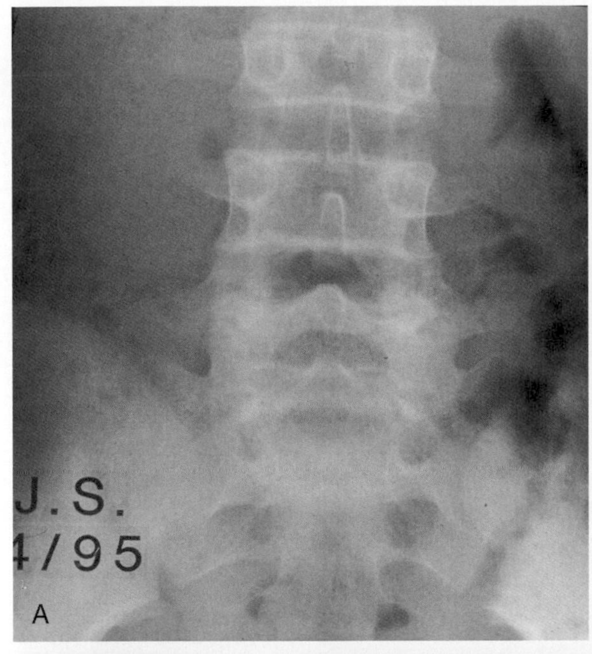

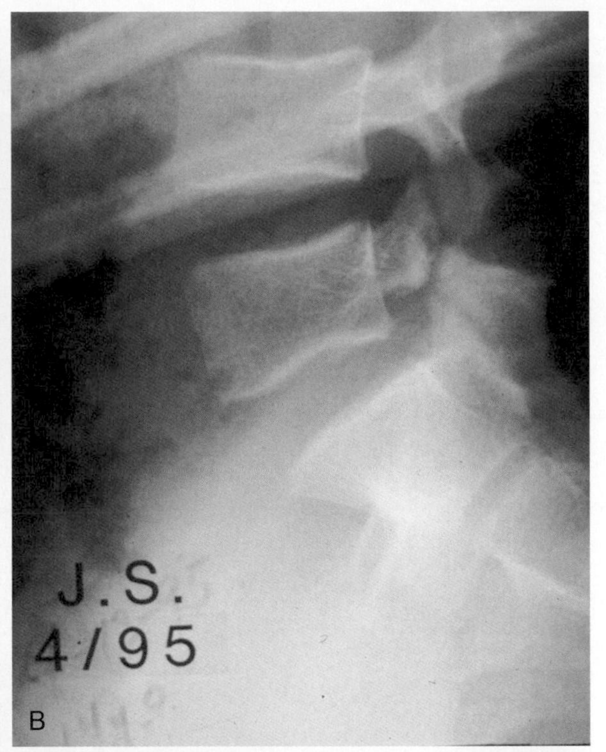

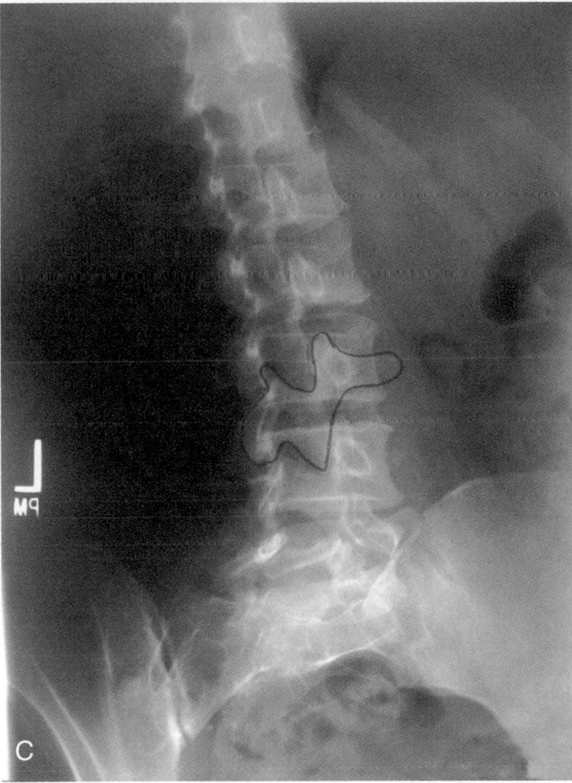

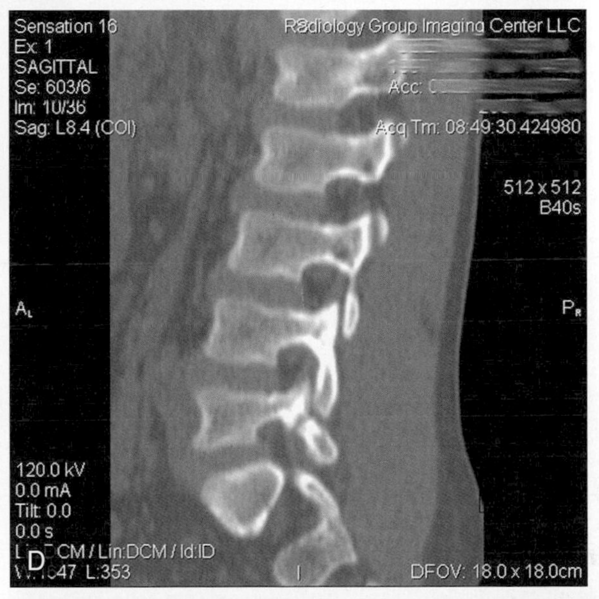

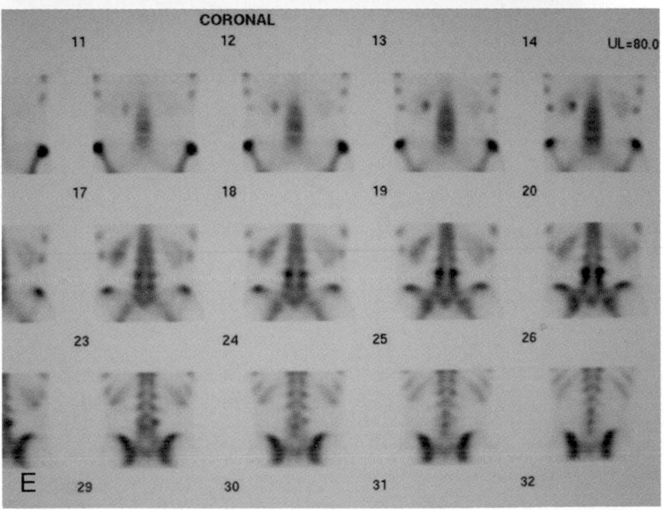

Figure 121-3 L5 spondylolysis. Anteroposterior (**A**), lateral (**B**), and oblique (**C**) radiographs. Note the lysis just inferior to the pedicle of L5 at the "neck of the Scotty dog." **D**, Sagittal computed tomography clearly demonstrates the lysis. **E**, Single-photon emission computed tomography images showing uptake at the pars interarticularis bilaterally at L5.

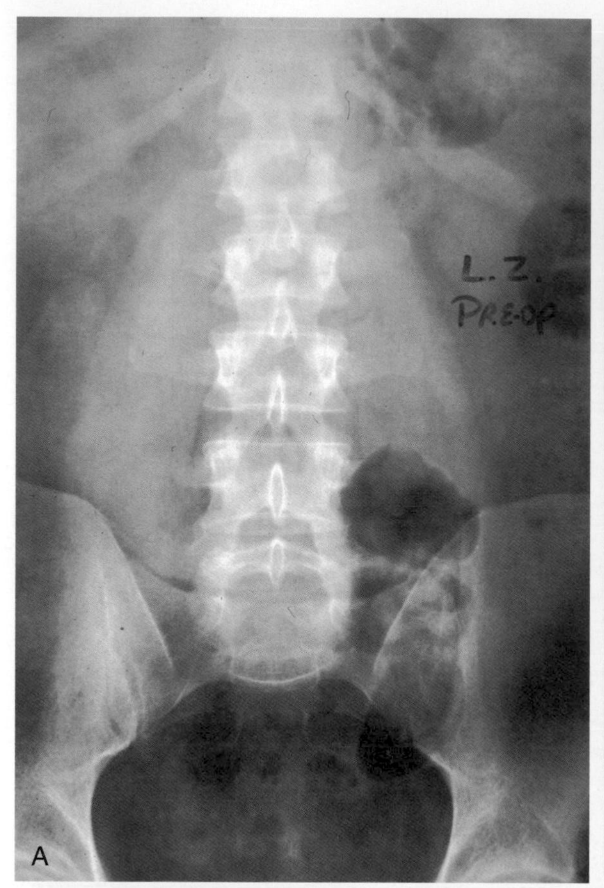

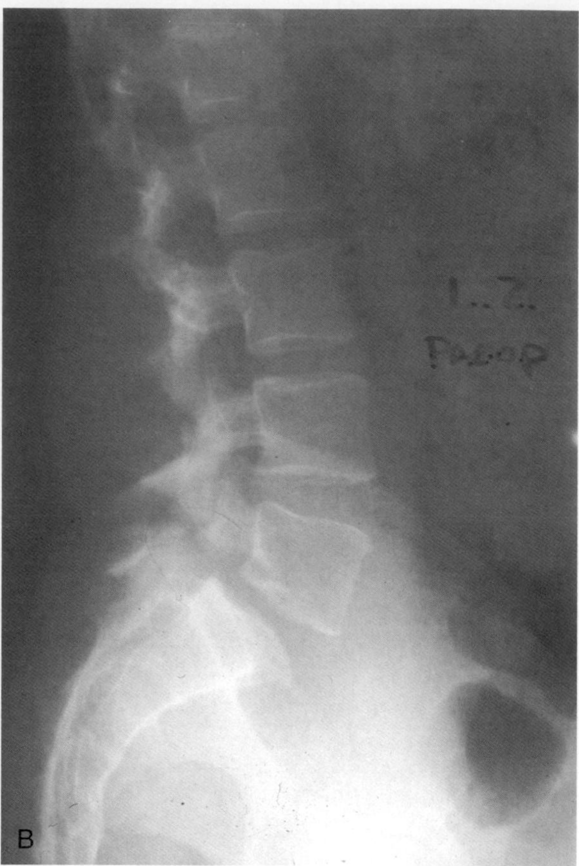

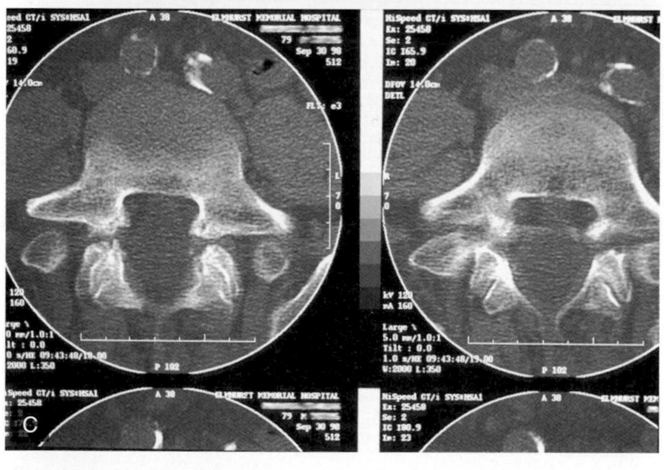

Figure 121-4 L5-S1 spondylolytic spondylolisthesis. Anteroposterior (**A**) and lateral (**B**) radiographs. Note the lack of dysplasia involving the L5 and S1 vertebrae. **C**, Axial computed tomography. Note the absence of central spinal stenosis due to separation of the lamina from the vertebral body.

Spondylolisthesis

- At diagnosis
  - Treatment is dependent on age and severity of the slip.
  - Nonoperative treatment includes nonsteroidal anti-inflammatory drugs, physical therapy, and consideration of bracing in the adolescent patient.
- Later
  - In adult patients, selective nerve blocks or epidural injections can be used in those with spondylolytic or degenerative spondylolisthesis, respectively.
  - Surgical treatment for patients in whom conservative management fails includes posterior spinal fusion with instrumentation in adolescent and adult patients (Fig. 121-6) and without instrumentation in pediatric patients.
  - Pediatric developmental high-grade spondylolisthesis (high risk of progression) requires surgical stabilization even in the absence of symptoms.

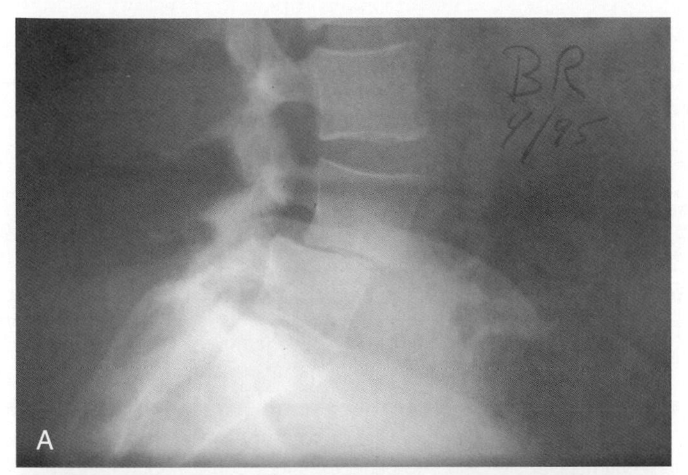

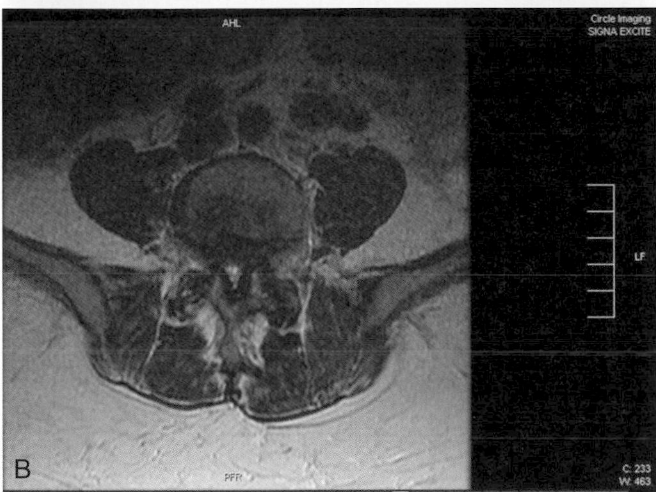

Figure 121-5 Degenerative spondylolisthesis. **A**, Lateral radiograph depicting the severity of slippage. **B**, Magnetic resonance imaging revealing the severity of the associated stenosis. Compare this with the lack of stenosis typically found in lytic spondylolisthesis as shown in Figure 121-4. Note the facet hypertrophy and anterior subluxation of the inferior facets resulting in the spinal stenosis.

When to Refer

- Refer patients younger than age 12 with spondylolisthesis, radiographic evidence of bony dysplasia, or higher-grade slips (grade 2 or higher).
- Adult and adolescent patients not responding to nonoperative treatment should also be referred for surgical discussion.

Prognosis

- In general, the prognosis for surgical treatment of spondylolisthesis for both adult and pediatric patients is good.
- The results of decompression and single-level posterior spinal fusion for degenerative spondylolisthesis are particularly successful.

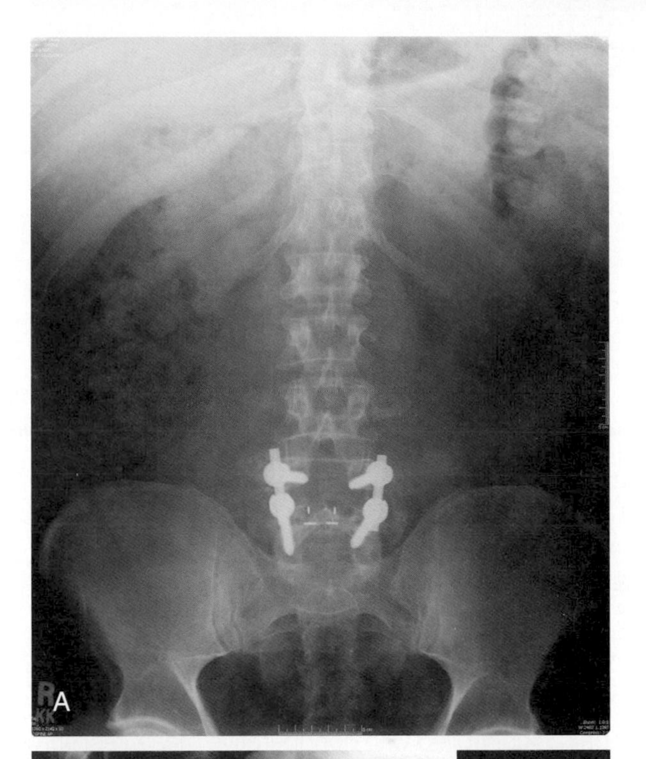

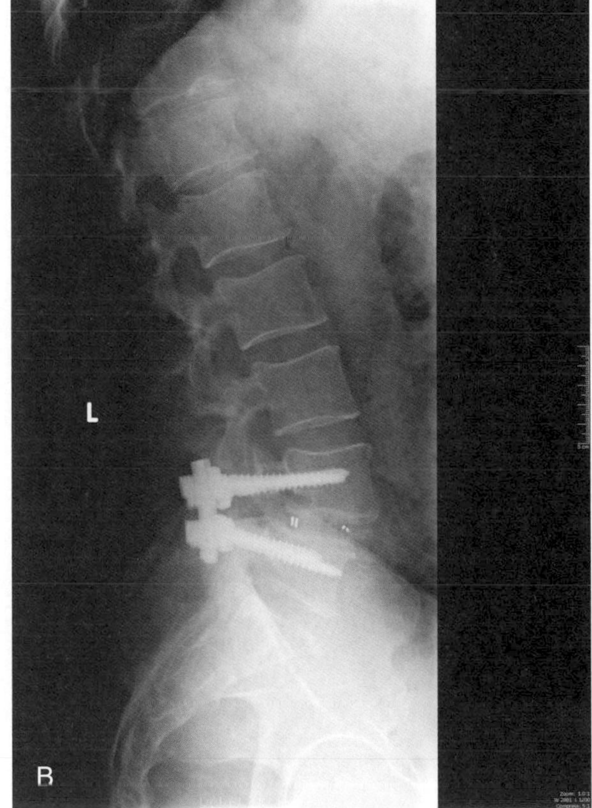

Figure 121-6 Posterior spinal fusion and instrumentation of an adult with spondylolytic spondylolisthesis at L4-5. Anteroposterior (**A**) and lateral (**B**) radiographs.

Troubleshooting

- Back pain in adolescents is unusual. If pain is significant or persistent, further workup is warranted.
- Often a change or cessation of a specific sport or activity will be sufficient to decrease pain and avoid surgery.
- When significant low back or radicular pain is continual, the benefits of surgical intervention become clear.
- Surgical risks include blood loss, infection, nerve root injury, pseudarthrosis, revision surgery, instrumentation failure (typically due to pseudarthrosis), and adjacent disc degeneration.

Patient Instructions

- Except for developmental highly dysplastic spondylolisthesis, patients with spondylolysis or spondylolisthesis can be treated based on symptoms. If the patient's pain is controlled with nonoperative measures, surgery can be avoided.

Suggested Reading

- Beutler WJ, Fredrickson BE, Murtland A, et al: The natural history of spondylolysis and spondylolisthesis: 45-year follow-up evaluation. Spine 2003;28:1027–1035.
- Carragee EJ: Single-level posterolateral arthrodesis, with or without posterior decompression, for the treatment of isthmic spondylolisthesis in adults. A prospective, randomized study. J Bone Joint Surg Am 1997;79A:1175–1180.
- Deguchi M, Rapoff AJ, Zdeblick TA: Posterolateral fusion for isthmic spondylolisthesis in adults: Analysis of fusion rate and clinical results. J Spinal Disord 1998;11:459–464.
- Fischgrund JS, Mackay M, Herkowitz HN, et al: Degenerative lumbar spondylolisthesis with spinal stenosis: A prospective randomized study comparing decompressive laminectomy and arthrodesis with and without spinal instrumentation. Spine 1997;22:2807–2812.
- Hammerberg KW: Spondylolysis and spondylolisthesis. In DeWald RL (ed): Spinal Deformities. The Comprehensive Text. New York: Thieme, 2003, pp 787–808.
- Herkowitz HN, Kurz LT: Degenerative lumbar spondylolisthesis with spinal stenosis. A prospective study comparing decompression and intertransverse process arthrodesis. J Bone Joint Surg Am 1991;73A:802–808.
- Hu SS, Tribus CB, Diab M, et al: Spondylolisthesis and spondylolysis: An instructional course lecture. American Academy of Orthopedic Surgeons. J Bone Joint Surg Am 2008;90A: 656–671.
- Molinari RW, Bridwell KH, Lenke LG, et al: Complications in the surgical treatment of pediatric high-grade isthmic dysplastic spondylolisthesis. A comparison of three surgical techniques. Spine 1999;24:1701–1711.
- Moller H, Hedlund R: Instrumented and noninstrumented posterolateral fusion in adult spondylolisthesis. A prospective randomized study: Part 2. Spine 2000;25:1716–1721.
- Sys J, Michielsen J, Bracke P, et al: Nonoperative treatment of active spondylolysis in elite athletes with normal X-ray findings: Literature review and review and results of conservative treatment. Eur Spine J 2001;10:498–504.

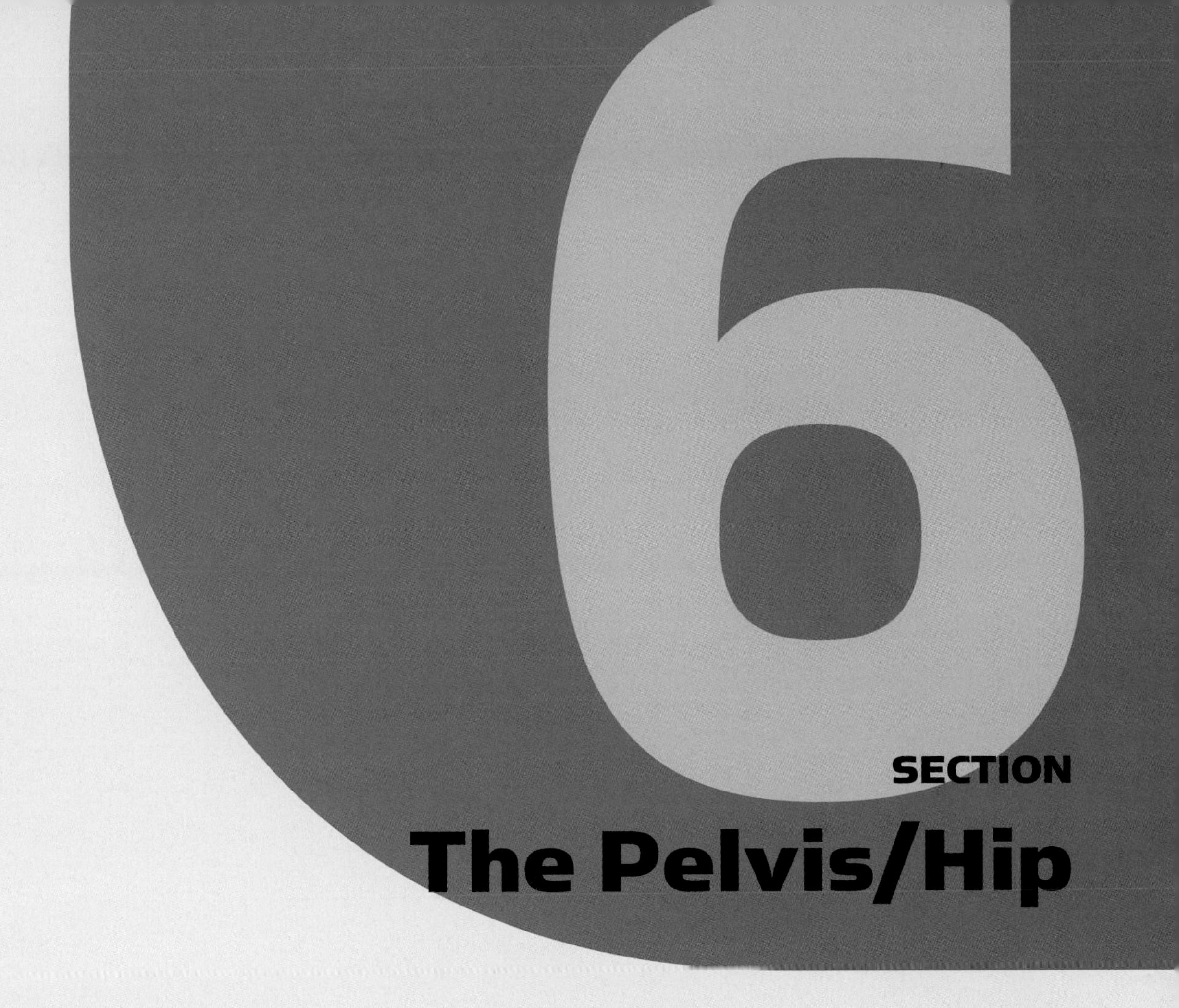

SECTION

6 The Pelvis/Hip

Chapter 122 Hip and Pelvis Overview

Paul Gubanich

Key Concepts

- The hip and pelvis serve many roles including the attachment site for the appendicular and axial skeleton, protector of vital internal organs, and structural support for locomotion.
- The hip and pelvis are commonly injured sites and account for approximately 5% to 24% of activity-related injuries in adults and children, respectively.
- The hip and pelvic areas are also often involved in referred pain from the lumbar spine and knee.
- The hip joint is a major weight-bearing joint (up to 3–5 times body weight with activity) and subject to both acute traumatic as well as chronic degenerative injury from repetitive loading.
- A thorough history, physical examination, and a good working knowledge of the anatomy of this region are essential for proficient diagnosis.
- Further evaluation such as the use of plain film radiographs, magnetic resonance imaging, and bone scan can be helpful to confirm the diagnosis.

Bones and Landmarks

- Coccyx (tailbone): Attached to the distal end of the sacrum, it consists of approximately three to five fused vertebrae. The coccyx is slightly concave ventrally and provides support to the rectum and pelvic floor but no significant structural support to the pelvis.
- Femur: The longest and strongest bone in the body, it is solely responsible for the distribution of body weight to the lower extremity.
  - Head: The spherical ball of the femur, the head articulates with the acetabulum and is lined with hyaline cartilage. In adults, the femoral neck is maintained in approximately 15 degrees of anteversion in relation to the axis of the knee.
  - Fovea capitis: A depression in the femoral head, it serves as the site of attachment for the ligament to the head of the femur.
  - Greater trochanter: Lateral prominence of the femur that serves as the site of attachment for a number of hip and pelvic muscles; it is also the most common site of bursitis of the hip
  - Lesser trochanter: Bony prominence located at the superomedial aspect of the femur, it is the site of insertion of the psoas major muscle.
  - Neck: The weakest portion of the femur, it connects the femoral head to the shaft. It is a common site for injury or fracture. The neck projects at an angle of approximately 120 degrees with the shaft and 15 degrees of anteversion.
- Ilium: One of the three bones (along with the ischium and pubis) that fuse to form the innominate.
- Innominate: The major bony structure of the pelvis; two innominate bones make up the ring-shaped pelvis. The ilium forms the most superior portion of the pelvis and consists of the body and large wing (ala).
- Anterior inferior iliac spine: Located inferior to the origin of the sartorius, it forms the upper rim of the acetabulum and is the site of attachment of the rectus femoris and iliofemoral ligament.
- Anterior superior iliac spine: Anterior margin of the iliac crest, this serves as the site of attachment for the iliacus, sartorius, and tensor fasciae latae muscles and inguinal ligament
- Arcuate line: Anatomic boundary between the true and false pelvis
- Greater sciatic notch: Located inferior to the posterosuperior iliac spine, the greater sciatic notch is a site of passage for many important structures from the pelvis including the piriformis, sciatic nerve, posterior femoral cutaneous nerve, pudendal nerve and vessels, and superior and inferior gluteal nerve and vessels. The notch is divided into the greater sciatic foramen and lesser sciatic foramen by the sacrospinous ligament.
- Iliac crest: The superior, lateral prominence of the wing (ala) of the ilium
- Iliac tuberosity: Posterior prominence of the iliac bone, it serves as the site of attachment for the sacroiliac ligament and the lower back muscles (erector spinae and multifidus).

- Posterior inferior iliac spine: Forms the superior boundary of the greater sciatic notch
- Posterosuperior iliac spine: The posterior margin of the iliac crest, it serves as a site of attachment for the sacrotuberous and sacroiliac ligaments.
- Ischium: One of the three bones (along with the ilium and pubis) that fuse to form the innominate. The ischium consists of a body and two rami and forms the posteroinferior portion of the pelvis.
  - Ischial ramus (inferior): The inferior margin of the obturator foramen, it serves as the anterior attachment to the pubic bone.
  - Ischial spine: Site of attachment for the sacrospinous ligament
  - Ischial tuberosity: The strongest part of the hip bone, this thickened area of the ischium is the major weight-bearing structure during sitting. It serves as the site of attachment of many muscles.
- Lesser sciatic notch: The obturator internus muscle and nerve and the pudendal vessels and nerve transgress the pelvis through this opening.
- Superior ramus: A posterior projection from the body, it contains the ischial tuberosity and serves as the site of attachment for the sacrotuberous ligament and the adductor magnus, biceps femoris (long), semimembranosus, and semitendinosus muscles.
- Pubis: One of the three bones (along with the ilium and ischium) that fuse to form the innominate. The pubis forms the anterior portion of the hip bone and consists of a body and two rami.
  - Inferior pubic ramus: It projects inferiorly from the superior ramus and forms part of the obturator foramen (along with the ilium) and also serves as a common site of attachment for several muscles including the adductor brevis and magnus, gracilis, and obturator internus and externus muscles.
  - Pubic tubercle: The medial prominence of the pubic bone, it serves as the site of attachment for the inguinal ligament.
- Superior pubic ramus: It forms part of the pubic symphysis and serves as a common site of muscle insertion for the adductor brevis and longus, gracilis, obturator internus and externus, and pectineus muscles.
- Shared structures
  - Acetabulum: It is a deep depression in the bony structure formed from the coalescence of the three pelvic bones (ilium, ischium, and pubis), is lined by hyaline cartilage, and articulates with the femoral head. A bony ridge deepens the cup superiorly while the labrum circumferentially provides stability and shock absorption.
  - Obturator foramen: Formed by the rami and body of the ischium and pubic bones, it is covered by the obturator membrane through which the obturator nerve and vessels exit the pelvis.
- Sacrum: Formed from the fusion of the five sacral vertebrae, the sacrum is a large triangle-shaped bone that forms the central posterior aspect of the pelvis ring.
  - Sacral promontory: This is the convex anterior prominence of the sacrum that forms the posterior margin of the pelvic inlet.
  - Anterior and posterior sacral foramina: These are four paired openings that allow transmission of the branches of the sacral plexus (anterior and posterior) and lateral sacral arteries (anterior).

Joints and Ligaments

- Hip joint (acetabulofemoral): The primary joint of the hip and pelvis, this ball-and-socket joint is composed of the femur and acetabulum. While still allowing multiaxial movement, the hip does not display as large a range of motion as the shoulder due to its increased inherent stability. Ligamentous and muscle constraints from the surrounding structures also add to both the static and dynamic stability. Dislocation of the hip joint is rare except in cases of severe trauma such as motor vehicle accidents. The complex relationship between the acetabulum, femoral neck, and femoral head determine force transmission through the hip to the lower extremities.
  - Acetabulum: The bony ridge located superiorly, depth of the acetabular cup, degree of acetabular anteversion, and degree of femoral head coverage all contribute to joint stability.
  - Femoral head: The size, shape, and angle affect joint mechanics and force transmission.
  - Joint capsule: It surrounds the acetabular rim to the femoral neck; its main components include the iliofemoral ligament. This strong V-shaped ligament provides anterior support to the joint capsule from the inferior border of the ilium (anterosuperior iliac spine and acetabular rim). It is the primary restraint in hip extension.
    - — Ischiofemoral ligament: Provides posterior support to the capsule from the ischium; it is the primary restraint in hip internal rotation
    - — Ligamentum orbicularis: Circumferential ligament that surrounds the hip capsule and reinforces other structures

    - Pubofemoral ligament: Provides inferior support to the capsule from the pubic bone and is the primary restraint in hip abduction
  - Acetabular labrum: Ring of fibrocartilage that deepens the cavity and helps to distribute stress
  - Ligament of the head of femur: Attaches the femoral head to the acetabulum; may play a role in stability in external rotation; also carries some of the arterial supply to the femoral head
  - Transverse acetabular ligament: Connects the ends of the acetabular notch and provides inferior reinforcement of the labrum and hip joint
- Pubic symphysis: The cartilaginous joint between the two superior rami of the pubic bones; a fibrocartilage disc also lines the joint.
  - Pubic ligaments (anterior, inferior, posterior, superior): Stabilize the pubic bones; the inferior ligament is the largest structure stabilizing the pubic arch
- Sacroiliac joint: Articulation between the lateral sacral wings and the ilium; both surfaces are lined with articular cartilage; motion at the sacroiliac joint is limited in all planes due to the joint's extensive ligamentous attachments
- Sacroiliac ligament (anterior, posterior): Attaches the anterior lateral sacrum to the ilium (anterior) as well as the posterior sacrum; these ligaments are responsible for the rotational and vertical stability of the pelvis; the posterior bands are the stronger and thicker of the two
  - Interosseous sacroiliac ligament: This lies deep to the posterior sacroiliac ligament and contributes to pelvic stability.
  - Sacrospinous ligament: Attaches the sacrum to the ischial spine ventrally; this ligament contributes to rotational stability and provides the boundary for the greater and lesser sciatic notches
  - Sacrotuberous ligament: Large ligament that attaches the sacrum to the ischial tuberosity; this ligament is a major pelvic stabilizer contributing to vertical stability and also forms the inferior border of the lesser sciatic notch
- Sacrococcygeal symphysis: This articulation between the apex of the sacrum and base of the coccyx allows little movement and also contains a small fibrocartilage disc.
  - Sacrococcygeal ligaments (anterior, posterior, lateral): Provide stability to the sacrococcygeal joint
- Lumbosacral joint: Articulation between the fifth lumbar vertebra and disc and the first sacral vertebra
  - Anterior longitudinal ligament: Strong band of connective tissue that stabilizes the spine from the axis to the sacrum; the fibers originate on the anterior portion of the vertebra
  - Ligamenta flava: Connect the vertebral laminae from C1 to S1 and help to stabilize the spine
  - Posterior longitudinal ligament: Connective tissue that stabilizes the spine from the axis to the sacrum; the fibers originate from the posterior portion of the vertebral body within the spinal canal
  - Supraspinal ligament: Strong band of fibrous tissue that stabilizes the spine; it connects the spinous processes from C7 through the sacrum and helps stabilize the lumbosacral articulation

Additional Ligaments

- Iliolumbar ligament: Attaches the transverse process of L5 to the iliac crest and works to stabilize the pelvis and the lumbar spine
- Inguinal ligament: Located between the anterosuperior iliac spine and pubic tubercle; a frequent site of hernia formation

Muscles

- A number of muscles are located in the pelvis or exert their influence here.
- Pelvic muscles generally provide stability to the trunk or function in the transmission of load to the lower extremities.
- The muscles of the hip are divided into four compartments: anterior (hip flexion), posterior (hip extension), medial (hip adduction), lateral (hip abduction).
- Table 122-1 lists the main muscles that exert action in the hip or pelvis.
- Origin, insertion, and main muscle activity with regard to function in the hip or pelvis are noted.

Soft Tissues

- Femoral triangle: Formed by the adductor longus (medially), sartorius (laterally), and inguinal ligament (superiorly).
  - The femoral artery and inguinal lymph nodes are palpable within the triangle.
  - The femoral nerve lies lateral to and the femoral vein lies medial to the femoral artery.
  - The organization of the structures can be remembered by the pneumonic NAVEL (lateral to medial for the structures): *n*erve, *a*rtery, *v*ein, *e*mpty space, *l*ymphatics.

TABLE 122-1 *Major Muscles of the Hip and Pelvis*

Muscle	Origin	Insertion	Action
Iliacus	Anterior iliac fossa	Lesser trochanter	Hip flexion
Psoas major	Vertebral body, transverse process, and discs T12-L4	Lesser trochanter	One of the primary hip flexors
Tensor fasciae latae	Iliac crest, anterosuperior iliac spine	Iliotibial band	Hip abduction, flexion, internal rotation
Gluteus medius	Posterior ilium	Greater trochanter (superior, lateral)	Primary hip abductor, internal rotation
Gluteus minimus	Posterior ilium	Greater trochanter (anterior, lateral)	Abduction > internal rotation
Gluteus maximus	Posterior ilium and sacrum	Femur, iliotibial band	Primary hip extensor, external rotation
Piriformis	Anterior sacrum	Greater trochanter (superior)	External rotation
Obturator externus	Ischiopubic rami, obturator membrane	Trochanteric fossa	External rotation
Obturator internus	Ischiopubic rami, obturator membrane	Greater trochanter (medial)	External rotation, abduction
Superior gemellus	Ischial spine	Greater trochanter (medial)	External rotation
Inferior gemellus	Ischial tuberosity	Greater trochanter (medial)	External rotation
Quadratus femoris	Ischial tuberosity	Intertrochanteric crest	External rotation
Sartorius	Anterosuperior iliac spine	Pes anserinus	Flexion, external rotation of hip
Rectus femoris	Anterosuperior iliac spine, acetabulum	Patella, tibial tuberosity	Flexion of hip, extension of knee
Vastus lateralis	Greater trochanter, femur	Patella (lateral), tibial tuberosity	Extends leg
Vastus intermedius	Femoral shaft	Patella, tibial tuberosity	Extends leg
Vastus medialis	Intertrochanteric line, femur	Patella (medial), tibial tuberosity	Extends leg
Adductor longus	Pubis	Femoral shaft	Adduction
Adductor brevis	Pubic body and rami (inferior)	Femoral shaft	Adduction
Adductor magnus	Ischiopubic ramus, ischial tuberosity	Femoral shaft, adductor tubercle	Adduction, flexion, extension
Gracilis	Pubic body and rami (inferior)	Pes anserinus	Adduction, flexion, internal rotation
Pectineus	Superior pubic ramus	Femoral shaft	Adduction, flexion
Semitendinosus	Ischial tuberosity	Pes anserinus	Extends thigh, flexes leg
Semimembranosus	Ischial tuberosity	Tibia (posterior, medial)	Extends thigh, flexes leg
Biceps femoris	Ischial tuberosity (long head)	Fibular head (long), fibula, tibia (lateral) (short)	Extends thigh, flexes leg
Quadratus lumborum	Iliac crest	Transverse process of upper lumbar vertebrae and 12th rib	Postural stability, lumbar extension (paired), lateral flexion (single)
Transversus abdominis	Iliac crest, last 6 ribs, inguinal ligament	Pubic crest, linea alba	Compresses abdomen

Neurovascular Structures and Bursae

- Lumbar plexi: Originate as roots from the anterior divisions of T12 nerve and lumbar nerves L1-L4. These further divide to form the upper and lower trunks in the case of L1 and L2 nerves or anterior and posterior branches in the case of L2-L4 nerves.
- Terminal branches of the anterior division supply flexor muscles, whereas the posterior division supplies extensor and abductor muscles.
- In addition, many of these terminal branches provide sensory innervation to the pelvis and lower extremities.
- A list of the many important nerves in this region along with their functions as they pertain to the hip and pelvis follows.

Anterior Division

- Iliohypogastric nerve: From lumbar trunk L1 (and T12); provides sensory innervation to the pubic region (anterior cutaneous branch) and posterior lateral buttocks (lateral cutaneous branch)

- Ilioinguinal: From lumbar trunk L1; provides sensory innervation to the inguinal region, scrotum, and base of the penis
- Genitofemoral: From lumbar trunks L1-L2, provides sensory innervation to the anteromedial thigh (lumbo-inguinal) as well as sensory function to the scrotum and pubic region and motor function for cremasteric function (external spermatic)
- Obturator: From the ventral portion of lumbar trunks L2-L4; provides sensory innervation to the inferior medial thigh (distal two thirds), and motor function to the external oblique, hip adductors (adductor longus, brevis, magnus, and gracilis), pectineus, and obturator externus through multiple terminal branches

Posterior Division

- Lateral femoral cutaneous nerve: From the dorsal division of lumbar trunks L2-L3; provides sensory innervation to lateral thigh through anterior and posterior branches
- Femoral: The largest nerve in the lumbar plexus, it is formed from the ventral lumbar trunks of L2-L4 and provides sensory innervation to the anteromedial thigh and motor innervation to the iliacus, pectineus, psoas, quadriceps (vastus lateralis, intermedius, medialis, and rectus femoris), and sartorius muscles.
- Sacral plexus: Provides important sensory and motor innervation in the pelvis and upper thigh and is formed by the anterior division of sacral nerves S1-S3 as well as the anterior division of the lumbar trunk (lumbar nerves L4-L5)
  - The anterior branches of the plexus supply the flexor muscles, and the posterior branches supply the extensor and abductor muscles of the limb.
  - The sacral plexus continues on to supply the lower extremities as the sciatic nerve, the largest nerve in the body.

Anterior Division

- Nerve to quadratus femoris: From lumbar (L4-L5) and sacral (S1) trunks, provides innervation to quadratus femoris and inferior gemelli
- Nerve to obturator internus: From lumbar (L5) and sacral (S1-S2) trunks, provides motor innervation to obturator internus and superior gemelli
- Tibial: A branch of the sciatic nerve, arising from lumbar (L4-L5) and sacral (S1-S3) trunks, provides motor innervation to biceps femoris (long head), semimembranosus, and semitendinosus as well as many branches in the lower leg and foot

Posterior Division

- Superior gluteal: From lumbar (L4-L5) and sacral (S1-S2) trunks, provides motor innervation to the gluteus medius, gluteus minimus, and tensor fasciae latae
- Common peroneal: From lumbar (L4-L5) and sacral (S1-S2) trunks, provides motor innervation to biceps femoris (short head); this is a branch of the sciatic nerve
- Inferior gluteal : From lumbar (L5) and sacral (S1-S2) trunks, provides motor innervation to the gluteus maximus
- Posterior femoral cutaneous nerve: With contributions from both the anterior and posterior divisions of sacral (S1-S3) trunks, provides sensory innervation to the posterior thigh, perineum, and gluteal areas
- Nerve to piriformis: From the sacral (S2) trunk, provides motor innervation to the piriformis
- Pudendal plexus: Formed from the anterior divisions of S2-S4 and the coccygeal nerve, provides sensory and motor supply to the deep pelvic muscles and perineum
  - Pudendal: From sacral (S2-S4) trunks, provides sensory innervation to the perineum and penis, urethral and anal sphincters

Arterial Supply

- The abdominal aorta divides approximately at the level of L4 into the common iliac artery (right and left), which further subdivides into its main branches, the internal and external iliac arteries (right and left).
- The internal iliac artery supplies most of the pelvic structures via its anterior and posterior divisions.
  - The anterior division supplies terminal branches to multiple pelvis organs (hemorrhoidal, iliac, inferior gluteal, uterine, vaginal, and vesical branches) and ultimately supplies the obturator and internal pudendal arteries.
  - The obturator artery bifurcates into anterior and posterior branches, which supply the hip adductors, femoral head, and, with additional small branches, the surrounding bone and musculature.
- The internal pudendal artery is the main blood supply to the perineum.
- The posterior division of the internal iliac artery supplies the superior gluteal, the iliolumbar, and the lateral sacral arteries, which provide multiple terminal branches.
- In addition, arterial supply to pelvic structures occurs from terminal branches of more proximal take-offs such as the superior hemorrhoidal artery, which

supplies the pelvic floor and anal region, and the internal spermatic, ovarian, and middle sacral arteries.

- The external iliac artery gives off two major branches: the deep circumflex iliac and the inferior epigastric arteries, before crossing the inguinal ligament and continuing as the femoral artery.
- The inferior epigastric artery supplies branches to the abdominal wall and musculature, spermatic cord, and pubic region.
- The deep circumflex iliac artery supplies branches to the surrounding musculature as well as anastomoses with more proximal branches.
- The femoral artery provides multiple branches (superficial epigastric, superficial iliac circumflex, superficial external pudendal, deep external pudendal, and profunda femoris branches) before continuing into the lower leg as the popliteal artery.
- The profunda femoris artery provides multiple branches to the hamstring and quadriceps muscles and femur through its circumflex and nutrient branches.

Bursae

- Bursae function as lubrication sacs to decrease friction between musculoskeletal structures. Because of excessive friction, poor biomechanics, or trauma, these sacs can fill with fluid and become painful (bursitis). Common areas of involvement in the hip and pelvis include the trochanteric, iliopectineal, and ischial bursae.

Hip and Pelvis Biomechanics

- Hip joint: range of motion
  - Abduction: 35 to 50 degrees (examine supine)
  - Adduction: 20 to 35 degrees (examine supine)
  - Flexion: 110 to 130 degrees (examine supine)
  - Extension: 30 degrees (examine prone)
  - Internal rotation: 30 to 35 degrees (examine with hip both extended and flexed)
  - External rotation: 45 to 50 degrees (examine with hip both extended and flexed)
- Biomechanical force generation by the hip and pelvis muscles is extremely complex. Muscle length, tension, and the degree of hip or knee flexion are but a few of the factors that determine force transmission.
  - Pubic symphysis: Motion at the pubic symphysis has been demonstrated to be very limited. Rotation is limited to 2 to 3 degrees, whereas translations of only 1 to 2 mm are common.
  - Sacroiliac joint: Motion at the sacroiliac joint does occur in all three planes, but is also extremely limited to approximately 2 to 4 degrees of rotation and 1 to 2 mm of translation. This may increase slightly during pregnancy.

History

- The examiner should attempt to discern the following before examining the hip and pelvis
  - Symptom onset: acute or chronic, duration
  - Quality, character, location of symptoms; groin pain (most commonly affects the hip joint), buttock or posterior thigh (spine), lateral thigh (trochanteric bursitis), anterior thigh (femur)
  - Exacerbating or relieving factors; pain with standing, ambulation, movement
  - Presence of night, exertional, or radiating pain
  - Paresthesia or weakness
  - Snapping, popping, slipping sensation
  - Muscle atrophy, fatigue
  - Clicking, catching, grinding
  - Edema, cyanosis, coolness in lower extremities
  - Trauma, falls, or overuse (premeditative loading) factors
  - Other joint involvement
- Other relevant historical information includes age, occupation, general medical health and medications, presence of connective tissue diseases, functional demands, and history of back pain, workers' compensation claim, or pending litigation.

Physical Examination

- The examination should be performed with the patient standing, sitting, lying down (supine, lateral, and prone) during various portions of the examination. Evaluation of the spine and knee should also be performed.
- A thorough examination of the hip and pelvis should include the following:
  - Inspection: atrophy, swelling, discoloration, skin changes, stance, posture, gait for limp, spine and pelvic alignment (anterosuperior iliac spine and iliac crests should be level), lumbar curvature
  - Palpation: bony structures (anterosuperior iliac spine, posterosuperior iliac spine, pubic tubercle, iliac tubercle, iliac crest, ischial tuberosity, greater trochanter), soft tissues (inguinal ligament, femoral pulse, lymph nodes); evaluate for focal tenderness, deformity, gaps, spasm
  - Range of motion: lumbar (flexion, extension, rotation, and bend) should be symmetrical; evaluate for compensatory changes and evaluate hip flexion, extension, internal/external rotation; examine both active and passive range of motion

TABLE 122-2 *Special Tests*

Test	Physical Maneuvers	Positive Test	Suggested Diagnosis
90-90 straight leg	Flex hip and knee 90 degrees, then extend knee	>20 degrees of hip flexion after full knee extension	Hamstring muscle involvement
Ely test	With patient prone, knee is flexed	Hip flexion	Rectus femoris tightness
FABER (Patrick's) test	Hip is flexed, abducted, and externally rotated, then placed into further abduction	Pain or asymmetry	Sacroiliac joint involvement
Gaenslen's test	With patient supine, flex one hip while extending the other	Pain	Lumbar or sacroiliac involvement
Leg length	Measure from anterosuperior iliac spine to medial malleoli	>1 cm of side-to-side difference	Leg length discrepancy
Log roll	With patient supine and hip extended, external/internal rotation of the hip	Loss of motion, pain	Hip osteoarthritis
Meralgia	Pressure placed medial to anterosuperior iliac spine	Pain, burning, reproduction of symptoms	Lateral femoral cutaneous nerve entrapment
Ober's test	With patient lying on side, flex knee 90 degrees, abduct hip	Leg stays in abduction when force removed	Iliotibial band
Piriformis	With patient on side, adduct hip	Pain in hip or pelvis	Piriformis involvement
Straight leg raise	With patient supine, passively extend knee and flex hip	Radiation of pain down leg (ipsilateral or contralateral)	Consider herniated disc with radiculopathy
Thomas test	With patient supine, bring knee to chest	Elevation of contralateral side	Flexion contracture
Trendelenburg's sign	With patient standing, have patient flex hip	Pelvis on ipsilateral side drops	Abductor or gluteus weakness
Pediatric tests			
Barlow	Hips flexed at 90 degrees, direct posterior force	Click	Hip instability
Ortolani	Hips flexed at 90 degrees, abduct hip	Click	Hip instability, maneuver reduces a dislocated hip

- Strength: assessed throughout the bilateral lower extremities, lower back; best accomplished in functional groups of flexion, extension, abduction, adduction and graded 0 to 5
- Neurovascular examination: test sensation in dermatomal distribution, pulses (femoral)

- Consider rectal or vaginal examination if trauma or indicated.

Additional Tests

- Please see Table 122-2 for a description of special physical examination components.

Suggested Reading

- Braly B, Beall DP, Martin HD: Clinical examination of the athletic hip. Clin Sports Med 2006;25:199–210.
- Cohen SP: Sacroiliac joint pain: A comprehensive review of anatomy, diagnosis, and treatment. Anesth Analg 2005;101:1440–1453.
- DeLee JC, Drez D Jr, Miller MD (eds): DeLee and Drez's Orthopaedic Sports Medicine: Principles and Practices, 2nd ed. Philadelphia: WB Saunders, 2002.
- Gray H: Anatomy of the Human Body. Philadelphia: Lea & Febiger, 1918.
- Griffin LY, Greene WB (eds): Essentials of Musculoskeletal Care, 3rd ed. Rosemont, IL: American Academy of Orthopaedic Surgeons, 2005.
- Hoppenfeld S: Physical Examination of the Spine and Extremities. Norwalk, CT: Appleton-Century-Crofts, 1976.
- Netter FH, Colacino S (eds): Atlas of Human Anatomy. Summit, NJ: CIBA-GEIGY, 1989.
- Thompson JC: Netter's Concise Atlas of Orthopaedic Anatomy. Philadelphia: WB Saunders, 2002.
- Tory MR, Schenker ML, Martin HD, et al: Neuromuscular hip biomechanics and pathology in the athlete. Clin Sports Med 2006;25:179–197.
- Walheim GG, Selvik G: Mobility of the pubic symphysis. In vivo measurements with an electromechanic method and a roentgen stereophotogrammetric method. Clin Orthop Relat Res 1984;191:129–135.

Chapter 123 Sacroiliac Joint

Per Gunnar Brolinson

Key Concepts

- The sacroiliac joint is a common source of low back pain in both the general (as many as 20%) and the athletic (as many as 50%) patient population.
  - The diagnosis and treatment of sacroiliac (SI) joint problems is controversial due to its complex anatomy and biomechanics.
  - There is no specific historical issue or single clinical examination technique that is both sensitive and specific for the diagnosis of SI dysfunction.
- The SI joint has been described as both a diarthrodial and synovial joint and has a well-defined L-shaped articulation with an upper long vertical pole and a shorter lower horizontal pole.
  - The sacropelvic region serves as a force transfer link between the spine and the lower extremities.
- There have been conflicting studies regarding the mobility of the SI joints. Clinicians now believe that motion occurs throughout life.
- Integral to the biomechanics of SI joint stability is the concept of a self-locking mechanism. The SI joint is the only joint in the body that has a flat joint surface that lies almost parallel to the plane of maximal load.

History

- Elements of the history should include the following factors
  - The age of the patient because many conditions occur within certain age ranges (ankylosing spondylitis versus osteoarthritis)
  - The type of sport or activity in which the patient is routinely involved
  - The acuteness or chronicity of the pain: Was there an acute traumatic injury or a chronic repetitive injury?
  - The mechanism of injury
  - For active pregnant women, remember that pregnancy causes laxity of the SI joint and predisposes women to pain or injury.
  - Identification of provocative and palliative measures
  - The duration and frequency of the pain
  - The quality and intensity of the pain as well as any radiation or referred pain (usually unilateral, dull, and deep, with radiation to buttock, posterior thigh, or groin)
  - Notation of previous low back injuries, with treatments and outcomes
  - The presence of red flags signaling more serious pathology including, but not limited to, weight loss, night pain and night sweats (cancer); fevers and chills (infection); dysuria and hematuria (nephrolithiasis); epigastric pain with nausea, vomiting, and/or heartburn (peptic ulcer disease or pancreatitis); left-sided abdominal pain with melena, hematochezia, diarrhea, and/or constipation (diverticular disease); pulsating abdominal pain with radiation to groin (abdominal aortic aneurysm); and numbness, tingling, weakness, and/or incontinence (radiculopathy or cauda equina syndrome)

Physical Examination

- Evaluate the patient in the standing, supine, and prone positions and assess the symmetry of the heights of the iliac crests, anterosuperior iliac spine, posterosuperior iliac spine, ischial tuberosities, gluteal folds, and greater trochanters, as well as symmetry of the sacral sulci, inferior lateral angles, and pubic tubercles.
- Determine whether there is any leg length discrepancy. Dynamic observation assesses for any asymmetry during both gait and specific motions characteristic of the patient's sport or usual activities.
- Always perform a thorough examination of the lumbar spine, hips, and knees because pathology in these areas can refer pain to the SI joint.
- A neurologic examination for radiculopathy should also be conducted, in addition to evaluating abdominal strength and overall flexibility.
- There have been numerous functional (motion) and provocative (pain-producing) tests reported in the literature; however, none have consistently been shown

to reliably diagnose SI joint dysfunction. A detailed discussion of the numerous tests described for diagnosing the SI joint is beyond the scope of this review.
- Common tests include standing forward flexion, sitting forward flexion, stork (Gillet), Gaenslen's, supine-to-sit, Patrick's (FABER [flexion, abduction, external rotation]) test, side-lying approximation, and supine gapping.
- Accurate diagnosis ultimately must be based on a combination of historic clues, along with findings from static palpatory examination, segmental and regional motion testing, overall functional biomechanical examination, and appropriate diagnostic testing.

Imaging

- There is no specific gold standard imaging test to diagnose the SI joint, largely because of the location of the joint and visualization difficulties due to overlying structures. However, standard radiographs taken at 25 to 30 degrees from the anteroposterior axis coupled with lateral views may show degenerative changes, ankylosis, demineralization, or fracture.
- Note that in adolescents, the SI joints may normally show widening and irregularity and therefore can make radiographic diagnosis more difficult.
- Bone scans identify osteoblastic activity and may signal infection, tumor, fracture, or a metabolic process.
- Computed tomography will identify fractures, osteoid osteomas, and degenerative changes.
- Magnetic resonance imaging helps to identify fractures, tumor, soft-tissue pathology, and lumbar disc disease and is most sensitive for identifying inflammatory sacroiliitis.

Additional Tests

- Doppler ultrasound imaging can capture SI motion in pregnant women with SI pain.

Differential Diagnosis

- The differential diagnosis is extensive and should include but not be limited to the following
  - Arthritis including ankylosing spondylitis
  - SI joint dysfunction (microinstability)
  - Lumbar radiculopathy
  - Tumor
  - Stress fracture
  - Facet syndrome
  - Degenerative disc disease
  - Abdominal aortic aneurysm
  - Nephrolithiasis
  - Diverticular disease
  - Referred pain from pelvic organs
  - Herpes zoster
  - Joint sepsis

Treatment

- Accurate diagnosis is the key to successful treatment, and pain relief is an important early goal.
- The use of nonsteroidal anti-inflammatory drugs, nonnarcotic and narcotic analgesics (acutely), as well as physical therapy modalities can be beneficial.
- Gross SI joint instability is rare, but microinstability is a relatively common component seen in patients with recurrent SI joint pain.
  - This microinstability often leads to chronic pain syndromes and must be identified and treated.
  - Instability often occurs as a result of the loss of the functional integrity of any of the systems of the lumbosacral and pelvic region that provide stability.
  - The myofascial, osteoarticular, ligamentous, and neural control components may be affected.
- Formal physical therapy can be helpful in both acute and chronic SI joint pain syndromes.
  - Rehabilitation must focus on the entire abdomino-lumbosacropelvic-hip complex addressing articular, muscular, neural, and fascial restrictions, inhibitions, and deficiencies.
  - A principle-centered, functional approach to evaluation and rehabilitation must be undertaken.
  - The transversus abdominis muscle has been shown to be the key muscle to functional core retraining due to its observed patterns of firing before and independent of the other abdominal muscles.
  - Exercise techniques that promote independent contraction of the transversus abdominis muscle have been shown to lower recurrence rates after an acute low back pain episode and lower pain and disability in chronic low back pain.
- Several joint mobilization or manipulative techniques can be used in the treatment of SI joint pain syndromes, including soft-tissue technique, muscle energy, myofascial release, functional technique, strain/counterstrain, craniosacral technique, and high-velocity/low-amplitude.
- Explanations of these techniques and their specific applications to the SI joint can be found in several excellent sources (see Suggested Reading).

Prognosis

- A comprehensive functional approach based on historic clues and appropriate diagnostic testing will lead to the best clinical result.
- Clinical experience is that a multimodal approach works best including aggressive pain control, functional therapeutic exercise, and potentially SI joint mobilization or manipulation.
- Identification and correction of functional or anatomic leg length discrepancy and optimization of posture are important but often overlooked clinical entities.

Troubleshooting

- Gravitational stress is a constant and greatly underestimated systemic stressor leading to postural imbalance, which is a systemic neuromuscular dysfunction.
- For patients with SI pain and dysfunction not responding to standard management, optimization of posture can be very beneficial; this can be achieved through the use of one or more of the following modes of treatment:
  - Contoured orthotics worn in the shoes to optimize foot and lower extremity biomechanics
  - A flat orthotic of sufficient thickness to correct anatomic leg length discrepancy and level the sacral base
  - Manipulation and/or mobilization directed to restore resilience to soft tissues and motion of restricted joint segment
  - Daily practice of therapeutic postural exercise for 20 minutes to counter the bias of soft tissues reflective of the initial posture
  - Use of pelvic belts (sacral belts) for sacropelvic support during the postural retraining process
- SI joint injections (local anesthetic with or without cortisone) have not been consistently shown to be effective, although they may at least help to diagnose the SI joint as the source of pain.
- Similarly, periarticular injections also show inconsistent results but can be clinically useful in the appropriately selected patient.

Patient Instructions

- Follow physician and physical therapist instructions closely with respect to the type and quantity of exercise and acceptable job-related activities.
- Home-based exercises including postural retraining are vital to overall management and should be performed diligently and regularly.
- Aggressively manage pain using physical therapy modalities as well as oral medications as appropriate.

Considerations in Special Populations

- Those caring for active patients will encounter this condition commonly and should be vigilant for its potential presence in any patient presenting with low back pain.
- One must be aware of this condition in the active pregnant female.
- For elderly patients, be particularly aware of issues potentially related to osteoporosis and be sure to screen for underlying occult malignancy.
- For adolescent patients, watch carefully for sacral and pelvic stress fractures as well as lumbar spondylolysis.

Suggested Reading

- Brolinson PG, Gray G: Principle-centered rehabilitation. In Garrett WE, Kirkendall DT, Squire DH (eds): Principles and Practice of Primary Care Sports Medicine. Philadelphia: Lippincott Williams & Wilkins, 2001, pp 645–652.
- Brolinson PG, Kozar AJ, Cibor G: Sacroiliac dysfunction in athletes. Curr Sports Med Rep 2003;2:47–56.
- Dreyfuss P, Dreyer S, Griffin J, et al: Positive sacroiliac screening tests in asymptomatic adults. Spine 1994;19:1138–1143.
- Greenman PE: Principles of Manual Medicine, 2nd ed. Baltimore: Williams & Wilkins, 1996.
- Richardson CA, Snijders CJ, Hides JA, et al: The relation between the transversus abdominis muscles, sacroiliac joint mechanics, and low back pain. Spine 2002;27:399–405.
- Slipman CW, Sterenfeld EB, Chou LH, et al: The predictive value of provocative sacroiliac joint stress maneuvers in the diagnosis of sacroiliac joint syndrome. Arch Phys Med Rehabil 1998;79:288–292.
- Van der Wurff P, Hagmeijer RHM, Meyne W: Clinical tests of the sacroiliac joint: A systematic methodological review. Part I: Reliability. Man Ther 2000;5:30–36.
- Van der Wurff P, Hagmeijer RHM, Meyne W: Clinical tests of the sacroiliac joint: A systematic methodological review. Part II: Validity. Man Ther 2000;5:89–96.
- Willard FH: The muscular, ligamentous and neural structure of the low back and its relation to back pain. In Vleeming A, Mooney V, Dorman T, et al (eds): Movement, Stability, and Low Back Pain: The Essential Role of the Pelvis. New York: Churchill Livingstone, 1997.

Chapter 124 Hip Pointer

Laura D. Goldberg

ICD-9 CODES
922.2 *Contusion, Iliac Region*

Key Concepts

- Hip pointer refers to a contusion of the iliac crest with an associated subperiosteal hematoma usually due to a direct blow.
- The iliac crest is relatively exposed, with little soft tissue covering it. The bruise is usually superficial, although it may be deep within muscle (Fig. 124-1).
- The term hip pointer is often misused to represent other conditions such as iliac crest avulsion fractures or strains of the muscles that attach to the iliac crest. These injuries usually result from bending or twisting motions or sudden force on the muscle. However, they may also result from a direct blow.
- Contusions to the soft tissues and bony prominences of the hip occur frequently in contact sports such as football, soccer, and ice hockey. The mechanism of injury involves a collision with another player, a player's equipment (i.e., helmet), or a playing surface.
- It is important to distinguish between a contusion, an apophyseal injury, a muscle strain, and a fracture.

History

- History of direct blow or fall (often acute but may present the next day)
- Localized pain and tenderness on the iliac crest (usually the anterior third)
- Localized swelling
- Bruising (immediate or delayed 24–48 hours)
- Painful gait
- Painful hip range of motion, specifically abduction and flexion
- Pain with coughing and sneezing due to abdominal muscle insertion

Physical Examination

- Observe gait (often has limp)
- Evaluate for swelling and ecchymosis.
- Evaluate for localized tenderness to palpation.
    - Usually on anterior third of the iliac crest (see Fig. 124-1)
    - If tender on the anterosuperior iliac spine or anteroinferior iliac spine, consider avulsion injury or muscle strain (Fig. 124-2).
- Evaluate active and passive range of motion.
- Evaluate for strength and pain with resisted motion.
    - Abdominal oblique muscles
    - Abduction
- A complete general hip and lower abdomen examination should be performed to rule out additional pathologies.

Imaging

- Radiographs are necessary to evaluate for fractures or avulsion injuries.
- Routine radiographic evaluation should include anteroposterior pelvis, iliac oblique, and frog-leg lateral views that include the entire iliac crest.
- Comparison views of the contralateral side may help identify an avulsion injury.

Additional Tests

- Additional testing is usually not required.
- If uncertain of the diagnosis, consider magnetic resonance imaging (MRI) to evaluate the surrounding soft tissues, muscles, and tendons. In the skeletally immature, closely examine the involved apophysis.
- Ultrasonography is also a good test in the hands of a skilled musculoskeletal sonographer to evaluate the apophysis; however, if the ultrasound scan is negative and the diagnostic question remains, MRI is a more definitive test.

Differential Diagnosis

- Muscle or soft-tissue contusion
- Avulsion fractures at origin of muscles
    - Tenderness on iliac crest, anterosuperior iliac spine, anteroinferior iliac spine (see Fig. 124-2)

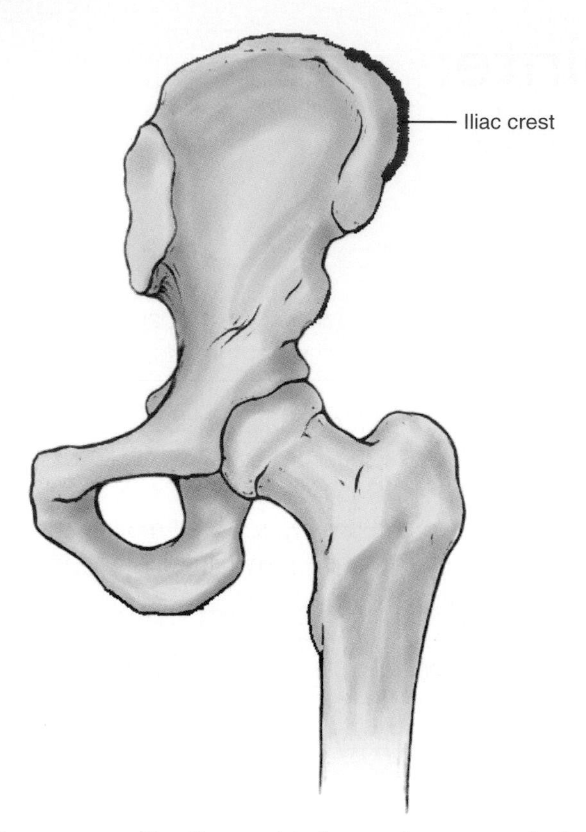

Figure 124-1 The iliac crest is the most common site for a hip pointer. (Image modified from Green N, Swiontkowski M [eds]: Skeletal Trauma in Children, 3rd ed. Philadelphia: Saunders, 2002, Fig. 2-42, p 50.)

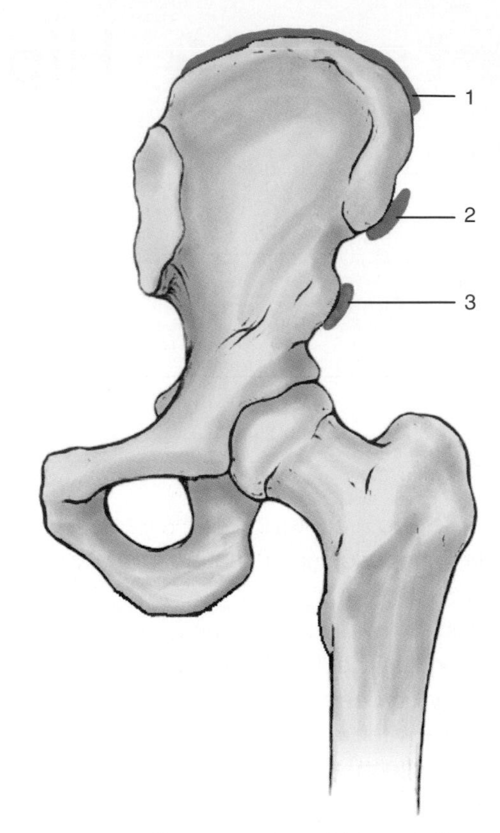

Figure 124-2 Common sites of injury. 1, iliac crest; 2, anterosuperior iliac crest; 3, anteroinferior iliac crest. (Image modified from Green N, Swiontkowski M [eds]: Skeletal Trauma in Children, 3rd ed. Philadelphia: WB Saunders, 2002, Fig. 2-42, p 50.)

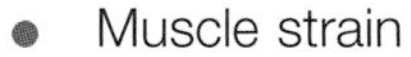

- Muscle strain
  - Most common in older sprinters, jumpers, and soccer or football players
  - Tenderness on anterosuperior iliac spine
    - — Origin of sartorius muscle and tensor fasciae latae muscles
    - — Usually occurs due to force on extended hip and flexed knee
  - Tenderness on anteroinferior iliac spine
    - — Origin of straight head of rectus femoris muscles
    - — Usually occurs due to kicking motion
  - Tenderness on iliac crest
    - — Insertion of obliquus externus abdominis muscles
    - — May occur from violent contraction of abdominal muscles or from direct blow
- Apophyseal avulsions (usually 14- to 25-year-olds)
  - May not be obvious on plain radiographs if ossification has not yet occurred; if increased suspicion, further ultrasonography or MRI studies are warranted
  - Iliac crest apophyseal avulsion
    - — Ossification begins at approximately 15 years, and fusion most often occurs by 18 years and 3 months.
  - Anterosuperior iliac spine apophyseal avulsion
  - Anteroinferior iliac spine apophyseal avulsion
    - — Increased frequently in younger patients because this apophysis ossifies earlier than the anterosuperior iliac spine or iliac crest
  - Tenderness and pain with resisted testing of involved muscle (see muscle strain)
- Iliac apophysitis
  - Injury to apophysis without avulsion or may be due to repetitive injury
  - Similar to apophysitis in other areas such as Osgood-Schlatter disease
  - Tenderness and pain with resisted testing of involved muscle
  - May have swelling and erythema
- If no preceding injury or repetitive activity, consider further testing to evaluate for other soft-tissue or bone pathology based on clinical suspicion.

Treatment

- Immediate (acutely painful)
    - Rule out other pathology.
    - Minimize pain and bleeding.
        - — Rest, ice, compression
        - — Crutches with protected weight bearing if painful gait
        - — Rarely, in an adult patient, a cortisone injection may help to decrease pain and disability and to hasten return to activity.
    - Maintain motion with gentle active and passive range of motion.
- Later, after 48 hours or after pain improved
    - Heat
    - Nonsteroidal anti-inflammatory medications
    - Physical therapy to improve range of motion and strength
- Return to play
    - Full, pain-free range of motion
    - Strength equal to that of opposite leg
    - Normal gait walking, sprinting, and changing directions
    - Evaluate protective padding for correct fit and location.
    - May initially benefit from extra padding until bony tenderness resolves
    - Premature return often leads to reinjury.

When to Refer

- Prolonged pain with inability to return to sport
- Excessive bleeding raises concern for bleeding disorder.

Prognosis

- Usually return to sport within 1 to 2 weeks, but bony tenderness may persist for months
- Apophyseal injury requires a longer rest period of 4 to 6 weeks.
- Rare long-term disability

Troubleshooting

- Avoid excessive activity.
- Avoid use of NSAIDs and heat in acute phase to minimize bleeding.
- Aspiration of hematoma is rarely successful in improving recovery.
- Avoid injury from premature return by testing for full, pain-free range of motion and strength as well as the ability to perform in controlled setting before returning to game play
- Counsel the patient that bony tenderness may persist for months.

Patient Instructions

- Initial treatment consists of rest, ice, compressive dressing, and pain medication to reduce bleeding and swelling, which contribute to prolonged symptoms.
- Heat, massage, and NSAIDs after 48 hours
- Early activity modification and stretching allow bruising to heal.
- Physical therapy or home exercises to speed return of strength and motion
- Protective padding may allow earlier return to activity.

Considerations in Special Populations

- In young athletes, one must consider injury or avulsion of an apophysis. These are most common between ages 14 to 25 years. Separation occurs in the cartilaginous area between the apophysis and the bone (see differential diagnosis section and Fig. 124-2)
- Avulsion injuries require protected weight bearing with an extended period of rest until pain-free range of motion has returned. Then progressive rehabilitation is started.

Suggested Reading

- Blankenbaker DG: The role of ultrasound in the evaluation of sports injuries of the lower extremities. Clin Sports Med 2006;25:867–897.
- LaBella CR: Common acute sports-related lower extremity injuries in children and adolescents. Clin Pediatr Emerg Med 2007;8(1): 31–42.
- Lombardo SJ, Retting AC, Kerlan RK: Radiographic abnormalities of the iliac apophysis in adolescent athletes. J Bone Joint Surg Am 1983;65A:444–446.
- Nuccion SL, Hunter DM, Finerman GAM: Hip and pelvis. In DeLee JC, Drez D Jr, Miller MD (eds): DeLee and Drez's Orthopaedic Sports Medicine, 2nd ed. Philadelphia: WB Saunders, 2002, pp 1443–1454.
- Ramachandran M, Skaggs DL: Physeal injuries. In Green N, Swiontkowski M (eds): Skeletal Trauma in Children, 4th ed. Philadelphia: WB Saunders, 2008, pp 19–38.

Chapter 125 Piriformis Syndrome

Edward J. Lewis and Thomas M. Howard

ICD-9 CODE
724.3 *Sciatica*

Key Concepts

- Definition: Sciatic nerve irritation caused by mechanical compression or chemical irritation of the sciatic nerve or its branches as it passes beneath or through the piriformis muscle.
- Often manifested as buttock pain that may radiate down the leg to the level of the knee
- There has been significant historical controversy as to whether piriformis syndrome exists as a distinct entity. Recent literature and medical opinion support the existence of piriformis syndrome.
- Functional anatomy of the piriformis muscle
  - Origin
    - — Anterior of the S2-S4 vertebrae
    - — Sacrotuberous ligament
    - — Upper margin of the greater sciatic foramen
  - Insertion
    - — Traverses greater sciatic notch to insert on the superior surface of greater trochanter of femur
  - Function
    - — Hip extended: primary external rotator of the femur
    - — Hip flexed: abductor of the hip
  - Relationship to sciatic nerve
    - — Six possible anatomic relationships as originally described by Beaton (Fig. 125-1)
- Epidemiology
  - Low back pain has an estimated lifetime incidence of more than 90% in the general population.
  - Piriformis syndrome has an estimated prevalence of six cases per 100 cases of sciatica.
  - 6:1 female-to-male ratio

History

- Chronic pain in the buttock
  - Pain may radiate to leg and worsens with squatting and walking.
  - Pain is worse with active external rotation or abduction of the femur.
  - Pain is often prominent as the patient gets out of bed when lying on asymptomatic side. This maneuver requires active abduction and external rotation of the affected extremity, selectively activating the piriformis muscle.
- History of trauma to the gluteal region in less than 50% of cases
  - Trauma is often subacute and may precede symptoms by months.
- Pain is often exacerbated by sitting on hard surfaces.
- May be manifest as painful bowel movements in both sexes and dyspareunia in women

Physical Examination

- Tenderness on palpation of the piriformis muscle or its origin on the sacrum
- Palpable gluteal mass, sometimes described as sausage-like
- Tenderness on palpation of lateral wall during rectal or pelvic examination
- Lack of lower extremity motor weakness or deep tendon reflex change
- Special attention should be paid to Morton foot, pes planus, and hyperpronation, which may lead to an overuse syndrome due to compensatory contraction of the piriformis muscle.
- Gluteus maximus hypertrophy may be present in advanced or severe cases.
- Beatty maneuver (Fig. 125-2)
  - Selectively contracts the piriformis muscle
  - The patient is placed in a side-lying position on the unaffected side.
  - The knee of the affected side is rested on the examination table.
  - The patient lifts the affected leg several inches off the table and holds this position, resulting in active abduction and external rotation of the lower extremity.
  - The test is positive when the maneuver is painful.

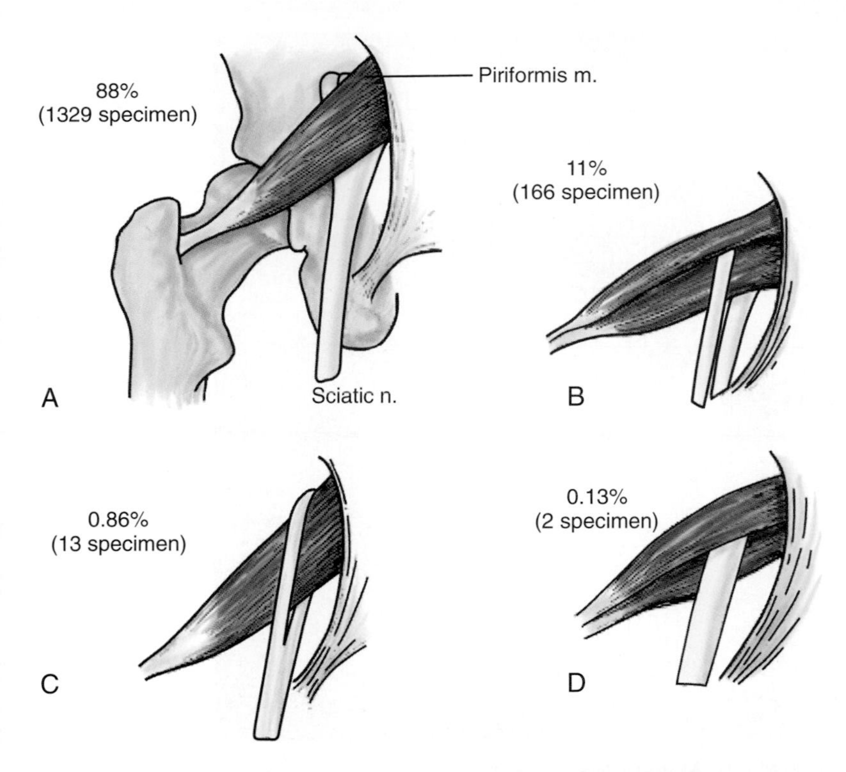

Figure 125-1 Beaton's classification of anatomic variation in the piriformis muscle and sciatic nerve. Relationship of the sciatic nerve to the piriformis muscle in 1510 extremities studies. **A,** Single-bodied piriformis muscle overlies sciatic nerve. **B,** One branch of underlying sciatic nerve penetrates bifurcated piriformis muscle. **C,** Single-bodied piriformis muscle penetrates sciatic nerve. **D,** Sciatic nerve penetrates bifurcated piriformis muscle.

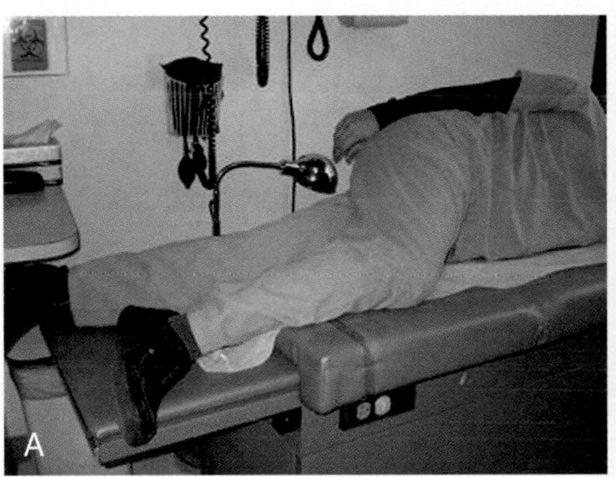

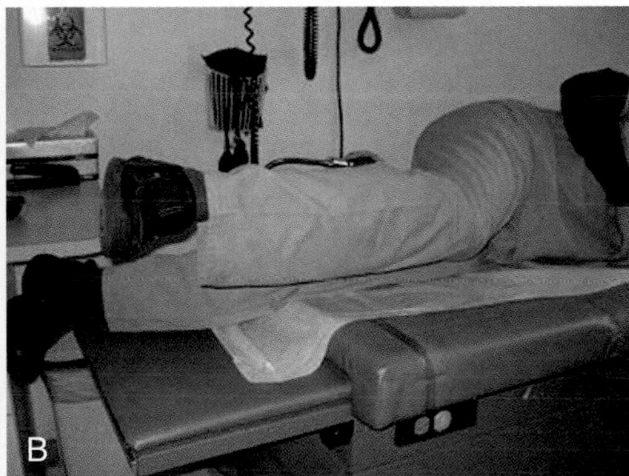

Figure 125-2 Beatty maneuver. Symptomatic leg resting (**A**) and actively lifted several inches (**B**).

- Pace test
  - The patient is placed in a seated position.
  - A positive test is marked by pain with resisted leg abduction.
- Freiberg test (Fig. 125-3)
  - The patient is placed in the supine position.
  - Pain upon passive internal rotation of the femur with hip extended/neutral

Imaging

- Magnetic resonance imaging
  - Useful to rule out tumor, herniated disc, and spinal stenosis
  - May demonstrate hypertrophy of the piriformis muscle on T1-weighted images; usually no signal change on T2-weighted images
- Computed tomography
  - Useful to characterize the degree of arthritis, assess for spinal stenosis
  - May identify mass anterior to the piriformis muscle
- Ultrasonography
  - May demonstrate painful hypertrophy of the piriformis muscle

Additional Tests

- Electromyography
  - Usually negative in piriformis syndrome
  - May demonstrate the specific pattern of gluteus maximus and piriformis abnormalities in piriformis syndrome
  - Positive tests usually indicate other diagnoses such as a herniated disc.

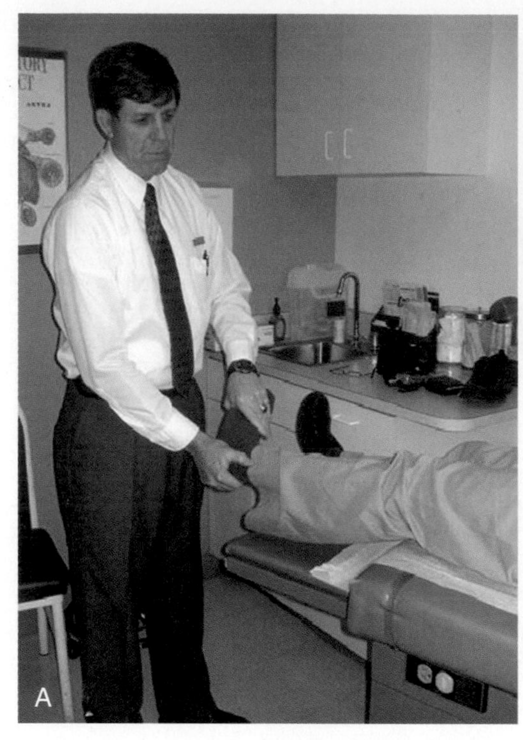

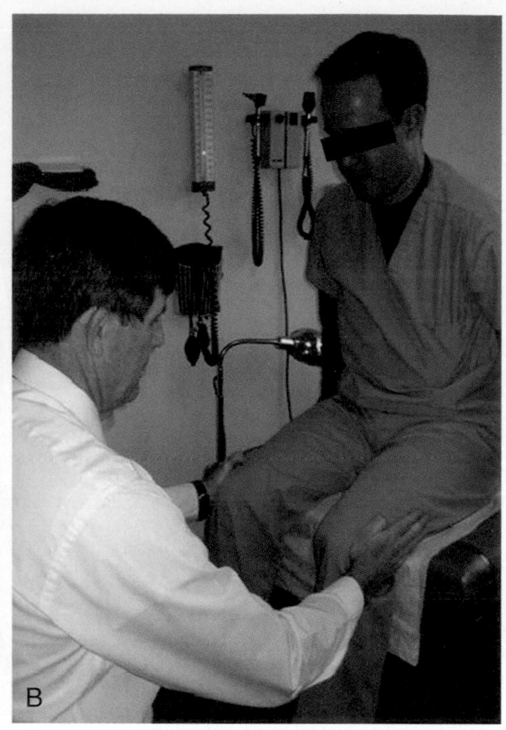

Figure 125-3 Freiberg (**A**) and Pace (**B**) tests.

- H-reflex
  - The Hoffman reflex, or H-reflex, elicits the Achilles reflex through stimulation of the sciatic nerve at the popliteal fossa.
  - An abnormal H-reflex in the anatomic position is usually indicative of disc herniation.
- FAIR test
  - The FAIR test compares the H-reflex in the anatomic position and in flexion, adduction, and internal rotation, stretching the piriformis muscle.
  - Prolongation of the H-reflex by 1.86 ms indicates pathologic compression of the sciatic nerve and is considered diagnostic of piriformis syndrome.
- Diagnostic injection
  - Diagnostic lidocaine injection of the piriformis muscle may be performed transcutaneously, transvaginally, or transrectally.
  - Relief of pain on provocative testing is suggestive of piriformis syndrome.

Differential Diagnosis

Please see Table 125-1.

Treatment

- At diagnosis
  - Avoid prolonged sitting and other exacerbating activities.
  - Home stretches, heat, ice, massage
  - Physical therapy
    - — Stretching, often preceded by moist heat or ultrasound
    - — Soft-tissue massage
    - — Myofascial release by therapist
    - — Cold packs or electrical stimulation after physical therapy
    - — Hip and core stability and flexibility exercises
- Later
  - Consider diagnostic or therapeutic injection
    - — Local anesthetic agents, steroids, and botulinum toxin have demonstrated efficacy.
  - Consider advanced imaging studies (e.g., electromyography) not already performed.

When to Refer

- Physical therapy
  - Consider immediate referral
- Neurologist
  - Consider referral for electromyography when diagnosis is unclear or the patient is not improving.
- Gynecologist
  - Consider referral for unclear diagnosis if pelvic pain is present.
- Surgery
  - Avoid surgical intervention with less than 6 months of conservative therapy.

TABLE 125-1 *Differential Diagnosis of Low Back and Buttock Pain*

Diagnosis	Differentiating Features	Chapter Reference
Piriformis syndrome	Positive Beatty maneuver, positive FAIR test, rule out other hip and spine pathology	N/A
Herniated lumbosacral disc	Motor weakness, altered deep tendon reflexes, radiology	118
Spinal stenosis	Neurogenic claudication, radiology	120
Lumbosacral discogenic pain syndrome	Pain with Valsalva maneuver	118
Spondylolysis or spondylolisthesis	Pain with back extension, radiology	121
Sacroiliac joint pain	Positive FABER (flexion, abduction, external rotation) test	123
Lumbosacral muscle or ligament sprain/strain	Pain with back flexion	117
Hamstring injury	Pain with resisted leg flexion	134
Facet pain	Pain with back extension, radiology	110
Pelvic or cord mass, tumor, or endometriosis	History, radiology	N/A
Gluteal abscess	Constitutional symptoms, radiology	N/A
Aneurysm of inferior or superior gluteal artery	Radiology	N/A
Bursitis: trochanteric, ischial, or obturator	Palpation, diagnostic injection	130
Strain or tendinitis of the gluteal muscles, obturator muscle, etc.	Provocative muscle testing	122

- Surgery has been demonstrated to be effective after failure of conservative therapy in select cases.
- Has shown greatest efficacy in posttraumatic piriformis syndrome

Prognosis

- As with most causes of low back pain, the majority of patients respond to conservative therapy.
- Symptoms often resolve with 6 weeks of conservative therapy.
- Less than 10% of patients require surgical evaluation.

Patient Instructions

- Counsel patients that this is rarely a disabling condition and typically responds well to conservative therapies.
- Provide instruction on active rest to include
  - Activity modification
  - Heat, ice, massage
  - Specific stretches for the piriformis muscle
  - Use of analgesics or nonsteroidal anti-inflammatory drugs
- Counsel patients regarding symptoms that may suggest an alternative diagnosis or require immediate evaluation.
  - Progressive weakness
  - Urinary retention
  - Constitutional symptoms

Considerations in Special Populations

- Sports medicine considerations
  - Look for abnormalities in the kinetic chain that may predispose to injury
  - Consider dynamic gait examination
  - Consider training habits that predispose to overuse injury with attention to frequency, intensity, duration, hill running, and so on.
  - Consider appropriate footwear.

Suggested Reading

- Beatty R: The piriformis syndrome: A simple diagnostic maneuver. Neurosurgery 1994;34:512–514.
- Benzon HT, Katz J: Piriformis syndrome: Anatomic considerations, a new injection technique, and a review of the literature. Anesthesiology 2003;98:1442–1448.
- Fishman LM, Konnoth C, Rozner B: Botulinum neurotoxin type B and physical therapy in the treatment of piriformis syndrome: A dose-finding study. Am J Phys Med Rehabil 2004;83:42–50.
- Foster M: Piriformis syndrome. Orthopedics 2002;25:821–825.
- Koes B, van Tulder M, Peul W: Diagnosis and treatment of sciatica. Br Med J 2007;334:1313–1317.
- Shah S, Wang T: Piriformis syndrome. Available at www.emedicine.com/sports/topic102.htm. Accessed December 12, 2008.

Chapter 126 Osteitis Pubis

Duane R. Hennion and Kevin deWeber

Key Concepts

- A self-limited inflammatory, overuse disorder of the pubic symphysis and surrounding tendinous attachments (Fig. 126-1)
- The pubic symphysis is composed of a nonsynovial amphiarthrodial joint that articulates through a fibrocartilaginous disc.
- It is hypothesized that shearing forces across the pubic symphysis cause inflammation of the joint and the surrounding periosteum.
- The exact mechanism of injury remains unclear; likely contributing biomechanical factors include
    - Repetitive adductor muscle contractions pull at their origins on the inferior pubic rami
    - Sacroiliac joint instability leading to a secondary stress reaction at the pubic symphysis
    - Limited hip motion with resultant shearing stress applied to the opposite hemipelvis
    - Excessive pelvic motion (frontal, up-and-down, or horizontal side-to-side sway)
- The disorder is common in sports that require rapid acceleration and deceleration, running, kicking, or rapid change of direction (i.e., running, hockey, soccer).
- It usually occurs during the third or fourth decade of life and is more common in men. The exact incidence is unknown.

History

- Gradual onset of progressively worsening unilateral or bilateral groin pain
- May be accompanied by pain in the lower abdomen, hip, thigh, testicle, or perineum
- Sharp, stabbing, or burning pain; less often described as dull or achy
- Exacerbated by activity, specifically running, pivoting, kicking, and frequent acceleration and deceleration maneuvers; sit-ups may cause pain; may have difficulty lying in bed at night
- If instability is present, may describe audible or palpable clicking sensation at the pubic symphysis with certain activities (e.g., arising from a seated position, turning in bed, walking on uneven surfaces)
- Typically no definitive history of injury

Physical Examination

- Tenderness to palpation over the pubic symphysis and adjacent areas of the superior and/or inferior pubic rami
- Passive hip abduction or resisted hip adduction may elicit pain (localized to the groin).
- May demonstrate decreased internal rotation of the hip
- The pubic spring test may be positive.
    - Apply pressure to both the left and right pubic rami to reproduce the pain at the pubic symphysis. Press the rami alternately to determine whether the pain lateralizes to one side.
- The lateral compression test may be positive.
    - Pain in the pubic symphysis area with lateral compression over the iliac wing with the patient in the lateral decubitus position
- In severe cases, the patient may develop a wide-based (antalgic) gait.

Imaging

Plain radiographs (anteroposterior and lateral) (Fig. 126-2)

- Radiographic abnormalities can lag behind clinical symptoms by 4 weeks and will likely be normal early in the disease course.
- Typical findings include symmetrical bone resorption at the medial ends of the pubic bones, widening of the pubic symphysis (>7 mm), and sclerosis along the pubic rami.
- Flamingo views (if instability of pubic symphysis suspected): one-legged, standing view; instability is defined as greater than 2 mm of vertical shift between the superior rami of the pubic symphysis.

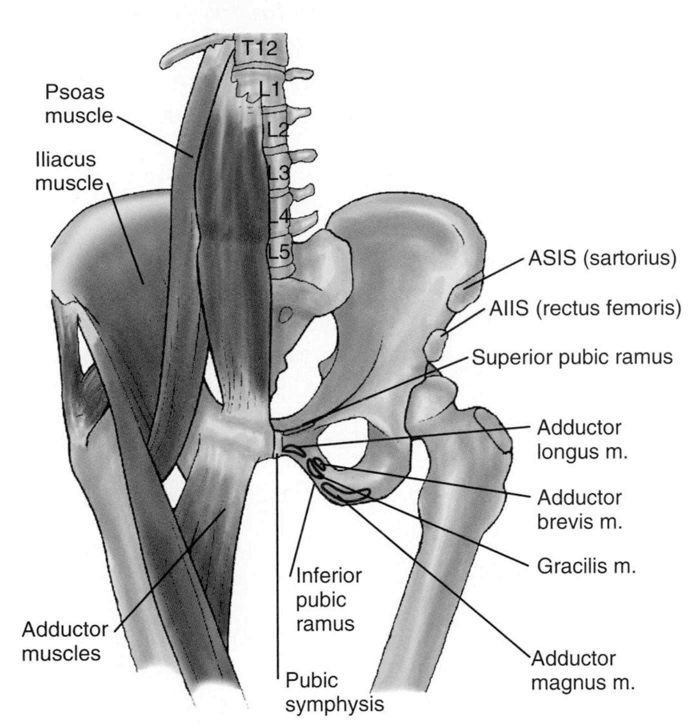

Figure 126-1 Muscles and muscle origins around the pubic symphysis. AIIS, anteroinferior iliac spine; ASIS, anterosuperior iliac spine; m, muscle.

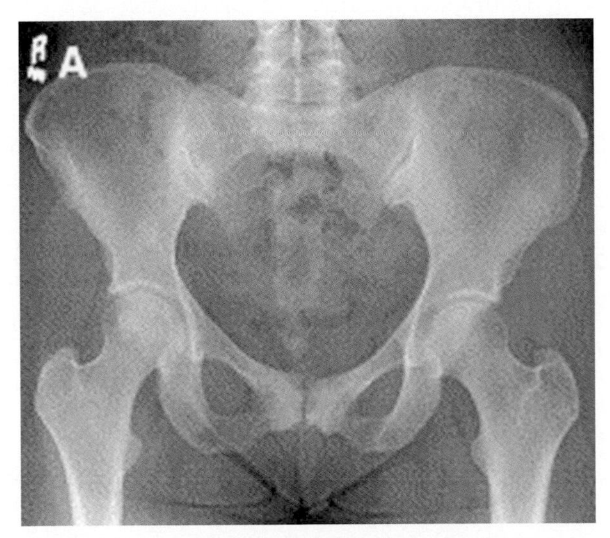

Figure 126-2 Anteroposterior radiograph demonstrating characteristic changes of osteitis pubis. (From Nelson EN, Kassarjian A, Palmer WE: MR imaging of sports-related groin pain. Magn Reson Imaging Clin N Am 2005;13:727–742.)

- Radionuclide bone scan
  - Increased uptake at the pubic symphysis, especially on the delayed views
  - May be positive early in the disease course
- Radiographic and radionuclide findings do not correlate well with severity or duration of disease.

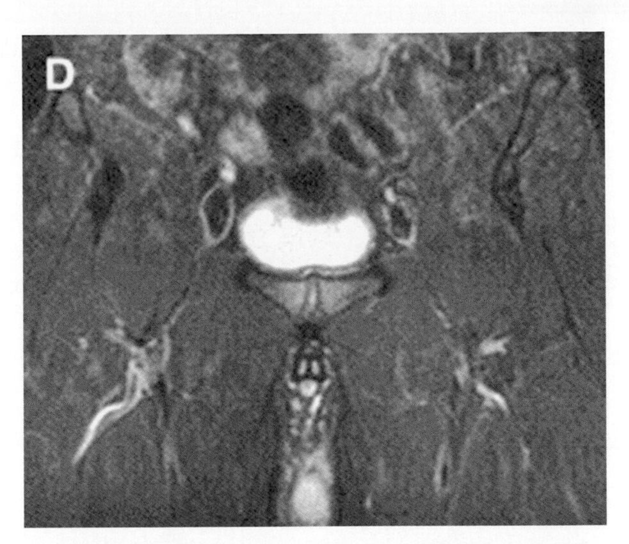

Figure 126-3 Magnetic resonance imaging demonstrating bone marrow edema on each side of the symphysis and fluid within the disc. (From Nelson EN, Kassarjian A, Palmer WE: MR imaging of sports-related groin pain. Magn Reson Imaging Clin N Am 2005;13:727–742.)

- Magnetic resonance imaging (MRI) (pelvis) (Fig. 126-3)
  - Ever-growing use in the diagnosis of osteitis pubis; consider MRI if symptoms are present for more than 6 weeks and not improving
  - Bone marrow edema, fluid in the pubic symphysis joint, and periarticular edema are reliable MRI findings of osteitis pubis of less than 6 months' duration. Subchondral sclerosis or resorption, bony margin irregularities, and osteophytes (or pubic "beaking") are reliable MRI findings of osteitis pubis present for more than 6 months.

Additional Tests

- If there is a sudden, atraumatic onset of signs and symptoms of osteitis pubis with subsequent development of a fever (or subjective chills), one must consider osteomyelitis of the pubic symphysis. A complete blood count with differential and an erythrocyte sedimentation rate are recommended as initial investigations. Consider urinalysis and blood cultures.

Differential Diagnosis

- Adductor strain (usually adductor longus muscle)
- Iliopsoas strain/bursitis
- Sports hernia
- Stress fracture (proximal femur, femoral neck, superior pubic ramus)

- Apophyseal avulsion fractures (skeletally immature athletes)
- Entrapment neuropathy (ilioinguinal nerve)
- Snapping hip syndrome
- Intra-articular hip pathology
- Inguinal hernia
- Lumbar disc disease
- Seronegative spondyloarthropathies (Reiter syndrome or ankylosing spondylitis)
- Osteomyelitis
- Urinary tract infection
- Prostatitis
- Urolithiasis
- Abdominal disorders

Treatment

- At diagnosis
  - Pain-producing activity should be avoided; encourage relative rest to maintain state of general fitness.
  - Course of nonsteroidal anti-inflammatory drug therapy
  - Consider a short course of oral corticosteroids for severe pain.
  - Physical rehabilitation is the cornerstone of therapy. Begin a graduated, stepwise approach to therapy (restore range of motion, strength exercises, sport-specific exercise) that emphasizes stretching and strengthening of the hip joint muscles (specifically hip adductors, flexors, and rotators).
  - Maintain a physical therapy program focusing on the muscles of the pelvis, back, and abdomen; include a core strengthening program.
- Later
  - The use of intra-articular steroid injections is controversial. Steroid injections have been used with variable results in case reports and small nonrandomized studies. Further well-designed study protocols are needed to evaluate treatment efficacy.
  - Any observed biomechanical abnormalities should be corrected.

When to Refer

- Chronic cases (>6 months' duration) that are unresponsive to conservative therapy and/or demonstrate vertical instability of the pubic symphysis may warrant operative treatment.
- Local débridement and arthrodesis of the pubic symphysis using bone grafting and compression plates have been described with successful results.

Prognosis

- Self-limited condition with average healing time of 3 to 12 months
- Successful symptom resolution occurs in 90% to 95% of cases with structured conservative rehabilitation program; the recurrence rate is 25%.
- Return to play when the patient is pain free with activity, has full range of motion of the hip, and strength greater than 90% of the contralateral hip/leg.

Troubleshooting

- Maintain a high index of suspicion for constitutional symptoms to help differentiate osteitis pubis from osteomyelitis of the pubic symphysis.

Patient Instructions

- This is a self-limited condition that typically resolves in 3 to 12 months with rest.
- Continue a fitness program that does not aggravate symptoms but provides cardiovascular fitness benefit.
- Flexibility training is a key component of therapy and should become a part of the athlete's daily routine.

Considerations in Special Populations

- In skeletally immature populations, consider apophyseal avulsion injuries.

Suggested Reading

- Andrews SK, Carek PJ: Osteitis pubis: A diagnosis for the family physician. J Am Board Fam Pract 1998;11:291–295.
- Disabella VN: Osteitis pubis. Available at www.emedicine.com/sports/topic90.htm. Accessed December 12, 2008.
- Fricker PA, Taunton JE, Ammann W: Osteitis pubis in athletes: Infection, inflammation, or injury? Sports Med 1991;12:266–279.
- Johnson R: Osteitis pubis. Curr Sports Med Rep 2003;2:98–102.
- Naticchia J, Kapur E: New technology, new injuries in the hip/groin. Clin Fam Pract 2005;7:267–278.
- Vitanzo PC, McShane JM: Osteitis pubis. Phys Sports Med 2001;29:33–38.

Chapter 127 Groin Strain (Adductor Injury)

Sarah McGinley

ICD-9 CODES
848.8 *Adductor Strain*
726.5 *Enthesopathy of the Hip Region (Glutei, Piriformis, Adductor Longus and Brevis)*

Key Concepts

- Groin (adductor) strain is a common injury in athletes, especially those in sports that involve cutting, such as soccer, football, ice hockey, basketball, and tennis.
- Among soccer players, the incidence rates range between 10% and 18%.
- High forces occur in the adductor tendons when an athlete moves from side to side or suddenly shifts directions. The adductor muscles contract to generate opposing forces to stabilize the hip and pelvis.
- Strains and adductor muscle/tendon ruptures result from repetitive contractions or a single forced contraction of the adductor muscles, while the thigh is in an externally rotated and abducted position (adductors are eccentrically contracted).
- The adductor muscle group is made up of the adductor magnus, minimus, longus, and brevis, along with the gracilis and pectineus. All the adductor muscles are innervated by the obturator nerve (L2-L4) except the pectineus (femoral nerve, L2-L4) and the adductor magnus (tibial nerve (L2-S3) (Fig. 127-1).
- Decreased abductor range of motion and decreased adductor strength have been associated with an increased incidence of adductor strains.
- Biomechanical abnormalities (i.e., excessive pronation or leg length discrepancy), imbalance of the surrounding hip and abdominal musculature, and muscular fatigue have also been postulated to increase the risk of adductor strain.
- Returning athletes to play before pain-free, sport-specific activities can be performed can lead to chronic injury.

History

- Groin pain localized to the adductors
- May be an insidious onset with progressive pain or a sudden, painful event, especially after a sudden change in direction or sudden increase in acceleration (stationary to sprinting)
- In an acute injury, the patient reports "ripping" or "stabbing" pain in the groin or the medial thigh that is intensified with passive abduction.
- In a chronic adductor injury, the pain is described as a diffuse dull ache that may radiate distally along the medial aspect of the thigh and/or proximally toward the rectus.
- Initial intense pain often lasts less than a second and is replaced by an intense dull ache.

Physical Examination

- Most strains occur at the musculotendinous junction of the adductor longus.
- Palpable tenderness, ecchymosis, and swelling can be observed at the superior medial thigh or along the course of the adductor muscles.
- With some adductor tears, a defect can be palpated.
- Marked tenderness directly over the pubis raises the possibility of an avulsion fracture.
- Pain is reproduced with resisted adduction and full passive abduction of the hip.
- To distinguish a pure hip adductor strain from other combined injuries involving the hip flexors (i.e., iliopsoas, rectus femoris), have the patient lie in the supine position. If more pain is elicited with resistive adduction when the knee and hip are extended than if the hip and knee are flexed, then a pure hip adductor strain can be assumed.
- A detailed and thorough examination, along with an understanding of the anatomy, will help distinguish

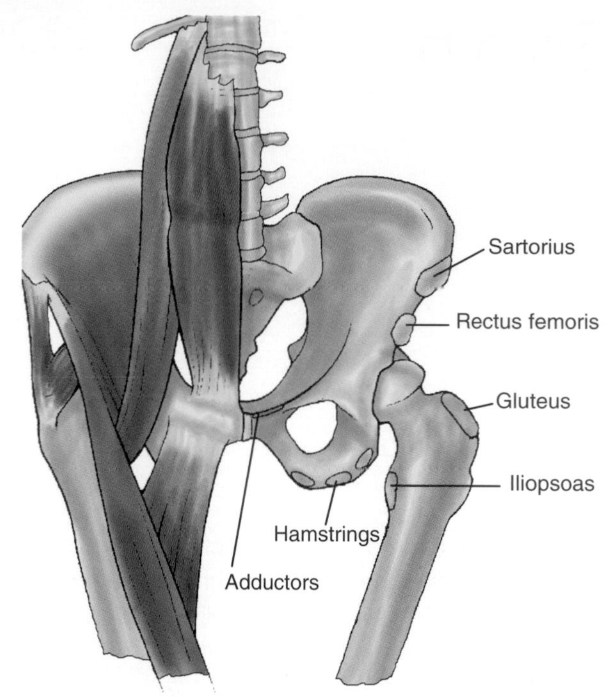

Figure 127-1 Applied anatomy of the groin. (From Morelli V, Weaver V: Groin injuries and groin pain in athletes: Part 1. Prim Care 2005;32:163–183, Fig. 1.)

adductor strains from other causes of groin pain (Table 127-1 and Fig. 127-2).

Imaging

- Plain radiographs can help distinguish adductor strain from late-stage osteitis pubis and/or confirm the presence of an avulsion fracture.
- Although rare, plain radiographs may show myositis ossificans of the adductor longus, indicating chronicity or previous injury to the muscle.
- Radiographs: The anteroposterior view with the athlete standing on one leg (flamingo view) helps to better evaluate the pubic symphysis.
- Ultrasonography is somewhat useful for diagnosing muscle and tendon tears as well as further evaluating a mass, but is less useful for strains.
- Magnetic resonance imaging can confirm muscle strains or tears as well as partial and complete tendon tears (Fig. 127-3).
- Magnetic resonance imaging can yield prognostic information about muscle tears: tears greater than 50% of the cross-sectional area, tissue fluid collection, and deep muscle tears may indicate more severe injury and a prolonged recovery.
- Computed tomography scans can also confirm complete or partial adductor tears as well as help distinguish acute from chronic injuries if calcium deposition within the muscle is present.
- Technetium-99m has no role in adductor strain diagnosis, but may be helpful if the physician is concerned about osteitis pubis or acute avulsion fracture (see Chapter 126).

Additional Tests

- None for adductor strain, but if genitourinary pathology is suspected, a urinalysis, complete blood count, and genital cultures may be pertinent
- The history and physical examination should guide the physician to order the appropriate tests and studies.

Differential Diagnosis

- Please see Table 127-1.

Treatment

- At diagnosis
  - Acute pain
    - — Protection and relative rest (avoid painful activities, can consider using crutches for a few days)
    - — Ice and compression
    - — Short course of nonsteroidal anti-inflammatory drugs can also be given
    - — Modalities such as electrical stimulation can help alleviate muscle spasm.
    - — Passive range of motion exercises can be started when the patient can perform these without pain; beginning stretches too early may result in chronic groin strain.
    - — Active range of motion exercises can be advanced slowly from isometric contractions without resistance to isometrics with resistance, progressing eventually to dynamic exercises when tolerated with little or no pain.
- Later
  - Pain has improved
    - — After passive and active range of motion has been achieved, rehabilitation should incorporate strengthening abdominal and hip flexor muscles.
    - — Coactivation of the abdominal muscles and the adductor muscles is a useful functional exercise.
    - — Completing several repetitions increases the endurance of the adductors; gradually progress to 30 to 40 repetitions.

TABLE 127-1 *Differentiating Groin Pain from an Adductor Strain*

Condition	Differentiating Features	Chapter Reference/Comments
Iliopsoas strain, iliopsoas bursitis	Occurs in activities requiring extensive use of hip flexors. Hip flexion against resistance is painful. Tenderness is difficult to localize due to the deep insertion of the iliopsoas on the femur. Magnetic resonance imaging can help determine the diagnosis.	122, 124
Osteitis pubis	Palpable tenderness at the symphysis pubis, possible loss of full rotation of one or both hips, positive gap test, positive lateral compression test. Radiographs, magnetic resonance imaging, and/or bone scan can help determine the diagnosis.	126
Conjoined tendon lesions: sportsman's hernia, groin disruption	The cause is multifactorial and thought to involve muscle imbalance with relatively strong adductors, weak lower abdominal musculature, increased shearing forces across the hemipelvis, overuse, and/or genetically weakened inguinal wall.	Hard to distinguish at times from adductor strains. If groin pain persists despite appropriate treatment of a strain, the physician should suspect a conjoined tendon lesion.
Sportsman's hernia	Controversy exists as to the presence of this condition. Insidious onset, gradually worsening deep groin pain. Pain increases with Valsalva maneuvers. Radiation of pain to testicles, inguinal ligament, perineum, and/or rectus muscles. Pain located more laterally and proximally than in groin disruptions (Fig. 127-2) and/or distal rectus strain. No true hernia is palpated; only the deep fascia is violated.	126; Imaging cannot help with this diagnosis, but can rule out other causes of groin pain. Exploratory surgery with repair will aid in a more definitive diagnosis. A trial of conservative treatment should be attempted before surgery. With proper surgical intervention, a 90% success rate has been reported.
Groin disruption	Encompasses distinct anatomic abnormalities of the posterior wall such as tears of the transversalis fascia, external oblique, conjoined tendon or aponeurosis, avulsion of fibers of the internal oblique at the pubic tubercle, abnormalities at the insertion of the rectus abdominis, or dehiscence of the conjoined and inguinal ligaments. Presents with groin pain on exertion; pain with the Valsalva maneuver is uncommon. Pain with resisted adduction often present, pain with palpation (see Fig. 127-3), and pain while athlete performs a half sit-up.	Imaging cannot help with this diagnosis, but can rule out other causes of groin pain. Exploratory surgery with repair will aid in a more definitive diagnosis. A trial of conservative treatment should be attempted before surgery. Surgical repair typically leads to 87% to 95% successful return to preinjury level, usually within 12 weeks.
Obturator neuropathy/nerve entrapment	Presents with a deep ache near the adductor origin of the pubic bone that worsens with exercise and often resolves with rest. Pain may radiate down medial thigh toward the knee. Spasm, weakness, and paresthesias can also occur. Positive Howship-Romberg sign (medial knee pain induced by forced hip abduction, extension, and internal rotation). Electromyography can be helpful if done by a neurologist familiar with this area. Obturator nerve block can also support the diagnosis if the athlete's symptoms resolve and reproduce the adductor weakness.	22, 129
Also can consider sacroiliac dysfunction, pelvic/femoral stress fracture, hip osteoarthritis		123, 133, 136, 137

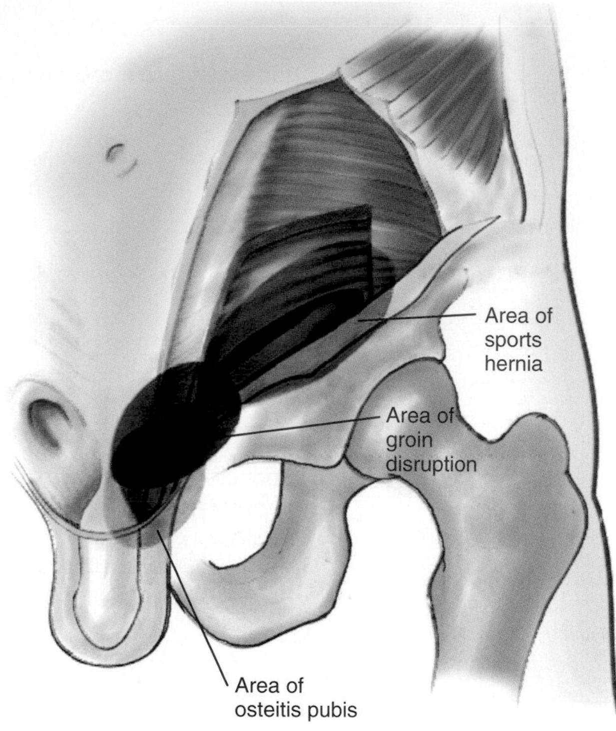

Figure 127-2 Landmarks for differentiating groin pain. (From Morelli V, Weaver V: Groin injuries and groin pain in athletes: Part 1. Prim Care 2005;32:163–183, Fig. 6.)

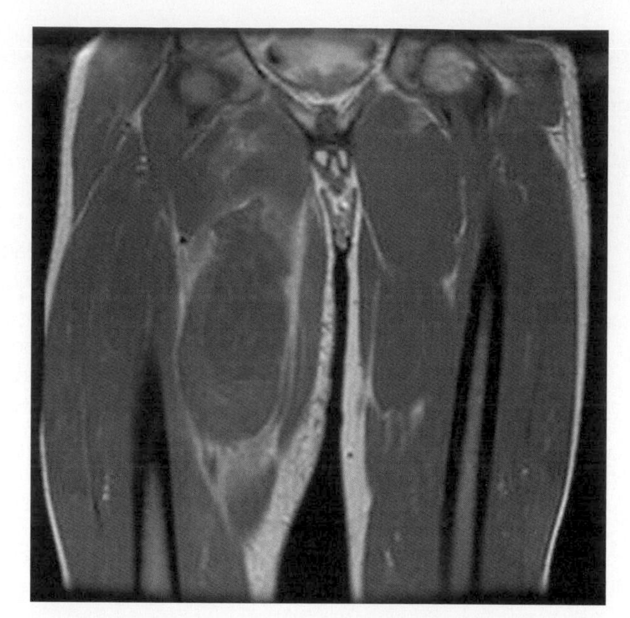
Figure 127-3 Coronal T1-weighted postgadolinium magnetic resonance image. Mass within adductor longus muscle, measuring 25 cm in length, 7.2 cm transversely, and 8.8 cm in width. This mass was consistent with a hematoma following a tear in the adductor longus muscle in a soccer player.

- — Fatigued muscle/tendon complex leaves it vulnerable to injury.
- — Proprioceptive exercises and stretches should also be incorporated at this stage.
- — Aquatic training can be helpful if it is available.
- — Sport-specific drills can be added after the patient has tolerated the described rehabilitation.
- — Assess for biomechanical abnormalities and correct those that are found.

When to Refer

- Patients with chronic adductor strains that fail to respond to at least 6 months of conservative treatment
- If a mass is palpated in the middle to upper thigh, consider a rupture of the musculotendinous structures and obtain imaging and refer to a surgeon.
- If obturator nerve entrapment is suspected, refer to a neurologist familiar with adductor injuries to obtain an electromyogram and assist with treatment.
- Appropriate referral is warranted if a medical condition is the cause of groin pain (i.e., gynecologist for ovarian pathology).

Prognosis

- Return to sports can take place when the athlete has restored at least 70% of strength and has pain-free full range of motion.
- Return to sports may take a few days to 8 weeks, depending on the severity of the injury (grade I, II, or II).
- In chronic adductor injuries, the rehabilitation may take 3 to 6 months before the patient can return to sports.
- If tendon repair is performed, the usual time to return to unrestricted sports activities is 10 to 12 weeks.

Troubleshooting

- Do not advance the patient too quickly back to his or her sport because this can lead to a chronic injury.
- Chronic strains are more difficult to manage and lead to a longer recovery time.
- The use of corticosteroid injections in adductor strains is controversial.
  - The potential for tendon rupture exists if the corticosteroid is injected into the tendon itself.
  - Some authorities advocate injection of a local anesthetic agent with or without corticosteroids into the tendon periosteal area if conservative treatment has been unsuccessful for 2 to 4 months.

- This treatment should be combined with 1 to 2 weeks of rest from activity after the injection.

Patient Instructions

- Follow physician, physical therapist, and/or athletic trainer instructions closely with respect to the type, quantity, and timing of exercises and activities that are acceptable.
- Home-based exercises, including stretching, are vital to overall management and should be performed regularly.
- Appropriate and aggressive pain management should be directed by a physician.

Considerations in Special Populations

- Those caring for athletes will commonly encounter this condition and should perform a thorough and careful history and physical examination and order appropriate tests to make the correct diagnosis and implement the right treatment plan.
- Treatment for athletes with adductor injuries requires a team approach and an understanding of the athlete's practice and competition schedule.
- It is important to emphasize that return to sports too soon can lead to chronic adductor strain.

Suggested Reading

- Ekstrand J, Gillquist J: The avoidability of soccer injuries. Int J Sports Med 1983;4:124–128.
- Hackney RG: The sports hernia: A cause of chronic groin pain. Br J Sports Med 1993;27:58–62.
- Harmon K: Evaluation of groin pain in athletes. Curr Sports Med Rep 2007;6:354–361.
- Martens MA, Hansen L, Mulier JC: Adductor tendinitis and musculus rectus abdominis tendopathy. Am J Sports Med 1987;15:353–356.
- Mens J, Inklaar H, Koes B, et al: A new view on adduction-related groin pain. Clin J Sports Med 2006;16:15–19.
- Morelli V, Weaver V: Groin injuries and groin pain in athletes: Part 1. Prim Care 2005;32:163–183.
- Morelli V, Weaver V: Groin injuries and groin pain in athletes: Part 2. Prim Care 2005;32:185–200.
- Tyler TF, Nicholas SJ, Campbell RJ, et al: The association of hip strength and flexibility with the incidence of adductor muscle strains in professional ice hockey players. Am J Sports Med 2001;29:124–128.
- Tyler TF, Nicholas SJ, Campbell RJ, et al: The effectiveness of a preseason exercise program to prevent adductor muscle strains in professional ice hockey players. Am J Sports Med 2002;30:680–683.

Chapter 128 Snapping Hip

Thomas A. Goodwin

Key Concepts

- Coxa saltans or snapping hip syndrome
- Most common in young, active women 15 to 40 years of age
- More common in sports that require repetitive hip flexion, extension, and abduction
    - Dancers, distance runners, rowers, and cyclists
    - Fifty percent to 90% of ballet dancers
- Three separate types have been defined: external, internal, and intra-articular (Table 128-1).
    - External
        - — Most common type
        - — Results when either a posteriorly thickened portion of the iliotibial band or thickened anterior fibers of the gluteus maximus muscle "snap" over the greater trochanter (Fig. 128-1)
    - Internal
        - — Occurs when the proximal portion of the iliopsoas tendon moves or snaps over a bony prominence, usually the iliopectineal eminence or femoral head; can cause resultant iliopsoas bursitis (Fig. 128-2)
    - Intra-articular
        - — Results from loose bodies, osteochondral fractures, labral tears, synovial chondromatosis, or underlying hip instability

History

- Patient reports audible and/or painful snapping, popping, or clicking sound/sensation with hip motion.
- Asymptomatic snapping is considered normal.
- External
    - Patients often report a snapping/popping/locking sensation in lateral hip.
    - Symptoms are exacerbated with repetitive hip flexion and extension.
    - Patients may have already adapted lifestyle modifications secondary to pain.
- Internal
    - Pain/snapping is anterior in nature
    - More painful than external
    - Symptoms are most common during exercise but may be present after it.
    - May progress from mildly painful snapping to debilitating pain
- Intra-articular
    - Painful clicking or grinding rather than audible snaps
    - Traumatic mechanism raises suspicion
    - Pain with adduction and internal rotation

Physical Examination

- Gait observation
    - Rule out muscular imbalance or neurologic impairment (i.e., Trendelenburg gait)
    - Patients often voluntarily demonstrate snapping.
- External
    - Tenderness over greater trochanter
    - Snapping is reproduced when the hip is flexed from an extended position.
    - Clicking/snapping is often audible and palpable over the greater trochanter.
    - If snapping is not demonstrated, tightening the iliotibial band with hip adduction and knee extension accentuates the snapping sensation.
    - Ober's test is frequently positive.
- Internal
    - Bringing the hip from the flexion, abduction, external rotation position to the extension, adduction, internal rotation position reproduces symptoms as the iliopsoas tendon snaps over the bony prominence (Fig. 128-3).
- Intra-articular
    - Pain with adduction and internal rotation
    - May note decreased internal rotation
    - The flexion, abduction, external rotation (FABER) test is often positive for inguinal pain.

Imaging

- Often unnecessary
- Plain radiographs typically normal unless underlying hip dysplasia or impingement

TABLE 128-1 *Differentiation of the Types of Snapping Hip*		
Type	**Anatomic Structure Implicated**	**Cause**
External	Greater trochanter	Iliotibial band or gluteus maximus muscle snapping over greater trochanter
Internal	Iliopsoas tendon	Iliopsoas tendon snapping over iliopectineal eminence or femoral head
Intra-articular	Hip joint	Loose bodies, osteochondral fractures, labral tears, synovial chondromatosis

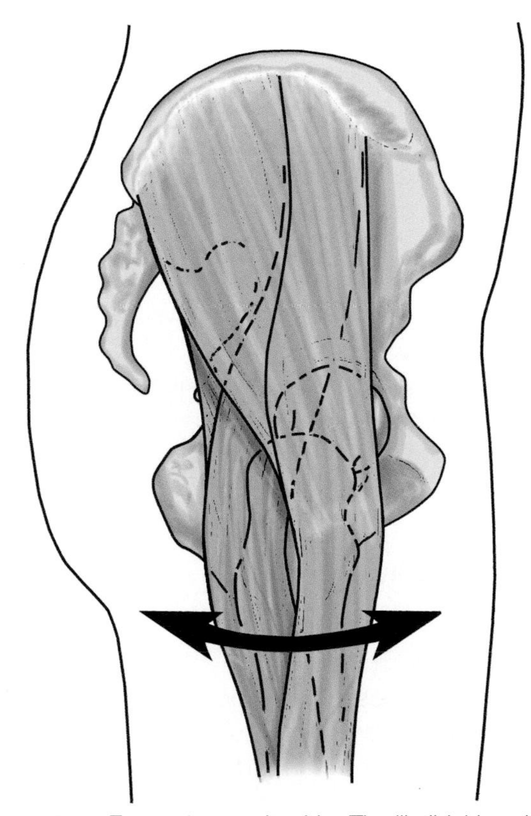

Figure 128-1 External snapping hip. The iliotibial band snaps back and forth over the greater trochanter, and the hip is moved between flexion and extension. (Adapted from Byrd JWT: Snapping hip. Oper Tech Sports Med 2005;13:46–54, Fig. 8.)

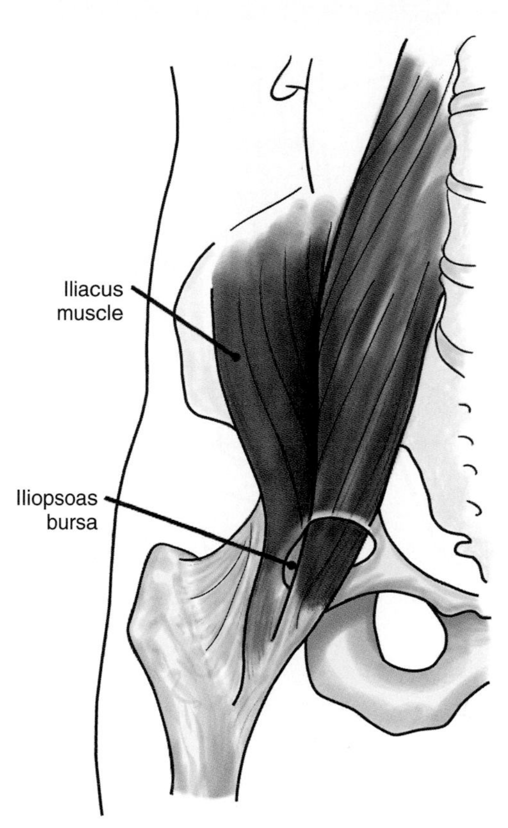

Figure 128-2 Iliopsoas bursa between the distal portion of the iliacus muscle and the psoas muscle. (Adapted from Morelli V, Weaver V: Groin injuries and groin pain in athletes: Part 1. Prim Care 2005;32:163–183, Fig. 3.)

- Dynamic ultrasonography preferred for external and internal varieties
  - May be able to view snapping of symptomatic tendon
  - May demonstrate tendinopathy
- Plain radiographs and computed tomography preferred if intra-articular pathology suspected
- Magnetic resonance arthrography if labral tear suspected
  - May also show signs of tendinopathy

Differential Diagnosis

- Iliotibial band syndrome
- Trochanteric bursitis
- Iliopsoas tendinitis/bursitis
- Osteoarthritis
- Femoral neck stress fracture
- Avascular necrosis
- Pediatric
  - Legg-Calvé-Perthes disease
  - Slipped capital femoral epiphysis
  - Inflammatory/infectious synovitis
  - Avulsion fracture

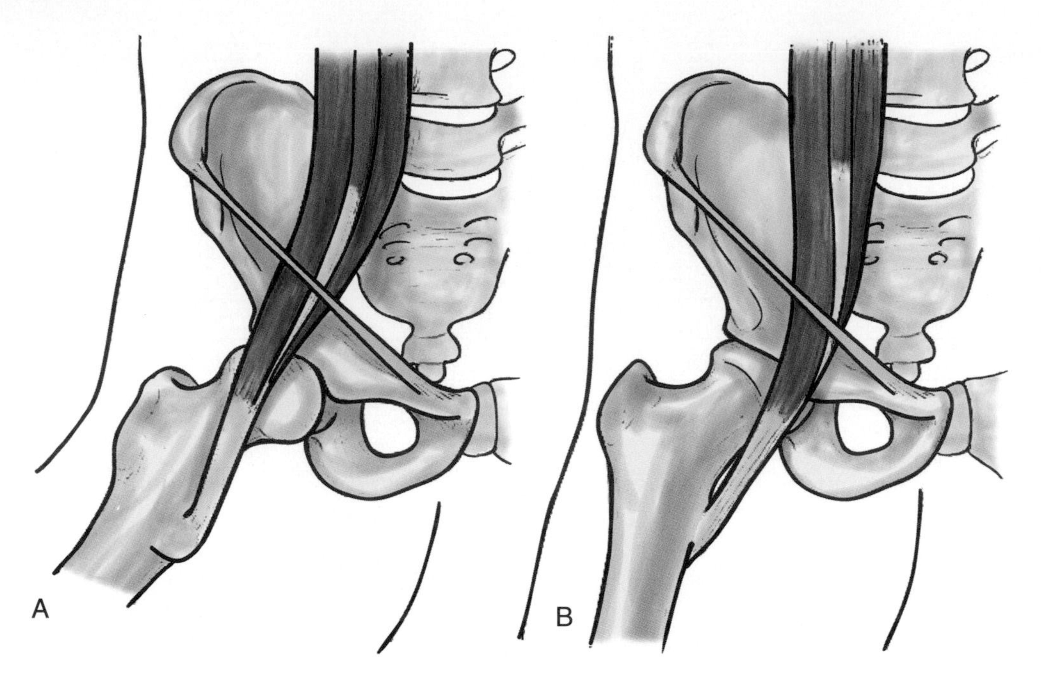

Figure 128-3 Internal snapping hip. The iliopsoas tendon snaps back and forth over the iliopectineal eminence. **A**, The hip shown in the FABER (flexion, abduction, external rotation) position. The iliopsoas tendon lies lateral to the center of the femoral head. **B**, The hip is brought into the EADIR (extension, adduction, internal rotation) position. The iliopsoas tendon snaps in the medial position. (Adapted from Byrd JWT: Snapping hip. Oper Tech Sports Med 2005;13:46–54, Fig. 1.)

Treatment

- At diagnosis
  - The primary goal is pain relief and correction of biomechanical factors.
  - Nonsteroidal anti-inflammatory drugs
  - Non–nonsteroidal anti-inflammatory analgesics
  - Manual medicine/osteopathic manipulation
    - — Conservative therapies are mainstay of treatment
  - Activity modification/relative rest
  - Formal physical therapy
    - — 6 to 8 weeks with aggressive stretching
    - — Ultrasound therapy, iontophoresis, cryotherapy, electrical stimulation as needed
  - Injection of trochanteric bursa (external) or iliopsoas bursa (internal) may be beneficial for diagnosis and treatment.
- Later
  - Aggressive, sport-specific physical therapy
  - Graded return to activity as symptoms allow

When to Refer

- Patients with symptoms after 3 to 6 months of conservative therapy
- Treatment considerations for external snapping hip include lengthening of the iliotibial band or Z-plasty, central excision or release of the iliotibial band, or excision of the trochanteric bursa.
- Treatment considerations for internal snapping hip include division or endoscopic release of the iliopsoas tendon.
- Strongly consider referral if intra-articular pathology discovered as often recalcitrant to conservative measures

Prognosis

- Excellent prognosis with few patients requiring surgical intervention
- Full return to activity likely after 6 to 8 weeks of appropriate conservative measures

Troubleshooting

- Internal and intra-articular snapping hips are difficult to distinguish clinically.
- Accurate diagnosis with appropriate modalities will ensure proper treatment.
- Correction of biomechanical factors may hasten recovery time.

Patient Instructions

- Continue stretching and strengthening exercises when pain subsides to minimize recurrence.
- Attempt to modify activity to avoid positions that predispose to hip snapping.
- If pain worsens with stretching and physical therapy, notify the physician immediately.

Considerations in Special Populations

- An external snapping hip can be seen in geriatric patients after hip arthroplasty due to lateral displacement of the greater trochanter.
- With pediatric patients, the presence of hip dysplasia and/or instability may predispose to intra-articular snapping hip.

Suggested Reading

- Anderson K, Strickland SM, Warren R: Hip and groin injuries in athletes. Am J Sports Med 2001;29:521–533.
- Byrd JWT: Snapping hip. Oper Tech Sports Med 2005;13:46–54.
- Dobbs MB, Gordon E, Luhmann SJ, et al: Surgical correction of the snapping iliopsoas tendon in adolescents. J Bone Joint Surg Am 2002;84A:420–424.
- Kelly BT, Williams RJ, Philippon MJ: Hip arthroscopy: Current indications, treatment options, and management issues. Am J Sports Med 2003;31:1020–1037.
- Morelli V, Smith V: Groin injuries in athletes. Am Fam Physician 2001;64:1405–1414.
- Wahl CJ, Warren RF, Adler RS, et al: Internal coxa saltans (snapping hip) as a result of overtraining: A report of 3 cases in professional athletes with a review of causes and the role of ultrasound in early diagnosis and management. Am J Sports Med 2004;32:1302–1309.
- Winston P, Awan R, Cassidy JD, Bleakney RK: Clinical examination and ultrasound of self-reported snapping hip syndrome in elite ballet dancers. Am J Sports Med 2007;35:118–126.

Chapter 129 Meralgia Paresthetica

Mark B. Rogers

ICD-9 CODE
355.1 *Meralgia Paresthetica*

Key Concepts

- Also known as lateral femoral cutaneous nerve compression, syndrome, or entrapment; Bernhardt-Roth disease, syndrome, or paresthesia; and British officer's cavalry disease
- Mononeuropathy of lateral femoral cutaneous nerve (from the primary ventral rami of L2 and L3 roots)
- Purely sensory nerve that innervates anterolateral thigh (Fig. 129-1)
    - Anterior branch innervates the anterior thigh to the knee
    - Posterior branch innervates the lateral thigh
- Diagnosis made primarily on history and physical examination; additional studies may help confirm the diagnosis
- Most common cause of damage is from entrapment at level of inguinal ligament
- Incidence rates reported three to four cases per 10,000 primary care patients
    - Male sex predominance
    - Obesity (body mass index ≥ 30)
    - Most prevalent in the fifth and sixth decades
    - Eighty percent of cases are unilateral
    - May have a genetic component
- Generally self-limiting over weeks to months

History

- Commonly presents with burning, numbness, tingling, and pain of the anterolateral thigh
- Although not absolute, standing and hip extension often aggravate symptoms, whereas sitting and hip flexion may relieve symptoms
- Mechanical causes
    - Direct trauma
    - Anatomic variants (Fig. 129-2)

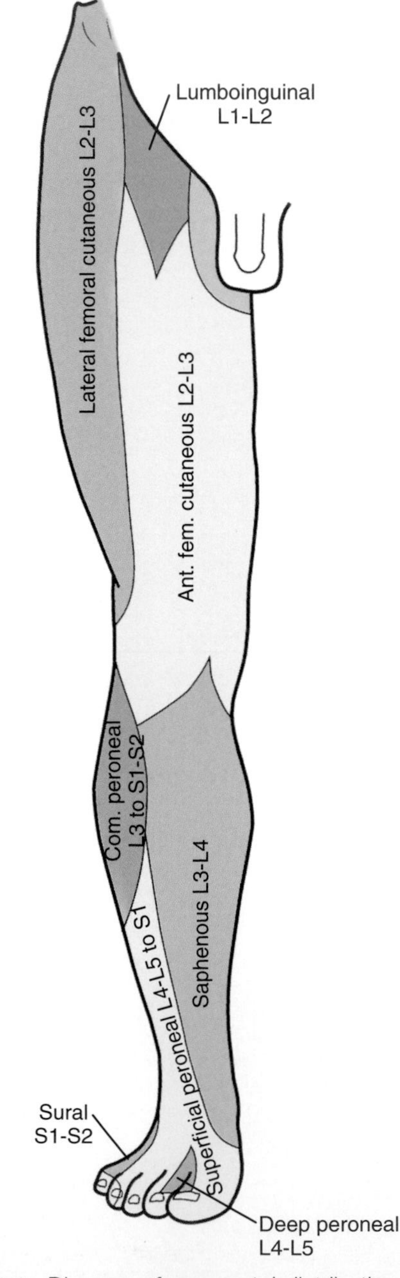

Figure 129-1 Diagram of segmental distribution of the cutaneous nerves of the right lower extremity. Front view.

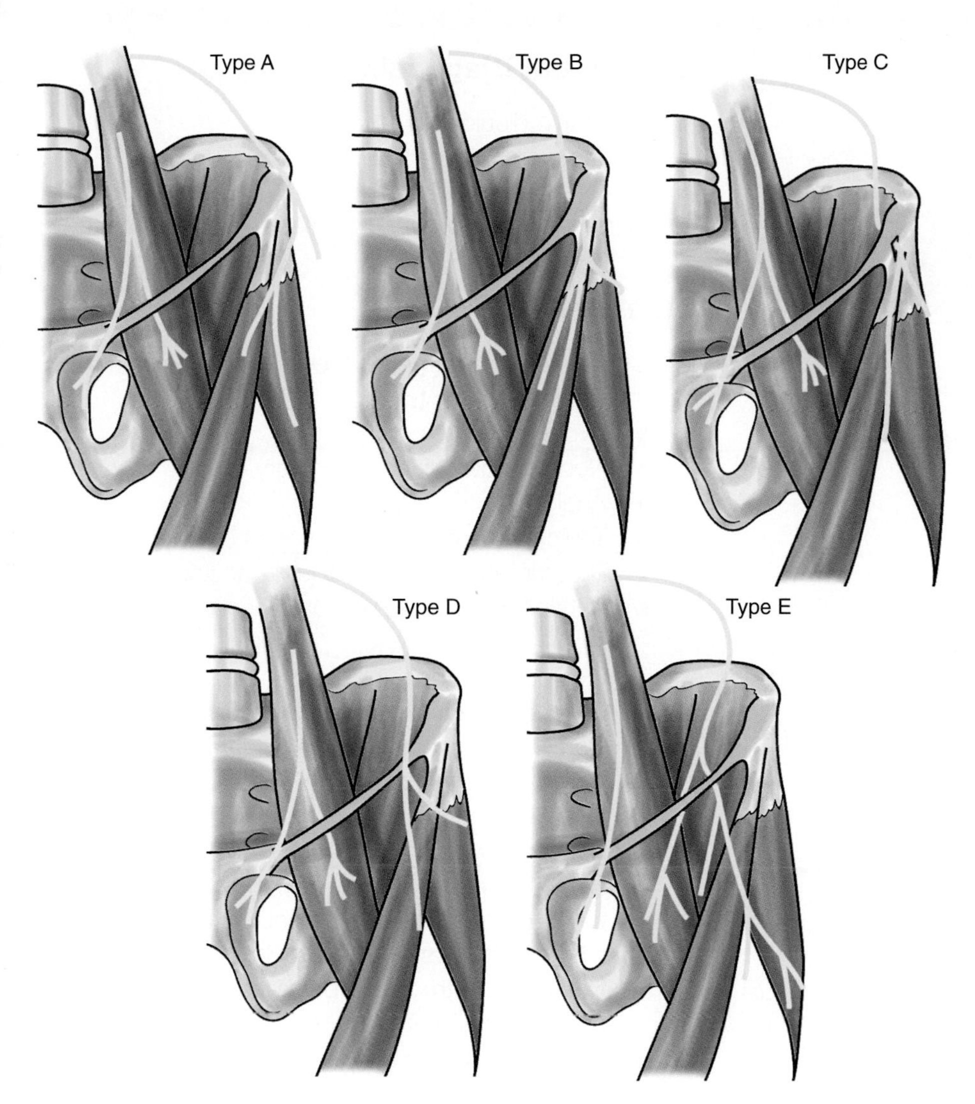

Figure 129-2 Variation of the course of the lateral femoral cutaneous nerve as it exits the abdomen. Type A (4%) courses across the iliac crest. In type B, it may be ensheathed by the inguinal ligament (27%). In type C (23%), it is ensheathed in the tendinous origin of the sartorius muscle. In type D (26%), it is deep to inguinal ligament and medial to sartorius muscle. In type E (20%), it is medial to iliopsoas muscle, contributing the femoral branch to the genitofemoral nerve. (Adapted with permission from Aszmann OC, Dellon ES, Dellon AL: Plast Reconstr Surg 1997;100:600–604.)

- Seatbelts
- Gun or hammer holsters
- Tight trousers
- Leg length discrepancy
- Pregnancy
- Obesity or rapid weight changes
- Intra-abdominal tumors
- Bone tumors
- Postsurgical (various surgeries and procedures reported in the literature)

- Metabolic causes
  - Diabetes, through one of two mechanisms: (1) abnormalities in metabolism of pyruvate, sorbitol, and lipids resulting in slowed nerve conduction or (2) swelling of the nerve due to decreased axoplasmic transport, making it more vulnerable to compression
  - Thyroid disease
  - Alcoholism
  - Inflammatory diseases (e.g., systemic lupus erythematosus)
  - Lead poisoning

Physical Examination

- The patient will not demonstrate gross motor deficits or reflex changes.
- Palpation over a point 1 cm inferior and 1 cm medial to the anterior superior iliac spine may reproduce symptoms or pain (depending on the anatomic course of the lateral femoral cutaneous nerve).
- The patient may have a positive Tinel's sign at this point as well.
- Positive pelvic compression test (Fig. 129-3)
- Appropriate physical examination to rule out lumbar disc disease (see appropriate section)

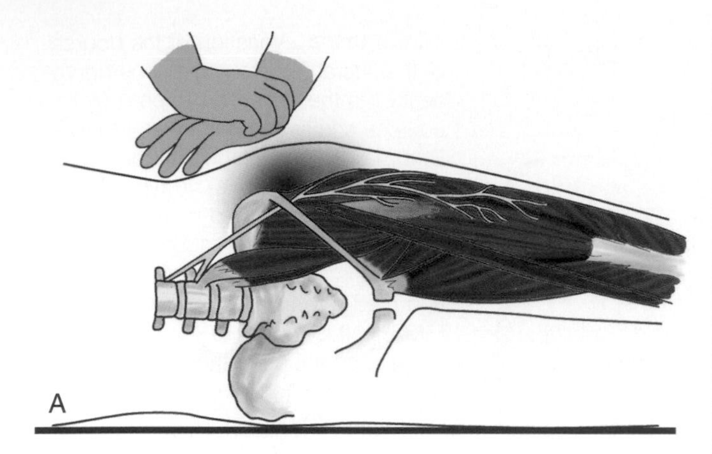

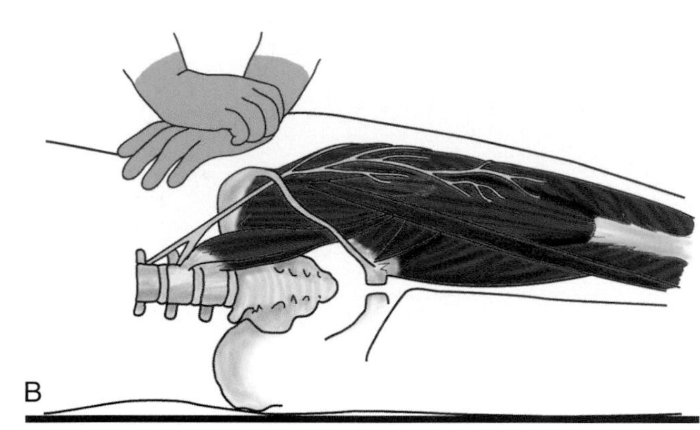

Figure 129-3 Pelvic compression test. **A**, The patient is positioned in the lateral recumbent position. **B**, Downward pressure is applied and maintained for approximately 45 seconds. A positive test result is when the patient's symptoms improve. (Adapted with permission from Nouraei SAR, Anand B, Spink G, O'Neill KS: A novel approach to the diagnosis and management of meralgia paresthetica. Neurosurgery 2007;60:696–700.)

Imaging

- Radiographs are often obtained to assess the lumbar and pelvic architecture and to rule out bony tumors.
- Ultrasonography may be useful to evaluate the course and morphology of the nerve.
- Magnetic resonance imaging may also be useful to further evaluate and rule out other etiologies.
- Additional tests
  - Complete blood count
  - Erythrocyte sedimentation rate
  - C-reactive protein
  - Complete metabolic panel
  - Urinalysis
  - Electromyography may help to rule out lumbar plexopathies.
  - Nerve conduction studies
  - Somatosensory evoked potentials

Differential Diagnosis

- Lumbar radiculopathy
- Lumbosacral plexopathies
- Femoral neuropathy
- Increased retroperitoneal pressure from a tumor

Treatment

- Conservative treatment relieves symptoms in more than 90% of patients.
  - Avoid compressive agents.
  - Nonsteroidal anti-inflammatory drugs
  - Analgesics
  - Topical creams (e.g., capsaicin)
  - Tricyclic antidepressants (e.g., amitriptyline)
  - Anticonvulsants (e.g., gabapentin, carbamazepine)
  - Five percent lidocaine patch
  - Local anesthetic injection with or without steroids
  - Osteopathic manipulation
  - Weight loss, if appropriate
  - Heel lift, if appropriate
- Surgical management
  - Refer for surgery as an option only when symptoms are intractable and disabling despite conservative measures for at least 6 months.
  - Neurolysis with decompression of lateral femoral cutaneous nerve
  - Resection of a portion of lateral femoral cutaneous nerve

Troubleshooting

- Typically, it is a benign, self-resolving disease; however, if there is no improvement despite conservative measures or if the history and physical examination suggest another etiology, consider further workup.

Patient Instructions

- Educate the patient about the typically benign nature of the diagnosis.
- Avoid compressive agents (e.g., hammer or gun holsters, cell phones, tight trousers, girdles).
- Weight loss, if indicated

Considerations in Special Populations

- In children, the course of symptoms may be more chronic, and symptoms are more often bilateral when compared with adults.

- They also frequently occur in those with a slimmer body habitus.

Suggested Reading

- Aszmann OC, Dellon ES, Dellon AL: Anatomical course of the lateral femoral cutaneous nerve and its susceptibility to compression and injury. Plast Reconstr Surg 1997;100:600–604.
- Ducic I, Dellon AL, Taylor NS: Decompression of the lateral femoral cutaneous nerve in the treatment of meralgia paresthetica. J Reconstr Microsurg 2006;22:113–117.
- Grossman MG, Ducey SA, Nadler SS, Levy AS: Meralgia paresthetica: Diagnosis and treatment. J Am Acad Orthop Surg 2001;9:336–344.
- Haim A, Pritsch T, Ben-Galim P, Dekel S: Meralgia paresthetica: A retrospective analysis of 79 patients evaluated and treated according to a standard algorithm. Acta Orthop 2006;77:482–486.
- Noureai SAR, Anand B, Spink G, O'Neill KS: A novel approach to the diagnosis and management of meralgia paresthetica. Neurosurgery 2007;60:696–700.
- Richer LP, Shevell MI, Stewart J, Poulin C: Pediatric meralgia paresthetica. Pediatr Neurol 2002;26:321–323.
- van Slobbe AM, Bohnen AM, Bernsen RM, et al: Incidence rates and determinants in meralgia paresthetica in general practice. J Neurol 2004;251:294–297.

Chapter 130 Trochanteric Bursitis

Howard McGowan and Kevin deWeber

ICD-9 CODE
726.5 *Bursitis of Hip, Trochanteric Area*

Key Concepts

- Trochanteric bursitis, a common cause of lateral hip pain, is associated with tenderness over or around the greater trochanter.
- There are at least three bursal sacs present around the greater trochanter area that can become inflamed (Fig. 130-1)
  - The subgluteus maximus bursa lying lateral to the greater trochanteric process of the femur and deep to the iliotibial tract
  - The subgluteus medius bursa superior and posterior to the greater trochanteric process beneath the gluteus medius tendon
  - The subgluteus minimus bursa lying anterior and superior to the proximal surface of the greater trochanteric process of the femur
- Trochanteric bursitis is commonly due to irritation of one or more of the bursal sacs.
- Ten percent to 20% of all patients presenting to primary care with hip problems have trochanteric pain.
- Incidence of 1.8 patients per 1000 per year
- The prevalence in patients with low back pain has been reported to be 20% to 35%.
- Affects women four times more frequently than men and peaks between the fourth and sixth decades
- Predisposing factors include
  - Gluteus medius dysfunction
  - Hip osteoarthritis
  - Degenerative disc disease of the lumbar spine
  - Iliotibial band syndrome
  - Leg length discrepancy
  - Gait abnormalities
  - Excessive pronation
  - Poor footwear
  - Increased or excessive training

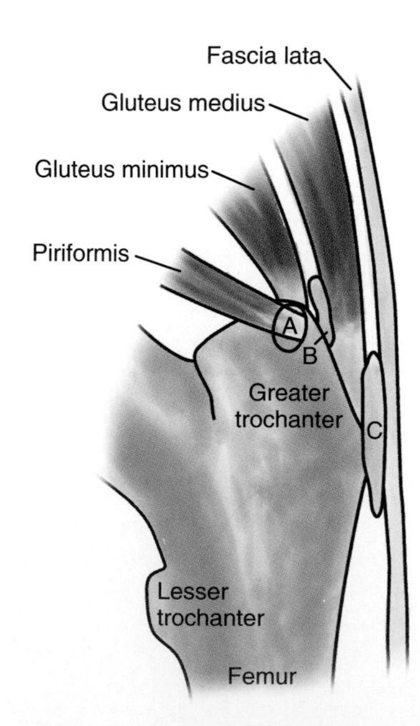

Figure 130-1 There are at least three bursal sacs present around the greater trochanter area that can become inflamed. A, Subgluteus minimus bursa; B, subgluteus medius bursa; C, subgluteus maximus bursa.

History

- The most common symptom is lateral hip pain.
- The pain worsens with direct pressure over the lateral hip.
- Running, climbing stairs, and transitioning from a lying or sitting to a standing position all exacerbate the pain.
- The pain can radiate down the medial or lateral thigh.

Physical Examination

- Localized tenderness over the greater trochanter is the most frequently encountered examination finding.
- Symptoms can be reproduced by abducting and externally rotating the hip.

- Passive and active range of motion of the hip should be assessed. Painful or limited range of motion, especially internal rotation, should alert the clinician to possible intra-articular pathology.
- Muscle strength testing of the hip should be assessed, and causes including lumbosacral pathology or gluteus medius or minimus tendon disruption should be explored if weakness is discovered.
- Ober's test may reveal a tight iliotibial band.
- A lumbosacral examination is essential to evaluate for lumbosacral disease.
- Gait assessment may reveal a leg length discrepancy, weak hip external rotation, or other mechanical problems.

Imaging

- Plain radiographs of the affected hip should be performed to evaluate for intra-articular pathology.
- Bone scintigraphy can help confirm disease and allow evaluation of other entities associated with trochanteric bursitis.
- Magnetic resonance imaging may be helpful in confirming disease and/or excluding other causes of lateral hip pain in patients not responding to therapy.

Additional Tests

- An injection of a local anesthetic agent into the trochanteric bursal area at the point of maximal tenderness should provide at least partial relief (Fig. 130-2).
- A complete blood count, erythrocyte sedimentation rate, or C-reactive protein test can be considered in patients with signs or symptoms of an infectious process.

Differential Diagnosis

- Degenerative disc disease
- Lumbar disc herniation
- Hip osteoarthritis
- Gluteus medius or minimus tear

Treatment

- At diagnosis (in early stages when acutely painful)
  - Pain relief is the primary goal.
    - — Nonsteroidal or non–nonsteroidal anti-inflammatory drugs
    - — Relative rest/activity modification
    - — Ice
    - — Gentle stretching
    - — An injection of a local anesthetic/corticosteroid solution into the affected bursa can provide rapid and long-lasting relief if the previously listed measures are inadequate (Table 130-1).
- Later (once pain free)
  - Correct precipitating factors to include muscular imbalance.
  - Hip rotational strengthening and more aggressive stretching
  - Graded return to desired level of activity

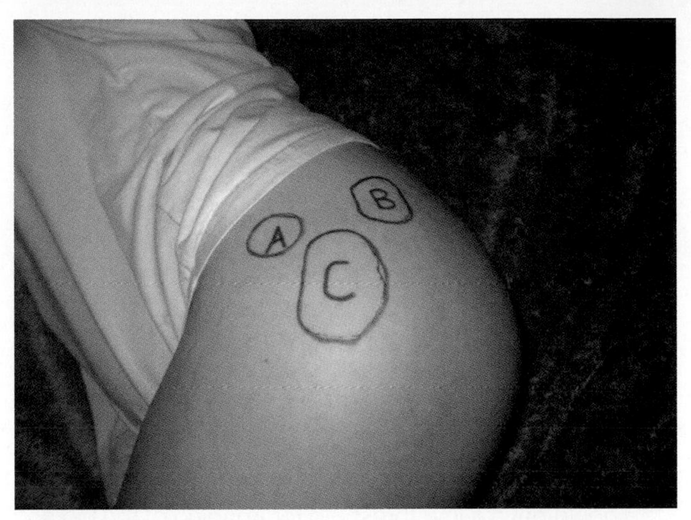

Figure 130-2 An injection of a local anesthetic solution into the trochanteric bursal area at the point of maximal tenderness. A, subgluteus minimus bursa; B, subgluteus medius bursa; C, subgluteus maximus bursa.

TABLE 130-1 *Components of Trochanteric Bursa Injection*

Syringe	Needle	Anesthetic Agent	Corticosteroid
10 mL	22 or 25 gauge, 1.5 inch or longer	3–5 mL total volume of 1% lidocaine with or without 0.25% or 0.5% bupivacaine	40 mg triamcinolone or 6 mg betamethasone

When to Refer

- Patients who fail to improve or have a chronic or relapsing course
- Patients with a tear of the gluteus tendons seen on imaging
- Surgical options include bursectomy, release of the iliotibial band, and tendon repair.

Prognosis

- Long-term studies are lacking, but a recovery rate of 90% at 2 years has been reported.
- Relapse is common as 36% and 29% of initial responders may have trochanteric pain at 1- and 5-year follow-up, respectively.
- Response rates from a corticosteroid injection have been reported at 70% after one injection and 90% after two injections, with a 25% relapse rate.

Troubleshooting

- If patients fail to respond to initial measures, clinicians should have a low threshold for imaging of the hip and low back areas.
- Follow-up is needed to ensure the adequacy of and compliance with recommended treatments and to evaluate for chronicity or relapse.
- Surgery is the final option in patients who are nonresponders to conservative treatments or those found to have correctable pathology.

Patient Instructions

- Adhere to prescribed therapeutic exercises.
- Exercises to include stretching and strengthening are essential and should be incorporated as part of a routine treatment plan even after resolution of symptoms.
- Alert the treating provider to any new, worsening, or persistent symptoms.

Considerations in Special Populations

- In elderly patients, assess for any associated osteoarthritis of the low back or hip area as a cause of or contributor to trochanteric pain.

Suggested Reading

- Baker CL, Massie V, Hurt WG: Arthroscopic bursectomy for recalcitrant trochanteric bursitis. Arthroscopy 2007;23:827–832.
- Bewyer DC, Bewyer KJ: Rationale for treatment of hip abductor pain syndrome. Iowa Orthop J 2003;23:57–60.
- Cohen SP, Narvaez JC, Lebovits AH: Corticosteroid injections for trochanteric bursitis: Is fluoroscopy necessary? A pilot study. Br J Anaesth 2005;94:100–106.
- Lequesne M: From "periarthritis" to hip "rotator cuff" tears: Trochanteric tendinobursitis. Joint Bone Spine 2006;73:344–348.
- Lievense A, Bierma-Zeinstra S, Schouten B: Prognosis of trochanteric pain in primary care. Br J Gen Pract 2005;55:199–204.
- Paluska SA: An overview of hip injuries in running. Sports Med 2005;35:991–1014.
- Segal NA, Felson DT, Torner JC: Greater trochanteric pain syndrome: Epidemiology and associated factors. Arch Phys Med Rehabil 2007;88:988–992.
- Walker P, Kannangara S, Bruce WJ, et al: Lateral hip pain. Clin Orthop Relat Res 2007;457:144–149.

Chapter 131 Hip: Labral Tear

Robert N. Royalty and Christian Lattermann

ICD-9 CODES

719.45 *Pain: Hip*
718.35 *Recurrent Dislocation of Joint*
718.85 *Other Joint Derangement Not Otherwise Classified*

Key Concepts

- The labrum of the hip is predominantly fibrocartilage and circumferentially covers the acetabular perimeter, making the depth of the acetabulum deeper and more stable.
- The labrum is triangular in shape, with thickness being greatest in the posterosuperior region.
- The labrum vascular supply originates from the obturator, superior gluteal, and inferior gluteal arteries with minimal vascular invasion from the surrounding synovial tissue and bony acetabular margin.
- A "sealing effect" is created by the labrum by limiting hip synovial fluid expression, which enhances hip joint stability by allowing atmospheric pressure to aid in maintaining anatomic joint reduction.
- Removing the acetabular labrum increases the frictional force between the femoral head and acetabulum by as much as 92% and shifts the center of contact toward the acetabular rim.
- Because the labrum enhances hip joint stability, labral pathology may lead to hip joint hypermobility and/or instability, creating excess capsular tissue that can generate abnormal load distribution with early degenerative joint disease of the hip as the final result.
- Isolated hip labral tears are rare, with approximately half of such injuries associated with articular damage of the hip joint.
- Mechanism of injury: sport dependent, but commonly twisting/pivoting injuries
- Most labral tears occur anteriorly with the labrum separating from the adjacent acetabular margin, especially in athletes involved in acute trauma or pivoting-type injuries; most posterior labral tears are associated with posterior hip dislocations.

History

- Mechanism of injury: twisting/pivoting injury
- Occupational/recreational history
- "C sign": characteristic of intra-articular hip joint pathology
  - Patients grip with the hand above the greater trochanter with the thumb over the posterior portion of the greater trochanter while at the same time cupping the fingers into the groin region.
- Insidious onset of symptoms
  - Hip pain
    - Sharp or dull pain
    - Groin pain (92%) with occasional radiation to knee
    - Activity-related pain (twisting, impact activities) most troublesome and straight plane activity well tolerated
  - Mechanical symptoms: catching, clicking, locking, "giving way"
    - Hip clicking sensation is a 100% sensitive and 85% specific clinical symptom of labral pathology
    - Painful mechanical locking
  - Prolonged duration of hip flexion (sitting) troublesome
  - Inclines and stairs more difficult to navigate than level surfaces

Physical Examination

- Impingement sign: groin pain with hip flexed to 90 degrees, adducted, and internally rotated, leads to approximation of abnormal contact between the femoral neck and the acetabular periphery

- Anterior labral tear: reproduction of symptoms (catching/clicking, pain) after moving from hip flexion, external rotation, and abduction to hip extension, internal rotation, and adduction
- Posterior labral tear
  - — Reproduction of symptoms (catching/clicking, pain) with hip flexion, internal rotation, and posterior loading
  - — Reproduction of symptoms (catching/clicking, pain) after moving from hip flexion, internal rotation, and adduction to hip extension, external rotation, and abduction
- Log rolling of the leg is the most specific physical examination test for intra-articular hip joint pathology.
- Forced flexion and internal rotation of the hip and forced abduction and external rotation of the hip are the most sensitive physical examination tests for intra-articular hip joint pathology.
  - The femoral head within the hip joint is rotated alone without stressing the surrounding anatomic structures.
- Reduced hip range of motion
- Antalgic gait

Imaging

- Anteroposterior view of the pelvis
- Anteroposterior/lateral view of the hip
- High-resolution magnetic resonance imaging
  - Significant variability in appearance of labrum in normal/asymptomatic labra
  - Limited for evaluating hip labrum because of the lack of inherent joint distention to outline tear
  - Presence of an effusion is a reliable indicator of intra-articular pathology.
- Magnetic resonance arthrography (gadolinium): sensitivity, 90%; accuracy, 91% (Fig. 131-1)

Additional Tests

- Fluoroscopically guided intra-articular hip injection of bupivacaine is a reliable indicator of intra-articular pathology if symptoms are temporarily alleviated.
  - Can be injected alone or concomitantly during magnetic resonance arthrography
  - The patient should perform activities that cause hip symptoms to truly evaluate response to injection.

Differential Diagnosis

- Please see Table 131-1.

Treatment

- At diagnosis
  - Rest (partial weight bearing for 4 weeks)
  - Anti-inflammatory medications
  - Activity modification: avoid extremes of hip range of motion
  - Physical therapy
    - — Exercises to strengthen hip muscles to stabilize joint
    - — Gentle hip range of motion, avoiding extremes of motion
    - — Therapeutic modalities to decrease pain and inflammation: cryotherapy, moist heat, ionto-

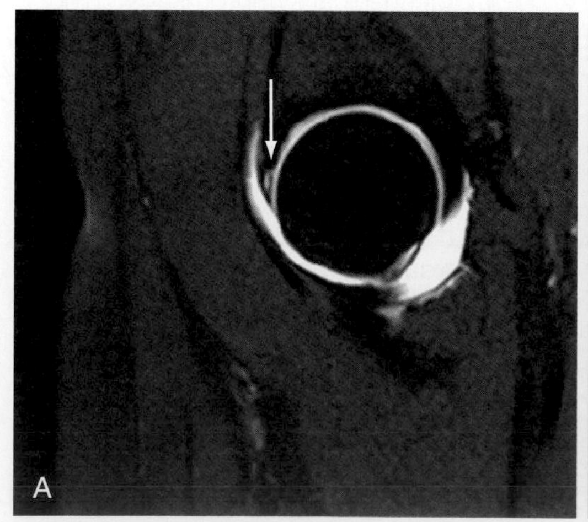

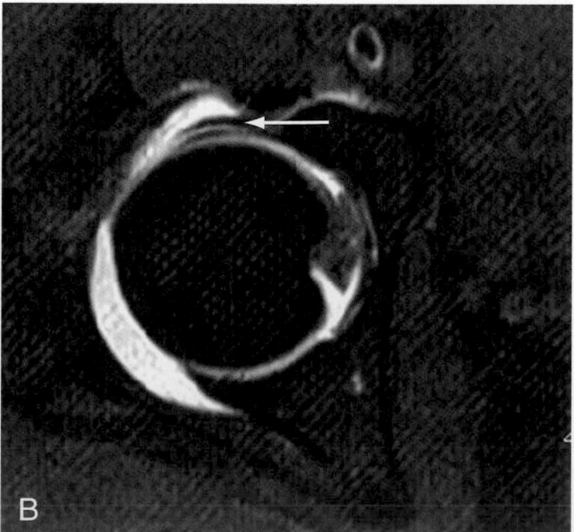

Figure 131-1 **A,** Saggital T1-weighted gadolinium contrast magnetic resonance image cut through a right hip. **B,** The corresponding axial cut. *Arrows* indicate the double contour of the labrum showing contrast agent between the two leafs of the labral tear.

TABLE 131-1 *Differential Diagnosis*

Acute Onset	
Various muscle strains	Hip dislocation/subluxation
Contusions	Hip joint loose bodies
Avulsions/apophyseal injuries	Proximal femur/acetabulum fractures
Insidious Onset	
Sports hernia/athletic pubalgia	Snapping hip syndrome
Osteitis pubis	Proximal femur stress fracture
Trochanteric bursitis	Degenerative joint disease
Other Disorders	
Spine pathology	
Femoral aneurysms	
Septic arthritis	
Avascular necrosis	
Renal abnormalities: nephrolithiasis, urinary tract infection, prostatitis	
Gynecologic abnormalities: ovarian cysts, pelvic inflammatory disease	
Compression neuropathies/nerve entrapment syndromes: ilioinguinal, genitofemoral, lateral femoral cutaneous	

phoresis, transcutaneous electrical nerve stimulation
  — Physical therapists identify activities that place excess stress on the hip joint and help patients to avoid those movements.
- Later
  - Aggressive physical therapy is initiated to maintain hip range of motion and strengthen hip rotators.
  - Return to high-demand athletics/activities should be delayed until the strength of the hip is nearly normal and the hip is pain free.

When to Refer

- Continued symptoms (clicking/locking, pain) despite adequate conservative treatment and equivocal radiographic studies or mechanical symptoms (clicking/locking) in high-level competitive athletes
- Treatment considerations
  - Hip arthroscopic labral débridement (Fig. 131-2)
    — Successful outcomes of hip arthroscopic labral débridement range from 68% to 82%.
  - A traumatic inciting event as the cause of symptoms is indicative of a likely successful outcome after surgical treatment with hip arthroscopy, whereas an insidious onset of symptoms suggests an underlying predisposition or degenerative process associated with a less certain prognosis after surgical treatment with hip arthroscopy.

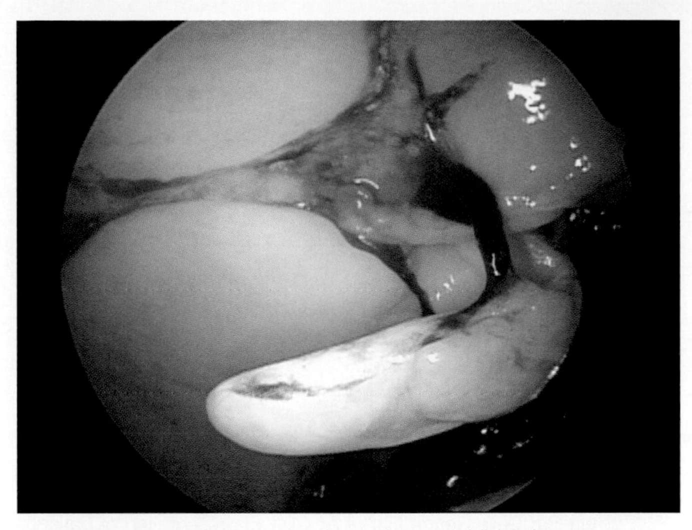

Figure 131-2 Arthroscopic view of a radial labral tear requiring debridement.

Troubleshooting

- The hip labrum has poor inherent vascularity, which means that conservative treatment modalities will commonly fail to improve symptoms if a hip labral tear is diagnosed; therefore, surgical modalities are viable alternatives especially in high-level competitive athletes.
- Intra-articular hip joint anesthetic injections that temporarily relieve hip symptoms reliably differentiate intra- and extra-articular sources of hip pain.

Patient Instructions

- Follow physical therapy instructions closely regarding range of motion and hip strengthening exercises.

Considerations in Special Populations

- Hip labral pathology is commonly seen in patients with hip dysplasia.
- Hip dysplasia leads to abnormal impingement between the femoral neck (secondary to proximal femoral dysplasia) and acetabular rim (secondary to abnormal version or overcoverage of the acetabulum).
- Hip dysplasia leads to hip degenerative joint disease in at least 50% of patients by the age of 50.
- A diagnosis of hip labral pathology in a patient with hip dysplasia and subsequent treatment with hip arthroscopy and labral débridement. The overgrown labrum destabilizes the hip joint and leads to rapid

progression of degenerative joint disease and worsening pain.

- Nonsurgical management (activity modification, nonsteroidal anti-inflammatory drugs, physical therapy) of a painful hip with labral pathology in patients with hip dysplasia is rarely successful because many of these patients are young and have a high activity level.
- Many patients with hip dysplasia and labral pathology would most benefit from femoroacetabular osteoplasty.

Suggested Reading

- Anderson K, Strickland SM, Warren R: Hip and groin injuries in athletes. Am J Sports Med 2001;29:521–533.
- Burnett SJ, Della Rocca GJ, et al: Clinical presentation of patients with tears of the acetabular labrum. J Bone Joint Surg Am 2006;88A:1448–1457.
- Byrd JW: Hip arthroscopy. J Am Acad Orthop Surg 2006; 14:433–444.
- Byrd JW: Hip arthroscopy: Patient assessment and indications. Instr Course Lect 2003;52:711–719.
- Byrd JW: Hip arthroscopy in athletes. Instr Course Lect 2003; 52:701–709.
- DeAngelis NA, Busconi BD: Assessment and differential diagnosis of the painful hip. Clin Orthop Relat Res 2003;406:11–18.
- McCarthy J, Noble P, Aluisio FV, et al: Anatomy, pathologic features, and treatment of acetabular labral tears. Clin Orthop Relat Res 2003;406:38–47.
- Newberg AH, Newman JS: Imaging the painful hip. Clin Orthop Relat Res 2003;406:19–28.
- Parvizi J, Leung M, Ganz R: Femoroacetabular impingement. J Am Acad Orthop Surg 2007;15:561–570.

Chapter 132 Hip Subluxation and Dislocation

Robert N. Royalty and Christian Lattermann

ICD-9 CODES

835.0 *Dislocation of Hip*
719.45 *Pain: Hip*
755.63 *Other Congenital Deformity of Hip (Dysplasia of Hip)*

Key Concepts

- The hip joint is intrinsically stable and requires significant force to dislocate.
- Ligaments of hip
  - Iliofemoral: anterior inferior iliac spine to intertrochanteric line
  - Pubofemoral: superior pubic ramus to femoral neck
  - Ischiofemoral: posterior acetabular/ischial rim to intertrochanteric crest
- The labrum is predominantly fibrocartilage and circumferentially covers the acetabular perimeter. The depth of the acetabulum is supplemented by the labrum, which makes the joint deeper and more stable and increases articular congruence. The labrum contributes approximately 10% to the coverage of the femoral head.
- The vascular supply to the femoral head arises from the medial and lateral circumflex arteries, which create a ring giving rise to the cervical vessels. A minor contribution comes from the obturator artery via the ligamentum teres.
- The sciatic nerve runs posterior to the hip joint and may be stretched or directly compressed with posterior dislocations.
- The obturator nerve runs through the superolateral obturator foramen and may be injured with anterior dislocation.
- The femoral nerve lies anterior and medial to the hip joint and may be injured with anterior dislocations.
- Mechanism of injury
  - Posterior dislocation: forward fall on the knee with a flexed hip or a blow from behind while down on all four limbs (i.e., knee driven into ground during football tackle)
  - Anterior dislocation: flexed hip vigorously forced into extreme abduction and concomitant external rotation (i.e., performing splits during gymnastics)
- The direction of the dislocation and associated injuries are dependent on the position of the hip and the direction of the force vector (Table 132-1).
- Posterior dislocations comprise more than 80% of traumatic dislocations and approximately 90% of those occurring during athletic competitions.
- Associated injuries are common, especially fractures of the femoral head and acetabulum. Ipsilateral injuries include the femoral head/neck/shaft fractures, pelvic fractures, acetabular fractures, knee ligamentous injuries, patellar fractures, and neurovascular injuries (sciatic nerve, obturator nerve, femoral nerve/artery).

History

- Posterior dislocation
  - Inability to ambulate
  - Relates a history of great force to a flexed hip and knee
  - Pain in the hip and/or buttock
  - Decreased sensation and abnormal motor strength in distribution of the sciatic nerve
- Anterior dislocation
  - Inability to ambulate
  - Relates a history of a direct blow to the posterior aspect of the hip or application of great force to abducted leg
  - Pain in the anterior hip/thigh
  - Decreased sensation and abnormal motor strength in distribution of the femoral or obturator nerves

TABLE 132-1 *Direction of the Dislocation and Associated Injuries Dependent on the Position of the Hip and Direction of the Force Vector*

Hip Position	Type of Dislocation
Flexion, adduction, internal rotation	Pure posterior dislocation
Partial flexion, less adduction, internal rotation	Posterior fracture-dislocation
Flexion, hyperabduction, external rotation	Anterior dislocation, obturator
Extension, hyperabduction, external rotation	Anterior dislocation, pubic

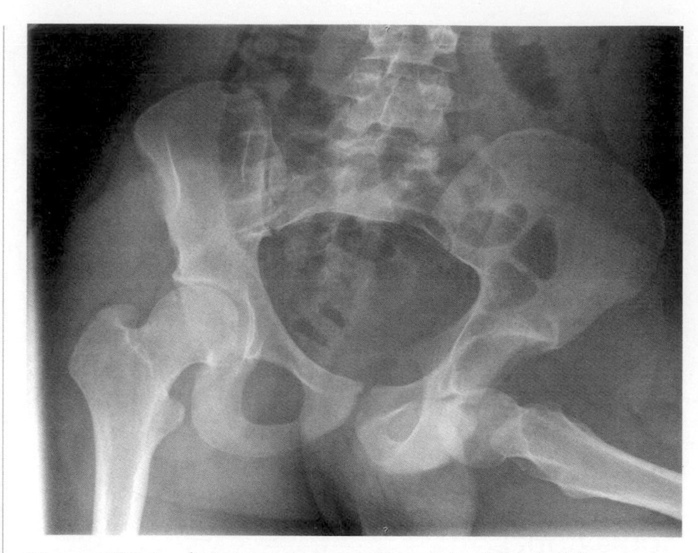

Figure 132-1 Anteroposterior radiograph of the pelvis: anterior hip dislocation.

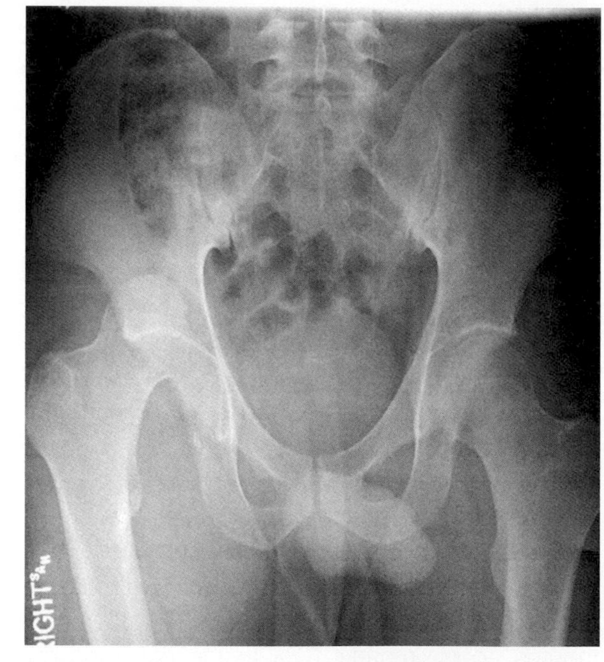

Figure 132-2 Anteroposterior radiograph of the pelvis: posterior hip dislocation.

Physical Examination

- Posterior dislocation: leg flexed, adducted, and internally rotated
- Anterior dislocation: leg flexed or extended, abducted, and externally rotated
- Complete neurovascular examination
  - Sciatic nerve
    - — Peroneal division: foot eversion/dorsiflexion, lateral leg sensation
    - — Tibial division: foot plantarflexion, posterior leg sensation
  - Femoral nerve: anteromedial thigh, leg extension
  - Obturator nerve: inferomedial thigh, thigh adduction
  - Dorsalis pedis artery
  - Posterior tibial artery

Imaging

- Single anteroposterior view of the pelvis for diagnosis (Figs. 132-1 and 132-2)
- Postreduction radiographs to identify associated injuries (femoral neck, acetabular fractures, loose bodies) and to verify concentric reduction
  - Anteroposterior view of the pelvis
  - Anteroposterior/lateral views of the hip
  - Judet views: obturator and iliac oblique views
- Computed tomography

Additional Tests

- Magnetic resonance imaging to evaluate labral pathology, femoral head contusions, and avascular necrosis or to evaluate unrelenting or new-onset hip pain during rehabilitation despite normal radiographs
  - Many recommend magnetic resonance imaging 2 to 6 weeks after hip dislocation to evaluate for femoral head ischemia, with the goal of intervening early to prevent complications of avascular necrosis.

Differential Diagnosis

- Acetabulum fracture with concomitant hip subluxation
- Femoral head fracture
- Femoral neck fracture
- Intertrochanteric/subtrochanteric femur fracture

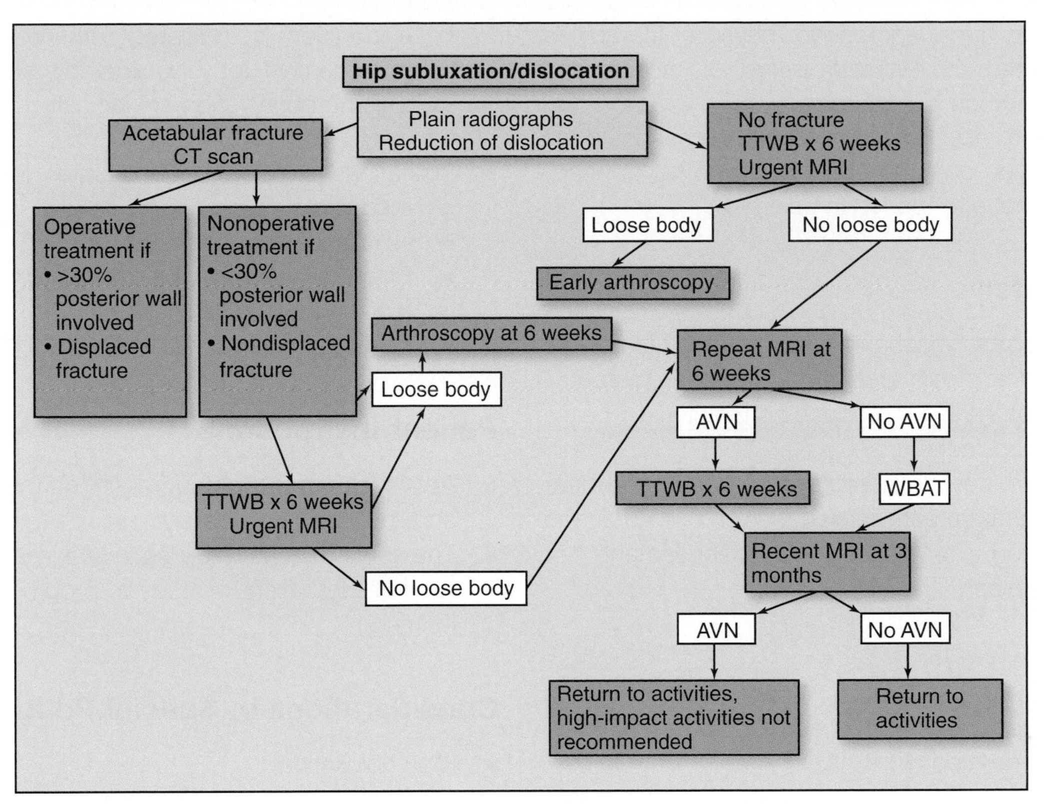

Figure 132-3 Algorithm for treatment of hip subluxation/dislocation. AVN, avascular necrosis; CT, computed tomography; MRI, magnetic resonance imaging; TTWB, toe-touching, weight-bearing; WBAT, weight bearing as tolerated.

Treatment (Fig. 132-3)

- At diagnosis
  - Urgent closed reduction: Allis technique of traction/countertraction
  - Posterior dislocation
    - — Sufficient patient sedation and muscle relaxation are necessities.
    - — Reduction is performed with the patient in the supine position using traction-countertraction techniques.
      - — An assistant stabilizes the hemipelvis by pushing down on the ipsilateral anterosuperior iliac spine.
      - — The hip and knee are flexed to relax the hamstring musculature.
      - — Steady axial traction to overcome muscular spasm and elastic restraints is then applied with the extremity in internal rotation and adduction.
      - — As the traction is applied, the leg is gently internally and externally rotated to achieve reduction.
  - Anterior dislocation
    - — Sufficient patient sedation and muscle relaxation are necessities.
    - — Reduction is performed with the patient in the supine position using traction-countertraction techniques.
      - — An assistant stabilizes the hemipelvis by pushing down on the ipsilateral anterosuperior iliac spine and simultaneously pushing laterally on the inner proximal thigh.
      - — Steady axial traction to overcome muscular spasm and elastic restraints are continuously applied in line with the deformity in association with gentle hip flexion, adduction, and internal rotation to achieve reduction.
- Later
  - Pure dislocations
    - — Active and passive hip range of motion should begin as soon as possible to avoid intra-articular adhesions and stiffness associated with immobilization.
    - — Standard anterior or posterior hip precautions should be applied during the first 6 weeks after the injury to allow capsular and soft-tissue restraints adequate time to heal.
    - — Toe-touch weight bearing progressing to weight bearing as tolerated by 6 weeks, during

which time aggressive physical therapy is initiated to maintain range of motion and strengthen hip rotators
    - Return to high-demand athletics should be delayed until the strength of the hip is nearly normal and the hip is pain free.

When to Refer

- Patient reports mechanical symptoms (catching, locking) or sharp pain localized to the hip region.
- Log rolling of the leg reproduces characteristic pain.
- Treatment considerations
    - Hip arthroscopy to address loose bodies and identify labral tears and cartilage lesions (femoral and acetabular) amenable to débridement or chondroplasty

Prognosis

- The outcome ranges from a normal hip to a severely painful/degenerated hip joint.
- The literature indicates that 48% to 95% of patients have a good or excellent outcome after pure posterior dislocations with outcomes varying depending on associated injuries (fractures).
- Arthritis
    - Most common complication after hip dislocation
    - Increased incidence after posterior dislocations and fracture-dislocations
    - Seen in approximately 50% of fracture-dislocations
- Avascular necrosis
    - Rates vary in the literature from 1% to 40%.
    - Increased incidence after posterior dislocation, which correlates with the duration of the dislocation
    - The literature suggests that reduction of the hip joint within 6 hours of dislocation reduces the rate to 0% to 10%.
    - Symptoms and/or radiographic findings may present years after a traumatic event.

Troubleshooting

- Sciatic nerve dysfunction
    - Occurs in 5% to 30% of posterior hip dislocations
    - If sciatic nerve injury occurs after closed reduction, then entrapment of the nerve is likely and surgical exploration is indicated; otherwise, nonsurgical management (physical therapy, ankle-foot orthosis) and observation are indicated for as long as 1 year.
- Indications for open reduction after hip dislocation
    - Irreducible dislocation
    - Nonconcentric reduction
    - Fractures of the acetabulum or femoral head requiring fixation
    - Ipsilateral femoral neck fracture

Patient Instructions

- Active and passive hip range of motion exercises should begin immediately.
- The ability to control the leg in space is a good indicator that the patient is ready to progress to full weight bearing.

Considerations in Special Populations

- Hip subluxation
    - Occurs when a patient falls on a flexed knee and hip or suddenly stops and pivots vigorously over the weight-bearing extremity causing the femoral head to sublux onto the acetabular rim and spontaneously reduce
    - Judet views may demonstrate a posterior acetabular lip fracture.
    - Magnetic resonance imaging triad
        - Posterior acetabular lip fracture
        - Rupture of the iliofemoral ligament
        - Hemarthrosis

Suggested Reading

- Anderson K, Strickland SM, Warren R: Hip and groin injuries in athletes. Am J Sports Med 2001;29:521–533.
- Byrd JW: Hip arthroscopy in athletes. Instr Course Lect 2003;52:701–709.
- Pallia CS, Scott RE, Chao DJ: Traumatic hip dislocation in athletes. Curr Sports Med Rep 2002;1:338–345.
- Tornetta P: Hip dislocations and fractures of the femoral head. In Bucholz RW, Heckman JD, Court-Brown C (eds): Rockwood and Green's Fractures in Adults, 6th ed. Philadelphia: Lippincott Williams & Wilkins, 2006, pp 1715–1752.

Chapter 133 Hip Joint Disorders: Osteoarthritis and Avascular Necrosis

Chris Pappas and Kevin deWeber

HIP OSTEOARTHRITIS

ICD-9 CODES
715.95 *Hip Osteoarthritis*
733.40 *Aseptic Necrosis of Bone*

Key Concepts

- Osteoarthritis (OA) of the hip, also known as degenerative joint disease, is common in patients older than 40 years of age and is the end-stage result of many different disorders.
- OA was once considered a normal process with aging, but is now recognized as a multifactorial process involving overuse, mechanical forces, joint integrity, cellular processes, local inflammation, and a possible genetic predisposition.
- The pathogenesis of OA is poorly understood, but probably begins with damage to articular cartilage by the mechanical forces of macrotrauma or repeated microtrauma. There is growing evidence that this damage leads to deranged chondrocyte metabolism. This in turn leads to thickening of the subchondral bone, abnormal bone structure (osteophytes), and synovial inflammation.
- OA can be broken down into primary (or idiopathic) and secondary osteoarthritis.
    - Risk factors for primary OA are shown in Box 133-1.
    - Risk factors for secondary OA are shown in Box 133-2.
- Hip OA can be diagnosed by hip pain plus two of the following:
    - Erythrocyte sedimentation rate less than 20 mm/hour
    - Radiographic evidence of femoral or acetabular osteophytes
    - Radiographic evidence of joint space narrowing (superior, axial, or medial)
        — This classification yields a sensitivity of 89% and specificity of 91%.
- Five percent of the population older than 65 years of age have radiographic evidence of hip osteoarthritis. There is an inconsistent relationship between clinical symptoms and radiographic evidence, resulting in underestimation of the true prevalence. Of note, nearly 200,000 total hip arthroplasties are performed annually.

BOX 133-1 *Risk Factors for Primary Osteoarthritis*

Older age
Female gender
Increased body mass index
Higher bone mass
Previous injury
Muscle weakness
Proprioceptive deficits
Sports activities (soccer)
Genetics
Occupations requiring heavy lifting or prolonged standing (farmers, construction workers)

BOX 133-2 *Risk Factors for Secondary Osteoarthritis*

Trauma (hip dislocation)
Avascular necrosis
Rheumatoid arthritis
Gout
Developmental disorders (congenital dysplasia, slipped capital femoral epiphysis)
Septic arthritis
Calcium pyrophosphate crystal deposition disease
Paget's disease
Legg-Calvé-Perthes disease
Diabetes mellitus
Hypothyroidism
Hyperparathyroidism
Acromegaly
Hemochromatosis
Hyperlaxity syndromes

History

- Hip pain aggravated by activity and relieved with rest
- Decreased range of motion of the hip joint
- Morning stiffness of the hip joint that resolves in 30 to 60 minutes
- As OA progresses, it may result in pain at rest or at night; this pain can radiate from the hip to the knee on the affected side.

Physical Examination

- Key findings on physical examination in advanced disease (note: the examination may be unremarkable in some patients)
    - Reduced internal rotation (<15 degrees)
    - Reduced hip flexion (<115 degrees)
    - Hip pain exacerbated by internal and external rotation with the knee in full extension

Imaging

- Key findings suggestive of OA, seen on weight-bearing anteroposterior pelvis plain radiographs (Fig. 133-1)
    - Joint space narrowing (normal is 4–5 mm)
    - Sclerosis along the joint space (subchondral sclerosis)
    - Osteophyte formation
    - Cyst formation

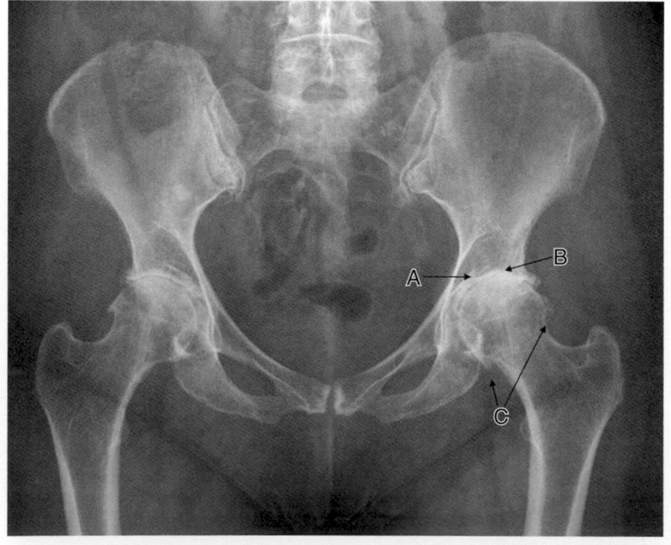

Figure 133-1 Weight-bearing anteroposterior plain radiograph of an 83-year-old woman with chronic hip osteoarthritis. Of note, only her left hip was symptomatic, yet the radiographic changes are present on the right as well. A indicates the severe joint space narrowing; B indicates the subchondral sclerosis; and C indicates the osteophytes.

- Magnetic resonance imaging is typically not warranted for the diagnosis of OA, but may be helpful when the diagnosis is in question.

Differential Diagnosis

- Please see Box 133-3.

Treatment

- At diagnosis
    - Pain relief and function preservation are the primary treatment goals. At present, there are no disease-modifying agents.
    - Acetaminophen (up to 4 g/day) is the first-line analgesic.
    - If acetaminophen is inadequate, add a nonsteroidal anti-inflammatory drug at the lowest effective dose (consider adding a proton pump inhibitor for gastrointestinal protection).
    - Consider adding oral glucosamine because it may benefit some patients and is generally considered safe to use.
    - In only the most severe flare-ups can opioids be recommended, with tramadol as the first-line opioid agent.
    - Arthritis education classes
    - Modification of risk factors and avoidance of high-impact activities
    - Exercise program to improve hip range of motion and leg muscle strength (aquatic therapy or physical therapy)
    - Weight loss
    - Use of assistive devices (e.g., cane, walker)
- Later
    - Steroid injections (under fluoroscopic guidance)

BOX 133-3 *Differential Diagnosis*

Trochanteric bursitis
Inflammatory arthritides
Septic joint
Avascular necrosis
Crystalline diseases
Lumbar radiculopathy
Lumbar spinal stenosis
Cancer (primary or metastatic)
Meralgia paresthetica
Iliotibial band syndrome
Vascular claudication

When to Refer

- When the patient experiences significant pain and/or disability despite conservative management, he or she may be a candidate for a total joint replacement (arthroplasty).
- Progressive limitation in activities of daily living
- Timing of arthroplasty is controversial, but the sixth or seventh decade is probably the best trade-off balancing life span and ability to recover from this significant surgery and its rehabilitation (6–12 months).

Prognosis

- Hip OA is a progressive disease.
- Total hip arthroplasty is effective for reducing pain and disability. Total hip arthroplasties have a failure rate of 1% per year over a period of 10 years according to population-based data.

Troubleshooting

- Counsel patients regarding the chronic nature of this condition.
- Counsel patients that they can slow the progression of this disease and delay (or avoid) the need for an arthroplasty if they modify their risk factors and restrict their exposure to high-impact activities.
- Counsel patients that surgery is probably best done in the sixth and seventh decades, but that there are significant risks associated with the surgery and its subsequent rehabilitation.

Patient Instructions

- Follow physician and physical therapist instructions closely with respect to the type and quantity of activities that are acceptable.
- Home- and community-based exercises are vital to the overall management of this disease process and should be performed diligently and regularly.
- Work to change those risk factors that are modifiable.

Suggested Reading

- Anderson BC: Evaluation of the adult with hip pain (online no. 15.3). UpToDate 2007. Available at www.UpToDate.com. Accessed October 16, 2007.
- DeLee JC, Drez D Jr, Miller MD (eds): DeLee & Drez's Orthopaedic Sports Medicine, 2nd ed. Philadelphia: WB Saunders, 2002, pp 1443–1479.
- Jude CM: Radiologic evaluation of the painful hip in adults (online no. 15.3). UpToDate 2007. Available at www.UpToDate.com. Accessed November 20, 2007.
- Kalunian KC: Clinical manifestations of osteoarthritis (online no. 15.3). UpToDate 2007. Available at www.UpToDate.com. Accessed October 16, 2007.
- Kalunian KC: Diagnosis and classification of osteoarthritis (online no. 15.3). UpToDate 2007. Available at www.UpToDate.com. Accessed October 16, 2007.
- Kalunian KC: Pathogenesis of osteoarthritis (online no. 15.3). UpToDate 2007. Available at www.UpToDate.com. Accessed November 20, 2007.
- Kalunian KC: Pharmacologic therapy of osteoarthritis (online no. 15.3). UpToDate, 2007. Available at www.UpToDate.com. Accessed October 16, 2007.
- Kalunian KC: Risk factors for and possible causes of osteoarthritis (online no. 15.3). UpToDate, 2007. Available at www.UpToDate.com. Accessed October 16, 2007.
- Lane NE: Osteoarthritis of the hip. N Engl J Med 2007;357:1413–1421.
- Recommendations for the medical management of osteoarthritis of the hip and knee: 2000 update. American College of Rheumatology Subcommittee on Osteoarthritis Guidelines. Arthritis Rheum 2000;43:1905–1915.
- Schenck RC, Barnes RP, Behnke RS, et al (eds): Athletic Training and Sports Medicine, 3rd ed. Sudbury, MA: Jones & Bartlett, 1999, pp 399–434.
- Zhang WB: Efficacy and safety evaluation of glucosamine hydrochloride in the treatment of osteoarthritis. Zhonghua Wai Ke Za Zhi 2007;45:998–1001.

HIP AVASCULAR NECROSIS

ICD-9 CODE
733.42 *Avascular Necrosis of the Femoral Head*

Key Concepts

- Avascular necrosis (AVN) is also known as aseptic necrosis, ischemic necrosis, osteochondritis dissecans, and osteonecrosis.
- AVN is a poorly defined pathologic process believed to result initially from a disruption in the blood supply to the femoral head. After this initial insult, the following occur in sequence: femoral head hyperemia, demineralization, trabecular thinning, and then architectural collapse. This results in progressive arthritis of the hip joint. If untreated, joint destruction occurs within 3 to 5 years. Causes of AVN fall under two major categories: traumatic and atraumatic.

BOX 133-4 *Atraumatic Causes*

Systemic corticosteroid use
Heavy alcohol use
Systemic lupus erythematosus
Gaucher's disease
Decompression (dysbarism) disease
Sickle cell disease
Chronic renal failure
Hemodialysis
Organ transplantation
Pancreatitis
Hyperlipidemia
Radiation
Thrombophlebitis
Cigarette smoking
Gout
Human immunodeficiency virus infection
Genetic predisposition (α chain of type II collagen [COL2A1])
Idiopathic

- Traumatic causes include
  - — Femoral neck fractures
  - — Hip dislocation (with or without fracture)
  - — Surgical complications
- Atraumatic causes are many and varied (Box 133-4).
- Possible mechanisms for steroid-induced AVN include alterations in venous endothelial cells, stasis, increased intraosseous pressure, alterations in circulating lipids, and/or microembolic phenomena.
- The prevalence of AVN is unknown, but an estimated 10,000 to 20,000 cases are newly diagnosed each year.
- AVN is implicated in approximately 10% of all total hip arthroplasties.
- The male-to-female ratio is 8:1.
- The majority of AVN cases are diagnosed in patients between 24 and 45 years of age.
- The key to an early diagnosis is a high level of suspicion and clarification of known risk factors. Early diagnosis is best, but most cases are diagnosed late in the disease process.
- Variants of AVN in children include idiopathic disease of the femoral neck (Legg-Calvé-Perthes disease) and that resulting from a slipped capital femoral epiphysis.

History

- Nonspecific hip, groin, thigh, and/or buttock pain
- Pain exacerbated with weight bearing and movement
- Rest pain occurs in two thirds of the patients with AVN.
- Night pain occurs in one third of the patients with AVN.

Physical Examination

- Pain is usually located in the anterolateral femoral head.
- Gait and hip range of motion are generally normal until an advanced stage.
- Once range limitations exist, they will primarily be seen with internal rotation and abduction.

Imaging

- Radiographic changes may be seen approximately 3 months after the inciting insult. Unfortunately, plain radiographs have a low sensitivity for detecting AVN in its earliest stages.
- Key findings on anteroposterior, lateral, and frog leg plain radiographs (Fig. 133-2):
  - Osteopenia or patchy areas of sclerosis and lucency of the femoral head, leading to a mottled appearance
  - The pathognomonic crescent sign (subchondral lucency) indicates collapse of trabeculae beneath the subchondral bone.
  - Later findings include collapse of the femoral head and/or loss of its sphericity, joint space narrowing, and degenerative changes of the joint.
- If plain radiographs are normal and the index of suspicion remains high, magnetic resonance imaging is sensitive and specific (both in the range of 97% to 100%) for this disease process. Magnetic resonance imaging is the study of choice for the early diagnosis of AVN. The classic finding is the double line sign at the border between the necrotic and reparative zones (Fig. 133-3). Magnetic resonance imaging of the bilateral hips and pelvis allows detection of additional lesions that may suggest a diagnosis other than AVN.
- Scintigraphy may be useful if magnetic resonance imaging is contraindicated or not available. Sensitivity of scintigraphy with single-photon emission computed tomography for detecting AVN is approximately 88%. An abnormal bone scan can be the result of a number of other conditions affecting the hip joint.

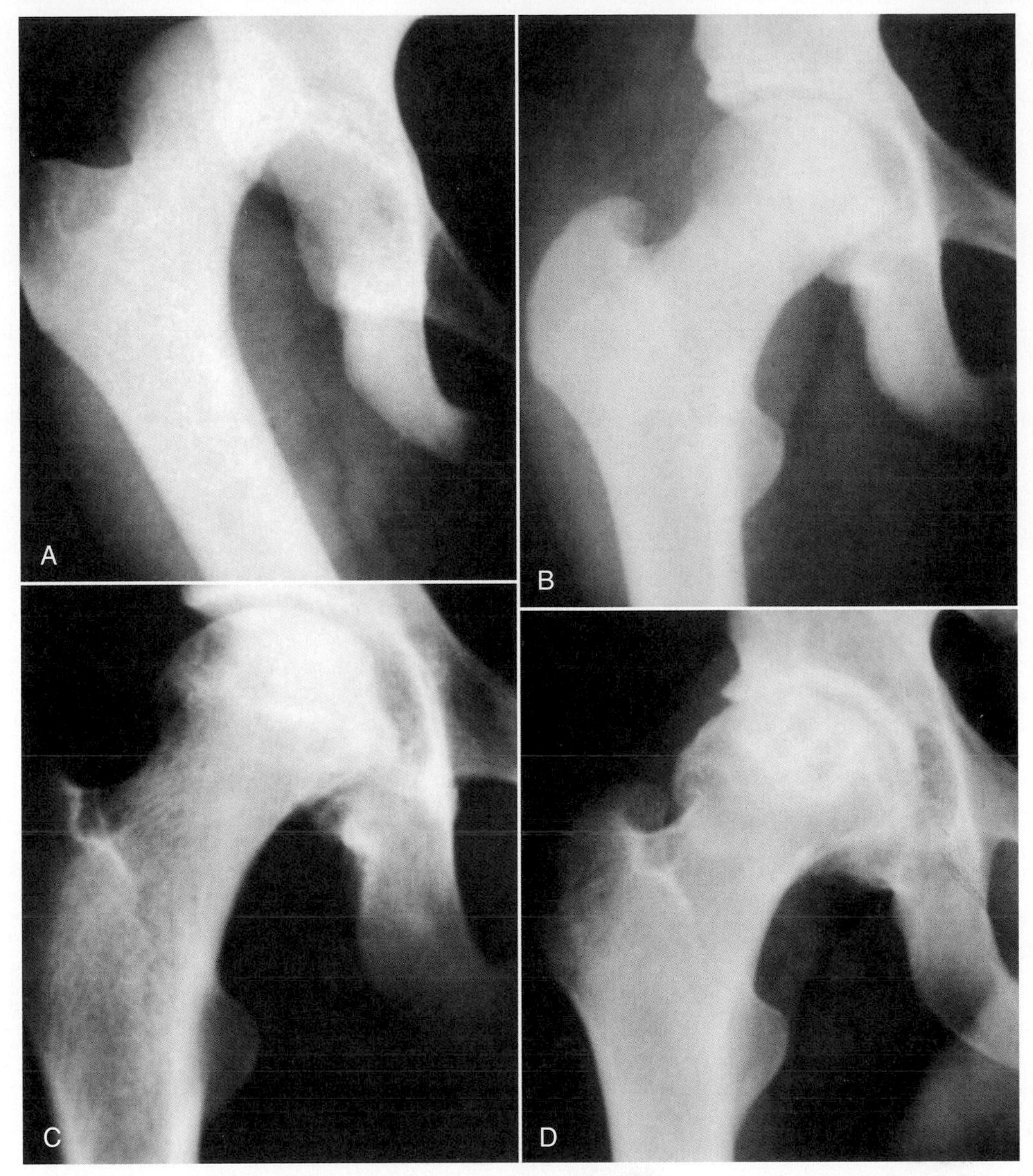

Figure 133-2 Avascular necrosis of the femoral head after hip dislocation. **A**, Traumatic dislocation in an older child. **B**, After satisfactory closed reduction. **C**, At 1 year after reduction, a suggestion of early avascular necrosis is seen. **D**, At 8 years after reduction, there is a cystic appearance of avascular necrosis. (From Canale ST [ed]: Campbell's Operative Orthopaedics, 10th ed. Philadelphia: Mosby, 2003, Fig. 33-118.)

Differential Diagnosis

- Trochanteric bursitis
- Inflammatory arthritides
- Septic joint
- Osteoarthritis
- Crystalline diseases
- Lumbar radiculopathy
- Lumbar spinal stenosis
- Cancer (primary or metastatic)
- Meralgia paresthetica
- Iliotibial band syndrome
- Vascular claudication

Treatment

- At diagnosis
  - The treatment of AVN is controversial. The primary goal is to preserve the native joint for as long as possible. Instruct the patient to remain non-weight bearing and refer to an orthopaedist.
  - Conservative measures (bed rest, protected weight bearing, medications) are generally ineffective in slowing the disease progression.
  - Asymptomatic lesions involving less than 15% of the femoral head may resolve without surgical intervention.

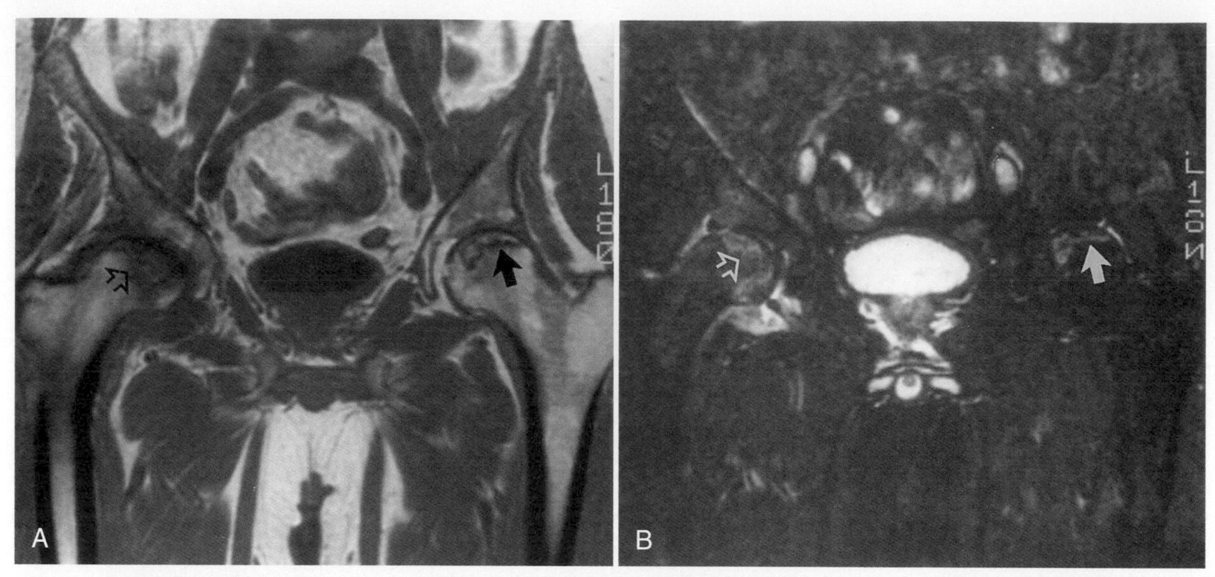

Figure 133-3 Coronal T1-weighted (**A**) and inversion recovery (**B**) images through both hips reveal the geographic focus of marrow replacement in the weight-bearing aspect of the left femoral head, indicating avascular necrosis (*solid arrows*). More advanced disease is seen in the right femoral head with collapse of the articular surface, adjacent marrow edema (*open arrows*), and effusion. (From Canale ST [ed]: Campbell's Operative Orthopaedics, 10th ed. Philadelphia: Mosby, 2002, Fig. 2-21.)

    - If asymptomatic lesions involve more than 30% of the femoral head, conservative management is appropriate, but with the expectation of a total hip arthroplasty at some point.
- Later
    - See previously

When to Refer

- At diagnosis

Prognosis

- Dependent on the stage of disease
- If diagnosed early (before femoral head collapse) and core decompression is performed (with or without bone grafting), the prognosis is better despite the various levels of reported success
- If extensive, total hip arthroplasty is the best treatment available
- It should be noted that failures are three to four times more common with this disease compared with joint replacements for OA

Troubleshooting

- Counsel patients regarding the progressive and chronic nature of this condition.
- Counsel patients that the treatment of AVN is controversial.

Patient Instructions

- Follow physician and physical therapist instructions closely with respect to the type and quantity of activities that are acceptable.
- Home- and community-based exercises are vital to the overall management of this disease process and should be performed diligently and regularly.
- Work to change those risk factors that are modifiable.

Considerations in Special Populations

- Legg-Calvé-Perthes disease (see Chapter 220)
- Slipped capital femoral epiphysis (see Chapter 221)

Suggested Reading

- Anderson BC: Evaluation of the adult with hip pain (online no. 15.3). UpToDate 2007. Available at www.UpToDate.com. Accessed October 16, 2007.
- DeLee JC, Drez D Jr, Miller MD (eds): DeLee & Drez's Orthopaedic Sports Medicine, 2nd ed. Philadelphia: WB Saunders, 2003, pp 1443–1479.
- Donohue JP: Osteonecrosis (avascular necrosis of bone) (online no. 15.3). UpToDate 2007. Available at www.UpToDate.com. Accessed October 31, 2007.
- Jackson SM, Major NM: Pathological conditions mimicking osteonecrosis. Orthop Clin North Am 2004;35:315–320, ix.
- Jude CM: Radiologic evaluation of the painful hip in adults (online no. 15.3). UpToDate 2007. Available at www.UpToDate.com. Accessed November 20, 2007.

- Kalunian KC: Clinical manifestations of osteoarthritis (online no. 15.3). UpToDate 2007. Available at www.UpToDate.com. Accessed October 16, 2007.
- Kalunian KC: Diagnosis and classification of osteoarthritis (online no. 15.3). UpToDate 2007. Available at www.UpToDate.com. Accessed October 16, 2007.
- Kalunian KC: Risk factors for and possible causes of osteoarthritis (online no. 15.3). UpToDate 2007. Available at www.UpToDate.com. Accessed October 16, 2007.
- Lane NE: Osteoarthritis of the hip. N Engl J Med 2007;357:1413–1421.
- Recommendations for the medical management of osteoarthritis of the hip and knee: 2000 update. American College of Rheumatology Subcommittee on Osteoarthritis Guidelines. Arthritis Rheum 2000;43:1905–1915.

Chapter 134 Hamstring Injury

Tracy Ray and Jeffrey W. Webb

ICD-9 CODES
843.8 *Sprain/Strain, Hip and Thigh*
843.9 *Sprain/Strain, Unspecified Site of Hip and Thigh*

Key Concepts

- Hamstring muscle strain is the most common muscle injury in running and sprinting athletes.
- Occurs in young and old, elite and "weekend warrior" athletes, and in a wide variety of sports
- Three muscles make up the hamstring muscle group (Fig. 134-1).
  - Biceps femoris
  - Semitendinosus
  - Semimembranosus
- Hamstring muscle injuries may be divided into proximal, central, and distal injuries.

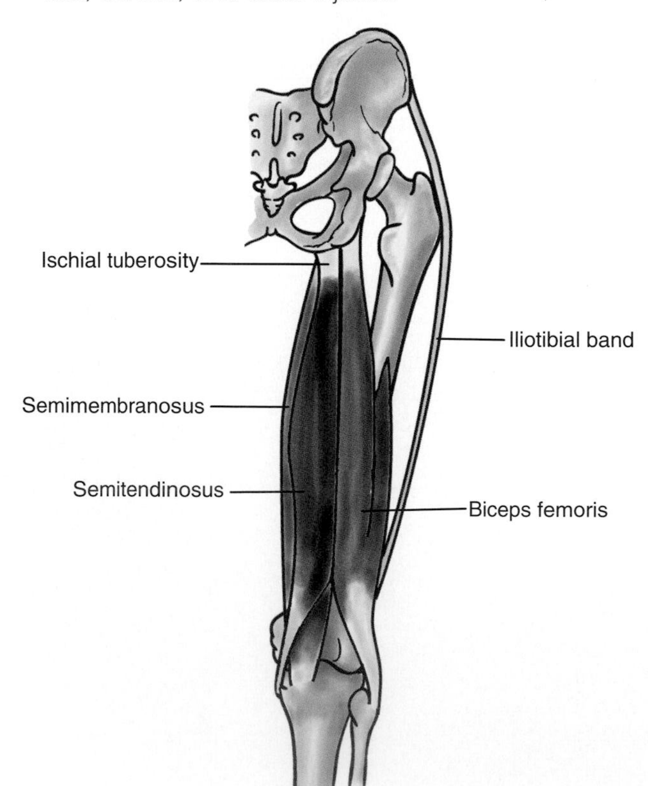

Figure 134-1 The muscles of the hamstring group.

  - Proximal injuries affect the origin at the ischial tuberosity and include complete tendon avulsion, partial tears, and apophyseal injuries in children.
  - Central injuries affect the proximal or distal musculotendinous junction.
  - Distal injuries affect the distal tendons and their insertions.
- The most common site for injury is the musculotendinous junction.
- Hamstring muscle strains, like other muscle strains, may be divided into grade I (minor injury), grade II (more significant partial tear), and grade III (complete tear).
- Injury usually occurs as a result of eccentric force as the muscle develops tension in lengthening during the swing phase of the gait.
- Injury may also occur with concentric force in the stance phase.
- Avulsion injuries usually occur with full hip flexion while the knee is extended.
- Most commonly cited factors in hamstring muscle strain are strength imbalances and lack of flexibility
  - Strength imbalance may be a difference between the hamstring muscle in each leg or imbalance between flexor and extensor muscle groups.
    - Imbalance of 10% or more between right and left hamstrings
    - Flexor-to-extensor strength ratio less than 0.5 to 0.6
- Fatigue, poor warm-up, poor running technique, and even psychosocial stress have been suggested as other risk factors for injury.
- The most common risk factor is a history of injury because hamstring muscle injuries are often slow to heal and reinjury rates are high.

History

- Sudden onset of pain in the posterior thigh during strenuous exercise
- Often described as a feeling of being kicked or stabbed in the thigh while running
- Frequently, an audible "pop"

- Athlete will often grab the thigh, which is often diagnostic
- Pain usually limits continuation of activity.
- May or may not fall to the ground
- For milder injuries, may describe tightness or "pull" in the thigh with exercise
- May have a history of fatigue or inadequate warm-up

Physical Examination

- Examine in the prone position with knee flexed to 90 degrees (Fig. 134-2)
- Palpate the entire length of the muscle from its origin at the ischial tuberosity to its insertion at the knee.
  - Feel for a defect in the muscle indicating a large tear, which is often difficult to find.
  - Palpate with the muscle fully relaxed and in mild flexion.
- Evaluate the range of motion of the hip and knee.
- Test the strength of the muscle group with hip extension and knee flexion.
- In a complete tendon rupture, there may be a mass of hamstring muscle with contraction similar to the "Popeye" appearance of a biceps rupture in the arm.
- Ecchymosis and edema may overlie the site of injury or be located in the dependent part of the thigh (Fig. 134-3).
- Evaluate the gait and neurovascular status.

Imaging

- Plain radiographs are of little help unless an avulsion fracture of the ischial tuberosity is suspected.
  - Radiographs should be obtained in pediatric patients due to the higher incidence of avulsion injury with open physes.
  - If concerned about avulsion injury, obtain an anteroposterior radiograph of the pelvis (Fig. 134-4)
- Magnetic resonance imaging may be useful to differentiate complete from partial tears; should be unnecessary with more minor injuries (Fig. 134-5)
- Ultrasonography is becoming a more common tool to identify a superficial tendon injury.
- A bone scan may be useful in more chronic overuse injuries to differentiate pelvic and femoral neck stress fractures.

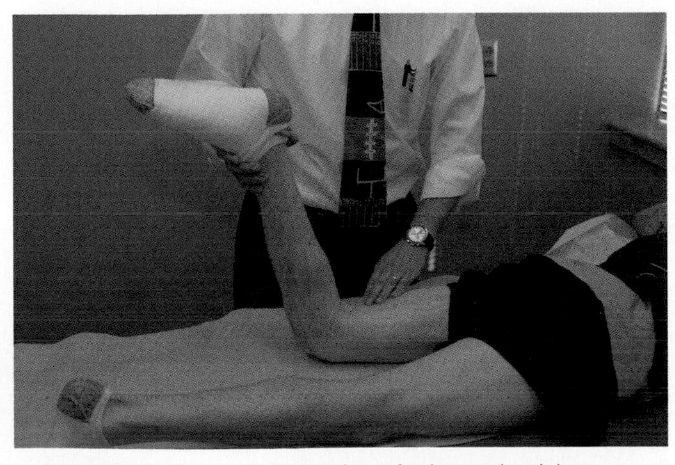

Figure 134-2 Examination of a hamstring injury.

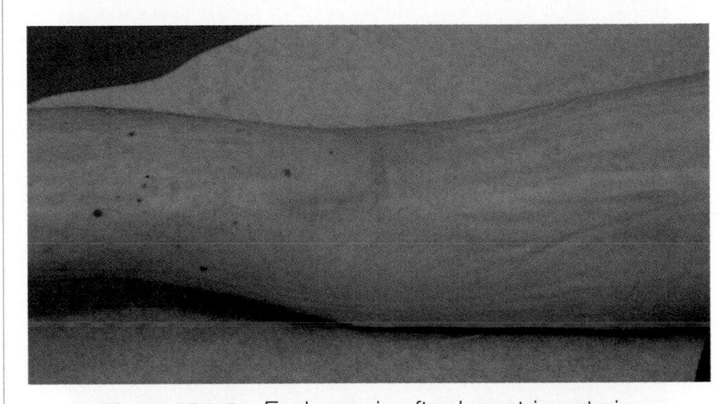

Figure 134-3 Ecchymosis after hamstring strain.

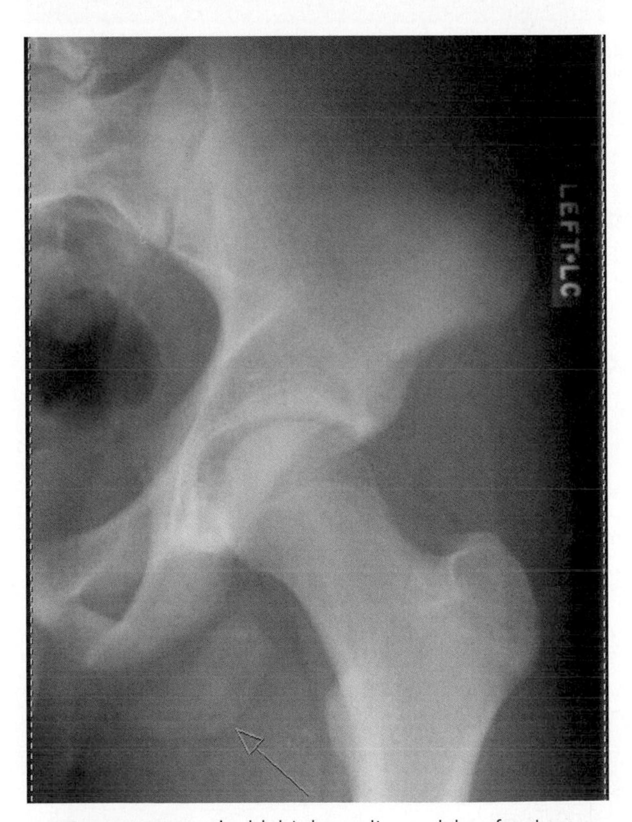

Figure 134-4 Ischial tuberosity avulsion fracture.

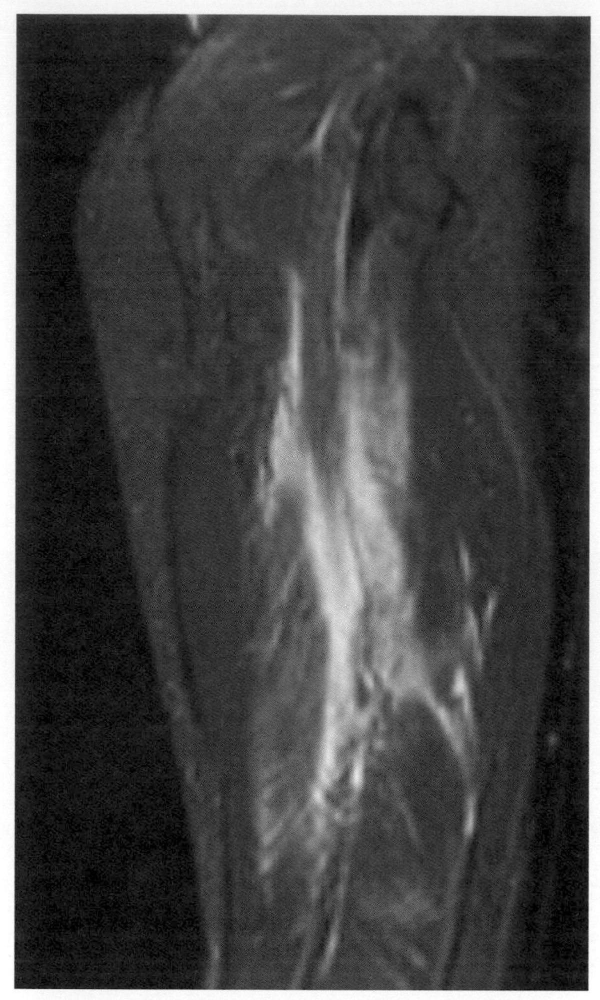

Figure 134-5 Magnetic resonance imaging of grade II hamstring strain. (Courtesy of D. Dean Thornton, MD.)

Differential Diagnosis

- See Table 134-1.

Treatment

- At diagnosis
  - Rest, ice, compression, and elevation
  - Nonsteroidal anti-inflammatory drugs
  - Early immobilization for 1 to 3 days may reduce hematoma development.
  - Mobilization should be initiated after this brief period to improve the range of motion.
  - Formal physical therapy
    - — Focus on edema and hematoma reduction in the acute period
    - — Advance to restoration of strength and range of motion
    - — Core strengthening may also be beneficial.

TABLE 134-1 *Differential Diagnosis*

Condition	Differentiating Feature	Chapter Reference
Sciatica	Neurologic symptoms, radiating pain from the back	118
Iliotibial band syndrome	Lateral pain at hip or knee, gradual onset	155
Stress fracture (femoral neck/ shaft/pelvis)	Seen on magnetic resonance imaging, overuse	136
Gluteus strain	More proximal injury	122
Ischial bursitis	More chronic pain, localized at ischial bursa	122

  - Stretching
    - — Both quadriceps and hamstring musculature
  - Immediate intramuscular corticosteroid injection is controversial, but has showed benefit in a retrospective noncontrolled study.
    - — More studies are needed before definitive recommendations can be made
- Later
  - Continued rehabilitation and gradual return to exercise/sport when pain free

When to Refer

- Complete rupture of the proximal or distal tendon
- Bony avulsion injury (surgery indicated if greater than 2 cm displacement)

Prognosis

- Wide variation in healing rate from days to months depending on patient and severity of injury

Troubleshooting

- Be aware that hamstring muscle injuries can be difficult to treat and that the recovery time varies on a case-by-case basis.
- The patient must be pain free with activity to return to sports.
- Counsel the patient that surgery, if necessary, carries a risk of neurologic injury.

Patient Instructions

- Follow physician and physical therapist instructions closely for a quick return to functionality.

- Be aware of the slow healing process and potential for recurrence.
- Stretch aggressively before activity.

Considerations in Special Populations

- Extremely common injury in sports medicine
- Athletes should be encouraged to stretch before exercise and develop well-balanced muscle groups.
- Return to play when pain free with activity.
- Hamstring muscle strains are less likely in the pediatric population due to increased flexibility, but apophyseal injuries including avulsions are more common and must be considered in proximal injuries.
    - Obtain radiographs in pediatric patients with proximal posterior thigh injury.

Suggested Reading

- Clanton T, Coupe K: Hamstring strains in athletes: Diagnosis and treatment. J Am Acad Orthop Surg 1998;6:237–248.
- Cohen S, Bradley J: Acute proximal hamstring rupture. J Am Acad Orthop Surg 2007;15:350–355.
- Drezner J: Practical management: Hamstring muscle injuries. Clin J Sports Med 2003;13:48–52.
- Lempainen L, Sarimo J, Mattila K, et al: Distal tears of the hamstring muscles: Review of the literature and our results of surgical management. Br J Sports Med 2007;41:80–83.
- Levine WN, Bergfeld JA, Tessendorf W, et al: Intramuscular corticosteroid injection for hamstring injuries: A 13-year experience in the National Football League. Am J Sports Med 2000;28:297–300.
- Mann G, Shabat S, Friedman A, et al: Hamstring injuries. Orthopedics 2007;30:536–540.
- Mason DL, Dickens V, Vail A: Rehabilitation for hamstring injuries. Cochrane Database Syst Rev 2007;24(1):CD004575.

Chapter 135 Quadriceps Contusions

Tracy Ray and Benson Scott

ICD-9 CODES
728.12 *Traumatic Myositis Ossificans*
924.00 *Contusion of Thigh*

Key Concepts

- A crush injury to the quadriceps musculature due to a direct blow causing either an intramuscular or intermuscular hematoma secondary to capillary damage
- Very common occurrence in contact sports (e.g., football, rugby, martial arts)
- Many contusions go unreported and untreated.
- An intermuscular hematoma usually disperses and results in significant ecchymosis.
- An intramuscular hematoma takes longer to resolve and may be associated with the major complications of the injury (e.g., myositis ossificans and acute compartment syndrome).
- Most often involves the anterior compartment (quadriceps femoris and sartorius muscles)
- Damaged tissue is replaced by a fibrous connective tissue scar that usually resolves, leaving no sign of injury after 3 to 4 weeks.
- Complications
  - Myositis ossificans: heterotopic bone formation within muscular tissue
    - — Pathogenesis still poorly understood
    - — Likelihood of occurrence increases with increasing grade of injury and with reinjury during recovery
    - — May reabsorb over time
    - — May be promoted by early surgery
  - Acute compartment syndrome: increased pressure within anterior compartment secondary to bleeding and edema causing secondary injury
    - — Pain out of proportion to injury
    - — Paresthesia distal to injury (later sign)
- Please see Table 135-1 and Figure 135-1.

History

- Symptoms
  - History of forceful blunt blow to anterior thigh
  - Painful anterior thigh with bruising
  - Painful to bear weight
  - Difficulty with knee flexion due to pain
  - Palpable hematoma
- May have insignificant symptoms initially with worsening over first 24 hours
- Include information on patient-reported symptoms, drawings that show the precise location of symptoms, and color photographs of the condition's appearance if appropriate.

Physical Examination

- Inspection
  - Observe gait.
  - Note any ecchymosis.
  - Measurement of girth (as much as a 4-cm difference can be normal)
- Palpation
  - Consider deferring to last piece of examination secondary to discomfort.
  - Note warmth and amount of tension in the thigh.
  - Examine for a muscular or quadriceps/patellar tendon defect.
  - Perform patellar range of motion.
  - Assess neurovascular status.

TABLE 135-1 *Quadriceps Contusion Grading*

Grade	Range of Motion	Symptoms/Presentation
1	>90 degree flexion	Minimal effect on ambulation No/minimal discomfort with resisted extension Feeling of "tightness" in the thigh Little, if any, swelling
2	45 to 90 degree flexion	Antalgic gait Pain reproducible with palpation Pain with resisted extension Likely, swelling
3	<45 degree flexion	Significant limp; crutches often required Immediate and significant swelling Quadriceps contraction with leg in extension is painful Unable to oppose resisted extension due to pain

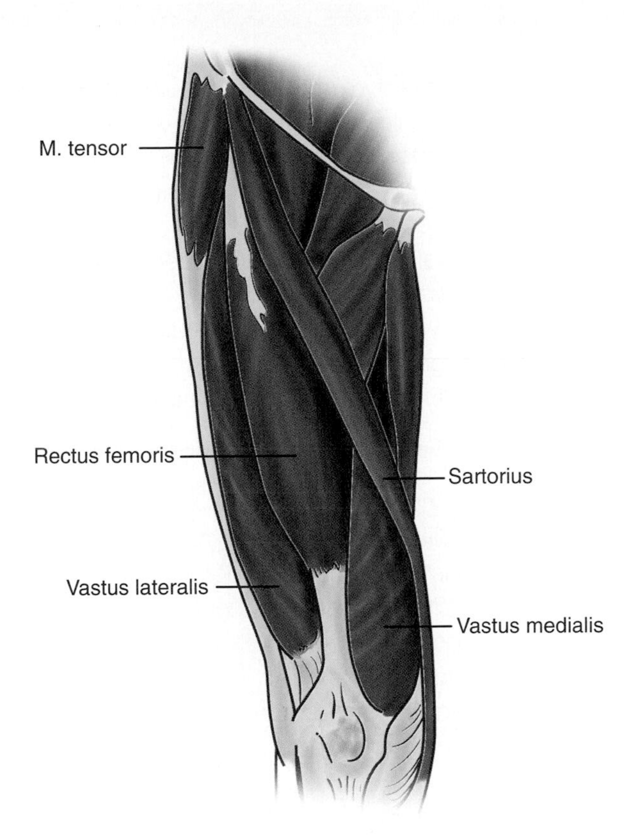

Figure 135-1 Thigh anatomy. M, musculus.

- Motion
  - Measure the flexion and extension of the knee.
  - Note the degree of passive flexion at which pain commences.
  - Perform straight leg raise (may be painful, but possible unless damage to extensor mechanism)
- Stability
  - Test ligamentous stability about the knee if swelling or effusion is present.

Imaging

- Radiographs should be obtained initially if there is any suspicion of bony injury; obtain additional radiographs if recovery is not progressing as expected (e.g., loss of flexion).
  - Radiographs may reveal myositis ossificans as early as 2 weeks post-injury (Fig. 135-2).
- No definite indication for magnetic resonance imaging unless considering a surgical procedure or for localization of unresolved or complicating hematoma or swelling
  - Abnormalities on magnetic resonance imaging may last longer than symptoms and functional impairment.

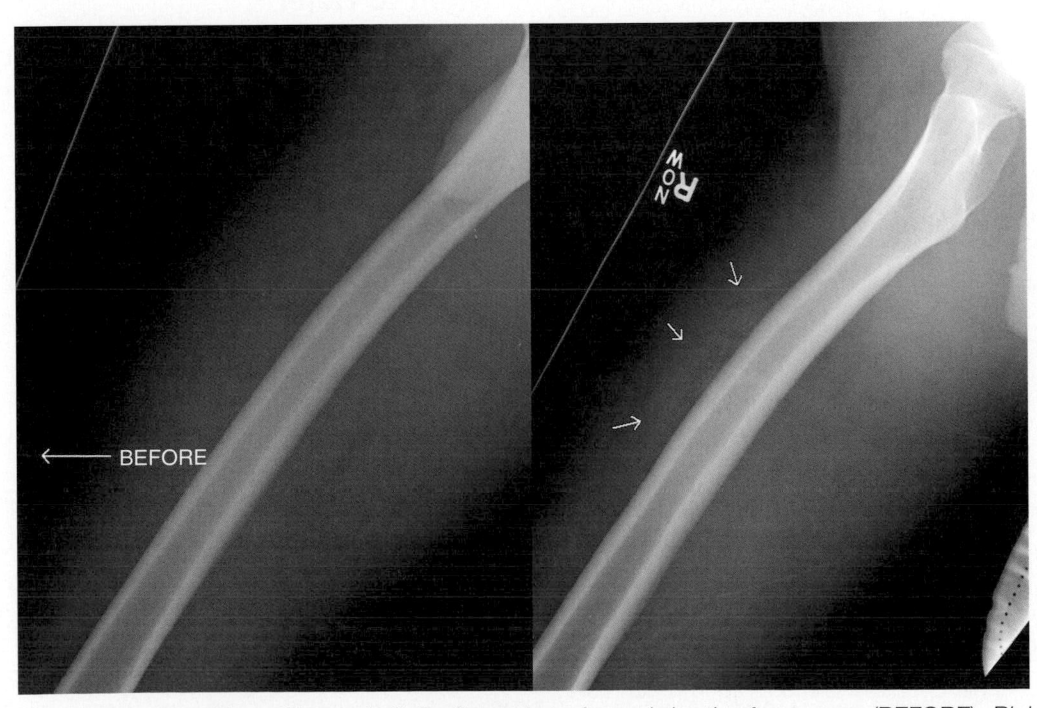

Figure 135-2 Radiograph of myositis ossificans. *Left,* Radiograph performed shortly after trauma (BEFORE). *Right,* Follow-up radiograph two weeks later shows the formation of myositis ossificans (*arrows*).

- Ultrasonography may be used to evaluate the size of the hematoma; however, this is not likely to change necessary treatment.

Differential Diagnosis

- Please see Table 135-2.

Treatment

- At diagnosis
  - Ice
  - Compression
  - Nonsteroidal anti-inflammatory medication
  - Immobilization of the knee in maximum painless flexion soon after injury may decrease the time to return to play; this should be maintained for 24 hours post-injury (Fig. 135-3).

TABLE 135-2 *Differential Diagnosis*

Diagnosis	Features	Chapter Reference
Quadriceps contusion	Swelling, ecchymosis, history of traumatic blow	
Myositis ossificans	Palpable mass, radiographic findings, decreased range of motion after period of improvement	
Compartment syndrome	Pain out of proportion, neurologic symptoms	
Quadriceps strain	No traumatic blow	

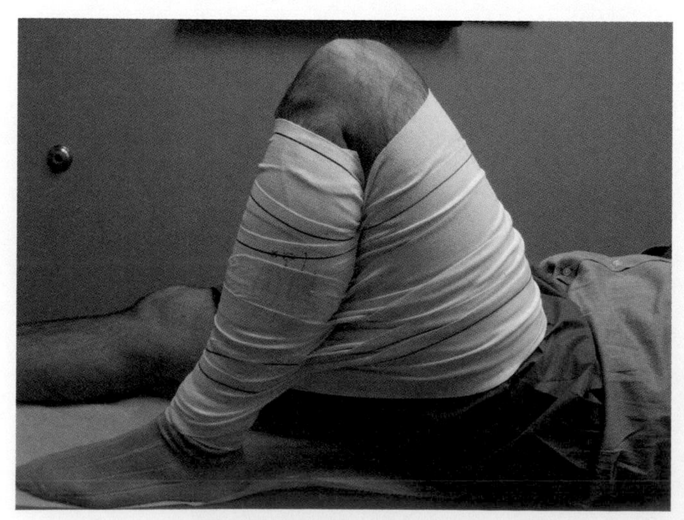

Figure 135-3 Example of patient immobilized in flexion using elastic wrap. Note that a postoperative or other locking knee brace can be used as well.

- Later
  - Active and passive painless range of motion stressing flexion multiple times daily as soon as immobilization is discontinued
  - Perform painless isometric strengthening exercises as soon as possible.
  - Nonsteroidal anti-inflammatory medication
- Myositis ossificans
  - Conservative treatment usually successful
  - Overly aggressive early therapy may stimulate growth of the ossification; avoid aggressive massage and forced motion and use pain as a guide.
  - Maintain range of motion
  - In adults with stable myositis ossificans, excision of the mass may be considered if the range of motion is significantly limited or pain is severe, but this can potentially result in recurrence and more extensive ossification.
- Acute compartment syndrome
  - Surgical emergency requiring a high level of clinical suspicion
  - Fasciotomy is sometimes performed, but a conservative approach involving rest, ice, compression, and elevation has shown promise.
  - If treating conservatively, monitor closely for muscular necrosis and renal compromise

When to Refer

- Considered emergently if any signs or symptoms of acute compartment syndrome arise
- Considered if development of myositis ossificans is accompanied by continuing symptoms that are affecting desired activities and/or significantly limiting range of motion
- Considered if hematoma fails to resolve

Prognosis

- Generally favorable because most patients are able to return to their previous level of activity without significant sequelae
- Surgery is usually unnecessary and recovery is usually complete.
- Return to play should be allowed when motion, strength, and skill have returned.
- Unrecognized compartment syndrome can lead to muscular death, scarring, limb contractures, and nerve damage.

- The future
  - Some evidence shows that corticosteroid injections may shorten the course of recovery and hasten the return to play.

Troubleshooting

- Early, aggressive massage and forced motion may worsen muscle damage and increase the chances of myositis ossificans.
- Counsel patients that surgery carries the risks of recurrence, infection, and extensor mechanism damage.
- Heat is not encouraged in early treatment.

Patient Instructions

- Maintaining the range of motion is imperative.
- Avoiding reinjury in the recovery/rehabilitation phase is of significant importance.
- Home therapy and patient initiative are required to allow the quickest return to activity.
- Close follow-up and communication between patient, physician, and therapist are needed.
- Take care not to return to activity too early; always discuss return to play with the physician.
- Inform the physician of worsening symptoms including neurologic symptoms.

Suggested Reading

- Aronen JG, Garrick JG, Chronister RD, McDevitt ER: Quadriceps contusions: Clinical results of immediate immobilization in 120 degrees of knee flexion. Clin J Sport Med 2006;16:383–387.
- Beiner JM, Jokl P: Muscle contusion injuries: Current treatment options. J Am Acad Orthop Surg 2001;9:227–237.
- DeLee JC, Drez D Jr, Miller MD (eds): DeLee & Drez's Orthopaedic Sports Medicine: Principles and Practice. Philadelphia: WB Saunders, 2003, Vol. 1, p 12 and Vol. 2, pp 1858–1860.
- Diaz JA, Fischer DA, Rettig AC, et al: Severe quadriceps muscle contusions in athletes. Am J Sports Med 2003;31:289–293.
- Newton M, Walker J: Acute quadriceps injury: A case report. Emerg Nurse 2004;12:24–29.

Chapter 136 Femoral Stress Fractures

George S. Edwards III, Brandon D. Bushnell, and Timothy N. Taft

ICD-9 CODE
733.95 *Stress Fracture of Other Bone*

Key Concepts

- Femoral stress fractures account for 7% to 12% of all stress fractures in athletes.
- The femur is the fourth most common bone to sustain a stress fracture. (The tibia is the most common bone.)
- Fracture may occur in any part of the femur: femoral head, neck, diaphysis, or distal femur. The femoral head and neck are the most common and the distal femur is the least common.
- Fractures are classified into two categories: fatigue and insufficiency.
  - Fatigue stress fractures
    - — An overuse problem
    - — Caused by repetitive excessive stresses on normal bone
    - — Running is the most common cause.
    - — Classically seen in military recruits and athletes who have recently increased their training
    - — Bone abnormalities, such as coxa vara, may increase the risk.
  - Insufficiency stress fractures
    - — Caused by normal activity on weak bone
    - — Often seen in elderly patients with osteoporosis or in those with medical conditions that cause weakened bone (e.g., Paget's disease, corticosteroid treatment, renal failure, irradiation, at sites of previous screw holes)
- Tension-side fractures of the femoral neck often require urgent surgical treatment and should be referred immediately (Fig. 136-1).

History

- Often there is no history of specific trauma, or the patient may describe minor trauma.
- The patient may describe pain in the hip, groin, or thigh that is gradually worsening.
  - Pain may not be as prominent with insufficiency fractures
  - Pain may become acutely worse if the fracture suddenly completes or displaces
- Location of pain depends on site of fracture; pain is often difficult to localize
- Pain is often relieved by rest.
- Exacerbated by exercise
- May report pain at night
- The index of suspicion for a stress fracture must be high due to the subtlety of symptoms and radiographs that are often normal (Fig. 136-2).

Physical Examination

- There is typically no obvious deformity in the area of the fracture.

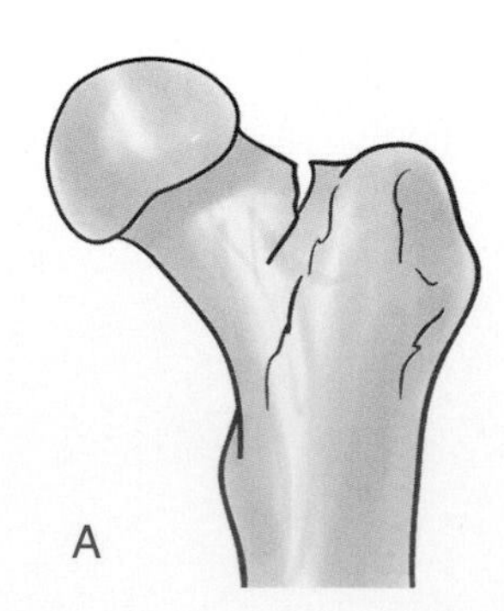

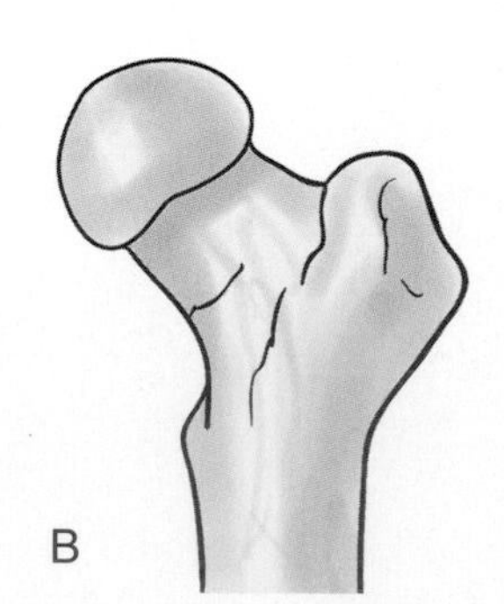

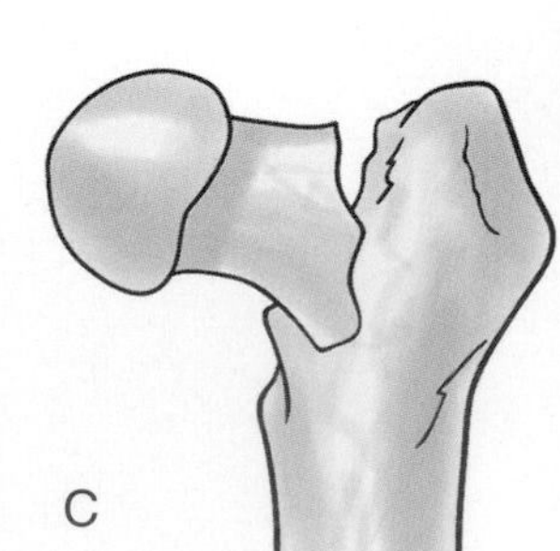

Figure 136-1 Fullerton and Snowdy classification of femoral neck stress fractures. **A**, Tension-type fracture; **B**, compression-type fracture; **C**, displaced type fracture. (Adapted from Canale ST [ed]: Campbell's Operative Orthopaedics, Vol. 3, 10th ed. Philadelphia: Mosby, 2003, p 2920, Fig. 52-58.)

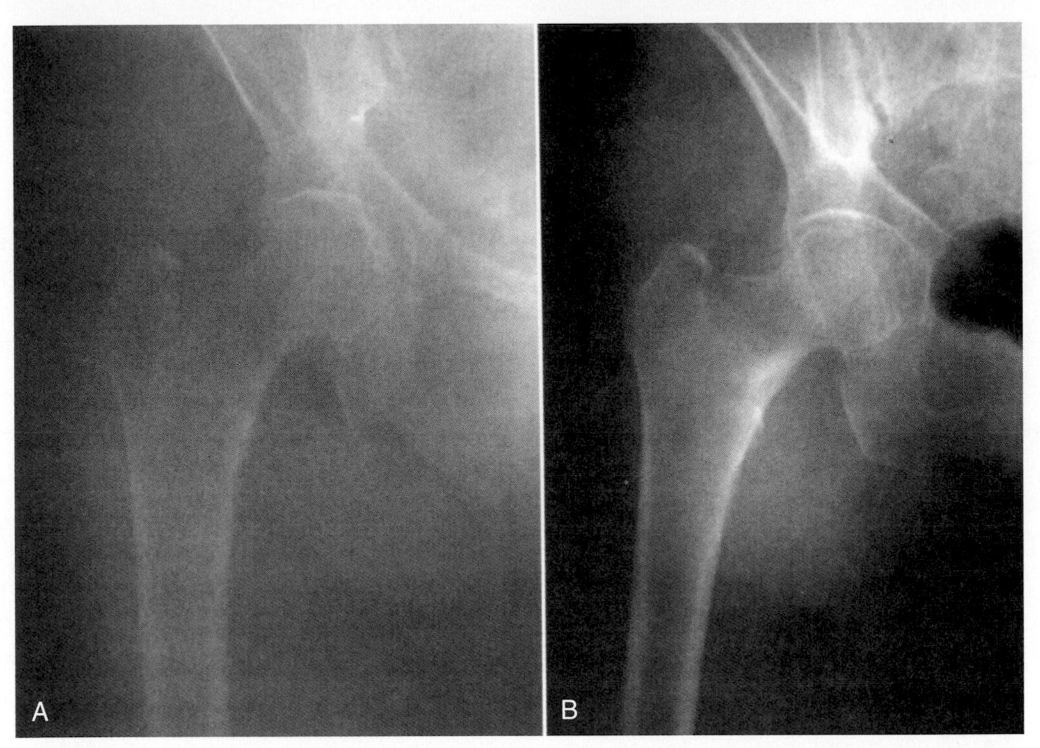

Figure 136-2 **A**, Radiograph demonstrating subtlety of a suspected femoral neck stress fracture. **B**, Radiograph taken 3 months later showing healed bone and increased bone density at site of injury. (From Canale ST [ed]: Campbell's Operative Orthopaedics, Vol. 3, 10th ed. Philadelphia: Mosby, 2003, p 2920, Fig. 52-57.)

- Often diffusely tender to palpation near the site of fracture, although an exact point of maximal tenderness often difficult to elicit because of the thick soft-tissue envelope surrounding the area
- Gentle hip range of motion may elicit groin pain, especially at the extremes of motion, if the fracture is in the femoral neck.
- Straight leg raise is often difficult for patients with femoral neck and shaft fractures.
- An antalgic gait pattern is often noted.

Imaging

- Obtain plain radiographs first because they often show the fracture and are relatively inexpensive.
- If no fracture is seen on plain radiographs but the patient continues to have pain, magnetic resonance imaging (Figs. 136-3 and 136-4) or a bone scan (Fig. 136-5) is the next test to order.
- Magnetic resonance imaging has been shown to be more accurate than a bone scan in diagnosing femoral neck stress fractures.
- However, a bone scan is the most sensitive test for femoral shaft stress fractures and is often less expensive.

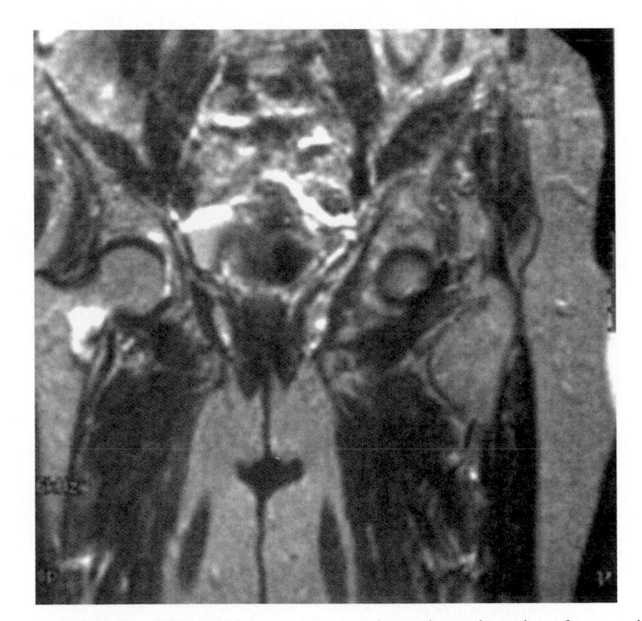

Figure 136-3 Magnetic resonance imaging showing femoral stress fracture of right femoral neck and ease of detection compared with plain radiograph in Figure 136-2. (From Canale ST [ed]: Campbell's Operative Orthopaedics, Vol. 3, 10th ed. Philadelphia: Mosby, 2003, p 2919, Fig. 52-56.)

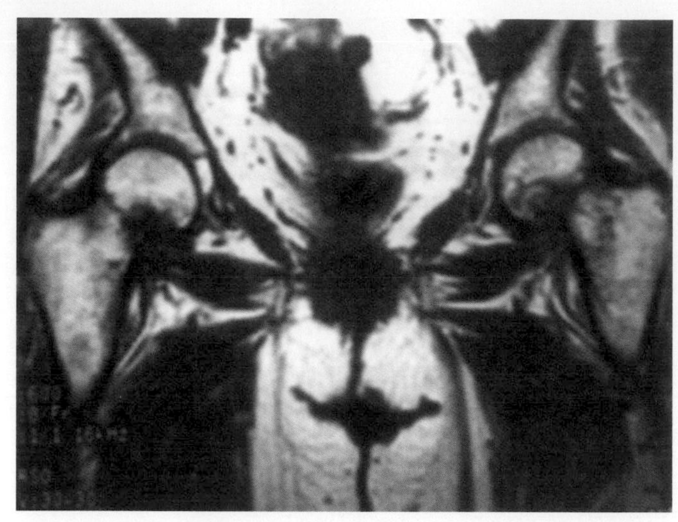

Figure 136-4 Bilateral insufficiency fractures in a patient with a long history of steroid use shown well on T2-weighted magnetic resonance imaging with diagnostic perifracture edema. The radiographs and bone scan were read as negative for this patient. (From Bucholz RW, Heckman JD, Court-Brown C, et al [eds]: Rockwood and Green's Fractures in Adults, 6th ed. Philadelphia: Lippincott Williams & Wilkins, 2005, p 670, Fig. 21-1.)

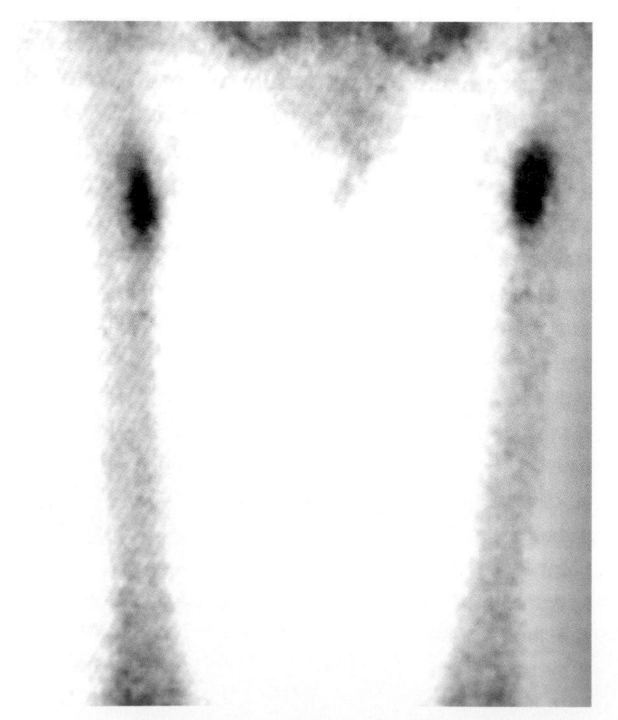

Figure 136-5 Bone scan demonstrating bilateral femoral shaft stress fractures. (From Bucholz RW, Heckman JD, Court-Brown C, et al [eds]: Rockwood and Green's Fractures in Adults, 6th ed. Philadelphia: Lippincott Williams & Wilkins, 2005, p 670, Fig. 21-1.)

- Radiographs of the contralateral side should be obtained to rule out a stress fracture of the contralateral femur because bilateral fractures can occur.

Additional Tests

- No additional laboratory tests are needed because they are usually normal in the setting of a stress fracture.

Differential Diagnosis

- Because the symptoms are often vague, the differential diagnosis is large but depends on the location of the pain.
- The differential diagnosis for femoral neck stress fractures should include all causes of hip pain, including musculoskeletal causes such as muscular, tendinous, ligamentous, intra-articular, osseous, and bursal disorders. Lower back, visceral, pelvic, and neurologic pathologies must also be considered.
- The differential diagnosis for femoral shaft stress fractures includes soft-tissue injuries, neoplasm, infection, nerve compression syndrome, and pain referred from the hip or knee.

Treatment

- Depends on location and amount of displacement
- Displaced stress fractures usually require operative treatment.
  - Children with displaced femoral neck fractures may be treated with a plaster spica cast for 6 weeks.
- Nondisplaced femoral head: Treatment is restricted weight bearing until symptoms resolve.
- Nondisplaced femoral neck: Treatment depends on whether the fracture is a tension-side or compression-side fracture.
  - Tension-side (superior neck) fracture: operative treatment is usually recommended because of increased risk of progression to displacement and possible nonunion; may be treated nonoperatively with protected weight bearing
  - Compression-side (inferior neck) fracture: may be treated nonoperatively with protected weight bearing
- Displaced femoral head or neck fractures may be treated with internal fixation or with total hip arthroplasty.
- Nondisplaced femoral shaft fractures: Some surgeons recommend nonoperative treatment with restricted

weight bearing for 1 to 4 weeks. Other sources recommend operative treatment with intramedullary nailing because nonoperative treatment can be painful, unsuccessful, and time-consuming.

When to Refer

- Refer if there are signs that the fracture may require operative management including displacement, if the fracture extends into a joint, if a tension-side fracture is present, or if there is evidence of nonunion.

Prognosis

- Nondisplaced femoral neck fractures heal well with conservative treatment and have no increased incidence of avascular necrosis or osteoarthritis.
- Displaced femoral neck fractures have a significant risk of nonunion and avascular necrosis of the femoral head.
- Femoral shaft fractures have a very good prognosis, assuming they are adequately treated.
- Femoral stress fractures in children, although rare, heal well. Rates approach 100%, regardless of the fracture location.

Troubleshooting

- Criteria for returning to full sports activity should include
  - Completion of rehabilitation protocol
  - Radiographic evidence of bone healing
  - Pain-free full range of motion
  - Normal gait in both running and walking
  - Equal muscle strength bilaterally

Patient Instructions

- It is important to follow the weight-bearing status set by the physician. Failure to do so may result in progression of the fracture or a prolonged healing time.

Considerations in Special Populations

- Female athletes: The female athlete triad of disordered eating, menstrual irregularities, and reduced bone density places female at risk of stress fractures.
- Paget's disease
  - The most common complication in Paget's disease is stress fracture.
  - Stress fractures are two times more likely to occur in the femur than the tibia in patients with Paget's disease.
  - Even though Paget's disease is more common in men, stress fractures in patients with Paget's disease are more common in women.
  - Treatment is similar to that of patients without Paget's disease. Treat nondisplaced stress fractures with symptomatic treatment and limited weight bearing and displaced fractures with internal fixation.

Suggested Reading

- Buckwalter JA, Brandser EA: Stress and insufficiency fractures. Am Fam Physician 1997;56:175–182.
- Burke G, Boissonnault WG, Andrews R: Differential diagnosis of a femoral neck/head stress fracture. J Orthop Sports Phys Ther 2005;36:80–88.
- Casterline M, Osowski S, Ulrich G: Femoral stress fracture. J Athletic Train 1996;31:53–56.
- Lee CH, Huang GS, Chao KH, et al: Surgical treatment of displaced stress fractures of the femoral neck in military recruits: A report of 42 cases. Arch Orthop Trauma Surg 2003;123:527–533.
- Pihlajamaki HK, Ruohola JP, Weckstrom M, et al: Long-term outcomes of undisplaced fatigue fractures of the femoral neck in young male adults. J Bone Joint Surg Br 2006;88B:1574–1579.

Chapter 137 Pelvic Fractures

Chancellor F. Gray, Brandon D. Bushnell, and Timothy N. Taft

Key Concepts

- Pelvic fractures, including acetabular fractures, are usually associated with high-energy trauma.
- Acetabular fractures, especially those involving the posterior wall, have a high association with hip dislocation.
- Major vascular and neurologic structures pass through the pelvic ring; there is great potential for serious complications or death with disruption.
- Large volumes of blood may be lost into the pelvis with no external evidence of bleeding. Hemodynamic instability requires immediate attention and treatment.
- Pelvic fractures are often separated into two groups, stable and unstable. This distinction determines much of the management and prognosis of the injury.
  - Stable injuries are those that will not deform in the presence of normal physiologic forces.
  - Unstable injuries may display vertical instability, rotational instability, or both.
- Other "lesser" fractures of the pelvis, such as nondisplaced iliac wing fractures, avulsion fractures, and coccygeal fractures, respond well to conservative treatment.
- Pelvic anatomy distortion after fracture can cause obstetric issues for women of child-bearing age, sometimes resulting in the need for a cesarean section.

Anatomy

- The pelvis is a ring structure composed of three bones: the sacrum and the left and right innominate bones (Fig. 137-1).
  - The innominate bone is composed of the ilium, ischium, and pubis.
  - The center of fusion of these three bones forms the acetabulum.
- The pelvis, in the sagittal plane, may be considered to have two functional columns: anterior and posterior.
  - The anterior column is also known as the iliopubic component and extends from the iliac crest to the pubic symphysis.
  - The posterior column, or ilioischial component, extends from the superior gluteal notch to the ischial tuberosity.
- The innominate bones join the sacrum posteriorly at the sacroiliac joint and join each other anteriorly at the symphysis pubis.
- The major sources of pelvic stability are the ligamentous structures posteriorly and anteriorly.
  - Posterior: the short and long sacroiliac ligaments, the sacrospinous and sacrotuberous ligaments; provide the main weight-bearing stability of the pelvis
  - Anterior: the symphysis pubis; provides rotational stability

History

- The most severe cases involve high-energy trauma, including motor vehicle collisions, vehicle-pedestrian impacts, crush mechanisms, or falls from height.
- Some low-energy fractures can also occur, often in athletic situations, and include patterns such as avulsions, coccygeal injuries, and minimal iliac wing fractures.
- Understanding the mechanism of injury will often aid in identifying and fully characterizing the fracture as injury patterns are typical to certain mechanisms.

Physical Examination

- Patients with higher-energy mechanisms require a full-scale trauma evaluation with primary, secondary, and tertiary surveys.

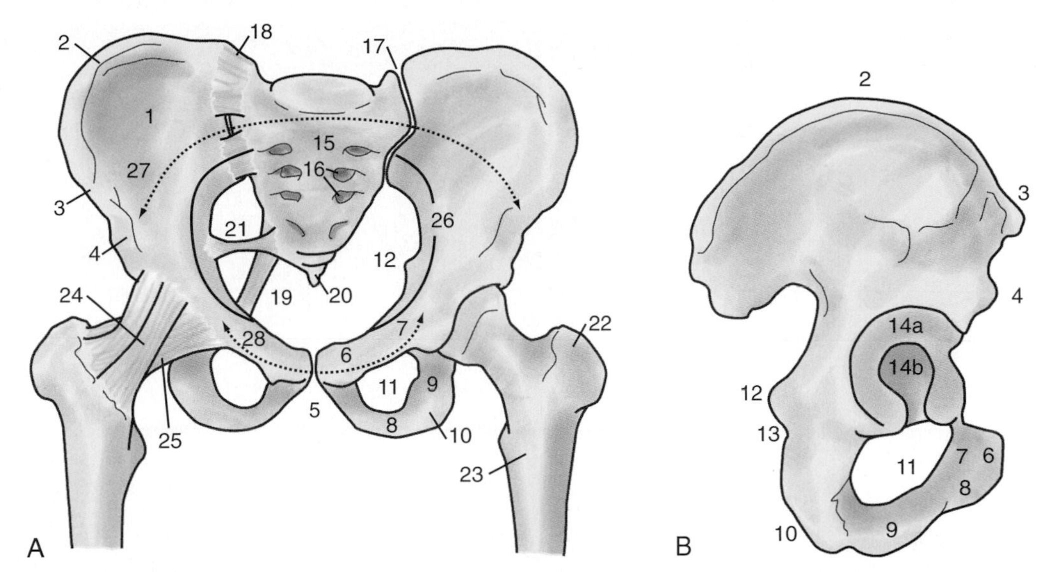

Figure 137-1 Pelvic anatomy. **A**, Anterior view of the pelvis; **B**, lateral view of the right innominate bone. 1, Iliac fossa; 2, iliac crest; 3, anterior superior iliac spine; 4, anterior inferior iliac spine; 5, symphysis pubis; 6, body of the pubis; 7, superior ramus of the pubis; 8, inferior ramus of the pubis; 9, ramus of the ischium; 10, ischial tuberosity; 11, obturator foramen; 12, ischial spine; 13, lesser sciatic notch; 14, acetabulum (14a, articular surface; 14b, fossa); 15, sacrum; 16, anterior sacral foramina; 17, sacroiliac joint; 18, anterior sacroiliac ligament; 19, sacrotuberous ligament (sacrum to ischial tuberosity); 20, coccyx; 21, sacrospinous ligament; 22, greater trochanter of the femur; 23, lesser trochanter of the femur; 24, iliofemoral ligament; 25, pubofemoral ligament; 26, arcuate line; 27, posterior or femorosacral arch through which main weight-bearing forces are transmitted; 28, anterior arch. (Adapted from Cwinn AA: Pelvis. In Marx JA (ed): Rosen's Emergency Medicine: Concepts and Clinical Practice, 6th ed. Philadelphia: Elsevier, 2006.)

- Early assessment of the neurovascular status is essential. Vessel rupture that can lead to major hemorrhage may be associated with loss of distal pulses and hemodynamic instability. A rectal examination checking for sphincter tone plays an important role in assessing the neurologic status of the patient.
- With inspection, the patient with a pelvic fracture may have a visible deformity, including a leg length discrepancy or an internally or externally rotated lower extremity.
  - Both patterns are suggestive of pelvic instability.
  - Ecchymosis may be present, especially anteriorly near the pubis or into the labia or scrotum.
- There may be tenderness to palpation over the site of the injury, and there may also be crepitus.
- A unique consideration in pelvic fracture is genitourinary injury, which occurs in approximately 15% of pelvic trauma cases, with higher rates reported in males.
  - Signs include blood at the urethral meatus or, in males, a "floating" prostate on rectal examination.
- Lower-energy injuries will have more localized and less severe findings, including mild tenderness, local ecchymosis, and pain with certain resisted motions (such as challenged hip extension with hamstring avulsion fractures).

Imaging

- Radiographs: Anteroposterior, inlet/outlet, and Judet views of the pelvis should be obtained (Fig. 137-2).
- If stability is unclear, stress views may be useful, with the patient under anesthesia. More than 0.5 to 1 cm of motion should be considered unstable. Other signs of instability include sacroiliac joint displacement of more than 5 mm and avulsion of the ischial spine.
- In cases of a suspected acetabular fracture, it is essential to get Judet views of the pelvis that include obturator and iliac oblique views.
- Computed tomography: Fine-slice computed tomography should also be performed (see Fig. 137-2). Recent studies have suggested that computed tomography scanning should be considered the gold standard for evaluation of bony injury to the pelvis and for defining the true extent of a fracture, especially injury to the iliac wing, sacrum, or coccyx.

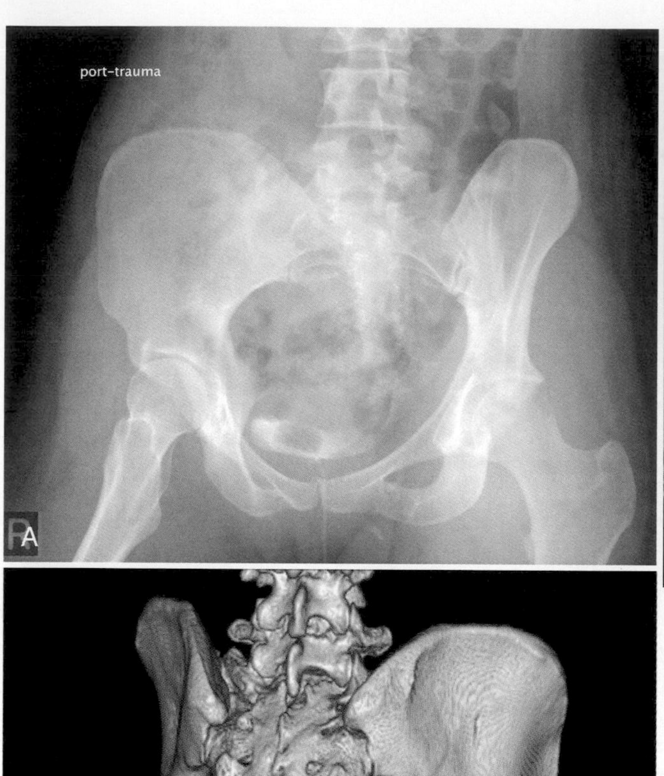

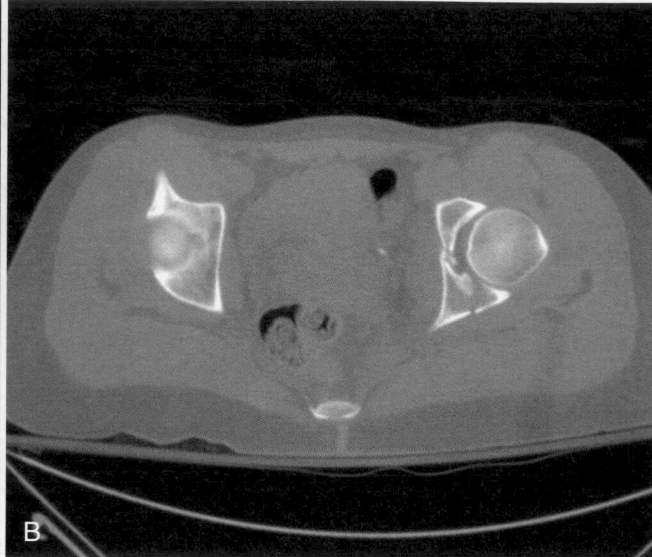

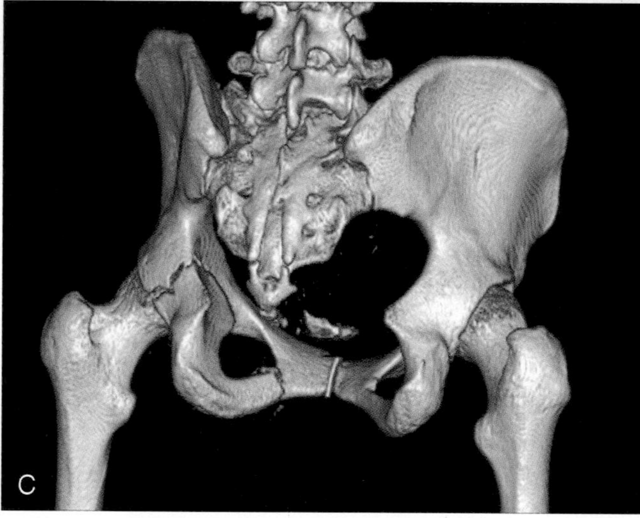

Figure 137-2 Separate images of the pelvis of a 24-year-old woman injured in a motor vehicle accident. Disruption of the left inferior pubic ramus can be seen as well as a fracture involving the left acetabulum. **A**, Plain radiograph taken in the Judet view. **B**, Axial computed tomography further reveals the nature of the acetabular fracture. **C**, Three-dimensional reconstruction computed tomography gives the best view of the fracture pattern, but may not be necessary in all situations.

Classification

- The most common classification system for pelvic injury is the Young and Burgess system (Box 137-1), which is based on the mechanism of injury.
- Tile also defined a classification system based on stability.
  - It is divided into types A, B, and C. Type A injuries are stable; type B injuries are rotationally unstable but vertically stable; and type C injuries are both rotationally and vertically unstable.
- The Letournel and Judet classification scheme (Table 137-1) is used to describe fractures involving the acetabulum and has two subdivisions, simple/elementary (Fig. 137-3) and complex/associated (Fig. 137-4).

BOX 137-1 *Young and Burgess Classification of Pelvic Injuries*

Lateral compression (LC): anterior injury rami fractures
- LC I: sacral fracture on side of impact
- LC II: crescent fracture on side of impact
- LC III: type I or II injury on side of impact with contralateral open-book injury

Anteroposterior compression (APC): anterior injury = symphysis diastasis/rami fractures
- APC I: minor opening of symphysis and sacroiliac (SI) joint anteriorly
- APC II: opening of anterior SI, intact posterior SI ligaments
- APC III: complete disruption of SI joint

Vertical shear (VS type): vertical displacement of hemipelvis with symphysis diastasis or rami fractures anteriorly; iliac wing or sacral fracture or SI dislocation posteriorly

Combination (CM type): any combination of above injuries

Additional Tests

- Retrograde urethrography or voiding cystourethrography if a genitourinary injury is suspected
- Angiography and possible intervention in the presence of uncontrolled hemorrhage

Differential Diagnosis

- Femoral head fracture
- Hip fracture
- Hip dislocation
- Femur fracture
- Hamstring strain
- Quadriceps strain
- Hip pointer (iliac wing contusion)

Treatment

- Treatment of a pelvic fracture will vary depending on the patient, the injury, and the institution.

TABLE 137-1 *Letournel and Judet Classification Scheme*

Simple/Elementary	Complex/Associated
Posterior wall	Transverse and posterior wall
Posterior column	Posterior column and posterior wall
Anterior wall	T-shaped
Anterior column	Anterior column/posterior hemitransverse
Transverse	Both columns

- The goals of treatment are to address/prevent life-threatening injuries, restore anatomy and function, and minimize long-term sequelae.
- The first decision to be made is determination of stability. Most stable injuries can be managed nonoperatively.
  - Associated injuries can alter the management picture. If the other injuries inhibit rehabilitation, operative management may be indicated.
  - Rehabilitation should focus on early mobilization with protected weight bearing initially. The patient

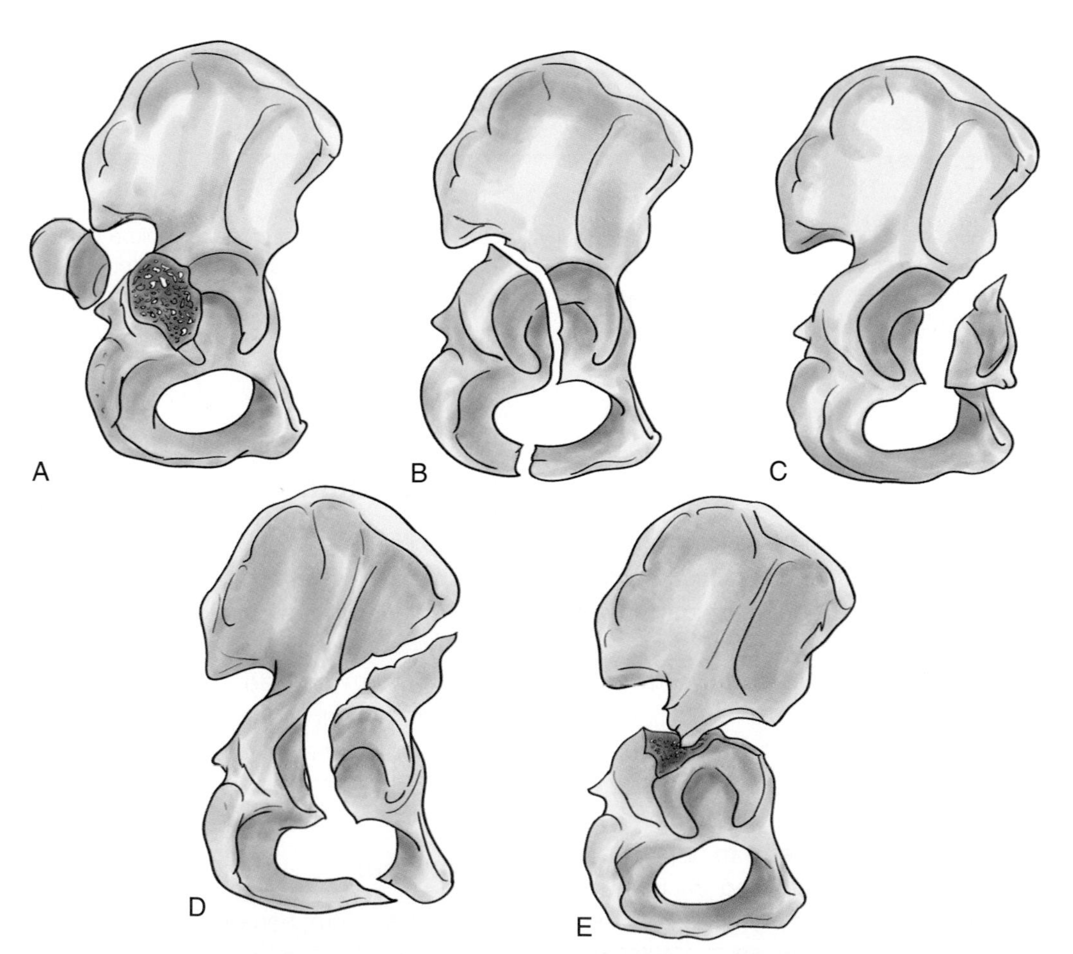

Figure 137-3 Letournel's classification of simple acetabular fractures. **A**, Posterior wall; **B**, posterior column; **C**, anterior wall; **D**, anterior column; **E**, transverse. (Adapted from Browner BD [ed]: Skeletal Trauma: Basic Science, Management and Reconstruction, 3rd ed. Philadelphia: Elsevier, 2003.)

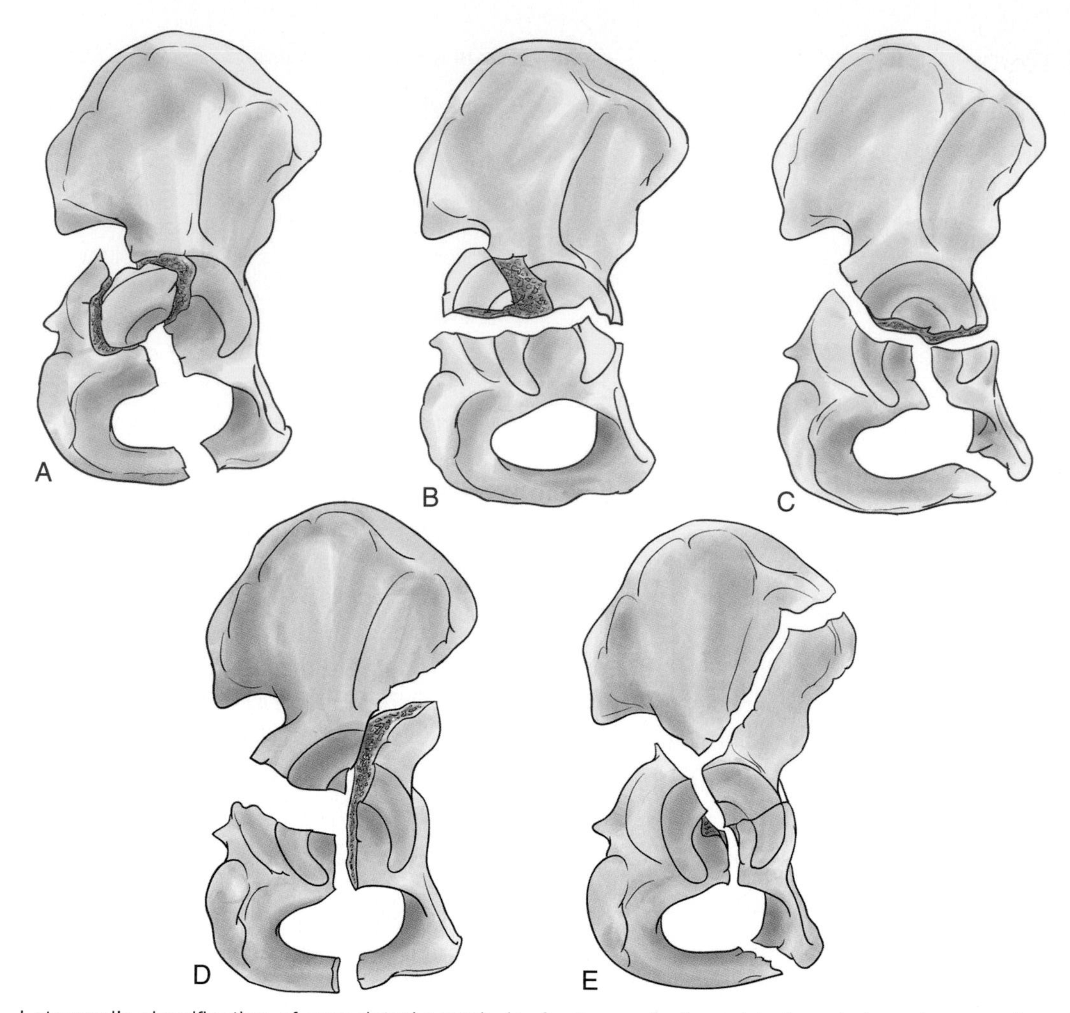

Figure 137-4 Letournel's classification of associated acetabular fractures. **A**, Associated posterior column and posterior wall fractures; **B**, associated transverse and posterior wall fractures; **C**, T-shaped fracture; **D**, associated anterior and posterior hemitransverse fractures; **E**, both-column fracture. (Adapted from Browner BD [ed]: Skeletal Trauma: Basic Science, Management and Reconstruction, 3rd ed. Philadelphia: Elsevier, 2003.)

should be followed with serial radiographs after mobilization.

- Unstable pelvic fractures should be treated with external fixation with or without skeletal traction, followed in some cases by open reduction and internal fixation.
- Acetabular fractures must be treated to minimize the risk of posttraumatic arthritis.
  - Initial management should include placement in skeletal traction.
  - Operative treatment should be used in certain circumstances, including fractures with displacement greater than 2 to 3 mm, displaced fractures that cannot be reduced by closed methods, and those in which a congruent joint cannot be maintained out of skeletal traction. Also, loose intra-articular fragments need to be removed operatively.

When to Refer

- Higher-energy pelvic and acetabular fractures should always be referred to an orthopaedic surgeon comfortable with the management of these fractures.
- Lower-energy avulsion fractures can be followed nonoperatively and do not mandate referral. Increased displacement of fracture fragments, however, should prompt referral.

Prognosis

- Open fracture, hemorrhagic shock on admission, and associated head and abdominal injuries have a poorer prognosis. In unstable fractures, posterior disruption has a higher incidence of mortality.

- Acetabular fracture: Injury to cartilage or bone of the femoral head reduces the likelihood of a good outcome by 20%.

Troubleshooting

- Several authorities recommend using a sheet or pelvic binder to emergently reduce open book–type pelvic instability and help control blood loss.

Considerations in Special Populations

- Heterotopic ossification may occur in as many as 70% of patients requiring fracture repair. The highest incidence is in young men and is worse with removal of muscle. Indomethacin is a useful preventive measure.

Suggested Reading

- Cwinn AA: Pelvis. In Marx JA (ed): Rosen's Emergency Medicine: Concepts and Clinical Practice, 6th ed. Philadelphia: Elsevier, 2006.
- Durkin A, Sagi HC, Durham R, Flint L: Contemporary management of pelvic fractures. Am J Surg 2006;192:211–223.
- Kellam JF, Mayo K: Pelvic ring disruptions. In Browner BD (ed): Skeletal Trauma: Basic Science, Management and Reconstruction, 3rd ed. Philadelphia: Elsevier, 2003.
- Koval KJ, Zuckerman JD: Handbook of Fractures, 3rd ed. Philadelphia: Lippincott Williams & Wilkins, 2006.
- Rice PL, Rudolph M: Pelvic fractures. Emerg Med Clin North Am 2007:25:795–802.

Chapter 138 Proximal Femur Fractures

Timothy D. Murphy, Brandon D. Bushnell, and Timothy N. Taft

ICD-9 CODES

820.09 *Other, Transcervical Fracture of Femur, Closed, Head*
820.8 *Fracture of Unspecified Part of Neck of Femur, Closed Hip NOS; Neck of Femur NOS*
820.9 *Fracture of Unspecified Part of Neck of Femur, Open*
820.21 *Fracture of Intertrochanteric Section of Femur, Closed*

Key Concepts

- Head fractures
  - Almost all are associated with posterior hip dislocations, with an incidence of 7% of all fractures involving the hip.
  - Rapid reduction is essential to prevent vascular compromise to the femoral head.
- Neck fractures
  - Most commonly occur in the elderly
  - When they do occur in younger patients, high-energy trauma is typically involved.
  - Femoral neck fractures are increasing in prevalence and are expected to double by the year 2040.
  - Higher risk in women, whites, the elderly, tobacco users, persions with low estrogen levels, athletes (stress fractures)
- Intertrochanteric fractures
  - Intertrochanteric fractures account for 50% of proximal femur fractures.
  - Timely management is essential to decrease morbidity and mortality, especially in younger patients or those with high-energy injuries.
  - Risk factors include osteoporosis, female gender, advanced age, and positive maternal history.

History

- Elderly patients
  - A history of a low-energy trauma, such as a fall from standing height, is involved. Delayed presentation is common.
- Younger patients
  - Most often present with a history of high-energy trauma such as a motor vehicle accident
  - Head fractures usually occur in association with a hip dislocation.

Physical Examination

- A shortened, externally rotated lower extremity, with pain on passive movement is the classic presentation for proximal femur fractures (Fig. 138-1).
- Patients with nondisplaced intertrochanteric fractures may have minor pain and be able to bear weight.
- A complete neurovascular examination should be performed.
- In younger patients, higher-energy injury is usually involved, and thus a full trauma workup is warranted.
- Elderly patients often have an upper extremity injury from the same fall.

Imaging

- An anteroposterior view of the pelvis and anteroposterior, frogleg, and cross-table lateral views of the hip should be obtained (Figs. 138-1 and 138-2).
- Computed tomography is commonly performed if associated fractures are suspected or in the setting of higher-energy injury.

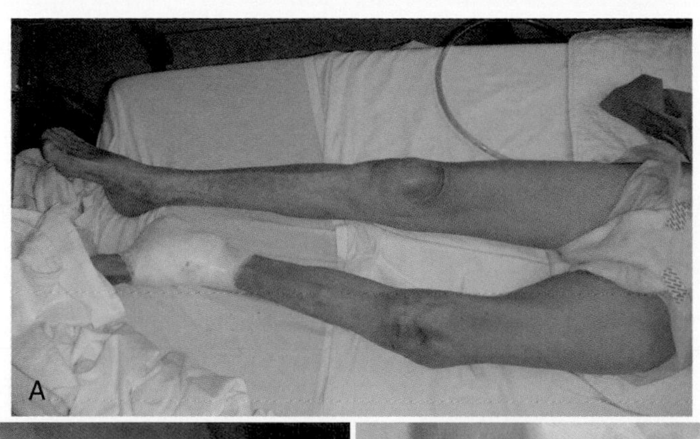

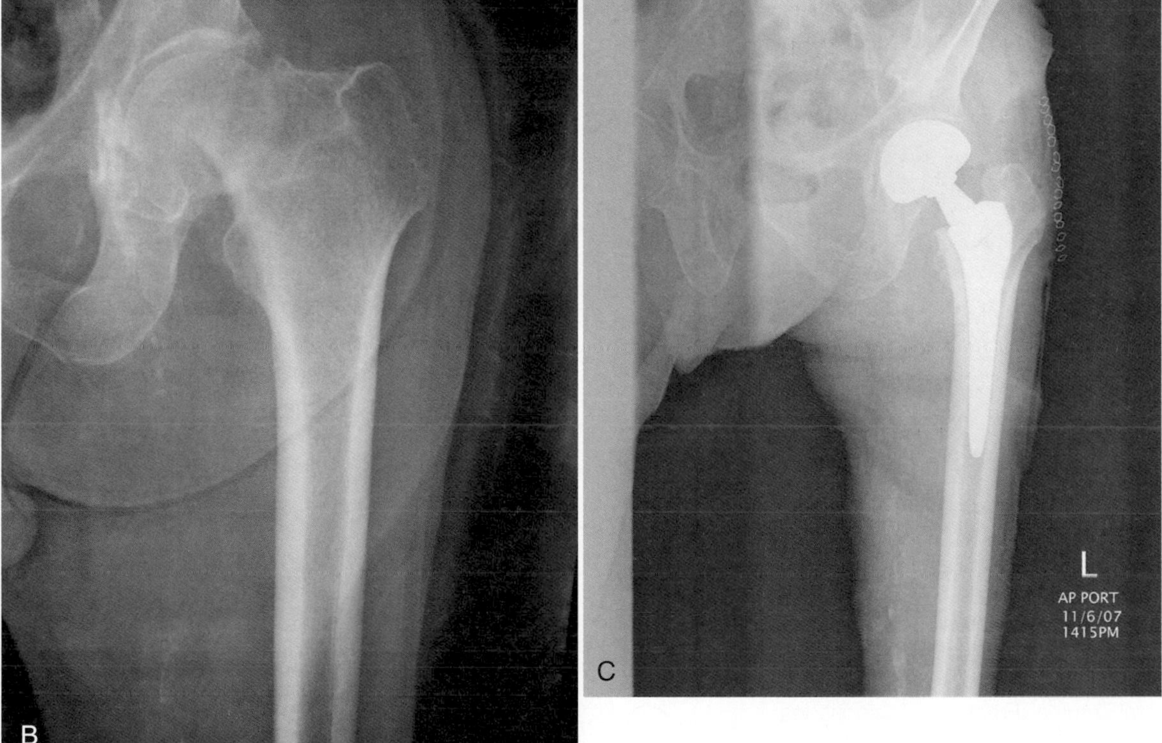

Figure 138-1 **A**, A patient with a left femoral neck fracture lying in a typical position with a shortened and externally rotated lower extremity. **B**, Preoperative anteroposterior radiograph. **C**, Postoperative anteroposterior radiograph after this patient was treated with a hemiarthroplasty.

Classification

- Head fractures
  - The Pipkin classification describes femoral head fractures associated with a posterior hip dislocation and gives some idea of the prognosis of the injury (Fig. 138-3).
- Neck fractures
  - Garden classification is the most commonly used. In general, increased displacement results in a higher risk of avascular necrosis and influences the choice of surgical treatment (Fig. 138-4).
  - More vertical fracture patterns have a higher risk of displacement.
- Intertrochanteric fractures
  - The Evans classification describes the fracture as stable versus unstable and helps guide treatment (Fig. 138-5).

Additional Tests

- Dual-energy x-ray absorptiometry is recommended in elderly individuals if they have not already been evaluated for osteoporosis.
- Elderly patients often require a workup for the cause of their fall, which can include syncope, heart disease, stroke, metabolic abnormality, delirium/dementia, and other medical conditions.

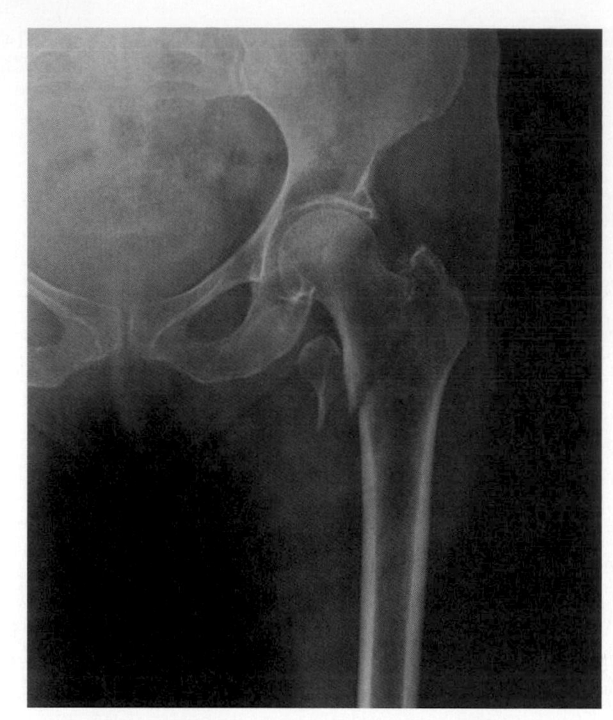

Figure 138-2 Anteroposterior view of an unstable intertrochanteric femur fracture.

Differential Diagnosis

- Hip dislocation
- Pelvic fracture
- Femoral shaft fracture
- Referred abdominal pain

Treatment

- Head fractures
  - Closed reduction of an associated hip dislocation should be promptly performed, followed by post-reduction computed tomography.
  - Nonoperative management with protected weight bearing is acceptable if reduction is maintained.
  - Operative management
    — Open reduction and internal fixation of a femoral head fracture and of associated femoral neck or acetabular fractures are required if reduction cannot be obtained or maintained by closed means.
- Neck fractures
  - Treatment usually involves surgery to obtain and maintain reduction.

Figure 138-3 Pipkin classification of femoral head fractures. **A**, Type I: below the fovea centralis. **B**, Type II: above the fovea centralis. **C**, Type III: either type I or II along with associated fracture of the femoral neck. **D**, Type IV: either type I or II along with associated acetabular fracture. (Adapted from Browner BD, Jupiter JB, Levine AM, Trafton PG [eds]: Skeletal Trauma: Fractures, Dislocations, Ligamentous Injuries. Philadelphia: WB Saunders, 1992, p 1339.)

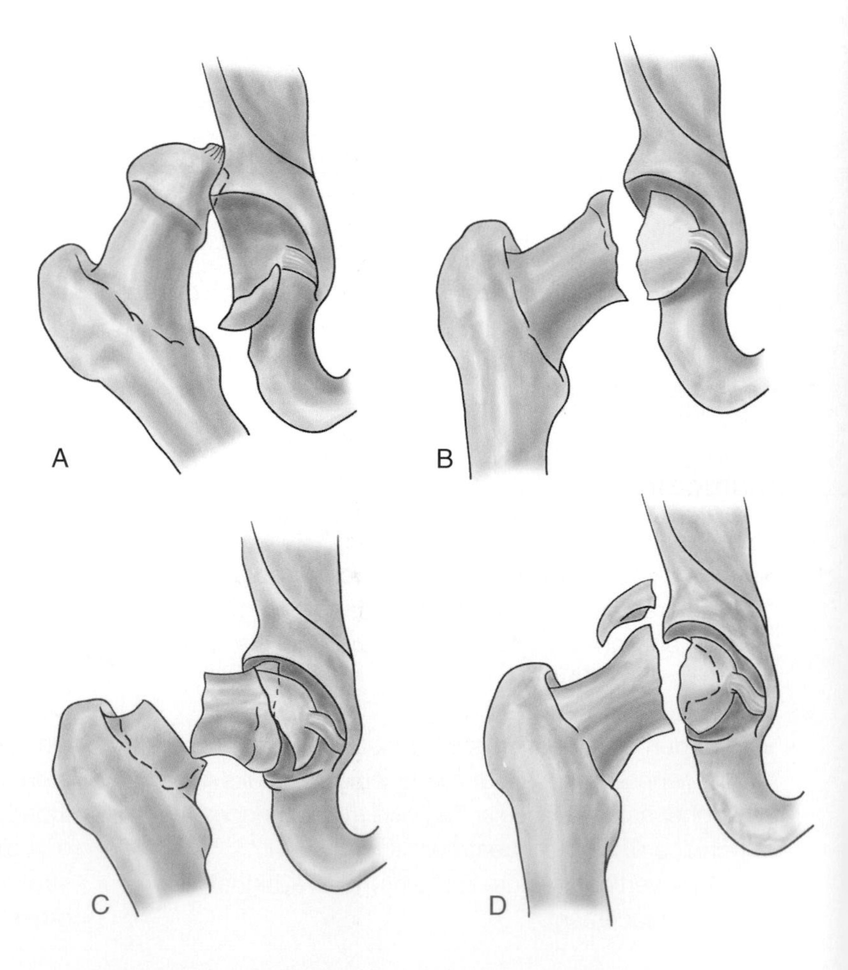

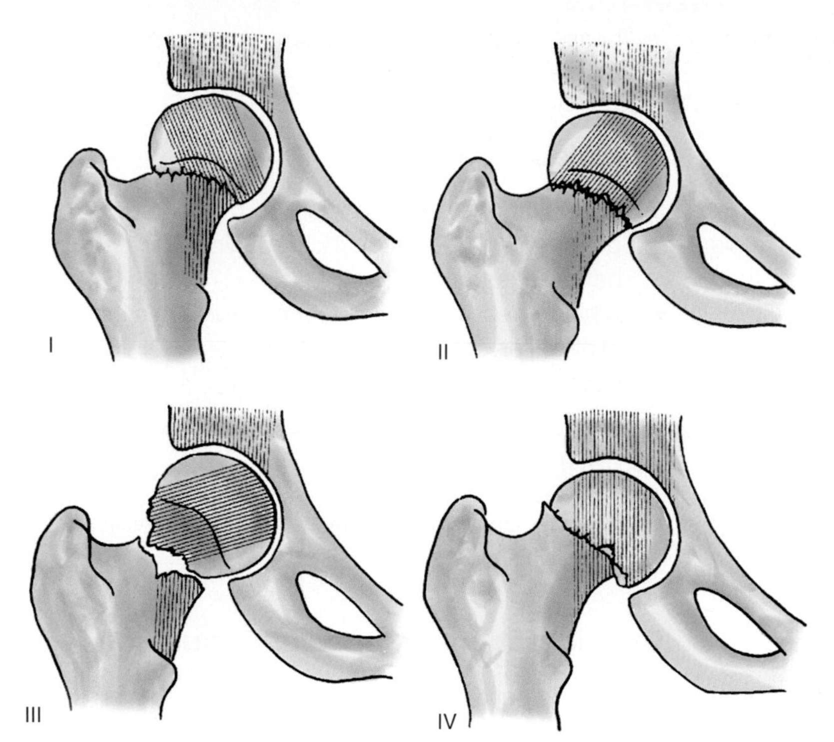

Figure 138-4 Garden classification of femoral neck fractures. Type I: incomplete fracture or valgus impaction. Type II: complete, nondisplaced fracture. Type III: complete, partially (<50%) displaced fracture. Type IV: complete, fully displaced fracture. (Adapted from Weissman BN, Sledge CB: Orthopedic Radiology. Philadelphia: WB Saunders, 1986, p 408.)

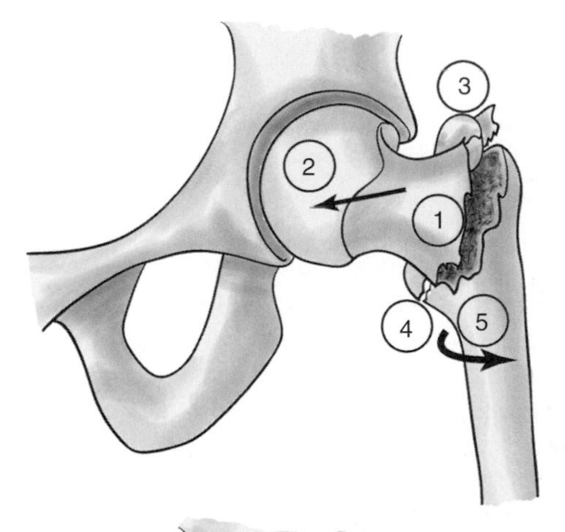

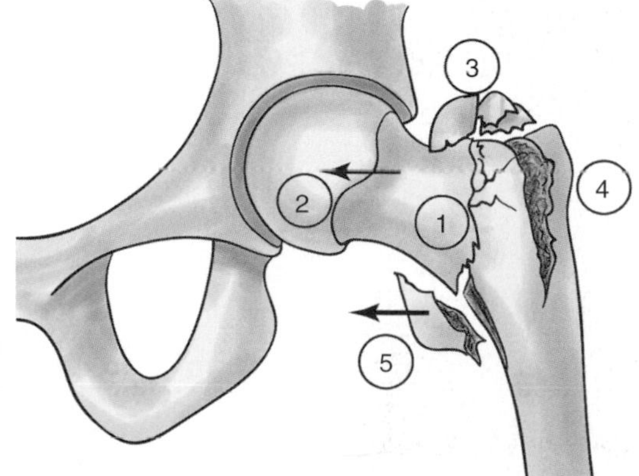

Figure 138-5 Simplified Evans classification of intertrochanteric femur fractures. *Top*, Stable oblique fracture. 1, Oblique intertrochanteric fracture line; 2, varus deformity; 3, greater trochanter involvement; 4, lesser trochanter involvement; 5, external rotation of the femur. *Bottom*, Unstable intertrochanteric fracture. 1, Fracture line is less oblique to reverse oblique; 2, varus deformity; 3, comminuted greater trochanter; 4, vertical fracture line through greater trochanter; 5, avulsion and displacement of lesser trochanter. (Adapted from Connolly JF [ed]: DePalma's The Management of Fractures and Dislocations, an Atlas, 3rd ed. Philadelphia: WB Saunders, 1981, p 1372.)

- Nonoperative management may be acceptable in cases of nondisplaced, minimally symptomatic fractures and in cases of extreme comorbidity for surgery.
- Younger patients (typically defined as younger than 50)
  - — Emergent open reduction and internal fixation are essential to try to preserve the integrity of the femoral head.
- Elderly patients (typically defined as older than 50)
  - — Nondisplaced fractures may be treated with internal fixation.
  - — Displaced fractures typically require hemiarthroplasty (replacement of the head).
- Intertrochanteric fractures
  - Nonoperative management is infrequent and usually only considered in patients who have a very high surgical risk or who are nonambulatory.
  - Operative management should proceed as soon as possible and usually involves open reduction and internal fixation with either a plate/screw construct or an intramedullary nail with screws into the femoral neck.

When to Refer

- Always

Prognosis

- Prognosis is generally related to the degree of injury and the timeliness of care as well as the age and medical status of the patient.
- Elderly patients have an extremely high rate of mortality within 1 year of a proximal femur fracture.
- Complications include avascular necrosis, nonunion, malunion, posttraumatic arthritis, deep venous thrombosis, pulmonary embolism, and other medical comorbidities.

Troubleshooting

- If radiographs are inconclusive, computed tomography or magnetic resonance imaging can help elucidate the pattern of injury.
- A high index of suspicion for fracture should be present in all cases of elderly patients with a history of a fall or hip/groin pain.

Patient Instructions

- Weight-bearing and activity restrictions will vary by situation.

Considerations in Special Populations

- Elderly patients warrant further investigation of the cause of their fall as well as for other associated fractures sustained at the same time.
- Ambulatory/functional status is a key point in planning the type of surgery for treatment of the fracture.

Suggested Reading

- Koval KJ, Zuckerman JD: Hip fractures: I. Overview and evaluation and treatment of femoral-neck fractures. J Am Acad Orthop Surg 1994;2:141–149.
- Koval KJ, Zuckerman JD: Hip fractures: II. Evaluation and treatment of intertrochanteric fractures. J Am Acad Orthop Surg 1994;2:150–156.
- Lu-Yao GL, Keller RB, Littenberg B, Wennberg JE: Outcomes after displaced fractures of the femoral neck—meta analysis of 106 published reports. J Bone Joint Surg Am 1994;76A:15–25.
- Parker MJ, Gurusamy K: Internal fixation versus arthroplasty for intracapsular proximal femoral fractures in adults. Cochrane Database Syst Rev 2006;4:CD001708.

Chapter 139 Femoral Shaft Fractures

George S. Edwards III, Brandon D. Bushnell, and Timothy N. Taft

Key Concepts

- Fractures of the femoral shaft and subtrochanteric area usually require urgent surgical treatment.
- In the acute setting, application of traction to the leg may result in life-saving control of blood loss.

History

- Both diaphyseal and subtrochanteric fractures follow a bimodal distribution
  - High-velocity or high-energy trauma in young patients
  - Low-energy falls in elderly patients
  - Subtrochanteric fractures are more common in the elderly than the young.
- A complete history includes the injury mechanism, any known associated injuries, and the time elapsed from the injury, as well as other comorbidities (such as visceral injuries, other fractures, vascular compromise, neurologic injury, and head injury) because this information may alter the treatment decision.

Physical Examination

- Patients will usually have obvious lower extremity rotational and angular deformity, swelling, and often ecchymosis.
- Any breakage of the skin should be noted and open fracture carefully ruled out.
- Examination must include the ipsilateral hip and knee for other fractures or soft-tissue injuries. Some portions of the examination may be limited by the injury (e.g., pain, instability for ligamentous testing).
- Femur fractures often limit the knee examination; thus, it is critical to re-examine the knee for ligamentous instability after treatment of the femur fracture.
- Full primary, secondary, and tertiary surveys are warranted in the multitrauma setting.

Imaging

- Radiograph of the entire femoral shaft with orthogonal views (usually anteroposterior/lateral views)
- Radiograph of the hip and knee to rule out associated injuries
- Contralateral femur films can be useful to determine preinjury femur length, which may help with operative planning.
- Computed tomography is often used to rule out associated femoral neck fractures.
- Appropriate imaging of associated injuries completes the workup of a multitrauma patient.

Classification

- Diaphyseal fractures
  - Winquist and Hansen classification rates severity of fracture based on amount of cortical contact of proximal and distal fragments (Fig. 139-1).
    - — Grade I: no or minimal comminution at the fracture site, does not affect stability after intramedullary nailing and may be treated as though it were not comminuted
    - — Grade II: cortical contact retained in more than 50% of shaft circumference at the fracture site, allowing control of length and rotation
    - — Grade III: cortical contact retained in less than 50% of shaft circumference at the fracture site; shortening, rotation, and translation may occur
    - — Grade IV: 0% of cortical contact retained; no intrinsic stability
- Subtrochanteric fractures
  - Defined as fractures between the lower border of the lesser trochanter and the isthmus of the diaphysis, approximately 5 cm below the lesser trochanter
  - Much less common than diaphyseal fractures

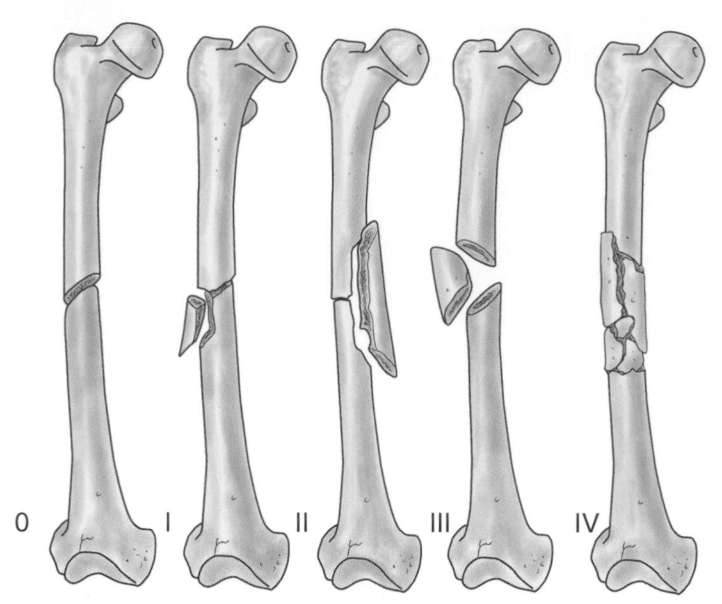

Figure 139-1 Winquist and Hansen classification of femoral shaft fractures. (Adapted from Bucholz RW, Heckman JD, Court-Brown CM [eds]: Rockwood and Greene's Fractures in Adults, 6th ed. Philadelphia: Lippincott Williams & Wilkins, 2006, p 1849.)

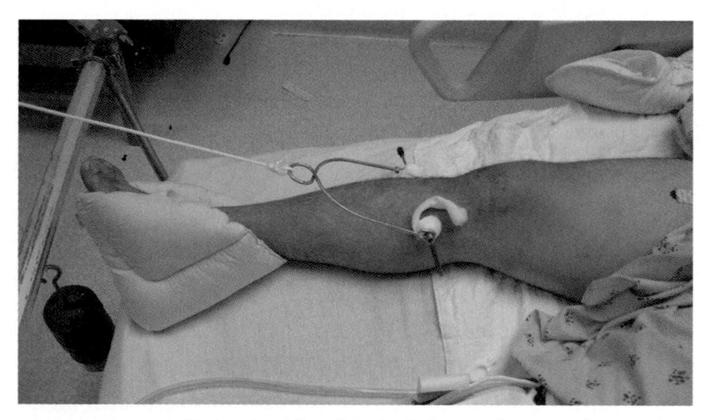

Figure 139-2 Patient with mid-shaft femur fracture in traction before operative fixation. (Photo courtesy of Tim Murphy, 2007.)

- There are several classifications, mostly based on the location of the fracture line relative to the lesser trochanter.

Differential Diagnosis

- The major component is associated injuries, especially of the hip or knee, which may be contributing to the lower extremity deformity.
- Pathologic fracture from neoplastic or metabolic disease; the subtrochanteric region most common site for pathologic fractures of the femur

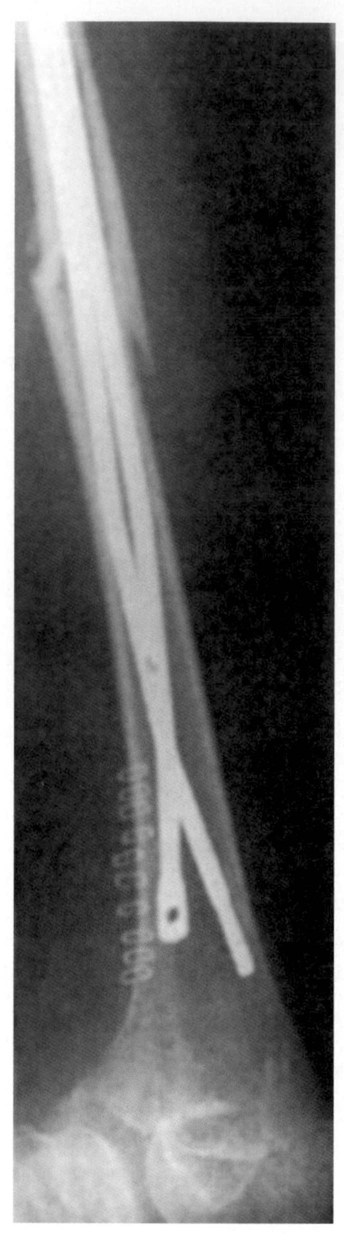

Figure 139-3 Percutaneous flexible ender nails used to treat femur fractures in skeletally immature patients to avoid the proximal and distal physes. (From Canale ST [ed]: Campbell's Operative Orthopaedics, 10th ed. Philadelphia: Mosby, 2003, p 1507.)

Treatment

- Stabilization by operative treatment within the first 24 hours reduces morbidity and mortality in patients with multiple injuries.
- Preoperative traction should be considered in all cases because there can be unforeseen delays in definitive treatment (Fig. 139-2).
- Nonoperative treatment is reserved only for isolated cases with extenuating circumstances that contraindicate surgery.

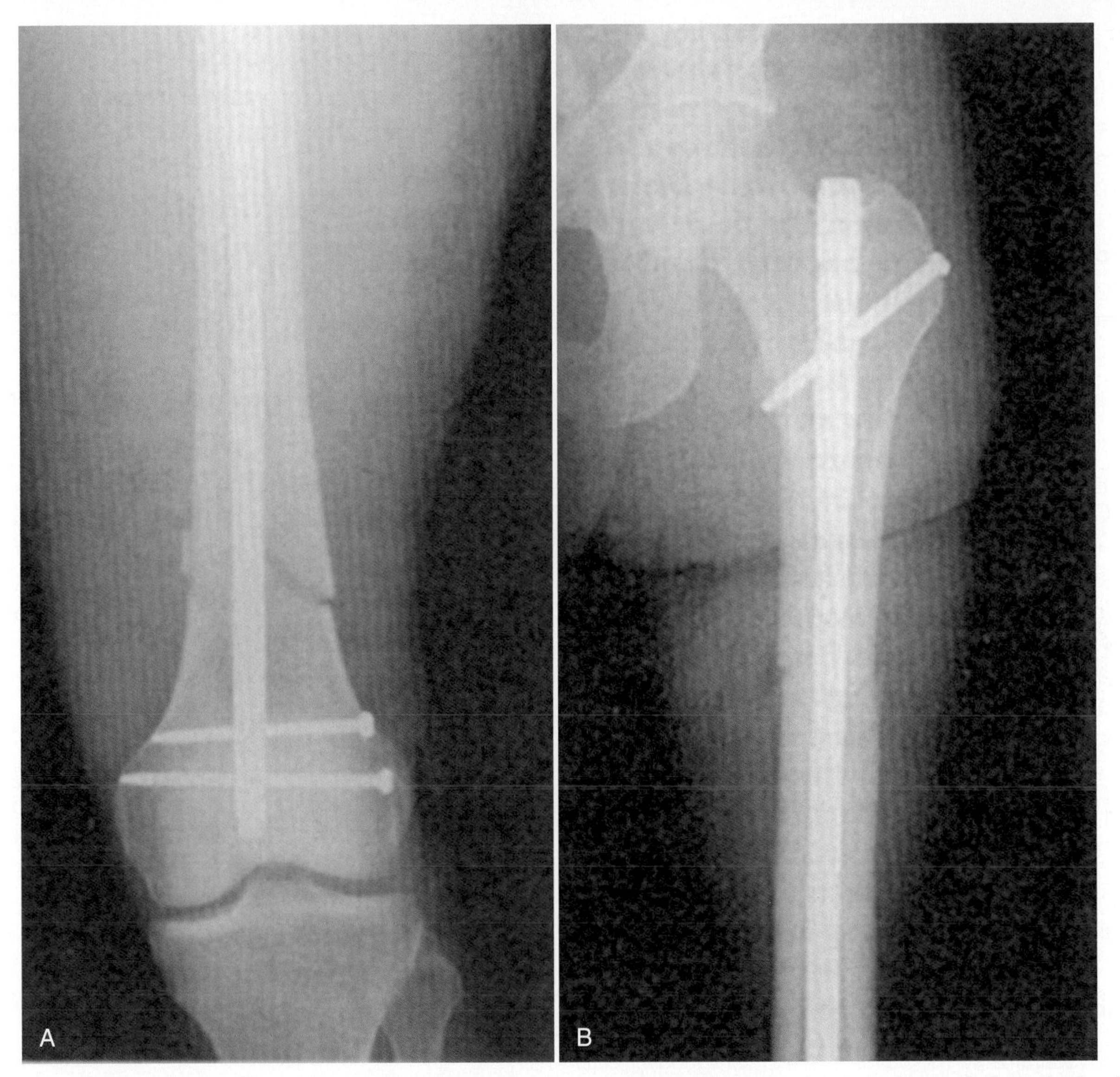

Figure 139-4 Anteroposterior (**A**) and lateral (**B**) radiographs of femur diaphyseal fracture treated with statically locked antegrade intramedullary nail. (From Bucholz RW, Heckman JD, Court-Brown CM [eds]: Rockwood and Greene's Fractures in Adults, 6th ed. Philadelphia: Lippincott Williams & Wilkins, 2006, p 1875.)

Diaphyseal Fractures

- In skeletally immature patients, closed treatment is often effective with immediate immobilization, closed reduction and traction, and then spica casting until healing occurs. Internal fixation with flexible nailing is another viable option, especially in older children who are not still growing (Fig. 139-3).
- For adults, operative treatment is most common because closed treatment usually requires traction for 6 to 8 weeks followed by spica casting for 3 to 4 months, with associated complications of prolonged immobilization.
    - Dynamic interlocked nailing, which allows compression at the fracture site, may be used if the fracture does not involve the isthmus and the fracture is intrinsically stable. This is often the case in grade I and II fractures with more than 50% circumferential cortical contact.
    - Static interlocked intramedullary nailing (Fig. 139-4), which preserves length and does not allow compression, is now the recommended treatment for most femoral shaft fractures because it prevents shortening and rotational malalignment in unstable situations such as grade III/IV fractures with less than 50% circumferential cortical contact.
- Intramedullary nailing is usually performed closed to reduce blood loss and soft-tissue damage. Open nailing is indicated when adequate reduction cannot be accomplished by closed means.

- The intramedullary nail provides anatomic alignment with stable fixation, permitting early mobilization and weight bearing.
- Plating of shaft fractures may also be performed in certain situations, but it is much less commonly used than intramedullary nailing.

Subtrochanteric Fractures

- Notoriously difficult to treat because of the mechanical forces that the muscles place on the fragments, pulling the proximal piece into a position of flexion, external rotation, and abduction
- Operative treatment is almost always indicated unless the patient's comorbidities mandate nonoperative treatment.
    - Operative treatment involves internal fixation using a combination of plates and screws or intramedullary nailing, depending on the configuration of the fracture and associated injuries.
    - With operative fixation, limited weight bearing is permitted and advanced with radiographic evidence of healing.
- Nonoperative treatment has a high risk of instability and resulting varus or rotational malalignment, as well as the complications associated with prolonged bed rest. Skeletal traction for 6 to 8 weeks is required with the hip and knee flexed at 90 degrees. Then, the hip and knee are progressively brought to neutral for another 6 to 8 weeks.

Prognosis

- Diaphyseal fractures have a good prognosis, with healing rates of 95% to 99% with intramedullary nailing.
- Subtrochanteric fractures have a worse prognosis, with a mortality rate reported as high as 20%.
    - The fracture usually heals within 3 to 4 months
    - Similar to hip fractures, subtrochanteric fractures often result in patients needing to use an assistive device (e.g., cane, walker) after treatment.

When to Refer

- Always

Troubleshooting

- Femur fractures are known for fat embolism and adult respiratory distress syndrome. Close observation for respiratory changes is critical in the acute recovery period.
- It is common for patients to lose several units of blood into the thigh after femur fractures. This is often difficult to detect by clinical examination, and thus close monitoring of the hemodynamic status should be maintained. Early traction application can help control blood loss.
- Neurovascular injury must be carefully evaluated and documented because compartment syndrome may develop.
- Later complications can include infection, deep venous thrombosis, and pulmonary embolus, malunion, leg length discrepancy, and joint stiffness.

Patient Instructions

- Weight-bearing status is critical and dependent on the individual factors of each case. Early range of motion and mobilization are key goals.

Considerations in Special Populations

- Fractures in children are often complicated by overgrowth of the injured leg, which occurs through the physes at each end of the bone. Thus, some overlap or shortening of the fracture fragments at the time of injury and treatment is actually encouraged.
- Fractures in the elderly create a unique situation because there is often a combination of osteopenic bone and multiple medical comorbidities that make fixation a challenge.

Suggested Reading

- Albert MJ: Supracondylar fractures of the femur. J Am Acad Orthop Surg 1997;5:163–171.
- Brumback RJ, Virkus WW: Intramedullary nailing of the femur: Reamed versus nonreamed. J Am Acad Orthop Surg 2000;8:83–90.
- Flynn JM, Schwend RM: Management of pediatric femoral shaft fractures. J Am Acad Orthop Surg 2004;12:347–359.
- Lundy DW: Subtrochanteric femoral fractures. J Am Acad Orthop Surg 2007;15:663–671.
- Nork SE: Fractures of the shaft of the femur. In Bucholz RW, Heckman JD, Court-Brown CM (eds): Rockwood and Greene's Fractures in Adults, 6th ed. Philadelphia: Lippincott Williams & Wilkins, 2006, pp 1846–1913.

Chapter 140 Trochanteric Bursa Injection

Tracy Ray and Ramon Ylanan

CPT CODE

20610 *Arthrocentesis, Aspiration and/or Injection; Major Joint or Bursa (e.g., Shoulder, Hip, Knee Joint, Subacromial Bursa)*

ICD-9 CODE

726.5 *Enthesopathy of Hip Region*

Equipment

- Sterile skin prep solution (Betadine)
- 10-mL syringe
- Needle (need a needle long enough to make contact with bone)
  - 20- or 22-gauge, 1.5-inch needle
  - Consider spinal needle for larger patients
- Ethyl chloride spray
- Gloves
- Medication
  - One percent lidocaine and/or 0.5% bupivacaine (Marcaine)
  - Corticosteroid: intermediate acting or methylprednisolone (Depo-Medrol) or triamcinolone acetonide (Kenalog)
  - Long acting: betamethasone sodium phosphate (Celestone)
- Sterile 4 × 4 adhesive bandage

Contraindications

- Specific allergies to medication used
- Skin disease (e.g., cellulitis, rash) overlying injection site
- Poorly controlled diabetes mellitus
- Underlying coagulopathy or if poorly controlled anticoagulant therapy

Instructions/Technique

- Informed consent
- Ask about the patient's allergies or reactions to medications.
- Risks
  - May develop allergic reaction to medication including anaphylaxis
  - Skin atrophy, depigmentation/hyperpigmentation
  - Local tissue necrosis
  - Systemic effects
    - — Transient hyperglycemia (in diabetic patients)
    - — Transient decreased cortisol production
    - — Infection
  - Bleeding (particularly with warfarin or other anticoagulant therapy)
- Steps (Figs. 140-1 to 140-5)
  - Place patient in lateral decubitus position with affected side up.
    - — Palpate point of maximal tenderness and mark before skin preparation.
  - Clean area of injection with sterile skin prep solution.
  - Maintain sterility (can use drapes and sterile gloves).
  - Topical anesthetic agent with ethyl chloride, optional
  - Insert needle perpendicular to skin until contact with greater trochanter is made.
  - Withdraw needle 1 to 2 mm (now in bursa); aspirate to make sure needle is not in a vascular structure.

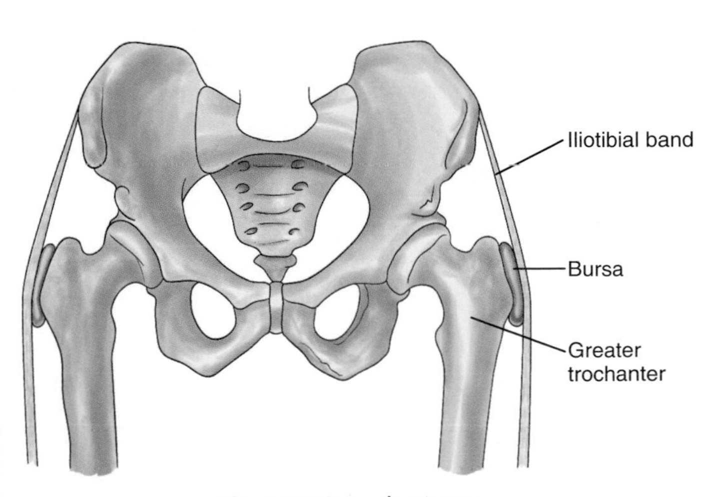

Figure 140-1 Anatomy.

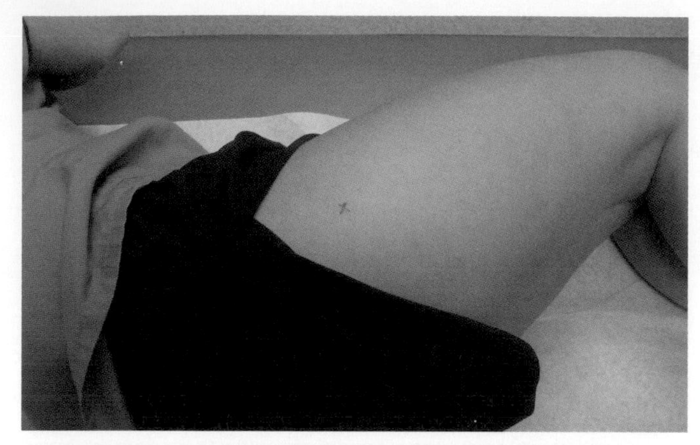

Figure 140-2 Patient in lateral decubitus position with affected side up. Area of tenderness marked.

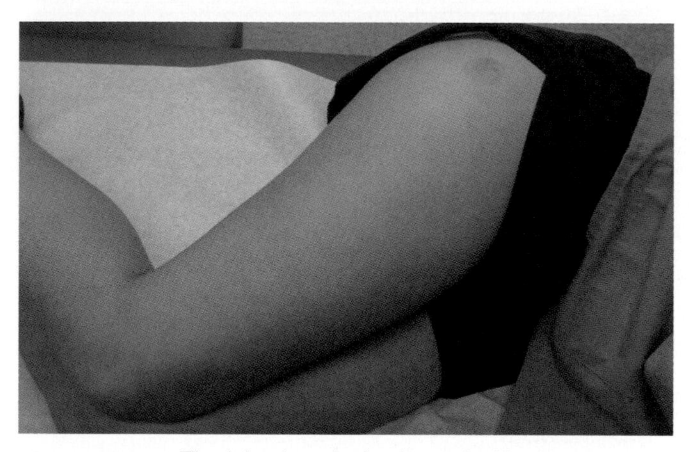

Figure 140-3 The injection site is cleaned with skin prep solution.

- Inject the mixture in 1- to 2-mL boluses beginning at the site of maximal discomfort and then fanning out to cover the surrounding area.
- Apply an adhesive dressing.

Considerations in Special Populations

- Diabetics: transient hyperglycemia
- Patients on warfarin
  - Ask about the last international normalized ratio or recent dose changes.

Troubleshooting

- Difficult injection
  - If the iliotibial band is tight, place a pillow between the patient's legs.

Patient Instructions

- Can be more sore transiently after injection
- Postinjection flare in 3% of patients; addressed well by ice, acetaminophen, or ibuprofen

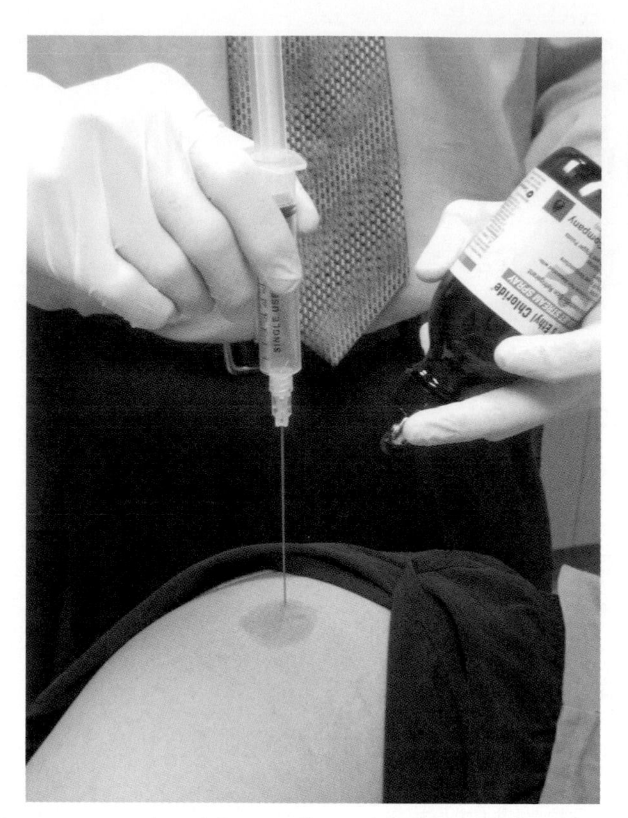

Figure 140-4 Insert the needle perpendicular to the skin until contact with bone is made.

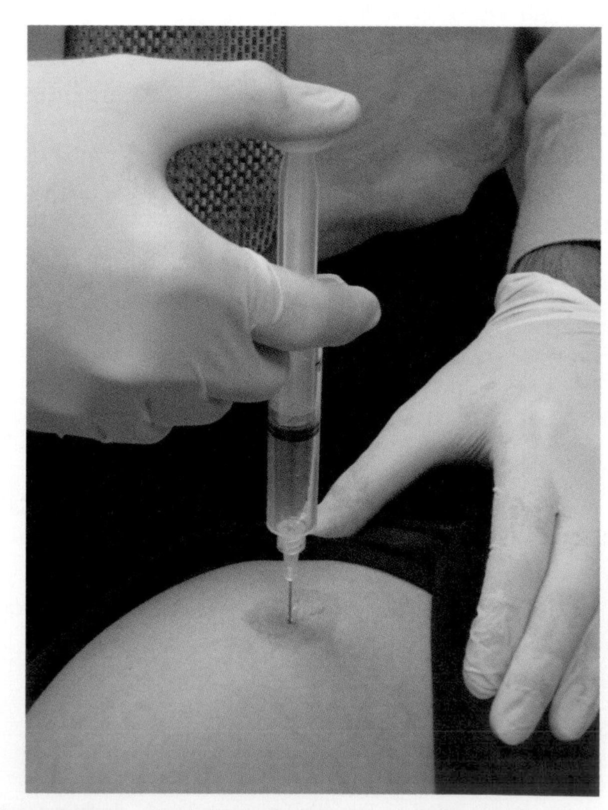

Figure 140-5 Aspirate to make sure that the needle is not in a vascular structure, and then inject.

- Steroid benefit will start in several hours or days, peaking at 48 hours.
- Ice for comfort

Suggested Reading

- Adkins SB, Figler RA: Hip pain in athletes. Am Fam Physician 2000;61:2109–2118.
- Cardone DA, Tallia AF: Diagnostic and therapeutic injection of the hip and knee. Am Fam Physician 2003;67:2147–2152.
- Cardone DA, Tallia AF: Joint and soft tissue injection. Am Fam Physician 2002;66:283–290.
- Griffin LY (ed): Trochanteric bursitis injection. In Essentials of Musculoskeletal Care, 3rd ed. Rosemont, IL: American Academy of Orthopaedic Surgeons, 2005, pp 464–465.

7

SECTION

The Knee and Lower Leg

Chapter 141 Overview of the Knee and Lower Leg

Mark D. Miller

Anatomy

Bones and Joint

- The knee joint is made up of the articulation of the distal femur and the proximal tibia and fibula (Fig. 141-1).
- This articulation allows flexion and extension of the joint as well as a rolling (screw home) motion during terminal extension.
- The patella, which is the largest sesamoid bone in the body, also articulates with the femur.

Femur

- The articular surface of the distal femur is composed of two condyles.
    - The medial condyle has a larger surface area, but the lateral condyle is longer.
- The intercondylar area serves as an attachment for the cruciate ligaments: the anterior cruciate ligament laterally and the posterior cruciate ligament medially.
- The medial epicondyle serves as the attachment for the medial collateral ligament.
- The lateral epicondyle serves as the attachment for the lateral collateral ligament.
- A groove distal to the epicondyle is where the popliteus tendon lies; it inserts distal and anterior to the lateral collateral ligament.

Tibia

- The tibia also has medial and lateral condyles.
    - The medial condyle is broad and concave.
    - The lateral condyle is smaller, more circular, and convex.
- The tibial eminences (spines) serve as the border of the anterior cruciate ligament.
- The posterior cruciate ligament lies between two bony prominences posteriorly, distal to the joint line.
- The patellar tendon inserts onto the tibial tuberosity.
- Gerdy's tubercle is the attachment site for the iliotibial band.

Fibula

- The fibula articulates with the tibia and serves as the attachment for the lateral collateral ligament.

Patella

- The patella has the thickest articular cartilage in the body.
- It has two facets: a larger lateral facet and a smaller medial facet, separated by a vertical ridge.
- The medial patellofemoral ligament originates near the medial epicondyle and inserts on the upper border of the medial patella; it is the primary restraint to lateral displacement of the patella.
- The knee is the largest joint in the body and includes the following structures
    - Ligaments
        - — Anterior cruciate ligament: resists anterior translation
        - — Posterior cruciate ligament: resists posterior translation
        - — Medial collateral ligament: resists valgus displacement
        - — Lateral collateral ligament: resists varus displacement
        - — Posteromedial and posterolateral corner structures: resist rotation
    - Menisci
        - — Medial: semicircular and broader posteriorly
        - — Lateral: more circular and covers a larger portion of the articular surface

Muscles

- A variety of muscles cross the knee and cover the leg (Fig. 141-2). These are perhaps best considered in groups or compartments.
    - Anterior thigh
        - — Quadriceps muscle (extends the leg)
        - — Vastus lateralis, intermedius, medialis, and rectus femoris muscles

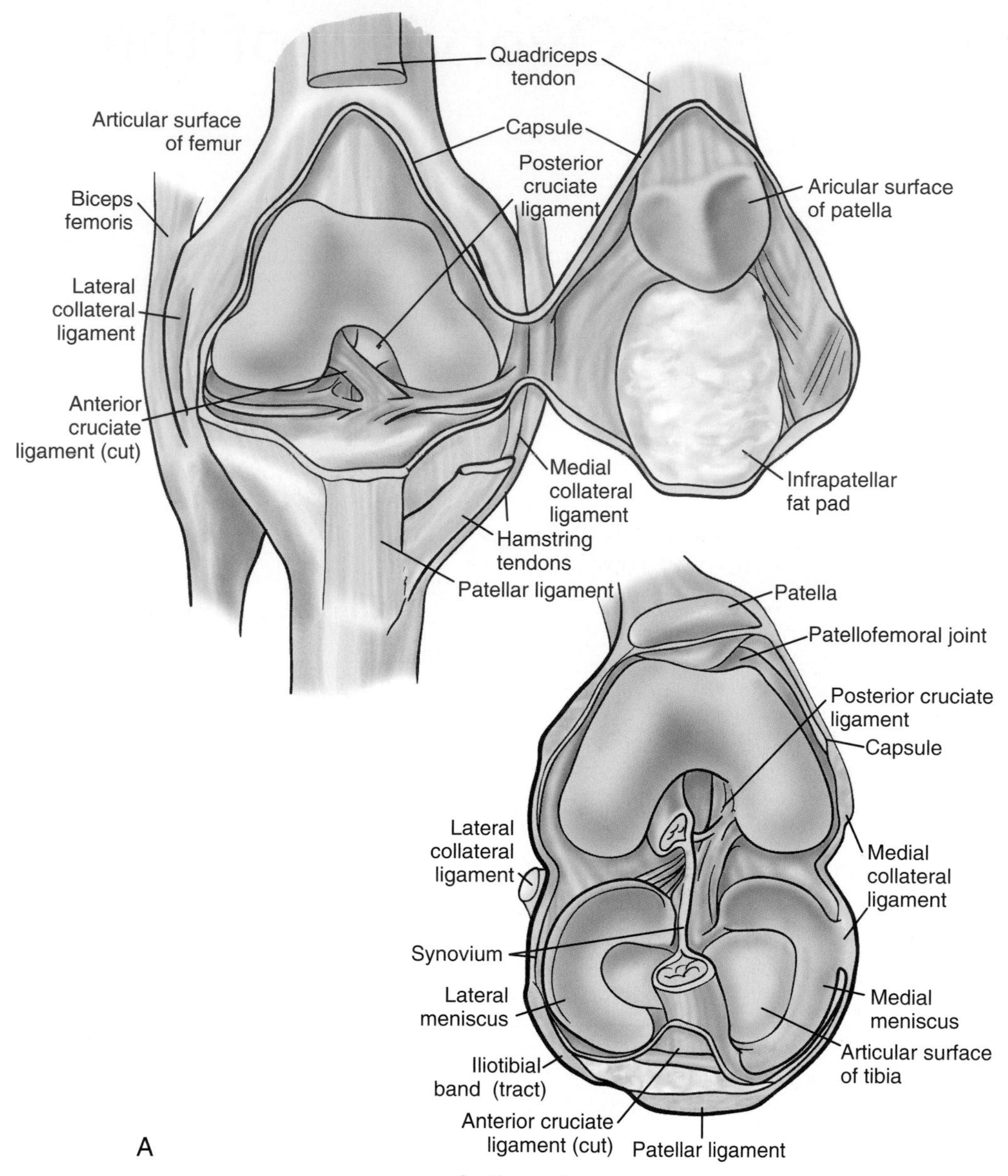

Figure 141-1 **A**, Knee joint structures.

- Posterior thigh
  - Hamstrings (flex the leg)
  - Lateral: biceps femoris muscle
  - Medial: semimembranosus, semitendinosus, sartorius, and gracilis muscles
- Medial thigh
  - Adductors (adduct the leg)
  - Adductor magnus, longus, and brevis muscles
- Anterior leg (extend/invert the foot/ankle)
  - Tibialis anterior, extensor hallucis longus, extensor digitorum longus muscles
- Posterior leg (flex the foot/ankle)
  - Gastrocnemius, soleus, flexor hallucis longus, flexor digitorum longus, tibialis posterior muscles
- Lateral leg (evert the foot/ankle)
  - Peroneus brevis, longus, and tertius muscles

Nerves

- The nerves that cross the knee and continue on into the leg are extensions of nerves from the lumbosacral plexus (Fig. 141-3).

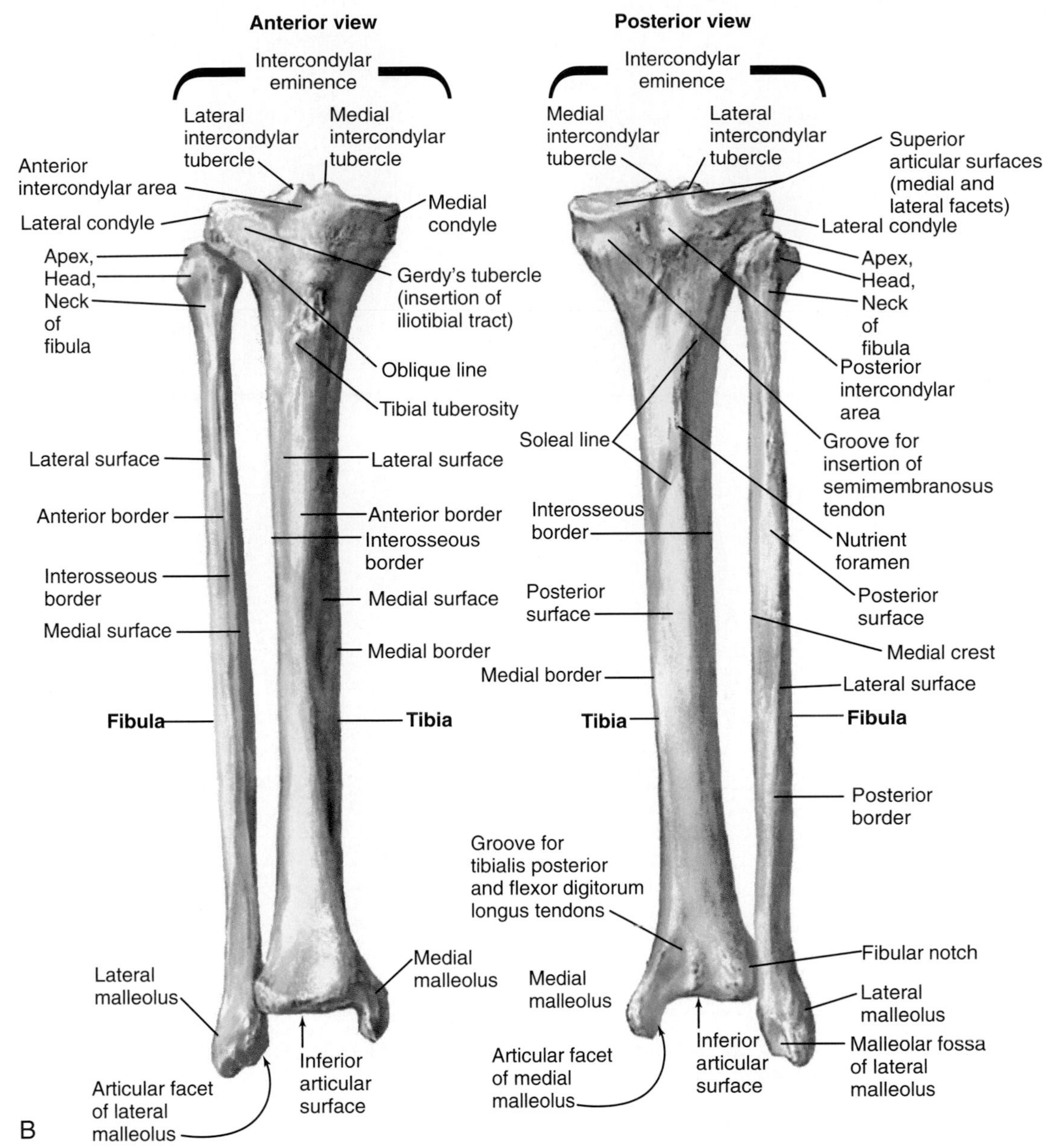

Figure 141-1, cont'd **B**, The tibia and fibula are the bones in the leg. (Adapted from Miller MD, Chhabra AB, Hurwitz SR, et al: Orthopaedic Surgical Approaches. Philadelphia: Saunders, 2008, p 426.)

- The femoral nerve (L2-L4 roots) innervates the quadriceps muscles.
- The obturator nerve (L2-L4 roots) innervates the adductors.
- The sciatic nerve (primarily S2-S4 nerve roots) innervates the hamstrings and divides in the mid-thigh into tibial and peroneal divisions.
- The tibial nerve continues distally to innervate the posterior compartments of the lower leg.
- The common peroneal nerve divides into superficial and deep branches after coursing around the fibular head.
- The superficial peroneal nerve innervates the lateral compartment of the leg and the deep peroneal nerve innervates the anterior compartment.

Vascularity

- The femoral artery divides in the thigh into deep (or profundus) and superficial branches.
- The artery passes posteriorly, becoming the popliteal artery as it passes between the origins of the gastrocnemius muscle and then bifurcates into the anterior and posterior tibial arteries.

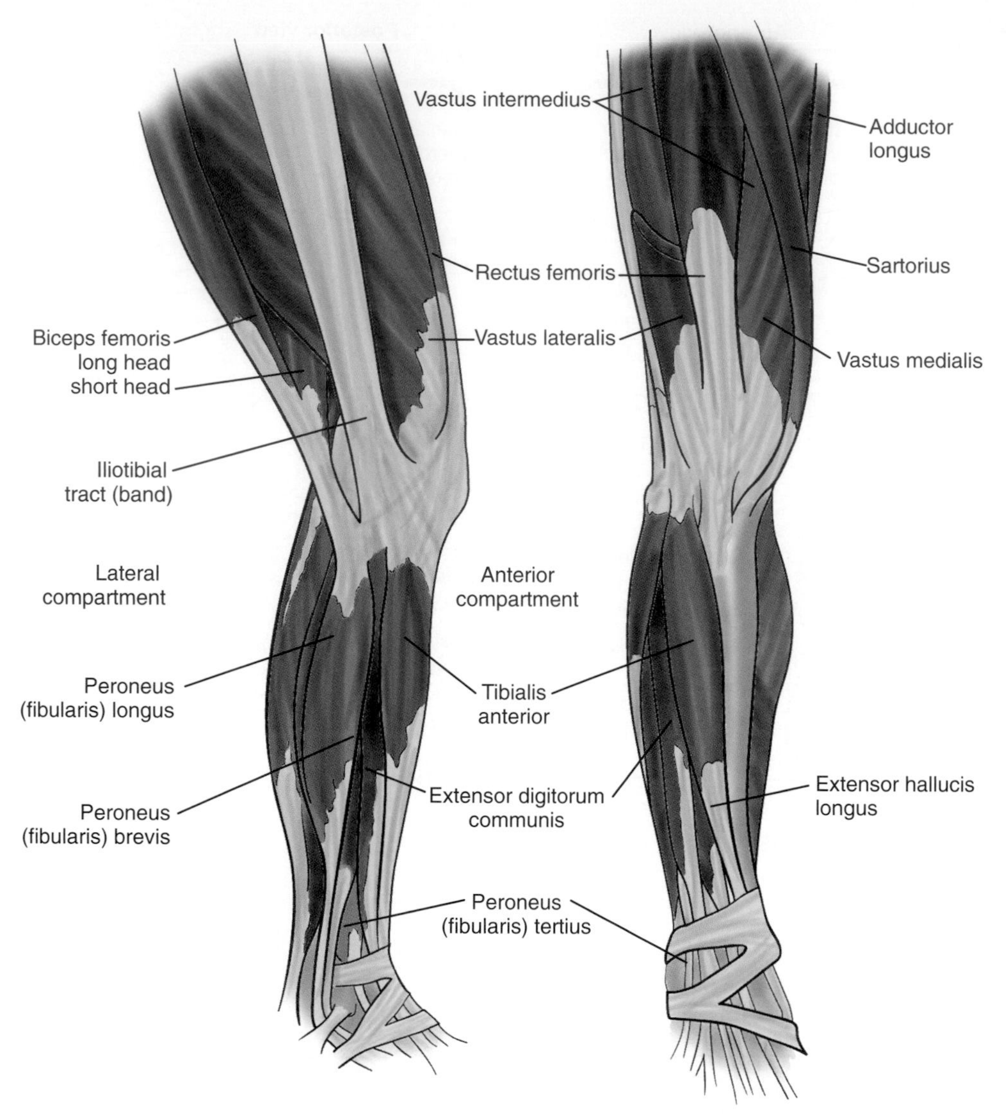

Figure 141-2 The muscles of the leg. (Adapted from Miller MD, Chhabra AB, Hurwitz SR, et al: Orthopaedic Surgical Approaches. Philadelphia: Saunders, 2008, p 432.)

- The peroneal artery is the first branch of the posterior tibial artery (Fig. 141-4).

Cross-sectional Anatomy

- It is often very helpful to have a good understanding of the cross-sectional anatomy of the thigh and especially the leg (Fig. 141-5).
- Three compartments are commonly recognized in the thigh and four in the leg:
  - Thigh
    - — Anterior compartment
      - — Vastus medialis, vastus intermedius, vastus lateralis, rectus femoris, sartorius muscles
      - — Superficial femoral artery and vein
      - — Femoral nerve branches
    - — Medial compartment
      - — Adductor longus, adductor brevis, adductor magnus, gracilis muscles
      - — Deep femoral artery and vein
      - — Femoral and obturator nerve branches
    - — Posterior compartment
      - — Biceps femoris, semitendinosus, semimembranosus muscles
      - — Sciatic nerve
  - Lower leg
    - — Anterior compartment
      - — Tibialis anterior, extensor hallucis longus, extensor digitorum longus muscles
      - — Deep peroneal nerve
      - — Anterior tibial artery and vein

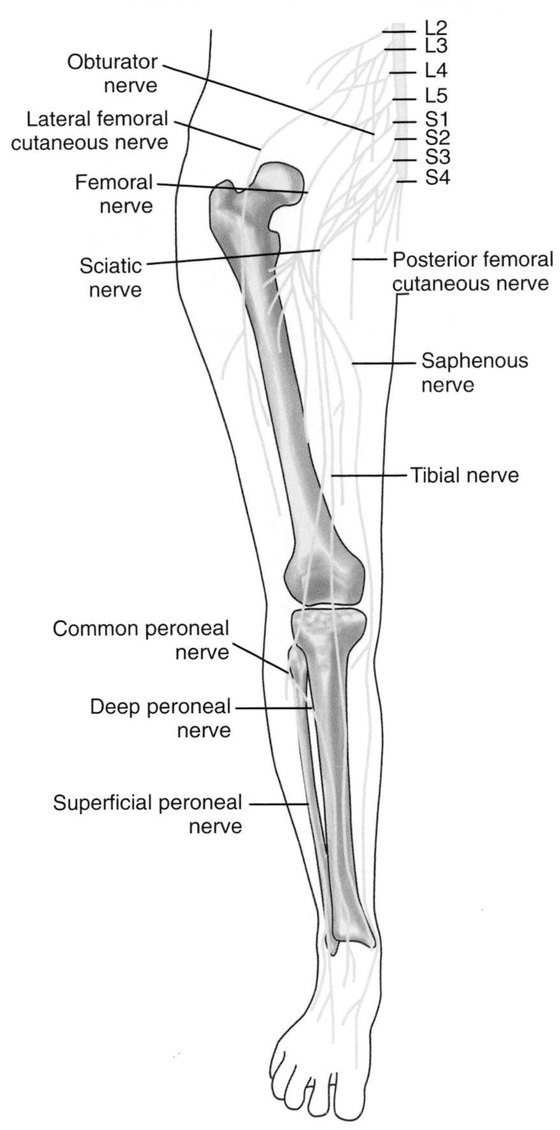

Figure 141-3 The nerves of the lower extremity. (Adapted from Miller MD, Chhabra AB, Hurwitz SR, et al: Orthopaedic Surgical Approaches. Philadelphia: Saunders, 2008, p 434.)

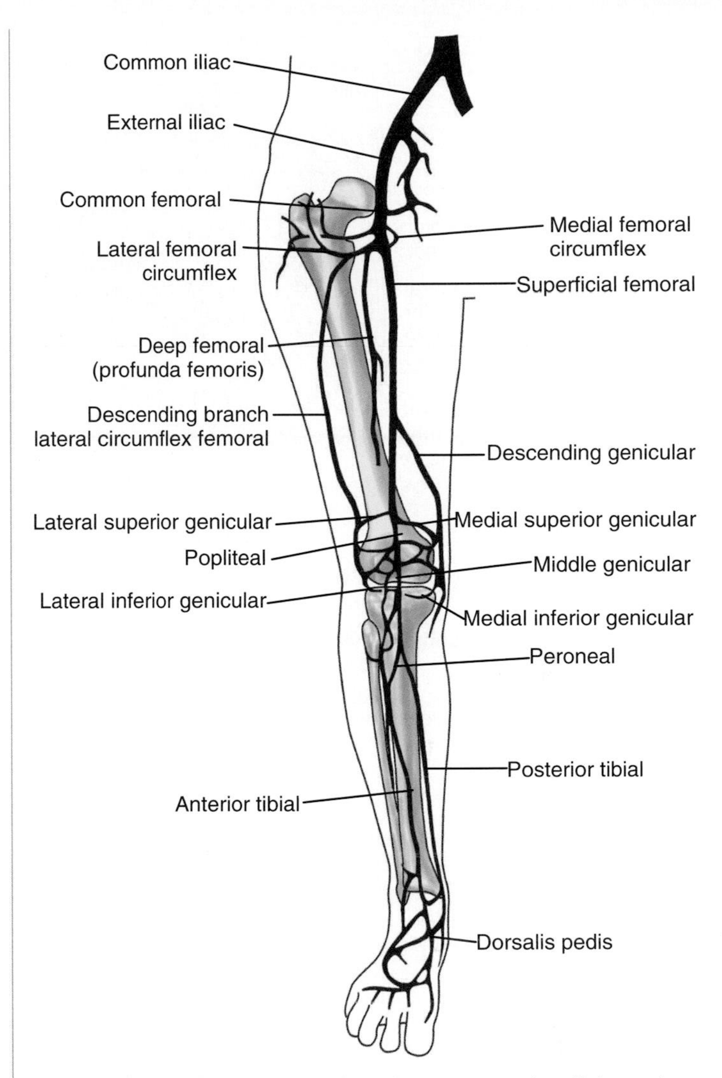

Figure 141-4 The arteries of the lower extremity. (Adapted from Miller MD, Chhabra AB, Hurwitz SR, et al: Orthopaedic Surgical Approaches. Philadelphia: Saunders, 2008, p 435.)

- Lateral compartment
  - Peroneus longus and brevis muscles
  - Superficial peroneal nerve
- Superficial posterior compartment
  - Gastrocnemius, soleus, plantaris muscles
- Deep posterior compartment
  - Flexor hallucis longus, flexor digitorum longus, tibialis posterior muscles
  - Tibial nerve
  - Posterior tibial artery and vein

Patient Evaluation

History

- In addition to demographic information, it is important to ask the patient about his or her symptoms.
- The injury history, duration of symptoms, exacerbating factors, pain, instability, mechanical symptoms, and a variety of other issues should be included.
- Some of the classic historical events and their significance are shown in Table 141-1.

Physical Examination

- It is important to observe the patient.
  - Look for asymmetry, skin lesions, effusions, and other findings.
  - Look grossly at the patient's mechanical alignment.
  - Observe the patient's gait.
  - Check for an antalgic (painful) gait, a lateral or medial thrust, or other abnormalities.
- Next, evaluate the patient's passive and active range of motion (typically full extension or as much as 10

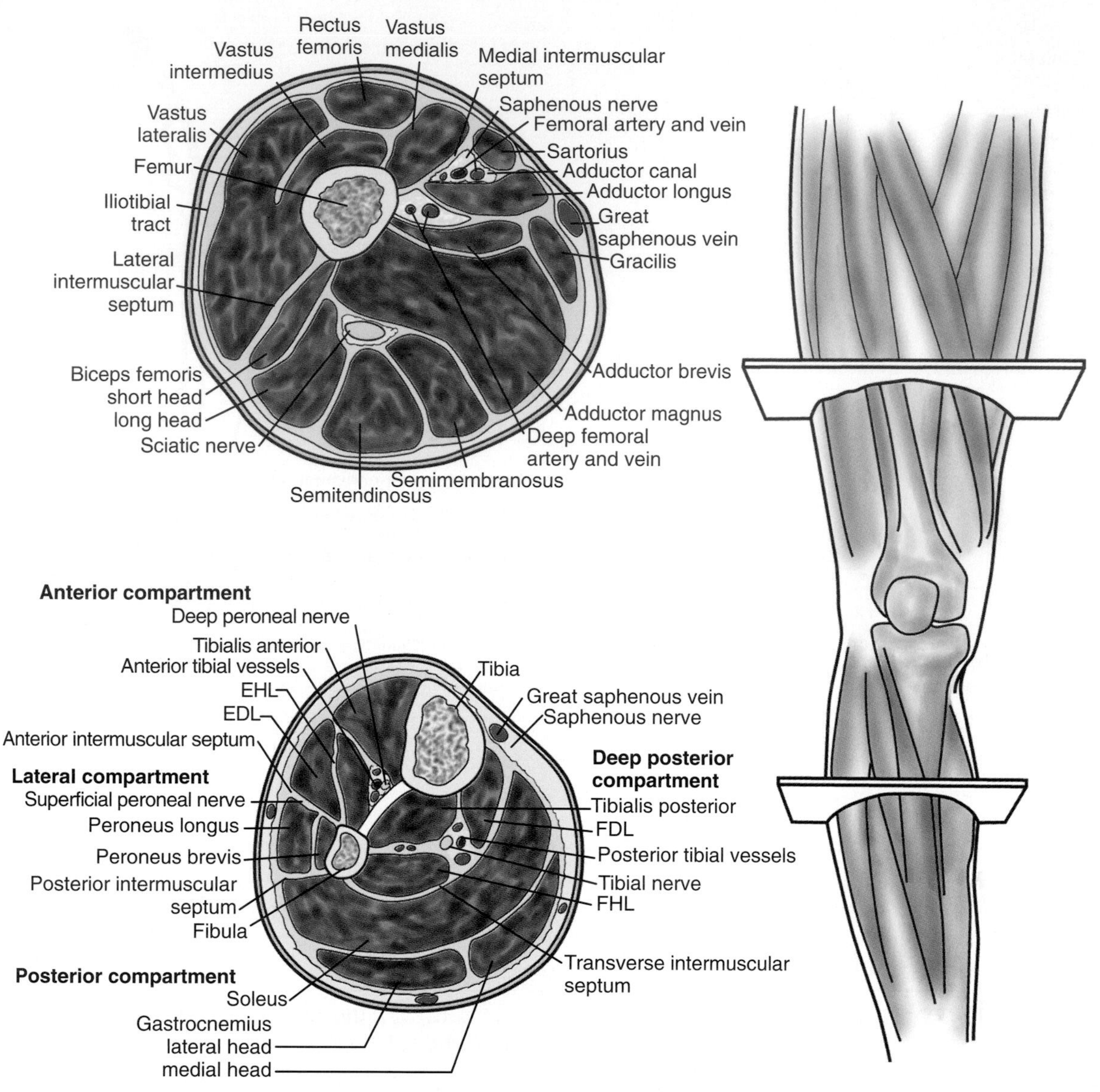

Figure 141-5 Cross-sectional anatomy of the thigh and leg. EDL, extensor digitorum longus; EHL, extensor hallucis longus; FDL, flexor digitorum longus; FHL, flexor hallicus longus. (Adapted from Miller MD, Chhabra AB, Hurwitz SR, et al: Orthopaedic Surgical Approaches. Philadelphia: Saunders, 2008, p 437.)

TABLE 141-1 *Key Knee Historical Points*

Historical Point	Significance
Noncontact pivoting injury with effusion	Anterior cruciate ligament tear
Blow to anterior tibia (dashboard injury)	Posterior cruciate ligament tear
Fall on leg with plantarflexed foot	Posterior cruciate ligament tear
Fall on leg with dorsiflexed foot	Patellar injury
Mechanical locking/catching	Meniscal tear
Pain with prolonged sitting/stair climbing	Patellofemoral syndrome

degrees of hyperextension and 130 to 140 degrees of flexion).

- Palpate the knee for an effusion (patellar ballottement or wave test) and locate the point of maximal tenderness (especially important in patients with meniscal tears).
- Attempt to displace the patella laterally and note whether the patient has apprehension (associated with patellar instability).
- Flex and rotate the knee and note whether the patient has popping (McMurray test) or increased joint line tenderness.
- Next, individual knee ligaments can be tested with specific examinations. The key maneuvers are shown in Table 141-2.

TABLE 141-2 *Key Knee Examination Findings*

Ligament/Structure	Examination
ACL	Lachman's test: anterior force applied to proximal tibia with knee in 30 degrees of flexion. A pillow under the knee will help the patient relax. Lachman's test is more specific than the anterior drawer test (Fig. 141-6). Pivot shift test: valgus force applied to the knee with foot internally rotated. As you flex the knee from full extension to approximately 30 degrees of flexion, it will "jump" or pivot as it reduces from a subluxed position. This examination is best done with the patient under anesthesia.
PCL	Posterior drawer test: posterior force applied to the proximal tibia with the knee flexed to 90 degrees. Grading is based on displacement in relation to the medial femoral condyle (I, anterior; II, flush; III, posterior) (Fig. 141-7).
MCL	Valgus stress test: valgus force with the knee flexed 30 degrees. Assess the medial opening. Note that if the knee opens in full extension, there is likely concurrent cruciate ligament injury (Fig. 141-8).
LCL	Varus stress test: varus force with the knee flexed 30 degrees. Assess lateral opening. Again, opening in full extension implies concurrent cruciate ligament injury (Fig. 141-9).
PLC	External rotation asymmetry: with the knees stabilized by an assistant, externally rotate the feet and compare the thigh-foot angle in both 30 and 90 degrees of knee flexion. If asymmetry (of ≥15 degrees) is present in 30 degrees of flexion only, it represents an isolated PLC injury (or an ACL-PLC injury). If the asymmetry is present at both 30 and 90 degrees of knee flexion, it represents a combined PCL-PLC injury (which can be confirmed with other tests) (Fig. 141-10).
PMC	Slocum test: an anterior drawer test with the foot in neutral is compared with an anterior drawer test with the foot in external rotation. Anterior displacement should be reduced with the foot in external rotation, unless there is a PMC injury. This is usually associated with a significant MCL injury and valgus laxity (Fig. 141-11).

ACL, anterior cruciate ligament; LCL, lateral collateral ligament; MCL, medial collateral ligament; PCL, posterior cruciate ligament; PLC, posterolateral corner; PMC, posteromedial corner.

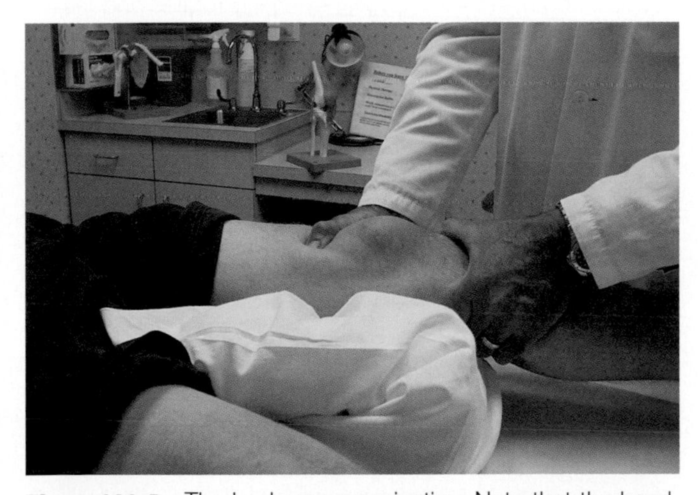

Figure 141-6 The Lachman examination. Note that the hand closest to the head of the patient grasps the thigh and the opposite hand performs the examination with the thumb close to the joint line. A pillow can be placed under the knee to help the patient relax.

Imaging

- Plain radiographs
  - Standard radiographs include orthogonal (anteroposterior and lateral) views and a patellar (sunrise or Merchant) view.

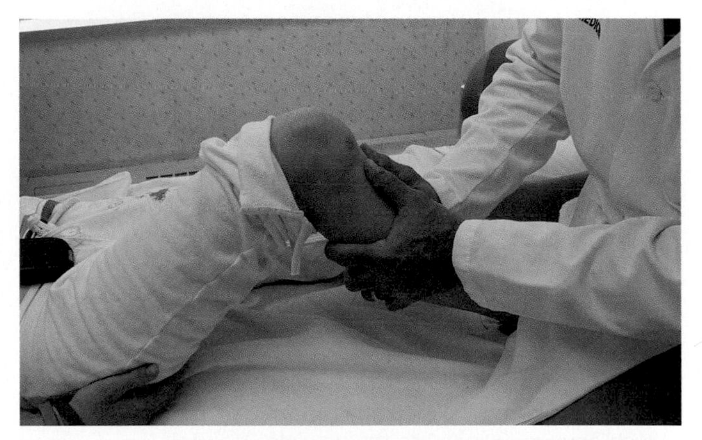

Figure 141-7 The posterior drawer examination. Note that the starting point is evaluated by palpating the medial tibial plateau in relation to the medial femoral condyle before applying a posteriorly directed force.

  - In older patients, it is very helpful to obtain a 45-degree posteroanterior flexion weight-bearing (Rosenberg) view (Fig. 141-12).
  - Radiographic findings may include those listed in Table 141-3 and are shown in Figure 141-13.
- Stress radiographs
  - Varus and valgus stress radiographs can be helpful in patients with open physes to determine whether there is a ligamentous or physeal injury.

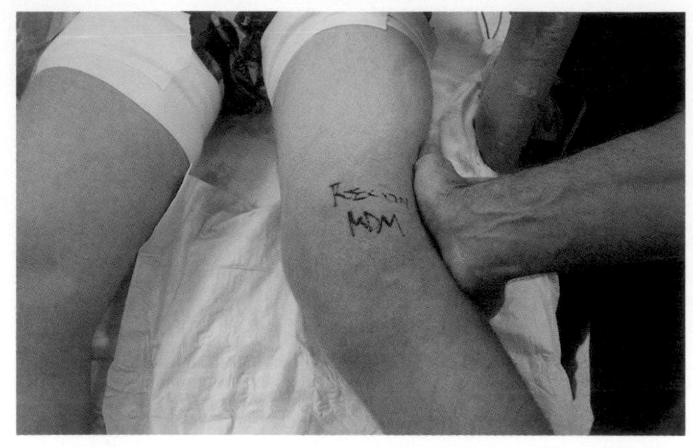

Figure 141-8 Valgus stress testing. A valgus stress is applied across the knee. This examination is done in both 30 degrees of knee flexion and full extension. Opening in full extension implies concurrent injury to the cruciate ligament(s).

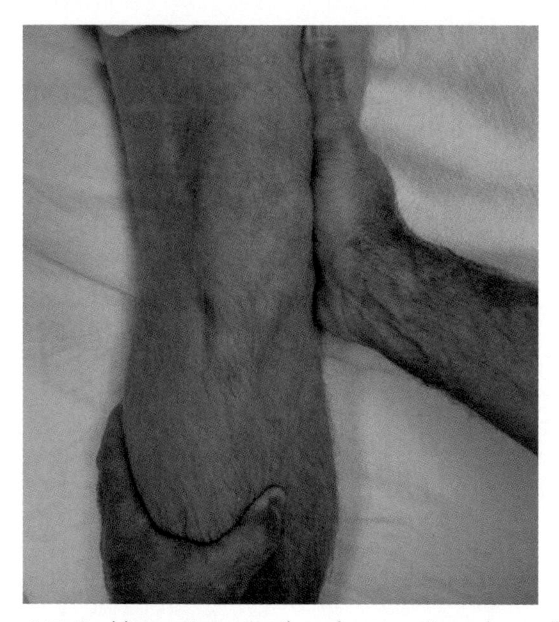

Figure 141-9 Varus stress testing. A varus stress is applied across the knee. This examination is done in both 30 degrees of knee flexion and full extension. Opening in full extension implies concurrent injury to the cruciate ligament(s).

- They can also be helpful in multiple ligament–injured knees when the collateral ligament status is unknown.
- Stress radiographs have also become the standard for reporting posterior cruciate ligament injuries and treatment.
  — A 15-kDa force is applied to the proximal tibia with the knee flexed 90 degrees and a lateral radiograph is obtained (Fig. 141-14).
  — Measurements are done posteriorly, and side-to-side comparisons are made.

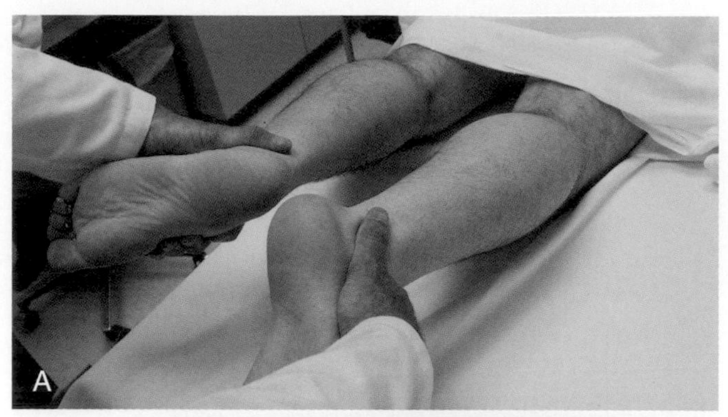

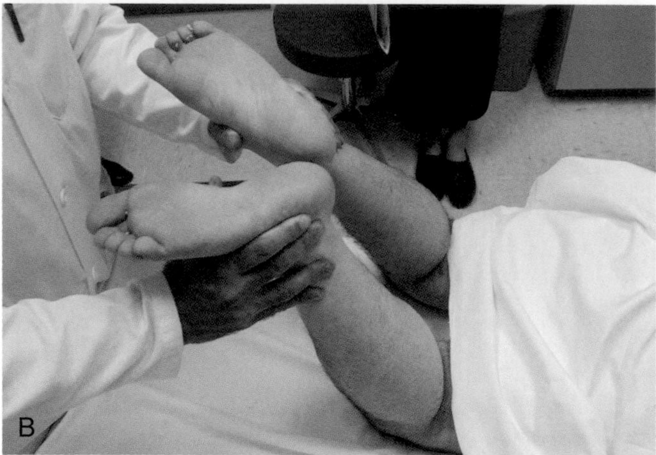

Figure 141-10 External rotation asymmetry. With the knees stabilized, both feet are passively externally rotated and the thigh-foot angle is measured. Asymmetry of 15 degrees or more implies injury to the posterolateral corner structures. The test is performed in both 30 degrees (**A**) and 90 degrees (**B**) of knee flexion. Asymmetry in both 30 and 90 degrees implies injury to both the posterolateral corner and the posterior cruciate ligament.

TABLE 141-3 *Key Knee Radiographic Findings*

Finding	Significance
Segond fracture (lateral capsular sign)	Highly associated with ACL tear (although it is not common)
Calcification of the proximal MCL (Pellegrini-Stieda)	Chronic MCL injury
Patella alta	Patellar instability
Patella baja	Arthrofibrosis (chronic stiff knee)
Squaring, ridging, narrowing (Fairbanks changes)	Post-medial meniscectomy DJD
Lucency lateral aspect MFC	Osteochondritis dissecans
Widened/cupping laterally	Discoid meniscus

ACL, anterior cruciate ligament; DJD, degenerative joint disease; MCL, medial collateral ligament; MFC, medial femoral condyle.

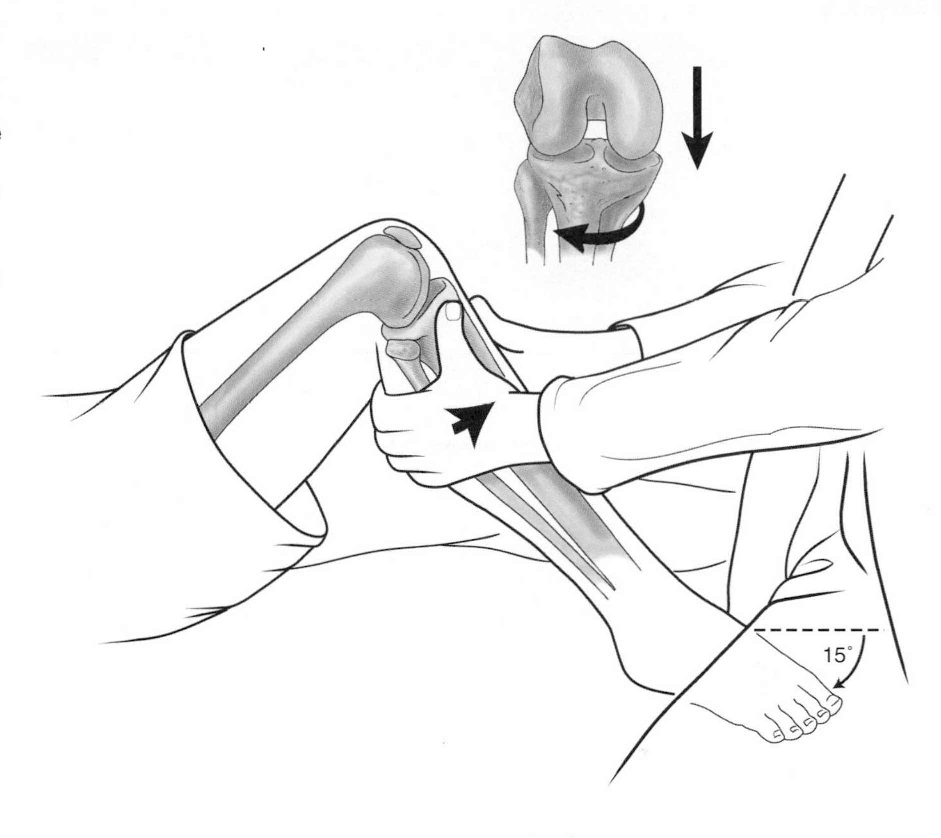

Figure 141-11 Slocum test. An anterior drawer is done in external rotation and the anterior translation is compared with the same test done with the foot in neutral. The displacement should decrease with the knee in external rotation; if it does not, then a posteromedial corner injury should be suspected. (Adapted from Tria AJ, Klein K: An Illustrated Guide to the Knee. New York: Churchill Livingstone, 1992.)

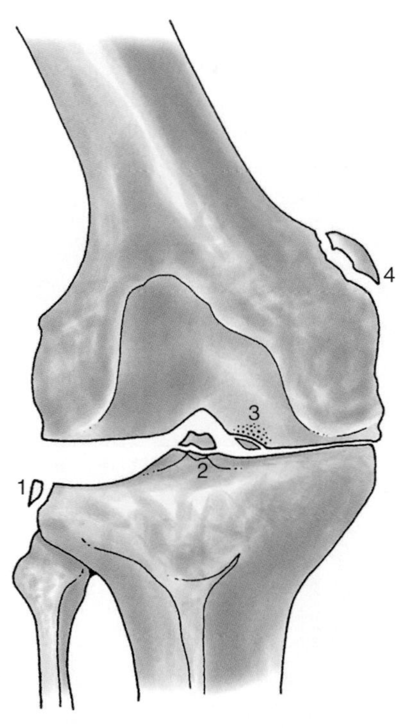

Figure 141-12 Illustration showing multiple radiographic findings. 1, Segond fracture (lateral capsular sign); 2, tibial emminence fracture; 3, osteochondritis dessicans; 4, Pelligrini-Stieda lesion. (Adapted from Miller MD: Sports medicine. In Miller MD (ed): Review of Orthopaedics, 3rd ed. Philadelphia: WB Saunders, 2000, p 200.)

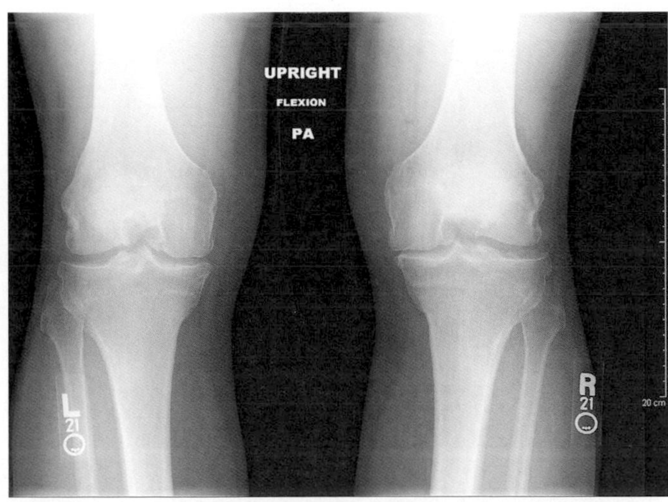

Figure 141-13 Flexion weight-bearing posteroanterior radiographs. This test is done in 45 degrees of flexion and demonstrates postmeniscectomy medial compartment arthrosis (right greater than left).

— Displacement of 10 mm implies an isolated posterior cruciate ligament injury. Displacement of 20 mm or more implies a combined posterior cruciate ligament–posterolateral corner injury.

- Magnetic resonance imaging
  - Unfortunately, most sports fans believe that the diagnosis of any sports injury must await the results of magnetic resonance imaging. In reality,

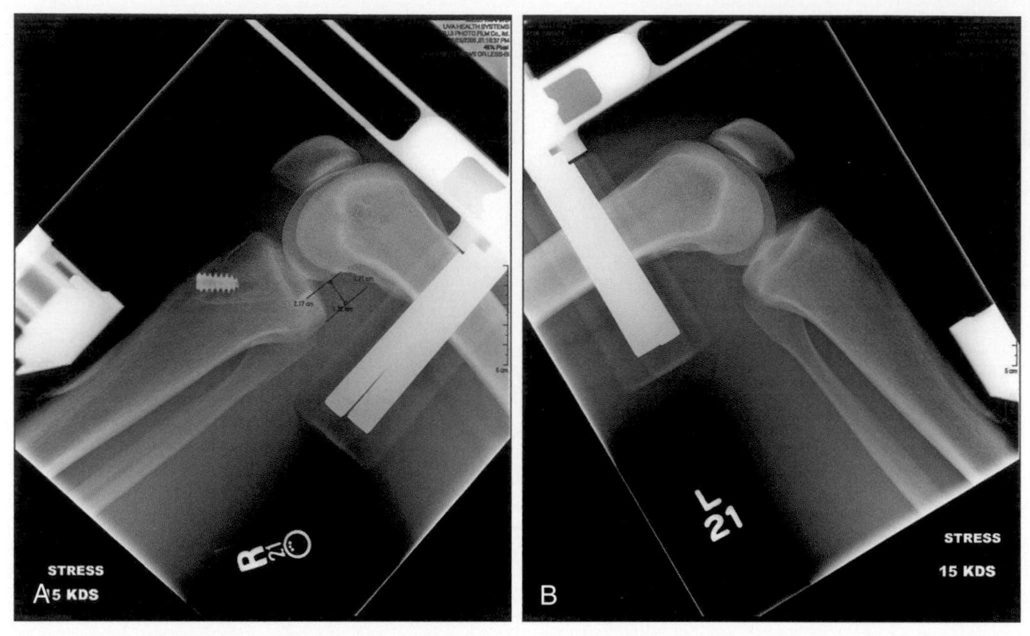

Figure 141-14 Telos stress radiograph with 15 kDa of force in a patient with a failed previous posterior cruciate ligament reconstruction (**A**). Note that the posterior displacement is measured and compared with the opposite normal knee (**B**).

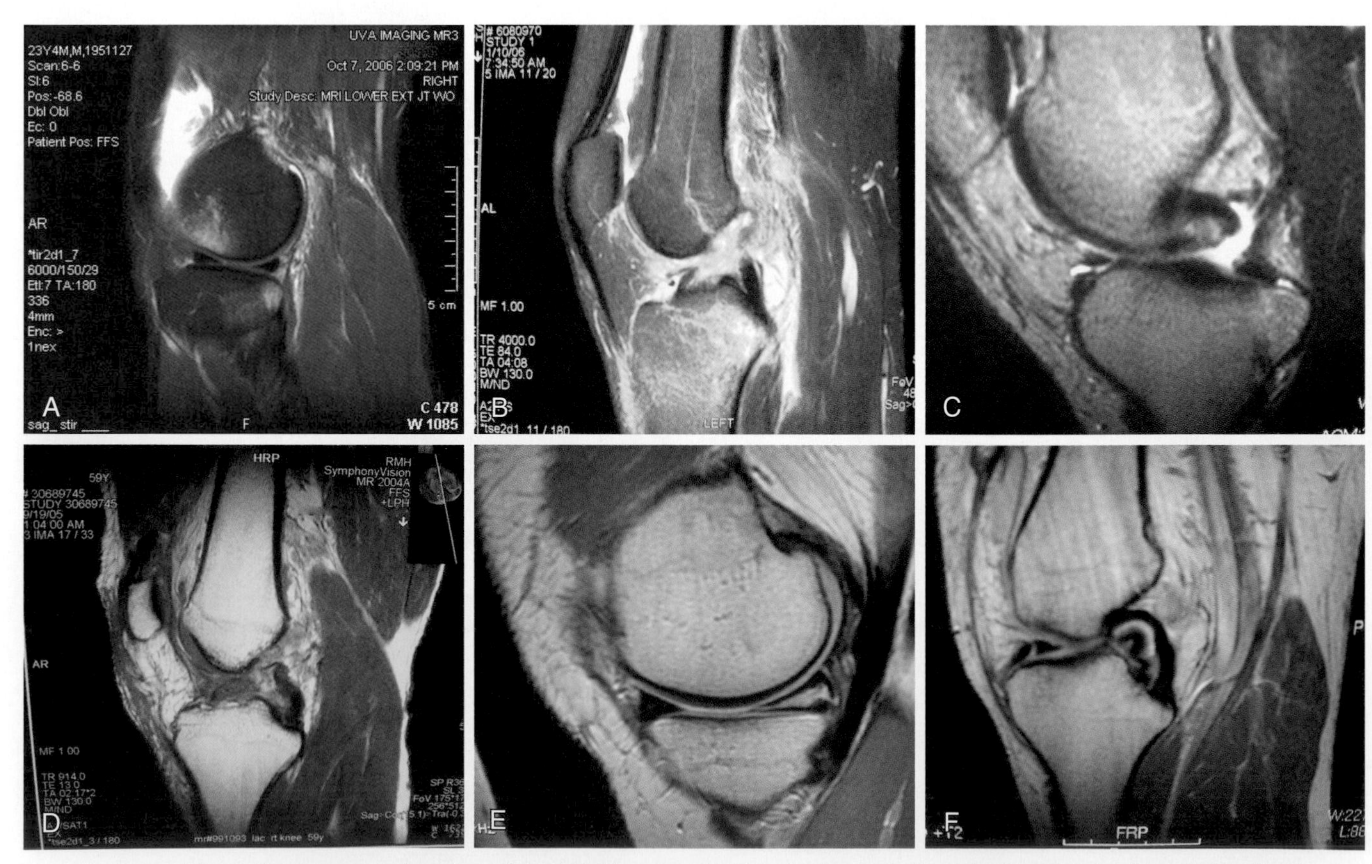

Figure 141-15 Magnetic resonance imaging of a typical bone contusion (bruise or trabecular microfracture) associated with an anterior cruciate ligament (ACL)–injured knee (**A**); an ACL injury with a linear fracture (**B**); a posterior cruciate ligament (PCL) injury (**C**); a combined ACL and PCL–injured knee (**D**); a complex posterior horn medial meniscal tear with a "picture frame" meniscus (**E**); and a displaced bucket-handle tear of the medial meniscus with a "double PCL sign" (**F**).

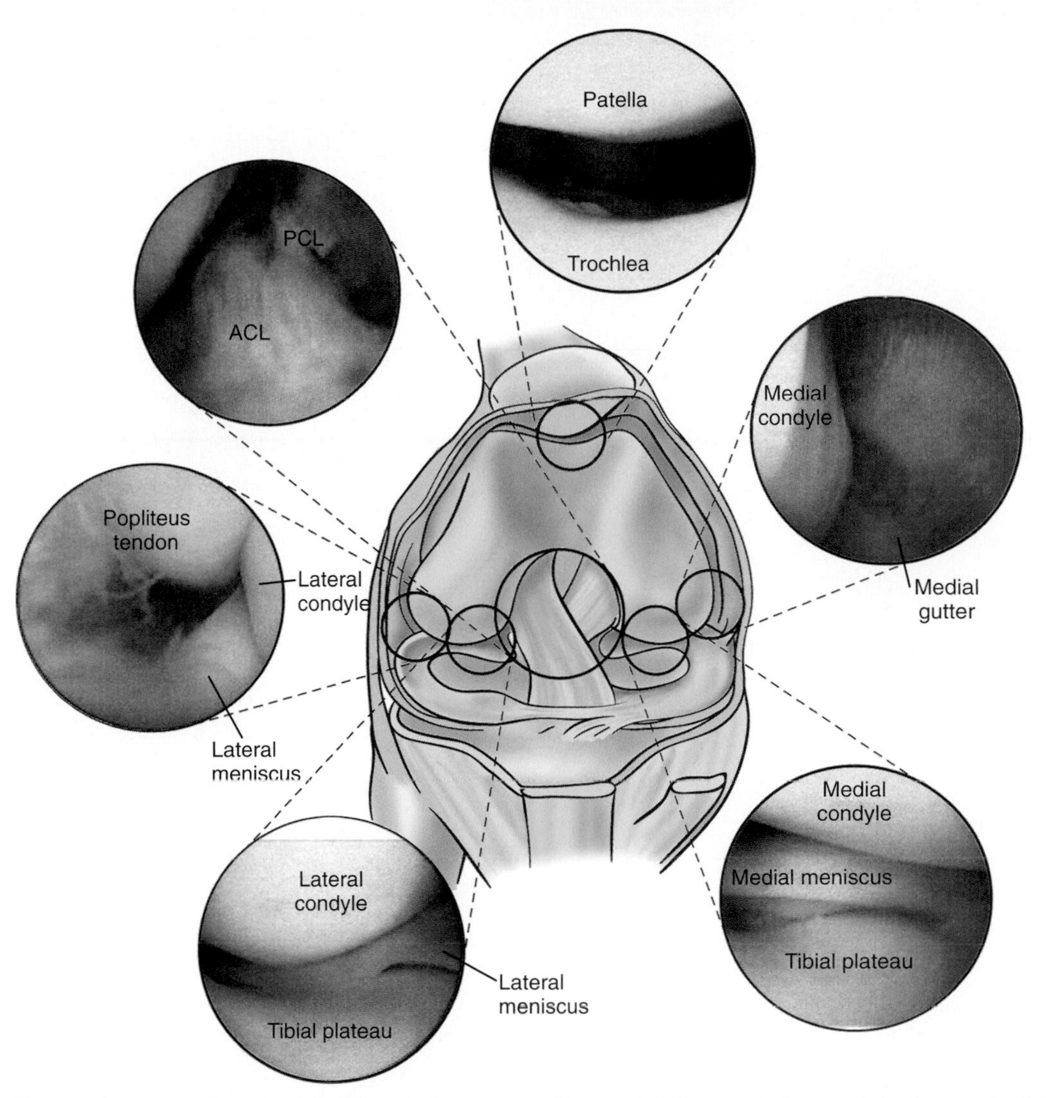

Figure 141-16 Diagnostic knee arthroscopy. ACL, anterior cruciate ligament; PCL, posterior cruciate ligament. (Adapted from Miller MD, Chhabra AB, Hurwitz SR, et al: Orthopaedic Surgical Approaches. Philadelphia: Saunders, 2008, p 486.)

magnetic resonance imaging should be a confirmatory examination.
- It is very accurate for ligament injuries, meniscal tears, and other problems (Fig. 141-15).
- Historically, it has not been as helpful for articular cartilage injuries, although techniques are improving.

- Computed tomography
  - Computed tomography can be useful for the evaluation of bony pathology (e.g., fractures, tumors, revision surgery with bone defects).
- Arthroscopy
  - Arthroscopy is typically done with the patient in the supine position with a leg holder or post.
  - The inferolateral portal is typically used for visualization and the inferomedial portal for instrumentation.
  - Additional portals are made as necessary.
  - A thorough and complete examination of the knee is performed and pathology addressed (Fig. 141-16).

Suggested Reading

- Ellis H: The applied anatomy of examination of the knee. Br J Hosp Med 2007;68:M60–M61.
- Hoppenfeld S: Physical Examination of the Spine and Extremities. Norwalk, CT: Appleton & Lange, 1976.
- Lubowitz JH, Bernardini BJ, Reid JB III: Current concepts review: Comprehensive physical examination for instability of the knee. Am J Sports Med 2008;36:577–594.
- Miller MD, Howard RF, Plancher KD: Surgical Atlas of Sports Medicine. Philadelphia: WB Saunders, 2003.
- Miller MD, Sekiya JK: Sports Medicine: Core Knowledge in Orthopaedics. Philadelphia: Elsevier, 2006.

- Post WR: Anterior knee pain: Diagnosis and treatment. J Am Acad Orthop Surg 2005;13:534–543.
- Slocum DB, Larson RL: Rotatory instability of the knee: Its pathogenesis and a clinical test to demonstrate its presence. J Bone Joint Surg Am 1968;50A:211–225.
- Tria AJ Jr: An Illustrated Guide to the Knee. New York: Churchill Livingstone, 1992.
- Wojtys EM, Chan DB: Meniscus structure and function. Instr Course Lect 2005;54:323–330.

Chapter 142 Anterior Cruciate Ligament Injury

Mark D. Miller

ICD-9 CODES
844.2 *Acute Anterior Cruciate Ligament Injury*
717.83 *Chronic Anterior Cruciate Ligament Injury*

Key Concepts

- The anterior cruciate ligament (ACL) is the primary restraint to anterior translation of the tibia.
- It also has a role in rotational stability of the knee.
- The ACL runs obliquely from just anterior to the center of the tibia to the inner portion of the lateral femoral condyle (Fig. 142-1).
- Injury to the ACL results in abnormal translation and rotation to the knee, leading to increased forces on other structures of the knee (e.g., menisci, articular cartilage), which can themselves be injured either acutely or chronically.
- Meniscal tears occur in approximately half of acute ACL injuries.
- A triad of injuries, including the ACL, the medial collateral ligament, and the lateral meniscus is not uncommon.
- ACL injuries can, uncommonly, be associated with other knee ligament injuries (multiple ligament injury) that may require reduction and careful neurovascular evaluation.

History

- Acute injury
  - Noncontact pivoting injury to the knee
  - "Pop"
  - Immediate swelling
  - Unable to continue in game or activity
- Chronic injury
  - Recurrent swelling with activity
  - Instability with pivoting sports

Physical Examination

- Observation
  - Abrasions
  - Deformity
  - Effusion (intra-articular swelling)
- Palpation
  - Patellar ballottement (effusion)
  - Tenderness
- Range of motion
  - Rule out a locked knee (lacking full extension) from an ACL tear in conjunction with a displaced bucket handle tear of the meniscus.
  - Loss of flexion can occur from an effusion.
- Special tests
  - Lachman's test (gold standard) (Fig. 142-2)
    - — Pull forward on the tibia with the knee in 20 to 30 degrees of flexion while stabilizing the femur.
  - Anterior and posterior drawer tests (rule out a posterior cruciate ligament injury)
    - — Flex the knee to 70 to 90 degrees of flexion, assess the starting point (the medial femoral condyle should be approximately 1 cm anterior to the medial tibial plateau) and apply a posterior (posterior cruciate ligament) and anterior (ACL, but not as reliable as the Lachman's test) force.
  - Pivot shift test
    - — A valgus force is applied as the knee is flexed and a rotational "clunk" may be appreciated.
  - McMurray's test (associated meniscal tear)
    - — Flexion and rotation of the knee may produce a clunk as the meniscus displaces.
  - Dial test (associated posterolateral corner [posterior cruciate ligament] injury)
    - — With the patient lying prone, rotate the foot externally with the knee flexed to 30 and 90 degrees.

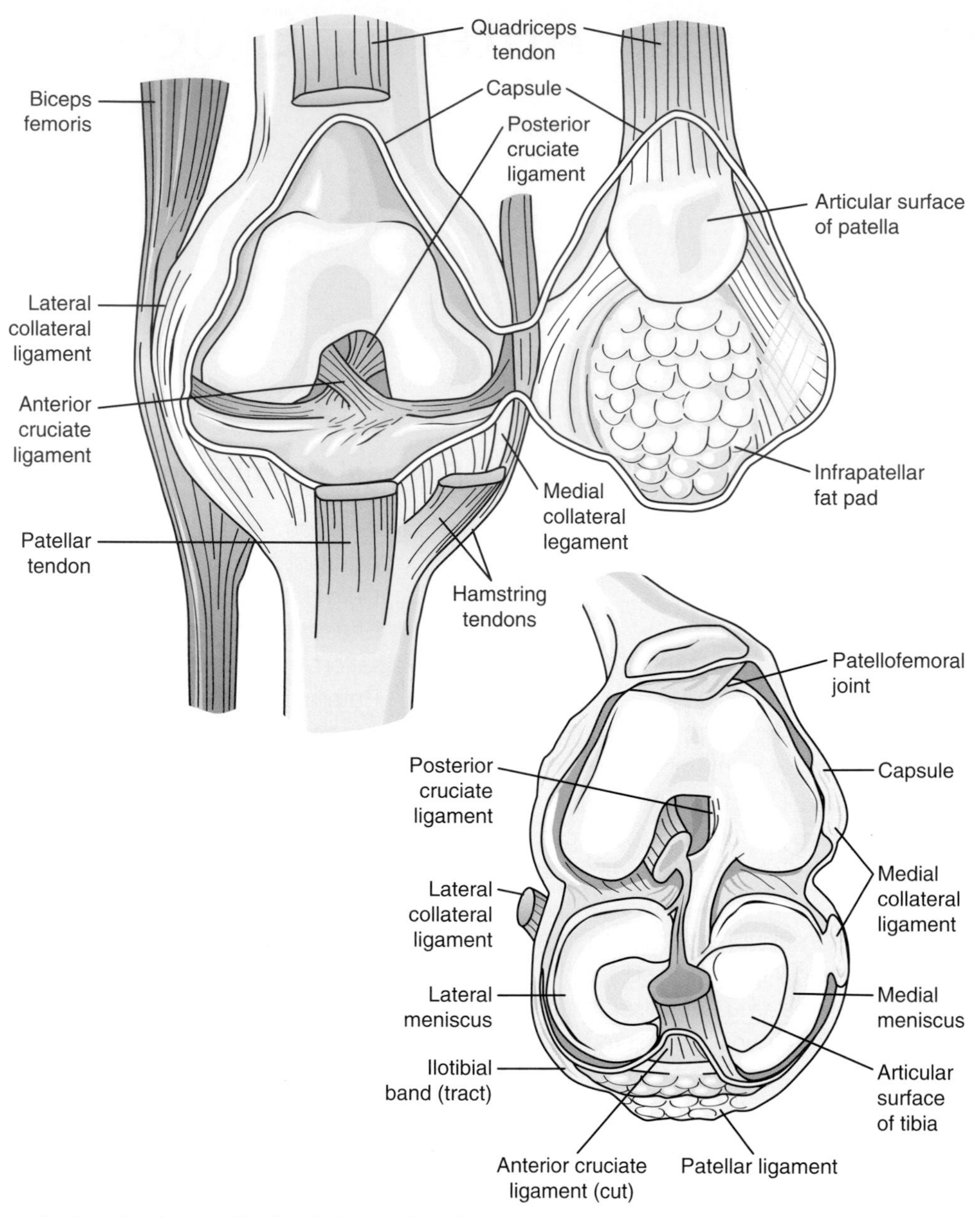

Figure 142-1 Front (*top*) and cut-away (*bottom*) views of the knee joint demonstrating the location of the anterior cruciate ligament.

- — Asymmetrical rotation in both 30 and 90 degrees of flexion suggests a combined posterolateral corner and posterior cruciate ligament injury.
- — Asymmetrical rotation in only 30 degrees of flexion suggests an isolated posterolateral corner injury (or a combined posterolateral corner and ACL injury).
- Patellar apprehension test (patellar instability may have a similar presentation)
  - — Attempt to displace the patella laterally and determine whether the patient is apprehensive.

Imaging

- Radiographs
  - Posteroanterior flexion weight-bearing view
    - — Check for arthritis (especially in older patients)
    - — Look for a lateral tibial avulsion (Segond fracture), which is highly associated with an ACL tear.
  - Lateral view
    - — Check for patellar height
    - — A high-riding patella (alta) may be associated with patellar instability or a patellar tendon rupture.

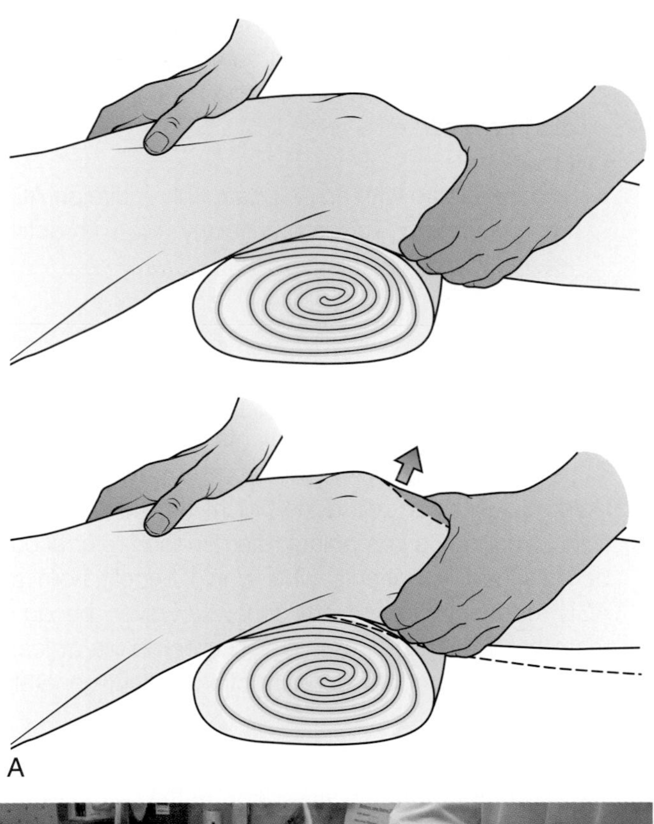

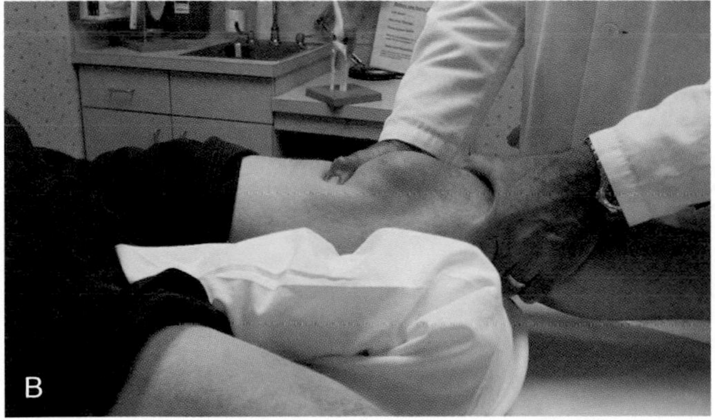

Figure 142-2 **A**, Lachman's test is the gold standard for evaluating an anterior cruciate ligament–injured knee. It is helpful to place a pillow under the knee to relax the hamstring muscle and gain the patient's confidence. **B**, Note that the examiner faces the injured knee and uses the hand that is closer to the patient's head to stabilize the thigh and the other hand to displace the tibia anteriorly.

 — A low-riding patella (baja) is associated with a stiff knee (arthrofibrosis).
- Sunrise view
 — Look for patellar subluxation/tilt.
 — Magnetic resonance imaging (Fig. 142-3)
 — Not required to make the diagnosis; confirmatory examination
 — Look for disruption of the ligament on the sagittal view
 — Look for the classic bone bruise pattern.

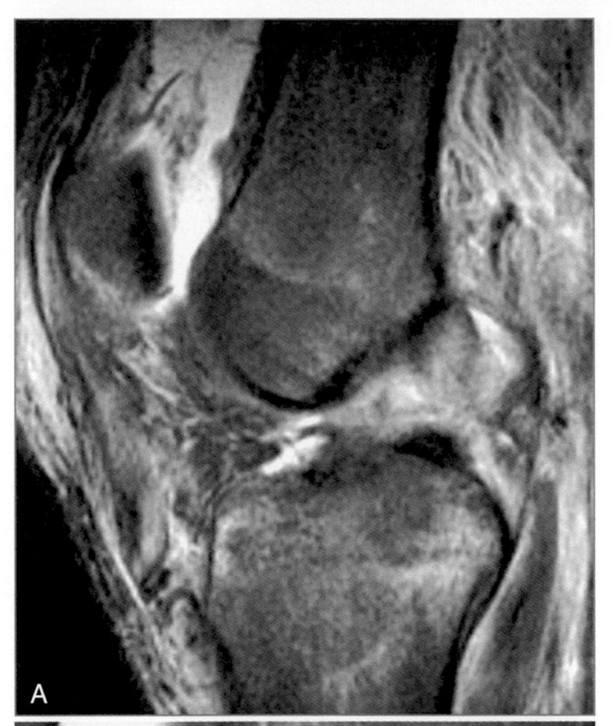

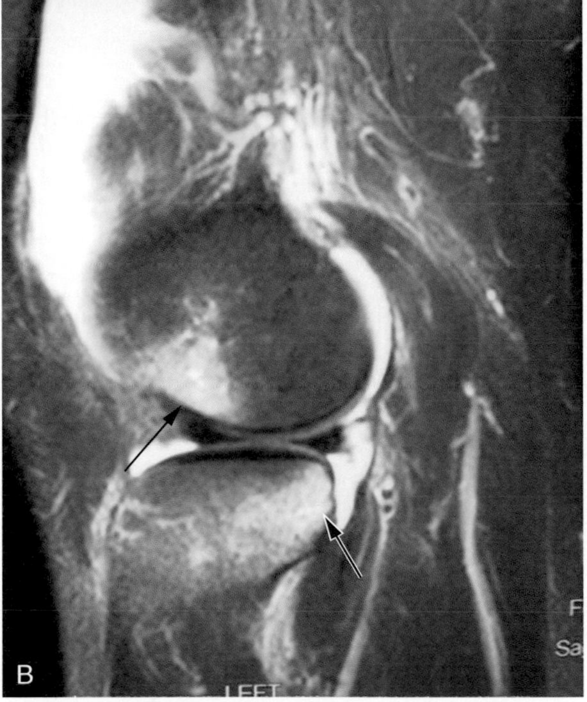

Figure 142-3 Sagittal magnetic resonance imaging demonstrating anterior cruciate ligament disruption (**A**) and classic bone bruise (**B**) (see *arrows*).

Additional Tests

- KT1000/KT2000
  - Optional test for objective measurement of anterior tibial translation
  - Often used by surgeons for objective evaluation after ACL reconstruction

Differential Diagnosis

- Patellar instability
  - Apprehension
  - Negative Lachman's test
  - Fat droplets may be present in aspiration
- Patellar or quadriceps tendon rupture
  - Patient unable to actively extend knee
- Posterior cruciate ligament rupture
  - Posterior drawer test (remember to assess starting point)
- Meniscal tear
  - Negative Lachman's test
  - Joint line tenderness

Treatment

- At diagnosis
  - The initial treatment of an ACL tear focuses on decreasing the effusion (consider aspiration, start therapy focusing on closed-chain quadriceps rehabilitation, use ice and compression). It is also important to work on motion, quadriceps tone, and pain control.
- Later
  - Most patients with an ACL tear will require an ACL reconstruction. This is particularly true with active patients and all athletes.

When to Refer

- All but sedentary, inactive patients
- If the examiner is confident that the patient has an isolated ACL tear and does not have a locked knee (which mandates immediate referral), then referral can be arranged in patients who would benefit from an ACL reconstruction at any time. However, because the rehabilitation process after surgery takes at least 4 to 6 months, then reconstruction should generally

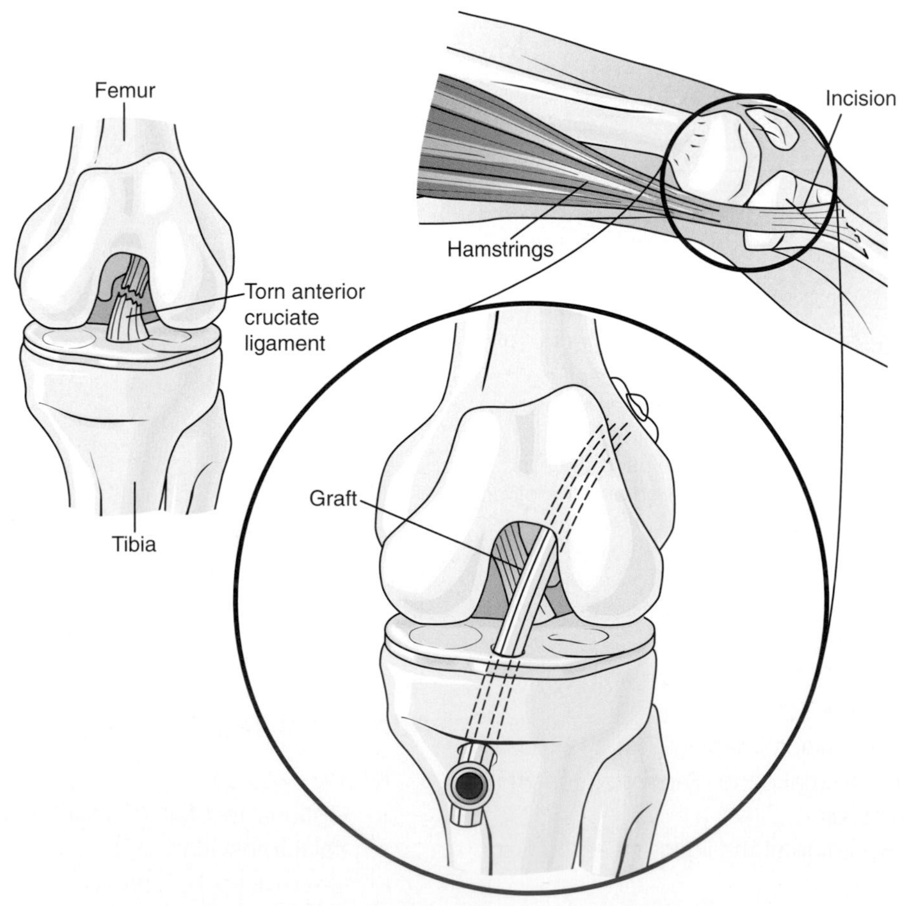

Figure 142-4 Anterior cruciate ligament reconstruction overview.

be scheduled after the effusion is under control, motion is regained, and quadriceps tone is restored.

Prognosis

- Good with ACL reconstruction
  - ACL reconstruction involves removing the torn ACL (the ends cannot simply be repaired because they are immediately coated with a myofibrinous cap) and replacing it with a tendon (autograft, typically the semitendinous and gracilis tendons folded in half or the central one third of the patellar tendon, or allograft from a cadaver). The tendon is passed through tunnel(s) in the tibia and femur and fixed with screws or other fixation devices (Fig. 142-4).
- If patients elect nonoperative treatment, recurrent instability may occur, often resulting in additional meniscal and/or articular cartilage injury (especially in active individuals).

Troubleshooting

- The patient should be counseled on the benefits and risks of surgery.
- Benefits (which usually far outweigh the risks of ACL reconstruction) include restoration of stability to the knee and (in most cases) successful return to sports.
- Risks include bleeding, infection, nerve injury (numbness is not uncommon after patellar tendon or hamstring harvesting from incision or retraction of the infrapatellar branches of the saphenous nerve), loss of motion, and recurrence. When patellar tendon autografts are used, there is also a slight risk of a patellar fracture and late anterior knee pain (typically with kneeling).

Patient Instructions

- It is important to achieve full range of motion prior to ACL reconstruction and immediately afterward. Patients should be encouraged to put a pillow or bolster under their heel rather than under their knee to maintain full extension.
- Swelling can be controlled with ice (apply for 15–20 minutes several times a day).
- Quadriceps strengthening (stationary cycle, eliptical trainer, etc.) is an important part of rehabilitation.
- Patients should avoid running and activities involving sudden changes in direction both pre-operatively and for at least 3 months after surgery.
- Patients should be able to return to sports after 6 months or longer for uncomplicated ACL reconstructions.

Considerations in Special Populations

- Inactive and sedentary patients should be treated nonoperatively. If they have associated meniscal tears, then sometimes arthroscopy can be considered for the meniscal tears and not for ACL reconstruction.
- Obese patients can make surgery challenging, but if they have instability, surgery should nonetheless be performed.

Suggested Reading

- Benjaminse A, Gokeler A, van der Schans CP: Clinical diagnosis of an anterior cruciate ligament rupture: A meta-analysis. J Orthop Sports Phys Ther 2006;36:267–288.
- Chhabra A, Starman JS, Ferretti M, et al: Anatomic, radiographic, biomechanical, and kinematic evaluation of the anterior cruciate ligament and its two functional bundles. J Bone Joint Surg Am 2006;33(Suppl 4):2–10.
- Clatworthy M, Amendola A: The anterior cruciate ligament and arthritis. Clin Sports Med 1999;18:173–198.
- Delfico AJ, Garret WE Jr: Mechanisms of injury of the anterior cruciate ligament in soccer players. Clin Sports Med 1998;17:779–785.
- Fithian DC, Paxton EW, Stone ML, et al: Prospective trial of a treatment algorithm for the management of the anterior cruciate ligament-injured knee. Am J Sports Med 2005;33:333–334.
- Iobst CA, Stanitski CL: Acute knee injuries. Clin Sports Med 2000;19:621–635.
- Kocher MS, DiCanzio J, Zurakowski D, Micheli LJ: Diagnostic performance of clinical examination and selective magnetic resonance imaging in the evaluation of intra-articular knee disorders in children and adolescents. Am J Sports Med 2001;29:292–296.
- O'Shea KJ, Murphy KP, Heekin RD, Herzwurm PJ: The diagnostic accuracy of history, physical examination, and radiographs in the evaluation of traumatic knee disorders. Am J Sports Med 1996;24:164–167.
- Sanders TG, Miller MD: A systematic approach to magnetic resonance imaging interpretation of sports medicine injuries of the knee. Am J Sports Med 2005;33:131–148.
- Solomon DH, Simel DL, Bates DW, et al: The rational clinical examination. Does this patient have a torn meniscus or ligament of the knee? Value of the physical examination. JAMA 2001;286:1610–1620.
- Utukuri MM, Somayaji HS, Khanduja V, et al: Update on pediatric ACL injuries. Knee 2006;13:345–352.

Chapter 143 Posterior Cruciate Ligament Injury

Michael J. Salata, Edward M. Wojtys, and Jon K. Sekiya

ICD-9 CODES
844.2 *Acute Posterior Cruciate Ligament Injury*
717.84 *Chronic Posterior Cruciate Ligament Injury*

Key Concepts

- The posterior cruciate ligament (PCL) is the primary restraint to posterior translation of the tibia.
- The PCL injury accounts for 3% to 20% of all knee ligament injuries.
- The PCL resists 85% to 100% of a posteriorly directed knee force at 30 and 90 degrees.
- The PCL runs obliquely, originating from the lateral border of the medial femoral condyle and inserting 1 to 1.5 cm inferior to the posterior rim of the tibia in a depression called the PCL fovea or facet (Fig. 143-1).
- There are two main bundles of the PCL, the anterolateral (stronger, larger) and the posteromedial, a concept important for reconstruction (Fig. 143-2).
- The PCL injury mechanism is usually trauma ("dashboard injury") or sports (fall on flexed knee with plantarflexed foot or isolated hyperflexion).
- Frequently injured in combination with other ligaments (posterolateral corner, anterior cruciate, collaterals); isolated injuries less than 50%
- Partial tears may heal due to their extrasynovial position and good blood supply.
- After PCL rupture, contact forces increase in the medial and patellofemoral compartments and may lead to arthritis.
- Results after reconstruction are encouraging, but surgery remains controversial in the setting of an isolated PCL injury.

History

- Acute injury
    - Minimal to large effusion
    - May complain of instability
    - In the setting of trauma, rule out associated injuries including occult knee dislocation.
    - Determine time from injury.
- Chronic injury
    - Anterior and/or medial knee pain
    - Feeling of instability, especially with twisting, impact activities, and stairs
    - Mild effusion, worsened with activities

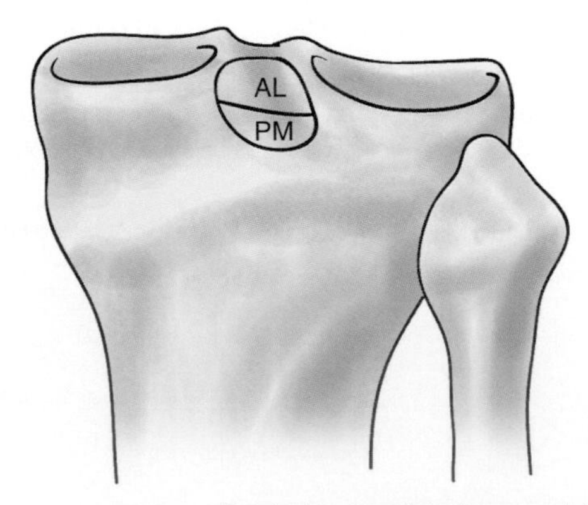

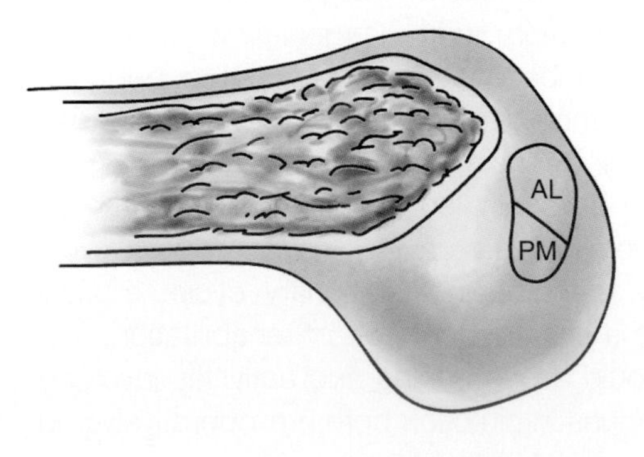

Figure 143-1 Posterior cruciate ligament insertion sites. AL, anterolateral; PM, posteromedial.

Physical Examination

- Observation
  - Effusion
  - Bruising or anterior abrasions
  - Deformity (rule out dislocation)
- Special tests
  - Lachman's test: rule out associated anteroposterior cruciate ligament injury
  - Posterior drawer test: impart a posterior force on the proximal tibia. Posterior translation is greatest at 70 to 90 degrees of knee flexion. The tibia must be reduced to its normal anatomic position before testing (Fig. 143-3).
    - — Grade I (0–5 mm): tibial condyles anterior to femoral condyles
    - — Grade II (5–10 mm): tibial condyles flush with femoral condyles, usually partial injury
    - — Grade III (10–15 mm): tibial condyles posterior to femoral condyles, complete tear, may indicate concomitant posterolateral corner injury
  - Posterior sag: hip and knee flexed to 90 degrees; gravity applies posterior force to tibia; look for "sag" of tibia on the injured side compared with the normal side (Fig. 143-4)
  - Passive external rotation (dial test): Test at 30 and 90 degrees, prone or supine, and compare with the other side. More than a 10-degree difference is positive.
    - — External rotation increased at 30 degrees only: isolated posterolateral corner injury
    - — External rotation increased at 90 degrees only: isolated PCL
    - — External rotation increased at both 30 and 90 degrees: PCL plus posterolateral corner injury

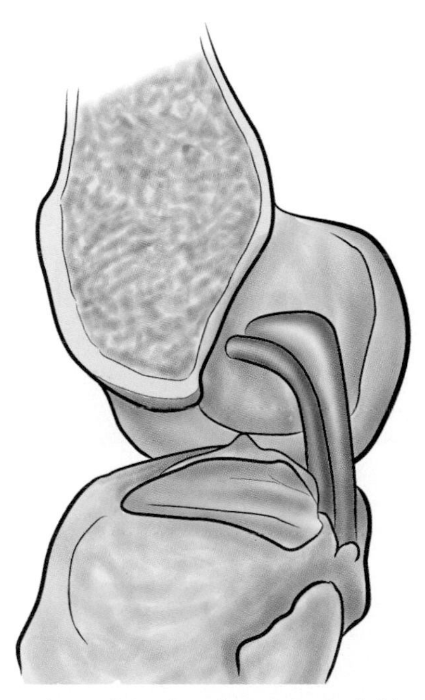

Figure 143-2 Anterolateral and posteromedial bundles of the posterior cruciate ligament.

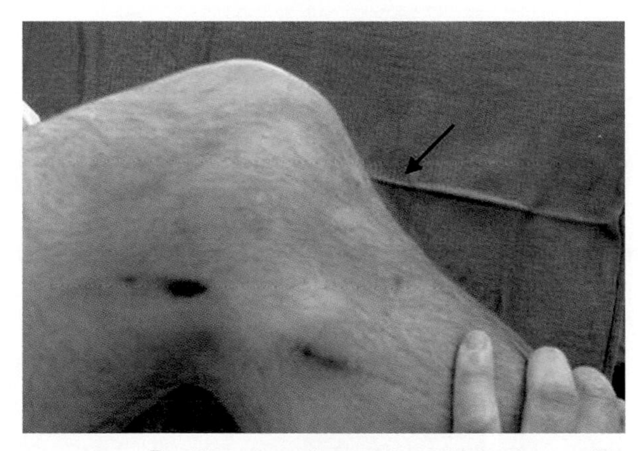

Figure 143-4 Positive posterior sag test. Note the position of the tibia (*arrow*).

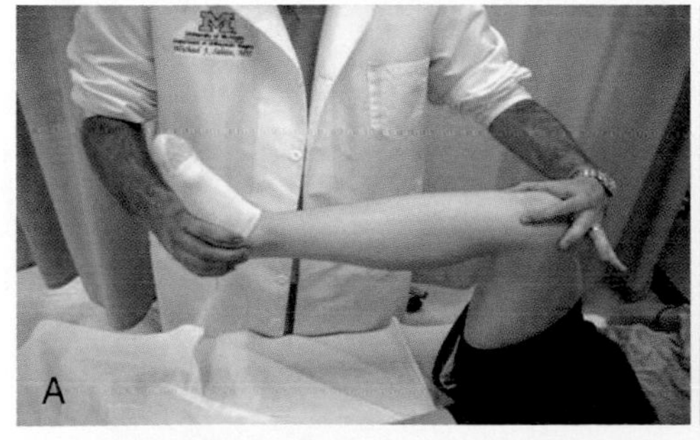

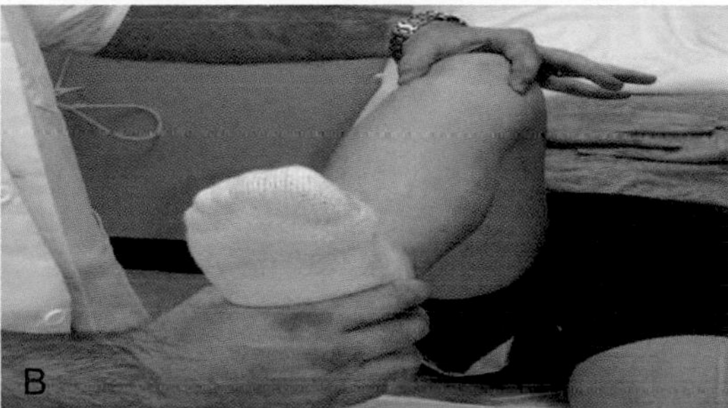

Figure 143-3 **A**, Hand position for the posterior drawer/sag test. **B**, The anterior joint line is palpated to determine the relationship of the proximal tibia to the femoral condyles.

Imaging

- Radiographs: weight-bearing anteroposterior, lateral, and merchant views
  - Look for PCL avulsion fragment in acute injuries (Fig. 143-5).
  - Evaluate for degenerative joint disease and osteochondral injury.
- Stress radiographs: taken with a posterior force applied to proximal tibia
  - A Telos device may be used to reliably reproduce this force.
  - Useful in suspected chronic injuries
- Magnetic resonance imaging (Fig. 143-6)
  - Useful to evaluate complete and partial PCL injuries
  - Identifies other associated ligament, meniscal, and chondral injuries
  - Magnetic resonance imaging should be used cautiously in the chronic setting; may interpret PCL as

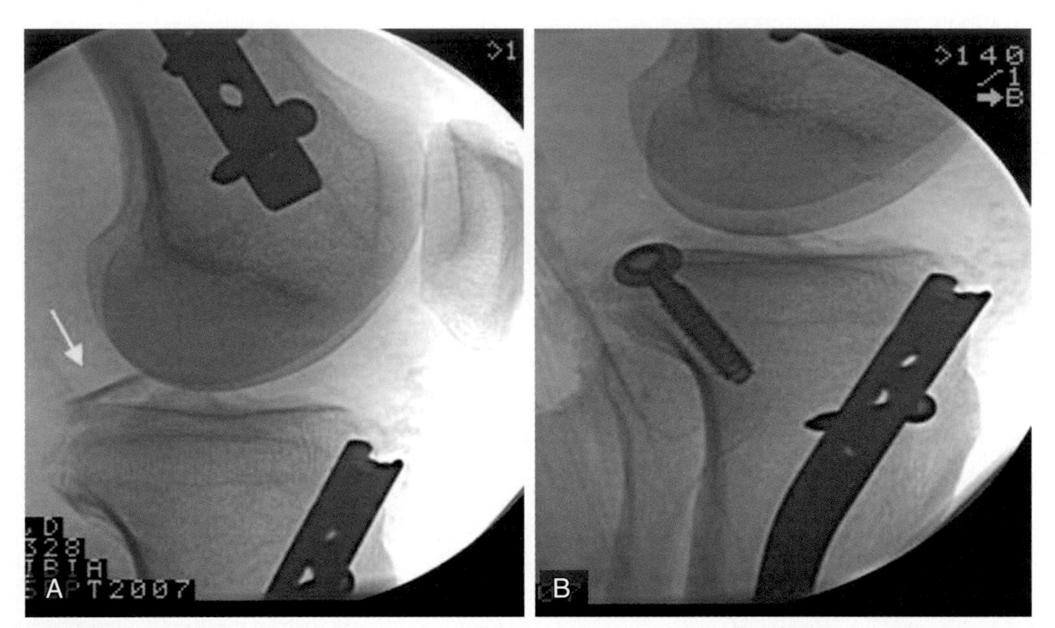

Figure 143-5 Radiographs depicting posterior cruciate ligament avulsion. **A**, *Arrow* denotes large bony avulsion fragment (also note the associated fractures). **B**, Same fragment after open reduction and internal fixation.

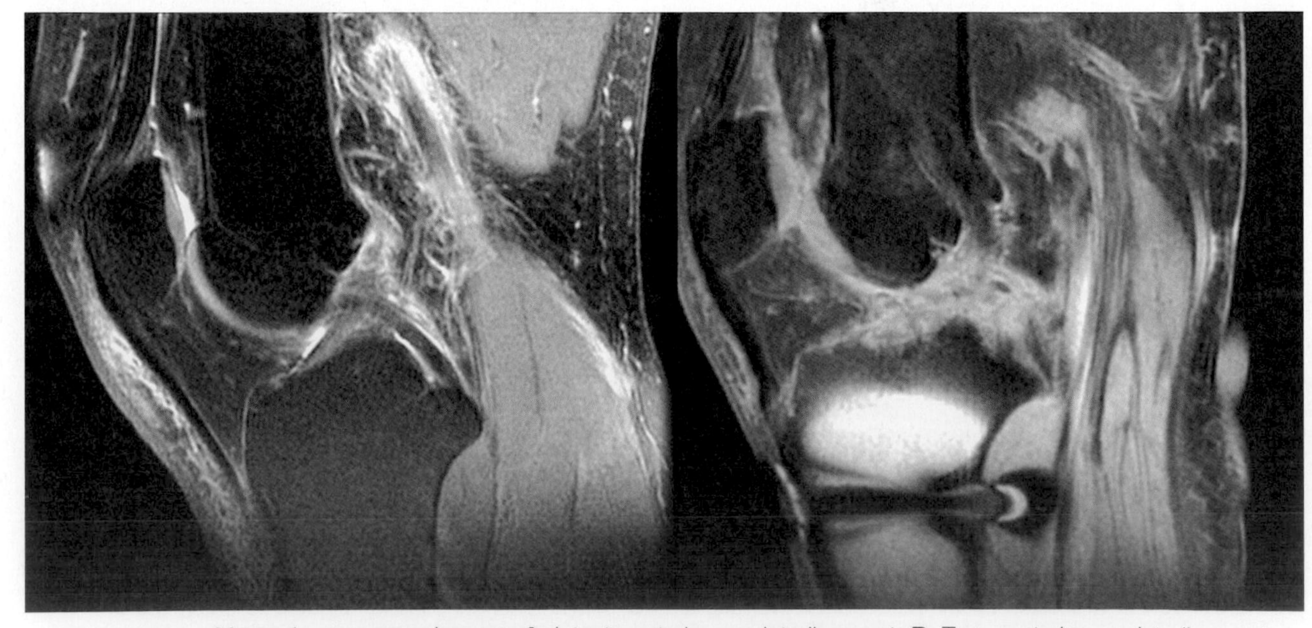

Figure 143-6 Magnetic resonance images. **A**, Intact posterior cruciate ligament. **B**, Torn posterior cruciate ligament.

healed in patient with clinical laxity due to postinjury lengthening of the ligament

Differential Diagnosis

- Anterior cruciate ligament rupture
- Occult knee dislocation (multiligamentous knee injury)
- Isolated posterolateral corner injury
- Tibial plateau fracture

Treatment

Isolated Posterior Cruciate Ligament Injuries

- At diagnosis (acute injuries)
  - Treatment is dependent on grade of injury and the presence or absence of avulsion fragment.
    - Grade I and II: no/small bony fragment
      - Nonoperative with aggressive rehabilitation program concentrating on quadriceps strengthening and range of motion
      - Return to play in approximately 1 month when quadriceps strength nearly normal
      - Children may require repair.
    - Grade I and II: large bony fragment
      - Refer for surgical fixation of fragment.
    - Grade III
      - Refer for operative consultation: Double- versus single-bundle reconstructions and arthroscopically assisted versus all-arthroscopic options exist.
- Later (chronic injuries)
  - Operative treatment is controversial.
  - Alignment and degree of joint degeneration must be taken into account.
  - Patients may require high tibial or sagittal plane osteotomy.

When to Refer

- Indications for referral include acute PCL injuries with large bony fragments amenable to fixation, grade III PCL injuries (must not be an isolated injury), and all multiligamentous knee injuries (see Chapter 145).

Prognosis

- The PCL has an increased healing capacity compared with the anterior cruciate ligament.
- A good therapy program focusing on quadriceps strengthening is successful in most cases.

Troubleshooting

- Large bony avulsions that are amenable to open reduction and internal fixation should be considered for acute operative intervention.
- Chronic injuries should be considered for surgery if nonoperative management has failed and the patient has persistent pain or instability.
- Careful examination is critical to rule out associated knee pathology and occult knee dislocation.

Patient Instructions

- Patients should be counseled that not all injuries require surgery.
- The prognosis is favorable in most cases with a good quadriceps strengthening program.
- The PCL-deficient knee may be at risk of developing a more rapid rate of medial compartment and patellofemoral arthrosis.

Suggested Reading

- Arnoczky SP, Grewe SR, Paulos LE, et al: Instability of the anterior and posterior cruciate ligaments. Instr Course Lect 1991;40:199–270.
- Campbell RB, Jordan SS, Sekiya JK: Arthroscopic tibial inlay for posterior cruciate ligament reconstruction. Arthroscopy 2007; 23:1356e1–1356e4.
- Campbell RB, Torrie A, Hecker A, et al: Comparison of tibial graft fixation between simulated arthroscopic and open inlay techniques for posterior cruciate ligament reconstruction. Am J Sports Med 2007;35:1731–1738.
- Miller MD, Bergfeld JA, Fowler PJ, et al: The posterior cruciate ligament injured knee: Principles of evaluation and treatment. Instr Course Lect 1999;48:199–207.
- Parolie JM, Bergfeld JA: Long-term results of nonoperative treatment of isolated posterior cruciate ligament injuries in the athlete. Am J Sports Med 1986;14:35–38.
- Sekiya JK, West RV, Ong BC, et al: Clinical outcomes after isolated arthroscopic single-bundle posterior cruciate ligament reconstruction. Arthroscopy 2005;21:1042–1050.
- Sekiya JK, Whiddon DR, Zehms CT, Miller MD: A clinically relevant assessment of PCL and posterolateral corner injuries. Part I: Evaluation of isolated and combined deficiency. J Bone Joint Surg Am 2008;90(8):1621–1627.
- Shelbourne KD, Davis TJ, Patel DV: The natural history of acute, isolated, nonoperatively treated posterior cruciate ligament injuries: A prospective study. Am J Sports Med 1999;27:276–283.
- Veltri DM, Warren RF: Isolated and combined posterior cruciate ligament injuries. J Am Acad Orthop Surg 1993;1:67–75.
- Whiddon DR, Zehms CT, Miller MD, et al: Double compared with single-bundle open inlay posterior cruciate ligament reconstruction in a cadaver model. J Bone Joint Surg Am 2008;90(9): 1820–1829.

Chapter 144 Medial Collateral Ligament Injury

Joy L. Long and James E. Carpenter

ICD-9 CODES
844.1 *Medial Collateral Ligament Sprain*
717.82 *Chronic Medial Collateral Ligament Tear*

Key Concepts

- The medial collateral ligament (MCL) is the primary restraint to valgus stress on the knee (Fig. 144-1).
- The MCL is the most commonly injured knee ligament.
- MCL injuries are classified as acute or chronic and graded as sprains: I (mild partial tear), II (moderate partial tear), III (complete tear).
- The "terrible triad" was classically described as injury to the MCL, anterior cruciate ligament, and medial meniscus after a twisting injury with valgus force.
- Lateral meniscus tears are actually more common with anterior cruciate ligament/MCL injuries.
- Most MCL injuries are treated nonoperatively in a hinged brace.

History

- Acute injury
  - Valgus force: contact or noncontact
  - Medial knee pain, with or without "pop"
  - May be able to walk
  - May feel unstable
- Chronic injury
  - Medial and/or lateral knee pain
  - Feeling of instability, especially with twisting and impact activities
  - Mild effusion, worsened with activities

Physical Examination

- Observation
  - Abrasions/contusions from blow on lateral side of knee
  - Swelling, ecchymosis, deformity
- Palpation
  - Mild effusion (if large, consider intra-articular injury)
  - Medial tenderness
- Range of motion
  - Flexion/extension: Swelling may limit extremes of motion.
  - Locked knee: associated bucket handle meniscal tear
- Special tests
  - Valgus stress in 30 degrees of flexion (Fig. 144-2A)
    - — Grade I: 1 to 4 mm laxity with endpoint
    - — Grade II: 5 to 9 mm laxity with endpoint
    - — Grade III: 10 to 15 mm laxity with no firm endpoint
  - Valgus stress in extension (Fig. 144-2B)
    - — Any laxity suggests grade III injury
    - — Consider concomitant cruciate injury

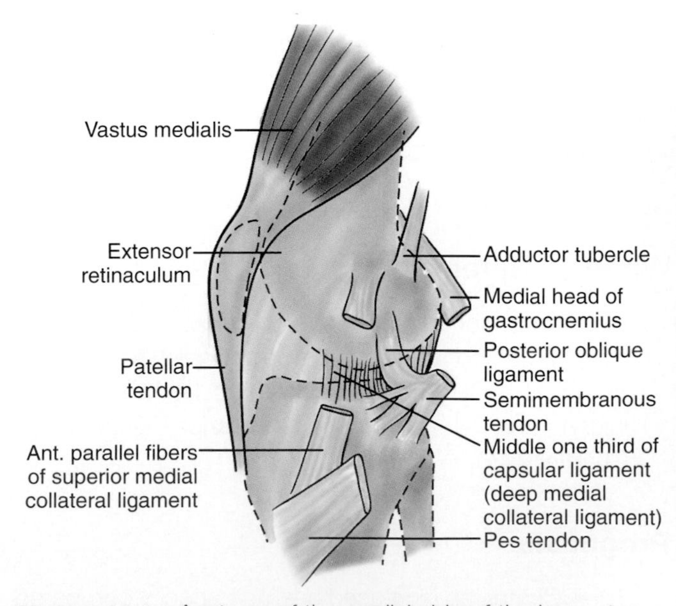

Figure 144-1 Anatomy of the medial side of the knee. Ant., anterior. (Adapted from DeLee JC, Drez D Jr, Miller MD [eds]: DeLee and Drez's Orthopaedic Sports Medicine, 2nd ed. Philadelphia: WB Saunders, 2002, p 1938.)

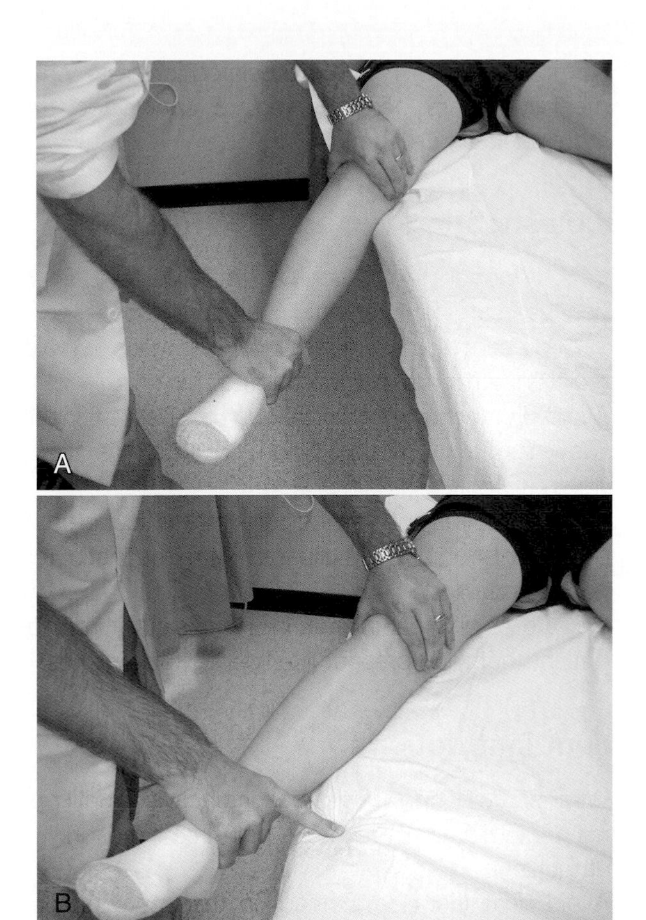

Figure 144-2 Valgus stress test performed at 30 degrees of flexion (**A**) and full extension (**B**). The examiner pulls the lower leg away from midline while stabilizing the femur. By palpating the joint line, the examiner can determine the amount of laxity and ensure assessment of true laxity rather than rotation.

- Lachman's/posterior drawer test: anterior/posterior cruciate ligaments
- McMurray test: meniscal tear
- Patellar apprehension test: Patellar dislocation/subluxation can occur along with MCL sprain; do not confuse pain over the medial patellofemoral ligament with an MCL injury.

Imaging

- Radiographs
  - Anteroposterior and lateral views: usually normal
  - Pellegrini-Stieda lesion is MCL calcification from a chronic injury (Fig. 144-3)
  - Posteroanterior flexion weight-bearing view to evaluate for degenerative changes
  - Patellofemoral view to evaluate for patellofemoral dislocation or avulsion fracture
- Magnetic resonance imaging
  - Not required unless additional pathology is suspected

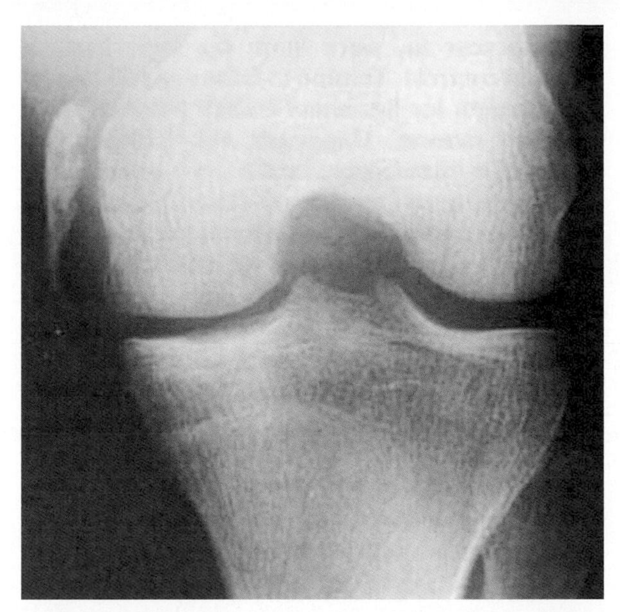

Figure 144-3 Pellegrini-Stieda lesion. Calcification of the medial collateral ligament due to traumatic injury. (From DeLee JC, Drez D Jr, Miller MD [eds]: DeLee and Drez's Orthopaedic Sports Medicine, 2nd ed. Philadelphia: WB Saunders, 2002, p. 1942.)

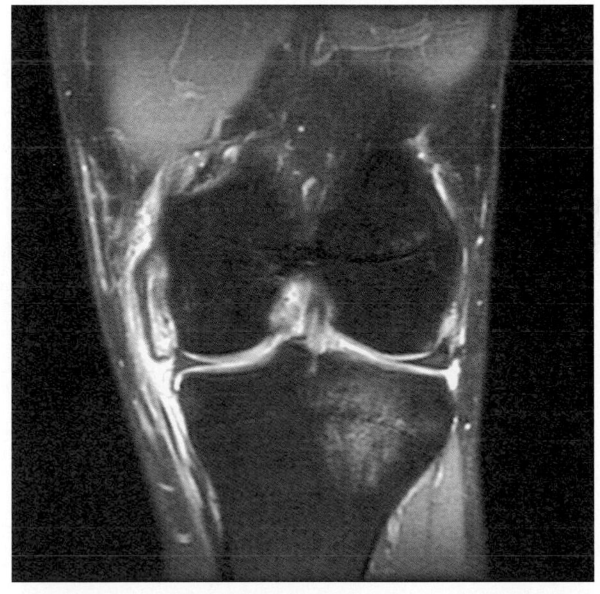

Figure 144-4 Coronal magnetic resonance imaging of distal medial collateral ligament avulsion.

  - Disruption of the MCL seen on coronal views (Fig. 144-4)
  - Bone bruises may be apparent in the lateral femoral condyle and lateral tibial plateau (Fig. 144-5).

Differential Diagnosis

- Patellar subluxation/dislocation
- Anterior cruciate ligament tear
- Medial meniscus tear

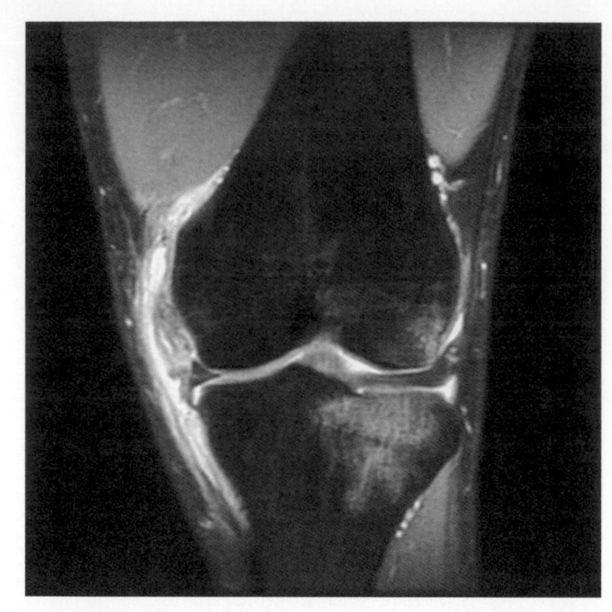

Figure 144-5 Coronal magnetic resonance imaging showing bone bruising in the lateral femoral condyle and lateral tibial plateau due to valgus impact force.

Treatment

- At diagnosis
  - Acute injuries are treated with ice and elevation for 48 hours, a compressive dressing, knee immobilization in slight flexion, and weight bearing as tolerated.
  - Begin motion and strengthening when pain subsides.
  - Usual return to play is based on severity: grade I, 10 days; grade II, 20 days; grade III, at least 4 weeks
- Later
  - For chronic injuries, bracing is the mainstay of treatment.
  - Late repair versus reconstruction is usually successful for symptomatic patients.
  - Osteotomies may be necessary in severe cases.

When to Refer

- Referral is indicated for MCL injuries with associated anterior cruciate ligament, posterior cruciate ligament, or lateral collateral ligament injury; locked knee; associated meniscal tear; grade III injuries; and chronically unstable knees.

Prognosis

- MCL injuries (including grade III) generally heal well with nonoperative treatment.
  - Some laxity may persist.
- Combined injuries with associated cruciate and/or meniscus tears generally require specialized treatment, including surgery.

Troubleshooting

- It is important to recognize multiligament injuries because surgical intervention is usually necessary.
- The presence of degenerative changes or valgus malalignment may complicate recovery.
- Avoid prolonged immobilization to prevent stiffness.
- Allow range of motion when pain permits, usually within a week.
- Persistent effusion may indicate intra-articular pathology that should be evaluated with magnetic resonance imaging.
- Beware of physeal injuries in the skeletally immature patient that may present like ligamentous injuries.

Patient Instructions

- Wear brace during weight-bearing activities until physical examination reveals pain-free motion and ambulation
- Avoid heat (use ice instead) in the acute phase of injury.

Considerations in Special Populations

- Patients with preexisting arthritis will have a higher risk of stiffness and may require formal physical therapy.
- Obtain stress radiographs in skeletally immature patients to rule out physeal injuries.
- Contact sport athletes may need a brace to return to play.

Suggested Reading

- Ellsasser JC, Reynolds FC, Omohundro JR: The non-operative treatment of collateral ligament injuries of the knee in professional football players. An analysis of seventy-four injuries treated non-operatively and twenty-four injuries treated surgically. J Bone Joint Surg Am 1974;56A:365–368.
- Hughston JC, Andrews JR, Cross MJ, et al: Classification of knee ligament instabilities. Part I. The medial compartment and cruciate ligaments. J Bone Joint Surg Am 1976;58A:159–172.
- Indelicato PA: Isolated medial collateral ligament injuries in the knee. J Am Acad Orthop Surg 1995;3:9–14.
- Indelicato PA, Linton RC: Medial ligament injuries in the adult. In DeLee JC, Drez D Jr, Miller MD (eds): DeLee and Drez's Orthopaedic Sports Medicine, 2nd ed. Philadelphia: WB Saunders, 2002, pp 1937–1949.

- LaPrade RF, Hauge Engebretsen A, Ly TV, et al: The anatomy of the medial part of the knee. J Bone Joint Surg Am 2007;89A:2000–2010.
- Quarles JD, Hosey RG: Medial and lateral collateral injuries: Prognosis and treatment. Prim Care 2004;31:957–975.
- Reider B, Sathy MR, Talkington J, et al: Treatment of isolated medial collateral ligament injuries in athletes with early functional rehabilitation. A five-year follow-up study. Am J Sports Med 1994;22:470–477.
- Sims WF, Jacobson KE: The posteromedial corner of the knee: Medial sided injury patterns revisited. Am J Sports Med 2004;32:337–345.
- Steadman JR: Rehabilitation of first- and second-degree sprains of the medial collateral ligament. Am J Sports Med 1979;7:300–302.
- Woo SLY, Vogrin TM, Abramowitch SD: Healing and repair of ligament injuries in the knee. J Am Acad Orthop Surg 2000;8:364–372.

Chapter 145 Lateral Collateral Ligament and Posterolateral Corner Injury

Joy L. Long and Bruce S. Miller

ICD-9 CODES
844.0 *Lateral Collateral Ligament Sprain*
717.81 *Chronic Lateral Collateral Ligament Tear*

Key Concepts

- The lateral collateral ligament (LCL), also known as the fibular collateral ligament, is the primary restraint to varus stress on the knee (see Figure 145-1 for anatomy).
- LCL sprains are classified as acute or chronic and graded as grade I (mild partial tear), II (moderate partial tear), and III (complete tear).
- The posterolateral corner (PLC) is a complex of ligamentous structures posterior to the LCL that resist external rotation of the knee.
- The PLC is rarely injured in isolation. Suspect concomitant cruciate and/or LCL injury in these patients.

History

- Acute injury
  - Varus force (inward bending), contact (hit from the inside) or noncontact
  - Lateral knee pain
  - Feeling of instability
  - May be able to walk
- Chronic injury
  - Medial and/or lateral knee pain
  - Feeling of instability, especially near extension and with cutting and stair climbing
  - Possible effusion, worsened with activities

Physical Examination

- Observation
  - Abrasions/contusions from medial force
  - Deformity
  - Swelling
  - Gait analysis: varus thrust may be present
  - Alignment: genu varum may be apparent
- Palpation
  - Effusion (should be mild; if large, consider intra-articular pathology)
  - Lateral tenderness
- Range of motion
  - Flexion/extension: swelling may limit extremes of motion
  - Locked knee, lacks full extension: likely bucket handle meniscal tear

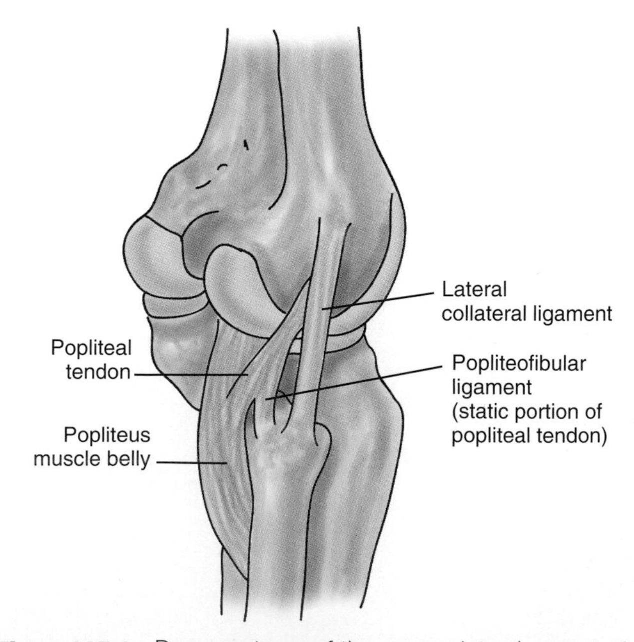

Figure 145-1 Deep anatomy of the posterolateral aspect of the knee. (Adapted from Larson RV, Tingstad E: Lateral and posterolateral instability of the knee in adults. In DeLee JC, Drez D Jr, Miller M [eds]: DeLee and Drez's Orthopaedic Sports Medicine, 2nd ed. Philadelphia: WB Saunders, 2002, pp 1968–1994, Fig. 28I1-5.)

- Special tests
  - Neurovascular examination
    - — Check for peroneal nerve injury (may be acute or chronic)
    - — Footdrop/weak dorsiflexion
    - — Variable sensory changes
    - — Tinel's sign at fibular neck
    - — Distal pulses
  - Knee ligaments and menisci examination
    - — LCL: varus stress in 30 degrees of flexion; if laxity in full extension, grade III LCL with or without concomitant cruciate injury (Fig. 145-2)
    - — PLC: dial test with increased external rotation at 30 degrees of flexion; if increased at 30 and 90 degrees of flexion, combined PLC/posterior cruciate ligament (PCL) injury (Fig. 145-3)
    - — Reverse pivot shift: valgus stress as knee is taken from 90 degrees of flexion to full extension with the foot externally rotated; a positive shift may indicate posterolateral rotatory instability (usually from PCL and PLC injury), but may also occur in normal patients
    - — Anterior cruciate ligament/PCL: Lachman's posterior drawer test

Figure 145-2 Perform the varus stress test at both 30 degrees and 0 degrees of flexion. The examiner is pushing the leg toward midline while stabilizing the femur with his other hand. By keeping his fingers along the joint line, the examiner can estimate laxity and ensure that he is assessing laxity rather than rotation.

Imaging

- Radiographs
  - Anteroposterior and lateral views: check for avulsion of fibular head
  - Posteroanterior flexion weight-bearing view: degenerative changes, particularly in the lateral compartment
  - Patellofemoral views: degenerative changes
- Magnetic resonance imaging
  - Highly recommended
  - Disruption of LCL seen on coronal views (Fig. 145-4)
  - PLC more difficult to image, but also usually seen on coronal views

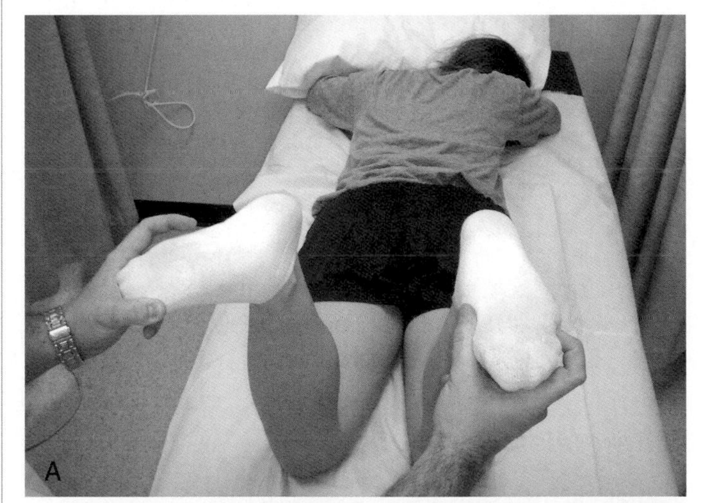

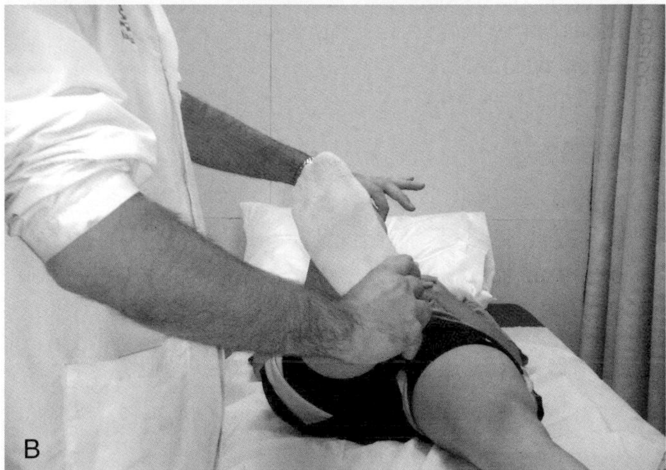

Figure 145-3 The dial test can be performed prone (**A**) or supine (**B**). Increased external rotation of the affected side at 30 degrees of knee flexion indicates posterolateral corner injury. Increased external rotation at 90 degrees indicates posterolateral corner and posterior cruciate ligament injury.

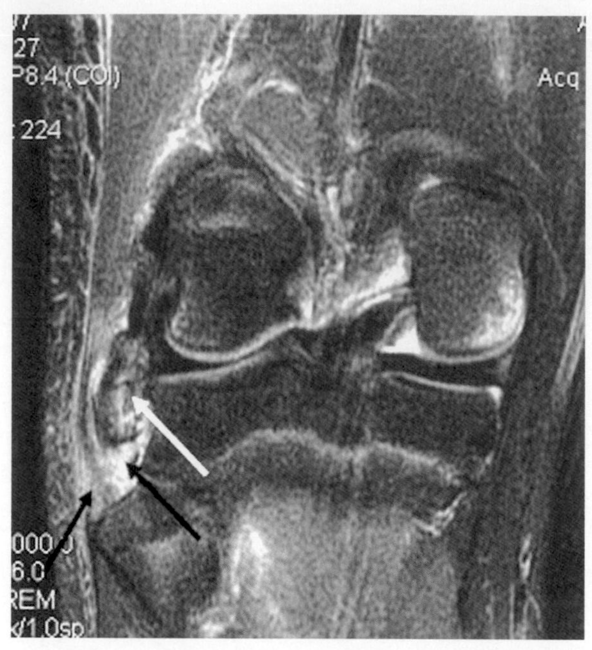

Figure 145-4 A completely torn lateral collateral ligament is seen on the coronal cuts of a magnetic resonance image (*white arrow*). The biceps femoris muscle (*black arrows*) is also injured. (From Beall DP, Googe JD, Moss JT, et al: Magnetic resonance imaging of the collateral ligaments and the anatomic quadrants of the knee. Radiol Clin N Am 2007;45:983–1002, Fig. 19.)

- Look for bone bruising in the medial femoral condyle and medial tibial plateau.
- Evaluate all knee ligaments for potential injury.

Differential Diagnosis

- Lateral meniscus tear
- Multiligamentous knee injury
- Knee dislocation

Treatment

- Acute
  - Rest, ice, compression, and elevation
  - Knee immobilization in extension or slight flexion
  - Toe touch or partial weight bearing for 2 to 4 weeks, followed by progressive rehabilitation for grade I and II injuries
  - Grade III injuries frequently require surgical intervention.
  - Surgery can often consist of repair rather than reconstruction if performed within 3 weeks.
- Chronic
  - Surgical reconstruction may be necessary.
  - A trial of bracing is reasonable.
  - Osteotomies may be necessary when malalignment is present.

When to Refer

- Grade III injuries should be referred right away because repair can only be performed within 3 weeks. In more chronic cases, reconstructive procedures are necessary.
- Vascular compromise is a true emergency.
- Peroneal nerve involvement
- Combined ligamentous injuries
- Locked knee/meniscal tear
- Chronically unstable knee
- Patients with varus alignment
- Avulsion fractures may be amenable to reduction and fixation and should be referred.

Prognosis

- Depends on the extent of the injury
- Isolated grade I or II injuries are likely to heal with nonoperative treatment.
- Complete LCL ruptures or combined ligament injuries often require surgical intervention. If untreated, these injuries can lead to chronic instability.
- The increase in risk of osteoarthritis after these injuries is unknown.

Troubleshooting

- The presence of degenerative changes or malalignment may complicate recovery.
- These injuries can become chronically disabling if not addressed appropriately.
- Beware of physeal injuries in the skeletally immature patient that may present like ligamentous injuries.

Patient Instructions

- Avoid heat (use ice instead) in the acute phase.
- Wear brace during weight-bearing activities for 2 to 4 weeks
- Report any episodes of giving way or instability.
- Seek medical attention for signs of deep venous thrombosis or vascular compromise.

Considerations in Special Populations

- High-level athletes may warrant referral to determine return to sporting activities.

- Patients with preexisting arthritis will likely have a higher risk of stiffness with immobilization. Be certain to prescribe physical therapy to maintain/regain motion in these patients.
- Obtain stress radiographs in the skeletally immature to rule out physeal fractures.
- Have a high index of suspicion for multiligamentous injury in high-energy trauma. Ensure that these patients have a normal vascular examination.

Suggested Reading

- Beall DP, Googe JD, Moss JT, et al: Magnetic resonance imaging of the collateral ligaments and the anatomic quadrants of the knee. Radiol Clin N Am 2007;45:983–1002.
- Chen FS, Rokito AS, Pitman MI: Acute and chronic posterolateral rotatory instability of the knee. J Am Acad Orthop Surg 2000;8:97–110.
- Cooper DE: Tests for posterolateral instability of the knee in normal subjects: Results of examination under anesthesia. J Bone Joint Surg Am 1991;73A:30–36.
- Hughston JC, Andrews JR, Cross MJ, Moschi A: Classification of knee ligament instabilities. Part II: The lateral compartment. J Bone Joint Surg Am 1976;58A:173–179.
- Kannus P: Nonoperative treatment of grade II and III sprains of the lateral ligament compartment of the knee. Am J Sports Med 1989;17:83–88.
- LaPrade RF, Terry GC: Injuries to the posterolateral aspect of the knee: Association of anatomic injury patterns with clinical instability. Am J Sports Med 1997;25:433–438.
- LaPrade RF, Wentorf F: Diagnosis and treatment of posterolateral knee injuries. Clin Orthop Relat Res 2002;402:110–121.
- Larson RV, Tingstad E: Lateral and posterolateral instability of the knee in adults. In DeLee JC, Drez D Jr, Miller M (eds): DeLee and Drez's Orthopaedic Sports Medicine: Principles and Practice, Vol. 2, 2nd ed. Philadelphia: WB Saunders, 2002, pp 1968–1994.
- Quarles JD, Hosey RG: Medial and lateral collateral injuries: Prognosis and treatment. Prim Care 2004;31:957–975.
- Veltri DM, Warren RF: Anatomy, biomechanics, and physical findings in posterolateral knee instability. Clin Sports Med 1994;13:599–614.

Chapter 146 Knee Dislocation

Michael J. Salata, Edward M. Wojtys, and Jon K. Sekiya

ICD-9 CODES
836.0 *Acute Knee Dislocation*
718.36 *Chronic Knee Dislocation*

Key Concepts

- Acute knee dislocations are a potentially limb-threatening emergency.
- Rare, accounting for less than 0.2% of all orthopaedic injuries
- Associated with vascular and neurologic injuries that can be devastating
  - The popliteal artery is tethered proximally by the adductor hiatus and distally by the soleus arch, making it at risk of injury.
- Multiligament knee injuries, involving three or more ligaments or a bicruciate injury, should be considered a spontaneously reduced knee dislocation (Figs. 146-1 and 146-2).
- Classified by involved structures, duration, or direction; anterior most common (40% knee hyperextension) followed by posterior (33% dashboard injury)
- Usually the result of high-energy trauma (e.g., motor vehicle accident, industrial accident)
- Can occur in sporting events (lower energy)
- Can occur with minimal trauma in obese patients (stepping off a curb)
- Extensor mechanism injury (quadriceps or patellar tendon) and patellar dislocation are also encountered in this injury pattern.

History

- Acute injury (<3 weeks)
  - Large effusion
  - Extreme pain
  - Obvious deformity
  - Determine time from injury.
- Chronic injury (>3 weeks)
  - Anterior or medial knee pain
  - Feeling of instability, especially with twisting and impact activities
  - Mild effusion, worsened with activities

Physical Examination

- Observation
  - Effusion
  - Bruising or abrasions
  - Deformity
- Special tests
  - Compartment syndrome evaluation
    - Unrelenting pain, pain with passive motion, tense compartments
    - Monitor compartment pressures if examination is equivocal (see Chapter 171).
    - Emergent surgical fasciotomies if high clinical suspicion or positive compartment pressures
  - Vascular examination (critical)
    - Serial examinations *mandatory* in the acute setting
    - Five percent to 45% incidence of popliteal artery injury; overall approximately 19%
    - Very low energy (obese) > high-energy motor vehicle accident > low energy (sports)
    - Delay of 6 to 8 hours of unrecognized arterial injury associated with high amputation rate
    - If symmetrical pulses on examination and ankle/brachial index more than 0.9 of contralateral side, arteriogram may not be needed; ankle/brachial indices less than 0.9 should have arteriogram
    - Arteriogram with venous runoff may also identify unrecognized intimal injury.
    - Prompt vascular surgery consultation should be obtained in the acute setting.

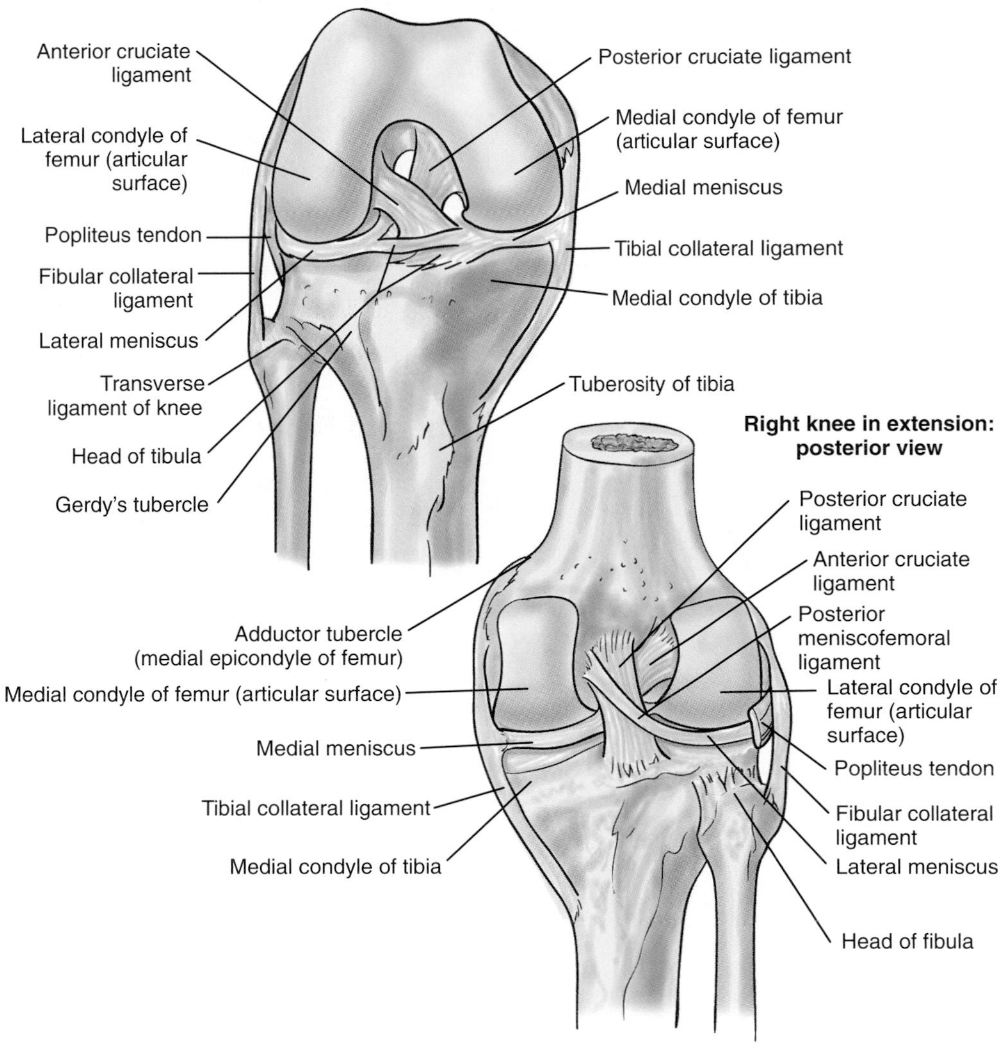

Right knee in flexion: anterior view

Anterior cruciate ligament
Lateral condyle of femur (articular surface)
Popliteus tendon
Fibular collateral ligament
Lateral meniscus
Transverse ligament of knee
Head of tibula
Gerdy's tubercle
Posterior cruciate ligament
Medial condyle of femur (articular surface)
Medial meniscus
Tibial collateral ligament
Medial condyle of tibia
Tuberosity of tibia

Right knee in extension: posterior view

Adductor tubercle (medial epicondyle of femur)
Medial condyle of femur (articular surface)
Medial meniscus
Tibial collateral ligament
Medial condyle of tibia
Posterior cruciate ligament
Anterior cruciate ligament
Posterior meniscofemoral ligament
Lateral condyle of femur (articular surface)
Popliteus tendon
Fibular collateral ligament
Lateral meniscus
Head of fibula

Figure 146-1 Anatomy of the cruciate and collateral knee ligaments.

- Neurologic examination (critical)
  - Sixteen percent to 40% incidence of nerve injury; overall approximately 20%
  - Most common after posterolateral dislocations
  - Peroneal nerve more commonly injured than tibial nerve
  - Even if the nerve is in continuity, function returns in only approximately 20% of patients.
- Knee ligaments: Lachman's test (anterior cruciate ligament), posterior drawer test (posterior cruciate ligament), varus/valgus stress test (lateral collateral ligament/medial collateral ligament), external rotation asymmetry test (posterolateral corner)

Imaging

- Radiographs: anteroposterior and lateral views of the knee
  - Used to evaluate direction of dislocation to aid in reduction
  - Look for posterior cruciate ligament avulsion fragment, Segond fragment, associated tibial plateau or distal femur fracture, fibular head avulsion fracture, and osteochondral injuries.
- Magnetic resonance imaging (Fig. 146-3)
  - Useful for preoperative planning
  - Not needed in the emergent setting, but should be obtained urgently

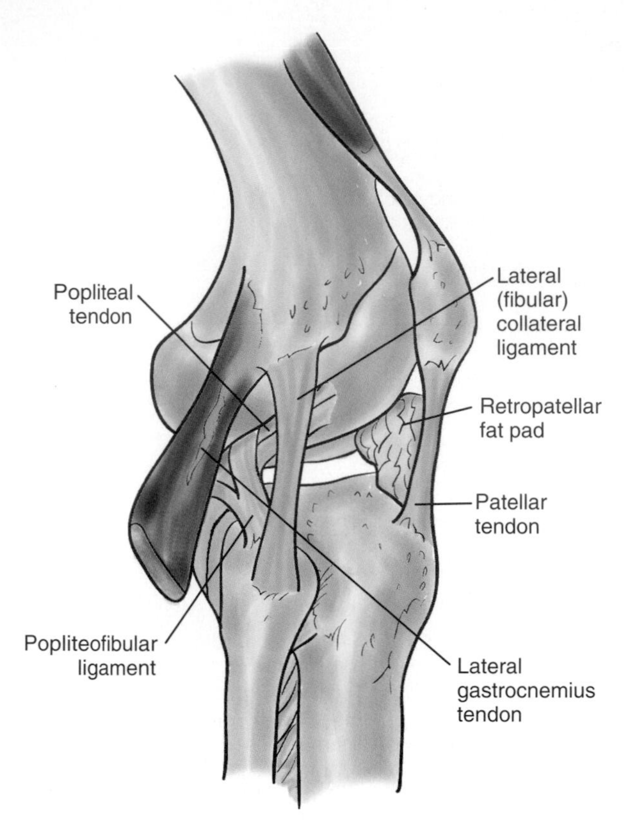

Figure 146-2 Anatomy of the posterolateral corner.

Differential Diagnosis

- Isolated cruciate ligament injury
- Distal femur or proximal tibia fracture

Treatment

- At diagnosis (acute injuries)
  - Reduction should always be attempted immediately and the patient transferred to an emergency department setting for workup.
  - Once reduced with good vascular examination, a long leg splint or knee immobilizer should be applied.
  - Ensure reduction is maintained with radiographs.
    - — Irreducible dislocations and those in which the vascular examination does not improve should be considered for emergent surgery.
    - — Nonsurgical management is often associated with dismal outcomes.
    - — Controversy exists about the timing of reconstruction.
    - — Unless contraindicated, delaying surgery for 1 to 2 weeks can help reduce the risk of postoperative stiffness, can allow the joint capsule to heal if surgery is to be performed arthroscopically assisted, and can reduce swelling and inflammation.
    - — Further delay may make surgery more difficult because of scarring, particularly if the posterolateral corner is involved.
    - — There is no consensus as to whether to perform acute or delayed multiligament knee reconstruction when surgery is elected.
- Later (chronic injuries)
  - Direct repair of the posterolateral structures difficult or impossible
  - Some authors believe that delay of reconstruction allows return of quadriceps strength and optimization of range of motion.

When to Refer

- Patients with acute knee dislocations should be sent to the emergency department and an orthopaedic surgeon notified.
- Stabilized acute and chronic injuries should be referred to an orthopaedic surgeon for reconstruction options (Fig. 146-4).
- Patients with associated arterial injuries should be promptly referred to a vascular surgeon.
- Patients with nerve injuries should be referred to an orthopaedic surgeon for potential tendon transfers in a delayed fashion.

Prognosis

- Devastating injury that usually precludes a normal knee
- Surgery can improve outcomes in terms of stability and function to a moderate degree.

Troubleshooting

- Potential limb-threatening injury should be treated in a time-sensitive manner.
- Clinical suspicion must be high for an occult knee dislocation when three or more ligaments are injured.

Patient Instructions

- Patients should be counseled early that a return to normal of the injured knee is unlikely.
- Expected outcomes postsurgically include improved stability.
- Overall risk of posttraumatic arthritis can be approximately 50% in the long term.
- Nerve injuries, even if intact, are likely to leave residual deficits.

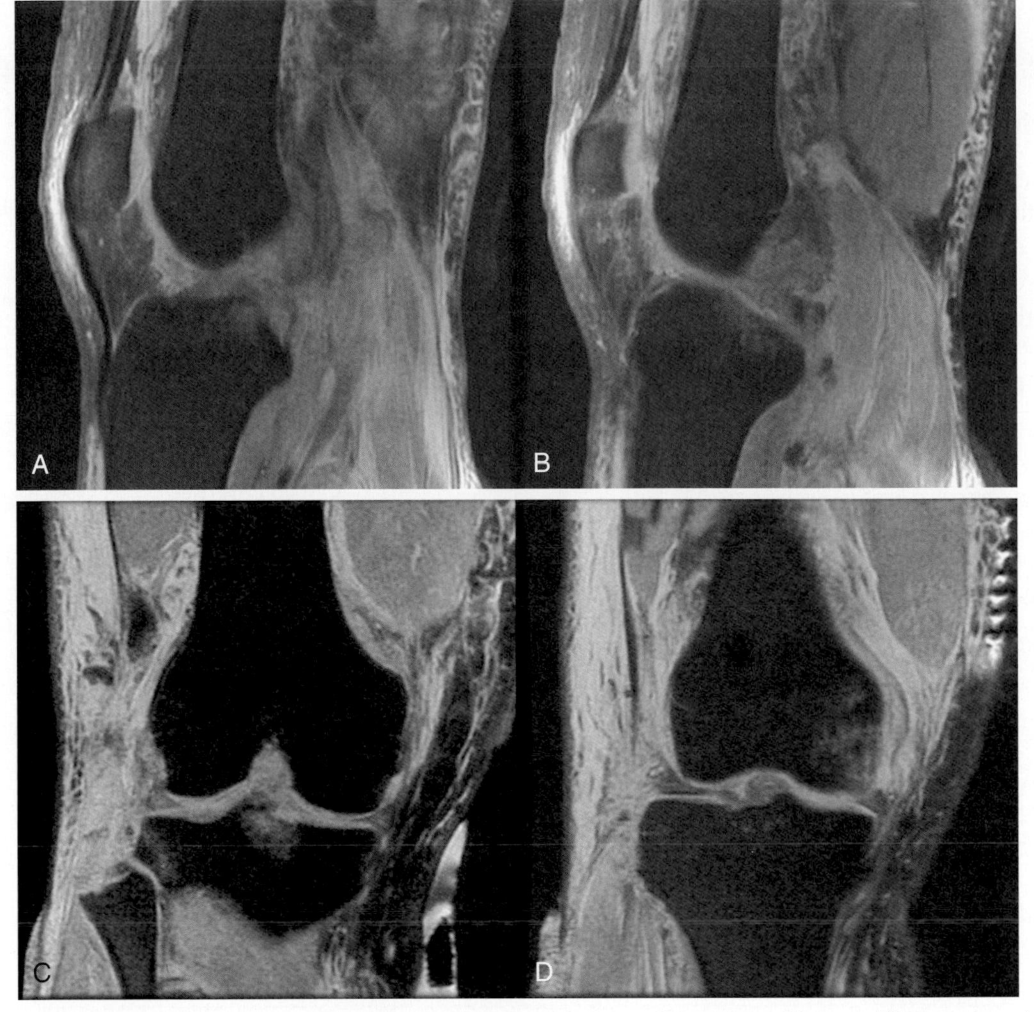

Figure 146-3 Magnetic resonance imaging of a patient after traumatic knee dislocation with a multiligamentous knee injury. **A**, Anterior cruciate ligament disruption. **B**, Posterior cruciate ligament disruption. **C**, Lateral collateral ligament and posterolateral corner ligament disruptions. **D**, Medial collateral ligament disruption.

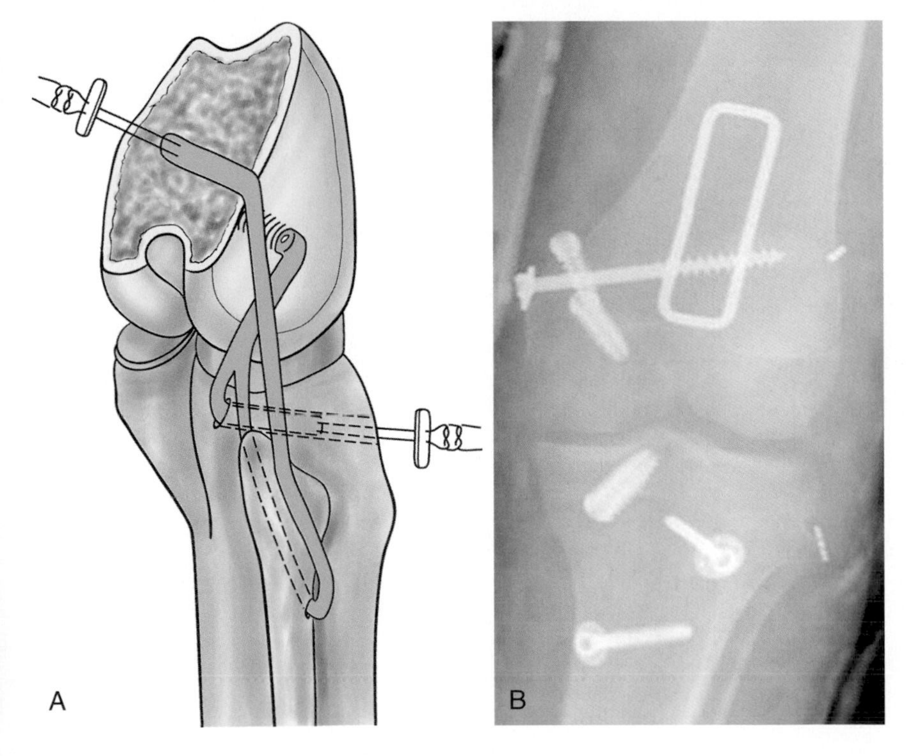

Figure 146-4 **A**, Reconstruction of the posterolateral corner. **B**, Postoperative radiograph after anterior cruciate ligament, posterior collateral ligament, lateral collateral ligament, and medial collateral ligament reconstruction.

Considerations in Special Populations

- Closed reduction and cast immobilization is indicated only for patients who are elderly or sedentary or have debilitating medical or posttraumatic comorbidities.
- Surgery in obese patients is very challenging, but if their comorbidities permit, it should be attempted.

Suggested Reading

- Chapman JA: Popliteal artery damage in closed injuries of the knee. J Bone Joint Surg Br 1985;67:420–423.
- Fanelli GC: The dislocated knee. J Knee Surg 2005;18:212–248.
- Green NE, Allen BL: Vascular injuries associated with dislocation of the knee. J Bone Joint Surg Am 1977;59A:236–239.
- Harner CD, Waltrip RL, Bennett CH, et al: Surgical management of knee dislocations. J Bone Joint Surg Am 2004;86A:262–273.
- McCoy GF, Hannon DG, Barr RJ, et al: Vascular injury associated with low-velocity dislocations of the knee. J Bone Joint Surg Br 1987;69B:285–287.
- Mills WJ, Barei DP, McNair P: The value of the ankle-brachial index for diagnosing arterial injury after knee dislocation: A prospective study. J Trauma 2004;6:1261–1265.
- Quinlan AG: Irreducible posterolateral dislocation of the knee with buttonholing of the medial femoral condyle. J Bone Joint Surg Am 1966;48A:1619–1621.
- Rinh JA, Cha PS, Groff YJ, et al: The acutely dislocated knee: Evaluation and management. J Am Acad Orthop Surg 2004;12:334–346.
- Robertson A, Nutton RW, Keating JF: Dislocation of the knee. J Bone Joint Surg Br 2006;88B:706–711.
- Shelbourne KD, Porter DA, Clingman JA, et al: Low velocity knee dislocation. Orthop Rev 1991;20:995–1004.

Chapter 147 Synovitis

Eric J. Gardner and Geoffrey S. Baer

ICD-9 CODES
727.00 *Synovitis*
719.20 *Proliferative Villonodular Synovitis*

Key Concepts

- Synovitis is inflammation of the synovial membrane or synovium.
- Nonspecific proliferative lesion
- Synovium lines the cavities of all synovial joints.
  - Composed of fibrous and vascular connective tissue
  - Produces synovial fluid that is a combination of fluid produced by the synovium and an ultrafiltrate of blood plasma
- Synovial fluid lubricates the joint and provides nutrients for the articular cartilage.
- Contains hyaluronic acid, proteinase, lubricin (glycoprotein and key lubricating component), prostaglandins, and collagenases
- Void of red blood cells, hemoglobin, and clotting factors

History

- Isolated to a single joint or involving multiple joints
- Acute injury
  - Jarring or twisting of joint
  - Pain and swelling
  - Knee ligaments stable
- Chronic injury (degenerative changes)
- Knee pain with or without swelling; worse with activity and at night

Physical Examination

- Observation
  - Effusion (intra-articular swelling)
  - Erythema (increased blood flow)
  - Quadriceps atrophy
  - Antalgic gait
- Palpation
  - Effusion/patellar ballottement (intra-articular swelling)
  - Nonspecific soft-tissue tenderness
  - Warmth (increased blood flow)
- Range of motion
  - Often decreased
    - — Painful due to inflamed synovium, distended joint
    - — Effusion may prevent full range of motion.
    - — Chronic underlying articular involvement may restrict range of motion due to degenerative changes (i.e., rheumatoid arthritis, osteoarthritis).
- Special tests
  - Crepitus with range of motion: degenerative changes
  - Joint line tenderness: meniscal tears or degenerative changes
  - McMurray's test: meniscal tears
  - Lachman's test, anterior/posterior drawer test, pivot shift test, reverse pivot shift test, dial test, varus/valgus stress test: ligamentous instability; may be associated with the synovitic process

Imaging

- Radiographs: bilateral weight bearing posteroanterior, 45 degrees of flexion posteroanterior (Rosenberg view), lateral, and 20 degrees of flexion patellofemoral view (Laurin view).
  - Typically normal, but may show soft-tissue swelling and effusion
- Magnetic resonance imaging
  - If clinical and laboratory studies are inconclusive for septic arthritis, magnetic resonance imaging can be used as a confirmatory test.
  - Pigmented villonodular synovitis can often be diagnosed based on the magnetic resonance imaging appearance (Fig. 147-1).
  - Allows better characterization of soft tissues and/or evaluation of soft-tissue mass (Fig. 147-2)

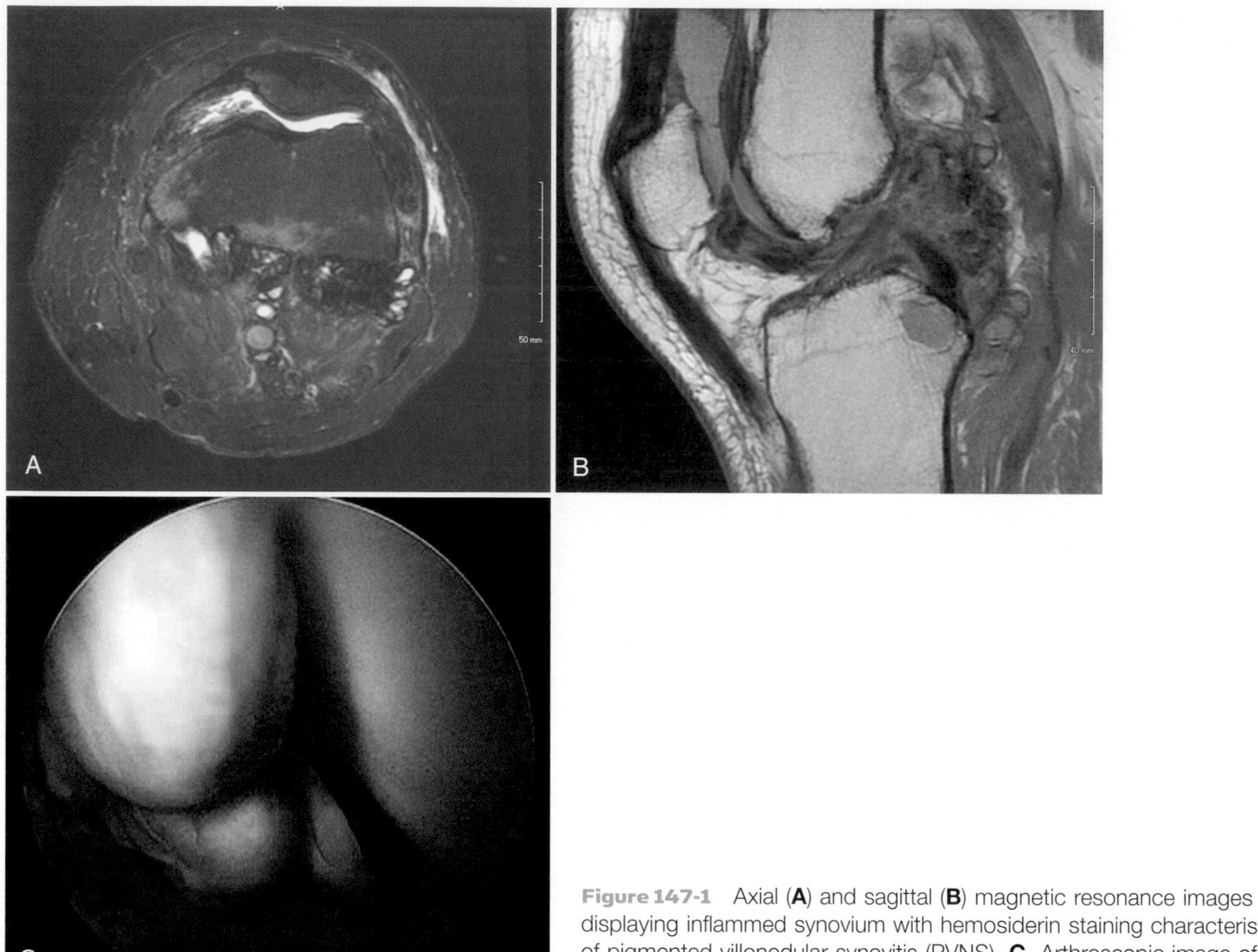

Figure 147-1 Axial (**A**) and sagittal (**B**) magnetic resonance images displaying inflammed synovium with hemosiderin staining characteristic of pigmented villonodular synovitis (PVNS). **C**, Arthroscopic image of a 51-year-old patient with diffuse PVNS.

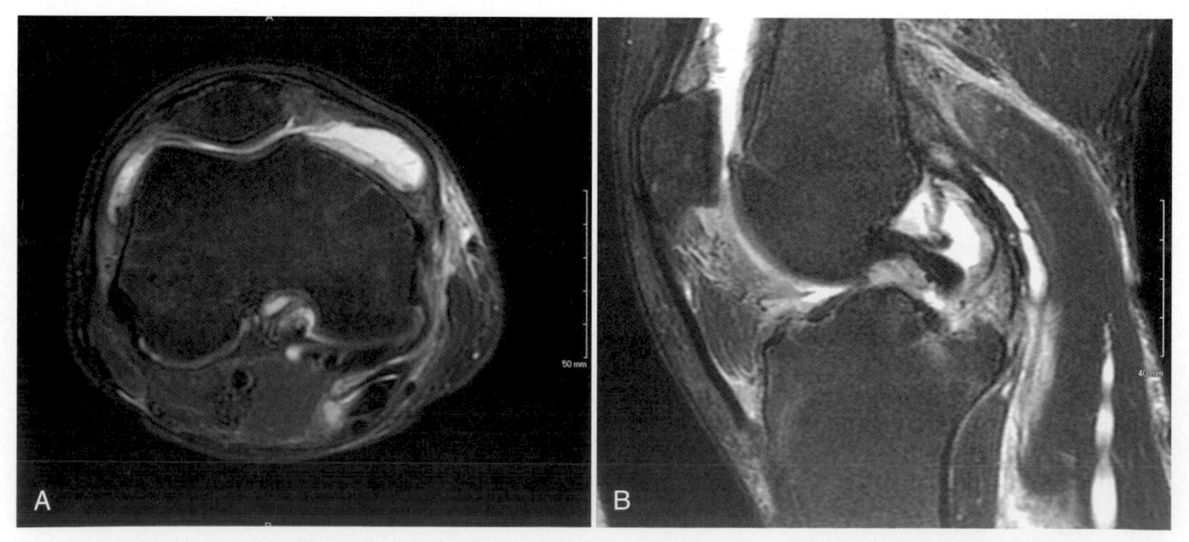

Figure 147-2 Axial (**A**) and sagittal (**B**) magnetic resonance images showing synovitis associated with gout in a 46-year-old patient.

- Bone scan
  - May identify other areas of involvement

Additional Tests

- Blood tests: complete blood count, erythrocyte sedimentation rate, C-reactive protein, serologic tests (i.e., rheumatoid factor)
- Aspiration: cell count, crystals, culture, and sensitivities

Differential Diagnosis

- Inflammatory arthritides: rheumatoid arthritis, juvenile rheumatoid arthritis, systemic lupus erythematosus, psoriatic arthritis, gout, pseudogout
- Infectious arthritides: septic arthritis, tuberculous arthritis, fungal arthritis, Lyme disease
- Noninflammatory arthritides: osteoarthritis, neuropathic joint
- Hemorrhagic arthritides: hemophilic arthropathy, sickle cell joint destruction, pigmented villonodular synovitis
- Others: toxic/transient synovitis, traumatic synovitis

Treatment

- At diagnosis
  - Rest, ice, compression, and elevation help decrease swelling and pain; acetaminophen and nonsteroidal anti-inflammatory drugs for pain control
- Later
  - Depending on the underlying cause of the synovitis, intra-articular corticosteroid, hyaluronic injections, or synovectomy may help treat symptoms. Most inflammatory and noninflammatory arthritides can be treated conservatively.

When to Refer

- Soft-tissue infections can be diagnosed and treated without surgical consultation. When intra-articular infection is determined to be present, urgent surgical evaluation is required. Some causes of synovitis, such as gout and hemophilic arthropathy, are amenable to synovectomy after exhaustion of conservative means (Figs. 147-3 and 147-4).
- Recurrence of synovitis after synovectomy is common.
- Patients with degenerative joint changes predisposing them to joint pain that interferes with quality of life can be sent for evaluation for total knee arthroplasty.
- Patients with pigmented villonodular synovitis should be seen for potential open versus arthroscopic synovectomy.
- Otherwise, most other patients can be treated effectively with conservative measures by primary care physicians, rheumatologists, or infectious disease doctors.

Prognosis

- The prognosis depends on the underlying etiology. Most causes of synovitis have excellent prognoses when the underlying cause is treated. The prognosis of joint infections depends on timely surgical evaluation, irrigation and débridement, and appropriate antibiotic therapy.

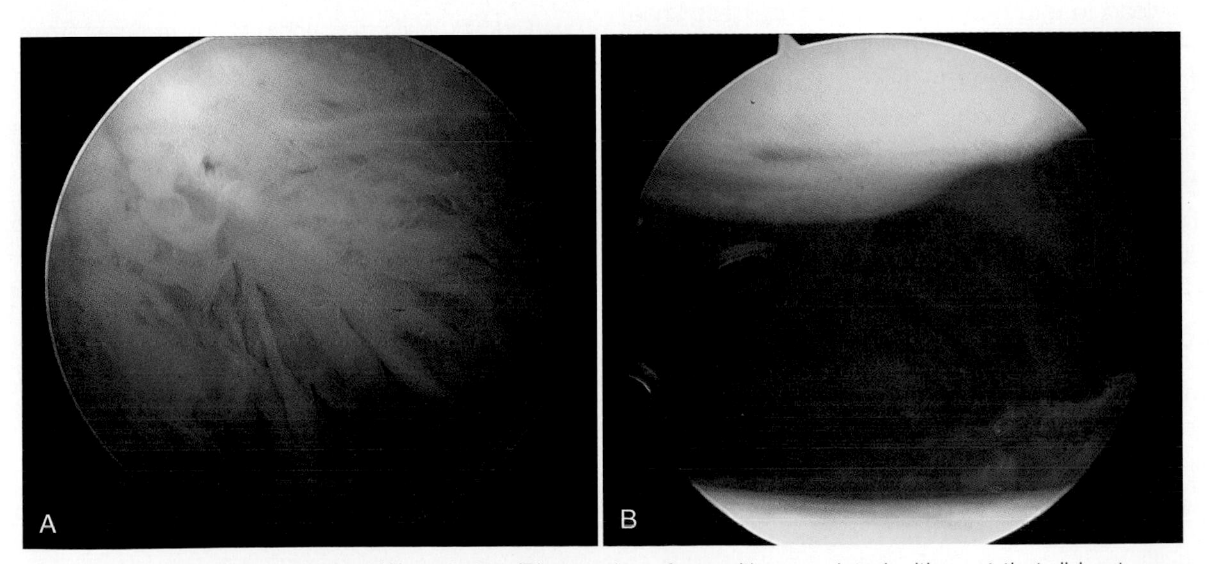

Figure 147-3 Arthroscopic images before (**A**) and after (**B**) resection of synovitis associated with gout that did not respond to conservative management.

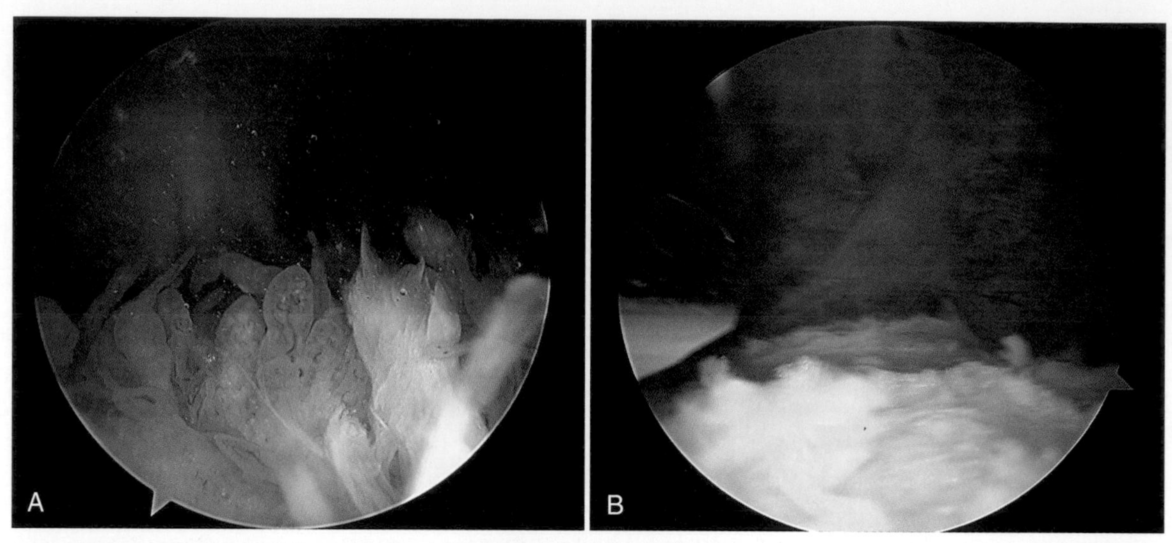

Figure 147-4 Arthroscopic images before (**A**) and after (**B**) resection of synovitis associated with advanced degenerative joint disease in a patient not interested in pursuing joint replacement.

Troubleshooting

- Aspiration should be performed in patients when there is concern for a septic joint.
  - The presence of purulent fluid, a positive Gram stain or cultures, or an elevated cell count suggestive of a septic joint are orthopaedic emergencies and demand immediate referral.

Patient Instructions

- The patient should be counseled on the risks and benefits of surgery to treat the underlying cause of synovitis.
  - Benefits: Treating the underlying cause of synovitis will lead to return of a nonswollen, painless knee.
  - Risks: Surgical management with arthroscopy or total knee arthroplasty risks bleeding, infection, nerve damage, and, of course, incomplete resolution of symptoms. Total knee arthroplasty adds the risks of prosthetic failure, deep venous thrombosis, pulmonary embolus, risks of anesthesia, and even death.

Considerations in Special Populations

- Young, highly active patients are not good candidates for total knee arthroplasty due to increased prosthetic wear and consequently early prosthetic failure.

Suggested Reading

- Carl HD, Klug S, Seitz J, et al: Site-specific intraoperative efficacy of arthroscopic knee joint synovectomy in rheumatoid arthritis. Arthroscopy 2005;21:1209–1218.
- Comin JA, Rodriguez-Merchan EC: Arthroscopic synovectomy in the management of painful localized post-traumatic synovitis of the knee joint. Arthroscopy 1997;13:606–608.
- De Ponti A, Sansone V, Malchere M: Results of arthroscopic treatment of pigmented villonodular synovitis of the knee. Arthroscopy 2003;19:602–607.
- Dines JS, DeBerardino TM, Wells JS, et al: Long-term follow-up of surgically treated localized pigmented villonodular synovitis of the knee. Arthroscopy 2007;23:930–937.
- Fiacco U, Cozzi L, Rigon C, et al: Arthroscopic synovectomy in rheumatoid and psoriatic knee joint synovitis: Long-term outcome. Br J Rheumatol 1996;35:463–470.
- Frick MA, Wenger DE, Adkins M: MR imaging of synovial disorders of the knee: An update. Radiol Clin North Am 2007;45:1017–1031.
- Gilbert MS, Radomisli TE: Therapeutic options in the management of hemophilic synovitis. Clin Orthop Relat Res 1997;343:88–92.
- Klug S, Wittmann G, Weseloh G: Arthroscopic synovectomy of the knee joint in early cases of rheumatoid arthritis: Follow-up results of a multicenter study. Arthroscopy 2000;16:262–267.
- Li TJ, Lue KH, Lin ZI, et al: Arthroscopic treatment for gouty tophi mimicking an intra-articular synovial tumor of the knee. Arthroscopy 2006;22:910.e1–910.e3.
- Wiedel JD: Arthroscopic synovectomy of the knee in hemophilia: 10 to 15 year follow-up. Clin Orthop Relat Res 1996;328:46–53.

Chapter 148 Meniscus Tears

David M. Marcu and Geoffrey S. Baer

ICD-9 CODES

717.3	*Old Tear of Medial Meniscus, Unspecified*
717.40	*Old Tear of Lateral Meniscus, Unspecified*
717.9	*Unspecified Internal Derangement of the Knee*
836.0	*Acute Tear of Medial Meniscus of the Knee*
836.1	*Acute Tear of Lateral Meniscus of the Knee*

Key Concepts

- Two C-shaped structures, consisting mainly of fibrocartilage, attached to the joint capsule at the periphery; the anterior and posterior horns of each meniscus also have ligamentous anchors to the tibial plateau
- Limited vascular supply and healing potential: outer third (red-red zone) is vascular, inner third (white-white zone) is avascular, middle third (red-white zone) is intermediate
- Critical for normal knee function: load sharing, shock absorption, stability, and proprioception
- Transmit 50% to 70% of load with knee extension and 85% to 90% with knee flexion
- Removing the entire meniscus causes the overall knee contact area to decrease, resulting in increased contact stress, degenerative joint disease, and pain.
- The medial meniscus is a secondary stabilizer to anterior tibial translation, making it critical for stability in an anterior cruciate ligament (ACL)–deficient knee.
- Meniscus tears can occur as an acute injury or as a result of degenerative joint disease.
- The most common location for a meniscal tear with an acute ACL tear is the lateral meniscus, whereas knees with ACL deficiency often result in medial meniscus injury over time.

History

- Acute injury
  - Twisting or hyperflexion mechanism
  - Acute pain with or without swelling
  - Pain recurs with deep knee bending or twisting.
  - Locking or catching (mechanical symptoms) may be present.
  - Associated injuries include ACL tears and collateral ligament sprains.
- Chronic (degenerative) injury
  - Older patients, associated with degenerative osteoarthritis
  - Atraumatic mechanism, like walking on uneven ground or bending at the knees
  - Chronic mild joint swelling, stiffness, joint line pain
  - Mechanical symptoms may be present.

Physical Examination

- Observation
  - Effusion (intra-articular swelling)
  - Quadriceps atrophy in subacute or chronic tears
  - Antalgic gait
- Palpation
  - Joint line tenderness: most sensitive examination finding (74%)
    - Assess with knee flexed.
    - Assess medial and lateral, anterior and posterior
  - Patellar ballottement (effusion)
- Range of motion
  - Displaced bucket handle tears may cause a block to full extension, a locked knee (Fig. 148-1).
  - Effusions may cause loss of flexion.
- Special tests
  - McMurray's test: flex and rotate the knee; positive if there is a palpable "clunk" at the joint line as the torn meniscus displaces
    - Most specific for meniscal tear (98%), but only 15% sensitive
    - Pain with McMurray's test without palpable clunk is more sensitive and more likely to be elicited, but less specific.

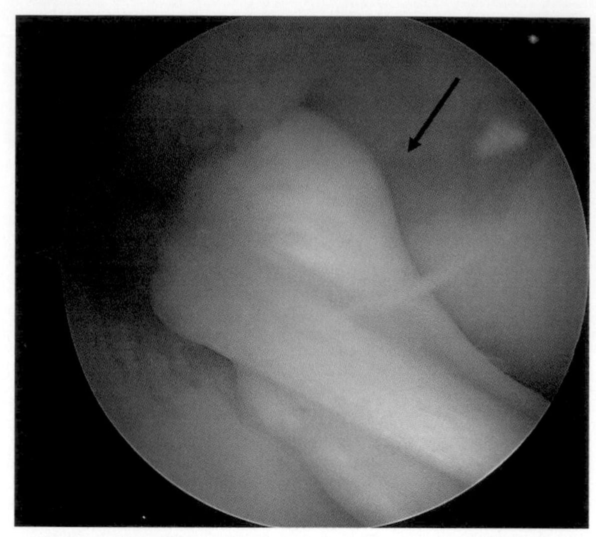

Figure 148-1 Displaced bucket handle tear (*arrow*) of the medial meniscus causing a mechanical block to full extension (locked knee).

- Squat test: posterior knee pain with squatting or inability to squat (anterior knee pain may reflect chondral defect of the patella or trochlea)
- Patellar apprehension test to rule out patellar instability
- Lachman's, anterior/posterior drawer, pivot shift, varus/valgus stress tests to rule out associated ligamentous injuries

Imaging

- Radiography
    - Bilateral weight bearing posteroanterior, lateral, 45 degrees of flexion posteroanterior (Rosenberg view), and 20 degrees of flexion in patellofemoral view (Laurin view)
        - — To rule out osteoarthritis, osteochondral fracture, osseous loose bodies, osteonecrosis of the femoral condyle, osteochondritis dissecans, plateau fracture, tibial eminence fracture, Segond fracture (ACL tear)
        - — Posteroanterior flexion weight-bearing view especially useful to look for osteoarthritis
        - — Laurin view to look for patellofemoral arthritis
- Magnetic resonance imaging
    - Sensitive and specific, accuracy approximately 95%
    - Meniscal tear pattern and displacement can often be determined by magnetic resonance imaging (MRI) (Figs. 148-2 to 148-4).

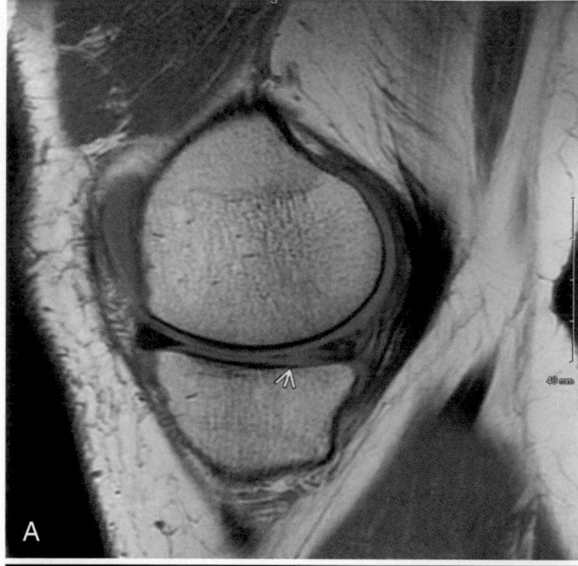

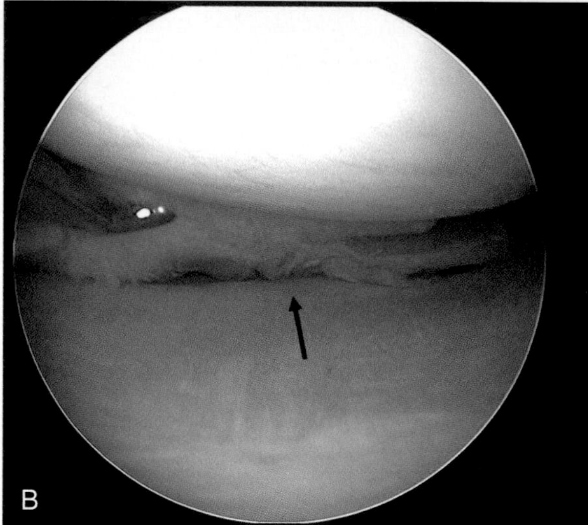

Figure 148-2 Complex tear of the medial meniscus (*arrows*). **A**, Sagittal magnetic resonance imaging. **B**, Arthroscopic view.

- — Vertical tears or displaced bucket handle tears require special attention because these often can be repaired (Fig. 148-5).

Differential Diagnosis

- Osteoarthritis: chronic stiffness, aching, joint space narrowed on radiographs
- Loose body: catching, mobile pain, osseous fragments on radiographs, cartilaginous fragments on MRI
- Patellar subluxation or dislocation: patellar apprehension test, pain at medial patella
- Osteochondritis dissecans: pain to palpation of condyle, seen on radiographs

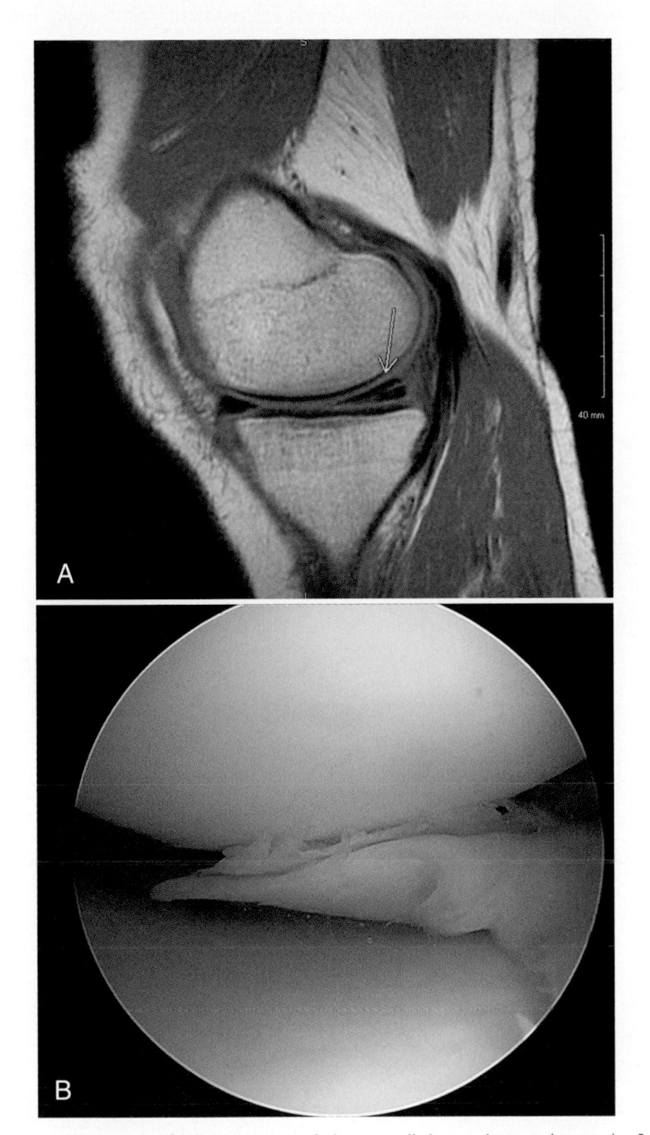

Figure 148-3 Oblique tear of the medial meniscus (*arrow*). **A**, Sagittal magnetic resonance imaging. **B**, Arthroscopic view of displaced fragment.

- Articular cartilage lesions: often associated with meniscal or cruciate injuries, seen on MRI
- Tibial plateau fracture: higher-energy injury, seen on radiographs or computed tomography scans
- ACL tear: positive Lachman's and anterior drawer tests, acute hemarthrosis, seen on MRI
- Collateral ligament sprain or tear: pain or instability to varus stress (lateral collateral ligament) or valgus stress (medial collateral ligament)
- Pes anserine bursitis: pain on medial side distal to the joint line
- Fat pad impingement syndrome: positive Hoffa's test (with knee in flexion, place pressure with thumbs along each side of patellar tendon; pain with knee extension indicates inflammation of the fat pad)

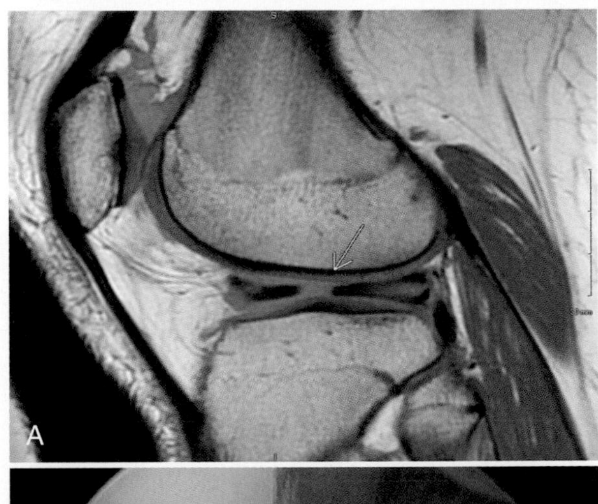

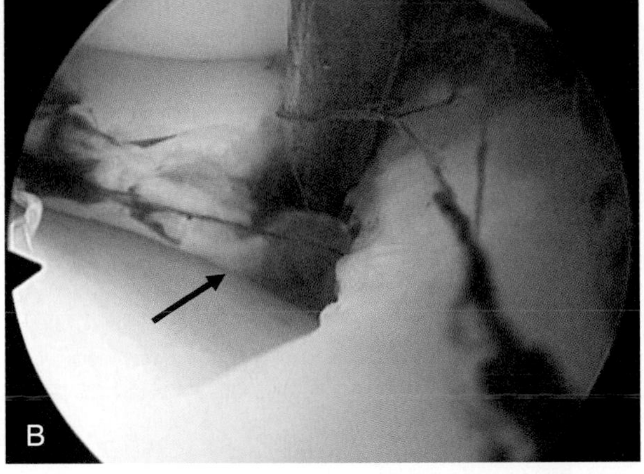

Figure 148-4 Radial tear of the lateral meniscus (*arrows*). **A**, Sagittal magnetic resonance imaging. **B**, Arthroscopic view.

- Symptomatic plica: painful snapping band across medial femoral condyle

Treatment

- At diagnosis
  - Young patients with acute meniscal tears and all patients with a locked knee should be referred to an orthopaedic surgeon. Otherwise, initial treatment is symptomatic.
  - Rest, ice, compression, and elevation are helpful to decrease swelling and pain.
  - Acetaminophen and/or nonsteroidal anti-inflammatory drugs are useful for pain control.
  - Physical therapy focused on restoring range of motion and reducing pain, while maintaining or improving muscle strength around the knee, is beneficial.
- Later
  - Patients with degenerative meniscal tears may require arthroscopic surgery for débridement

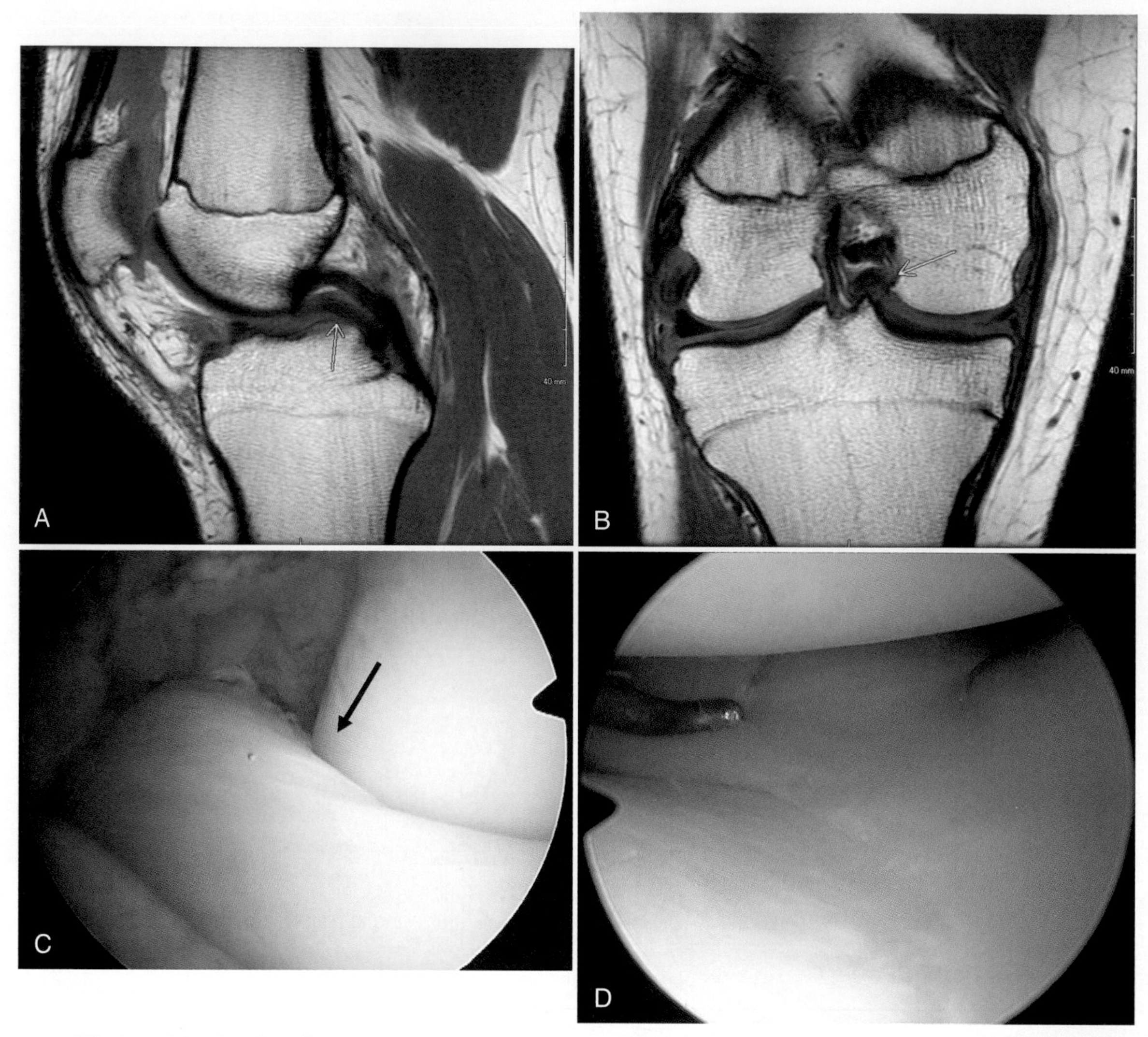

Figure 148-5 Displaced bucket handle tear of the medial meniscus. **A**, Sagittal magnetic resonance imaging (MRI). Note double posterior cruciate ligament sign (*arrow*). **B**, Coronal MRI. Note meniscus displaced into the notch (*arrow*). **C**, Arthroscopic view of displaced meniscus draped over medial femoral condyle (*arrow*). **D**, Arthroscopic view of meniscus after reduction and inside-out meniscal repair.

(partial meniscectomy) if symptoms are not responsive to conservative treatment.

When to Refer

- It is appropriate to refer patients with clinical and MRI evidence of a meniscus tear, particularly those who have pain, swelling, and feelings of apprehension that significantly limit their lives after a diligent trial of conservative treatment.
- The threshold for referral should be lower for acute tears, younger patients, and those with more active lifestyles.
- Patients with vertical tears in the vascular zone of the meniscus should be referred early for meniscal repair (see Fig. 148-5C and D). Note that many asymptomatic tears are picked up on MRI, especially in older individuals with arthritis. MRI findings should be correlated with the history and examination before referral.

Prognosis

- The prognosis of partial meniscectomy is excellent when no concomitant cartilage damage is present.
- The results remain good if associated cartilage lesions are addressed appropriately.
- The prognosis of meniscal repair is also very good, depending on the location and vascularity of the tear, and it improves when repair is performed in conjunction with ACL reconstruction.

Troubleshooting

- Patients with degenerative meniscal tears and arthritic change may benefit from corticosteroid or hyaluronic acid injections. These patients may also continue to have arthritis-related pain after knee arthroscopy.

Patient Instructions

- The patient should be counseled on the benefits and risks of surgery.
  - The benefits include restoration of a smooth range of motion, decrease in pain, and return to sports, exercise, and activities of daily living.
  - The risks are minimal with arthroscopic surgery, but include bleeding, infection, and nerve injury (particularly with inside-out meniscal repairs requiring a separate incision).

Considerations in Special Populations

- Sedentary patients should be given a trial of nonoperative management. However, if symptoms are adversely affecting daily activities, it is reasonable to perform arthroscopy.

Suggested Reading

- Andersson-Molina H, Karlsson H, Rockborn P: Arthroscopic partial and total meniscectomy: A long-term follow-up study with matched controls. Arthroscopy 2002;18:183–189.
- Burks RT, Metcalf MH, Metcalf RW: Fifteen-year follow-up of arthroscopic partial meniscectomy. Arthroscopy 1997;13:673–679.
- Ericsson YB, Roos EM, Dahlberg L: Muscle strength, functional performance, and self-reported outcomes four years after arthroscopic partial meniscectomy in middle-aged patients. Arthritis Rheum 2006;15:946–952.
- Fox MG: MR imaging of the meniscus: Review, current trends, and clinical implications. Radiol Clin North Am 2007;45:1033–1053.
- Hegedus EJ, Cook C, Hasselblad V, et al: Physical examination tests for assessing a torn meniscus in the knee: A systematic review with meta-analysis. J Orthop Sports Phys Ther 2007;37:541–550.
- Higuchi H, Kimura M, Shirakura K, et al: Factors affecting long-term results after arthroscopic partial meniscectomy. Clin Orthop Relat Res 2000;377:161–168.
- Lee SJ, Aadalen KJ, Malaviya P, et al: Tibiofemoral contact mechanics after serial medial meniscectomies in the human cadaveric knee. Am J Sports Med 2006;34:1334–1344.
- Matsusue Y, Thomson NL: Arthroscopic partial medial meniscectomy in patients over 40 years old: A 5- to 11-year follow-up study. Arthroscopy 1996;12:39–44.
- Ryzewicz M, Peterson B, Siparsky PN, et al: The diagnosis of meniscus tears: The role of MRI and clinical examination. Clin Orthop Relat Res 2007;455:123–133.
- Wheatley WB, Krome J, Martin DF: Rehabilitation programs following arthroscopic meniscectomy in athletes. Sports Med 1996;21:447–456.

Chapter 149 Chondral Injuries of the Knee

David M. Marcu and Geoffrey S. Baer

ICD-9 CODES
718.0 *Articular Cartilage Disorder*
719.9 *Derangement, Internal, Knee, Unspecified*
717.6 *Loose Body of the Knee*

Key Concepts

- Chondral lesions can be purely articular cartilage defects or articular cartilage and subchondral bone defects (osteochondral lesions).
- Articular (hyaline) cartilage is uniquely suited for joint functions, such as axial loading and shear forces.
- Articular cartilage is composed mainly of type II collagen and has very limited regenerative potential; it is avascular.
- When a chondral defect is created, that gap does not simply heal and fill in.
- Osteochondral lesions violate the subchondral bone and create a bleeding healing response, causing the lesion to be partially filled with fibrocartilage (mainly type I collagen; poor mechanical properties compared with those of hyaline cartilage).
- Cartilage damage predisposes the joint to further degeneration with time.
- Cartilage defects (chondral lesions) may be asymptomatic and symptoms/signs of chondral lesions overlap with those of other knee conditions (meniscal tears, arthritis, loose bodies).
- Treatment is a spectrum from symptomatic control through cartilage transplantation or regeneration.

History

- Acute injury
    - Athletic injury: often associated with anterior cruciate ligament (ACL), meniscus, or collateral ligament injury
    - Patellar dislocation: chondral injury to lateral femoral condyle and patellar facets
    - Dashboard injury or other high-energy trauma: The patella is forced into the trochlea or an external object directly traumatizes the femoral condyles.
    - Acute pain with or without swelling
    - Hemarthrosis if the subchondral bone is fractured
    - Pain recurs with weight bearing or flexion-extension.
    - Locking or catching (mechanical symptoms) may be present, indicating an unstable cartilage flap or a loose body.
    - Symptomatic loose bodies often accompany acute chondral lesions; articular cartilage fragments are displaced into the joint.
- Chronic (degenerative) lesion
    - Older patients with no traumatic mechanism; associated with degenerative osteoarthritis
    - Chronic mild joint swelling, stiffness, joint line pain
    - Mechanical symptoms may be present, especially if there are loose bodies or unstable flaps of articular cartilage.

Physical Examination

- Observation
    - Effusion (intra-articular swelling); large hemarthrosis if subchondral fracture present
    - Skin abrasions or ecchymoses in direct trauma to the knee
    - Quadriceps atrophy for subacute or chronic symptomatic lesions
    - Antalgic gait
- Palpation
    - Assess joint line tenderness with knee flexed (possible meniscus tear).
    - Assess medial and lateral, anterior and posterior
    - Tenderness over the femoral condyles or behind the patella

- Range of motion
  - Loose body, released from site of articular lesion, may cause block to extension and/or flexion.
  - Effusions may cause loss of flexion.
  - Crepitus with motion may indicate a large area of chondral damage.
  - A "clunk" with motion may indicate a displaced fragment.
  - Special tests to identify other pathology or narrow the differential
  - McMurray test, squat test, and joint line tenderness for meniscal pathology
  - Patellar facet tenderness and apprehension
  - Ligament testing for cruciate or collateral ligament injury

Imaging

- Radiographs: weight-bearing posteroanterior, lateral, 45 degrees of flexion posteroanterior (Rosenberg view), 20 degrees of flexion patellofemoral (Laurin), and tunnel posteroanterior views
  - Rule out osteochondral fracture, osseous loose body, osteoarthritis, osteonecrosis of the femoral condyle, osteochondritis dissecans, plateau fracture, tibial eminence fracture, and Segond fracture (ACL tear).
  - Posteroanterior flexion weight-bearing view especially useful to look for osteoarthritis
  - Laurin view to look for patellofemoral arthritis
  - Tunnel view helpful to look for osteochondritis dissecans lesions
- Magnetic resonance imaging (MRI)
  - Sensitive for cartilage injury, but underestimates damage (Fig. 149-1)
  - Bone edema may indicate local subchondral overloading in an area with chondral defect.
  - Identifies associated pathology of the meniscus, cruciates, collateral ligaments, and patellar retinaculum
- Computed tomography (CT)
  - Sensitive for identifying fractures as well as the size of bone fragments
  - Reconstructions give accurate depiction of injury.

Differential Diagnosis

- Osteoarthritis: chronic stiffness, aching, narrow joint space on radiographs
- Loose body without significant chondral defect: catching, mobile pain, osseous fragments on radiographs, cartilaginous fragments on MRI

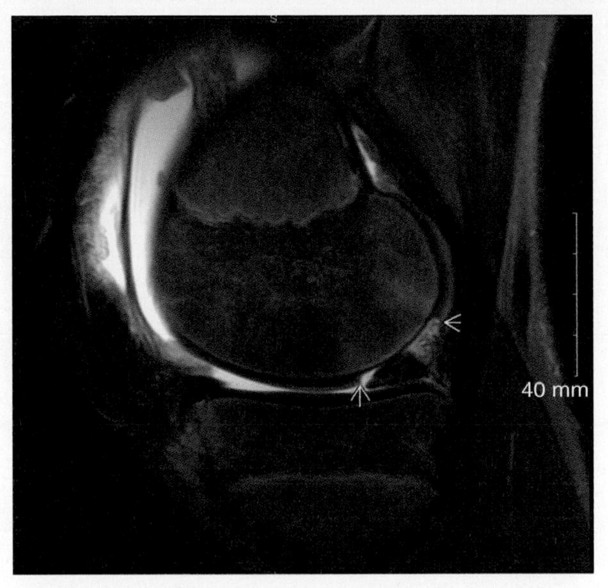

Figure 149-1 Sagittal magnetic resonance imaging of a displaced osteochondritis dissecans lesion of the medial femoral condyle (*arrows* indicate anterior and posterior extent of full thickness defect).

- Patellar subluxation or dislocation: patellar apprehension, pain at the medial patella
- Osteochondritis dissecans: pain to palpation of the condyle, seen on radiographs, MRI, or CT
- Tibial plateau fracture: high-energy injury, seen on radiographs or CT
- ACL tear: positive Lachman's/anterior drawer tests, acute hemarthrosis, seen on MRI
- Collateral ligament sprain or tear: pain or instability to varus stress (lateral collateral ligament) or valgus stress (medial collateral ligament)
- Pes anserine bursitis: pain on medial side distal to the joint line
- Fat pad impingement syndrome
- Symptomatic plica: painful snapping band across medial femoral condyle

Treatment

- At diagnosis
  - Traumatic injuries in which there is significant concern for fracture, unstable knee joint, or open knee require the consultation of an orthopaedic surgeon
  - Acute chondral injuries from athletics or other activities, including those associated with tears of the cruciate or collateral ligaments, also warrant referral to an orthopaedic surgeon.
  - Young patients with potentially unstable chondral lesions should be referred to an orthopaedic surgeon for close evaluation and early intervention

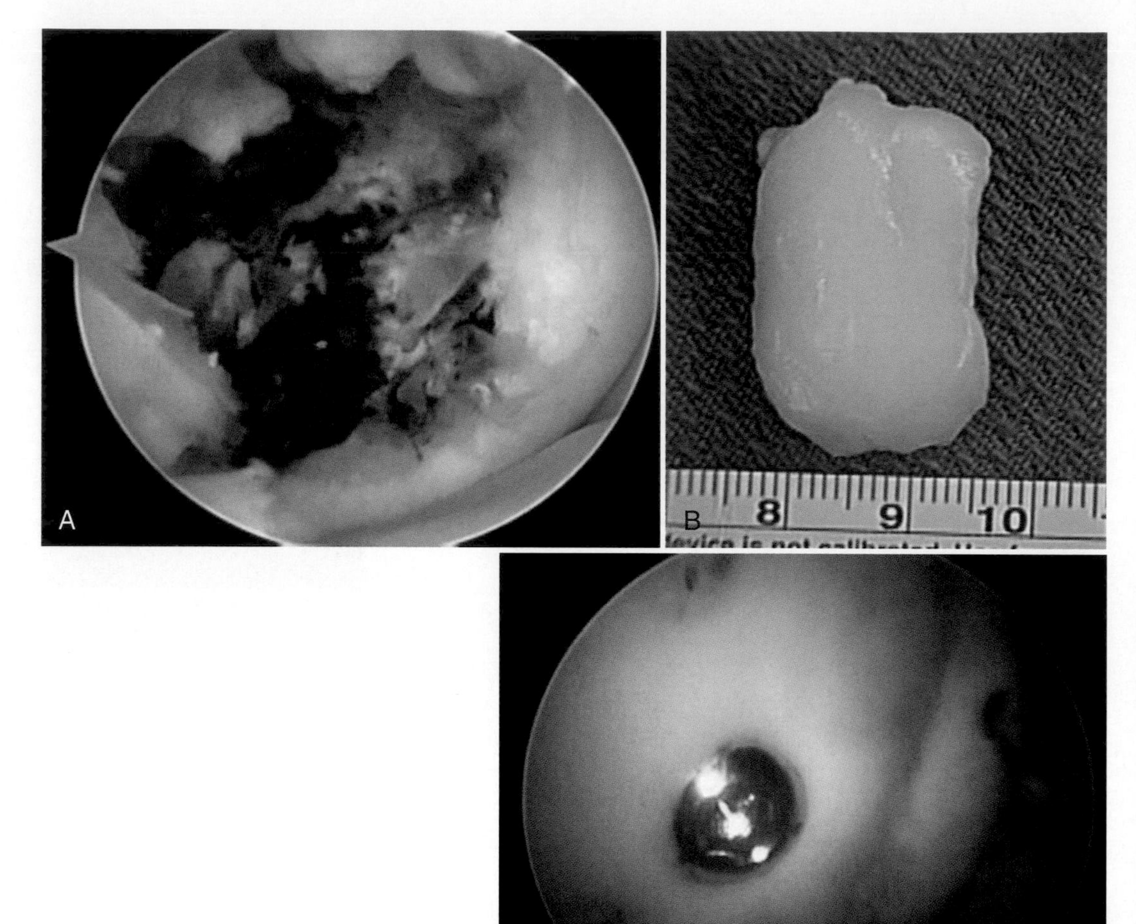

Figure 149-2 Acute osteochondritis dissecans (OCD) lesion of the medial femoral condyle. **A**, Crater base of acutely displaced OCD lesion. **B**, Displaced fragment before reimplantation. **C**, Primary repair of the displaced OCD fragment with screw and bioabsorbable pin fixation.

should the lesion become unstable or displace (Fig. 149-2).

- Otherwise, for chondral lesions found by radiological evaluation for knee pain, initial treatment is symptomatic.
  - — Rest, ice, compression, and elevation are helpful to decrease swelling and pain.
  - — Acetaminophen and/or nonsteroidal anti-inflammatory drugs are useful for pain control.
  - — Physical therapy focused on restoring range of motion and reducing pain while maintaining or improving muscle strength around the knee is beneficial.
  - — If there is malalignment and overloading of the medial or lateral compartment, an unloader brace or heel wedge may be helpful.
- Later
  - If symptoms are not responsive to conservative treatment or if mechanical symptoms persist, the patient may be a surgical candidate.
    - — Arthroscopic options include chondroplasty (débridement) and loose body removal, microfracture, cartilage transfer (osteochondral autograft or allograft transfer), or autogenous chondrocyte implantation (Figs. 149-3 and 149-4).

When to Refer

- Acute injuries with a concern for fracture or articular cartilage injury should be referred immediately for orthopaedic evaluation.

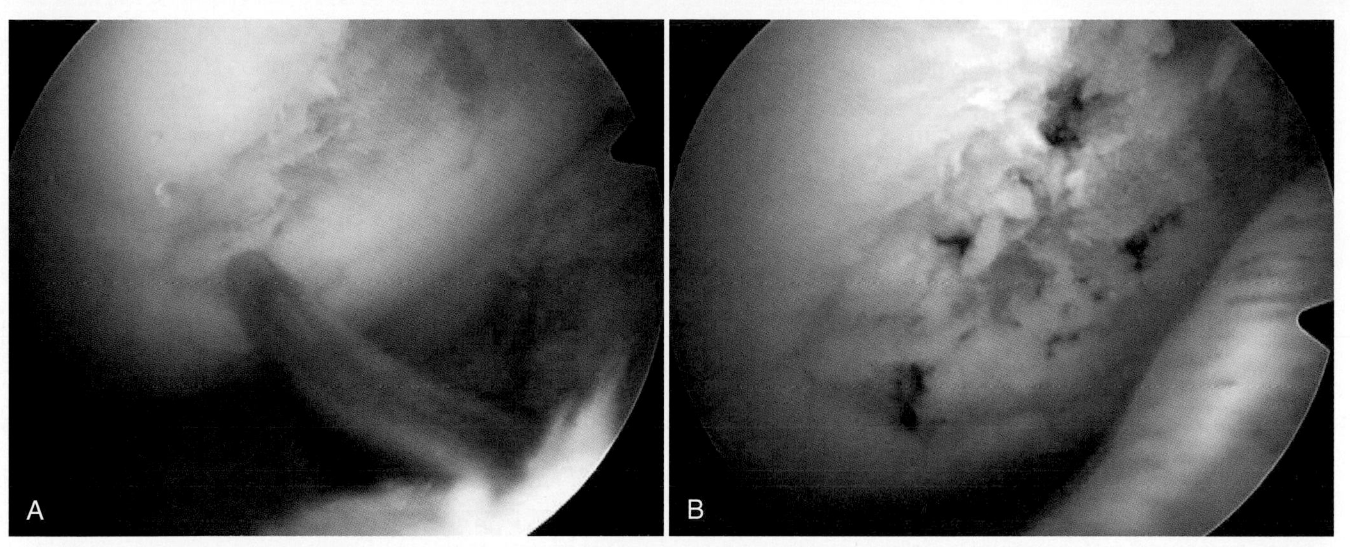

Figure 149-3 Full thickness chondral lesion treated with microfracture. **A**, Calcified layer is débrided, and a microfracture awl is used to penetrate the subchondral bone. **B**, Multiple microfracture holes are made in the defect to facilitate healing of the defect with fibrocartilaginous tissue.

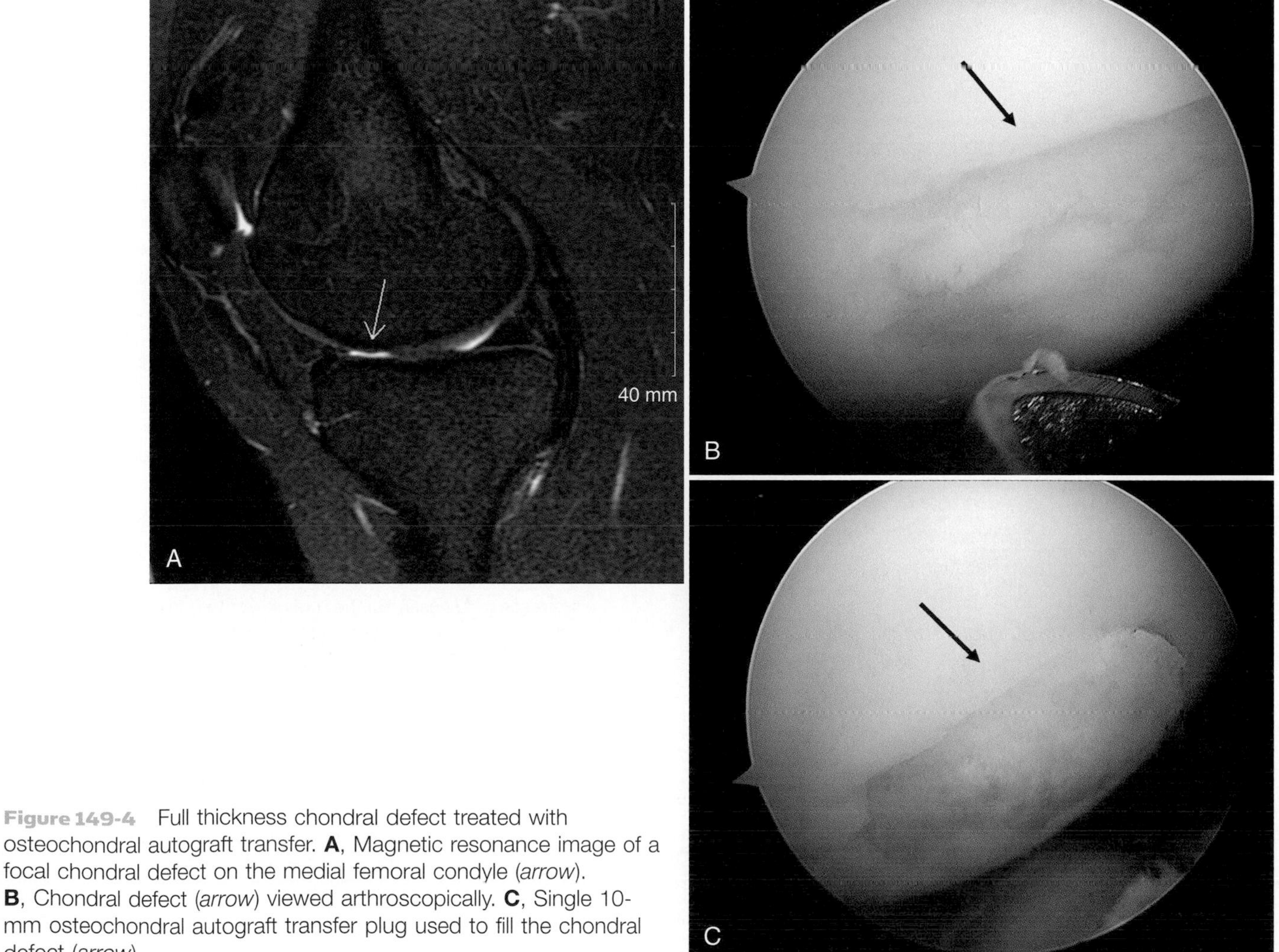

Figure 149-4 Full thickness chondral defect treated with osteochondral autograft transfer. **A**, Magnetic resonance image of a focal chondral defect on the medial femoral condyle (*arrow*). **B**, Chondral defect (*arrow*) viewed arthroscopically. **C**, Single 10-mm osteochondral autograft transfer plug used to fill the chondral defect (*arrow*).

- Older patients with continued mechanical symptoms in whom conservative management has failed should also be referred.

Prognosis

- Many patients with symptomatic chondral lesions will improve with conservative therapy only.
- Patients with mechanical symptoms often respond well to arthroscopy for loose body removal and chondroplasty of loose cartilage flaps.
- Marrow stimulation techniques (microfracture) for cartilage defects have shown positive results, especially in the short term.
- Osteochondral autograft transplantation has shown a high percentage of good to excellent results and in limited studies was found to produce better results than microfracture for larger lesions.
- Autogenous chondrocyte implantation results are mixed, but generally positive.

Troubleshooting

- The patient should be counseled on the benefits and risks of surgery.
  - Benefits include restoration of smooth range of motion and decrease in pain with return to sports, exercise, and activities of daily living. Restoration of a more anatomic joint surface and joint mechanics will likely decrease the rate of progression to posttraumatic arthritis.
  - Risks are minimal with arthroscopic débridement and loose body removal, but symptomatic relief cannot be guaranteed and may be only temporary.
  - Microfracture, osteochondral autograft or allograft transfer, and autogenous chondrocyte implantation require an extended period of non–weight bearing for 6 to 8 weeks with results that are variable. Return to full activities often requires 6 to 12 months of rehabilitation.
  - High-impact activities should be discouraged in patients with significant chondral injuries.

Patient Instructions

- Physical therapy focused on strengthening and range of motion can help improve the return to activities.
- Low-impact activities should be encouraged in patients with chondral injuries.
- Young patients with osteochondritis dissecans lesions should be aware that a sudden loss in motion may indicate a displaced fragment that may require surgery.

Considerations in Special Populations

- Sedentary patients should be given a trial of nonoperative management. However, if symptoms are adversely affecting daily activities, it is reasonable to perform arthroscopy for chondroplasty, loose body removal, and potentially marrow stimulation techniques or grafting.
- It is important to match the individual patient and his or her physical demands with the treatment for the chondral lesion.

Suggested Reading

- Alford JW, Cole BJ: Cartilage restoration, part 1: Basic science, historical perspective, patient evaluation, and treatment options. Am J Sports Med 2005;33:295–306.
- Alford JW, Cole BJ: Cartilage restoration, part 2: Techniques, outcomes, and future directions. Am J Sports Med 2005; 33:443–460.
- Gudas S, Kalesinskas RJ, Kimtys V, et al: A prospective randomized clinical trial of mosaic osteochondral autologous transplantation versus microfracture for the treatment of osteochondral defects of the knee in young athletes. Arthroscopy 2005;21:1066–1075.
- Hangody L, Fules P: Autologous osteochondral mosaicplasty for the treatment of full-thickness defects of weight-bearing joints: Ten years of experimental and clinical experience. J Bone Joint Surg Am 2003;85A:25–32.
- Mandelbaum BR, Browne JE, Fu F, et al: Articular cartilage lesions of the knee. Am J Sports Med 1998;26:853–861.
- Marcacci M, Kon E, Zaffagnini S, et al: Multiple osteochondral arthroscopic grafting (mosaicplasty) for cartilage defects of the knee: Prospective study results at 2-year follow-up. Arthroscopy 2005;21:462–470.
- Messner K, Maletius W: The long-term prognosis for severe damage to weight-bearing cartilage in the knee. Acta Orthop Scand 1996;67:165–168.
- Peterson L, Minas T, Brittberg M, et al: Two- to 9-year outcome after autologous chondrocyte transplantation of the knee. Clin Orthop Relat Res 2000;374:212–234.
- Sharpe JR, Ahmed SU, Fleetcroft JP, et al: The treatment of osteochondral lesions using a combination of autologous chondrocyte implantation and autograft: Three-year follow-up. J Bone Joint Surg Br 2005;87B:730–735.
- Steadman JR, Briggs KK, Rodrigo JJ, et al: Outcomes of microfracture for traumatic chondral defects of the knee: Average 11-year follow-up. Arthroscopy 2003;19:477–484.

Chapter 150 Osteonecrosis of the Knee

Eric J. Gardner and Geoffrey S. Baer

ICD-9 CODES
733.40 *Aseptic Necrosis of Bone, Unspecified Site*
733.43 *Aseptic Necrosis of Bone, Medial Femoral Condyle*

Key Concepts

- Osteonecrosis (ON) or avascular necrosis refers to bone death.
- Medial femoral condyle typically involved, being called spontaneous osteonecrosis of the knee
- Etiology: two theories
  - Vascular theory: Interference of microcirculation to subchondral bone leads to edema and increased compartmental pressure resulting in bone ischemia. If blood supply restored before subchondral collapse, the lesion may heal and symptoms resolve.
  - Traumatic theory: Minor trauma results in microfractures of weak subchondral bone in osteoporotic patients. Resulting edema leads to increased pressure and bone ischemia with ultimate ON/spontaneous osteonecrosis of the knee.
- Primary ON is idiopathic; secondary ON is due to trauma, long-term steroid therapy, renal transplantation, systemic lupus erythematosus, sickle cell anemia, or Gaucher's disease.
- Typically women older than 60 years of age (female-to-male ratio, 3:1)
- As blood supply to bone is lost, subchondral bone necrosis leads to segmental collapse of the subchondral bone.
- Osteoarthritis is typically the end stage of ON.
- Always consider in elderly patient with painful knee that appears normal radiographically

History

- Sudden onset of pain
  - Occasionally after specific activity or minor trauma
  - Pain from subchondral fracture or injury to articular cartilage
- Typically unilateral (bilateral symptoms <20%)
- Pain worse at night in the acute phase (6–8 weeks)
- Pain may resolve or become chronic depending on the size and stage of the lesion.

Physical Examination

- Observation
  - Antalgic gait
  - Usually benign unless history of minor trauma
- With trauma, minor abrasions or ecchymoses may be present.
- Knee typically not red
- Slight swelling possible (intra-articular effusion)
- Palpation
  - Patellar ballottement (effusion)
  - Tenderness to palpation over affected area (medial femoral condyle) or joint line (secondary degenerative changes)
  - Crepitus: degenerative changes
- Range of motion
  - Acute phase: decreased due to pain, effusion, or synovitis
  - Chronic phase: decreased due to degenerative changes

Imaging

- Radiographs: bilateral weight-bearing posteroanterior, lateral, 45 degrees of flexion posteroranterior (Rosenberg), and 20 degrees of flexion patellofemoral (Laurin) views
  - Long-cassette posteroanterior weight-bearing views may be helpful to assess limb alignment.
  - Radiographic staging of ON/spontaneous osteonecrosis of the knee
    - — Stage I: radiograph normal (positive bone scan)

- Stage II: subtle flattening of articular surface
- Stage III: typical lesion with radiolucent area in subchondral bone and a sclerotic halo
- Stage IV: collapse of subchondral bone
- Stage V: collapse with secondary degenerative changes (Fig. 150-1).

- Bone scan
  - Confirmatory test for suspected stage I and II lesions
  - Static phase shows intense area of radioisotope uptake over affected area
  - Uptake on both sides of joint (tibia and femur) is more indicative of osteoarthritis than ON

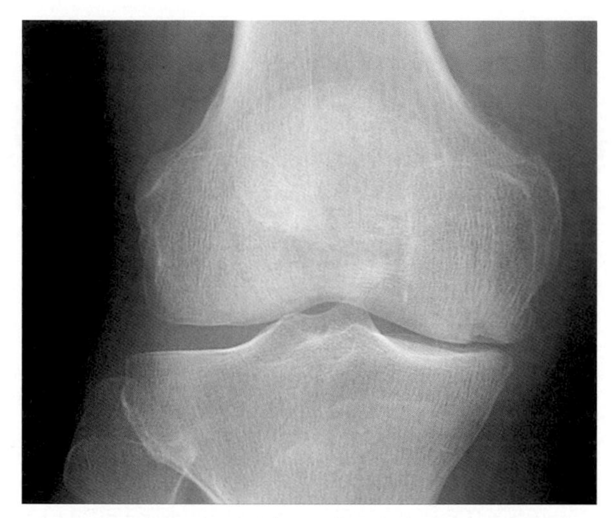

Figure 150-1 Anteroposterior radiograph depicting early stage V spontaneous osteonecrosis of the knee lesion with osseous collapse and medial joint space narrowing in a 66-year-old woman.

- Magnetic resonance imaging
  - Confirmatory test to delineate extent of pathology: lesions often more extensive than appreciated on radiographs (Fig. 150-2)

Differential Diagnosis

- Meniscal tear: joint line tenderness, swelling, mechanical symptoms, evident on magnetic resonance imaging
- Osteoarthritis: chronic stiffness, aching, often tricompartmental involvement on radiographs
- Osteochondritis dissecans: location of tenderness, sex, age
- Pes anserine bursitis: location of tenderness below the medial joint line
- Iliotibial band tendinitis: lateral pain with positive Ober's test

Treatment

- At diagnosis
  - Stages I and II treated conservatively with analgesics and protected weight bearing until the lesion has been defined (may take as long as 6 months).
  - Glucosamine chondroitin sulfate supplements may provide some symptomatic relief (benefits may not be noticed for 6–9 weeks).
  - Corticosteroid or hyaluronic acid injections may be considered in patients who do not respond.
  - Unloader braces, conditioning programs to restore strength and endurance, and activity modifications all help to alleviate pain.

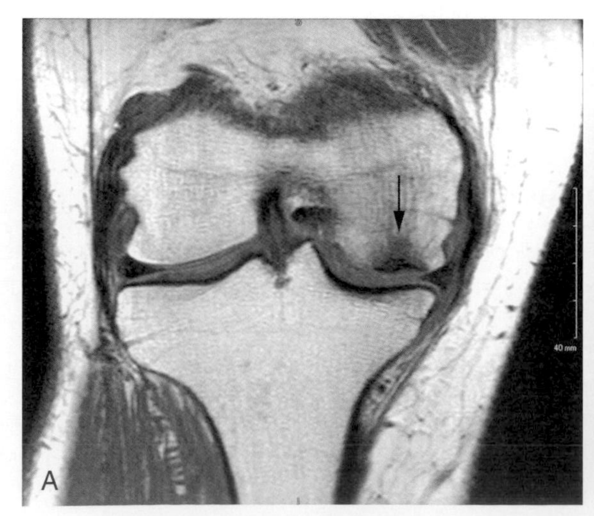

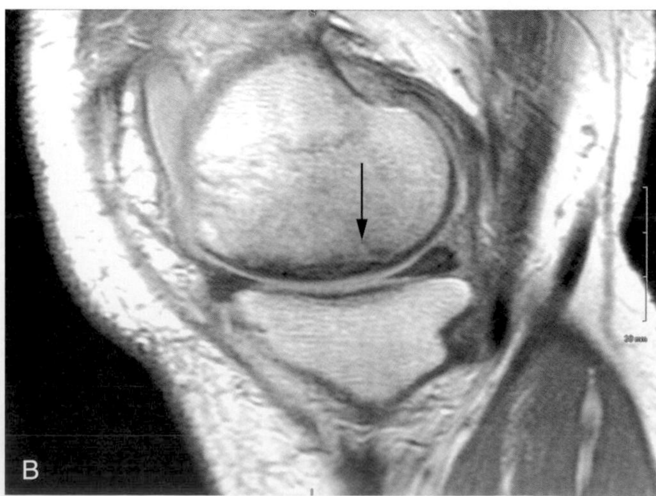

Figure 150-2 Coronal (**A**) and sagittal (**B**) T1-weighted magnetic resonance imaging of bone marrow edema and subchondral collapse involving the medial femoral condyle in a 66-year-old woman.

- Later
  - Larger stage I and II lesions that do not respond to conservative treatment may be considered for surgical intervention.

When to Refer

- Magnetic resonance images should be correlated with clinical symptoms before referral.
- Patient with pain that is not responsive to conservative modalities (lifestyle changes, nonsteroidal anti-inflammatory drugs, acetaminophen, steroid injections, hyaluronic acid injections) and significantly interferes with everyday activities should be referred.
- Patients with large lesions and those of stages III through V should also be referred for surgical consideration. Options include
  - Arthroscopic chondroplasty (débridement)
  - Microfracture, drilling, or core decompression (with or without grafting)
  - High tibial osteotomy
  - Unicompartmental knee arthroplasty (UKA)
  - Total knee arthroplasty (TKA)

Prognosis

- Small lesions do well, but mild degenerative changes may develop.
- Ultimately, the prognosis depends on the size of the initial lesion.
- Lesions that involve more than 50% of the condyle have a poor prognosis; these tend to deteriorate progressively to osteoarthritis.

Troubleshooting

- The patient should be counseled on the benefits and risks of surgery.
  - Benefits include pain relief, restoration of quality of life, and slowing degenerative changes (drilling, grafting, high tibial osteotomy). UKA and TKA remove degenerative joint surfaces to more closely approximate normal anatomy and function.
  - Risks include bleeding, infection, blood clots, and neurovascular injury. Risk are minimal with arthroscopic chondroplasty; however, it is also least likely to prevent further degenerative changes. Microfracture, drilling, decompression, and high tibial osteotomy may slow changes, but will not reverse damage or stop progression. UKA and TKA halt the progression of degenerative changes by replacing articular surfaces with prostheses. The risks of arthroplasty also include early prosthetic failure, infection, and the possibility of revision surgery. Pain relief with UKA and TKA, as with the other procedures described, is not guaranteed.

Patient Instructions

- Patients should be counseled on the findings of ON. The size of the lesion and expectations for outcome should be discussed.
- Options for initial conservative management and possible surgical interventions—débridement, with arthroscopic drilling, cartilage replacement, and joint replacement surgery—should be discussed with the patient, depending on the size and location of the lesion.
- Weight loss should be encouraged in obese patients in an effort to protect the knee and increase the likelihood of success with future surgical intervention.
- Physical therapy programs should be encouraged in patients to help improve strength and function.

Considerations in Special Populations

- Younger, more active patients are not candidates for UKA and TKA due to increased prosthetic wear and early failure. Conservative means of treatment should be exhausted before seeking surgical intervention.
- Older, sedentary patients typically have degenerative changes far too advanced to benefit from surgical procedures aside from UKA or TKA. Even then, conservative measures should be exhausted first.

Suggested Reading

- Akgun I, Kesmezacar H, Oqut T, et al: Arthroscopic microfracture treatment for osteonecrosis of the knee. Arthroscopy 2005;21:834–843.
- Kim JY, Finger DR: Spontaneous osteonecrosis of the knee. J Rheumatol 2006;33:1416.
- Marulanda G, Seyler TM, Sheikh NH, et al: Percutaneous drilling for the treatment of secondary osteonecrosis of the knee. J Bone Joint Surg Br 2006;88B:740–746.
- Mont MA, Baumgarten KM, Rifai A, et al: Atraumatic osteonecrosis of the knee. J Bone Joint Surg Am 2000; 82A:1279.
- Myers TG, Cui Q, Kuskowski M, et al: Outcomes of total and unicompartmental knee arthroplasty for secondary and spontaneous osteonecrosis of the knee. J Bone Joint Surg Am 2006;88A:76–82.
- Pape D, Seil R, Kohn D, et al: Imaging of early stages of osteonecrosis of the knee. Orthop Clin North Am 2004; 35:293–303.

- Patel DV, Breazeale NM, Behr CT, et al: Osteonecrosis of the knee: Current clinical concepts. Knee Surg Sports Traumatol Arthrosc 1998;6:2–11.
- Soucacos PM, Johnson EO, Soultanis K, et al: Diagnosis and management of the osteonecrotic triad of the knee. Orthop Clin North Am 2004;35:371–381.
- Valenti Nin JR, Leyes M, Schweitzer D: Spontaneous osteonecrosis of the knee: Treatment and evolution. Knee Surg Sports Traumatol Assoc 1998;6:12–15.
- Yates PJ, Calder JD, Stranks GJ, et al: Early MRI diagnosis and non-surgical management of spontaneous osteonecrosis of the knee. Knee 2007;14:112–116.

Chapter 151 Osteoarthritis of the Knee

David M. Marcu and Geoffrey S. Baer

ICD-9 CODES

715.16	*Osteoarthrosis, Localized, Primary, Lower Leg*
715.26	*Osteoarthrosis, Localized, Secondary, Lower Leg*
716.9	*Arthritis, Degenerative Joint Disease, Nonspine*
716.16	*Traumatic Arthropathy, Lower Leg*
717.7	*Knee Chondromalacia*
718.0	*Articular Cartilage Disorder*

Key Concepts

- Primary osteoarthritis (OA) is the most common cause of knee pain in the older adult; approximately 85% of people older than 65 years of age have radiographically detectable OA.
- Age-related articular cartilage degeneration, often called wear and tear arthritis
- Obesity and jobs/lifestyles that require intense or repetitive loading of the knees may accelerate the disease and exacerbate symptoms.
- Articular (hyaline) cartilage is uniquely suited for joint functions (axial loading and shear forces) and has very limited regenerative potential (avascular).
- Secondary OA may occur at any age and is secondary to damage of the protective anatomy of the joint or the cartilage itself, which predisposes to further degradation. Examples of preceding events include intra-articular fracture, osteochondral defect, ligament instability, meniscus tear/meniscectomy, gout, pseudogout, or septic joint.

History

- Primary OA
  - Older patients, often obese
  - Chronic mild joint swelling, stiffness, joint line pain with periodic flares
  - Pain worse with weight-bearing activity; relief with rest and nonsteroidal anti-inflammatory drugs
  - More severe disease will cause pain even at night or at rest.
  - The medial compartment is the most commonly affected, but tricompartmental disease in the older adult with OA is very common (Fig. 151-1).
  - Mechanical symptoms (catching, locking), especially if there are loose bodies, unstable articular cartilage flaps, or meniscal tears
- Secondary OA
  - Often younger patients
  - Posttraumatic (Fig. 151-2): previous knee injury (cruciate/collateral ligament injury, meniscal tear requiring subtotal meniscectomy, intra-articular fracture, osteochondral lesion) or previous injury that is remote from the knee but causes mechanical malalignment (slipped capital femoral epiphysis, hip fracture, femur fracture, tibia fracture, physeal injury with subsequent growth disturbance)
  - Degenerative joint disease of the knee can also be secondary to a history of gout, pseudogout (calcium pyrophosphate dihydrate deposition syndrome), or a septic knee joint.

Physical Examination

- Observation
  - Varus malalignment with medial compartment OA (Fig. 151-3); valgus with lateral compartment OA
  - Quadriceps atrophy in chronic symptomatic knees
  - Antalgic gait, use of cane or walker
  - Effusion
- Palpation
  - Effusion, osteophytes, crepitus
  - Tenderness secondary to reactive synovitis
  - Joint line tenderness (may have associated meniscal pathology)
  - Loose bodies (may cause decreased range of motion)

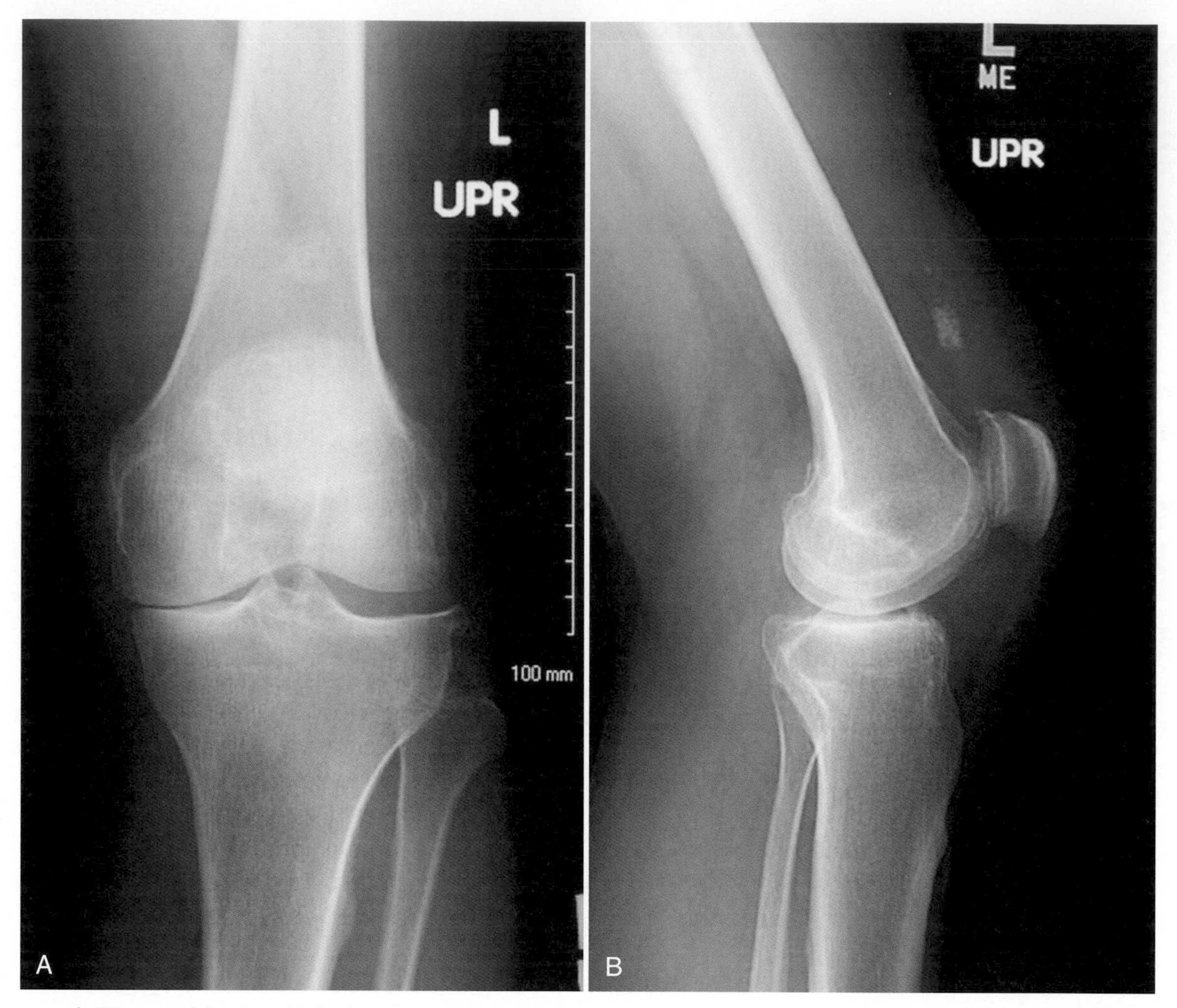

Figure 151-1 A 55-year-old man with isolated medial compartment pain. Anteroposterior (**A**) and lateral (**B**) radiographs reveal medial compartment degenerative joint disease.

- Range of motion
  - Decreased compared with contralateral knee
  - Lack of full extension is common presentation

Imaging

- Radiographs: bilateral weight-bearing posteroanterior, lateral, 45 degrees of flexion posteroanterior (Rosenberg), and 20 degrees of flexion patellofemoral (Laurin) views
  - Posteroanterior flexion weight-bearing view especially useful to look for OA
    - — Cartilage degeneration leads to loss of joint space, subchondral sclerosis, cyst formation, osteophyte formation, and flattening of femoral condyles.
    - — May be more advanced on posterior condyles early in the disease
  - Long cassette posteroanterior weight-bearing views can be helpful to assess limb alignment (see Fig. 151-3).
- Magnetic resonance imaging
  - Usually unnecessary and costly
  - Bone edema may indicate local subchondral overloading.

Differential Diagnosis

- Rheumatoid arthritis: Look for other signs of rheumatoid arthritis or autoimmune disease.
- Septic arthritis: fever; elevated white blood cell count, erythrocyte sedimentation rate, C-reactive protein; hot knee; intense pain with range of motion
- Meniscal tear: mechanical symptoms; often associated with OA

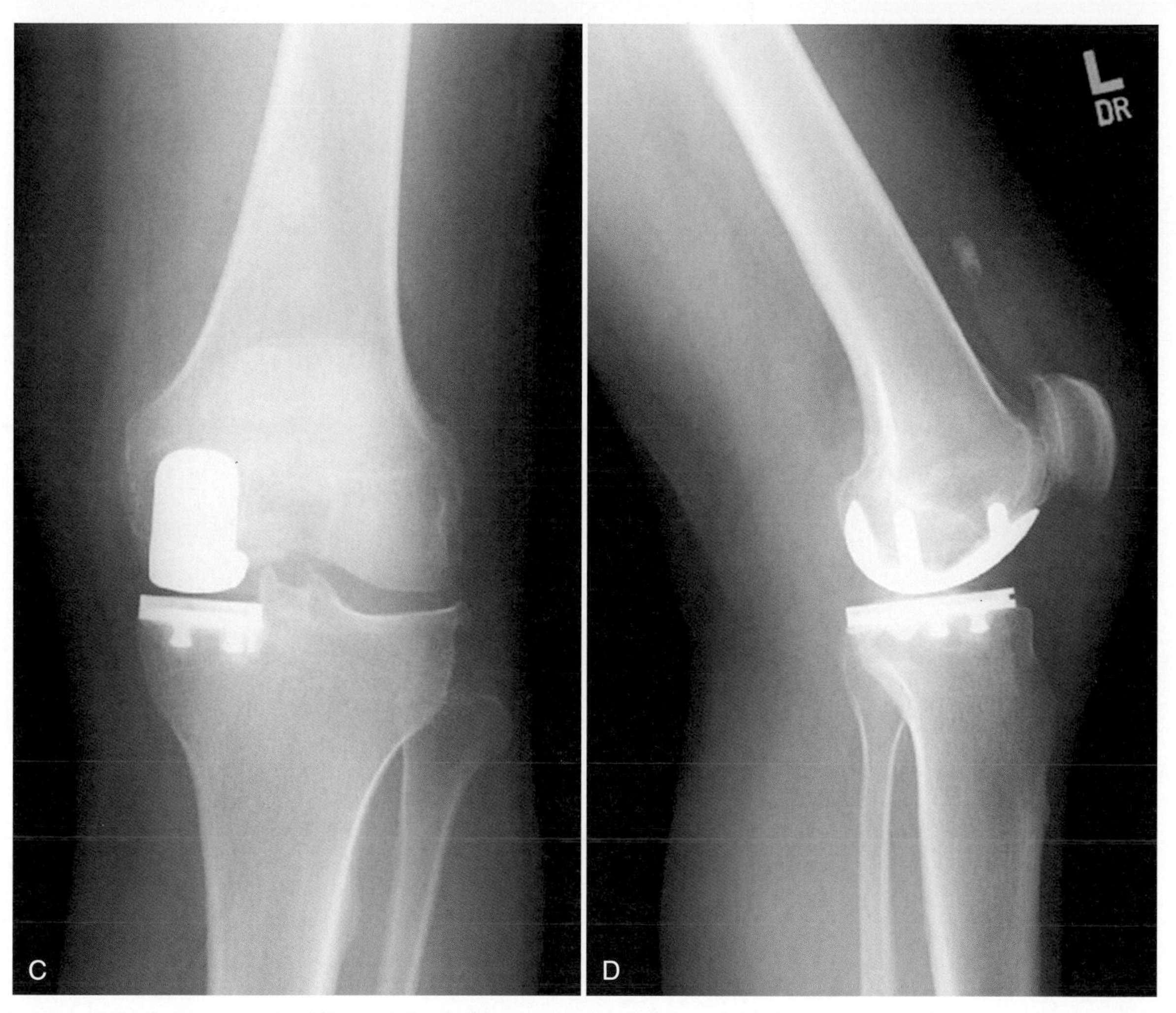

Figure 151-1, cont'd Anteroposterior (**C**) and lateral (**D**) radiographs after medial unicompartmental knee replacement.

- Tibial plateau or femoral condyle fracture: history of fall or other trauma
- Osteonecrosis of the femur or tibia: older, steroid use, female, blood dyscrasia
- L3-L4 radiculopathy: worse with straining/coughing, positive femoral stretch test
- Pigmented villonodular synovitis: recurrent hemarthroses
- Patellar tendinitis (jumper's knee)
- Prepatellar bursitis: palpable fluid collection superficial to patella
- Iliotibial band syndrome: lateral pain, worse with repetitive activity like cycling
- Pes anserine bursitis: pain distal to the medial joint line
- Hip OA: pain with rotation and flexion of the hip, often groin pain but may be referred to the knee

Treatment

- At diagnosis
  - Treatment of OA follows a stepwise progression, depending on symptomatic response to treatment.
    - Lifestyle modifications: Formal physical therapy is often helpful, especially in those patients who are less motivated or less able to initiate an appropriate exercise routine.
    - Medications: Acetaminophen is the first-line analgesic. Nonsteroidal anti-inflammatory drugs can be added with caution (gastrointestinal/renal abnormalities with long-term use). Narcotics are not recommended. Glucosamine (1500 mg) and chondroitin sulfate (1200 mg) as daily dietary supplements

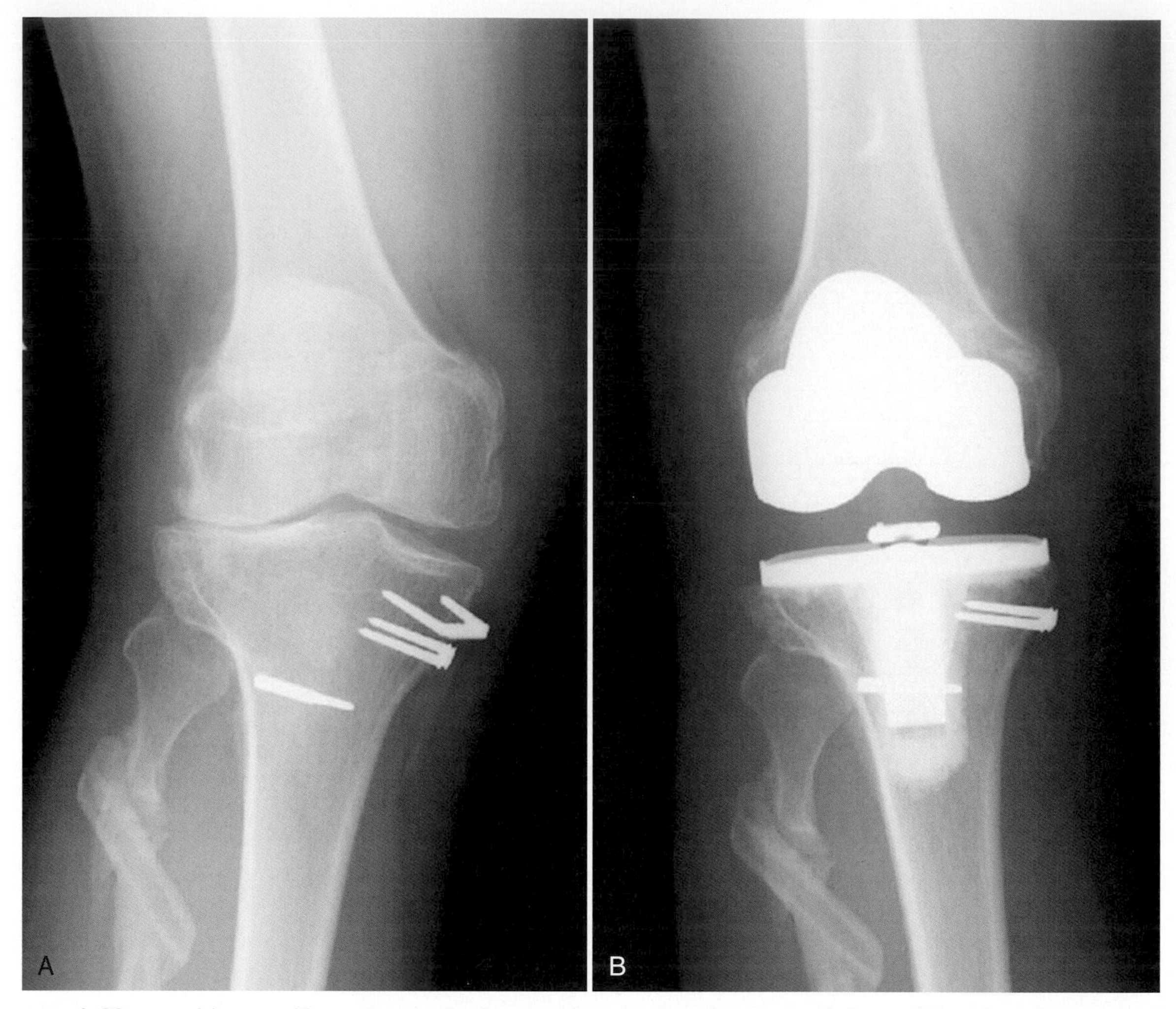

Figure 151-2 A 60-year-old man with posttraumatic degenerative change after traumatic knee dislocation. **A**, Preoperative radiograph with tricompartmental degenerative change. **B**, Postoperative radiograph after total knee arthroplasty.

have shown some analgesic effect with few to no side effects.
    - Intra-articular injections: Corticosteroid injections are limited to three per year, but can significantly reduce symptoms. A series of hyaluronic acid injections carries less risk and is effective as a lubricant and local analgesic.
    - Orthotics: Heel wedges and unloader braces may be effective in unloading isolated compartment arthritis.
- Later
  - Surgical options are available for patients in whom conservative measures fail.
    - Arthroscopic débridement may be helpful as a temporizing measure. Ideal candidates have mechanical symptoms and radiographic/magnetic resonance imaging evidence of loose bodies, meniscal tears, or cartilage flaps, along with the OA.
    - High tibial osteotomy: Young, active patients with isolated medial or lateral compartment degenerative joint disease (see Fig. 151-3)
    - Unicompartmental knee arthroplasty (partial knee replacement): older, low-demand patients with isolated medial or lateral compartment degenerative joint disease (see Fig. 151-1)
    - Total knee arthroplasty: gold standard for knee arthritis (see Fig. 151-2)

When to Refer

- Those patients who have significant symptoms from knee OA despite the previously listed therapies should be presented with surgical options and referred to an orthopaedic surgeon.
- Loss of range of motion is also an indication for referral because it can significantly limit a patient's way of life and is usually progressive.

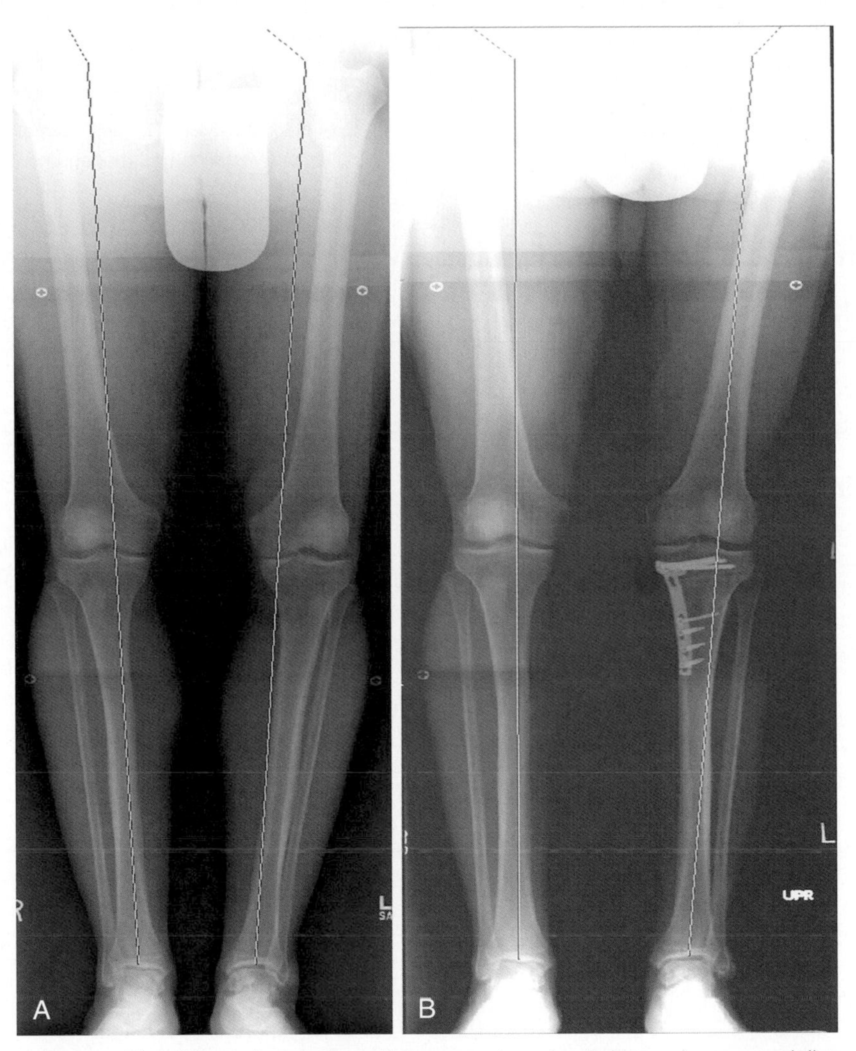

Figure 151-3 A 39-year-old man with left knee isolated medial compartment arthritis and varus malalignment. **A**, Long cassette alignment radiograph depicting varus malalignment (mechanical axis shown). **B**, Long cassette alignment after medial opening wedge high tibial osteotomy with correction of mechanical axis into the lateral compartment (mechanical axis shown).

Prognosis

- The overall success rate of total knee arthroplasty is generally excellent for relief of pain and restoration of range of motion.

Troubleshooting

- Patients should be counseled on the benefits and risks of surgery.
  - Benefits include pain relief, restoration of knee motion, and return to nonimpact exercise and activities of daily living.
  - Risks are minimal with arthroscopic débridement, but include infection and nerve injury. The patients should be counseled that symptomatic relief cannot be guaranteed and will likely be temporary if it occurs. Unicompartmental and total knee arthroplasty, especially in an older population, carry a risk of intraoperative and postoperative medical complications such as deep venous thrombosis, pulmonary embolism, myocardial infarction, stroke, and even death. Arthroplasty also carries the risk of revision surgery.

Patient Instructions

- Overweight patients should be instructed on need for weight control to help relieve pain as well as make them better candidates for joint replacement surgery.
- Avoiding high-impact activities (running, jumping) and participating in low-impact exercise (cycling, swimming, elliptical training) can be helpful in decreasing stiffness and improving pain control.
- Patients should be instructed on quality-of-life issues. Realistic expectations of activity level after joint

replacement surgery should be clearly explained. Younger patients should exhaust conservative measures before progression to unicompartmental or total knee arthroplasty because the life span for joint replacement is limited.

Considerations in Special Populations

- In the truly sedentary patient with knee OA, the cost and risks of operative treatment are rarely warranted, unless it is determined that the reason for the sedentary status is primarily the arthritis itself.

Suggested Reading

- Amin AK, Patton JT, Cook RE, et al: Unicompartmental or total knee arthroplasty? Results from a matched study. Clin Orthop Relat Res 2006;451:101–106.
- Backstein D, Morag G, Hanna S, et al: Long-term follow-up of distal femoral varus osteotomy of the knee. J Arthroplasty 2007;22:2–6.
- Bin SI, Lee SH, Kim CW, et al: Results of arthroscopic medial meniscectomy in patients with grade IV osteoarthritis of the medial compartment. Arthroscopy 2008;24:264–268.
- Clegg DO, Reda DJ, Harris CL, et al: Glucosamine, chondroitin sulfate, and the two in combination for painful knee osteoarthritis. N Engl J Med 2006;23:795–808.
- Cole BJ, Harner CD: Degenerative arthritis of the knee in active patients: Evaluation and management. J Am Acad Orthop Surg 1999;7:389–402.
- Crevoisier X, Munzinger U, Drobny T: Arthroscopic partial meniscectomy in patients over 70 years of age. Arthroscopy 2001;17:732–736.
- Felson DT, Zhang Y, Anthony JM, et al: Weight loss reduces the risk for symptomatic osteoarthritis in women: The Framingham Study. Ann Intern Med 1992;116:535–539.
- Leopold SS, Redd BB, Warme WJ, et al: Corticosteroid compared with hyaluronic acid injections for the treatment of osteoarthritis of the knee: A prospective, randomized trial. J Bone Joint Surg Am 2003;85A:1197–1203.
- Naal FD, Fischer M, Preuss A, et al: Return to sports and recreational activity after unicompartmental knee arthroplasty. Am J Sports Med 2007;35:1688–1695.
- Poolsup N, Suthisisang C, Channark P, et al: Glucosamine long-term treatment and the progression of knee osteoarthritis: Systematic review of randomized control trials. Ann Pharmacother 2005;39:1080–1087.

Chapter 152 Baker Cyst (Popliteal Cyst)

Eric J. Gardner and Geoffrey S. Baer

ICD-9 CODE
727.51 *Popliteal Cyst*

Key Concepts

- Most common synovial cyst found in the knee
- Small cysts are typically asymptomatic and found incidentally.
- Develops from the popliteal bursa in the posteromedial knee between the semimembranosus muscle and medial head of the gastrocnemius muscle
- The popliteal bursa normally communicates with the knee joint.
- Any condition that causes synovitis or increases the production of synovial fluid can cause the bursa to enlarge including arthritis (rheumatoid arthritis, osteoarthritis), meniscal tears, anterior cruciate ligament rupture, gout, and other causes of synovitis.
- The propensity of cysts to enlarge is common, and they may dissect down the calf.
- The flow of synovial fluid from the cyst back into the knee joint is prevented due to a soft-tissue one-way valve.
- Commonly mistaken for deep venous thrombosis when it ruptures, causing severe pain
- Rupture typically occurs in older patients, as well as those with rheumatoid and degenerative arthritis.

History

- Fullness, mass, or swelling in the back of the knee without any obvious trauma
  - Noticed grossly or during exercise
  - Fullness noted on flexion or extension
- Associated with pain and tenderness
- Possible severe calf pain (ruptured cyst)

Physical Examination

- Observation
  - Effusion (intra-articular swelling)
  - Enlarged, swollen calf (ruptured cyst)
  - Fullness of popliteal space
- Palpation
  - Mass in posteromedial aspect of knee with or without tenderness
  - Patellar ballottement (effusion)
  - Pain in calf (ruptured cyst)
  - Joint line tenderness (meniscal tear)
- Range of motion
  - Usually normal; may be decreased if associated with underlying arthritis or a large cyst that limits flexion
  - Ankle motion may be decreased in the presence of a ruptured cyst with an enlarged calf.

Imaging

- Radiographs: bilateral weight-bearing posteroanterior, lateral, 45 degrees of flexion posteroanterior (Rosenberg), and 20 degrees of flexion patellofemoral (Laurin) views
  - May reveal underlying degenerative changes, soft-tissue swelling, effusion
- Ultrasonography
  - Noninvasive; distinguishes solid and cystic lesions
- Arthrography
  - Shows communication of cyst with knee joint
- Magnetic resonance imaging
  - May help distinguish a popliteal cyst from other space-occupying lesions (Fig. 152-1)
  - May demonstrate rupture of a cyst (Fig. 152-2)

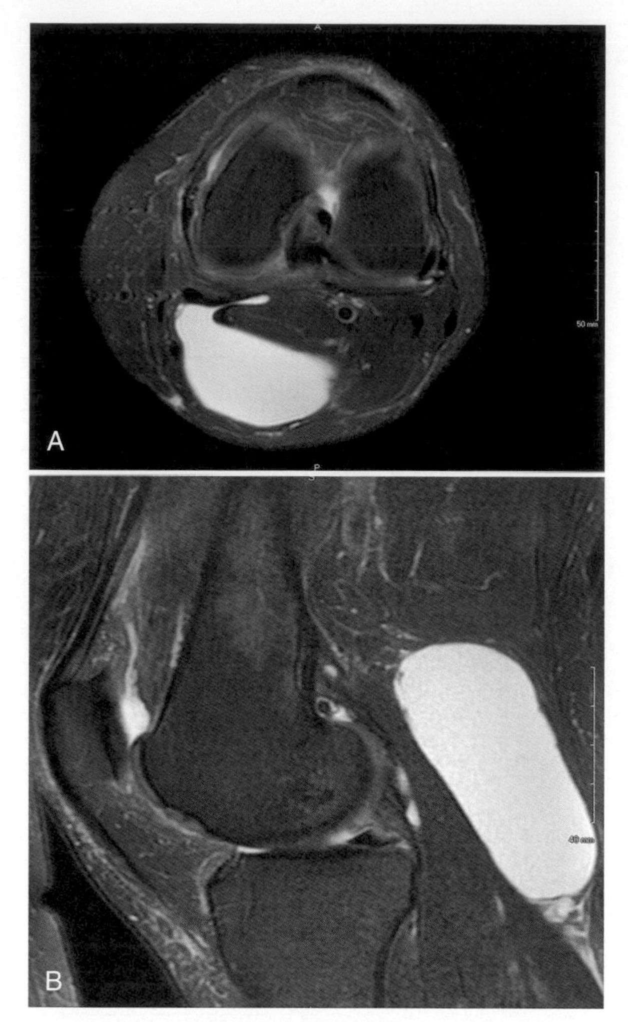

Figure 152-1 Axial (**A**) and sagittal (**B**) T2-weighted magnetic resonance imaging of a large Baker cyst in a 49-year-old man with fullness in the popliteal space.

Differential Diagnosis

- Deep venous thrombosis: ultrasonography or venography
- Exertional compartment syndrome: history and examination findings
- Inflammatory arthritis: positive serologic test results
- Medial gastrocnemius muscle strain: physical examination
- Soft-tissue tumor: magnetic resonance imaging
- Superficial phlebitis: tenderness with negative venography or ultrasonography results

Treatment

- At diagnosis
  - If there is clinical concern for deep venous thrombosis, an ultrasound scan should be performed.

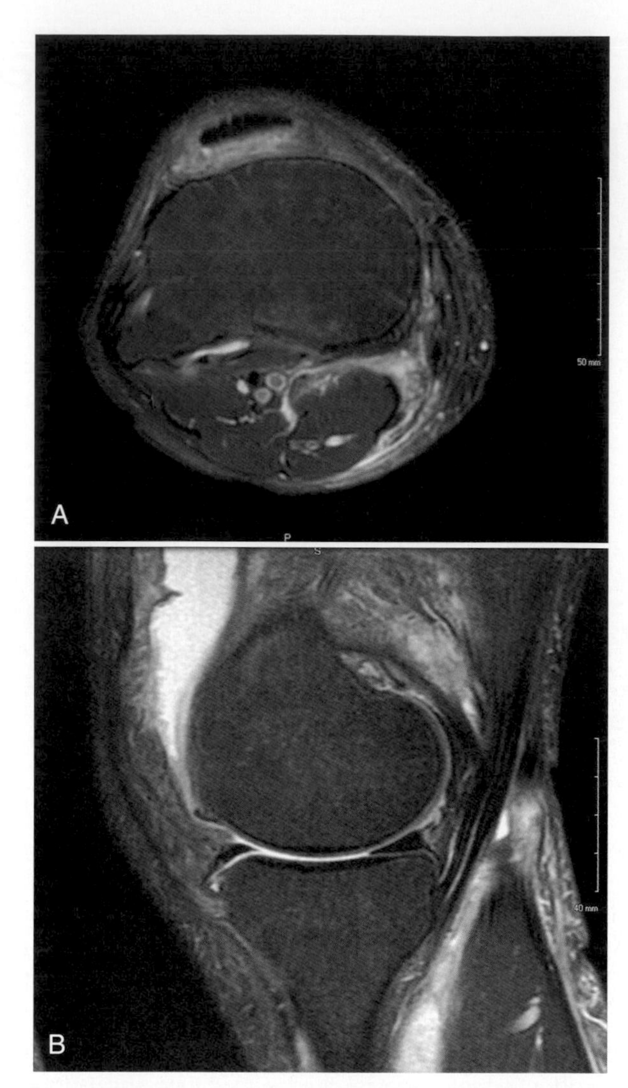

Figure 152-2 Axial (**A**) and sagittal (**B**) T2-weighted magnetic resonance imaging of a ruptured Baker cyst in a 46-year-old man with calf pain.

- Cysts generally recur unless the underlying cause for the cyst is addressed.
  - Some have advocated aspiration of the cyst fluid or even injecting corticosteroids. These measures result in temporary relief as the fluid eventually reaccumulates. Frequently, the cystic fluid is gelatinous and not easily aspirated. Caution should be taken with cyst aspiration due to the proximity of neurovascular structures.
  - With or without rupture, cysts can be treated conservatively. Elevation and compression with a knee sleeve or Ace wrap help decrease swelling. Nonsteroidal anti-inflammatory drugs and acetaminophen help alleviate pain.

- Later
  - Complete resolution of the cyst may be obtained by determining and treating the underlying cause of the cyst.
  - Meniscal pathology can be treated with arthroscopy.
  - Cysts due to inflammatory or degenerative arthritis resolve with knee replacement if otherwise indicated.
  - Open or arthroscopic cyst excision can be performed as well, but recurrence is common.

When to Refer

- Popliteal cysts associated with underlying causes that are amenable to surgical treatment as discussed previously
- Other symptoms, such as fevers, chills, night sweats, and weight loss, need further evaluation for a neoplastic process.

Prognosis

- Treated or not, popliteal cysts have a good prognosis.
- Rarely will a cyst compress surrounding neurovascular structures to produce motor or sensory changes or even venous occlusion.

Troubleshooting

- Fullness in the popliteal space is not always a Baker cyst. The popliteal space should be palpated to ensure that a popliteal aneurysm is not present. Soft-tissue sarcomas or tumors of the distal femur may also cause fullness within the popliteal space.
- Magnetic resonance imaging or ultrasonography can often distinguish between other lesions and a Baker cyst.
- Ultrasonography can be used to aspirate the cyst to prevent injury to surrounding neurovascular structures.

Patient Instructions

- The patient should be counseled on the benefits and risks of surgery.
  - The benefit of aspiration, injection, or excision of the cyst is temporary resolution of the mass; recurrence is likely. When a cyst is associated with a treatable underlying cause (meniscal tear, osteoarthritis, rheumatoid arthritis), complete resolution of the cyst can be accomplished.
  - The risks of treating a popliteal cyst without addressing the underlying cause are temporary relief and/or recurrence. Aspiration and/or injection risks damage to neurovascular structures located in the posterior aspect of the knee. Arthroscopic risks include bleeding, infection, and nerve damage. Open excision also risks damage to surrounding neurovascular structures. Arthroplasty risks include infection, bleeding, neurovascular damage, deep venous thrombosis, pulmonary embolus, prosthetic failure, risks of anesthesia, and death.

Considerations in Special Populations

- In the pediatric population, cysts are usually self-limited and should be treated conservatively.
- In all age groups, when the cyst is asymptomatic, treatment should not be undertaken as the risks outweigh the benefits.

Suggested Reading

- Ahn JH, Yoo JC, Lee SH, et al: Arthroscopic cystectomy for popliteal cysts through the posteromedial cystic portal. Arthroscopy 2007;23:559.e1–e4.
- Curl WW: Popliteal cysts: Historical background and current knowledge. J Am Acad Orthop Surg 1996;4:129–133.
- Damron TA, Sim FH: Soft tissue tumors about the knee. J Am Acad Orthop Surg 1997;5:141–152.
- Dinham JM: Popliteal cysts in children: The case against surgery. J Bone Joint Surg Br 1975;57B:69–71.
- Fritschy D, Fasel J, Imbert JC, et al: The popliteal cyst. Knee Surg Sports Traumatol Arthrosc 2006;14:623–628.
- Rupp S, Seil R, Jochum P, et al: Popliteal cysts in adults. Prevalence, associated intra-articular lesions, and results after arthroscopic treatment. Am J Sports Med 2002;30:112–115.
- Van Rhijn LW, Jansen EJ, Pruijs HE: Long-term follow-up of conservatively treated popliteal cysts in children. J Pediatr Orthop 2000;9:62–64.

Chapter 153 Patellofemoral Pain Syndrome

Richard D. Parker

ICD-9 CODES

717.7 *Chondromalacia of Patella*
717.9 *Unspecified Internal Derangement of Knee*
307.80 *Psychogenic Pain, Site Unspecified*

Key Concepts

- Patellofemoral pain syndrome is defined as retropatellar or peripatellar pain resulting from physical and biomechanical changes in the patellofemoral joint.
- Spectrum of pathology from soft-tissue inflammation to severe arthritic changes
- Often associated with significant disability
- Also commonly referred to as anterior knee pain
- History and physical examination are imperative.
- Initial treatment is usually nonoperative.

History

- Recurring anterior knee pain, interferes with work/sports and occasionally with activities of daily living, such as climbing and descending stairs
- When asked to localize pain, patients point to the anterior knee in a general sense, although they may report more pain laterally.
- Pain may be noted when rising from a seated position or at night. Patients typically deny pain with walking on level surfaces.
- The etiology is often multifactorial and may include muscular (weak quadriceps/vastus medialis obliquus muscles) (Fig. 153-1), biomechanical (foot pronation, knee valgus) (Fig. 153-2), tight iliotibial band, and overuse issues.
- Can be associated with psychosocial issues, such as depression

Physical Examination

- Observation
  - Gait
  - Lower extremity alignment (knee valgus, foot pronation)
  - Q angle (Fig. 153-3)
  - Localized swelling may be noted.

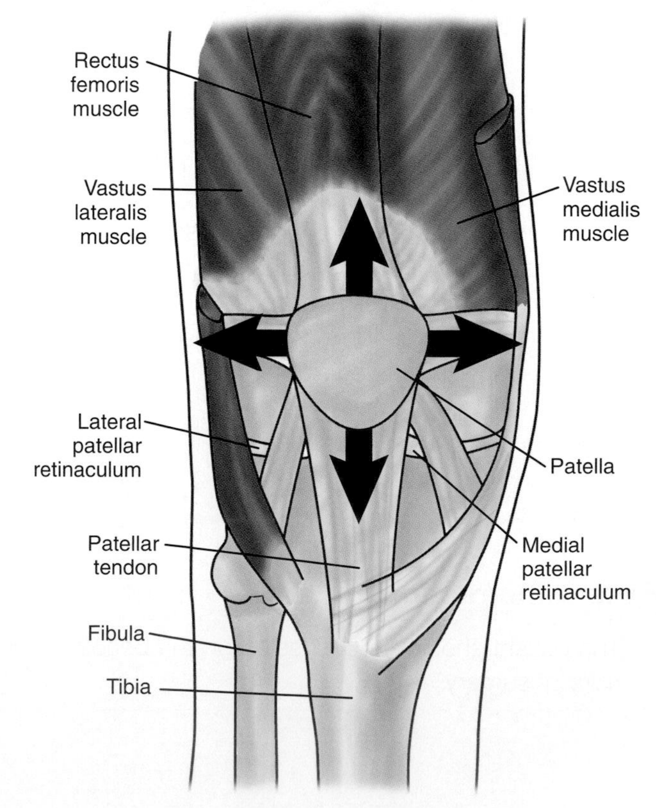

Figure 153-1 The patella is stabilized by dynamic (muscles) and static (retinaculum and tendon) restraints.

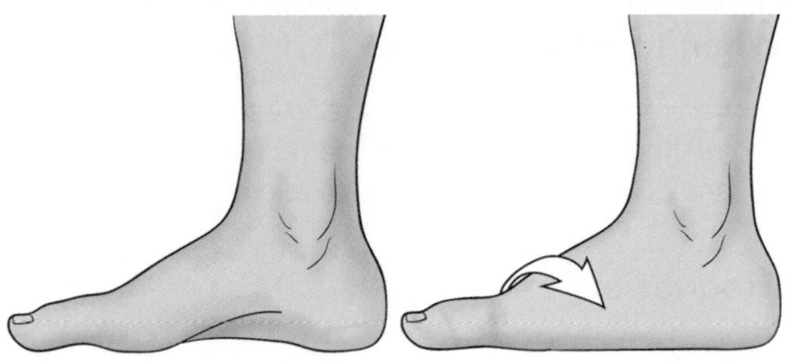

Figure 153-2 Pes planus, or "flatfoot," in a nonweight-bearing state (*left*). Loss of the medial arch with weight bearing (*right*) causes the ankle to "roll" medially. To compensate, the femur or tibia rotates internally, increasing valgus and stressing the patellofemoral mechanism. Arch supports can help with this problem.

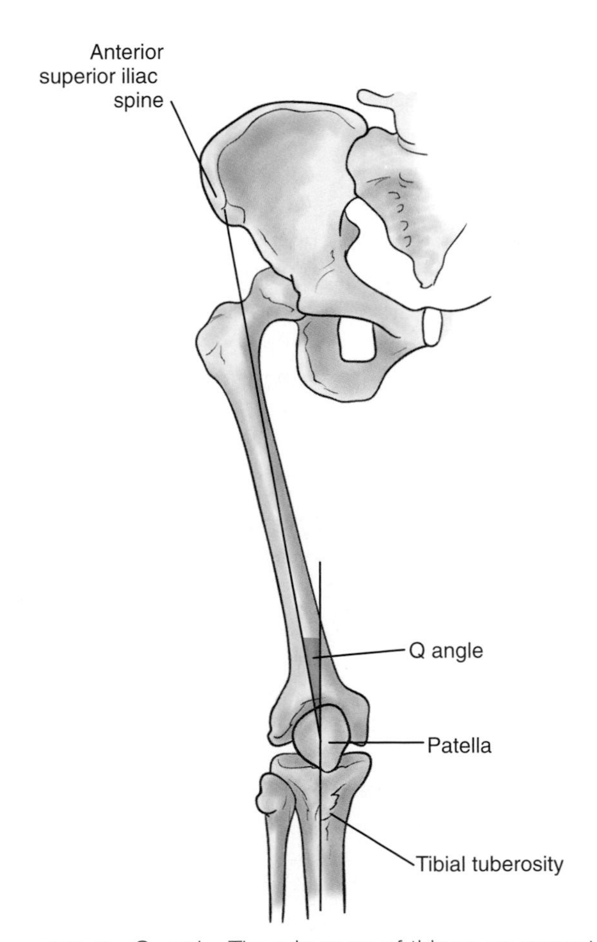

Figure 153-3 Q angle. The relevance of this measurement in patients with patellofemoral pain syndrome has been questioned.

- Palpation
  - Tenderness
  - With or without tight lateral retinaculum (Fig. 153-4)
  - No effusion

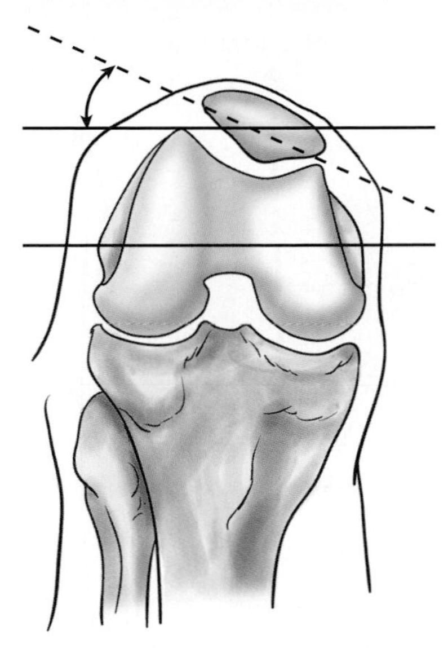

Figure 153-4 Patellar tilt evaluates the tightness of the lateral retinaculum.

- Range of motion
  - Assess patellar mobility (Fig. 153-5).
  - Crepitus
- Special tests
  - Patellar alignment and tracking: tilt, grind, glide, and Q angle
  - Knee ligament stability testing

Imaging

- Radiographs: anteroposterior, lateral, and patellofemoral views of the knee
  - May show tilting of the patella or patellar arthritis
- Magnetic resonance imaging
  - Typically not necessary; consider in cases of refractory symptoms
  - Effusion and patella chondral changes

Differential Diagnosis

- Patellofemoral arthritis
- Hip arthritis, medial/lateral knee arthritis
- Patellar instability
- Stress fracture patella
- Chondral lesion/osteochondritis dissecans patella or trochlea
- Iliotibial syndrome
- Medial plica syndrome
- Meniscus tear
- Patellar tendinitis

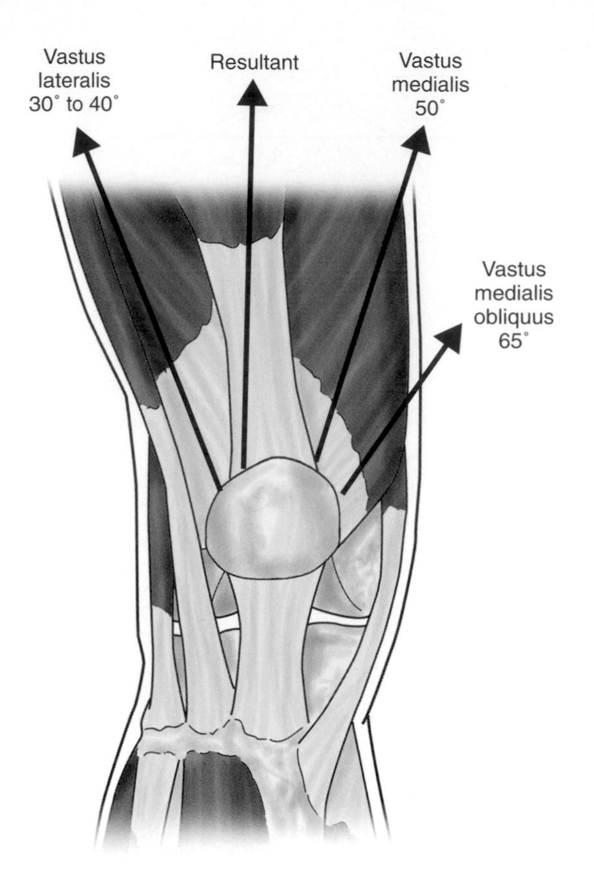

Figure 153-5 The quadriceps muscle influences the patella throughout its range of motion.

Treatment

- At diagnosis
  - Rest and nonsteroidal anti-inflammatory drugs are first-line treatment.
  - Physical therapy including stretching and strengthening exercises, ice, ultrasound, and electrical stimulation is beneficial.
  - McConnell taping and orthotics (to address foot pronation) may also be useful.
  - Obesity should be addressed in cases in which it is a contributing factor.
- Later
  - Surgical intervention is considered a last resort after failure of extensive conservative management including a formal physical therapy program.
  - Surgical procedures typically include arthroscopy to rule out other conditions in the differential diagnosis, débridement of the patella, and possible lateral release if there is a documented tight lateral retinaculum and no hypermobility of the patella.

When to Refer

- Failure of 3 to 6 months of appropriate conservative treatments, including rest, ice, activity modifications, and physical therapy warrants referral.

Prognosis

- Good
- Typically a self-limiting condition
- The majority of patients obtain symptom resolution with conservative management.

Troubleshooting

- Consider magnetic resonance imaging in patients with refractory symptoms.
- Remember that there can be a psychogenic component to this condition.

Patient Instructions

- Listen to your physician and rehabilitation team regarding the importance of rehabilitation.
- Notify your physician if symptoms of instability, loose body sensations, or mechanical symptoms such as locking and catching develop.

Suggested Reading

- Brukner P, Khan K: Clinical Sports Medicine. Sydney, Australia: McGraw-Hill, 1993, pp 372–391.
- Cutbill JW, Ladly KO, Bray RC, et al: Anterior knee pain: A review. Clin J Sport Med 1997;7:40–45.
- Finestone A, Radin EL, Lev B, et al: Treatment of overuse patellofemoral pain. Prospective randomized controlled clinical trial in a military setting. Clin Orthop Relat Res 1993;293:208–210.
- Koh TJ, Grabiner MD, De Swart RJ: In vivo tracking of the human patella. J Biomech 1992;25:637–643.
- McConnell JS: The management of chondromalacia patellae: A long-term solution. Aust J Physiother 1986;32:215–223.
- Reid DC: Sports injury assessment and rehabilitation. New York: Churchill Livingstone, 1992, pp 345–398.
- Thomee R, Renstrom P, Karlsson J, et al: Patellofemoral pain syndrome in young women. I. A clinical analysis of alignment, pain parameters, common symptoms and functional activity level. Scand J Med Sci Sports 1995;5:237–244.
- Tria AJ Jr, Palumbo RC, Alicea JA: Conservative care for patellofemoral pain. Orthop Clin North Am 1992;23:545–554.

Chapter 154 Patellar Instability

Richard D. Parker

ICD-9 CODES
836.3 *Dislocation of Patella, Closed*
836.4 *Dislocation of Patella, Open*

Key Concepts

- The chief symptom is instability, not chronic pain.
- Treatment varies depending on all components of the history, physical examination, and previous treatment.
- Can occur secondary to severe trauma or with minimal trauma
- The medial patellofemoral ligament is an important restraint to lateral instability of the patella.

History

- Acute trauma with or without abnormal alignment, hypermobility of patella
- Acute patellar instability (dislocation) commonly results in a tense, bloody effusion (hemarthrosis).
- Acute patellar instability is the second leading cause of acute, traumatic hemarthrosis (anterior cruciate ligament tear is most common).
- Patients typically present with the fear that the patella will dislocate again.
- The patient should be able to describe the first injury. Note whether the patella is subluxed, dislocated and spontaneously reduced, or has to be manually reduced.
- Can present as acute, subacute, or chronic patellar instability
- Inquire about loose body symptoms, duration of pain and swelling associated with instability episodes, number and frequency of instability events, and the degree of trauma required for recurrent dislocations.

Physical Examination

- Observation
  - Gait
  - Lower extremity alignment
- Palpation
  - Effusion, tenderness
- Range of motion
  - Crepitus
  - Assess for generalized ligamentous laxity.
- Special tests
  - Patellar alignment and tracking
    - — Tilt: lateral retinaculum (see Fig. 153-4).
    - — Grind: crepitus
    - — Glide/apprehension: mobility/instability (Fig. 154-1).
    - — J sign: tracking (Fig. 154-2)
    - — Q angle: alignment
  - Knee ligament stability examination

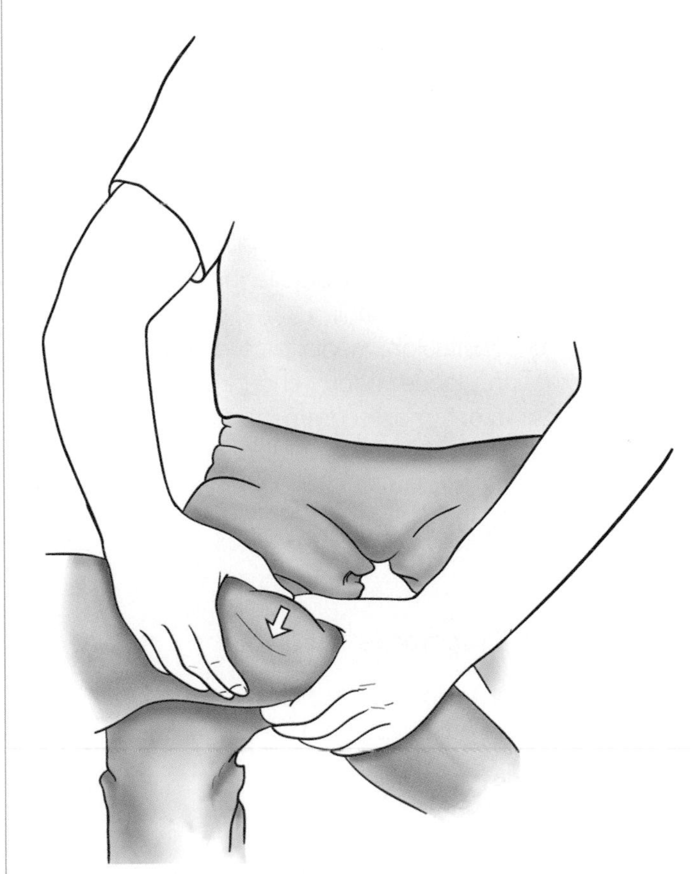

Figure 154-1 Patellar glide assesses the degree of patellar translation with medial/lateral stress of the patella with the knee in slight flexion. Apprehension is present when the patient has a sense/fear of instability with lateral stress on the patella.

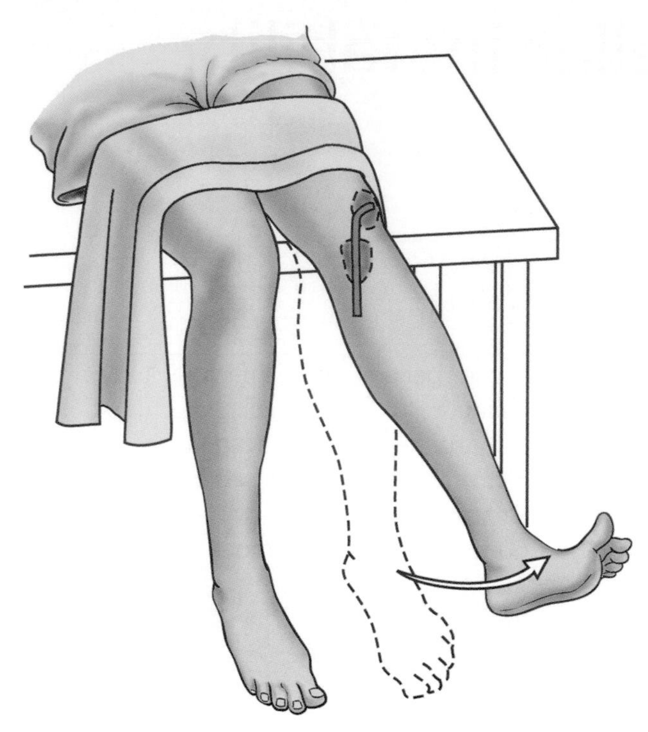

Figure 154-2 The J sign is positive when the patella suddenly shifts laterally when the knee is extended.

Imaging

- Radiographs: anteroposterior, lateral, and patellofemoral views of the knee
  - May show shallow trochlea, patellar subluxation, tilting of the patella, or patellar arthritis
- Magnetic resonance imaging
  - May show effusion, medial patellofemoral ligament disruption, loose body, chondral injury (medial patellar facet most common), and subchondral edema of the lateral femoral condyle and medial patella (secondary to the dislocation/relocation episode)

Differential Diagnosis

- Anterior cruciate ligament rupture
- Patellofemoral pain syndrome
- Loose body

Treatment

- At diagnosis
  - First, ensure that the patella is reduced with physical examination and radiographs.
  - Aspiration may be indicated if severe effusion exists and is affecting rehabilitation.
  - Initial immobilization is controversial, but may be helpful in patients with severe swelling or pain for a short period.
  - Physical therapy has traditionally focused on strengthening of the vastus medialis obliquus/quadriceps muscles to realign the patella.
  - Strengthening of the hip abductors and hip flexors (so-called pelvic stabilization exercises) offers better control of the patella.
  - Bracing and taping may provide symptomatic relief, but are not long-term solutions.
  - Better footwear may also improve symptoms by decreasing pressure on the patella.
- Later
  - Immediate surgery is reserved for a loose body, osteochondral fracture, gross malalignment, and possibly first-time dislocations in athletes (controversial).
  - Patients with recurrent dislocations and pain for whom appropriate physical therapy failed may be candidates for surgical intervention as well.
  - Arthroscopy is helpful to treat loose bodies and chondral pathology; however, open surgery is required to stabilize the patella.
  - Proximal realignment ranges from medial soft-tissue reefing and lateral retinaculum release (indicated only in the setting of an associated tight lateral retinaculum, not isolated instability) to medial patellofemoral ligament repair or reconstruction. Distal realignment (tibial tubercle osteotomy) is reserved for laterally located tibial tuberosity (increased Q angle).

When to Refer

- Patients with recurrent dislocations and failure of rehabilitation should be referred for possible surgical intervention.
- Athletes should be referred after a first-time dislocation.

Prognosis

- Good if the cause of the patellar instability episode occurred during an activity that is not part of the athlete's sport
- If surgery is required, instability can be eliminated, but not always pain.

Troubleshooting

- Beware of a loose body.
- Look for osteochondral fracture on magnetic resonance imaging.
- Important to consider and address underlying anatomic predispositions

Patient Instructions

- Patients should be instructed to complete the nonoperative rehabilitation protocol because this is effective in preventing recurrence in many patients.
- Patients should be instructed to report any recurrent episodes of instability or recurrent sensations of apprehension.

Suggested Reading

- Aglietti P, Buzzi R, Insall J: Disorders of the patellofemoral joint. In Insall J, Scott W (eds): Surgery of the Knee, 3rd ed. New York: Churchill Livingstone, 2001, pp 878–912.
- Ahmad C, Stein B, Matuz D, Henry J: Immediate surgical repair of the medial patellar stabilizers for acute patellar dislocation. A review of eight cases. Am J Sports Med 2000;28:804–810.
- Arendt E, Fithian D, Cohen E: Current concepts of lateral patella dislocation. Clin Sports Med 2002;21:499–519.
- Atkin D, Fithian D, Marangi K, et al: Characteristics of patients with primary acute lateral patellar dislocation and their recovery within the first 6 months of injury. Am J Sports Med 2000;28:472–479.
- Buchner M, Baudendistel B, Sabo D, et al: Acute traumatic primary patellar dislocation. Long term results comparing conservative and surgical treatment. Clin J Sports Med 2005;15:62–66.
- Cash J, Hughston J: Treatment of acute patellar dislocation. Am J Sports Med 1988;16:244–249.
- Cofield R, Bryan R: Acute dislocation of the patella: Results of conservative treatment. J Trauma 1977;17:526–531.
- Desio S, Burks R, Bachus K: Soft tissue restraints to lateral patellar translation in the human knee. Am J Sports Med 1998;26:59–65.
- Harilainen A, Sandelin J: Prospective long-term results of operative treatment in primary dislocation of the patella. Arthroscopy 1993;1:100–103.
- Mäenpää H, Lehto M: Patellar dislocation. The long-term results of nonoperative management in 100 patients. Am J Sports Med 1997;25:213–217.

Chapter 155 Iliotibial Band Syndrome

Richard D. Parker

ICD-9 CODES

727.2 *Specific Bursitides Often of Occupational Origin*

726.60 *Enthesopathy of Knee, Unspecified*

Key Concepts

- Involves the distal iliotibial band (ITB) and lateral femoral epicondyle (Fig. 155-1)
- With flexion/extension, the ITB rubs on the lateral femoral epicondyle.

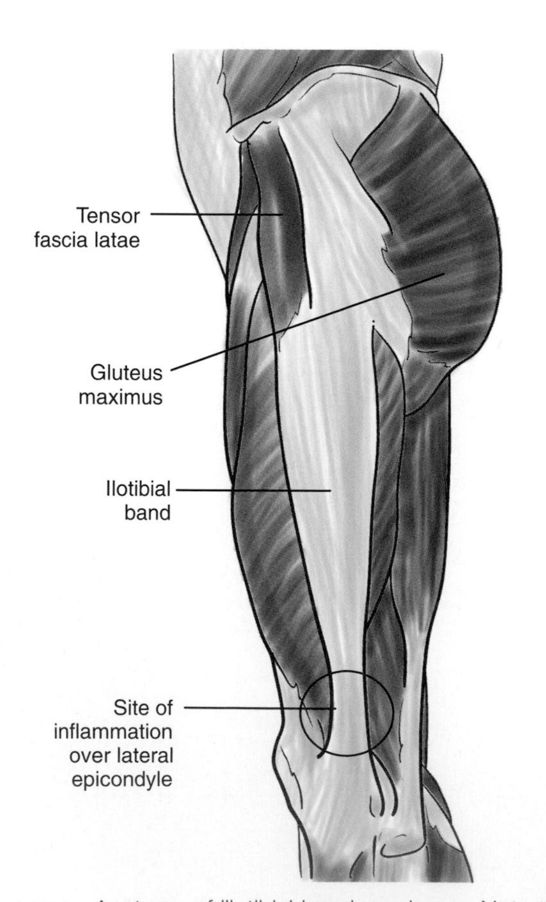

Figure 155-1 Anatomy of iliotibial band syndrome. Note the area of involvement over the lateral femoral epicondyle.

- Occurs primarily as an overuse injury in sports such as long distance running, bicycling, and cross-country skiing
- The differential diagnosis includes lateral meniscus tear, posttraumatic arthritis, patellofemoral pain, patellofemoral instability, and osteochondroma of the lateral femoral condyle.
- Medical management consists of rest, ice, nonsteroidal anti-inflammatory drugs, stretching, and cortisone injection.
- Surgery requires arthroscopy to rule out intra-articular knee pathology, open exploration of the area with elliptical excision or fenestration of the ITB, and débridement of the inflamed bursa or synovium.
- Slow return to sport

History

- Insidious onset
- Worsens with activity and responds initially to rest
- Patient can point to exact area of involvement over the lateral femoral epicondyle.

Physical Examination

- Observation
  - Swelling over area of tenderness with soft-tissue thickening
- Palpation
  - Minimal to no knee effusion
  - No lateral joint line tenderness
- Range of motion
  - Tight ITB
- Special tests
  - Ober's test: With patient on his or her side (involved extremity up), the hip is extended and adducted. The knee is then flexed and extended. Pain indicates a positive test.
  - Negative McMurray's test
  - Stable knee ligament examination
  - Benign patella examination

Imaging

- Radiographs and magnetic resonance imaging are negative.

Additional Tests

- ITB injection (see Chapter 170); may be diagnostic and therapeutic
  - Lidocaine (1%) injection test: Injecting 5 mL to the lateral femoral epicondyle provides pain relief in the physician's office.
  - Bupivacaine (0.25%) injection test: Have the patient perform the aggravating activity (running) after the injection to determine whether symptoms are relieved.

Differential Diagnosis

- Patellofemoral pain
- Patellofemoral instability
- Lateral meniscus tear
- Posttraumatic knee arthritis
- Lateral femoral condyle osteochondroma
- Hip disease
- Stress fracture

Treatment

- At diagnosis
  - Conservative measures are the mainstay of treatment and include rest, ice, physical therapy for stretching and strengthening, orthotics, and cross-training.
  - Corticosteroid injections to the area of maximal tenderness may also provide significant relief.
- Later
  - If all conservative measures have failed and the patient is unwilling to change sports/activities, surgical intervention may be considered.
  - Surgery typically involves knee arthroscopy to rule out differential diagnoses, followed by open exploration of the area, with débridement of the synovium or bursa, shaving of any bony prominences, and excision or fenestration (piecrusting) of the ITB over the lateral femoral condyle (Fig. 155-2).
  - Postsurgical rehabilitation is focused on slow strengthening, core strengthening, ITB stretching, orthotics, and slow return to sport.

When to Refer

- Patients in whom a minimum of 6 weeks of conservative treatment, including formal physical therapy, fail are appropriate for referral.

Prognosis

- Good with rest, time, and stretching

Patient Instructions

- Patients should be aware that this is a diagnosis of exclusion, and recovery (after nonoperative or operative treatment) is slow.

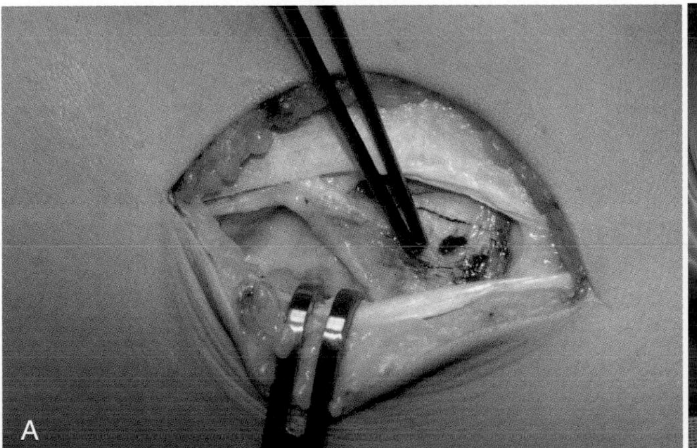

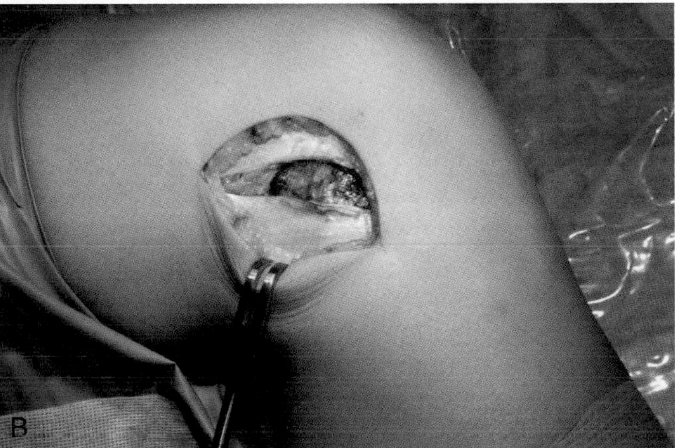

Figure 155-2 **A**, Bursitis at the lateral femoral condyle. **B**, After removal of bursitis, shaving of the lateral femoral epicondyle and excision of a portion of the iliotibial band is performed.

Suggested Reading

- Biundo JJ Jr, Irwin RW, Umpierre E: Sports and other soft tissue injuries, tendinitis, bursitis, and occupation-related syndromes. Curr Opin Rheumatol 2001;13:146–149.
- DeLee JC, Drez D Jr, Miller M (eds): DeLee and Drez's Orthopaedic Sports Medicine: Principles and Practice, 2nd ed. Philadelphia: WB Saunders, 1994.
- Drogset JO, Rossvoll I, Grontvedt T: Surgical treatment of iliotibial band friction syndrome. A retrospective study of 45 patients. Scand J Med Sci Sports 1999;9:296–298.
- Ekman EF, Pope T, Martin DF, et al: Magnetic resonance imaging of iliotibial band syndrome. Am J Sports Med 1994;22:851–854.
- Fredericson M, Cookingham CL, Chaudhari AM, et al: Hip abductor weakness in distance runners with iliotibial band syndrome. Clin J Sport Med 2000;10:169–175.
- Fredericson MF, Guillet M, DeBenedictis L: Quick solutions for iliotibial band syndrome. Phys Sports Med 2000;28:53–68.
- Greenman PE: Principles of Manual Medicine. Philadelphia: Lippincott Williams & Wilkins, 1996.
- Krivickas LS: Anatomical factors associated with overuse sports injuries. Sports Med 1997;24:132–146.

Chapter 156 Quadriceps and Patellar Tendinitis

Richard D. Parker

ICD-9 CODES
726.64 *Patella Tendinitis*
727.65 *Quadriceps Tendinitis*

Key Concepts

- Quadriceps and patellar tendinitis are usually secondary to overuse.
- Physical examination often reveals tight musculature and tenderness at the site of tendinitis.
- Magnetic resonance imaging can be helpful to isolate the area of discomfort.
- Treatment must include modification of activities.
- Surgery is indicated in very specific instances.

History

- Usually associated with overuse; may occur with increasing or changing workouts
- Gradual onset
- Symptoms improve with short periods of rest, but recur.
- Nonsteroidal anti-inflammatory drugs provide relief initially.
- Can affect sports performance

Physical Examination

- Observation
  - Focal swelling
  - Shoewear
- Palpation
  - Identify areas of tenderness.
  - Minimal to no effusion
- Range of motion
  - Look for loss of flexibility in hamstring, quadriceps, and Achilles tendons.
- Special tests
  - Confirm that the extensor mechanism is intact.
  - Knee ligament examination
  - Evaluate core strength.

Imaging

- Radiographs: anteroposterior, lateral, and patellofemoral views of the knee
  - Rule out fracture
  - Look for patellar alta (high) or baja (low) on lateral view.
  - Evaluate for malalignment and arthritis.
- Magnetic resonance imaging
  - Allows localization of the tendinitis (Fig. 156-1).
  - Can rule out complete tear or other structural abnormalities, such as stress fracture
- Ultrasonography
  - May also localize tendinitis
- Bone scan
  - May be useful adjunct in difficult cases (Fig. 156-2)

Differential Diagnosis

- Quadriceps or patellar tendon rupture
- Partial tendon tear
- Patellofemoral pain syndrome
- Prepatellar bursitis

Treatment

- At diagnosis
  - Rest for 4 to 6 weeks is the mainstay of treatment, followed by gradual return to activity and rehabilitation.
  - Local modalities such as ultrasound, ice, and electrical stimulation are appropriate.
  - Rehabilitation concentrates on stretching of hip, quadriceps, hamstring, and Achilles tendons. Core strength and endurance training is imperative. High-frequency shock wave treatment has been advocated.
- Later
  - Surgical intervention is indicated only if rest, rehabilitation, and activity modification have failed.

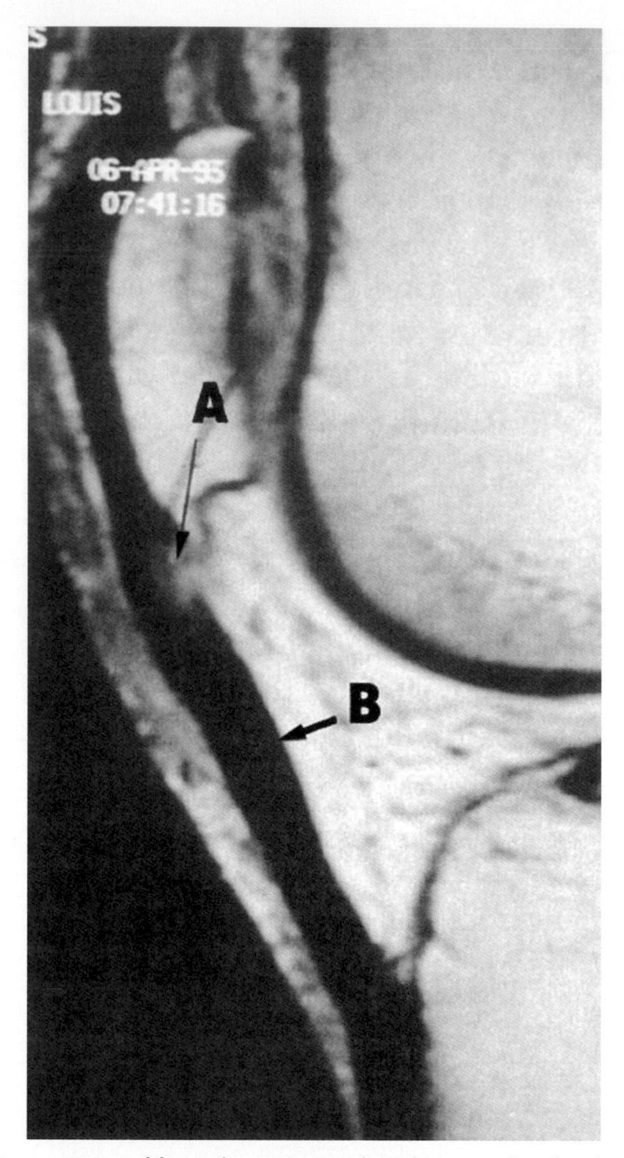

Figure 156-1 Magnetic resonance imaging revealing focal area of patellar tendinosis (A) compared with normal tendon signal (B). Note the area of tendinosis is located at the bone-tendon junction.

- In addition, the history, physical examination, and imaging studies must all be in concordance before surgery is considered.
- Surgery consists of débriding the areas of tendinosis and removal of the bone-tendon interface.
- After surgery, the rehabilitation outlined previously is instituted.

When to Refer

- Referral is indicated after failure of appropriate conservative treatment for a minimum of 3 months.

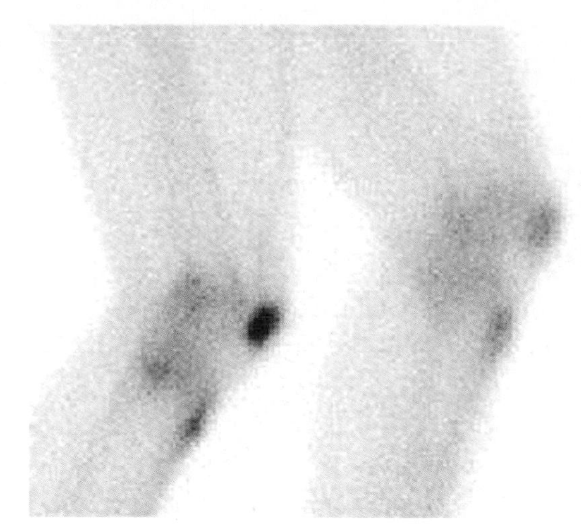

Figure 156-2 Bone scan revealing a focal area of involvement at the bone-tendon junction.

Prognosis

- Good when recognized early and completely treated

Troubleshooting

- Beware of associated metabolic diseases.
- Do not underestimate the value of rest and core strengthening.

Patient Instructions

- Patients should be encouraged to adhere to the treatment regimen.
- Stretching and modification/correction of training errors are imperative.

Suggested Reading

- Basso O, Johnson DP, Amis AA: The anatomy of the patellar tendon. Knee Surg Sports Traumatol Arthrosc 2001;9:2–5.
- Hyman J, Rodeo SA, Wickiewicz T: Patellofemoral tendinopathy. In DeLee JC, Drez D Jr, Miller MD (eds): DeLee and Drez's Orthopaedic Sports Medicine: Principles and Practice, 3rd ed. Philadelphia: WB Saunders, 2002, pp 184–186.
- Nordin M, Frankel VH: Biomechanics of the knee. In Nordin M, Frankel VH (eds): Basic Biomechanics of the Musculoskeletal System. Philadelphia: Lea and Febiger, 1980, pp 115–134.
- Petersen W, Stein V, Tillmann B: Blood supply of the quadriceps tendon [in German]. Unfallchirurg 1999;102:543–547.
- Simon SR, Alaranta H, An KN, et al: Kinesiology. In Buckwalter JA, Einhorn TA, Simon SR (eds): Orthopaedic Basic Science. Rosemont, IL: American Academy of Orthopaedic Surgeons, 2000, pp 789–797.

Chapter 157 Prepatellar Bursitis

Richard D. Parker

ICD-9 CODE
726.65 *Prepatellar Bursitis*

Key Concepts

- Prepatellar bursitis involves inflammation of the anterior knee bursa (Fig. 157-1).
- May be the result of direct trauma to the anterior knee (fall) or repetitive, overuse injury (excessive kneeling)
- In acute cases, the bursa may be very swollen secondary to trauma (Fig. 157-2).
- In chronic cases, the bursa may be thickened.
- Septic bursitis involves an infection (typically *Staphylococcus aureus*) of the inflamed bursa, usually from a break in the skin.
  - May be mistaken for septic/pyogenic arthritis

History

- Anterior knee pain
- Difficulty with ambulation and inability to kneel on the affected side
- Relief of pain with rest
- History of repetitive, overuse injury, or occupation requiring excessive kneeling

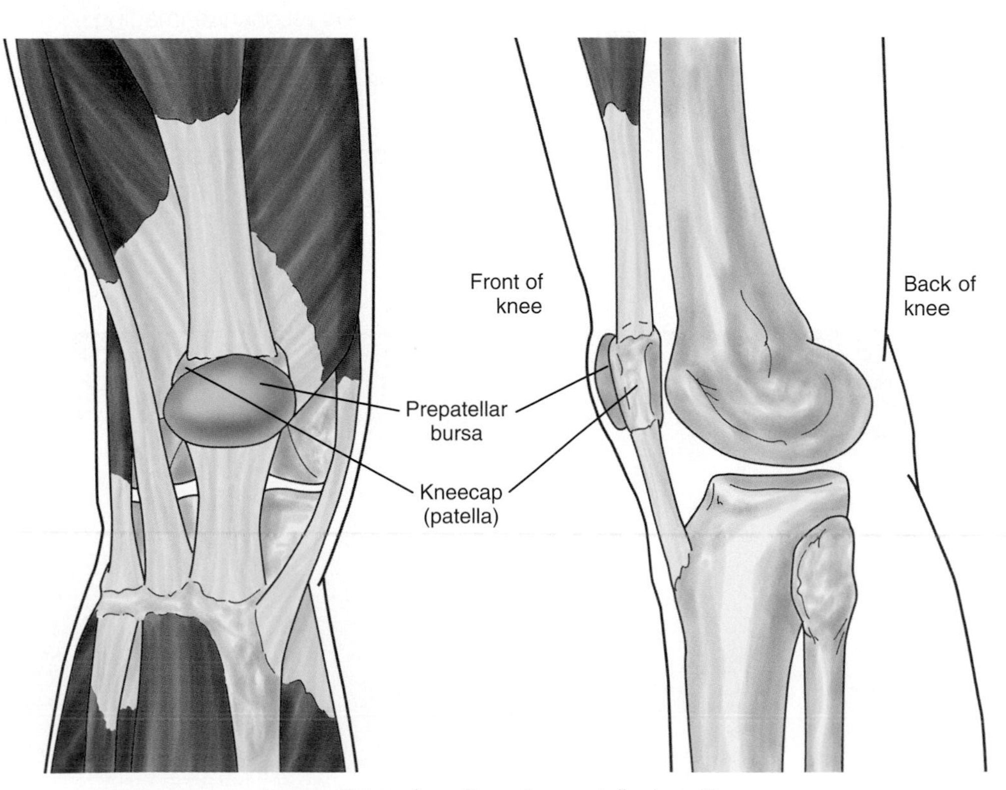

Figure 157-1 Location of prepatellar bursitis.

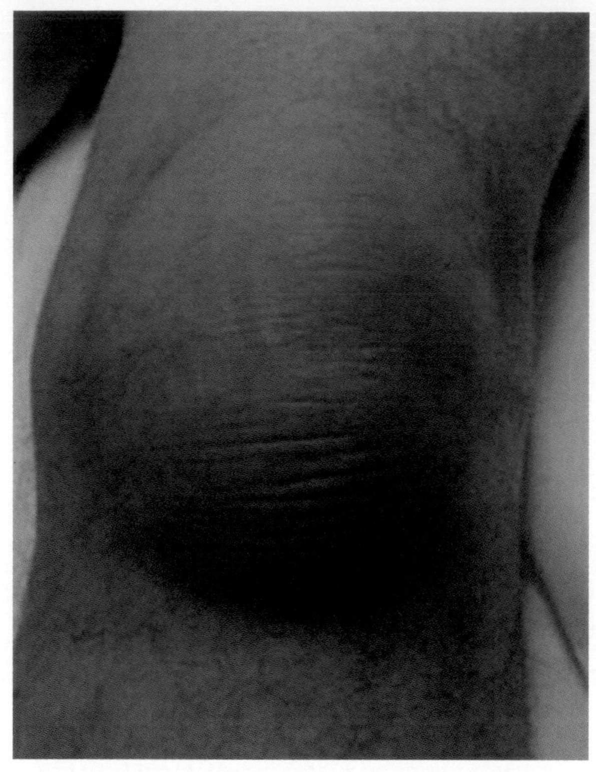

Figure 157-2 Patient with acute prepatellar bursitis.

- History of a fall on the knee or blunt trauma to the knee (with presentation of symptoms as long as 10 days after the incident)
- Septic bursitis is more common in children.
- Inquire about history of gout, pseudogout, hemophilia, warfarin use, and inflammatory conditions.

Physical Examination

- Observation
  - Swelling and erythema
- Palpation
  - Tenderness over the patella
  - Fluctuant edema over the lower pole of the patella
  - Crepitus
- Range of motion
  - Decreased flexion secondary to pain
- Special tests
  - Aspiration is not indicated for the diagnosis of prepatellar bursitis. However, if infection is suspected, then aspiration is recommended, and fluid should be sent for analysis because the bursa is a common site of infection.
  - Findings consistent with septic bursitis include a white blood cell count greater than 5000/μL, elevated protein and lactate, decreased glucose, and bacteria seen on Gram stain.
  - Crystal analysis may reveal monosodium urate crystals (gout), calcium pyrophosphate crystals (pseudogout), or cholesterol crystals (rheumatoid bursitis).
  - Laboratory tests (erythrocyte sedimentation rate, C-reactive protein) are performed as well.

Imaging

- Radiographs: anteroposterior, lateral, and patellofemoral views of the knee
  - Negative except for anterior soft-tissue swelling
- Magnetic resonance imaging
  - An axial view may demonstrate fluid in the area of the prepatellar bursa (Fig. 157-3).

Differential Diagnosis

- Patella fracture
- Patellar tendinitis

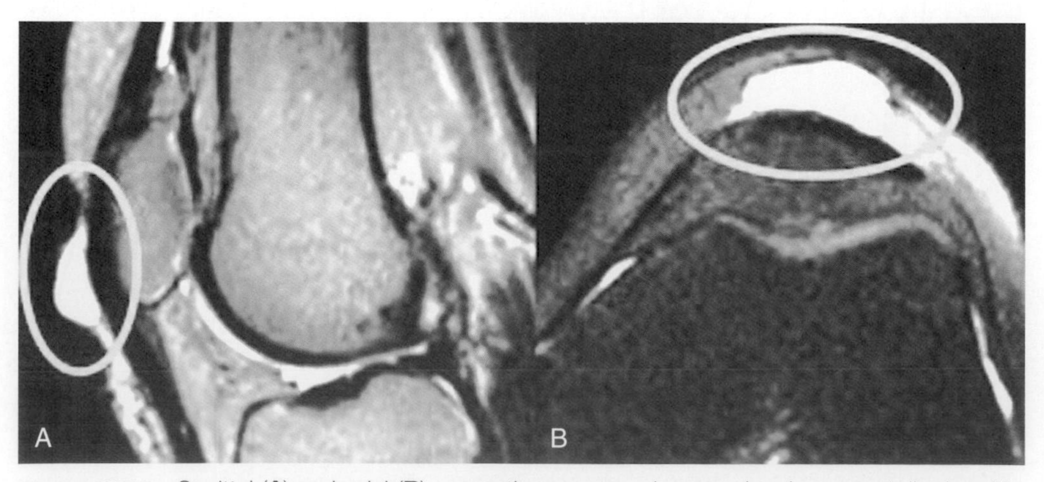

Figure 157-3 Sagittal (**A**) and axial (**B**) magnetic resonance images showing prepatellar bursitis.

- Patellofemoral pain syndrome
- Morel-Lavallé lesion (traumatic injury to the tissue planes secondary to shear)

Treatment

- At diagnosis
  - Conservative measures include avoidance of the precipitating cause, use of knee pads, and time.
  - Aspiration of the bursa may be indicated if pain and warmth are greater than expected.
  - If infection is excluded, may consider corticosteroid injection into the bursa (see Chapter 168)
- Later
  - Surgical intervention is reserved for infections and recalcitrant, symptomatic prepatellar bursitis.
  - Surgical options include open or arthroscopic excision of the bursa.

When to Refer

- Referral is indicated in cases of septic bursitis and in patients in whom a course of conservative treatment including rest, ice, and activity modification has failed.

Prognosis

- The prognosis good if the bursitis is recognized early and treated. Even in cases of septic bursitis, long-lasting sequelae are rare with proper treatment.

Troubleshooting

- Remember infection and beware of methicillin-resistant *S. aureus*.
- Complications of injection include infection; bleeding; postinjection inflammation, pain, and erythema; tendon rupture; and subcutaneous atrophy.

Patient Instructions

- If swelling becomes more painful and warm, contact your physician.
- Complete the treatment course of antibiotics (if infected) regardless of symptoms and appearance.
- Avoid the cause of the bursitis to avoid chronic swelling.

Suggested Reading

- Bellon EM, Sacco DC, Steiger DA, et al: Magnetic resonance imaging in “housemaid’s knee” (prepatellar bursitis). Magn Reson Imaging 1987;5:175–177.
- Dawn B, Williams JK, Walker SE: Prepatellar bursitis: A unique presentation of tophaceous gout in a normouricemic patient. J Rheumatol 1997;24:976–978.
- Donahue F, Turkel D, Mnaymneh W, et al: Hemorrhagic prepatellar bursitis. Skeletal Radiol 1996;25:298–301.
- Garcia-Porrua C, Gonzalez-Gay MA, Ibanez D, et al: The clinical spectrum of severe septic bursitis in northwestern Spain: A 10 year study. J Rheumatol 1999;26:663–667.
- Kaalund S, Breddam M, Kristensen G: Endoscopic resection of the septic prepatellar bursa. Arthroscopy 1998;14:757–758.
- Kerr DR: Prepatellar and olecranon arthroscopic bursectomy. Clin Sports Med 1993;12:137–142.
- Wilson-MacDonald J: Management and outcome of infective prepatellar bursitis. Postgrad Med J 1987;63:851–853.

Chapter 158 Pes Anserine Bursitis

Richard D. Parker

ICD-9 CODE
726.61 *Pes Anserine Tendinitis or Bursitis*

Key Concepts

- Pes anserine bursitis (tendinitis) involves inflammation of the bursa at the insertion of the pes anserine tendons on the medial proximal tibia (Fig. 158-1).
- The pes anserine is composed of the sartorius, gracilis, and semitendinosus tendons.
- The superficial medial collateral ligament inserts onto the proximal tibia deep to the pes insertion.
- Symptoms include medial pes swelling, pain to touch, warmth, and pain with hamstring activation.
- The cause is usually overuse.
- Treatment involves modification of activities, icing, and stretching.
- Treatment usually resolves this condition.

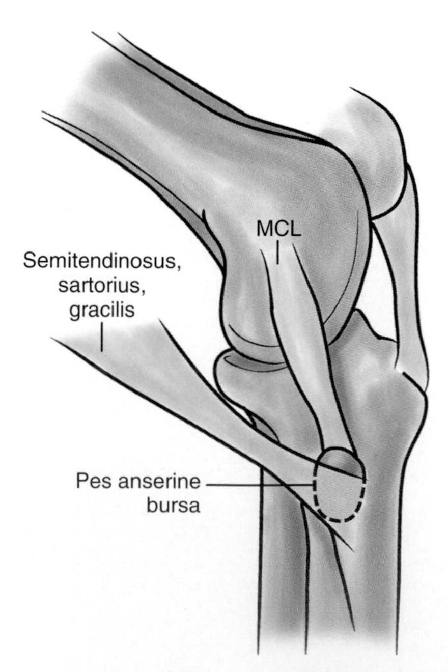

Figure 158-1 Location of the pes anserine bursa on the medial side of the knee. MCL, medial collateral ligament.

History

- Acute trauma to the medial knee, athletic overuse, chronic mechanical (pes planus) process, or degenerative process
- Pain, tenderness, and localized swelling over the medial knee
- Worse on ascending and, possibly, descending stairs and when rising from a seated position; typically deny pain with walking on level surfaces
- May have chronic, refractory pain in setting of arthritis or obesity
- More common in sports requiring side-to-side movements and cutting
- May have coexistent medial collateral ligament pathology (tenderness superior and posterior to the pes bursa)
- Bilateral symptoms in one third of patients

Physical Examination

- Observation
  - Localized swelling
- Palpation
  - Tenderness over the proximal medial tibia at the insertion of the pes anserine, approximately 2 to 5 cm distal to the anteromedial joint line
  - Bursa usually not palpable unless effusion and thickening present
  - Crepitus over the bursa occasionally present
  - Absence of joint line pain
  - Exostosis of the tibia may contribute to chronic symptoms in athletes.
- Range of motion
  - May have pain with resisted internal rotation, resisted flexion, and valgus stress (especially in athletes)

Imaging

- Radiographs: anteroposterior, lateral, and patellofemoral views of the knee

- Negative, except for possible degenerative changes
- Magnetic resonance imaging
  - Axial view may demonstrate fluid in the area of the pes anserine bursa.
  - Rule out meniscus tears and medial collateral ligament pathology.

Additional Tests

- Injections may be diagnostic and therapeutic (see Chapter 169).
  - Lidocaine (1%) injection test: Injecting 5 mL into the pes anserine bursa provides pain relief in the physician's office.
  - Bupivacaine (0.25%) injection test: Have the patient perform the aggravating activity (running) after the injection to determine whether symptoms are relieved.

Differential Diagnosis

- Medial meniscus tear
- Medial compartment osteoarthritis
- Medial tibial stress (insufficiency) fracture
- Semimembranosus tendinitis or bursitis
- Superficial medial collateral ligament sprain at tibial insertion
- Patellar tendinitis
- Patellofemoral pain
- Proximal medial tibia osteochondroma

Treatment

- At diagnosis
  - Rest and nonsteroidal anti-inflammatory drugs are first-line treatment.
  - Physical therapy including stretching and strengthening (Fig. 158-2), ice, ultrasound, and electrical stimulation may be beneficial.
  - A small cushion placed between the thighs for sleeping is also useful.
  - Address obesity in cases in which it is a contributing factor.
- Later
  - Resection may be appropriate in refractory cases, such as those causing 6 to 8 weeks of limitation among athletes, especially if mature exostosis is present and causing irritation.
    - — The operation includes excision of the bursa and bony exostosis (if present).

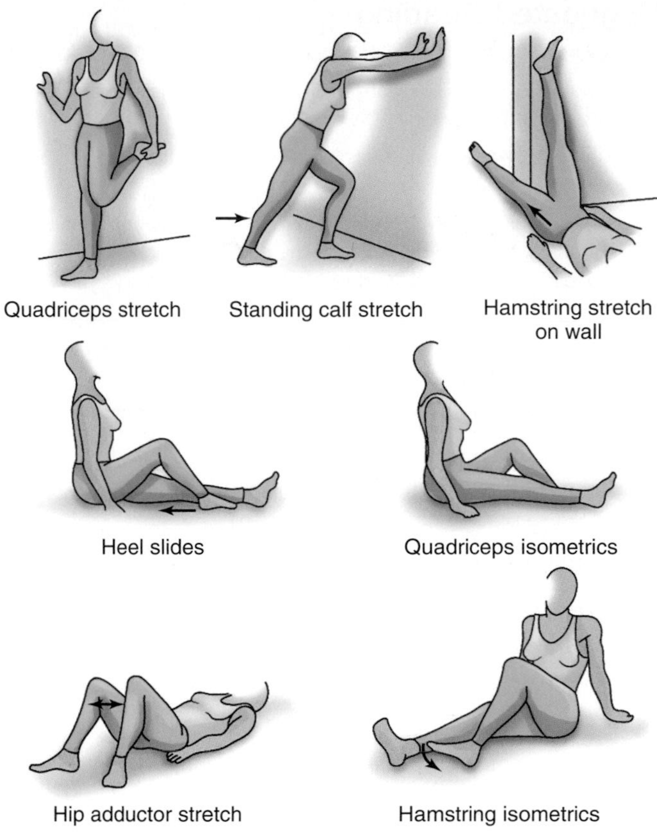

Figure 158-2 Exercises for pes anserine (knee) bursitis.

    - — Rupture or impending rupture of any of the pes anserine tendons is also addressed.
    - — Postoperatively, the knee is immobilized in extension or slight flexion for 1 to 2 weeks.

When to Refer

- Referral is indicated after failure of conservative treatment including rest, ice, and activity modification.
- Corticosteroid injections should be given 6 weeks to assess their effectiveness before referral.

Prognosis

- Good

Troubleshooting

- If symptoms persist, magnetic resonance imaging is helpful to rule out differential diagnoses.

Patient Instructions

- If symptoms worsen, contact your physician.
- Modification of activities is the most important component of the treatment.

Suggested Reading

- Abeles M: Anserine bursitis. Arthritis Rheum 1986;29:812–813.
- Forbes JR, Helms CA, Janzen DL: Acute pes anserine bursitis: MR imaging. Radiology 1995;194:525–527.
- Handy JR: Anserine bursitis: A brief review. South Med J 1997;90:376–377.
- Hemler DE, Ward WK, Karstetter KW, et al: Saphenous nerve entrapment caused by pes anserine bursitis mimicking stress fracture of the tibia. Arch Phys Med Rehabil 1991;72:336–337.
- Larsson LG, Baum J: The syndrome of anserine bursitis: An overlooked diagnosis. Arthritis Rheum 1985;28:1062–1065.
- Muchnick J, Sundaram M: Radiologic case study. Pes anserine bursitis. Orthopedics 1997;20:1092–1094.
- Rennie WJ, Saifuddin A: Pes anserine bursitis: Incidence in symptomatic knees and clinical presentation. Skeletal Radiol 2005;34:395–398.

Chapter 159 Extensor Tendon Rupture

Richard D. Parker

ICD-9 CODES
727.66 *Rupture of Tendon, Patellar Tendon*
727.67 *Rupture of Tendon, Quadriceps Tendon*

Key Concepts

- Patellar tendon rupture is usually due to a sports injury in patients younger than 40 years old.
- Quadriceps tendon rupture is relatively infrequent and typically occurs in patients older than 40 years of age.
- Bilateral rupture of either tendon is uncommon and usually results from systemic disease (inflammatory disease, diabetes, chronic renal failure) and previous degenerative changes.
- A palpable defect at the site of injury is often found.
- With contraction of the quadriceps, the patella may (patellar tendon rupture) or may not (quadriceps tendon rupture) travel proximally.
- Surgical repair is usually indicated.

History

- Acute traumatic injury: stumble, fall, or a giving way of the knee
- Severe pain, immediate disability, and swelling
- Cannot lift leg and feel wobbly
- With or without history of knee pain/tendinosis
- Inquire about history of steroid injections and anabolic steroid use.

Physical Examination

- Observation
  - Diffuse, tender swelling and ecchymosis of anterior knee
- Palpation
  - Effusion and tenderness
  - Palpable defect at level of rupture (Fig. 159-1)
- Range of motion
  - Active extension may be completely lost and the patient is unable to maintain the passively extended knee against gravity.
  - Quadriceps rupture: The patella does not move with quadriceps contraction.
  - Patella tendon rupture: The patella moves with quadriceps contraction.
- Special tests
  - Knee ligament examination

Imaging

- Radiographs: anteroposterior, lateral, and patellofemoral views of the knee
  - Rule out fracture and assess patella position: alta/baja (Figs. 159-2 and 159-3)
- Magnetic resonance imaging
  - Recommended for documentation, localization of the tear, and identification of additional injuries (Fig. 159-4)
- Ultrasonography
  - May also document and localize tear

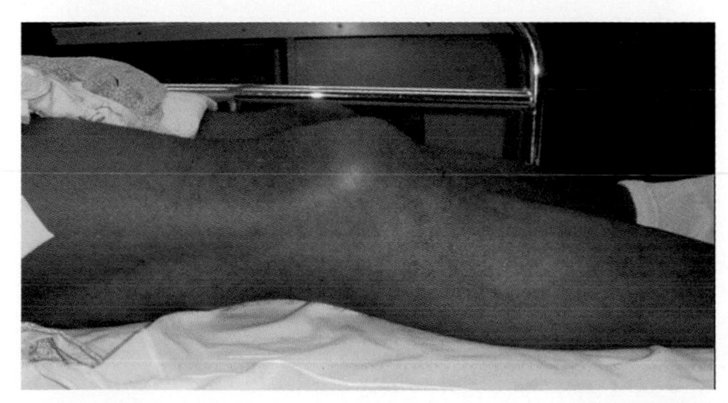

Figure 159-1 Clinical photograph of superior patellar swelling associated with quadriceps rupture.

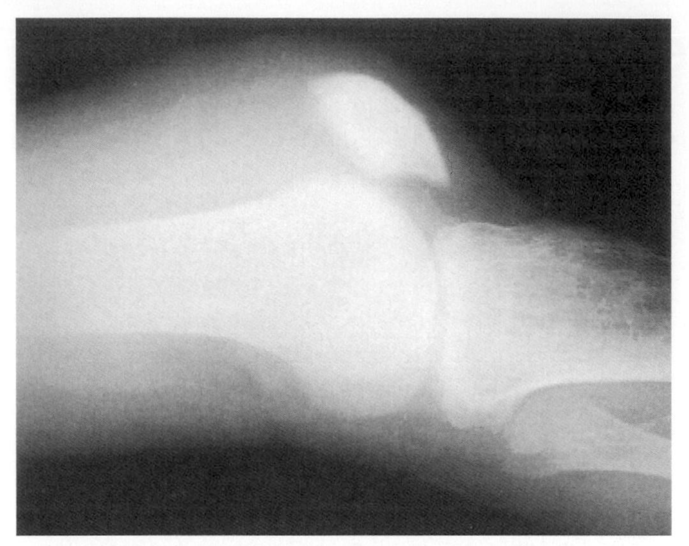

Figure 159-2 Lateral radiograph revealing soft-tissue swelling superior to the patella and patella baja consistent with quadriceps rupture. (Copyright 2006 by Elsevier, Inc.)

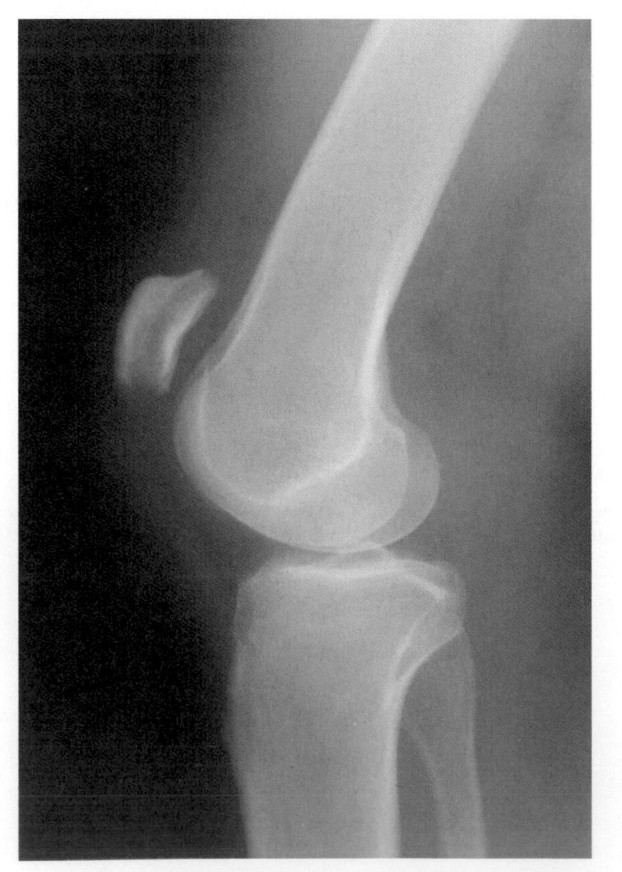

Figure 159-3 Lateral radiograph revealing patella alta (high riding), consistent with patellar tendon rupture.

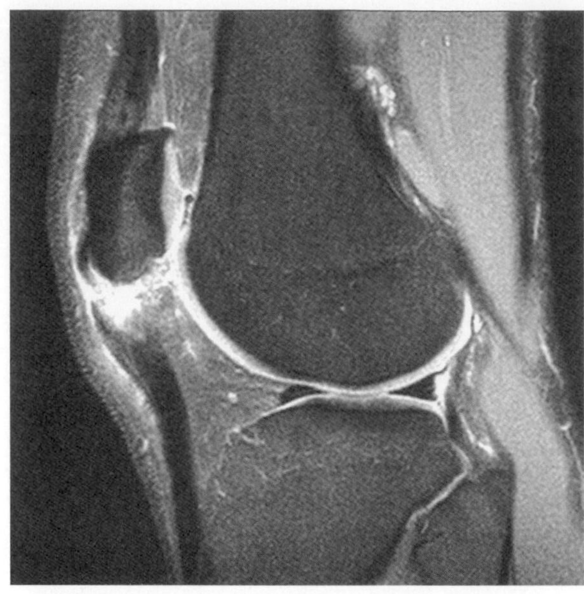

Figure 159-4 Sagittal magnetic resonance image of a patellar tendon rupture at the inferior pole of the patella.

Differential Diagnosis

- Quadriceps or patellar tendinitis
- Patellar fracture
- Partial tendon tear
- Metabolic disease

Treatment

- At diagnosis
  - Surgical repair is indicated in all but the most medically unstable patients for optimal return of function.
  - Patients should be immobilized in extension, instructed in crutch use with weight bearing as tolerated in extension, and referred for surgical intervention.
- Later
  - Surgery is best performed as soon as possible and certainly within 3 weeks.
  - Repair of the patella or quadriceps tendon is performed with anchors or bone tunnels in the patella.

When to Refer

- All patients with quadriceps or patellar tendon rupture should be referred on presentation and diagnosis of the rupture.

Prognosis

- Good for function, but often have residual discomfort and loss of flexion

Troubleshooting

- Beware of associated metabolic diseases.

Patient Instructions

- Avoid smoking during the postoperative period (3 months).
- Commit to postoperative rehabilitation.
- Adhere to postoperative deep venous thrombosis prevention exercises (ankle pumps).

Suggested Reading

- Albitar S, Chuet C: Bilateral spontaneous avulsion of quadriceps tendons. Nephrol Dial Transplant 1998;13:817.
- Kannus P, Józsa L: Histopathological changes preceding spontaneous rupture of a tendon. J Bone Joint Surg Am 1991;73:1507–1525.
- Webb LX, Toby EB: Bilateral rupture of the patella tendon in an otherwise healthy male patient following minor trauma. J Trauma 1986;26:1045–1048.
- Woo SL, Maynard J, Butler D: Ligament, tendon, and joint capsule insertions to bone. In Woo SL, Buckwalter JA (eds): Injury and Repair of the Musculoskeletal Soft Tissues. Park Ridge, IL: American Academy of Orthopaedic Surgeons, 1988, pp 133–166.

Chapter 160 Medial Tibial Stress Syndrome (Shin Splints)

Jason Blackham and Ned Amendola

ICD-9 CODE
844.9 *Shin Splints*

Key Concepts

- Medial tibial stress syndrome (MTSS) is characterized by pain and tenderness over the posteromedial middle and/or distal third of the tibia.
- Shin splints is a broad, nonspecific term that has been used to describe exertional leg pain over the anterior or medial tibia, anterior compartment, or lateral compartment.
- MTSS is one of the most common causes of exertional leg pain with an incidence of 13% to 17% of running injuries and 4% to 35% of military recruits in basic training.
- It is most common in repetitive running and jumping activities such as running, volleyball, basketball, and soccer. It is a cumulative overuse syndrome; symptoms become more severe with continued repetitive activity.
- The medial soleus muscle and crural fascia originate from the medial tibia in the area of symptoms. The flexor digitorum longus muscle also originates in the area and has been implicated in MTSS.
- The etiology of MTSS is not well understood. Theories include inflammation/periostitis, traction injury from the medial soleus muscle, and bone stress reaction.
- A benign stress fracture of the distal third of the tibia may be a continuum in severe recalcitrant cases of MTSS as a result of the bone stress reaction.
- Risk factors for MTSS include foot pronation during gait, rapid increase in training or training errors, training on hard surfaces, improper shoe wear, muscle imbalance between dorsiflexors and plantar flexors with decreased dorsiflexion, and a history of MTSS. The risk in women is twice that of men.

History

- Dull pain over the middle and/or distal third of the posteromedial tibia (Fig. 160-1). With increasing severity, the tenderness extends proximally over the soleal bridge.
- Early in MTSS, pain occurs at the beginning and/or end of exercise and resolves with rest.
- In severe cases, pain is more pronounced and persists throughout exercise.

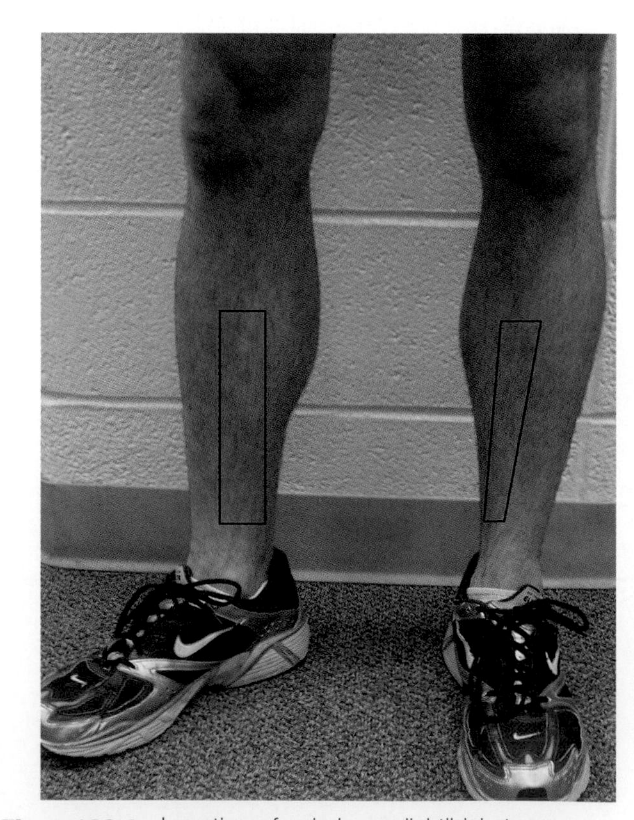

Figure 160-1 Location of pain in medial tibial stress syndrome along the posteromedial aspect of the middle and distal thirds of the tibia (*area shown by black boxes*). The right leg is externally rotated for clarity.

TABLE 160-1 *Differential Diagnosis for Exercise-related Leg Pain*

	MTSS	Stress Fracture	Exertional Compartment Syndrome	Popliteal Artery Entrapment
Pain	Exercise +/− rest	Exercise, rest, night	Exercise, gone 20 min after	Exercise: Claudication
Palpation	Diffuse	Focal	+/− with exercise	+/− with exercise
Percussion	Negative	Positive	Negative	Negative
Range-of-motion pain	Positive or negative	Positive or negative	Negative, +/− with exercise	Negative
Neurovascular	Normal	Normal	+/− with exercise	+/− with exercise
Bone scan	Diffuse	Focal	Negative	Negative
Magnetic resonance imaging	Bone diffuse	Bone focal	+/− in muscle compartment after exercise	Magnetic resonance arthrography or angiography

MTSS, medial tibial stress syndrome.

- Pain may be present with ambulation and at rest, not completely resolving after exercise, which is in contrast to exertional compartment syndrome, which usually subsides with rest (Table 160-1).

Physical Examination

- Observation
  - Evaluate for pes planus, hindfoot valgus, and foot pronation during stance.
- Palpation
  - Diffuse tenderness over the middle and/or distal third of the posteromedial tibia
  - With increasing severity, tenderness may extend proximally.
- Range of motion
  - Pain with stretching of the soleus muscle during passive ankle dorsiflexion or contraction of the soleus muscle during resisted ankle plantarflexion, standing toe raises, or jumping
  - With pes planus, tibialis posterior tendon tenderness may be present with resisted inversion.

Imaging

- Radiographs
  - Usually normal
  - Rarely, cortical hypertrophy or scalloping in the area of pain
- Bone scan and magnetic resonance imaging help differentiate stress fracture, stress reaction, and MTSS.
- Triple phase bone scan
  - Diffuse, longitudinal linear uptake along the posteromedial tibia in the delayed phase (Fig. 160-2)
- Magnetic resonance imaging
  - Periosteal edema, periosteal reaction, bone marrow edema, fascia or muscle inflammation (Figs. 160-3 and 160-4)

Differential Diagnosis (see Table 160-1)

- Exertional compartment syndrome
- Tibial stress fracture
- Popliteal artery entrapment
- Fascial hernia

Treatment

- At diagnosis
  - Conservative treatment is effective in most cases.
  - Modification of activity, with relative rest by cross-training and decreasing running volume, is the mainstay of therapy.
  - If pain continues to inhibit training, cease activity (absolute rest) until pain has disappeared, which may take 3 days to 3 weeks.
  - Correct training errors by decreasing mileage and modifying the training surface to avoid harder surfaces.
  - Modalities to decrease inflammation include ice, nonsteroidal anti-inflammatory drugs, local transcutaneous anti-inflammatory modalities, leg wraps, and ultrasound.

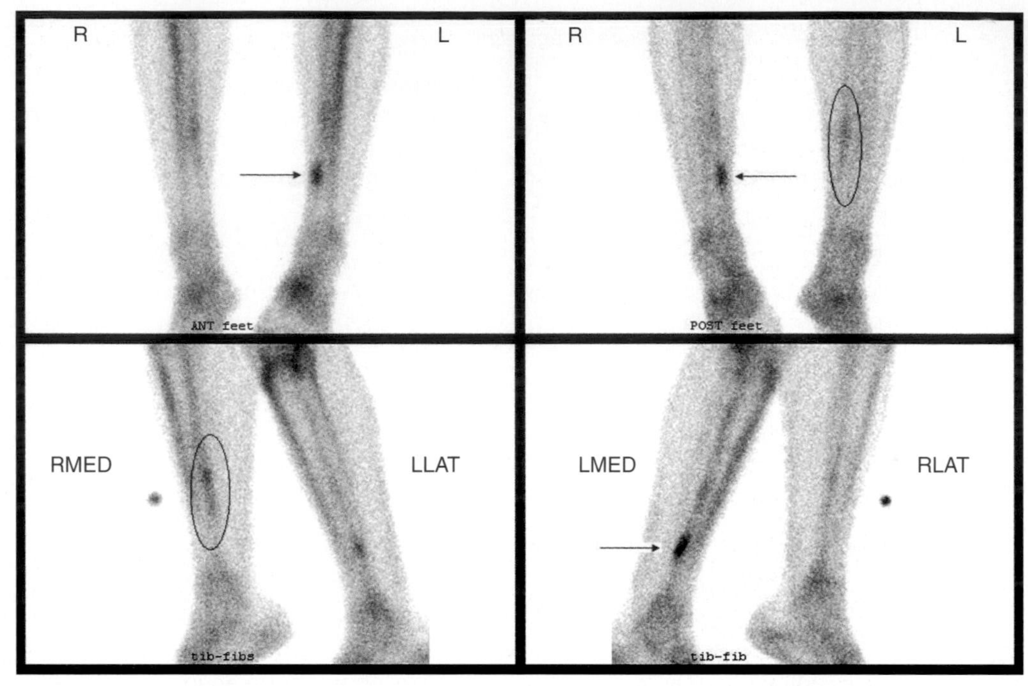

Figure 160-2 Delayed phase of triple-phase bone scan showing the difference between medial tibial stress syndrome (*right*) and stress fracture (*left*). The right posteromedial middle third of the tibia has diffuse linear uptake (*red circle*). The left distal posteromedial tibia has focal uptake (*arrows*). ANT, anterior view; fib, fibula; L, left; LLAT, left lateral view; LMED, left medial view; POST, posterior view; R, right; RLAT, right lateral view; RMED, right medial view; tib, tibia.

- Correct foot pronation with orthotics, supportive shoe wear, or taping.
- Stretching and global strengthening of the gastrocsoleus muscle, ankle dorsiflexors and plantarflexors, and foot invertors and evertors
- Later
  - Gradually increase mileage or activity with no more than 10% increase per week as long as asymptomatic

When to Refer

- If conservative treatment fails after 6 to 12 months, consider referral. Operative therapy with fasciotomy of the medial deep posterior compartment and periosteal stripping can be beneficial for cases in which conservative management has failed.

Prognosis

- Good with graduated rehabilitation program
- The majority will be able to return to the previous level of activity.
- Pain improves in more than 70% of those undergoing surgery.

Troubleshooting

- Avoid rapid conditioning, especially on hard surfaces.
- Pain may improve with taking a week off, and then gradually increasing activity.
- Imaging may be used when the diagnosis is in question and to distinguish between other entities.

Patient Instructions

- Discuss proper shoe wear, training modifications, and training errors.
- Cross-training can maintain cardiovascular fitness. However; if pain continues, absolute rest is indicated, followed by gradual progression of activity.
- Pain may recur in the future, especially after a period of inactivity (e.g., off-season followed by initiating training at the beginning of the next season).

Considerations in Special Populations

- MTSS may be more common in obese individuals.

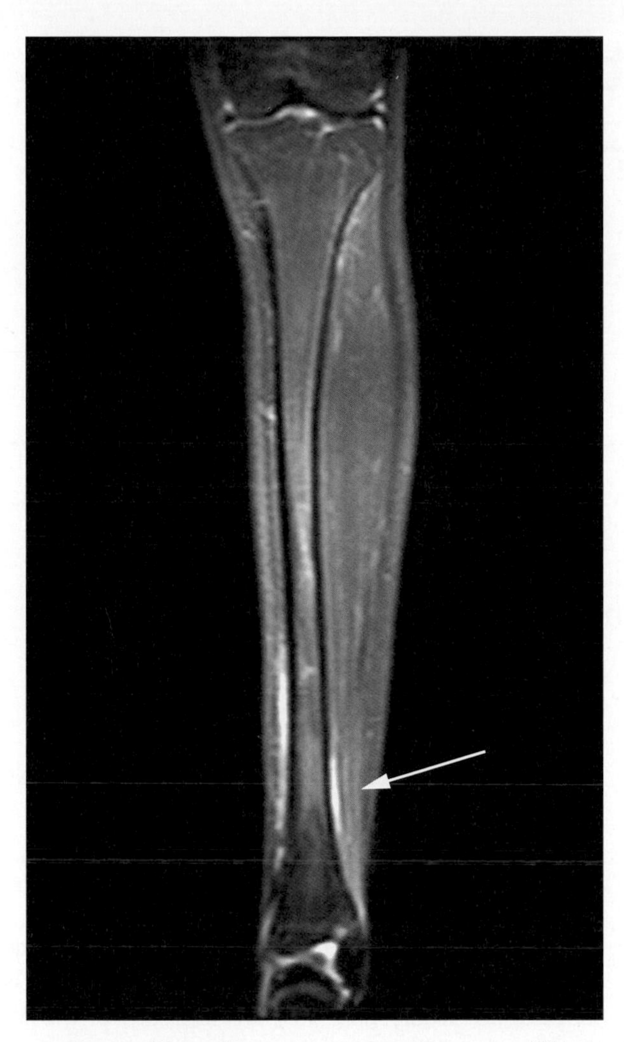

Figure 160-3 Magnetic resonance imaging coronal T1 short tau inversion recovery image of medial tibial stress syndrome. Note the periosteal and bone marrow edema (*arrow*) in the posteromedial middle and distal thirds of the tibia on the left side of the image.

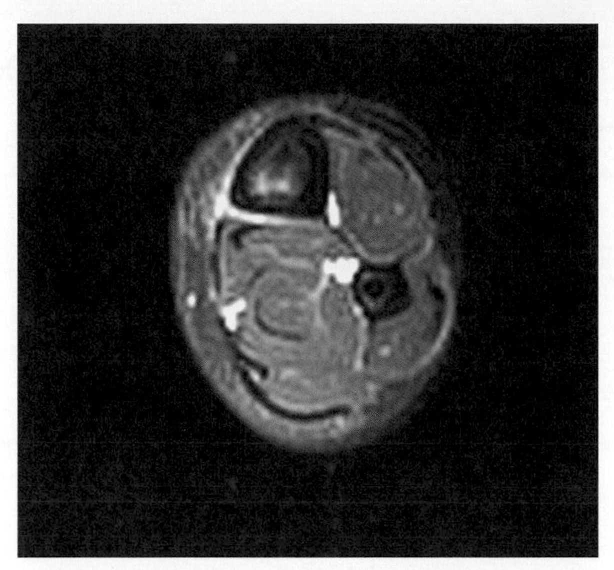

Figure 160-4 Magnetic resonance imaging axial T2-weighted fat-saturated image of medial tendon stress syndrome with periosteal edema at posteromedial corner of the tibia, posterior bone marrow edema, and soft-tissue edema medial to the tibia.

Suggested Reading

- Andrish JT, Bergfeld JA, Walheim J: A prospective study on the management of shin splints. J Bone Joint Surg Am 1974;56A:1697–1700.
- Batt ME, Ugalde V, Anderson MW, et al: A prospective controlled study of diagnostic imaging for acute shin splints. Med Sci Sports Exerc 1998;30:1564–1571.
- Beck BR, Osternig LR: Medial tibial stress syndrome: The location of muscles in the leg in relation to symptoms. J Bone Joint Surg Am 1994;76A:1057–1061.
- Detmer DE: Chronic shin splints. Classification and management of medial tibial stress syndrome. Sports Med 1986;3:436–446.
- Kortebein PM, Kaufman KR, Basford JR, et al: Medial tibial stress syndrome. Med Sci Sports Exerc 2000;32:S27–S33.
- Plisky MS: Medial tibial stress syndrome in high school cross-country runners: Incidence and risk factors. J Orthop Sports Phys Ther 2007;37:40–47.
- Van Mechelen W: Running injuries: A review of the epidemiological literature. Sports Med 1992;14:320–335.
- Yates B, Allen, MJ, Barnes MR: Outcome of surgical treatment of medial tibial stress syndrome. J Bone Joint Surg Am 2004;85A:1974–1980.
- Yates B, White S: The incidence and risk factors in the development of medial tibial stress syndrome among naval recruits. Am J Sports Med 2004;32:772–780.

Chapter 161 Exertional Compartment Syndrome

Robert P. Wilder

Key Concepts

- Chronic exertional compartment syndrome is defined as reversible ischemia secondary to a noncompliant osseofascial compartment that is unresponsive to the expansion of muscle volume that occurs with exercise.
- Most commonly seen in the lower leg, exertional compartment syndrome in athletes has also been described in the thigh and medial compartment of the foot.
- Several factors contribute to increased compartment pressures during exercise.
  - Enclosure of compartment contents in an inelastic fascial sheath
  - Increased volume of skeletal muscle due to blood flow and edema
  - Muscle hypertrophy
  - Myofiber damage from eccentric exercise causes release of protein-bound ions and subsequent increase in osmotic pressure.
- Increased compartment pressures have been identified in athletes taking creatine.
- There are four major compartments in the leg: the anterior compartment is most frequently involved, followed by the deep posterior, lateral, and superficial posterior compartments.
- Chronic compartment syndrome left untreated can develop into an acute syndrome.
- Resting intracompartmental pressure greater than 30 mmHg is associated with diminished blood flow and resultant muscle and nerve ischemia.
- Women may be more susceptible to chronic lower leg compartment syndrome.

History

- Tight, cramplike, squeezing pain localized over a specific compartment
- Symptoms typically occur at a well-defined and reproducible point of exercise (distance, time, or intensity) and increase if training persists. Relief of symptoms occurs with cessation of activity.
- Neurologic symptoms (paresthesias, weakness) may or may not occur.
- In some cases, the classic exertional component is not as evident and patients report pain at rest or with daily activities.

Physical Examination

- Observation
  - Swelling
- Palpation
  - Tightness and tenderness over involved compartments
  - Fascial hernia may be present.
- Special tests
  - Neurologic findings may be present.
- Anterior compartment: weakness of ankle dorsiflexion or toe extension (may include transient or persistent footdrop), sensory changes over dorsum of the foot (numbness in first web space)
- Deep posterior compartment: weakness of toe flexion and foot inversion, sensory changes on the plantar foot
- Lateral compartment: weakness of ankle eversion, sensory changes in the anterolateral leg
- Superficial posterior compartment: weakness of foot plantarflexion and sensory changes in dorsolateral foot

Imaging

- Radiographs, bone scan, or magnetic resonance imaging may identify stress fractures that may coexist with compartment syndrome.

Additional Tests

- Diagnosis based solely on clinical presentation can lead to misdiagnosis and therefore should be confirmed with exercise challenge and documentation of pressure elevation.
- Intracompartment pressure measurements are obtained at rest and after an exercise challenge (see

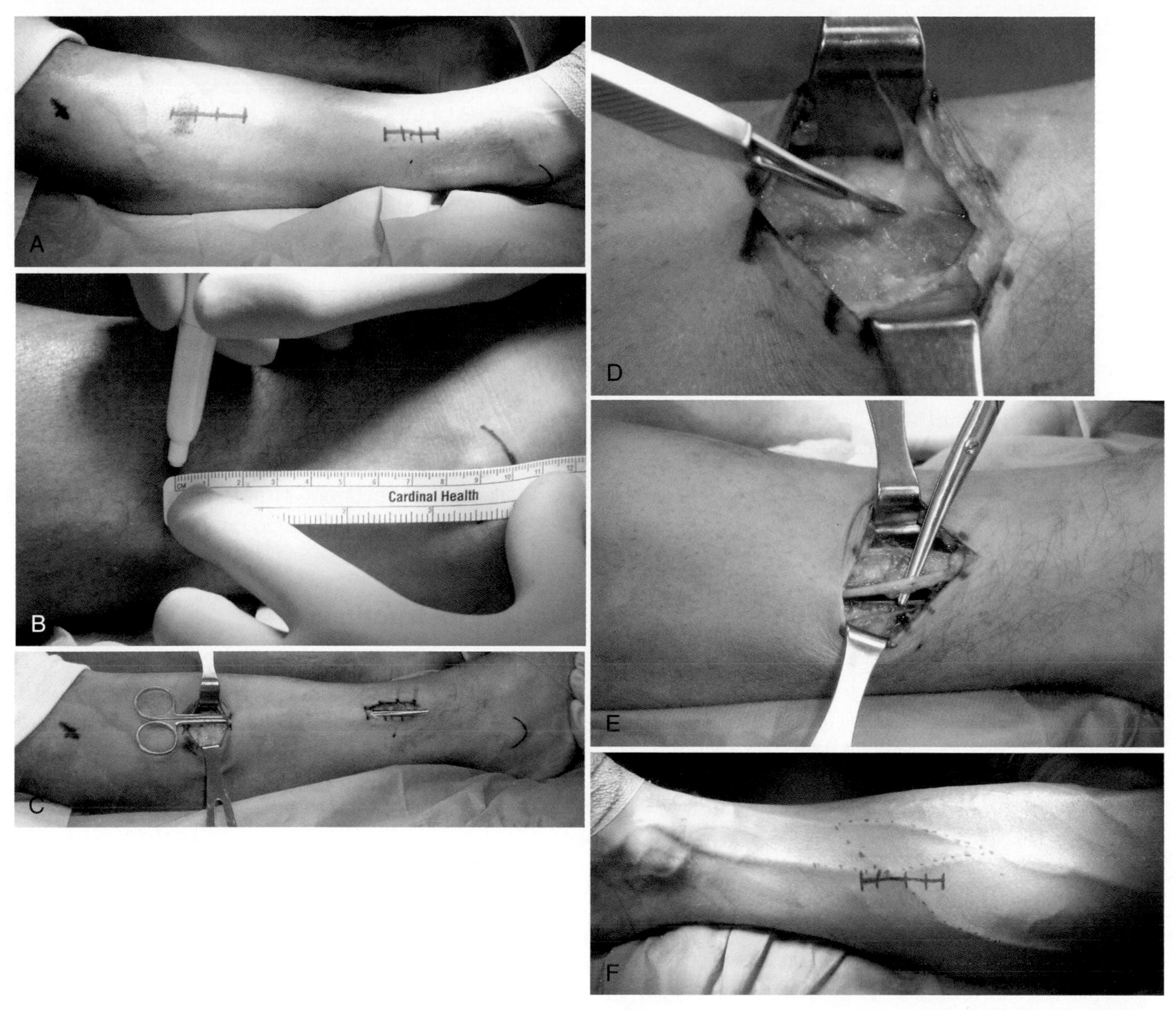

Figure 161-1 Surgical fasciotomy. **A**, Dual lateral incisions for release of the anterior and lateral compartments. **B**, The distal lateral incision is centered 10 to 12 cm proximal to the tip of the distal fibula, at the site where the superficial peroneal nerve penetrates the fascia. **C**, Blunt dissection produces subcutaneous connection of the incisions to allow adequate release of the compartments throughout their lengths. **D**, Anterior compartment fascial incision. The fascial incision is then extended proximally and distally under direct visualization. **E**, Superficial peroneal nerve after release of the anterior and lateral compartments. It is important to freely mobilize the nerve. **F**, Medial incision for release of the superficial and deep posterior compartments.

Chapter 171). Generally accepted pressure criteria suggesting compartment syndrome: before exercise, ≥15 mmHg; 1 minute after exercise, ≥30 mmHg; 5 minutes after exercise, ≥20 mmHg

Differential Diagnosis

- Shin splints
- Stress fracture
- Entrapment neuropathy
- Lumbar radiculopathy
- Spinal stenosis
- Popliteal artery entrapment syndrome
- Arterial insufficiency
- Deep venous thrombosis

Treatment

- At diagnosis
  - Conservative measures include relative rest (limiting activity to the level that avoids significant symptoms), anti-inflammatory drugs, stretching and strengthening of the involved muscles, and orthotics (particularly in cases of excessive pronation).

  - Some athletes may simply choose to refrain from the causative activity, which is a viable option provided they remain neurovascularly intact.
- Later
  - Surgical fasciotomy may alleviate persistent symptoms (Fig. 161-1). Single incision, double incision, and endoscopic techniques have been described. Fasciectomy has also been described and is used more often in revision surgery.
    - — Regardless of the technique chosen, fascial hernias must be included in the fascial incision and the superficial peroneal nerve must be released.
    - — Due to the high rate of coexistence, some authors advocate release of the lateral compartment whenever the anterior compartment is released.
    - — When performing deep posterior compartment release, attention must be given to adequate decompression of the tibialis posterior muscle.

When to Refer

- Referral for pressure measurements should be made when symptoms are present with daily activities, fail to abate with rest from athletic activity and conservative care, or in the presence of neurologic symptoms.
- Surgical remediation should be considered if symptoms persist despite 6 to 12 weeks of conservative care and in cases of extreme pressure elevation (resting pressures > 30 mmHg) or focal motor weakness.

Prognosis

- Early diagnosis and management are critical to minimize the risk for muscle necrosis or permanent neurologic deficit.
- Good to excellent results have been reported in 60% to 96% of patients after fasciotomy.
- The best results are obtained if surgery is performed within 12 months of symptom onset.
- Patients undergoing anterior release have a higher rate of satisfactory results than those undergoing deep posterior release.
- For unclear reasons, women may respond less favorably to fasciotomy than men.

Troubleshooting

- All potentially involved compartments must be tested; failure to identify all involved compartments is a cause for failure of surgical remediation.
- Potential complications may include bleeding, damage to neurologic structures, and recurrent symptoms.
- Patients with recurrent symptoms may require fasciectomy in addition to fasciotomy.

Patient Instructions

- Activity should be limited to the level at which symptoms are considered mild and abate within minutes of activity cessation.
- Activity should not produce weakness or limping.
- Cross-training may be substituted for running when necessary.

Suggested Reading

- Glorioso J, Wilckens J: Compartment syndrome testing. In O'Connor F, Wilder R (eds): The Textbook of Running Medicine. New York: McGraw-Hill, 2001, pp 95–100.
- Glorioso J, Wilckens J: Exertional leg pain. In O'Connor F, Wilder R (eds): The Textbook of Running Medicine. New York: McGraw-Hill, 2001, pp 181–198.
- Pedowitz RA, Hargens AR, Mubarak SJ, et al: Modified criteria for the objective diagnosis of chronic compartment syndrome of the leg. Am J Sports Med 1990;18:35–40.
- Wilder R, Sethi S: Overuse injuries: Tendinopathies, stress fractures, compartment syndrome, and shin splints. Clin Sports Med 2004;23:55–81.

Chapter 162 Medial Gastrocnemius Rupture (Tennis Leg)

Jason Blackham and Ned Amendola

ICD-9 CODES

844.9 *Sprain and Strain, Unspecified Site of Knee and Leg*

728.84 *Rupture of Muscle, Nontraumatic*

Key Concepts

- Tennis leg is a complete or partial tear of the medial head of the gastrocnemius muscle at the distal musculotendinous junction (Fig. 162-1).
- It usually occurs in running or jumping, with sudden cutting or stopping.
- The term is attributed to the tennis motion of fully extending the knee with sudden ankle dorsiflexion causing maximum eccentric stress on the calf.
- It is most common in men in the fourth to sixth decades and in the poorly conditioned sports enthusiast.

History

- Eccentric load to the medial gastrocnemius muscle with the knee extended and the ankle dorsiflexed
- Sharp pain in the calf with or without audible "pop"
- Often describe feeling of being hit in the calf by an object such as a ball
- At least 20% of patients have calf pain for 1 to 2 days before the acute injury.
- Ambulation after the injury causes pain.

Physical Examination

- Observation
  - Swelling and ecchymosis over the gastrocnemius muscle within 24 to 48 hours
  - Antalgic gait
  - Ankle held in plantarflexion
- Palpation
  - Point of tenderness over the medial head of the gastrocnemius muscle
  - Palpable defect at the musculotendinous junction (see Fig. 162-1)
- Range of motion
  - Passive ankle dorsiflexion elicits pain.
  - Ankle plantarflexion and single leg toe raise are weak and painful.

Imaging

- Clinical diagnosis: Imaging may be performed when the diagnosis is in question.
- Ultrasonography
  - Identifies disruption of the musculotendinous junction and may be used to document healing progression
  - Distinguishes deep venous thrombosis

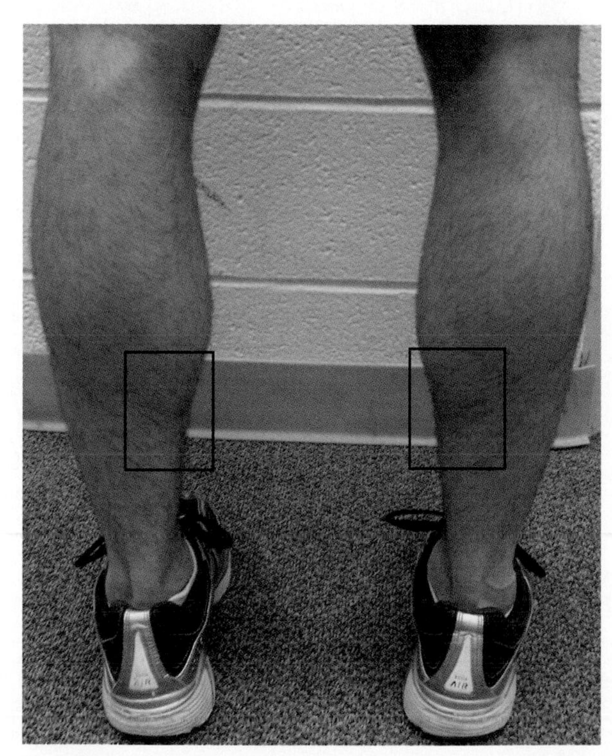

Figure 162-1 Location of medial gastrocnemius strain or tear (tennis leg) as demarcated by *boxes.*

- Magnetic resonance imaging
  - May also be used for diagnosis
  - In chronic cases, local scarring may be visualized.

Differential Diagnosis

- Deep venous thrombosis
- Thrombophlebitis
- Posterior compartment syndrome
- Plantar tendon rupture
- Achilles tendon rupture

Treatment

- At diagnosis
  - Conservative management is the mainstay of treatment.
  - Rest, ice, compression, and elevation for 24 to 72 hours. Compression has been shown by ultrasonography to decrease the fluid collection between the soleus and gastrocnemius muscles, allowing a quicker return to ambulation.
  - If pain with ambulation, crutches or heel lift recommended until pain free (usually 3 days to 2 weeks); weight-bearing ambulation should be started as soon as tolerated.
  - When able to perform range of motion without pain, progress to passive stretching exercises and then to standing stretching.
  - Other authors endorse keeping the ankle in a position of maximal dorsiflexion without pain as a means of increasing the rate of healing.
- Later
  - When able to perform pain-free stretching, usually by 2 weeks, begin plantarflexion and dorsiflexion strengthening exercises; may also begin stationary cycling, electrical stimulation, and cross-frictional massage
  - As strength and range of motion improve to nearly normal, advance to sport-specific activities.
  - After recovering full range of motion and strength of at least 90% compared with the opposite side, return to sport participation.

When to Refer

- If continued pain beyond the expected 2 to 6 weeks, or recurrent injury, consider referral
- In the acute setting, if any clinical suspicion of compartment syndrome, refer for measurement of compartment pressures and possible fasciotomy

Prognosis

- The prognosis after medial gastrocnemius injury for recovery and return to participation with a staged rehabilitation program is good with a low recurrence rate.

Troubleshooting

- Healing is quicker, resulting in less time lost from sport, if treated within the first 48 hours.
- Avoid using nonselective nonsteroidal anti-inflammatory drugs in the first 48 hours of injury, because these drugs may lead to increased bleeding and swelling in the area.
- Heel lifts help relieve pain in the initial stages of healing. Gradually taper the thickness of the heel lift until it is no longer needed.
- If rehabilitation is inadequate, scar tissue (which is weaker than muscle) may become reinjured, resulting in chronic or repeated strains.
  - Cross-frictional massage, stretching, and eccentric strengthening may be beneficial in reducing scar tissue.

Patient Instructions

- If the patient is seen in the initial 48 hours, tell the patient that extensive ecchymosis and swelling will likely occur.
- Expect approximately 2 weeks for a minor strain and at least 6 weeks for a major injury before return to full participation.
- Discuss the rehabilitation process so that the patient knows what to expect during recovery.
- The patient should continue strengthening and stretching exercises for several months after the injury to avoid re-injury.
- Re-tears are uncommon, although they do occur. The injury may also occur in the contralateral leg.

Considerations in Special Populations

- Geriatric patients may sprain or tear the medial gastrocnemius muscle by stepping out of a car or out of bed.
- The injury is not common in athletes younger than 19 years old.

Suggested Reading

- Delgado GJ, Chung CB, Lektrakul N, et al: Tennis leg: Clinical US study of 141 patients and anatomic investigation of four cadavers with MR imaging and US. Radiology 2002;224:112–119.

- Fromison AI: Tennis leg. JAMA 1969;209:415–416.
- Garrick JG: Tennis leg: How I manage gastrocnemius strains. Phys Sports Med 1992;20:203–207.
- Hutchinson MR, Laprade RF, Burnett QM, et al: Injury surveillance at the USTA boys' tennis championships: A 6-year study. Med Sci Sports Exerc 1995;27:826–830.
- Kwak HS, Lee KB, Han YM: Ruptures of the medial head of the gastrocnemius ("tennis leg"): clinical outcomes and compression effect. J Clinical Imaging 2006;30:48–53.
- Miller AP: Strains of the posterior calf musculature ("tennis leg"). Am J Sports Med 1979;7:172–174.
- Shields CL, Redix L, Brewster CE: Acute tears of the medial head of the gastrocnemius. Foot Ankle 1985;5:186–190.

Chapter 163 Stress Fractures of the Tibia and Fibula

Jason Blackham and Ned Amendola

ICD-9 CODE
733.93 *Stress Fracture of the Tibia or Fibula*

Key Concepts

- The tibia is the most common site of stress fracture (25% to 46%), followed by the fibula (5% to 12%).
- Most tibia stress fractures occur in the proximal third (volleyball, basketball), followed by the distal and middle thirds (runners).
- The "dreaded black line" is a mid-shaft anterior tibia stress fracture seen on the lateral radiograph. It is notorious for delayed healing, with a high nonunion rate, and represents the majority of operatively treated stress fractures (Fig. 163-1).
- Most stress fractures of the fibula occur in the distal third.
- High-risk stress fractures in the leg (under tension) include the anterior tibia and medial malleolus. Low-risk areas (under compression) include the posteromedial tibia and fibula.
- The pathophysiology of stress fractures involves accumulated stress to the bone without adequate time for repair, causing failure of bone remodeling.
- A stress reaction is a precursor to stress fracture with periosteal and bone marrow edema but no fracture line.
- Risk factors include younger age, white race, female gender, exercise-induced amenorrhea, recent increase in intensity/duration of exercise, previous inactivity, foot pronation, training on hard or uneven surfaces, previous stress fracture, and narrow intramedullary canal.

History

- Exertional pain of insidious onset after a change in activity level
- Exercise makes the pain worse, but the pain does not go away with rest.
- Night pain possible
- Pain localized over a discrete area of bone
- Important to ask about a history of stress fractures

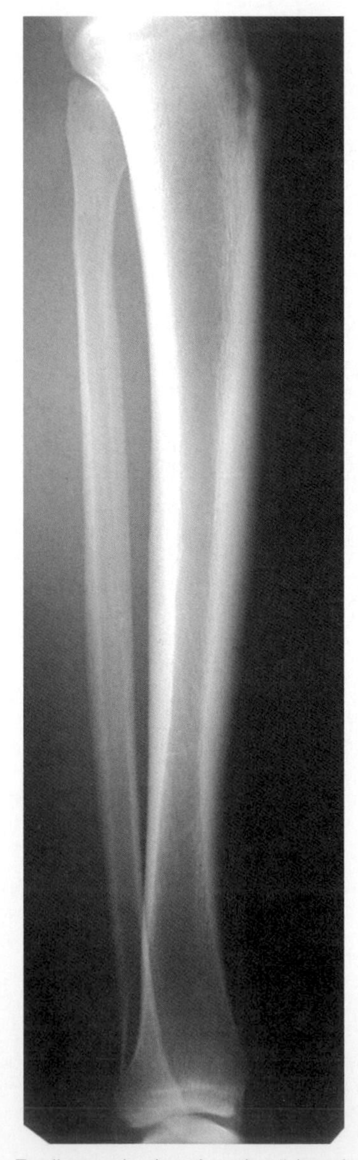

Figure 163-1 Radiograph showing the "dreaded black line" of an anterior tibia stress fracture with a thickened anterior cortex and a lucent line.

Physical Examination

- Observation
  - Antalgic gait with walking or running
  - Focal swelling over the fracture site
- Palpation
  - Localized point tenderness
  - Periosteal edema or palpable bump
- Special tests
  - Hop test: Hopping on one leg causes pain at the site of stress fracture.
  - Tuning fork test: Vibration causes pain over the fracture site.
  - Percussion test: Percussion of the bone at a site distant from the injury causes pain.
  - Neurovascular examination is normal.

Imaging

- Radiographs
  - Only 20% to 30% positive at presentation; 50% later in the course
  - Focal sclerosis, periosteal reaction, and cortical thickening (Fig. 163-2)
  - Dreaded black line: linear transverse lucency in the anterior tibial cortex on the lateral view (see Fig. 163-1)
  - If negative, consider repeating in 2 to 4 weeks or obtain additional studies.
- Bone scan
  - Focal area of uptake (versus diffuse linear uptake in medial tibial stress syndrome)
  - Gold standard for diagnosis: highly sensitive, less specific
  - More radiation exposure and more time-consuming than magnetic resonance imaging
- Magnetic resonance imaging
  - Periosteal edema, bone marrow edema, and fracture line (Figs. 163-3 to 163-6)
  - Distinguishes between soft-tissue and bone injury
- Computed tomography
  - May be used to define fracture lines or distinguish a fracture from other diagnoses
  - May show evidence of healing with resolution of the lucency or bone sclerosis

Differential Diagnosis (see Table 160-1)

- Medial tibial stress syndrome
- Exertional compartment syndrome
- Fascial hernia

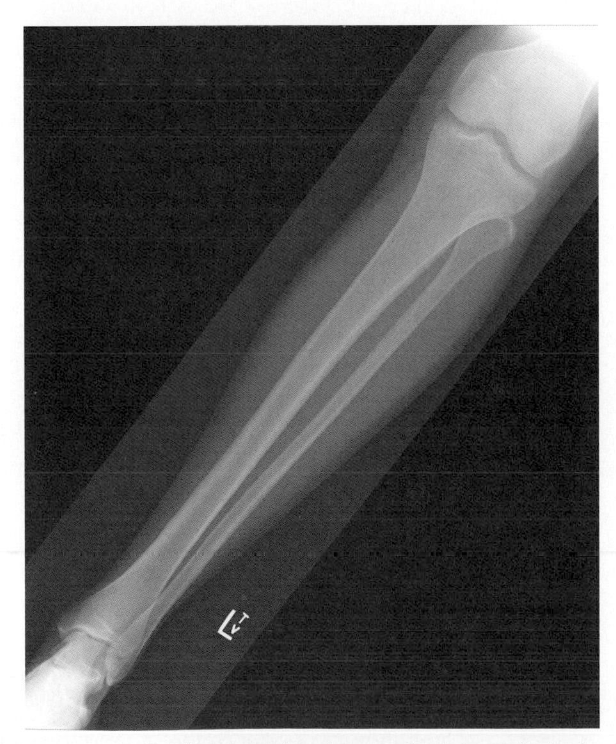

Figure 163-2 Radiograph showing scalloping, periosteal thickening, and cortical thickening at the medial distal tibia consistent with a stress fracture.

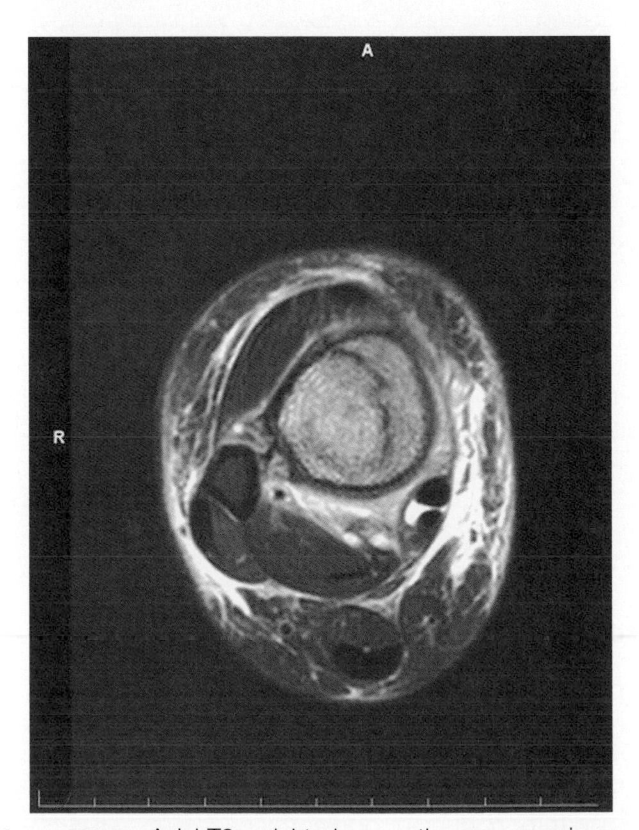

Figure 163-3 Axial T2-weighted magnetic resonance image showing a tibia stress fracture with the fracture line and severe periosteal and bone marrow edema.

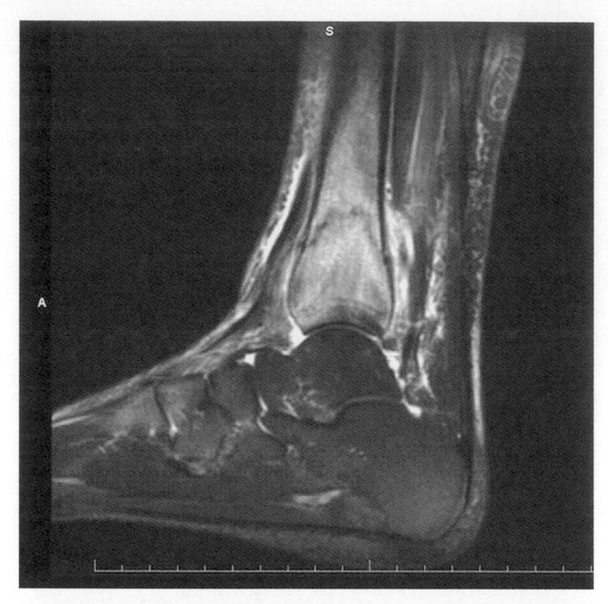

Figure 163-4 Sagittal T2-weighted magnetic resonance image showing a tibia stress fracture with the fracture line and severe periosteal and bone marrow edema.

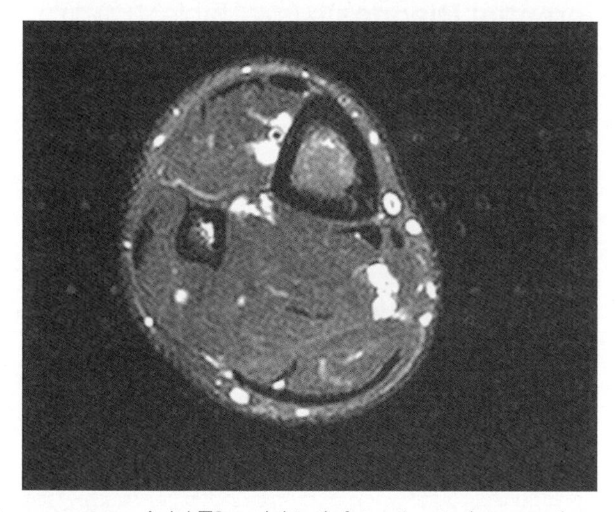

Figure 163-5 Axial T2-weighted, fat-saturated magnetic resonance image showing bone marrow edema with adjacent cortical thickening of the lateral fibula consistent with stress reaction.

- Neoplasm
- Nerve entrapment

Treatment

- At diagnosis
  - Treatment varies depending on the fracture site.
  - Less aggressive treatment of high-risk stress fractures may result in progression to complete fracture, nonunion, or recurrence.
  - Low-risk stress fractures tend to heal with activity modification and nonaggressive treatment.

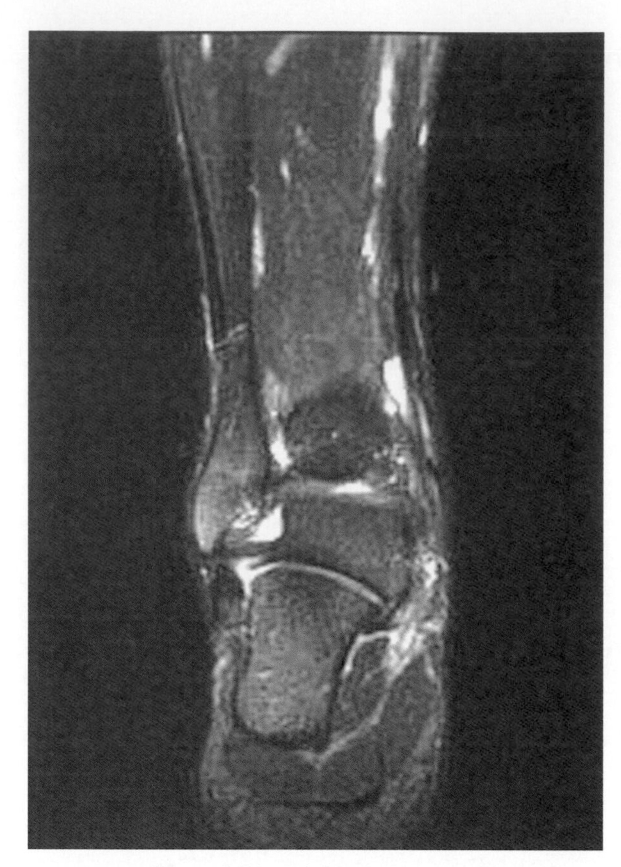

Figure 163-6 Coronal T2-weighted, fat-saturated magnetic resonance image showing bone marrow edema with cortical thickening of the lateral fibula consistent with stress reaction.

- Nonsteroidal anti-inflammatory drugs and physical therapy modalities help control pain.
  - — Anterior tibia (high-risk): strict avoidance of weight bearing; use crutches, casting, or bracing for 3 to 12 weeks
    - — If there is a clear fracture line or failed nonoperative treatment, operative treatment is indicated with intramedullary nailing.
    - — Other surgical techniques include drilling or excising the fracture site with or without bone grafting and tension-band plating.
  - — Posteromedial tibia or fibula (low risk): Treatment depends on the athlete's goals, functional limitations, and timing of the season.
    - — If no limitations and pain not progressive, activity level may be continued to complete the season
    - — If functional limitation due to pain, activity modification with relative rest (cross-training)
    - — If limitations in walking due to pain, bracing or crutches may be used with cross-training to remain pain free

- Later
  - Anterior tibia stress fractures should be healed and have painless activity before return to sport (typically 3–6 months).
  - After surgical management, the patient may weight bear as tolerated.
  - Crutches and bracing are discontinued as soon as symptoms allow, followed by a gradual progression of activity based on symptoms.
  - For low-risk stress fractures, gradually advance activity as tolerated to remain pain free.
    - If fracture does not heal with activity modification, implement complete rest, immobilization, or surgical treatment.

When to Refer

- Patients with high-risk stress fractures, low-risk stress fractures with progressive pain despite conservative treatment, and recurrent stress fractures should be referred.

Prognosis

- An anterior tibia stress fracture may take 6 to 12 months to heal, even with surgery and can be a career-ending injury for a high-performance athlete.
  - Complications of intramedullary nailing include anterior knee pain, recurrent fracture, progression to complete fracture, nonunion, and infection.
- Fibula and posteromedial tibia stress fractures generally heal in 4 to 9 weeks with appropriate-level rest.
- Stress reactions (no definite fracture line) usually heal more quickly in 3 to 6 weeks.

Troubleshooting

- Worsening pain at a previously comfortable level should prompt investigation for progression of the fracture.
- Search for training errors that may be changed to avoid future injury because training errors are the most common cause of stress injuries.
- Pneumatic leg braces may be effective in speeding healing, decreasing pain, and returning to activity earlier.
- Bone stimulators may help to heal stress fractures.

Patient Instructions

- For an anterior tibia stress fracture, counsel the patient about the risk of progression to complete fracture and the prolonged recovery period so that activity is not advanced too early.

Considerations in Special Populations

- Stress fractures in female athletes require assessment for female athletic triad including menstrual history, nutritional assessment, and consideration of bone density testing.
- For recurrent stress fractures, consider a laboratory workup for metabolic bone disease, bone density testing, and nutritional assessment.

Suggested Reading

- Bennell KL, Malcolm SA, Thomas SA, et al: The incidence and distribution of stress fractures in competitive track and field athletes. A twelve-month prospective study. Am J Sports Med 1996;24:211–217.
- Brukner P, Bradshaw C, Khan KM, et al: Stress fractures: A review of 180 cases. Clin J Sport Med 1996;6:85–89.
- Fredericson M, Bergman AG, Hoffman KL, et al: Tibial stress reaction in runners. Correlation of clinical symptoms and scintigraphy with a new magnetic resonance imaging grading system. Am J Sports Med 1995;23:472–481.
- Iwamoto J, Takeda T: Stress fractures in athletes: Review of 196 cases. J Orthop Sci 2003;8:273–278.
- Jones BH, Thacker SB, Gilchrist J, et al: Epidemiol Rev 2002; 24:228–247.
- Kaeding CC, Yu JR, Wright R, et al: Management and return to play of stress fractures. Clin J Sport Med 2005;15:442–447.
- Rome K, Handoll HHG, Ashford R: Interventions for preventing and treating stress fractures and stress reactions of bone of the lower limbs in young adults. Cochrane Database Syst Rev 2005;2:CD000450.
- Swensen EJ, DeHaven KE, Sebastianelli WJ, et al: The effect of pneumatic leg brace on return to play in athletes with tibial stress fractures. Am J Sports Med 1997;25:322–328.
- Varner KE, Younas SA, Lintner DM, et al: Chronic anterior midtibial stress fractures in athletes treated with reamed intramedullary nailing. Am J Sports Med 2005;33:1071–1076.

Chapter 164 Distal Femur and Proximal Tibia Fractures

Franklin D. Shuler and Claire F. Beimesch

ICD-9 CODES

821.23 *Supracondylar Fracture of Femur, Closed*
821.33 *Supracondylar Fracture of Femur, Open*
823.00 *Tibia Condyles or Tuberosity Fracture, Closed*
823.10 *Tibia Condyles or Tuberosity Fracture, Open*

Key Concepts

- Supracondylar femur fractures involve the distal femoral metaphysis with or without intra-articular extension.
- Tibial plateau fractures are intra-articular fractures of the proximal tibia.
- Radiographs and computed tomography are essential to characterize intra-articular extension (Fig. 164-1).
- Supracondylar femur fractures occurring proximal to total knee arthroplasty components are classified as periprosthetic fractures (Fig. 164-2).
- Open supracondylar femur fractures are frequently associated with an additional coronal (Hoffa) fracture of the femoral condyle (Fig. 164-3).
- Tibial plateau fractures are classified as lateral (most common), medial, or bicondylar plateau fractures. The Schatzker classification is most helpful (Fig. 164-4).
- High-energy tibial plateau fractures can be associated with neurovascular injuries or compartment syndrome; both are indications for immediate surgical referral.
- Knee ligament and meniscal injuries are common.
- All periarticular knee fractures require referral to an orthopaedic surgeon.

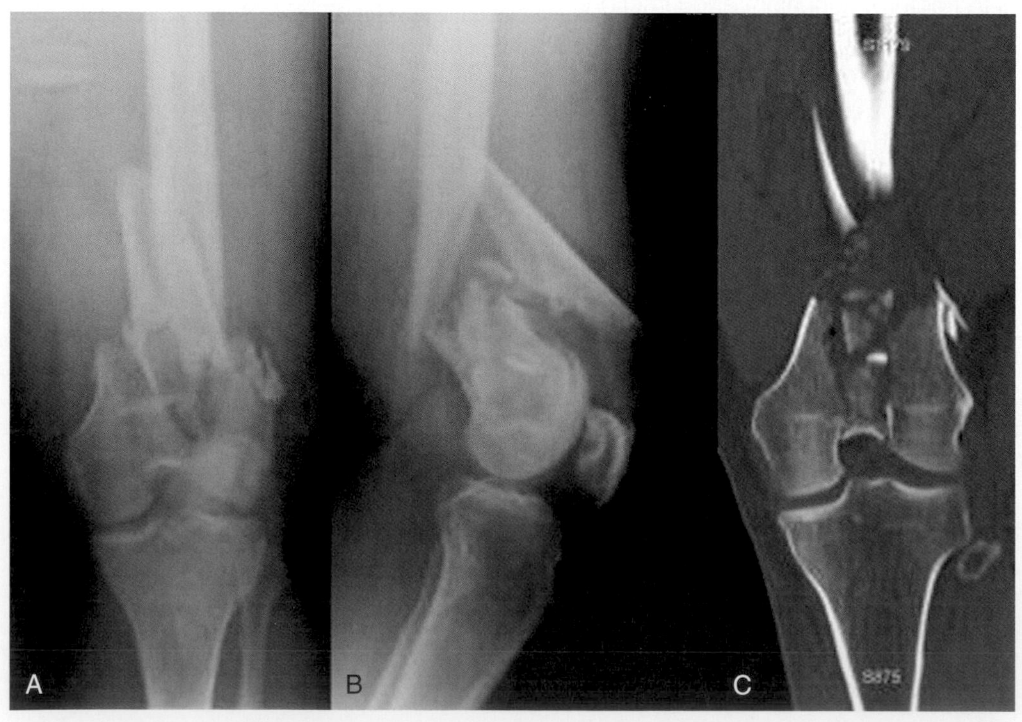

Figure 164-1 Open comminuted supracondylar femur fracture with intercondylar extension. Anteroposterior (**A**) and lateral (**B**) radiographs. **C**, Computed tomography demonstrating the intra-articular extension.

History

- High-energy mechanism (e.g., motor vehicle collision, polytrauma) in young patients
- Low-energy mechanisms are common in older patients (see Fig. 164-2).
- Pain, swelling, and inability to bear weight
- Possible neurovascular symptoms
- If previous total knee arthroplasty, history of postoperative course is critical (infection, deep venous thrombosis, pulmonary embolism, range of motion, ambulatory ability, pain, instability)

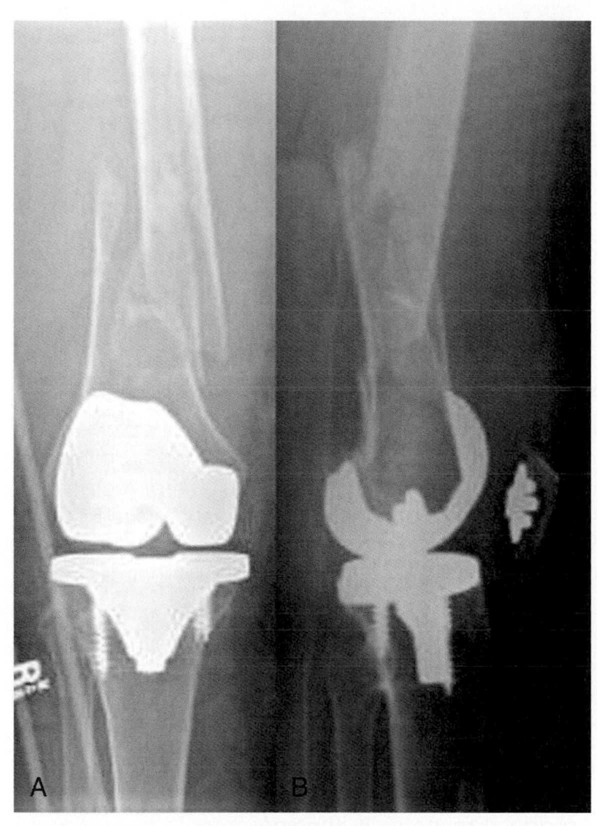

Figure 164-2 Periprosthetic distal femur fracture. Anteroposterior (**A**) and lateral (**B**) radiographs demonstrating fracture above a well-fixed total knee arthroplasty.

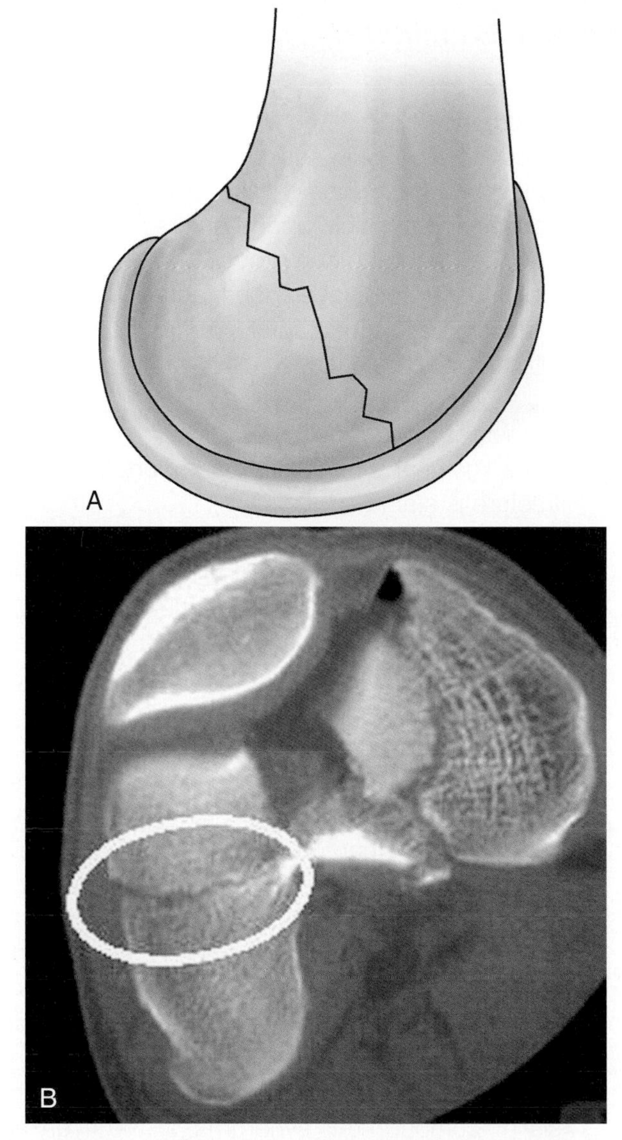

Figure 164-3 Hoffa fracture. Coronal shear injury of the femoral condyle, common in open fractures. **A**, Lateral diagram of fracture orientation. **B**, Computed tomography image of an open supracondylar femur fracture showing the coronal fracture fragment (*circle*).

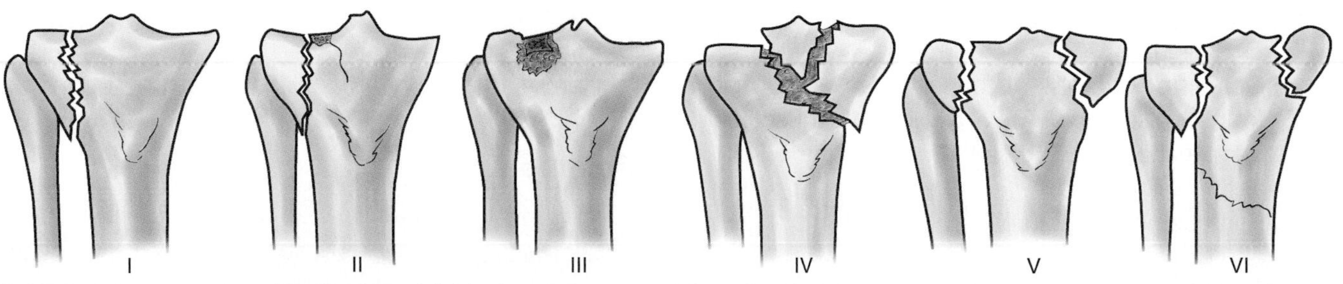

Figure 164-4 Schatzker classification of tibial plateau fractures. I, lateral split; II, lateral split depression; III, lateral isolated depression; IV, medial; V, bicondylar; VI, bicondylar with metadiaphyseal dissociation.

Physical Examination

- Observation
  - Deformity
  - Circumferential skin assessment: Any blood, lacerations, or surrounding skin trauma must raise concern for possible open fracture.
  - Fracture blisters: A compromised soft-tissue envelope (i.e., blisters, lacerations, abrasions, previous surgical incision for a total knee arthroplasty) can alter the surgical plan.
- Palpation
  - Tenderness and crepitus
  - Knee ligament examination is important after the fracture is stabilized.
- Special tests
  - Advanced Trauma Life Support protocol when indicated in a trauma setting, including secondary survey to assess for additional skeletal trauma and complete neurovascular examination.
  - Posterior tibial and dorsalis pedis pulses: use Doppler if nonpalpable
  - The ankle-brachial index measures systolic pressure at the ankle compared with the upper extremity. Values less than 0.9 indicate a high probability of arterial injury, possibly requiring arteriography and/or vascular surgery consultation (Fig. 164-5). There is a 2% to 3% incidence of vascular disruptions in the fractures.
  - The neurologic examination may be compromised in an obtunded patient.
  - Compartment syndrome evaluation: If the diagnosis of compartment syndrome of the thigh and bone is established, emergent fasciotomy is recommended.

Imaging

- Radiographs: anteroposterior, lateral, and 45-degree oblique views of the knee
  - Traction (manual or external fixator) will aid in fracture visualization (Fig. 164-6).
  - Evaluate fracture displacement and intra-articular extension.
  - Obtain radiographs of the joint above and below for associated injuries. A proximal tibia fracture in combination with a distal femur fracture is known as a floating knee.
  - Periprosthetic fractures require full-length femur and/or tibia radiographs.
  - The Schatzker classification system is commonly used for tibial plateau fractures (see Fig. 164-4).

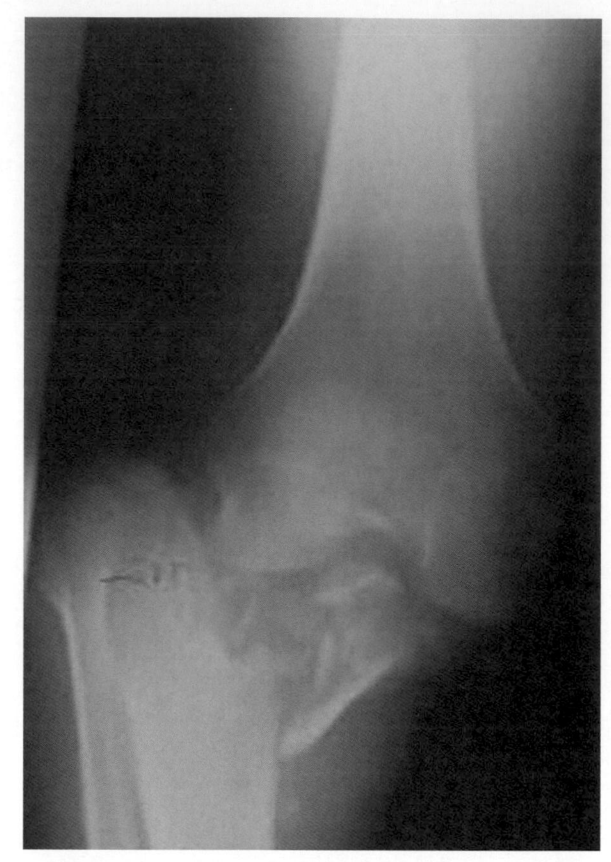

Figure 164-5 Anteroposterior radiograph of comminuted, high-energy, medial tibial plateau fracture (Schatzker grade IV). The patient had a vascular injury at the level of the popliteal fossa that was detected after reduction and ankle-brachial index determination (ankle-brachial index < 0.9). This patient required hospital admission and urgent orthopaedic referral.

- Computed tomography with coronal and sagittal reconstructions
  - Mandatory to characterize intra-articular extension and articular depression (see Figs. 164-1 and 164-3).
- Magnetic resonance imaging detects associated ligamentous and meniscal injuries.

Differential Diagnosis

- Distal femoral or proximal tibial shaft fracture
- Knee dislocation
- Pathologic fracture
- Compartment syndrome without fracture

Treatment

- Initial management
  - Reduce and stabilize fracture to limit further soft-tissue injury with a padded, well-molded, long leg splint.

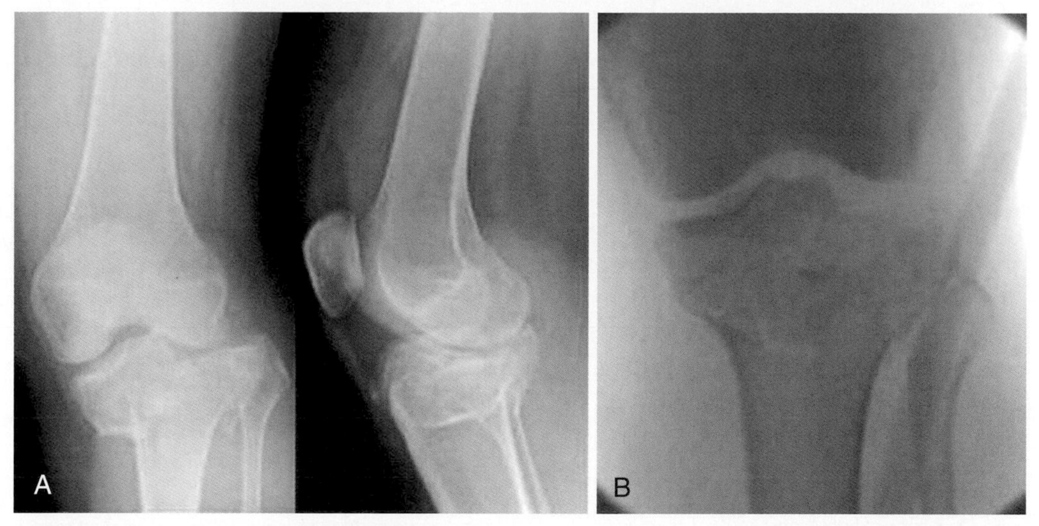

Figure 164-6 Bicondylar tibia plateau fracture (Schatzker grade V). **A**, Anteroposterior and lateral radiographs demonstrating subluxation of the knee. **B**, Radiograph obtained after application of temporizing external fixation (traction). This image assists with preoperative planning. Computed tomography should also be performed with the knee in a reduced position.

- Open fractures first require a sterile saline dressing in addition to appropriate antibiotic and tetanus prophylaxis (Tables 166-2 and 166-3). Do not irrigate or probe the wound, remove bone fragments, apply tourniquets or clamps for vascular injury (address with direct pressure), or perform wound closure. After splint application, repeat physical examination and obtain radiographs and perform computed tomography. Patients with high-energy fractures should be admitted and monitored for compartment syndrome with serial examinations for 24 hours.
- Definitive management
  - Definitive treatment is determined by consulting an orthopaedic surgeon.
  - Nonoperative treatment is indicated for isolated, nondisplaced, extra-articular distal femur fractures and isolated lateral tibial plateau fractures with less than 3 mm of articular step-off and less than 10 degrees of varus/valgus instability.
    - — A locked hinged knee brace and no weight bearing for 6 to 12 weeks are required.
    - — Knee range of motion is initiated at 2 to 4 weeks.
    - — Occasionally, nonoperative treatment is also selected for nonambulatory patients with advanced medical conditions.
    - — Physical therapy is essential as are serial radiographs to ensure proper alignment.
    - — Consider deep venous thrombosis prophylaxis with injectable low molecular weight heparin or aspirin.
  - Operative treatment is required for all other distal femur and tibial plateau fractures.
    - — Temporizing external fixation is performed on all fractures with residual knee subluxation after traction and splinting.
    - — The duration of temporizing fixation ranges from 1 to 6 weeks and is generally dictated by the soft tissues (i.e., fracture blisters).
    - — When the soft tissues improve, the treating surgeon will decide between definitive open reduction and internal fixation versus other treatment methods.

When to Refer

- All patients with supracondylar femur or tibial plateau fractures require referral.
- Delayed referral can be considered in patients with low-energy injuries, adequate reduction, soft compartments, and intact neurovascular status.
- Emergent orthopaedic surgical consultation is required for open fractures, neurovascular injury, severe fracture displacement (e.g., Schatzker grade IV, V, VI) or knee subluxation requiring external fixation (see Figs. 164-5 and 164-6), and/or impending or established compartment syndrome.

Prognosis

- Varies from simple fracture patterns with minimal soft-tissue damage to severe limb-threatening injuries associated with neurologic, vascular, muscle, and skin damage

- The prognosis also varies depending on patient comorbidities.
- Timely antibiotic administration in open fractures is considered to improve the prognosis.

Troubleshooting

- Delayed unions should be evaluated for the presence of infection (complete blood count with differential, erythrocyte sedimentation rate, and C-reactive protein) and are often associated with high-energy injuries and poor host factors (i.e., nicotine use, diabetes).
- Fracture complications include malunion, nonunion, posttraumatic arthritis, nerve injury, vascular injury, deep venous thrombosis, pulmonary embolism, fat embolism, pain, weakness, and knee stiffness. Additional surgery-related complications include infection, hardware failure, and wound-healing issues.

Patient Instructions

- Patients should be counseled on weight-bearing restrictions, splint care, extremity elevation, and deep venous thrombosis prophylaxis.
- Patients should return or call if increased pain, swelling, or neurovascular changes.

Considerations in Special Populations

- Individuals who are at high risk of complication from anesthesia may benefit from non-operative management.
- Non-operative treatment may be considered in patients with low functional demands (i.e., non-ambulatory patients).

Suggested Reading

- Barei DP, Nork SE, Mills WJ, et al: Functional outcomes of severe bicondylar tibial plateau fractures treated with dual incisions and medial and lateral plates. J Bone Joint Surg Am 2006;88A:1713–1721.
- Bennett WF, Browner B: Tibial plateau fractures: A study of associated soft tissue injuries. J Orthop Trauma 1994;8:183–188.
- Browner B, Jupiter J, Levine A, et al (eds): Skeletal Trauma: Basic Science, Management, and Reconstruction, 3rd ed. Philadelphia: Elsevier, 2003.
- Canadian Orthopaedic Trauma Society: Open reduction and internal fixation compared with circular fixator application for bicondylar tibial plateau fractures. Results of a multicenter, prospective, randomized clinical trial. J Bone Joint Surg Am 2006;88A:2613–2623.
- Miller M (ed): Review of Orthopaedics, 4th ed. Philadelphia: Elsevier, 2004.
- Nork SE, Segina DN, Aflatoon K, et al: The association between supracondylar-intercondylar distal femoral fractures and coronal plane fractures. J Bone Joint Surg Am 2005;87A:564–569.
- Okike K, Bhattacharyya T: Trends in the management of open fractures: A critical analysis. J Bone Joint Surg Am 2006;88A:2739–2748.
- Patzakis MJ, Wilkins J: Factors influencing infection rate in open wounds. Clin Orthop Relat Res 1989;243:36–40.
- Weigel DP, Marsh JL: High-energy fractures of the tibial plateau: Knee function after longer follow-up. J Bone Joint Surg Am 2002;84A:1541–1551.

Chapter 165 Patella Fractures

Franklin D. Shuler and Barry C. Davis

ICD-9 CODES

822.0 *Closed Fracture of Patella*

822.1 *Open Fracture of Patella*

Key Concepts

- Patella fractures are uncommon, comprising approximately 1% of all fractures.
- Patella fractures are twice as common in males.
- The diagnosis is made with physical examination and confirmed with radiographs.
- Fractures are classified by the orientation of the fracture line(s) on radiographs (Fig. 165-1), the degree of displacement, and whether the fracture is open or closed.
- Displaced fractures have more than 2-mm articular step-off and/or 3-mm separation between fragments.
- Patella fractures are rarely bilateral; bilateral radiographic findings may represent a bipartite patella.
- Patella fractures disrupt the extensor mechanism and may result in an inability to actively extend the knee (Fig. 165-2).
- In fractures with an intact medial/lateral retinacula, active knee extension may be possible. In this situation, focus on the knee extension lag.

History

- Direct (e.g., knee striking dashboard) or indirect trauma
- Pain and swelling
- Ambulatory capacity may be limited or absent.
- Active knee extension may be reported as limited or absent.

Physical Examination

- Observation
  - Visible defect with displaced fractures
  - Effusion (hemarthrosis)
  - Circumferential skin assessment: Any blood, lacerations, or surrounding skin trauma must raise concern for a possible open fracture with traumatic knee arthrotomy. Perform a saline load test if in doubt (see later).

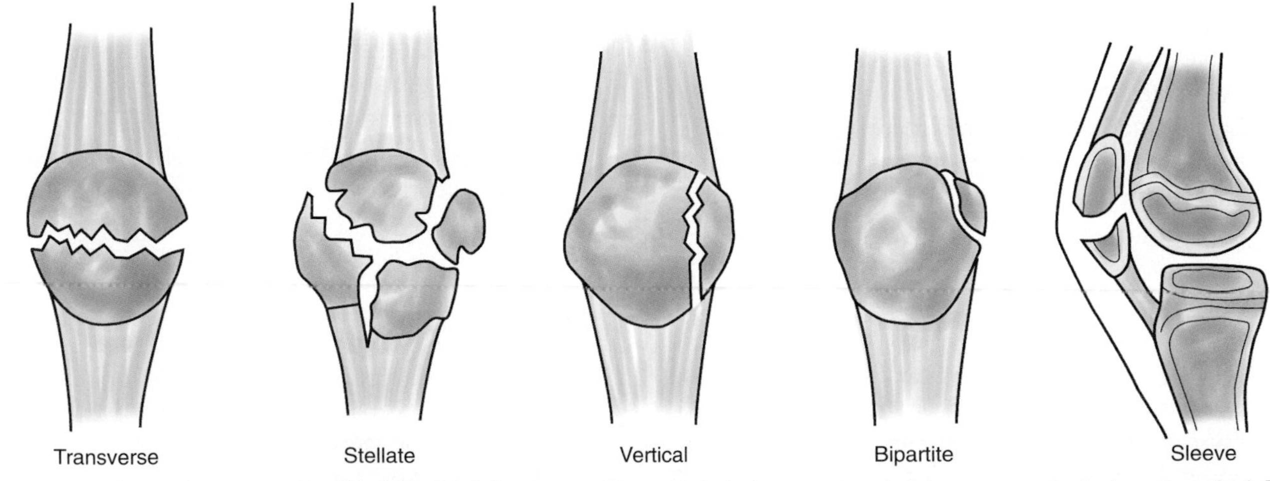

Figure 165-1 Patella fracture classification. Adult fracture patterns include transverse, stellate or comminuted, and vertical. The bipartite patella is frequently confused with a patella fracture. Patellar sleeve fractures are the most common patella fracture in the pediatric population.

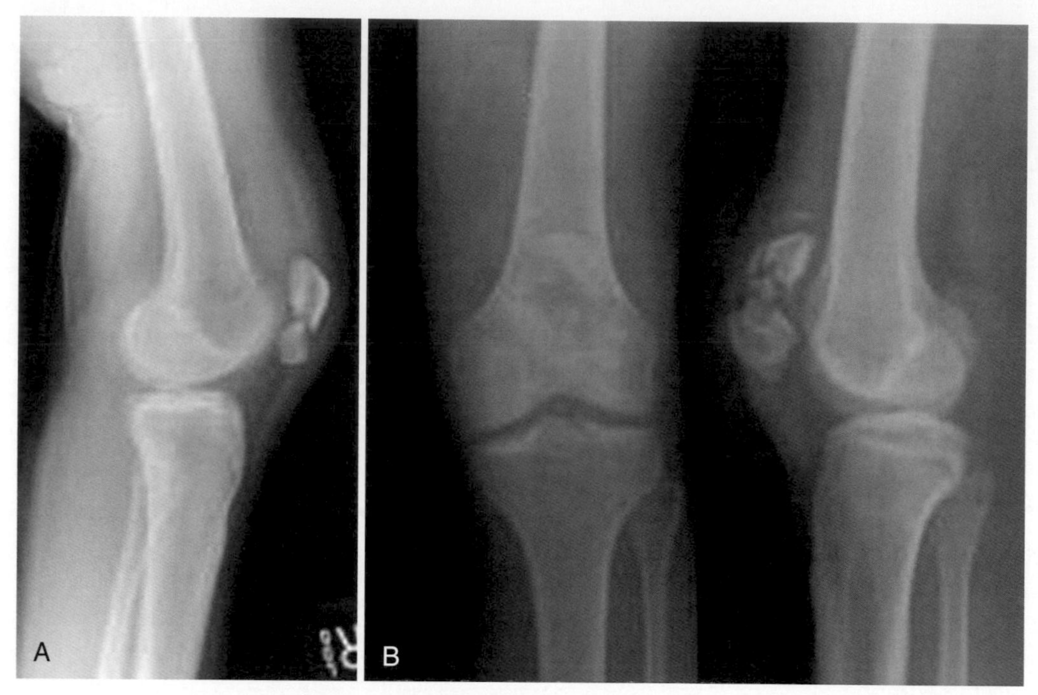

Figure 165-2 Radiographs of displaced patella fractures. **A**, Lateral view of transverse patella fracture associated with loss of active knee extension. Note knee effusion and fracture displacement. The superior fragment is pulled by the quadriceps muscle while the inferior pole of the patella is pulled by the patellar ligament. **B**, Anteroposterior and lateral views of stellate (comminuted) open patella fracture in a patient with loss of active knee extension.

- Palpation
  - Palpable defect with displaced fractures
  - Tenderness
  - Effusion
- Range of motion
  - Document active knee extension as either absent, intact, or with extension lag.
- Special tests
  - Advanced Trauma Life Support protocol when indicated in trauma setting, including secondary survey to assess for additional skeletal trauma and complete neurovascular examination
  - Saline load test: sterile arthrocentesis followed by intra-articular injection of at least 60 mL of sterile saline with or without methylene blue
    - — Extravasation of fluid from the open wound confirms the presence of an open fracture with communication to the knee joint (traumatic arthrotomy).
    - — Any remaining fluid is aspirated to decrease capsular distention and resultant patient pain.
  - Avoid routine aspiration of hematomas or instillation of intra-articular lidocaine to minimize the risk of iatrogenic septic arthritis.

Imaging

- Radiographs: Anteroposterior and lateral rediographs are required. Some consideration can be given to Merchant/sunrise knee views; however, knee flexion is required and can be painful for the patient.
  - Evaluate fracture orientation (transverse, stellate, or vertical), displacement, presence of effusion, presence of foreign materials or free air, and patella alta (indicating patella ligament avulsion).
  - Obtain radiographs of the joint above and below (tibia/ankle, femur/hip).
- Magnetic resonance imaging
  - May be helpful in the diagnosis of extensor mechanism (retinacular) injuries and osteochondral injuries

Differential Diagnosis

- Bipartite patella: round, smooth bony fragment at the superolateral corner of the patella with sclerotic borders (see Fig. 165-1)
- Femoral condyle fracture or chondral injury (Fig. 165-3)

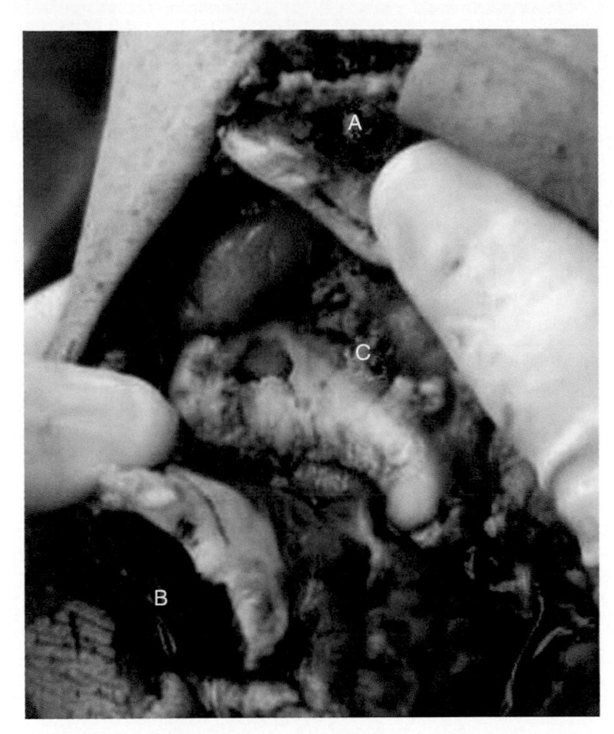

Figure 165-3 Intraoperative photograph of transverse patella fracture. This patient had direct patella trauma striking the dashboard during a motor vehicle collision. Superior patella fracture fragment (A). Inferior patella fracture fragment (B). Femoral condyle impaction fracture with articular cartilage damage and loss (C).

- Quadriceps tendon or patella ligament disruption
- Patella sleeve fracture (see Fig. 165-1).

Treatment

- Initial management
  - Stabilize fracture with a padded long leg splint or knee brace to limit further soft-tissue injury.
  - For open injuries
    - — First apply sterile saline gauze and administer appropriate antibiotic and tetanus prophylaxis (see Tables 166-2 and 166-3).
    - — Do not irrigate or probe the wound, remove bone fragments, or perform wound closure.
- Definitive management
  - Definitive treatment determined by consulting orthopaedic surgeon
  - For operative and non-operative management, consider deep venous thrombosis prophylaxis with injectable low–molecular-weight heparin or aspirin.
  - Nonoperative treatment is indicated for closed, nondisplaced, or minimally displaced fractures with an intact extensor mechanism.
    - — Patients may weight bear as tolerated with the knee immobilized in extension. Instruct the patient on the use of crutches or walker.
  - Operative treatment is indicated for open or displaced fractures.
    - — The goal is to reconstruct the extensor mechanism and patellar joint surface.
    - — Options include open reduction and internal fixation, partial patellectomy, and total patellectomy (as a last resort).

When to Refer

- All patients with patella fractures generally require referral to an orthopaedic surgeon.
- Closed, nondisplaced, or minimally displaced fractures with an intact extensor mechanism may be referred within 1 to 2 weeks.
- Displaced fractures should be referred more acutely.
- Emergent orthopaedic surgical consultation is required in patients with open fractures or traumatic arthrotomy.

Prognosis

- Varies based on fracture type, associated injuries, and patient comorbidities including obesity, nicotine use, diabetes, vascular disease, clotting disorders, osteoporosis, and preexisting knee arthritis, among other factors
- Timely antibiotic administration in open fractures is considered to improve the prognosis.
- In general, fracture healing can be seen on radiographs 8 to 12 weeks after injury.
- Hardware associated with fracture fixation is typically not removed unless there is irritation (common), nonunion, or infection.

Troubleshooting

- Patients should be informed of possible complications including loss of reduction or fixation requiring repeat surgery, nonunion or malunion, knee stiffness, persistent extensor lag, and posttraumatic arthritis.

Patient Instructions

- Patients should be instructed on the importance of strict adherence to range of motion restrictions and bracing.
- Physical therapy is vital to the outcome and will be dictated by the treating orthopaedist.

Considerations in Special Populations

- After anterior cruciate ligament reconstruction with a patellar tendon autograft, patients may be at risk of a patella fracture.
- Patellar sleeve (osteochondral) fractures are the most common patella fracture in pediatric patients and require prompt reduction; internal fixation is usually necessary.

Suggested Reading

- Bostrom A: Fracture of the patella: A clinical study of 422 patellar fractures. Acta Orthop Scand 1921;143:1–80.
- Browner B, Jupiter J, Levine A, Trafton P (eds): Skeletal Trauma: Basic Science, Management, and Reconstruction, 3rd ed. Philadelphia: Elsevier, 2003.
- Carpenter JE, Kasman R, Matthews LS: Fractures of the patella. J Bone Joint Surg Am 1993;75A:1550–1561.
- Catalano JB, Iannacone WM, Marczyk S, et al: Open fractures of the patella: Long-term functional outcome. J Trauma 1995; 39:439–444.
- Hunt DM, Somashekar N: A review of sleeve fractures of the patella in children. Knee 2005;12:3–7.
- Miller M (ed): Review of Orthopaedics, 4th ed. Philadelphia: Elsevier, 2004.
- Okike K, Bhattacharyya T: Trends in the management of open fractures. A critical analysis. J Bone Joint Surg Am 2006; 88A:2739–2748.
- Stein DA, Hunt SA, Rosen JE, et al: The incidence and outcome of patella fractures after anterior cruciate ligament reconstruction. Arthroscopy 2002;18:578–583.

Chapter 166 Tibial and Fibular Shaft Fractures

Franklin D. Shuler and Matthew J. Dietz

ICD-9 CODES

823 *Fracture Tibia and Fibula (Fifth-Digit Subclassification Is for Use with 823.X0 Tibia Alone; 823.X1 Fibula Alone; 823.X2 Fibula with Tibia)*
823.0 *Upper End, Closed*
823.1 *Upper End, Open*
823.2 *Shaft, Closed*
823.3 *Shaft, Open*
823.4 *Torus Fracture*
823.8 *Unspecified Part, Closed*
823.9 *Unspecified Part, Open*

Key Concepts

- The tibia is the major weight-bearing bone of the lower leg. Although the fibula is not significant in weight bearing (6% to 17%), it does serve an important role in ankle stability.
- Tibial shaft fracture is the most common long bone diaphyseal fracture.
- Fracture of the tibial shaft is the most common open fracture (25%). Timely tetanus and antibiotic prophylaxis is critical, along with immediate surgical referral.
- Tibia fractures are most frequently associated with fibula fractures (80%); they may also be associated with ligamentous injuries of the knee and ankle.
- High-energy tibia fractures may result in neurovascular injuries or compartment syndrome; both are indications for immediate surgical referral.

History

- Acute injury
  - Direct or indirect trauma
  - Low-energy (fall) or high-energy (motor vehicle collision) trauma (Fig. 166-1)
  - Low- versus high-velocity penetrating injuries (gunshot wounds)
  - Pain and inability to bear weight

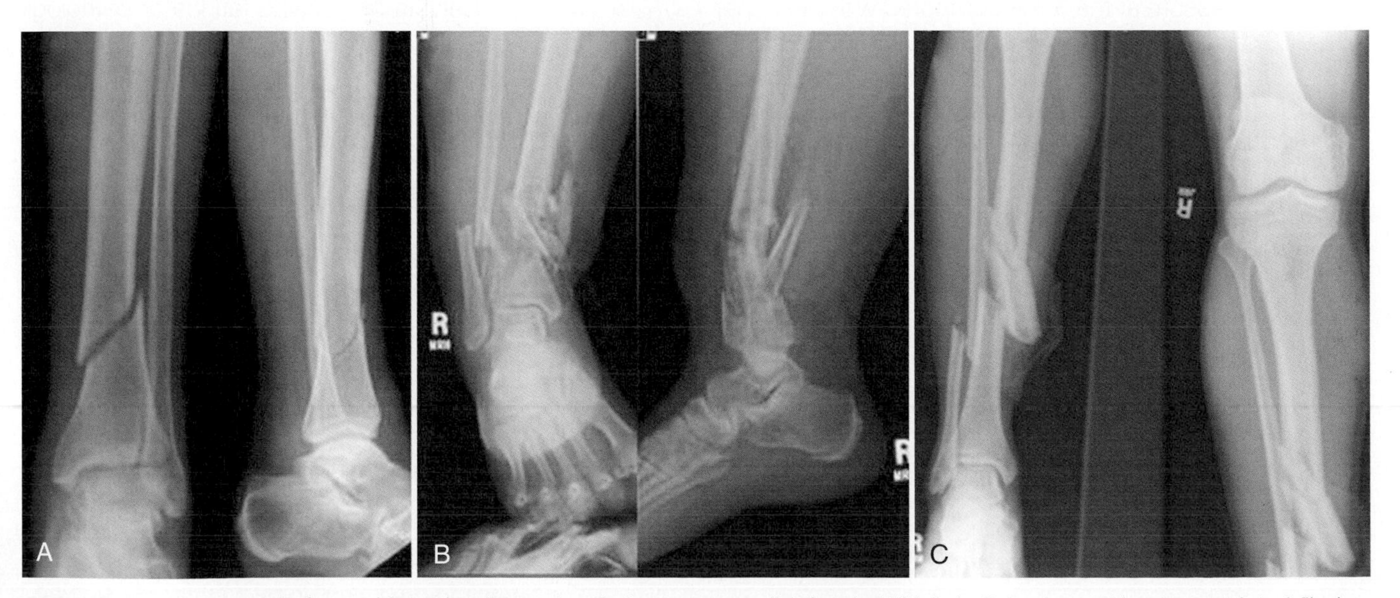

Figure 166-1 Anteroposterior and lateral radiographs. **A**, Low-energy, distal, spiral tibial shaft fracture without associated fibula fracture. **B**, High-energy, distal, comminuted, open tibial shaft fracture with associated fibula fracture. **C**, High-energy, mid-shaft, segmental, comminuted, open tibial shaft fracture with associated fibula fracture.

- Chronic injury
  - Soldiers, dancers, and runners are susceptible to fatigue fractures.
  - Pathologic fractures may result from a tumor causing mechanical weakening in the bony architecture.

Physical Examination

- Observation
  - Deformity
  - Circumferential skin assessment: Any blood, lacerations, or surrounding skin trauma must raise concern for possible open fracture.
  - Fracture blisters: A compromised soft-tissue envelope (i.e., fracture blisters, abrasions) can alter the surgical plan.
- Palpation
  - Tenderness, crepitus
  - Manual compression of leg compartments (see later in the chapter)
- Range of motion
  - Assess for injuries to the knee and ankle after stabilizing the fracture.
- Special tests
  - Advanced Trauma Life Support protocol when indicated in a trauma setting, including secondary survey to assess for additional skeletal trauma and complete neurovascular examination
    - — Posterior tibial and dorsalis pedis pulses: Doppler scan if nonpalpable
    - — The ankle-brachial index measures systolic pressure at the ankle compared with the upper extremity. Values less than 0.9 indicate a high probability of arterial injury and warrant vascular consultation and possible arteriography.
    - — Neurologic examination (Table 166-1) may be compromised in obtunded patients. Proximal fibula fractures (bumper injuries), in particular, may be associated with injury to the common peroneal nerve as it courses around the fibular neck.
  - Compartment syndrome evaluation
    - — Elevated compartment pressures are common after skeletal leg trauma. Maintain a high index of suspicion. Firmness to manual compression is a cause for concern.
    - — Pain with passive motion can be difficult to assess due to the presence of fracture-related pain.
    - — Compartment pressures should be obtained at the level of the fracture. ΔP (diastolic blood pressure – compartment pressure) of less than 30 mmHg warrants emergent fasciotomy of all four leg compartments.

TABLE 166-1 *Neurologic Examination of a Tibial Shaft Fracture*

Nerve	Motor Function	Sensory Distribution
Sural	Foot plantarflexion	Lateral heel
Saphenous	None	Medial leg and ankle
Superficial peroneal	Foot eversion	Dorsum of foot including great toe
Deep peroneal	Great toe dorsiflexion	First web space of the foot
Tibial	Toe plantarflexion	Sole of foot

Imaging

- Radiographs: anteroposterior and lateral views of the tibia and fibula
  - Obtain radiographs with traction and no plaster to better characterize the fracture pattern (see Fig. 166-1B).
  - Obtain radiographs of the joint above and below.
  - Evaluate postreduction radiographs for fracture location, comminution, malalignment, and the presence of foreign materials or free air.
- Bone scan or computed tomography
  - May be useful in diagnosing fatigue or pathologic fractures

Differential Diagnosis

- Intra-articular fracture of the knee (plateau) or ankle (pilon)
- Compartment syndrome without fracture
- Pathologic, osteopenic, or stress fracture

Treatment

Tibial Shaft Fractures

- Initial management
  - Reduce and stabilize the fracture to limit further soft-tissue injury with a padded, well-molded, long leg splint.
  - For open fractures, first apply a sterile saline dressing and administer appropriate tetanus and antibiotic prophylaxis (Tables 166-2 and 166-3).

TABLE 166-2 *Current Centers for Disease Control and Prevention Recommendations Regarding Tetanus Prophylaxis*

	Clean Minor Wounds <6 Hours Old		All Other Wounds	
Previous Doses of Absorbed TT	**Tdap or Td**	**TIG**	**Tdap or Td**	**TIG**
Unknown or <3	Yes	No	Yes	Yes
≥3	No*	No	No†	No

The preferred vaccine preparation depends on the age of the child or adolescent:
<7 yr: DTaP
7–11 yr: Td
11–64 yr: Tdap for those who have never received Tdap.
Td is preferred to TT for those who received Tdap previously, when Tdap is not available, or for persons >64 years.
*Yes, if ≥10 years since last TT-containing vaccine dose.
†Yes, if ≥5 years since last TT-containing vaccine dose.
DTap, diphtheria-tetanus-acellular pertussis; Td, adult tetanus; Tdap, booster tetanus toxoid-reduced diphtheria toxoid-acellular pertussis; TIG, human tetanus immune globulin; TT, tetanus toxoid.
Data from Centers for Disease Control and Prevention.

TABLE 166-3 *Recommended Antibiotic Prophylaxis for Open Fractures*

Open Fracture Type	Definition	Antibiotic
Grade I	<1 cm skin opening	First-generation cephalosporin
Grade II	Between 1- and 10-cm skin opening	First-generation cephalosporin
Grade III	A = 10 cm B = 10 cm requiring soft-tissue coverage C = vascular injury requiring repair	First-generation cephalosporin + gentamicin
Special circumstances		
High-velocity gunshot, shotgun close range, segmental fracture, open wound >8 hr	Defined as a grade III	First-generation cephalosporin + gentamicin
Farm injury or grossly contaminated	Defined as a grade III	Cefazolin, gentamicin + penicillin G (12 million U/day q4h)
Freshwater-, saltwater-, or brackish water–related open fracture	Define using Gustilo-Anderson classification	Consider the addition of fluoroquinolone

    - Do not irrigate or probe the wound, remove bone fragments, apply tourniquets or clamps for bleeding (address with direct pressure), or perform wound closure.
    - Patients with high-energy injuries should be admitted and monitored for compartment syndrome with serial examinations for 24 hours.
- Definitive management
    - Definitive treatment determined by consulting orthopaedic surgeon
    - Nonoperative treatment indicated for closed, stable fractures with acceptable alignment including angulation less than 5 degrees, shortening less than 12 mm, and translation less than 50% (see Fig. 166-2)
        - — Splint immobilization is converted to a long leg cast in 1 to 2 weeks as swelling improves.
        - — Protected brace or cast weight bearing is initiated within 6 weeks.
    - Operative treatment is indicated for most tibial shaft fractures.
        - — Surgical intervention varies based on fracture type and condition of the soft-tissue envelope.
        - — Options include intramedullary rod fixation, plate fixation, external fixation (temporary stabilization or definitive management), and possible amputation for the most severe nonviable extremity injuries.

Isolated Fibular Shaft Fractures

- Immobilize in a short leg splint or prefabricated air-splint and instruct the patient to be nonweight bearing with crutches.
- Proximal third fibula shaft fractures, without an associated tibia shaft fracture, may represent a Maisonneuve injury.
    - These fractures result from an external rotation injury to the ankle, causing a disruption of the

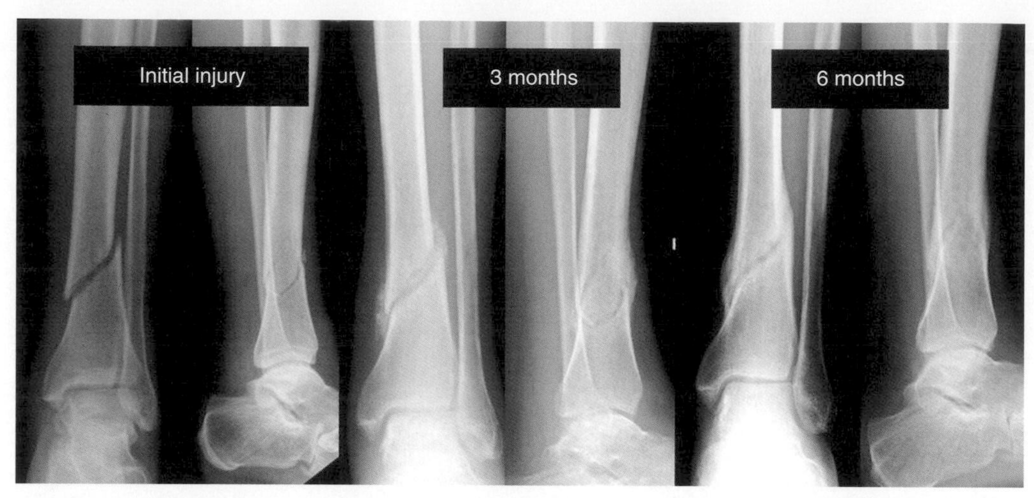

Figure 166-2 Nonoperative management: anteroposterior and lateral radiographs. Callus formation is noted in the 3-month radiograph, with healed fracture and acceptable alignment demonstrated 6 months after injury.

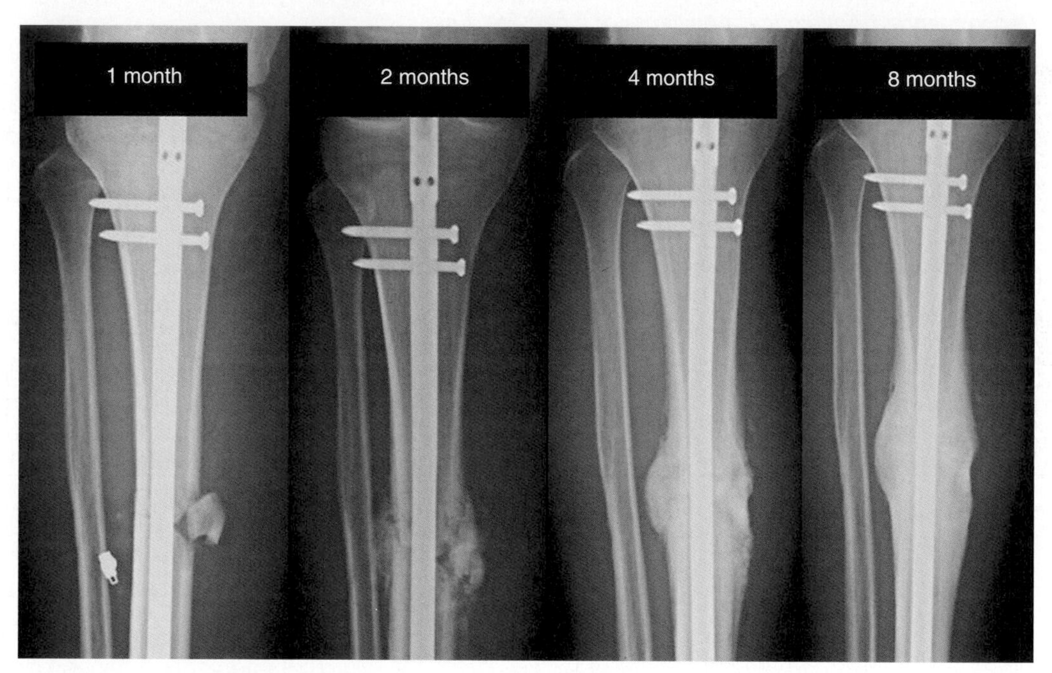

Figure 166-3 Operative management with intramedullary fixation: anteroposterior radiographs. Callus formation is noted in the 2-month postoperative radiograph. Note that surgery does not change the overall time required for fracture healing.

ligamentous connection between the tibia and fibula (syndesmosis) and typically require surgical intervention.
- Isolated fibular shaft fractures are otherwise typically treated conservatively.

When to Refer

- All patients with a tibial or fibular shaft fracture generally require referral.
- Emergent orthopaedic surgical consultation is required in open fractures, neurovascular injury, and impending or established compartment syndrome.

Prognosis

- Varies from simple fracture patterns with minimal soft-tissue damage to severe limb-threatening injuries with associated neurovascular, muscular, and/or skin damage (see Fig. 166-1)
- Timely antibiotic administration in open fractures is considered to improve prognosis
- In general, fracture healing can be seen radiographically 4 to 12 weeks after injury (Figs. 166-2 and 166-3).
- Normal tensile strength of bone is not restored until 8 to 12 months after fracture healing.

Troubleshooting

- Delayed unions should be evaluated for the presence of infection (complete blood count with differential, erythrocyte sedimentation rate, and C-reactive protein) and are often associated with high-energy injuries and poor host factors (i.e., nicotine use, diabetes).
- Fracture complications include malunion, nonunion (10%), neurovascular injury, deep venous thrombosis, pulmonary embolism, fat embolism, pain, weakness, and knee/ankle stiffness.
- Additional cast-related complications include skin irritation, skin breakdown, and cast saw burns.
- Additional surgery-related complications include infection, hardware failure, and wound healing issues.

Patient Instructions

- Patients should be instructed on the importance of weight-bearing restrictions, splint or cast care, extremity elevation, and deep venous thrombosis prophylaxis.
- Patients should call the physician if any increased pain, swelling, or neurovascular changes are noted.
- Frequently, due to changes in swelling or patient noncompliance issues (i.e., wet cast), adjustment or reapplication of the splint or cast is required.

Suggested Reading

- Bhandari M, Guyatt GH, Swiontkowski MF, et al: Treatment of open fractures of the shaft of the tibia. J Bone Joint Surg Br 2001;83B:62–68.
- Browner B, Jupiter J, Levine A, Trafton P: Skeletal Trauma: Basic Science, Management, and Reconstruction, 3rd ed. Philadelphia: Elsevier, 2003.
- Court-Brown CM, McBirnie J: The epidemiology of tibial fractures. J Bone Joint Surg Br 1995;77B:417–421.
- Fletcher N, Sofianos D, Berkes M, et al: Prevention of perioperative infection. J Bone Joint Surg Am 2007;89A: 1605–1618.
- Gustilo RB, Anderson JT: Prevention of infection in the treatment of one thousand and twenty-five open fractures of long bones: Retrospective and prospective analyses. J Bone Joint Surg Am 1976;58A:453–458.
- Miller MD: Review of Orthopaedics, 4th ed. Philadelphia: Elsevier, 2004.
- Okike K, Bhattacharyya T: Trends in the management of open fractures. A critical analysis. J Bone Joint Surg Am 2006;88A:2739–2748.
- Patzakis MJ, Wilkins J: Factors influencing infection rate in open wounds. Clin Orthop Relat Res 1989;243:36–40.
- Shuler FD, Obremskey WT: Tibial shaft fractures. In Stannard JP, Schmidt AH, Kregor PJ (eds): Surgical Treatment of Orthopaedic Trauma. New York: Thieme, 2007 pp 742–766.
- White TO, Howell GE, Will EM, et al: Elevated intramuscular compartment pressures do not influence outcome after tibial fracture. J Trauma 2003;55:1133–1138.

Chapter 167 Knee Aspiration and/or Injection Technique

Jennifer A. Hart

CPT CODE
20610 *Aspiration and/or Injection, Large Joint*

Procedure Name

- Knee aspiration (arthrocentesis) and injection

Equipment

- 25-gauge needle if local anesthesia planned
- Injection needle (21 gauge)
- Large-bore aspiration needle (16- to 18-gauge)
- Stopcock, optional for combined aspiration and injection
- Injection syringe (5–10 mL)
- Aspiration syringe (30 mL)
- Local anesthetic
- Sterile cup and/or appropriate laboratory tubes for aspiration
- Sterile tray
- Sterile gloves
- Sterile prep solution (e.g., povidone-iodine)
- Ethyl chloride, optional
- Injectable agent (steroid, hyaluronic acid)
- Sterile gauze and bandage

Indications

- Aspiration
  - Suspected joint infection
  - Gouty arthritis
  - Large painful effusion
  - Loss of motion secondary to effusion
- Injection
  - Osteoarthritis
  - Rheumatoid arthritis
  - Pseudogout
  - Patellar chondromalacia

Contraindications

- Aspiration
- Generalized sepsis without evidence of infected joint
- Injection
- Active or recent joint infection
- Overlying skin disease
- Impending surgical procedure

Technique

- Verbal patient consent is obtained and the correct knee is identified.
- The medication is prepared on a sterile tray with a stopcock and extra syringe available if aspiration is indicated.
- Ethyl chloride, if used, should be administered topically before sterile skin preparation (Fig. 167-1).
- With sterile gloves in place, the skin is prepared with a sterile prep solution (Fig. 167-2).
- If an effusion is present, a small needle is used to infiltrate the skin with local anesthetic before inserting the larger needle for aspiration (Fig. 167-3).

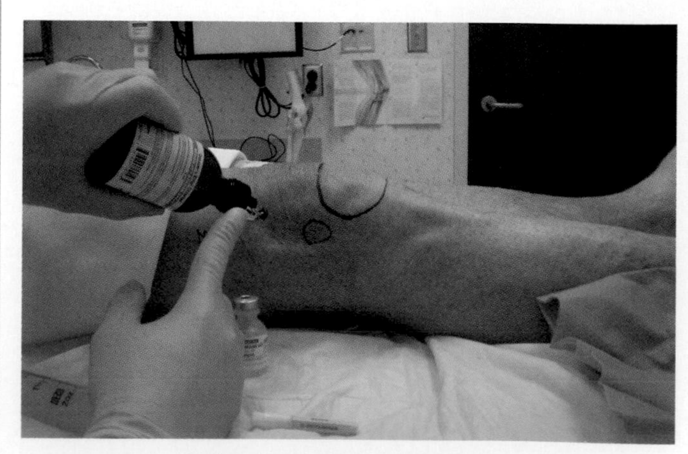

Figure 167-1 Optional use of ethyl chloride for anesthetizing the skin.

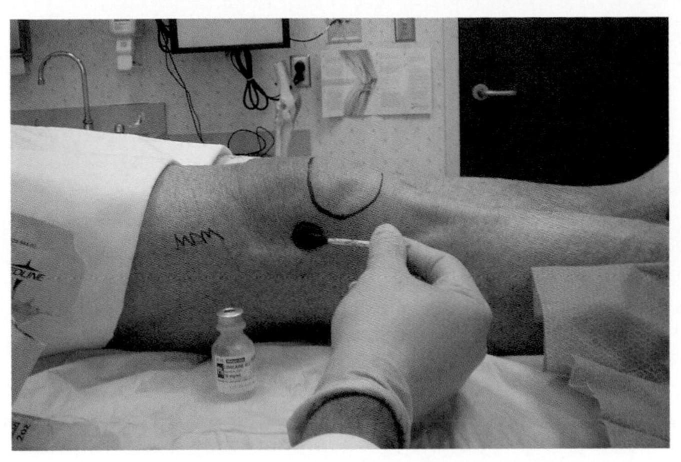

Figure 167-2 Skin preparation begins.

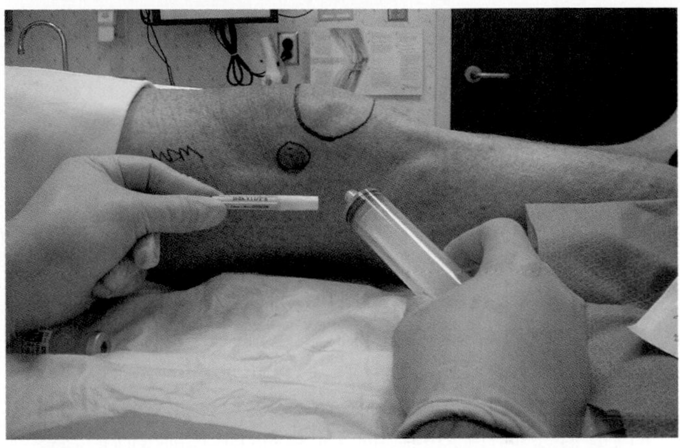

Figure 167-4 A large-bore needle and large syringe are prepared for arthrocentesis.

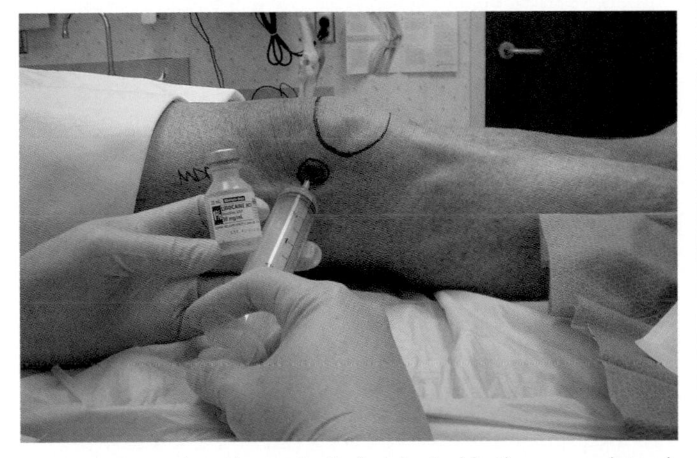

Figure 167-3 Local anesthetic is injected in the superolateral space.

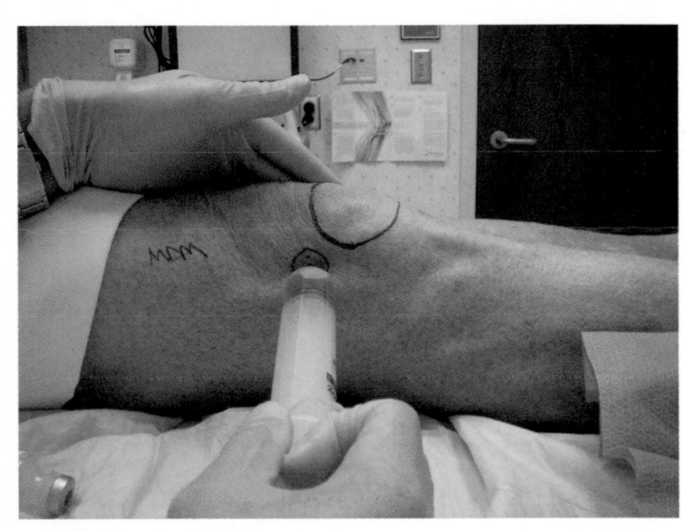

Figure 167-5 The plunger of the syringe is pulled back with gentle pressure for aspiration.

- A large-bore aspiration needle is passed into the superolateral pouch at a site just proximal and lateral to the superolateral border of the patella (Fig. 167-4).
- After feeling the needle pass into the joint capsule, apply gentle pressure to the plunger of the syringe to aspirate the fluid (Fig. 167-5).
- Using a stopcock will allow the same needle to be used for the injection after the aspiration is complete.
- After ensuring that the needle tip is unobstructed and in place inside the joint capsule, turn the stopcock and inject the steroid or hyaluronic acid preparation. Alternatively, the injection can be done without the use of a stopcock by using a second needle and syringe (Fig. 167-6).
- Apply dressing as per routine

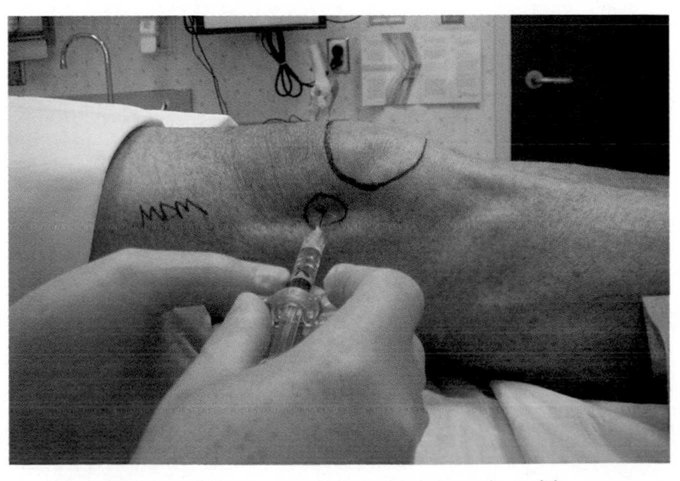

Figure 167-6 Injection of hyaluronic acid.

Considerations in Special Populations

- Multiple approaches have been described but the superolateral approach (described here) and the direct lateral approach have been found to be the most accurate.
- Injections of morbidly obese patients may be made easier by using an inferomedial or inferolateral approach with the knee flexed to 90 degrees. This is also useful for patients who are unable to lie fully prone secondary to conditions such as back pain or orthopnea.
- If joint infection is suspected, synovial fluid obtained during aspiration should be sent for cell count, crystal analysis, Gram stain, and aerobic/anaerobic cultures.

Troubleshooting

- "Bumping" bone: Gently redirect the needle superiorly to enter the suprapatellar pouch above the femur.
- No fluid on aspiration: Make sure that the needle is in the synovial capsule and push the plunger back in to clear any obstructions in the needle tip.
- Not all fluid removed**:** Gently "milk" the knee with your other hand, directing the fluid medially to laterally.

Patient Instructions

- The patient may remove the dressing the following day.
- Use ice to treat any local soreness at the injection site.
- Call the physician's office immediately if any redness, warmth, increased swelling, severe increase in pain, fever, or chills develop.
- Diabetic patients may notice slight transient elevations in the blood glucose level.

Chapter 168 Prepatellar Bursa Aspiration and/or Injection Technique

Luke S. Choi and Mark D. Miller

CPT CODE

20610 *Arthrocentesis, Aspiration, or Injection of Major Joint or Bursa*

Procedure Name

- Prepatellar bursa aspiration and injection

Equipment

- 25-gauge needle if local anesthesia planned
- Injection needle (21-gauge)
- Injection syringe (5–10 mL)
- Large-bore aspiration needle (16- to 18-gauge)
- Aspiration syringe (30 mL)
- Local anesthetic agent
- Sterile tray
- Sterile gloves
- Sterile prep solution (e.g., povidone-iodine)
- Ethyl chloride, optional
- Injectable agent (steroid, anesthetic)
- Sterile gauze and bandage

Indications

- Acute or chronic prepatellar bursitis refractory to conservative management

Contraindications

- Overlying cellulitis or skin disease

Technique

- Verbal patient consent is obtained and the correct knee is identified.
- The medication is prepared on a sterile tray with an extra syringe available if aspiration is planned.
- The patient is placed in the supine position with the knee resting in a comfortable position. A small pillow may be placed under the knee for comfort and support (Fig. 168-1).
- The area over the patella is palpated for fluctuance (Fig. 168-2).
- Prepare the skin site by anesthetizing with ethyl chloride (Fig. 168-3) and sterilizing with povidone-iodine solution (Fig. 168-4).

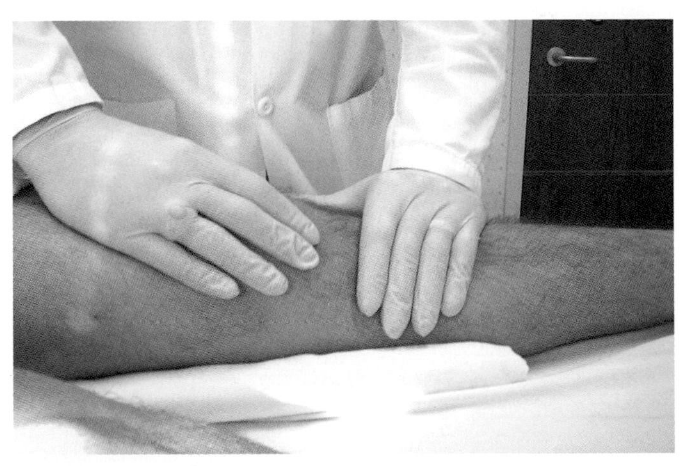

Figure 168-1 The patient is placed supine with a small support under the knee for comfort.

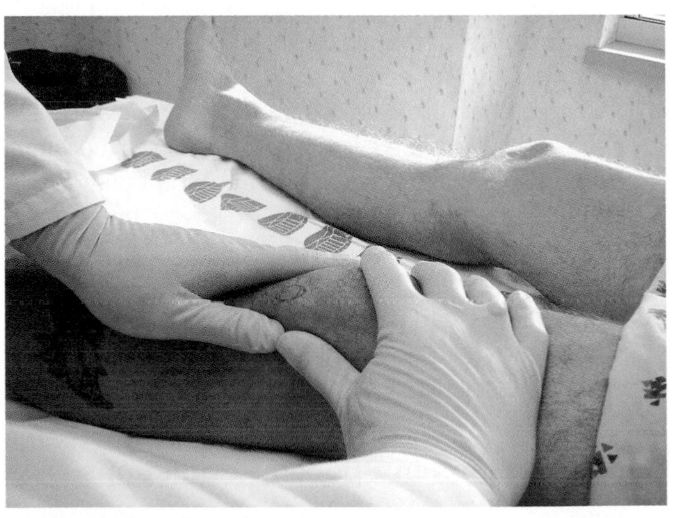

Figure 168-2 The prepatellar bursa is palpated and the injection site determined.

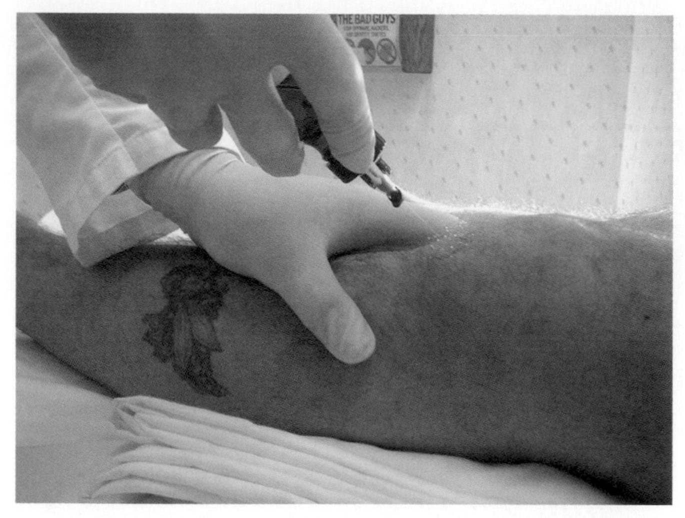

Figure 168-3 Optional use of ethyl chloride for anesthetizing the skin.

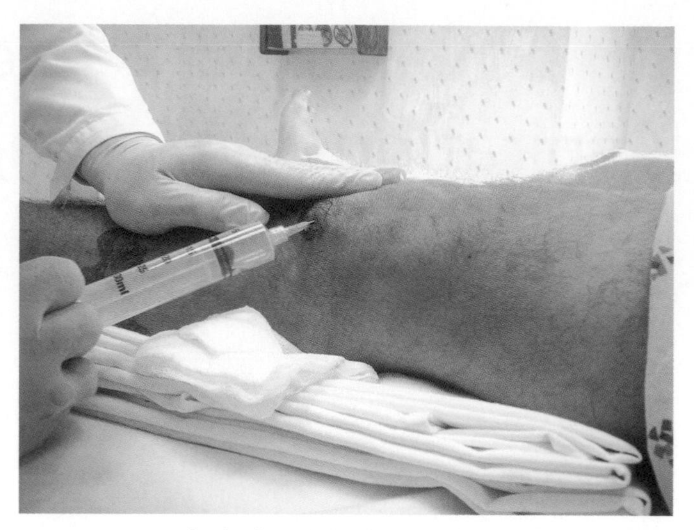

Figure 168-5 Aspiration of the bursa with large-bore needle.

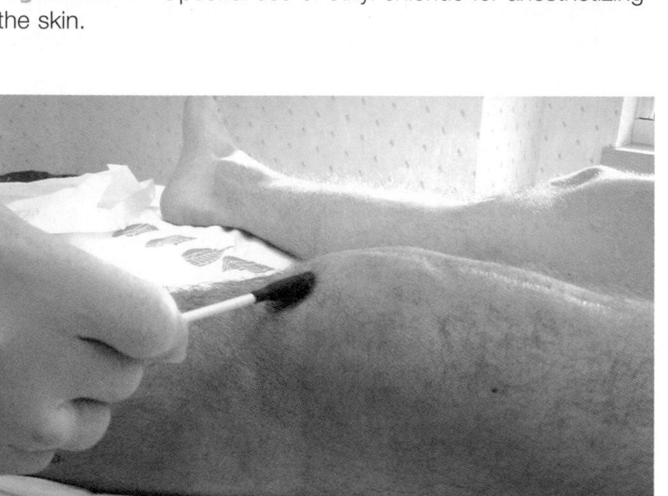

Figure 168-4 Sterile skin preparation.

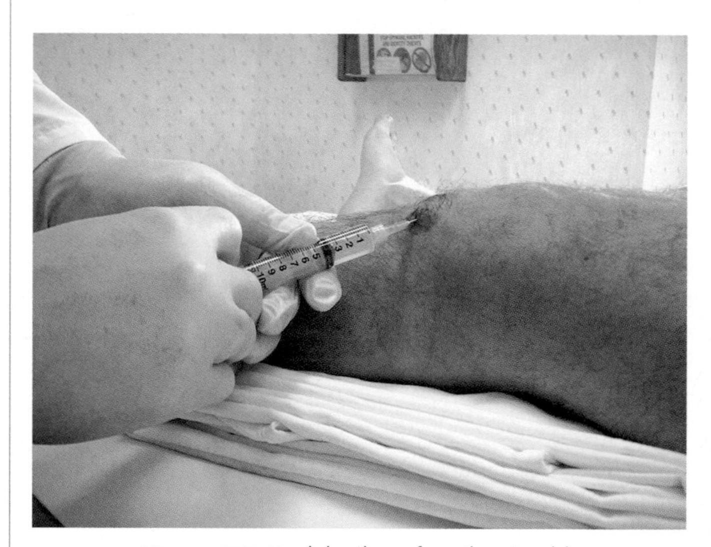

Figure 168-6 Injection of corticosteroid.

- If aspiration is planned, a small needle is used to infiltrate the skin with local anesthetic before inserting the larger aspiration needle.
- Aspiration and injection are performed by placing the needle directly into the fluid-filled bursa from the lateral side. Fluid should be aspirated from the bursa with a large-bore needle (Fig. 168-5) followed by injection with a corticosteroid (Fig. 168-6). If injecting, a hemostat is used to hold the needle in place while changing the syringe. Alternatively, a separate needle and syringe may be used for injection.
- Apply dressing per routine

Considerations in Special Populations

- In the evaluation of a patient with prepatellar bursitis, the physician should be aware of possible underlying infection, fracture of the patella, or an associated intra-articular injury of the knee.
- Bursitis-related prepatellar swelling must be differentiated from an intra-articular effusion.
- If infection is suspected, bursal fluid obtained during aspiration should be sent for a cell count, a Gram stain, and aerobic/anaerobic cultures.

Patient Instructions

- The dressing may be removed the following day.
- Use ice to treat any local soreness at the injection site.
- Call the physician's office if any redness, warmth, increased swelling, fever, or chills develop.

Chapter 169 Pes Anserine Bursa Injection Technique

Luke S. Choi and Mark D. Miller

CPT CODE
20610 *Aspiration or Injection of Major Joint or Bursa*

Procedure Name

- Pes anserine bursa injection

Equipment

- 25-gauge needle if local anesthesia planned
- Injection needle (21-gauge)
- Injection syringe (5–10 mL)
- Local anesthetic agent
- Sterile tray
- Sterile gloves
- Sterile prep solution (e.g., povidone-iodine)
- Ethyl chloride, optional
- Injectable agent (steroid, anesthetic)
- Sterile gauze and bandage

Indications

- Pes anserine bursitis

Contraindications

- Overlying cellulitis or skin disease

Technique

- Verbal patient consent is obtained and the correct extremity is identified.
- The medication is prepared on a sterile tray.
- The patient is placed in the supine position with the knee slightly flexed.
- Identify the tendinous border of the medial hamstring muscle and follow it distal to the joint line to its insertion at the pes anserine. The pes anserine bursa is located at this site, along the medial aspect of the knee approximately 2 cm below the joint line.
- Prepare the skin site by anesthetizing with ethyl chloride and sterilizing with povidone-iodine solution (Fig. 169-1).
- The needle is inserted perpendicular to the tibia into the point of maximal tenderness. The needle is gently advanced to bone and then withdrawn 2 to 3 mm to perform the injection (Fig. 169-2).
- Apply a dressing per routine

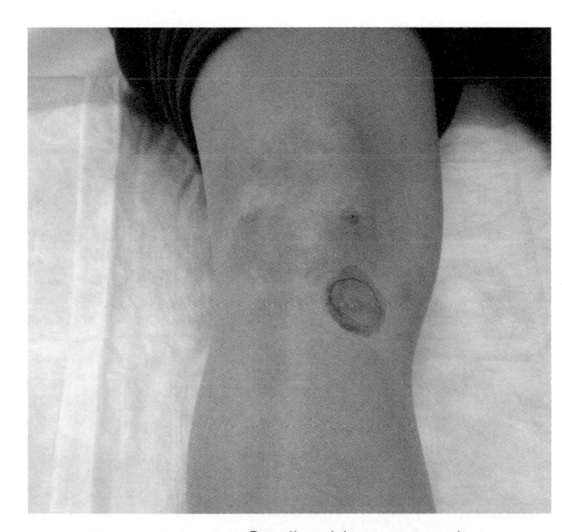

Figure 169-1 Sterile skin preparation.

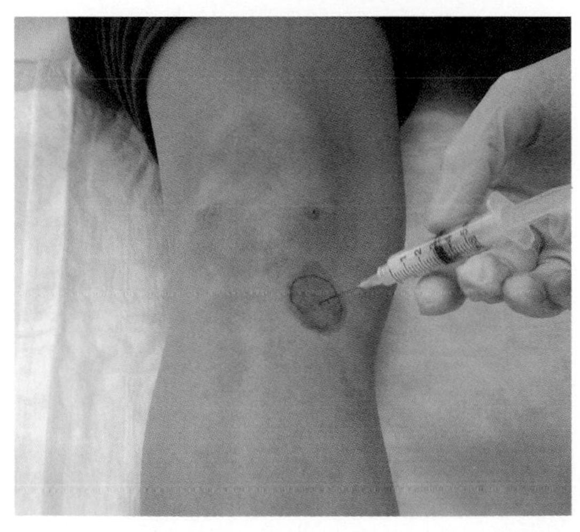

Figure 169-2 Injection of corticosteroid into the pes anserine bursa distal to the medial joint line.

Considerations in Special Populations

- Injection in this condition is often performed early in the course of treatment rather than after an extended trial of other modalities.

Patient Instructions

- The dressing may be removed the following day.
- Use ice to treat any local soreness at the injection site.
- Call the physician's office if any redness, warmth, increased swelling, fever, or chills develop.

Chapter 170 Iliotibial Band Injection Technique

Luke S. Choi and Mark D. Miller

CPT CODE
20610 *Aspiration or Injection of Major Joint or Bursa*

Procedure Name

- Iliotibial band injection technique

Equipment

- 25-gauge needle if local anesthesia planned
- Injection needle (21-gauge)
- Injection syringe (5–10 mL)
- Local anesthetic agent
- Sterile tray
- Sterile gloves
- Sterile prep solution (e.g., povidone-iodine)
- Ethyl chloride, optional
- Injectable agent (steroid, anesthetic)
- Sterile gauze and bandage

Indications

- Iliotibial band syndrome

Contraindications

- Overlying cellulitis or skin disease

Technique

- Verbal patient consent is obtained and the correct extremity is identified.
- The medication is prepared on a sterile tray.
- The patient is placed in the lateral decubitus position with the knee flexed 20 to 30 degrees (Fig. 170-1).
- Palpate the course of the iliotibial band along the lateral thigh to its insertion at Gerdy's tubercle on the proximal tibia. Determine the site of maximal tenderness (Fig. 170-2).
- Prepare the skin site by anesthetizing with ethyl chloride (Fig. 170-3) and sterilizing with povidone-iodine solution (Fig. 170-4).
- The needle is inserted at the point of maximal tenderness in the region of the lateral femoral condyle and the corticosteroid is injected (Fig. 170-5).
- Apply a dressing per routine

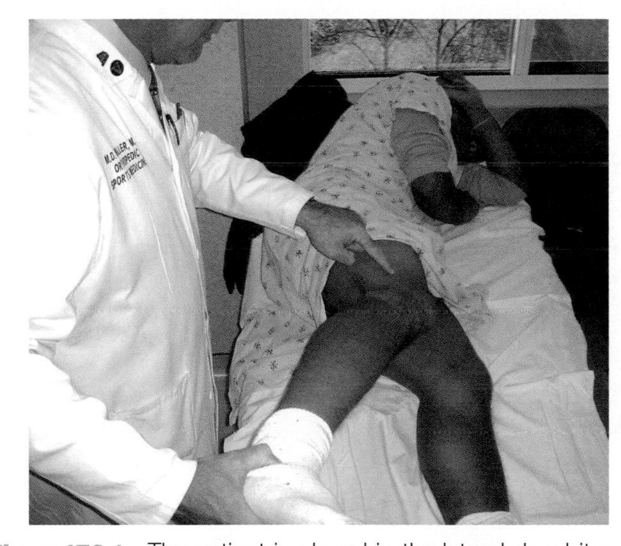

Figure 170-1 The patient is placed in the lateral decubitus position with the knee slightly flexed.

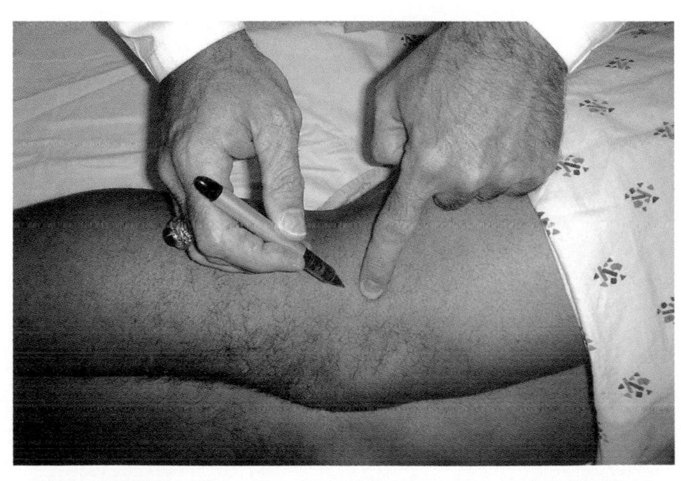

Figure 170-2 The site of maximal tenderness is identified.

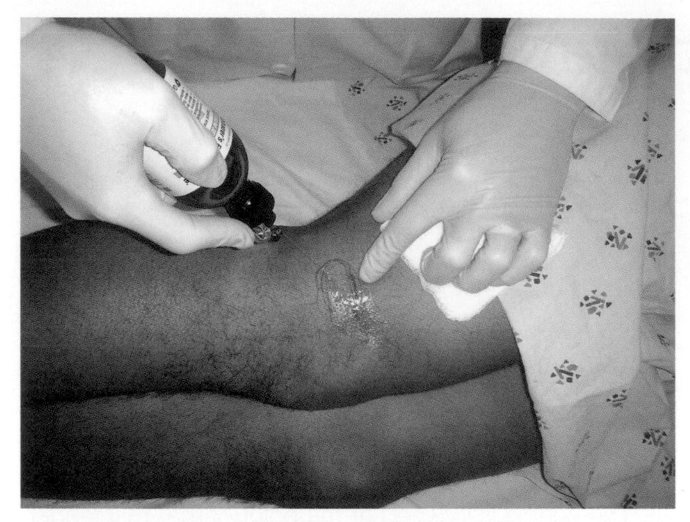

Figure 170-3 Optional use of ethyl chloride for anesthetizing the skin.

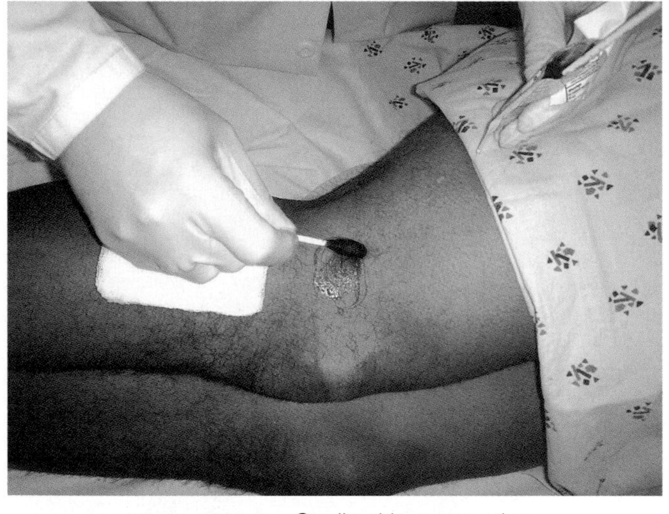

Figure 170-4 Sterile skin preparation.

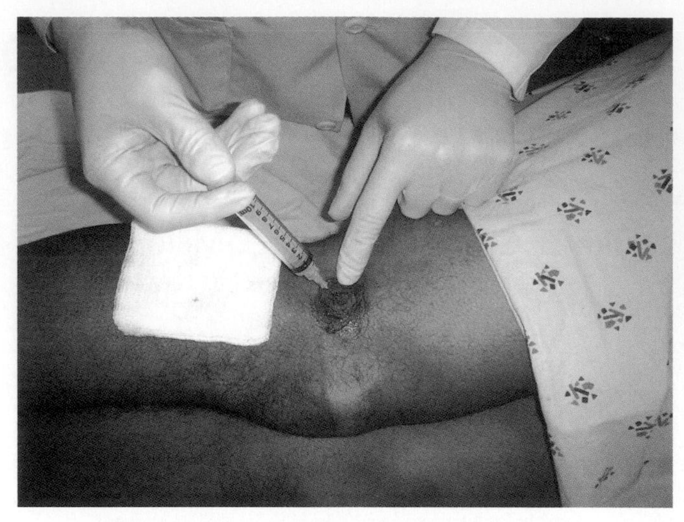

Figure 170-5 Injection of the corticosteroid.

Considerations in Special Populations

- Injection is typically reserved for patients in whom a program of iliotibial band stretching, hip abductor strengthening, and activity modification has failed.

Patient Instructions

- The dressing may be removed the following day.
- Use ice to treat any local soreness at the injection site.
- Call the physician's office if any redness, warmth, increased swelling, fever, or chills develop.

Chapter 171 Technique for Measuring Compartment Pressures

Robert P. Wilder

CPT CODE

20950 *Monitoring of Interstitial Fluid Pressure, Muscle Compartment Syndrome*

Procedure Name

- Intramuscular compartment pressure monitoring

Equipment

- Sterile prep solution (e.g., alcohol, iodine)
- Local anesthetic agent
- Aspiration needle for local and injection needle (25-gauge) for local
- Ethyl chloride
- Sterile gloves
- Sterile gauze
- Adhesive bandages
- Stryker hand-held pressure monitor (Fig. 171-1)
- Quick pressure monitor set (see Fig. 171-1)
  - 3-mL sodium chloride fluid-filled syringe
  - Sterile monitor pack (large-bore needle and monitor hub)

Indications

- Suspected compartment syndrome

Contraindications

- Local infection or overlying skin disease
- Anticoagulation (relative contraindication)

Technique

- Informed consent is obtained and the correct extremity identified.
- The needle, hub, and syringe of the quick pressure monitor set are attached to each other, maintaining sterility of the needle and hub. The hub is then placed into the port on the manometer. Saline is gently pushed through the apparatus until a drop is visualized at the tip of the needle.
- To avoid damage to neurovascular structures, each compartment should be approached with an understanding of anatomic contents (Table 171-1).
  - Anterior: Needle insertion is made into the muscle belly of the tibialis anterior muscle just lateral to the anterior tibial border at the level of the middle third of the tibia (Fig. 171-2).
  - Lateral: Needle insertion is into the bellies of the peroneus longus and brevis muscles midway between the fibular head and lateral malleolus (see Fig. 171-2).
  - Deep posterior: Needle insertion is posterior to the posteromedial tibia in its middle aspect, closely approximating the posterior aspect of the bone. The needle will first enter the flexor digitorum longus muscle and, when guided deeper, will enter the posterior tibial muscle. As long as the needle

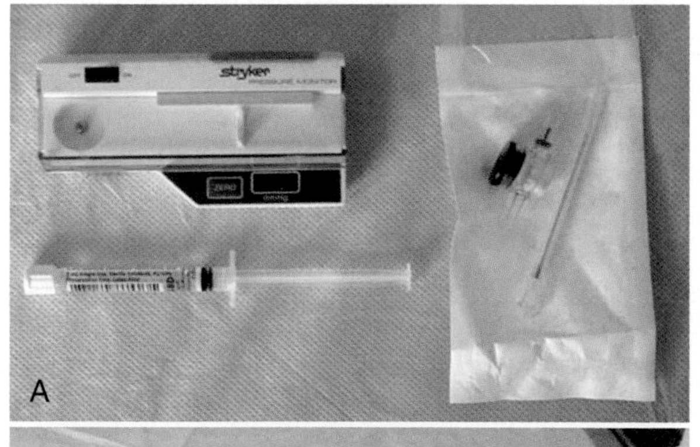

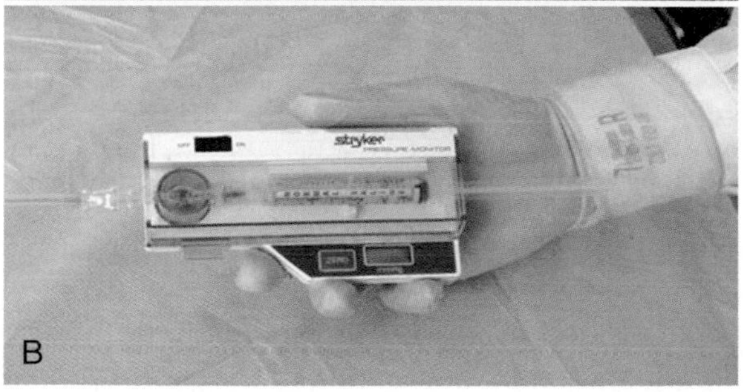

Figure 171-1 Stryker hand-held monitor and quick pressure monitor set. **A,** Preassembly. **B,** Postassembly.

TABLE 171-1 *Neurovascular Contents of Lower Leg Compartments*

Compartment	Neurovascular Structures
Anterior	Deep peroneal nerve, tibial artery
Lateral	Superficial peroneal nerve
Deep posterior	Peroneal artery/vein, tibial nerve/artery
Superficial posterior	Sural nerve, saphenous vein

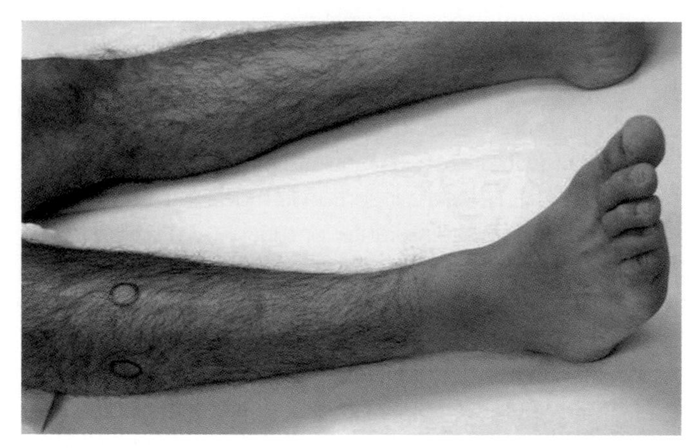

Figure 171-2 Insertion sites for anterior and lateral compartments.

is not driven too deeply, this method will keep the needle anterior and medial to the neurovascular structures (Fig. 171-3).

- Superficial posterior: Needle insertion is made into the muscle bellies of the gastrocnemius and soleus muscles just medial to the midline (Fig. 171-4).

- Needle insertion sites are marked and cleansed with alcohol. Topical anesthesia is achieved with ethyl chloride spray. Local anesthesia is then achieved with 1 mL of 1% lidocaine injected subcutaneously at each site.
- Each of the test insertion sites is then thoroughly prepped with alcohol and iodine.
- Before insertion, the needle is placed perpendicular to the insertion site and the monitor zeroed. The needle is inserted into the muscle compartment and 0.3 mL of saline is injected. The pressure reading will slowly decrease. Measurement is recorded as the value at which the pressure stops decreasing or after the pressure vacillates up and down a few times. After the resting test, the areas are cleansed with alcohol and adhesive bandages are placed.
- In suspected exertional compartment syndrome, the athlete then exercises until symptoms are reproduced. Athletes should perform the specific exercise that typically causes their symptoms, to the point at which they would normally have to stop or to a level of 8 out of 10.
- After exercise, each of the areas is again cleansed with alcohol and testing is repeated for each of the compartments, entering the same insertion sites as used pre-exercise. The sites are then again thoroughly cleansed with alcohol, antibiotic ointment is applied (as long as it is not contraindicated), and adhesive bandages are placed.

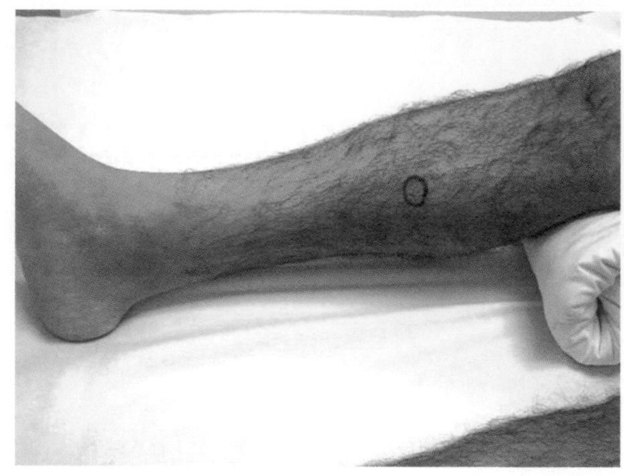

Figure 171-3 Insertion site for deep posterior compartment.

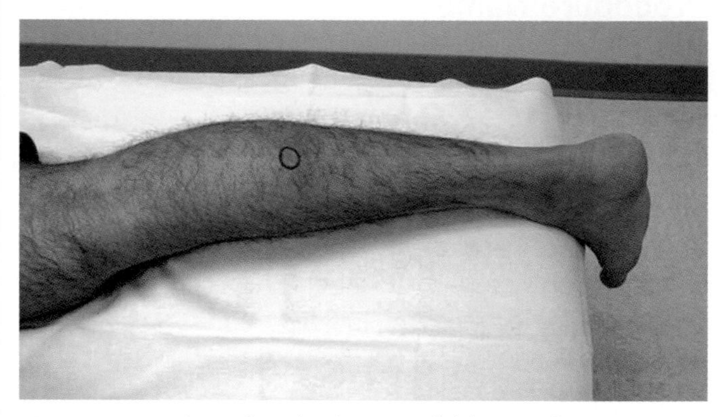

Figure 171-4 Insertion site for superficial posterior compartment.

Considerations in Special Populations

- Static (most common) and dynamic testing can be performed. Dynamic testing requires continuous monitoring with an indwelling catheter, which limits testing to a single compartment, requires the athlete to remain in one setting, and may result in the catheter failing to remain in place during the procedure.
- It is advised that anticoagulated patients be removed from anticoagulants before pressure measurements whenever possible.

Troubleshooting

- Several factors will ensure accurate pressure measurements.
    - Leg positioning, particularly of the knee and ankle, must be identical before and after exercise.
    - Exercise using the same activity that normally causes symptoms.
    - No contact should be made with the limb tested other than with the pressure monitor.
    - Patients are instructed to relax to prevent additional muscle contraction (which can result in an artificially high reading).
    - All potentially involved compartments must be tested. Failure to identify all involved compartments is a cause of surgical remediation failure.

Patient Instructions

- Ice for 10 minutes three times daily for 3 days.
- Perform local wound care daily (alcohol wipe, antibiotic ointment if not contraindicated, and adhesive bandages) for 3 days.
- Call the physician's office if you experience swelling, severe pain, neurologic sequelae, or symptoms suggestive of infection.

Suggested Reading

- Glorioso J, Wilckens J: Compartment syndrome testing. In O'Connor F, Wilder R (eds): The Textbook of Running Medicine. New York: McGraw-Hill, 2001, pp 95–100.
- Glorioso J, Wilckens J: Exertional leg pain. In O'Connor F, Wilder R (eds): The Textbook of Running Medicine. New York: McGraw-Hill, 2001, pp 181–198.
- Pedowitz RA, Hargens AR, Mubarak SJ, et al: Modified criteria for the objective diagnosis of chronic compartment syndrome of the leg. Am J Sports Med 1990;18:35–40.
- Wilder R, Sethi S: Overuse injuries: Tendinopathies, stress fractures, compartment syndrome, and shin splints. Clin Sports Med 2004;23:55–81.

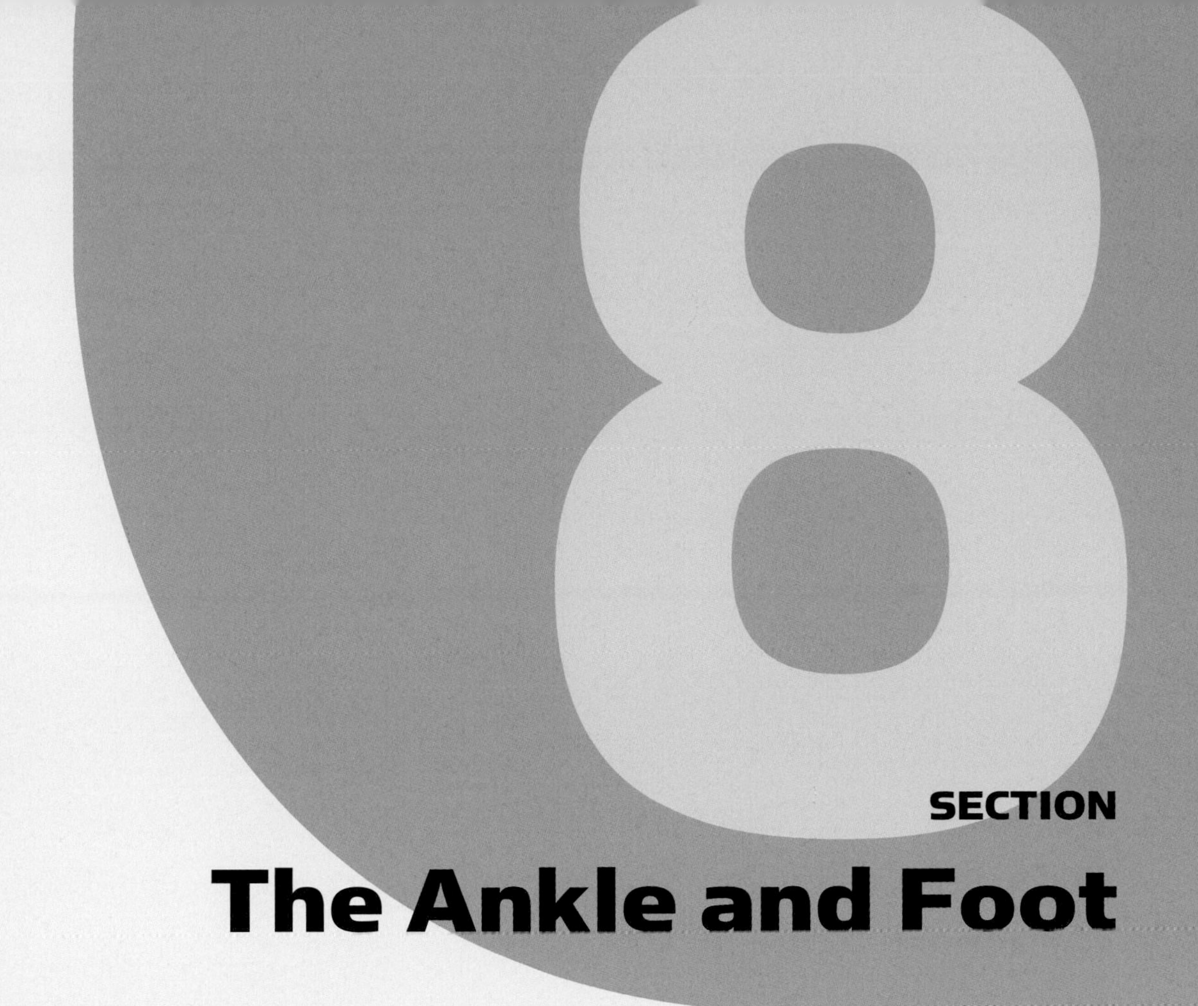

SECTION

8 The Ankle and Foot

Chapter 172 Overview of the Ankle and Foot

Anish R. Kadakia

Key Concepts

- The ankle and foot are a continuation of the locomotor system of the body that allows efficient ambulation.
- The most important aspect in the treatment of ankle and foot disorders is obtaining the correct diagnosis.
- A thorough history and physical examination are often all that is required to elucidate the diagnosis.
- Supplemental imaging, such as magnetic resonance imaging, computed tomography, technetium-99m bone scan, and ultrasonography are frequently not required and deferral to the specialist is appropriate for ordering these examinations.
- The treatment of many ankle and foot conditions can be initiated in the office, minimizing the delay inherent in referral to a specialist.

Anatomy

Bones and Joints

- The primary articulation between the foot and the appendicular skeleton is the ankle joint.
- The joint is composed of the distal tibia and fibula and their respective articulations with the talus.
- The foot itself consists of 28 bones: talus, calcaneus, navicular, cuboid, cuneiforms (3), metatarsals (5), proximal phalanges (5), middle phalanges of the lesser toes (4), distal phalanges (5), and sesamoids of the great toe (2) (Figs. 172-1 to 172-5).
- The multiple joints in the foot can be divided into three distinct divisions: hindfoot, midfoot, and forefoot.
  - Hindfoot: talocalcaneal (subtalar), talonavicular, and calcaneocuboid joints
  - Midfoot: Naviculocuneiform and metatarsocuneiform (tarsometatarsal or Lisfranc) joints
  - Forefoot: Metatarsophalangeal, proximal interphalangeal, and distal interphalangeal joints

Ligaments

- Multiple ligaments in the ankle and foot impart the stability required for weight bearing.
- Those most commonly injured include the anterior talofibular ligament, calcaneofibular ligament, deltoid ligament, Lisfranc ligament, and spring ligament (Table 172-1).

Muscles

- The muscular and tendinous structures that cross the ankle and foot can be divided into two groups: intrinsic and extrinsic muscles.
  - Extrinsic muscles are those that originate superior to the ankle joint and insert in the foot.
  - Intrinsic muscles originate and insert in the foot.

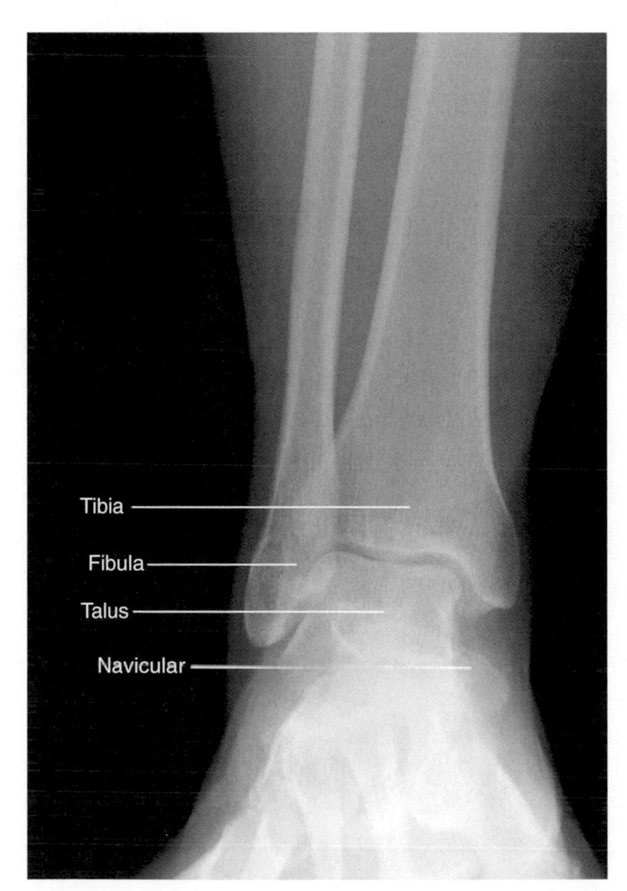

Figure 172-1 Anteroposterior weight-bearing radiograph of the ankle.

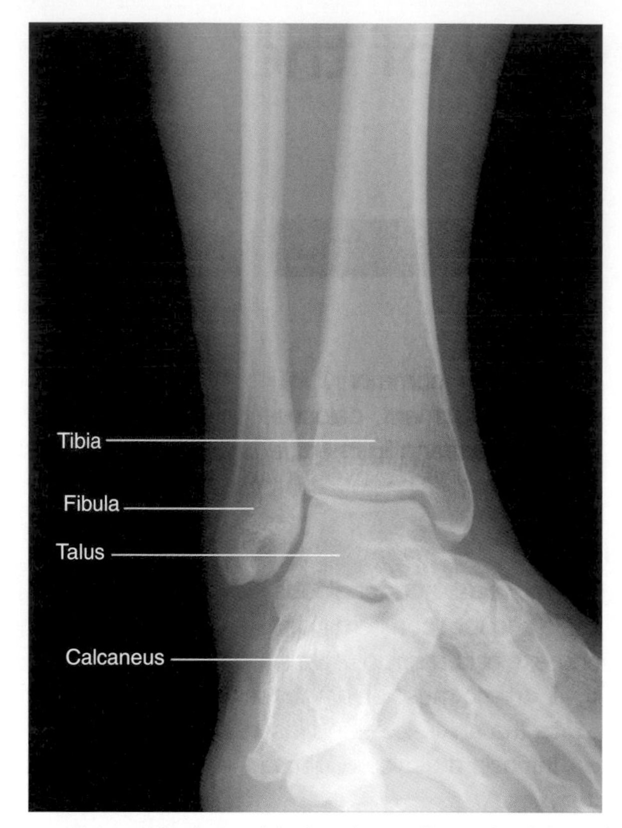

Figure 172-2 Mortise weight-bearing radiograph of the ankle.

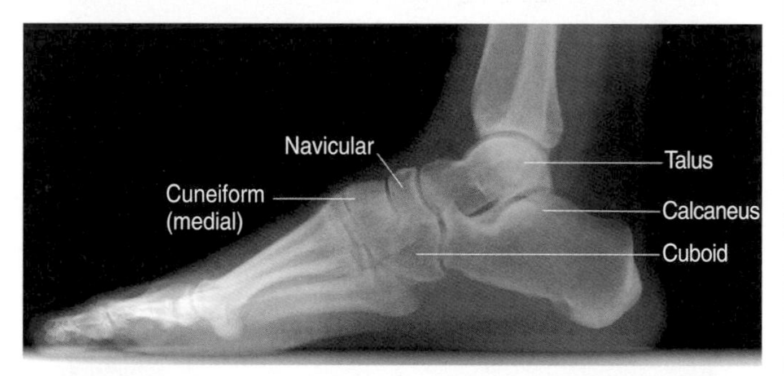

Figure 172-3 Lateral weight-bearing radiograph of the ankle and foot.

TABLE 172-1 *Ligaments of the Foot and Ankle*

Ligament	Origin	Insertion
ATFL	Tip of the fibula	Talus
CFL	Tip of the fibula	Calcaneus
Deltoid	Tip of the medial malleolus	Talus and calcaneus
Lisfranc	Medial cuneiform	Base of the second metatarsal
Spring	Sustentaculum tali of calcaneus	Navicular

ATFL, anterior talofibular ligament; CFL, calcaneofibular ligament.

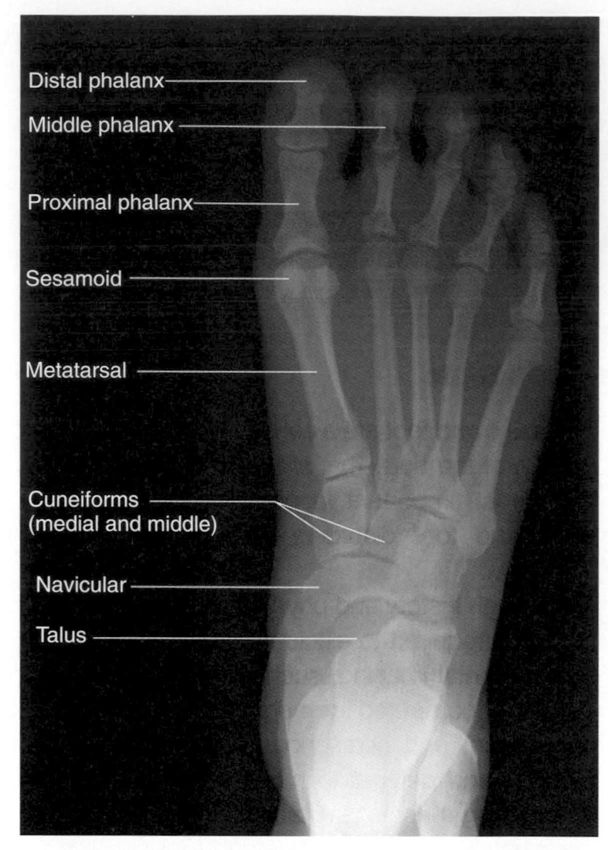

Figure 172-4 Anteroposterior weight-bearing radiograph of the foot.

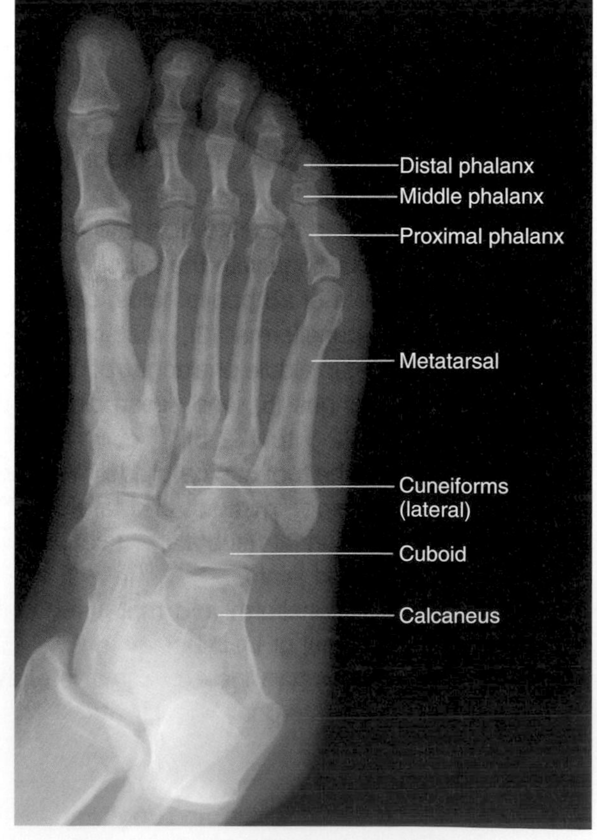

Figure 172-5 Internal oblique view radiograph of the foot.

- The most common tendon pathologies of the foot and ankle involve the extrinsics.

Extrinsic
- Anterior: tibialis anterior, extensor hallucis longus, extensor digitorum longus, peroneus tertius
- Posterior: Achilles tendon
- Posterolateral: peroneus brevis and peroneus longus
- Posteromedial: tibialis posterior, flexor digitorum longus, flexor hallucis longus

Intrinsic
- Dorsum of foot: extensor digitorum brevis, extensor hallucis brevis
  - The extensor hallucis brevis is the medial portion of the extensor digitorum brevis, which originates from the anterior calcaneus. Innervation is by the deep peroneal nerve.
- Plantar foot: There are four layers of intrinsic muscles plantarly that are innervated by the medial and lateral plantar nerves (terminal branches of the tibial nerve)
  - Layer 1 (superficial): abductor hallucis, flexor digitorum brevis, abductor digiti minimi
  - Layer 2: quadratus plantae, lumbricals (four)
  - Layer 3: adductor hallucis, flexor hallucis brevis, flexor digiti minimi brevis
  - Layer 4 (deep): dorsal interossei (four), plantar interossei (three)

Nerves
- The sensation to the foot is provided by six terminal extensions of the lumbosacral plexus (Table 172-2).

Patient Evaluation

History
- The critical step in the diagnosis and treatment of foot and ankle disorders is obtaining a thorough history.
  - Injury history, duration of symptoms, exacerbating factors, pain, instability, mechanical symptoms, and a variety of other issues should be included.

TABLE 172-2 *Superficial Nerve Distribution of the Ankle and Foot*

Nerve	Sensory Distribution
Superficial peroneal	Dorsum of ankle and foot
Deep peroneal	First web space
Saphenous	Medial ankle
Sural	Lateral aspect of heel and foot
Medial plantar	Plantar foot (medial 3½ toes)
Lateral plantar	Plantar foot (lateral 1½ toes)

- Pain is a primary presenting symptom and can provide a wealth of information when analyzed critically. The common types of pain and their significance are presented Table 172-3.
  — Instruct the patient to localize the source of the pain with one finger; this will allow a focused examination of the anatomic structures within the area, facilitating diagnosis.
- Instability or "giving out" can be associated with recurrent ankle sprains and incompetence of the lateral collateral ligaments (anterior talofibular ligament and calcaneofibular ligament) or osteochondral lesions (paroxysmal instability).
- In addition to the focused musculoskeletal history, evaluation for peripheral vascular disease, diabetes, inflammatory arthropathy, and neuropathy may aid in diagnosis and affect the course of treatment.

Physical Examination
- Standing position: The physical examination begins with observing the patient's gait to assess alignment, asymmetry, limp, knee thrust (varus, valgus, recurvatum), and foot position at heel strike. Evaluate for uneven shoe wear and assess the shape of the shoe compared with the shape of the foot. Examination with the patient in a standing position allows a true assessment of the longitudinal arch, heel alignment (varus or valgus), and position of the toes (Figs. 172-6 and 172-7). During a single limb heel rise (Fig. 172-8), failure of heel inversion, lack of a rise of the longitudinal arch, and external rotation of the leg are indicative of a pathologic process such as posterior tibial tendon dysfunction or an Achilles tendon disorder.
- Sitting position: A systematic examination begins with the skin, evaluating for edema, callosities, ecchymo-

TABLE 172-3 *Pain Type and Clinical Correlation*

Type of Pain	Significance
Start-up pain (at the initiation of activity)	Arthritis, fasciitis
Night pain (at the end of the day after activity)	Arthritis, impingement
Activity-related pain	Tendinitis, osteochondral lesions, impingement, stress fractures, trauma
Burning or tingling pain	Morton's neuroma, tarsal tunnel, neuropathy
Shoe wear–related pain	Hallux valgus, hallux rigidus, claw or hammer toes, midfoot arthritis (osteophytes and deformity), accessory navicular, nail disorder

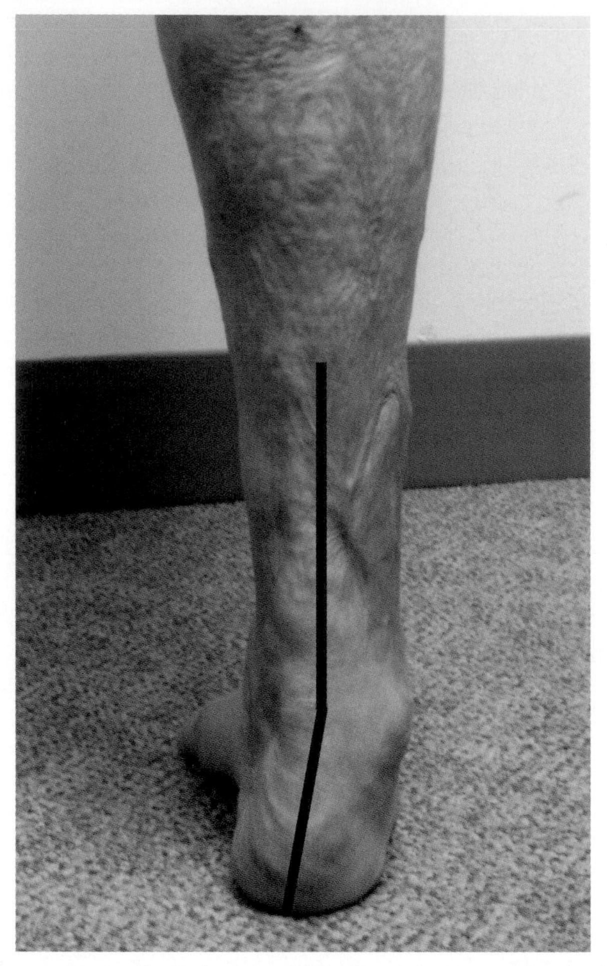

Figure 172-6 Posterior view of the heel demonstrating heel varus. Note how the heel turns toward the midline. Associated with stress fractures of the fifth metatarsal, instability, or hereditary sensory motor neuropathy.

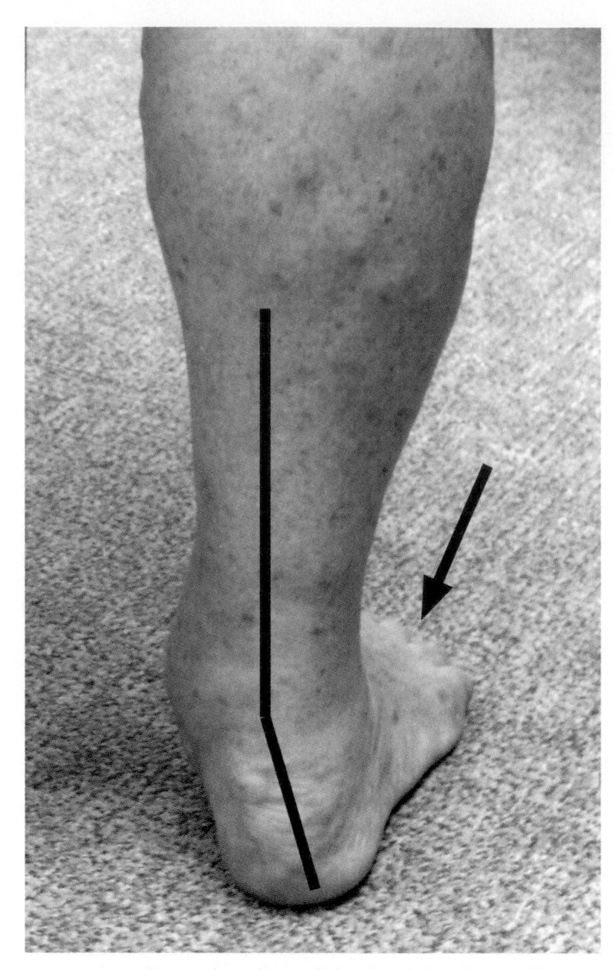

Figure 172-7 Posterior view of the heel demonstrating heel valgus. Note how the heel turns outward, away from the midline. "Too many toes" sign (*arrow*). Less than 5 degrees is physiologic; if more, it can be associated with pes planovalgus (flatfoot), midfoot arthritis, or posterior tibial tendinitis.

sis, erythema, ulcers, or previous incisions. The two palpable pulses are the dorsalis pedis (dorsum of foot) and the tibialis posterior (posterior to medial malleolus).

- The inability to palpate the pulses or loss of hair can indicate peripheral vascular disease.
- The most sensitive test for the presence of neuropathy is the failure to sense a Semmes-Weinstein 5.07 monofilament. These are commercially available and should be a routine part in the examination of diabetic patients.
- Systematic palpation is very effective at localizing the source of the pain given the superficial location of the bony, ligamentous, and tendinous structures of the foot and ankle.
- Some of the classic anatomic locations and their significance are shown in Table 172-4.
- Range of motion is extremely helpful in understanding the pathologic process.

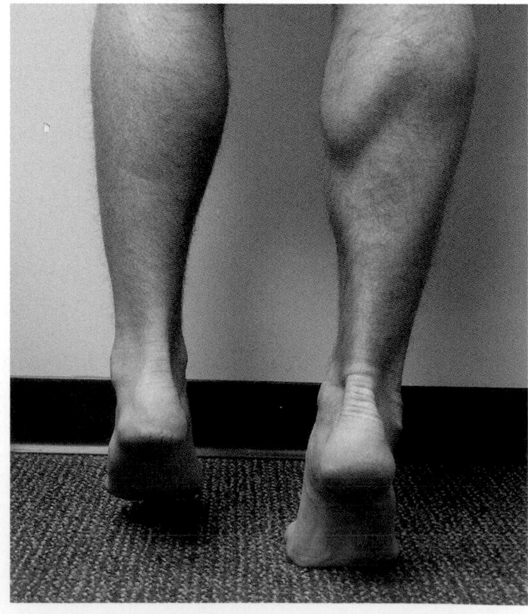

Figure 172-8 Single limb heel rise with slight inversion of the heel and normal longitudinal arch.

TABLE 172-4 *Pain Location and Clinical Correlation*

Location	Significance
Anterior ankle	Ankle arthritis, osteochondral lesion of the talus
Posteromedial ankle	Posterior tibial tendon dysfunction
Posterolateral ankle	Peroneal tendinitis
Posterior ankle: superficial	Achilles tendinitis or rupture (acute)
Posterior ankle: deep	Os trigonum or flexor hallucis longus tendinitis
Dorsal midfoot	Midfoot arthritis or Lisfranc injury
Inferior to the fibula	Ankle sprain
Between the tibia and fibula	High ankle sprain (syndesmotic injury)
Heel tenderness	Calcaneal stress fracture, fat pad atrophy, insertional Achilles tendinitis or rupture
Plantar foot	Plantar fasciitis
Great toe	Hallux rigidus or hallux valgus
Lesser toes	Synovitis or neuroma (burning/tingling)

- — Asymmetry between extremities or pain at the extremes of motion is more relevant than the absolute value.
- — Maximal range of motion of the ankle is 10 to 23 degrees of dorsiflexion and 23 to 48 degrees of plantarflexion (Figs. 172-9 and 172-10).
- — Maximal range of subtalar inversion is 5 to 50 degrees and eversion is 5 to 26 degrees (Figs. 172-11 and 172-12).
- — Maximal range of motion for the first metatarsophalangeal joint (great toe) is 45 to 90 degrees of dorsiflexion and 10 to 40 degrees of plantarflexion (Figs. 172-13 and 172-14).

- Motor strength should be tested with the patient actively firing the muscle group to be tested (Table 172-5).
  - — The examiner then attempts to move the foot against the patient's resistance.
  - — At full strength, the examiner should not be able to overcome the patient.
- The gastrocnemius/soleus complex is best tested with single limb heel rise (see Fig. 172-8). The posterior tibial tendon can be isolated from the anterior tibial tendon using the figure 4 position (Fig. 172-15).

Imaging

- Plain radiographs are critical in the evaluation of foot and ankle pathology.
- All views should be weight bearing when possible.

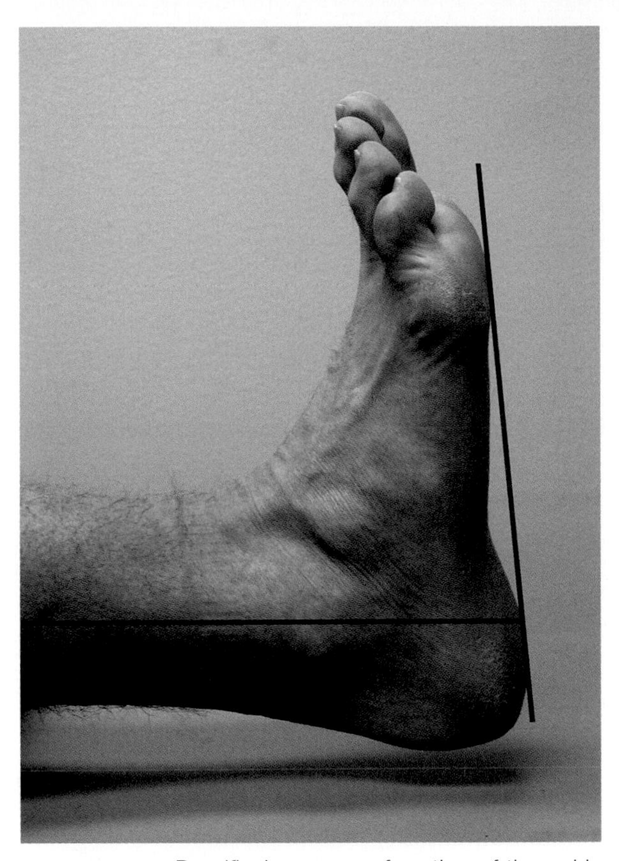

Figure 172-9 Dorsiflexion range of motion of the ankle.

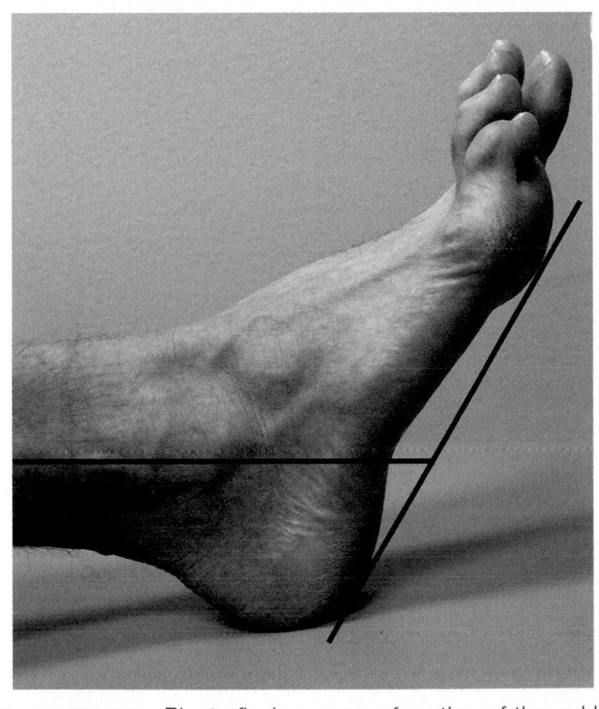

Figure 172-10 Plantarflexion range of motion of the ankle.

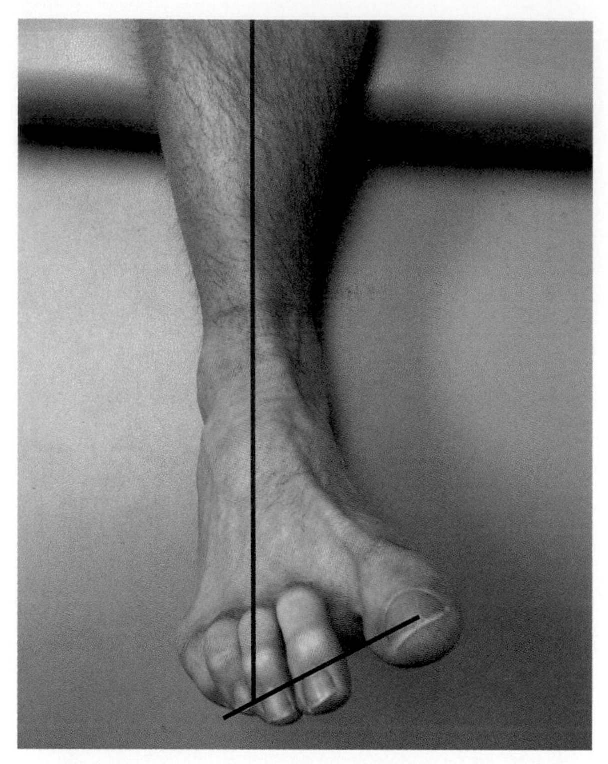

Figure 172-11 Inversion range of motion of the hindfoot.

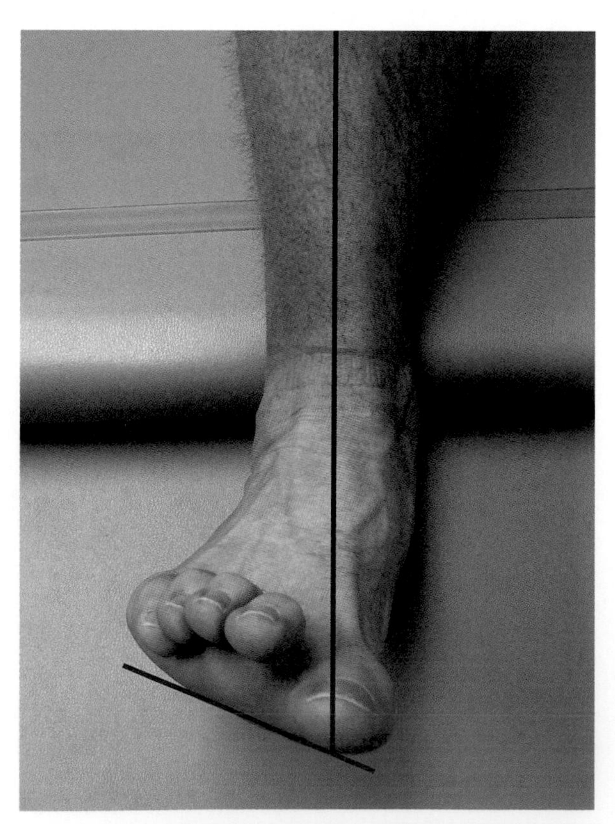

Figure 172-12 Eversion range of motion of the hindfoot.

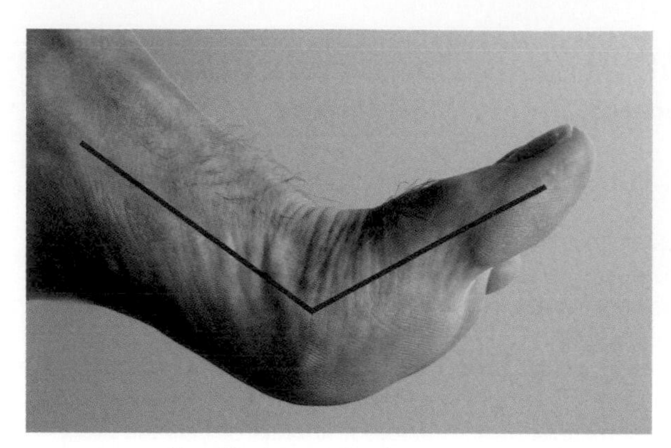

Figure 172-13 Dorsiflexion of the first metatarsophalangeal joint.

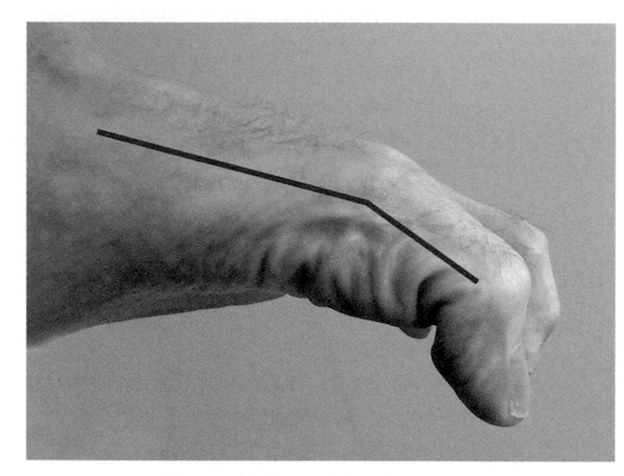

Figure 172-14 Plantarflexion of the first metatarsophalangeal joint.

TABLE 172-5 *Motor Examination of the Ankle*

Muscle Group	Motion
Anterior tibialis	Dorsiflexion
Gastrocnemius/soleus (Achilles)	Plantarflexion
Posterior tibial tendon	Inversion
Peroneal tendons	Eversion

- The ability to detect subtle alignment and arthritic conditions is improved with weight-bearing views.
- Standard views of the ankle include anteroposterior (see Fig. 172-1), mortise (15 degrees of internal rotation) (see Fig. 172-2), and lateral (see Fig. 172-3).
- Standard views of the foot include anteroposterior (see Fig. 172-4), internal oblique (see Fig. 172-5), and lateral (Fig. 172-3).
- Radiographic findings may include those shown in Table 172-6.

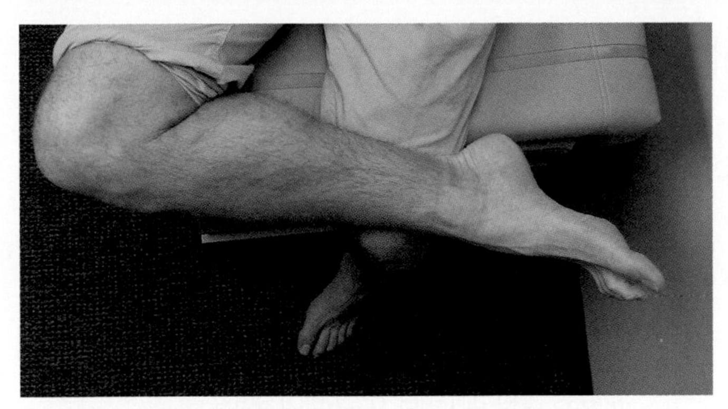

Figure 172-15 The figure 4 position to assess the strength of the posterior tibial tendon. Test-resisted inversion with the patient's foot in the plantarflexed position.

Suggested Reading

- Baumhauer JF, Parekh SL, Lee T: Internet resources for foot and ankle care. J Am Acad Orthop Surg 2004;12:288.
- Coughlin MJ, Mann RA, Saltzman CL (eds): Surgery of the Foot and Ankle, 8th ed. St Louis: Mosby, 2006.
- Myerson MS (ed): Foot and Ankle Disorders. Philadelphia: WB Saunders, 2000.

TABLE 172-6 *Clinical Relevance of Common Radiographic Findings*

Finding	Significance
Lucency in the talus	Osteochondral lesion of the talus
Small bone medial to the navicular	Accessory navicular (associated with posterior tibial tendon dysfunction)
Calcaneal spur (superior)	Insertional Achilles tendinitis
Calcaneal spur (inferior)	Fasciitis (spur does not require removal)
Dorsal spur on first metatarsophalangeal	Hallux rigidus
Fleck at the base of the second metatarsal	Lisfranc injury

Chapter 173 Chondral Injuries

Gerardo Juan Maquieira and Norman Espinosa

ICD-9 CODE
732.7 *Osteochondritis Dissecans*

Key Concepts

- Injury to articular cartilage can result in progressive osteoarthritis.
- Articular cartilage damage ranges from softening or fibrillation to separation and detachment from the underlying subchondral bone.
- Chondral lesions of the talus or distal tibia may occur after acute or cumulative trauma to the ankle joint.
- High incidence of chondral injuries in ankle fractures
- The most common cause of chondral injury is acute trauma, such as an ankle sprain.
- The talar dome is more often injured than the tibial plafond.

History

- Acute injury
  - Ankle sprain and/or fracture
  - Pain around ankle joint
  - Locking or popping
- Chronic injury
  - Continued or worsening symptoms despite prolonged period of conservative treatment
  - Recurrent swelling and pain with activity
  - Limited ankle range of motion

Physical Examination

- Observation
  - Effusion (intra-articular swelling)
  - Deformity
- Palpation
  - Anteromedial and/or anterolateral ankle tenderness
- Range of motion
  - Loss of dorsiflexion/plantarflexion can occur from effusion.
  - Possible locking or popping in conjunction with displaced articular cartilage fragment
- Special tests
  - Assessment of lateral ankle stability with inversion stress and anterior drawer tests
  - Varus/valgus stress to the hindfoot may produce medial or lateral talar dome pain.

Imaging

- Radiographs: weight-bearing anteroposterior, lateral, and mortise views of the ankle
  - Check for medial or lateral talar dome avulsions or displaced fragments
  - Chronic injuries may have medial or lateral cystic lesions in the talus (Fig. 173-1).
  - Look for preexisting osteophytes on the anterior distal tibia or talar neck ("talar nose" on lateral view) (Fig. 173-2).
- Magnetic resonance imaging
  - Often required to diagnose the chondral lesion
  - Look for the classic bone bruise pattern (Fig. 173-3).
  - Look for additional ligamentous or syndesmosis lesions.
- Computed tomography
  - Gadolinium arthrography computed tomography often reveals the articular cartilage defect.
  - Reveals size and location of osteochondral lesions most accurately
  - Look for underlying cystic lesions to the bone (Fig. 173-4).

Additional Tests

- Optional infiltration of the ankle joint with local anesthetic and/or cortisone may be used as a diagnostic and therapeutic measure (see Chapter 200).

Differential Diagnosis

- Ankle instability: tenderness over ligaments, possible varus/valgus hindfoot deformity, ligament laxity compared with contralateral side
- Avascular necrosis: often pain at rest; differentiate on magnetic resonance imaging

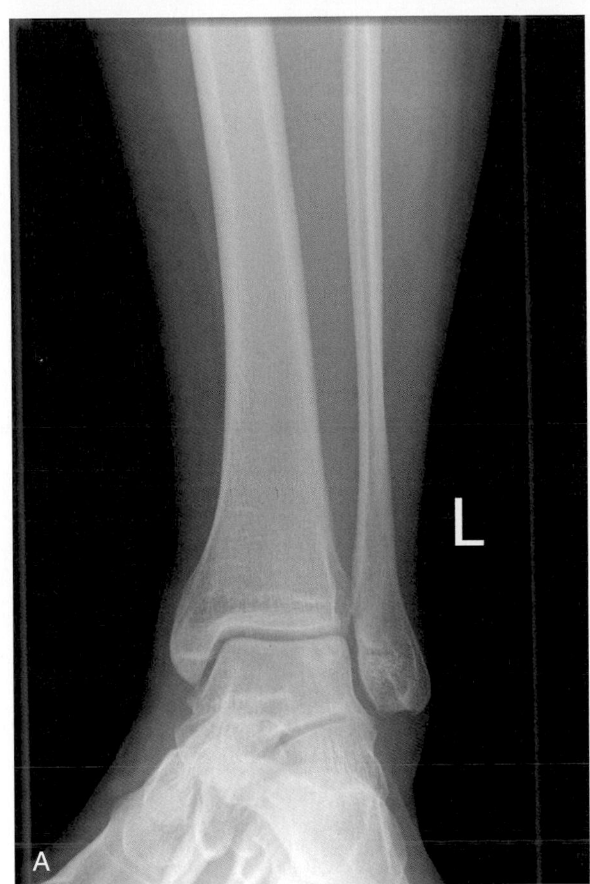

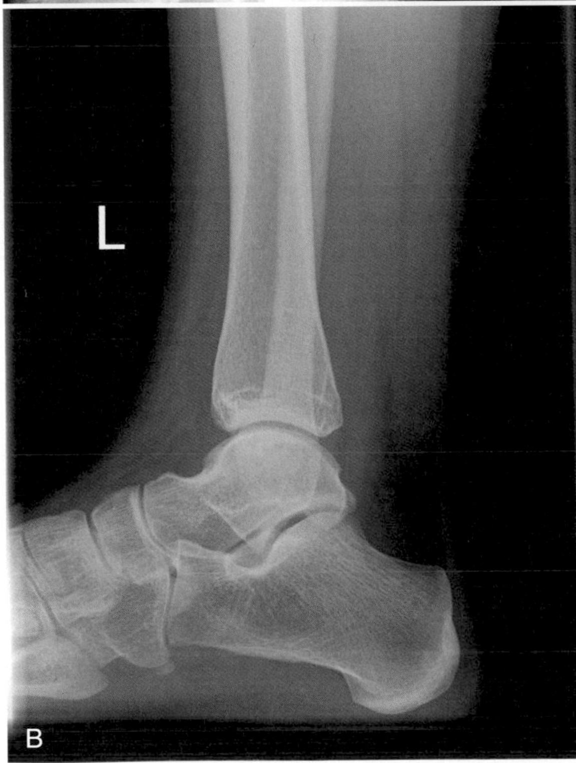

Figure 173-1 **A**, Mortise view of the ankle showing a subchondral osteolytic lesion on the lateral talar dome. **B**, The lesion is not visible on the lateral view.

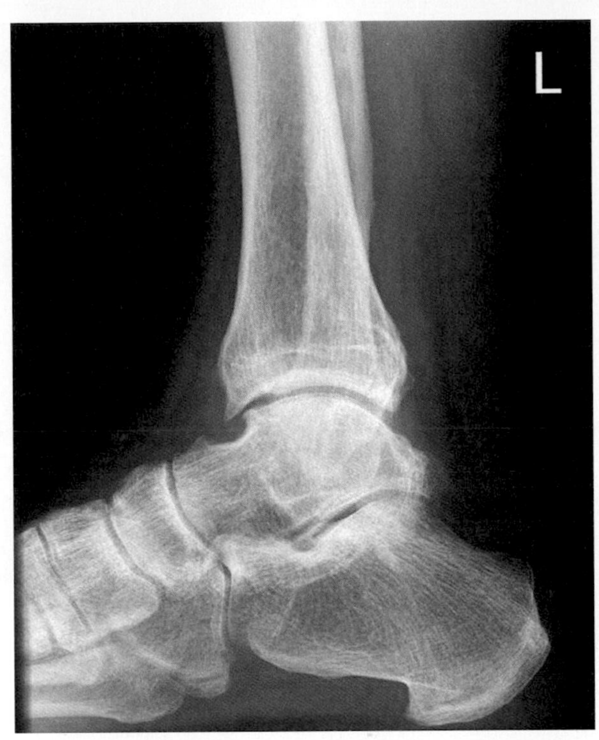

Figure 173-2 Osteophytes on anterior distal tibia and superior talar neck.

- Osteoarthritis: joint line tenderness, decreased range of motion
- Ankle impingement: anterolateral tenderness, pain with forced dorsiflexion

Treatment

- At diagnosis
  - Initial treatment of chondral injuries includes immobilization of the ankle and non-weight bearing on the involved extremity combined with analgesia.
  - Ankle arthroscopy is recommended acutely in the case of intra-articular step-off or loose body.
  - The treatment of choice for an acute chondral injury is open reduction and internal fixation if the fragment is displaced and greater than 5 mm in size.
  - In the case of avulsion fractures or loose fragments, débridement is standard.
- Later
  - Most symptomatic osteochondral lesions are amenable to ankle arthroscopy.
  - The entire articular surface of the talus and tibia should be gently probed to detect changes in surface texture and consistency (Fig. 173-5).

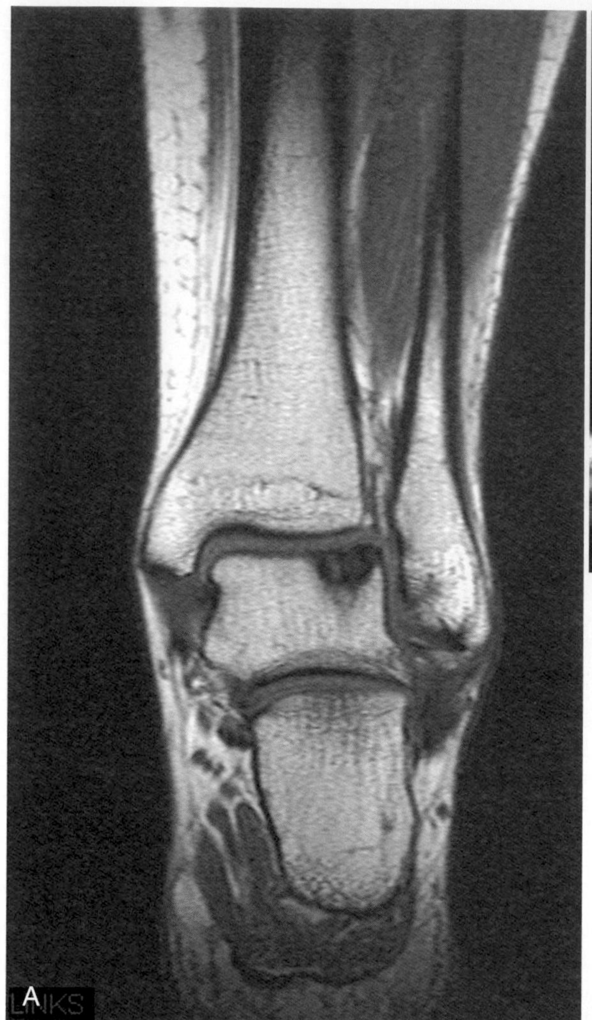

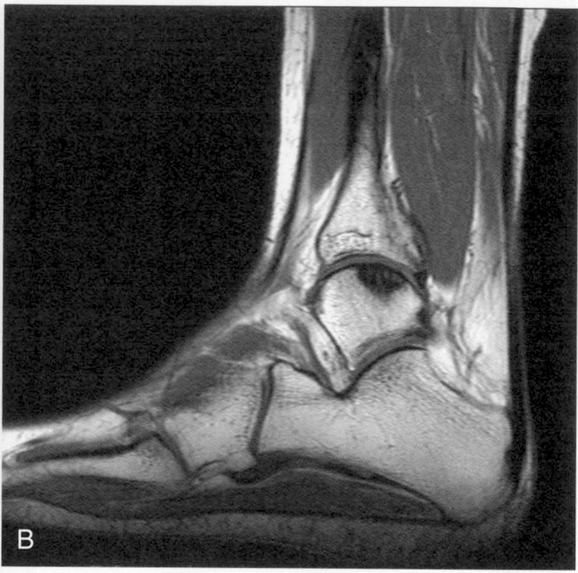

Figure 173-3 **A**, T2-weighted coronal magnetic resonance imaging with chondral irregularity and subchondral bone bruise on lateral talus. **B**, T2-weighted sagittal magnetic resonance imaging.

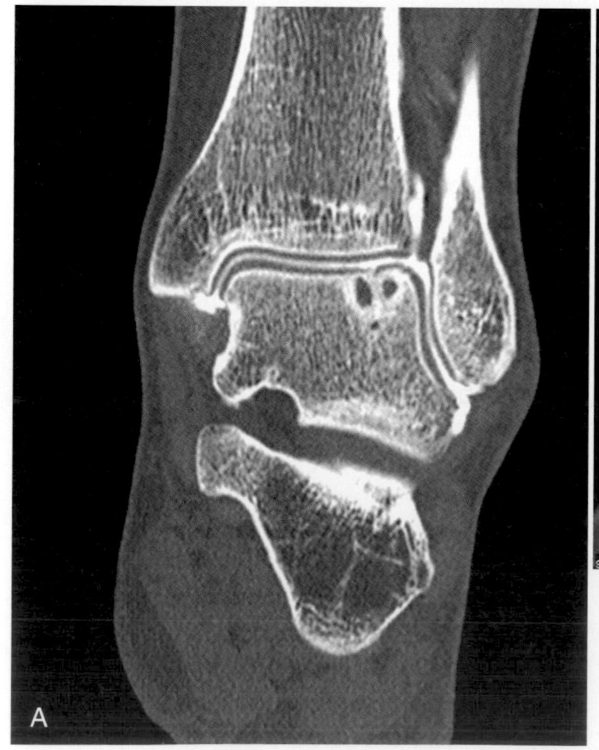

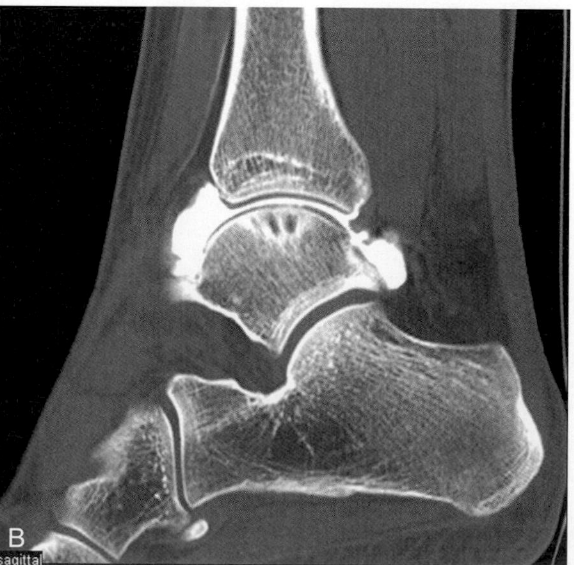

Figure 173-4 **A**, Coronal arthrography computed tomography with cartilage lesion (gadolinium entrance) and multicystic subchondral lesion. **B**, Sagittal view.

Continued

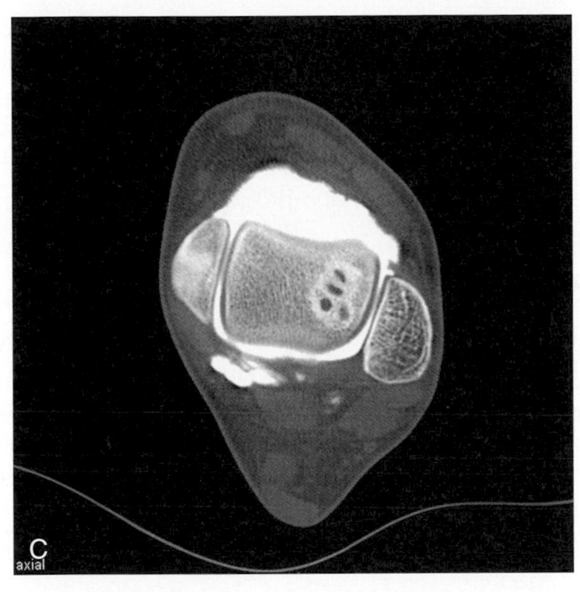

Figure 173-4, cont'd **C**, Axial view.

- If subchondral bone is exposed, débridement, drilling, or microfracture is generally recommended to establish vascular channels with eventual formation of a fibrocartilage surface.
- Patients with persistent symptoms after arthroscopy attributed to chondral lesions may be candidates for restorative techniques, such as autologous chondrocyte implantation or osteochondral grafting (Fig. 173-6).

When to Refer

- All but sedentary, inactive patients should be referred.
- In the case of an isolated osteochondral injury without a locked ankle (which mandates immediate referral), referral can be arranged at any time.

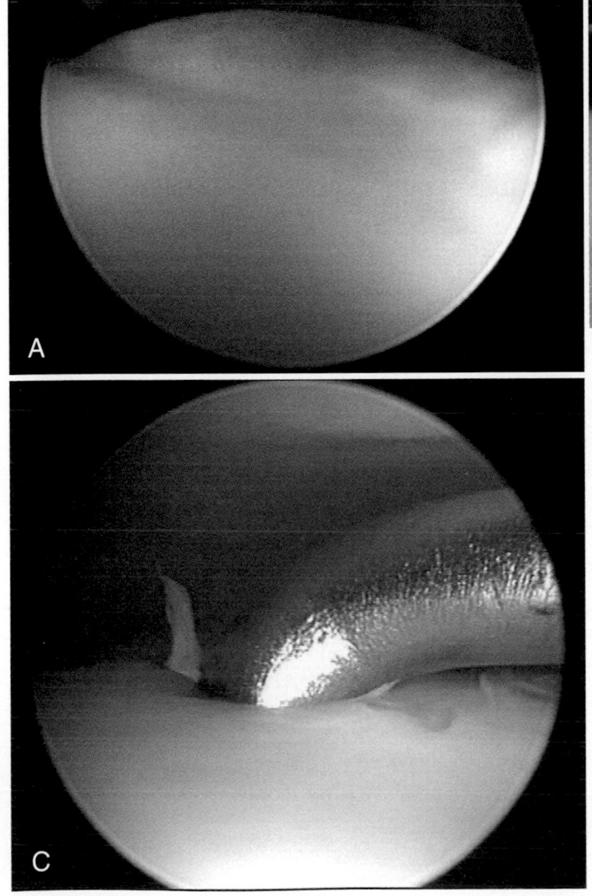

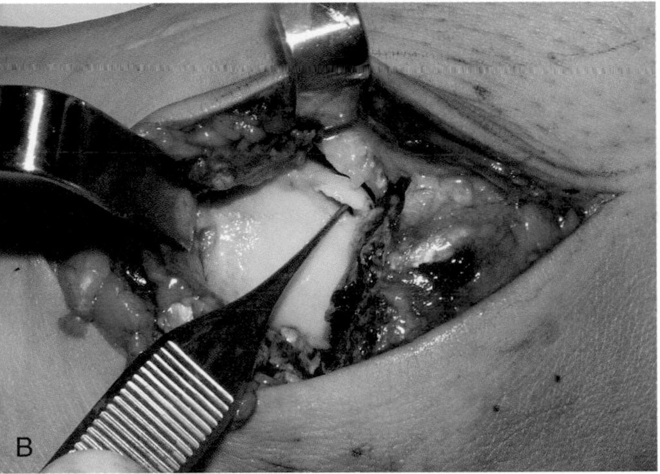

Figure 173-5 **A**, Arthroscopic view of talar cartilage irregularity. **B**, Cartilage instability of same patient after anterolateral arthrotomy. **C**, Arthroscopic view of talar cartilage lesion.

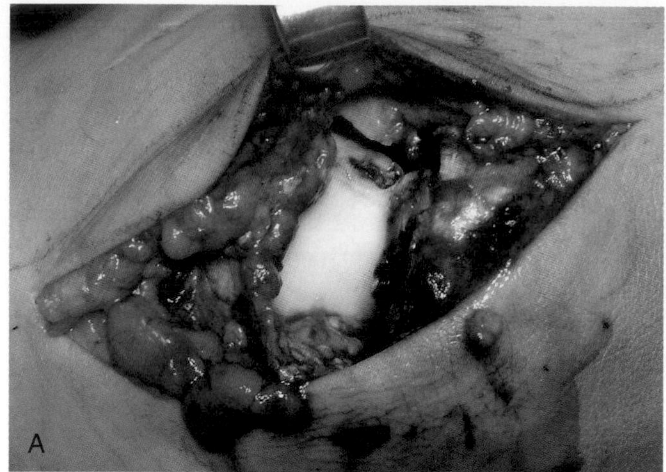

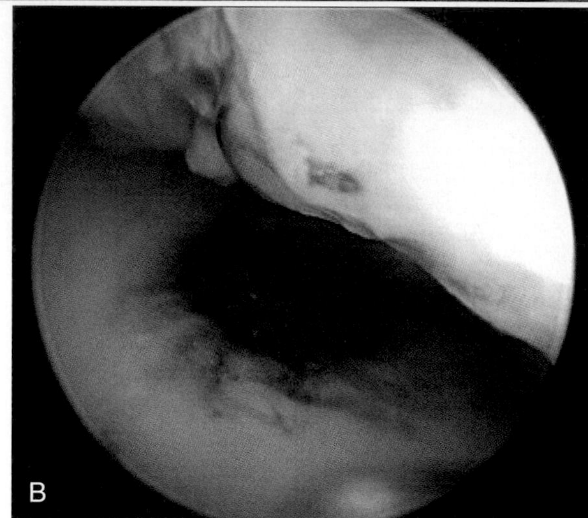

Figure 173-6 **A,** Talar cartilage lesion after open débridement and drilling. **B,** Talar cartilage lesion after débridement and autogenous bone grafting.

- However, because rehabilitation after restorative cartilage techniques requires 6 weeks of non-weight bearing, the referral should be made in a timely fashion to allow for appropriate planning.

Prognosis

- Good, if osteochondral lesions are small (<6 mm)
- Persistent radiologic osteochondral lesions after nonoperative or operative treatment may be asymptomatic.
- Progressive osteoarthritis of the ankle is more likely in larger osteochondral injuries after trauma.

Troubleshooting

- The patient should be counseled on the benefits and risks of surgery.
  - Benefits may include restoration of ankle mobility and reparation of the cartilage surface with successful return to sports and resolution of pain.
  - Risks include bleeding, infection, nerve injury, loss of motion, persistent pain, recurrence of the osteochondral lesion, and progressive osteoarthritis.

Patient Instructions

- In nonoperative treatment of an acute osteochondral injury, patient education is focused on decreasing the effusion (consider aspiration, start therapy with passive and active ankle motion, use ice and compression).
- Weight bearing is usually started 6 weeks after injury.
- If surgery is planned, follow the instructions of your surgeon.

Considerations in Special Populations

- Inactive, sedentary patients should be treated nonoperatively. If they have persistent pain, arthroscopic débridement can be considered.
- Obese patients should be motivated to lose weight before surgery so that the osteochondral lesion is relieved and the prognosis is improved.

Suggested Reading

- Buckwalter JA, Mankin HJ: Articular cartilage: Degeneration and osteoarthritis, repair, regeneration and transplantation. Instr Course Lect 1998;47:487–504.
- Farmer JM, Martin DF, Boles CA, et al: Chondral and osteochondral injuries. Diagnosis and management. Clin Sports Med 2001;20:299–320.
- Gobbi A, Francisco RA, Lubowitz JH, et al: Osteochondral lesions of the talus: Randomized controlled trial comparing chondroplasty, microfracture and osteochondral autograft transplantation. Arthroscopy 2002;22:1085–1092.
- Hintermann B, Regazzoni P, Lampert C: Arthroscopic findings in acute fractures of the ankle. J Bone Joint Surg Br 2000; 82B:345–351.
- Japour C, Vohra P, Giorgini R, et al: Ankle arthroscopy: Follow-up study of 33 ankles—effect of physical therapy and obesity. J Foot Ankle Surg 1996;35:199–209.
- Loren GJ, Ferkel RD: Arthroscopic assessment of occult intraarticular injury in acute ankle fractures. Arthroscopy 2002;18:412–421.
- Toth AP, Easley ME: Ankle chondral injuries and repair. Foot Ankle Clin 2000;5:799–840.
- Ueblacker P, Burkart A, Imhoff AB: Retrograde cartilage transplantation of the proximal and distal tibia. Arthroscopy 2004;20:73–78.

Chapter 174 Arthritis of the Ankle

Andrew Moore and Anish R. Kadakia

ICD-9 CODES

714.0 *Rheumatoid Arthritis*
715.17 *Osteoarthritis, Localized, Primary, Ankle, and Foot*
715.27 *Osteoarthritis, Localized, Secondary, Ankle, and Foot*
716.17 *Traumatic Arthritis*

Key Concepts

- Primary arthritis of the ankle is rare (Fig. 174-1).
- Trauma is the most common cause of ankle arthritis (ankle fractures, 37%; instability, 15%).

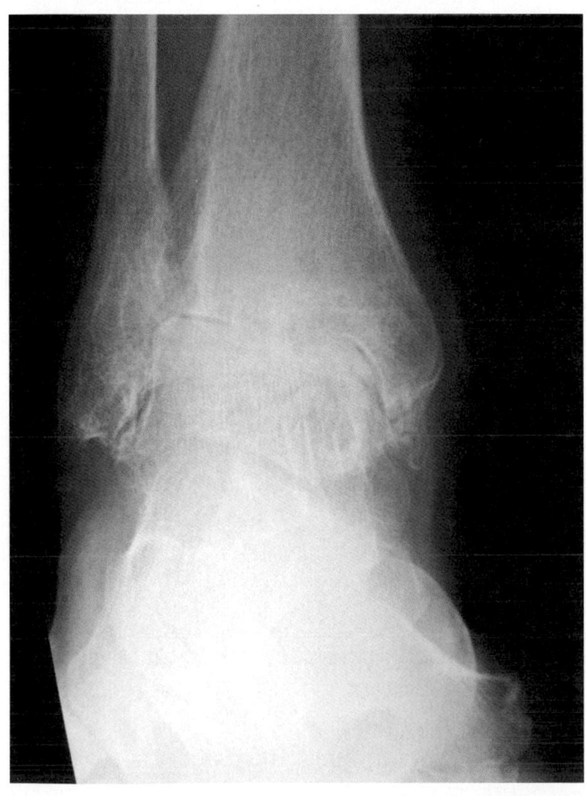

Figure 174-1 Anteroposterior ankle radiograph of a patient with end-stage ankle arthritis. Note the nearly total narrowing of the tibiotalar joint space. Medial and lateral osteophytes are also present.

- Many patients with ankle arthritis can be effectively managed without surgery.
- Ankle arthrodesis is the current gold standard for surgical treatment of ankle arthritis in which conservative measures have failed (Fig. 174-2).
- Ankle replacement may be a viable option for end-stage ankle arthritis in carefully selected patients, although long-term results are less predictable (Fig. 174-3).

History

- Ankle stiffness, swelling, and pain
- Most often unilateral
- Difficulty with inclines and stairs secondary to impingement
- Often report history of trauma or instability

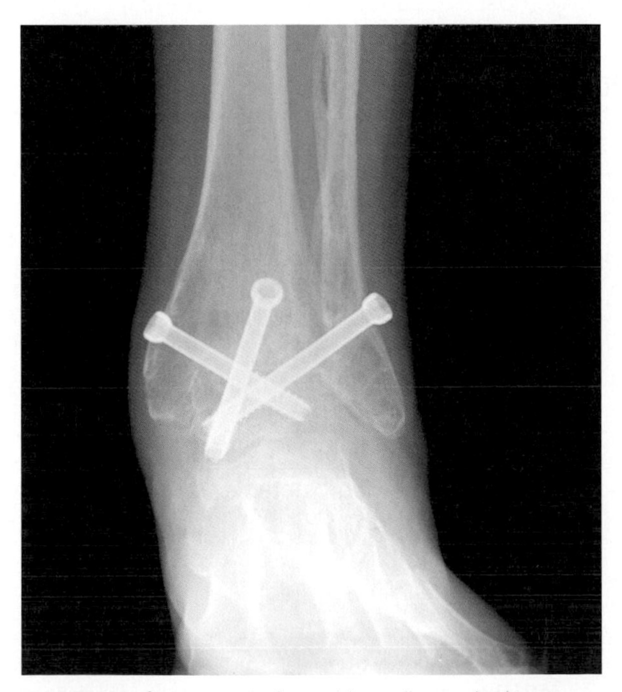

Figure 174-2 Anteroposterior ankle radiograph demonstrating a common three-screw technique for ankle arthrodesis.

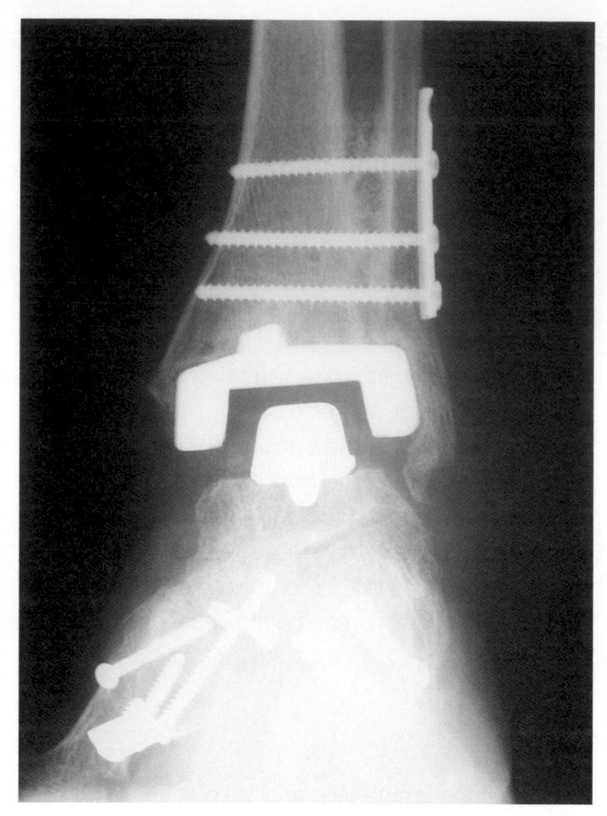

Figure 174-3 Anteroposterior ankle radiograph depicting the Agility total ankle arthroplasty.

- Less commonly, history of inflammatory arthropathy, infection, or bleeding disorder
- History of swelling, erythema, or warmth without significant pain suggests Charcot's (neuropathic) arthropathy, most frequently related to diabetes.

Physical Examination

- Observation
  - Effusion/swelling
  - Surgical scars
  - Deformity, limb/hindfoot malalignment
  - Gait
- Palpation
  - Tenderness at anterior ankle joint line
  - Lateral hindfoot pain indicates subtalar involvement.
- Range of motion
  - Ankle (dorsiflexion/plantarflexion); compare with contralateral side
  - Hindfoot motion (inversion/eversion); assess for concomitant hindfoot (subtalar) arthritis
- Special tests
  - Diagnostic injection: Injection of local anesthetic into the ankle or subtalar joint can help differentiate ankle from subtalar joint pain.

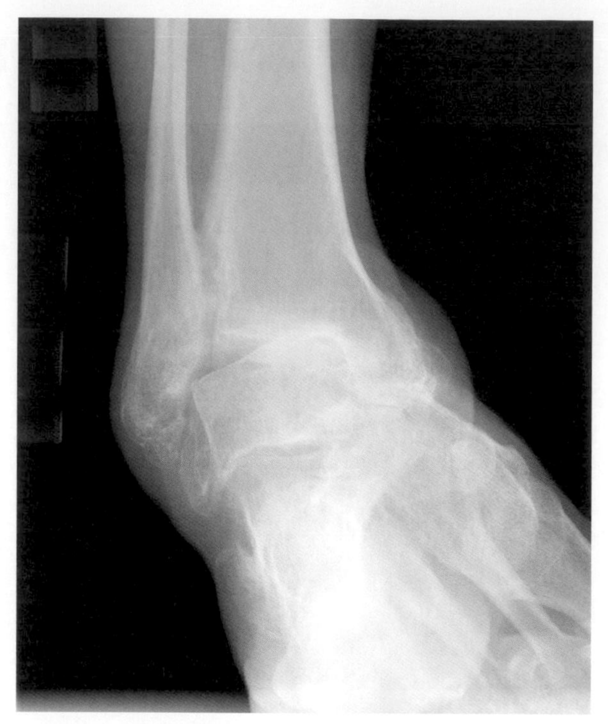

Figure 174-4 Mortise ankle radiograph of a patient with end-stage ankle arthritis. Secondary to chronic instability, the patient developed a severe varus deformity with subchondral sclerosis and obliteration of the medial joint line.

    — Use of contrast and fluoroscopy can ensure appropriate placement of the injection.
    — Addition of steroid can provide short-term relief.

Imaging

- Radiographs
  - Anteroposterior and mortise (15-degree oblique) views of the ankle (Fig. 174-4)
    — Assess for loss of joint space, syndesmosis widening, angular deformity, subchondral sclerosis, evidence of previous trauma.
  - Lateral view of the ankle (Fig. 174-5).
    — Anterior or posterior osteophytes result in impingement.
    — Assess subtalar joint
  - Anteroposterior, oblique, and lateral weight-bearing views of the foot
    — Assess for concomitant degenerative changes, malalignment
- Computed tomography
  - Not required to make the diagnosis
  - Study of choice to assess subtalar arthritis
- Magnetic resonance imaging
  - Useful to assess for localized osteochondral lesions of the talus or associated tendon disorders, but

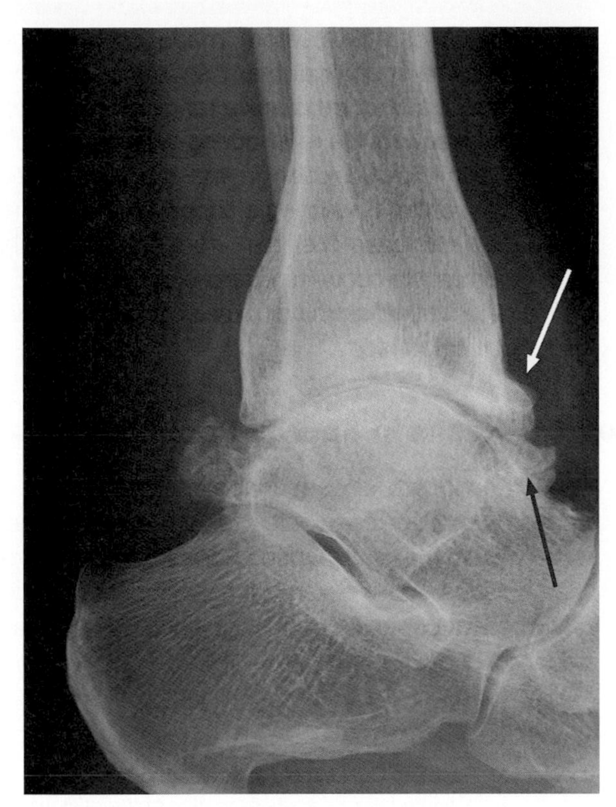

Figure 174-5 Lateral ankle radiograph of an arthritic ankle with large anterior tibial (*white arrow*) and talar (*black arrow*) osteophytes.

generally not required in cases of advanced ankle arthritis

Differential Diagnosis

- Charcot's (neuropathic) arthropathy: swelling, minimal pain in relation to the destructive changes on radiographs
- Acute gouty arthritis: acute onset, history of gout, joint effusion
- Subtalar arthritis: pain walking on uneven surfaces, limited and painful hindfoot inversion/eversion, pain localized laterally over sinus tarsi (inferior to the tip of the fibula); diagnostic injection if source of pain is unclear
- Osteochondral lesion of the talus: paroxysmal pain with locking, catching, or instability; focal defect noted on plain radiographs; magnetic resonance imaging to further evaluate

Treatment

- At diagnosis
  - Initial management is nonoperative.
  - Lifestyle modifications include weight loss in obese patients (joint reactive forces in the ankle are estimated at five times the body weight during normal gait), termination of vigorous activities, and changing to a more sedentary job, if possible.
  - Anti-inflammatory medications and intra-articular steroids may be useful for symptomatic management, particularly for acute exacerbations.
- Later
  - Chronic arthritic pain may be managed with modified footwear or a brace.
  - Shoe modifications with a rocker-bottom sole and solid ankle cushioned heel may improve gait dynamics and symptoms.
  - A custom polypropylene ankle–foot orthosis or Arizona ankle-foot orthosis brace may provide symptomatic relief, particularly in the setting of deformity or instability.
  - Finally, a trial of immobilization in a short-leg walking cast may provide symptomatic relief and simulate an ankle fusion for patients contemplating surgery.

When to Refer

- Patients with radiographic or clinical evidence of anterior impingement, loose bodies, or osteochondral lesions that may be amenable to open or arthroscopic débridement should be referred.
- Patients with radiographic or clinical malalignment (e.g., previous malunited tibia fracture) may be candidates for surgical realignment procedures.
- Finally, all patients who have end-stage arthritis and debilitating symptoms despite adequate nonoperative management should be referred for consideration for arthrodesis (fusion), joint replacement, or operative joint distraction procedures.

Prognosis

- The use of a rigid custom brace (ankle-foot orthosis or Arizona ankle-foot orthosis) can be a very successful treatment choice for patients who are compliant with brace use.
  - Common complaints include difficulty donning the brace, restricted range of motion, shoe wear difficulty, cosmetic appearance, and pain when out of the brace.
- Ankle arthrodesis is the most reliable surgical intervention with a high rate of fusion and pain relief using current surgical techniques.
  - Despite successful fusion, patients can have difficulty with uneven ground, stairs, driving, prone

sleeping, and increased risk of arthritis in adjacent joints.
- Recent gait analysis has shown a more symmetrical gait with reduced limp in patients with ankle replacement compared with fusion.
- The benefits of an improved gait must be weighed against the less predictable longevity of ankle replacement and the higher complication rate.

Troubleshooting

- Patients should be counseled on risks and benefits of surgery.
  - Fusion results in predictable relief of pain and good preservation of function in many patients. Permanent stiffness results from the fusion.
  - Smokers (high risk of fusion failure) and patients with involvement of the subtalar joint are less likely to have a successful outcome with surgery.
  - Despite recent advances, ankle replacement is in its infancy compared with total knee and hip replacement, with far less predictable results, and patients should adjust their expectations accordingly.

Patient Instructions

- There are multiple lifestyle modifications that can be made to help alleviate the pain from ankle arthritis.
  - Activities such as swimming, elliptical biking, and seated weight lifting are excellent for physical fitness yet minimize the impact on the ankle.
  - Avoidance of running, uneven ground (sand, grass, and gravel), inclines, and stairs will minimize the discomfort.
  - Walking is encouraged and will not cause the arthritis to worsen.
  - Use of shoes with a rocker bottom is very helpful to relieve pain.
    - — These can be custom made or purchased over-the-counter at many shoe stores.
    - — Use of a boot limits ankle range of motion and will also provide relief during walking.
    - — Given the restriction in the range of motion from arthritis, wearing a shoe with a small heel can decrease the pain from the spurs that commonly occur in the front of the ankle.
- Ice and anti-inflammatory medications can help reduce discomfort.

Considerations in Special Populations

- Patients who are obese, diabetic, dysvascular, or smokers are poor candidates for ankle replacement surgery given the risk of wound complications and risk of amputation. Ankle fusion is the procedure of choice in this patient population, although each case is evaluated individually.

Suggested Reading

- Coester LM, Saltzman CL, Leupold J, et al: Long-term results following ankle arthrodesis for post-traumatic arthritis. J Bone Joint Surg Am 2001;83:219–228.
- Coughlin MJ, Mann RA (eds): Surgery of the Foot and Ankle, 8th ed. St Louis: Mosby, 2006.
- Knecht SI, Estin M, Callaghan JJ, et al: The Agility total ankle arthroplasty. Seven- to sixteen-year follow-up. J Bone Joint Surg Am 2004;86:116–171.
- Myerson MS (ed): Foot and Ankle Disorders. Philadelphia: WB Saunders, 2000.
- Soohoo NF, Zingmond DS, Ko CY: Comparison of reoperation rates following ankle arthrodesis and total ankle arthroplasty. J Bone Joint Surg Am 2007;89A:2143–2149.
- Thomas R, Daniels TR, Parker K: Gait analysis and functional outcomes following ankle arthrodesis for isolated ankle arthritis. J Bone Joint Surg Am 2006;88A:526–535.
- Thomas RH, Daniels TR: Ankle arthritis. J Bone Joint Surg Am 2003;85A:923–936.

Chapter 175 Ankle Sprain

Norman Espinosa and Victor Valderrabano

ICD-9 CODES
845.02 *Fibulocalcaneal Sprain*
845.09 *Talofibular Sprain*

Key Concepts

- Approximately 85% of all ankle sprains involve the lateral structures.
- Most common injury in sports and dance
- Occurs commonly in the general population
- Bony and ligamentous structures provide proprioception, stability, and proper kinetics and kinematics.
- Typically, ankle sprains occur when the foot is in plantarflexion, adduction, and inversion.
- The anterior talofibular ligament (ATFL) is most prone to injury, followed by the calcaneofibular ligament (CFL).
- Approximately 20% of all patients develop chronic lateral ankle instability.

History

- Acute injury
  - Popping or tearing sensation in the ankle
  - Sometimes audible "pop" reported (rare)
  - Swelling and pain on the lateral (medial less common) aspect of the ankle
  - Patient may report inversion and plantarflexion mechanism.
- Chronic injury
  - Recurrent ankle sprains with increasingly less severe trauma

Physical Examination

- Observation
  - Effusion (intra-articular swelling)
  - Hindfoot alignment: A cavovarus foot can be a risk factor for ankle sprain.
- Palpation
  - Anterolateral (ATFL) and inferior (CFL) ankle tenderness
  - Keep in mind that in the acute phase, the specificity of tenderness is reduced (repeat examination 3–5 days after initial injury).
  - Possible tenderness along the peroneal tendons
  - Possible tenderness at the tip of the fibula
- Range of motion
  - Loss of dorsiflexion/plantarflexion/inversion due to effusion
  - Analyze potential hypermobility of joints
- Special tests (not possible to perform in the acute phase)
  - Anterior drawer test: ATFL (Fig. 175-1)
  - Inversion stress test: CFL (Fig. 175-2)
  - External rotation stress test: syndesmosis (Fig. 175-3)

Imaging

- Radiographs: weight-bearing anteroposterior, mortise, and lateral views of the ankle
  - Check for avulsion fractures and osteochondral lesions.

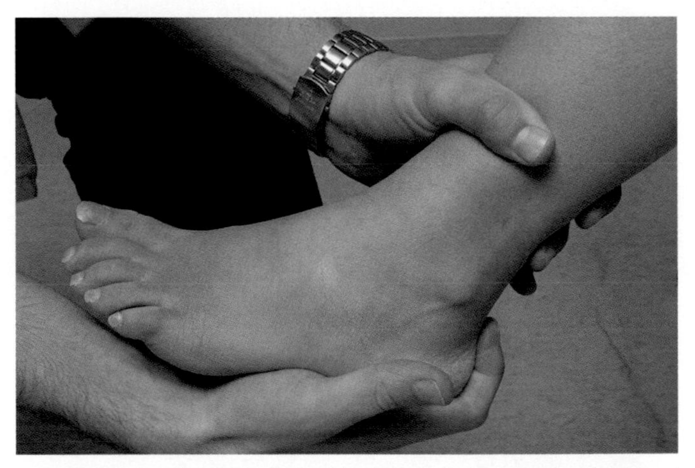

Figure 175-1 Anterior drawer test (anterior talofibular ligament [ATFL]). The hindfoot is grasped with the nondominant hand and the foot is held in plantarflexion. The calcaneus is then pulled anteriorly. Any significant difference when compared with the contralateral side indicates the possibility of ATFL rupture.

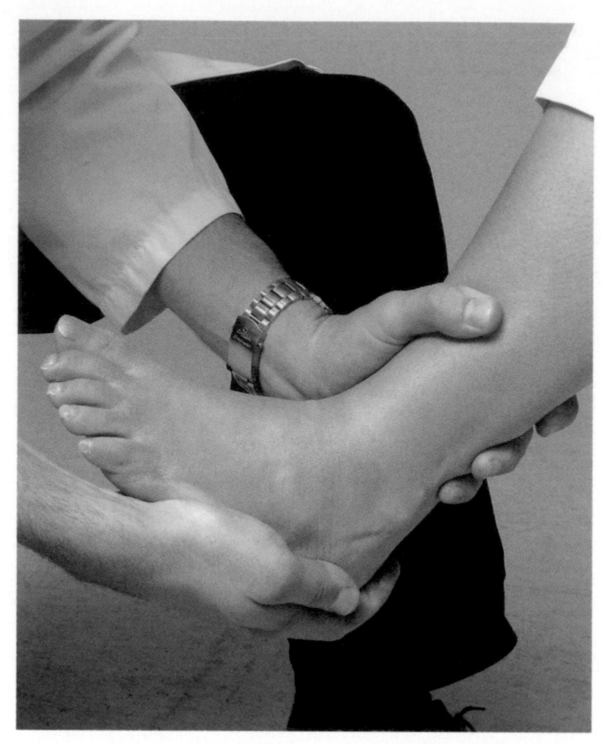

Figure 175-2 Inversion stress test (calcaneofibular ligament). The hindfoot is grasped with the dominant hand and the ankle is held in dorsiflexion. Inversion is performed and talar tilting noted.

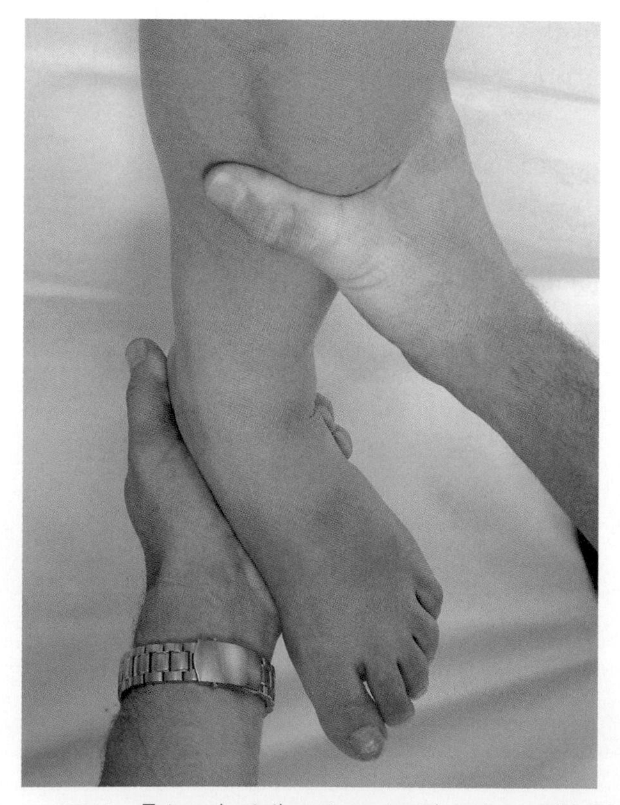

Figure 175-3 External rotation stress test (syndesmosis). The patient is seated with the knee flexed 90 degrees. The tibia is held with the nondominant hand and the foot is externally rotated. Pain provoked in the upper front of the ankle indicates syndesmotic injury.

- Ottawa ankle rules: Radiographs should be obtained in patients with tenderness at the posterior edge of the distal tibia/fibula or at the tip of the medial/lateral malleolus, inability to bear weight, or pain at the base of the fifth metatarsal.
- Stress radiographs
  - Talar tilt stress: Talar tilt greater than 15 degrees compared with the contralateral side is suspicious for complete tear of the CFL.
  - Anterior drawer stress: Anterior translation of the talus greater than 5 mm is considered a tear of the ATFL.
- Magnetic resonance imaging (MRI; not required in the acute phase of injury)
  - Often required to diagnose a chondral lesion
  - Look for classic bone bruise pattern and occult fractures.
  - Look for ligamentous or syndesmotic injury (Fig. 175-4).
  - Look for possible peroneal tendon involvement.
  - Define the extent of the lesions.

Differential Diagnosis

- Acute fracture of the fibula, talus, or calcaneus: tenderness, pain provoked by motion, inability to bear weight, swelling, hematoma, effusion, crepitus, deformity
- Partial tibial or talar avascular necrosis: often pain at rest; define on MRI
- Osteochondral fracture of the talar dome: similar to other acute fractures
- Peroneal tendon subluxation: swelling and pain along the course of the peroneal tendons; subluxation occurs when everting foot against resistance
- Congenital tarsal fusion/coalition: hindfoot stiffness, fixed deformity
- Osteoarthritis: joint line tenderness, decreased range of motion
- Ankle impingement: anterolateral tenderness, pain with forced dorsiflexion

Treatment

- At diagnosis
  - Rest, ice, compression, and elevation until swelling decreases (usually 3–5 days)
  - Nonsteroidal anti-inflammatory medication reduces pain.
  - After swelling has subsided, stability of the joint is re-evaluated, and a short ankle soft cast (in neutral position) is applied.

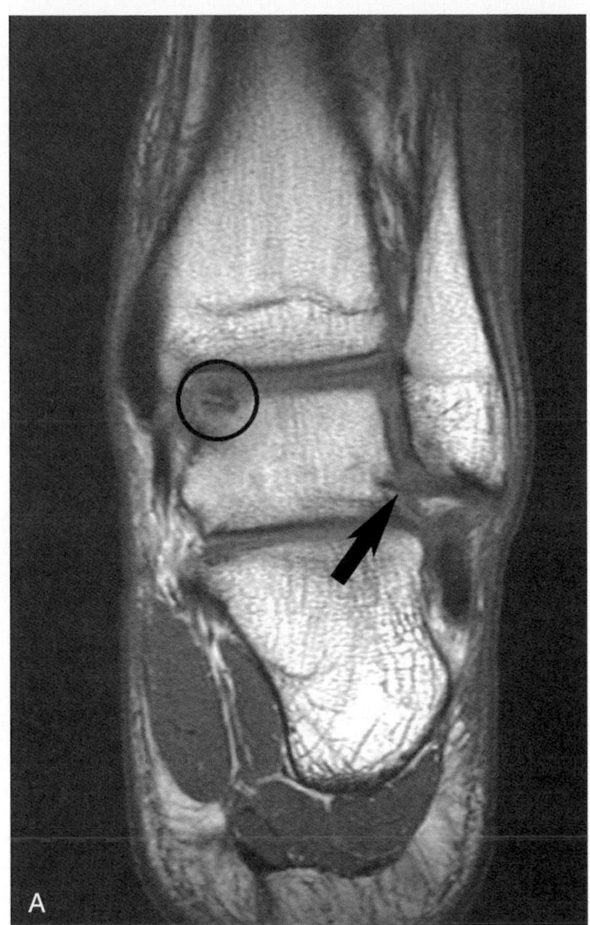

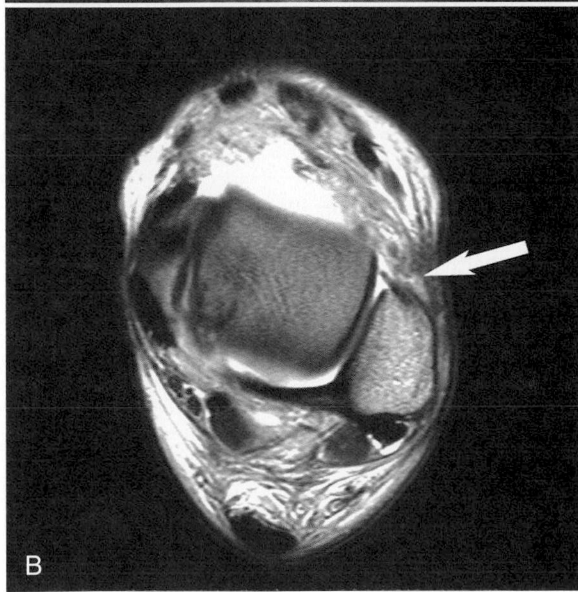

Figure 175-4 **A,** Coronal magnetic resonance imaging reconstruction of the hindfoot in a patient who sustained an ankle sprain. Note the lesion of the lateral ligamentous complex (*arrow*) and the talar dome fracture (*circle*). **B,** Axial MRI of the hindfoot of the same patient. The anterior talofibular ligament and calcaneofibular ligament are completely torn (*arrow*).

- — Alternatively, a lace-up ankle brace, stirrup brace, walking boot, or taping can be used for 4 to 6 weeks.
  — The patient is allowed to ambulate as tolerated.
  - Rehabilitation is started with proprioceptive training, range-of-motion exercises, peroneal and ankle dorsiflexor strengthening, and Achilles tendon stretching.
- Later
  - Repetitive ankle sprains, even on flat surfaces, indicate the presence of chronic lateral ankle instability.
  - Physical therapy that corrects deficits in proprioception, strength, and flexibility is usually sufficient to relieve disabling symptoms.
  - Other nonsurgical treatment options include activity and shoe modification (lower heels, stiffer soles, lateral heel wedge), an ankle-foot orthosis with ankle (and perhaps subtalar) support, and orthoses with a lateral heel wedge.

When to Refer

- Young to middle-aged, active patients in whom a well-designed nonoperative physical therapy program for chronic lateral ankle instability has failed are candidates for surgery and should be referred to an orthopaedic surgeon for further evaluation.
  - These patients are likely to require a lateral ankle ligament reconstruction.
  - Options include anatomic reconstruction by suturing the injured ligament stumps together (Broström-Gould procedure) and nonanatomic reconstruction of the ATFL and CFL by means of a gracilis tendon graft or by using the peroneus brevis tendon or other tendon transfer (modified Chrisman-Snook procedure). The latter reconstruction spans the tendon over the ankle and subtalar joints resulting in maximal stability but also stiffness of the hindfoot.

Prognosis

- Nonoperative treatment generally produces good to excellent results, but approximately 30% of patients have pain and swelling for at least 6 months.
- Functional impairment, including in sports activities at the desired level in athletes, is reported by 72% of subjects with residual disability.
  - Repeated inversion sprains or so-called chronic ankle instability occurs in 20%. In these patients,

the overall outcome after lateral ligament reconstruction has been reported to be good to excellent as well.

Troubleshooting

- Risks of nonoperative treatment include persisting pain for a poorly defined period, recurrent sprains, and persistent instability.
- Risks of surgical treatment include bleeding, infection, sural nerve injury, loss of motion at the ankle and subtalar joint (especially when choosing a nonanatomic reconstruction), and recurrence.
- Physical therapy is important for successful outcomes after nonoperative or operative treatment.

Patient Instructions

- The patient is allowed to ambulate and bear weight as tolerated.
- Non-weight bearing over a prolonged period is not advised.
- Once physical therapy has started, the patient should get precise instruction on how to perform the proprioceptive training at home.
- If the patient cannot bear any weight on his or her foot or has chronic pain (even at night), an additional diagnostic workup (MRI for occult fractures, osteonecrosis) should be considered.
- If surgery is considered, follow the instructions of the orthopaedic surgeon.

Considerations in Special Populations

- Inactive, sedentary patients should be treated nonoperatively.
    - If there is persistent pain, surgery must be tailored to the patient's needs (often nonanatomic reconstructions).
- Obese patients should be motivated to lose weight before surgery.
- Patients with hyperlaxity are better treated with nonanatomic lateral ankle ligament reconstructions because this type of surgical intervention stiffens up the hindfoot and produces increased stability.

Suggested Reading

- Alonso A, Khoury L, Adams R: Clinical test for ankle syndesmosis injury: Reliability and prediction of return to function. J Orthop Sports Phys Ther 1998;27:276–284.
- Anderson KJ, LeCocq JF, Clayton ML: Athletic injury to the fibular collateral ligament of the ankle. Clin Orthop Relat Res 1962;23:146–160.
- Attarian DE, McCrackin HJ, DeVito DP, et al: Biomechanical characteristics of human ankle ligaments. Foot Ankle 1985;6:54–58.
- Bröstrom L: Sprained ankles. I. Anatomic lesions in recent sprains. Acta Chir Scand 1964;128:483–495.
- Espinosa N, Smerek JP, Kadakia AR, et al: Operative management of chronic ankle instability: Reconstruction with open and percutaneous methods. Foot Ankle Clin 2006; 11:547–565.
- Henning CE, Egge LN: Cast brace treatment of acute unstable ankle sprain: A preliminary report. Am J Sports Med 1977; 5:252–255.
- Hertel J: Functional instability following lateral ankle sprain. Sports Med 2000;29:361–371.
- Hintermann B: Arthroscopic findings in patients with chronic ankle instability. Am J Sports Med 2002;30:402–409.
- Lynch S: Assessment of the injured ankle in the athlete. J Athl Train 2002;37:406–412.
- Yeung MS, Chan KM, So CH, et al: An epidemiological survey on ankle sprain. Br J Sports Med 1994;28:112–116.

Chapter 176 Achilles Tendon Disorders

Scott Van Aman and M. Truitt Cooper

ICD-9 CODES
845.09 *Achilles Tendon Rupture (Acute)*
726.71 *Achilles Tendinitis*
727.81 *Achilles Contracture*

Key Concepts

- Acute injuries commonly occur in middle-aged men participating in athletics, resulting from concentric (push-off) or eccentric (landing) contraction of the gastrocsoleus complex.
- Acute ruptures are missed initially in as many as 25% of patients.
- Most active patients benefit from operative treatment of the rupture, although success may be obtained nonoperatively.
- Achilles tendinitis has been classified based on the presence of paratendinitis (inflammation of tissue lining the tendon), tendinosis (noninflammatory, atrophic degeneration of the tendon itself), or both.
- Tendinitis may also be classified based on location as insertional (often older, inactive, overweight individuals) or noninsertional (overuse in runners/athletes).
- Conservative treatment of tendinitis has a success rate of approximately 90%.

History

- Acute injury (rupture)
  - Eccentric contraction of the gastrocsoleus complex (landing from jump) or, less commonly, strong concentric contraction
  - Sensation of being shot or kicked in the back of the heel often described
  - Pain, ecchymosis, cramping, inability to bear weight
  - Sedentary individuals may describe a history of chronic pain before the acute injury, which may be a minor trauma.
  - Fluoroquinolone use may predispose to rupture.
  - Patients may also sustain direct laceration of the tendon.
- Chronic injury (tendinitis/tendinosis)
  - Insidious onset of pain with activity; may progress to constant pain
  - Pain located in posterior/posterolateral heel (insertional) or proximal (noninsertional)
  - Noninsertional tendinitis occurs most commonly in young, active patients, whereas insertional tendinitis may occur in young, active patients or older, obese patients.
  - Athletes may note recent increase in intensity/volume of training.
  - History of spondyloarthropathy, gout, corticosteroid use, or diffuse idiopathic skeletal hyperostosis may predispose to insertional tendinitis.

Physical Examination

- Observation
  - Limp or inability to bear weight
  - Ecchymosis with acute injury
  - Calf atrophy, common with chronic disease; may occur rapidly after acute rupture
  - Forefoot varus: risk factor for chronic tendinitis
- Palpation
  - Palpable defect in the Achilles tendon (usually 2–7 cm proximal to insertion) in cases of acute rupture; may be subtle, particularly after several days, due to hematoma formation (Fig. 176-1).
  - Tenderness with heel squeeze or pressure over posterior/posterolateral calcaneal tuberosity in tendinitis
  - Swelling/tenderness of distal Achilles tendon substance
  - Palpable osteophytes at Achilles insertion
  - Nodules may be present in long-standing tendinosis.

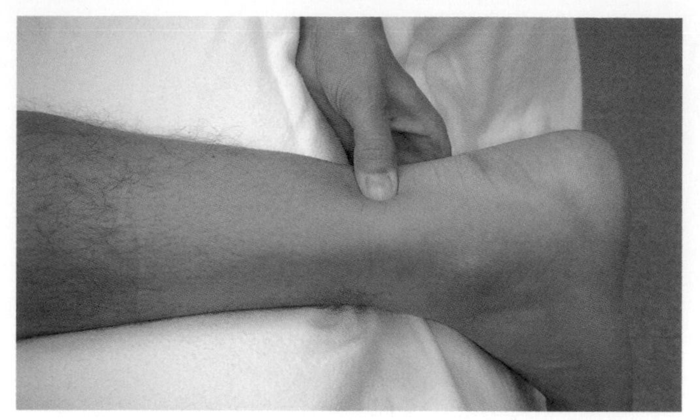

Figure 176-1 Palpation of the Achilles tendon in a patient with an acute injury reveals a defect approximately 5 to 7 cm proximal to the calcaneal tuberosity.

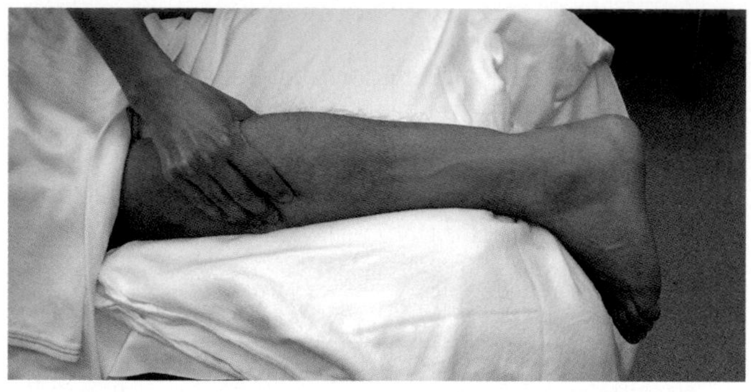

Figure 176-2 Thompson's test. As the calf muscles are squeezed proximally, the examiner watches for plantarflexion of the foot. In a positive test, as shown here, there is no plantarflexion, indicating a discontinuity between the insertion and the muscle due to acute rupture.

- Range of motion
  - Increased ankle dorsiflexion with acute injury
  - Decreased dorsiflexion with insertional tendinitis due to contracture of calf muscles
  - With severe tendinopathy, lengthening may occur, leading to an increase in dorsiflexion.
  - Patients with acute rupture usually have residual ability to weakly plantarflex because the toe flexors and posterior tibialis are intact, but they are unable to perform single heel raise.
- Special tests
  - Thompson's test
    - — The patient is placed prone with the knee flexed; the calf is squeezed to assess for plantarflexion of the foot (Fig. 176-2).
    - — No flexion is considered positive for complete rupture of the Achilles tendon.
    - — A false negative may result from squeezing the long toe flexor muscles or posterior tibialis.

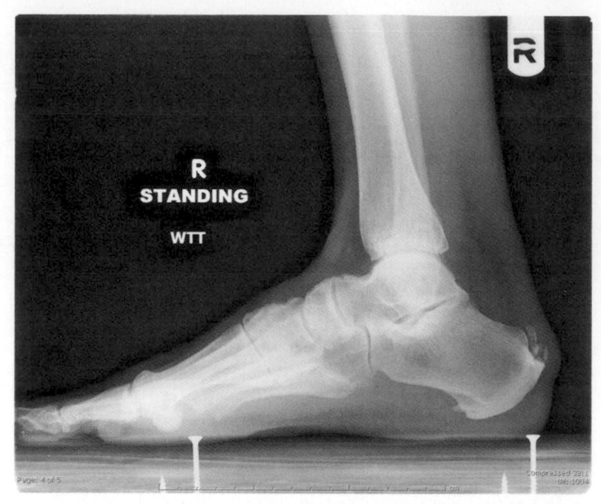

Figure 176-3 Lateral radiograph demonstrates a calcific spur that has formed on the posterior aspect of the calcaneus.

  - Knee flexion sign
    - — The patient is prone and brings the knee from an extended position to 90 degrees of flexion.
    - — If the foot falls to neutral dorsiflexion or beyond, considered positive for rupture

Imaging

- Rarely necessary; diagnosis of acute and chronic injuries is primarily clinical
- Radiographs
  - Lateral view of the foot may demonstrate a spur on the posterior margin of the calcaneus in insertional tendinitis (Fig. 176-3).
  - Calcification within the tendon may be visible on lateral and oblique views of the foot.
- Magnetic resonance imaging
  - Unnecessary for most acute ruptures and for nonoperative treatment of tendinitis
  - Useful for determining severity of disease and amount of tendon involved if planning surgical treatment in recalcitrant cases (Fig. 176-4)

Differential Diagnosis

- Retrocalcaneal bursitis: increased fluid in retrocalcaneal space on ultrasonography/magnetic resonance imaging
- Haglund's disease: erythema and posterolateral calcaneal pain
- Calcaneal stress fracture: pain over medial or lateral border of calcaneus
- Sever's disease: usually adolescent males with pain at the Achilles insertion

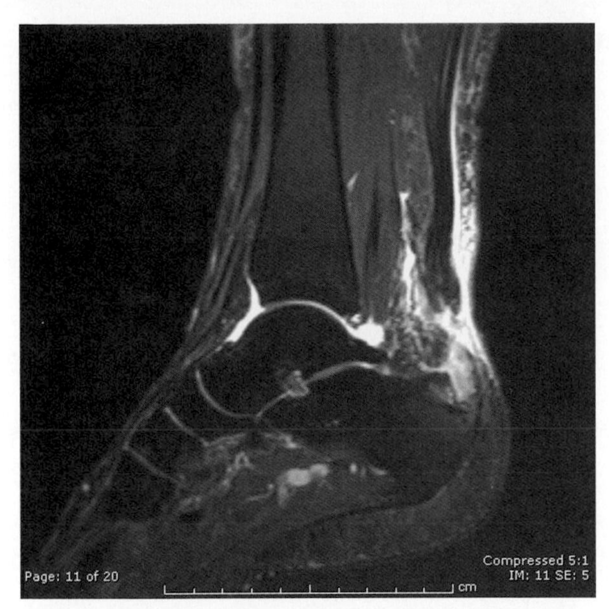

Figure 176-4 T2-weighted sagittal magnetic resonance imaging demonstrates insertional rupture of the Achilles tendon through chronic tendinosis. Note the edema around the Achilles tendon with discontinuity of the tendon as well as the bony prominence on the superior margin of the calcaneus.

- Spondyloarthropathy: HLA-B27 positive; diagnosis of psoriasis, Reiter syndrome, or ankylosing spondylitis
- Posterior tibial, peroneal, or flexor hallucis longus tendinitis: pain along tendon, exacerbated by resisted inversion, eversion, or great toe flexion, respectively

Treatment

- At diagnosis
  - Acute ruptures
    - Splint in position of comfort with foot plantarflexed 30 degrees
    - Non-weight bearing, ice/elevation to decrease swelling, and oral analgesics
    - Most patients benefit from surgical repair, with lower rerupture rates and improved plantarflexion strength.
    - Alternatively, nonoperative treatment consists of serial casting over several weeks, gradually bringing the foot from plantarflexion to neutral.
  - Tendinitis
    - Activity modifications, eccentric stretching of the gastrocsoleus complex, 1-cm heel lift, and nonsteroidal anti-inflammatory drugs
- Later
  - Chronic ruptures
    - Splint and non-weight bearing
    - Most of these patients also benefit from surgical intervention.
    - Sedentary patients may be treated long term with an ankle-foot orthosis.
  - Chronic tendinitis
    - Physical therapy modalities and night splint or full-time use of walking boot with rocker-bottom sole
    - If mechanical abnormality (cavus foot, hyperpronation) is present, a semirigid orthosis can be used.
    - Activity is gradually reinstituted on a pain-free basis.
    - Corticosteroid injections are discouraged due to reports of rupture.

When to Refer

- Acute ruptures should be referred promptly because repairs are most successful if performed within 2 weeks of injury. Direct repair is usually possible. If degeneration was present before rupture, grafting or tendon transfer (flexor hallucis longus) may be necessary.
- Patients with chronic ruptures should also be referred for surgical evaluation.
  - Treatment frequently involves débridement of the diseased tendon in combination with lengthening procedures or flexor hallucis longus transfer.
- Patients with recalcitrant tendinitis, despite several months of conservative treatment, may be referred for possible surgical treatment including débridement of diseased tissue, resection of a small portion of the calcaneal tuberosity, and possibly tendon transfer.

Prognosis

- Good and excellent outcomes have been demonstrated for both operative and nonoperative treatment of acute ruptures, with most patients returning to normal activity levels and sports by 6 months.
- The prognosis for chronic rupture is not as good. The primary goal of surgery is a return to normal activities of daily living. There is a 90% success rate with nonoperative treatment of tendinitis, and most athletes return to their previous level of participation.

Troubleshooting

- Risks of surgical treatment include wound complications (which can be severe) and nerve injury (sural nerve most common).

- Risks of nonoperative treatment of acute rupture include residual weakness and a significantly higher risk of rerupture.

Patient Instructions

- Patients with acute ruptures should be informed early that recovery is lengthy, frequently requiring as long as 6 months to return to normal activity.
- Patients with Achilles tendinitis must be instructed to avoid the offending activities. Conservative management is the mainstay of treatment.

Considerations in Special Populations

- In patients unfit for surgery, nonoperative treatment should be continued indefinitely and may include ankle-foot orthoses, even for ruptures.
- Diabetic patients and patients who smoke are at significantly increased risk of wound complications with surgery, but this is not a strict contraindication to repair.

Suggested Reading

- Angermann P, Hovgaard D: Chronic Achilles tendinopathy in athletic individuals: Results of nonsurgical treatment. Foot Ankle Int 1999;20:304–306.
- Hakan A: Conservative management of Achilles tendinopathy: New ideas. Foot Ankle Clin 2005;10:321–329.
- Inglis AE, Scott WN, Sculco TP, et al: Ruptures of the tendo achillis. An objective assessment of surgical and non-surgical treatment. J Bone Joint Surg Am 1976;58A:990–993.
- Kocher MS, Bishop J, Marshall R, et al: Operative versus non-operative treatment of Achilles tendon ruptures. Am J Sports Med 2002;30:783–790.
- Moller M, Movin T, Granhed H, et al: Acute rupture of tendon Achilles. A prospective randomized study of comparison between surgical and non-surgical treatment. J Bone Joint Surg Br 2002;83B:843–848.
- Silbernagel KG, Thomee R, Eriksson BI, et al: Continued sports activity using a pain-monitoring model during rehabilitation in patients with Achilles tendinopathy: A randomized controlled study. Am J Sports Med 2007;35:897–906.

Chapter 177 Posterior Tibial Tendon Disorders

Jonathan Smerek

ICD-9 CODE
726.72 *Posterior Tibialis Tendon Insufficiency*

Key Concepts

- The posterior tibial tendon (PTT) courses posterior to the medial malleolus to insert onto the navicular tuberosity and the plantar midfoot (Fig. 177-1).
- The PTT is the main invertor of the hindfoot, initiating heel rise during gait.
- Chronic insufficiency of the tendon leads to progressive collapse of the longitudinal arch and weakness during heel rise.
- PTT insufficiency (PTTI) is more common in women and in individuals with hypertension and obesity.
- The cause of the tendon insufficiency is not well understood, but may be related to long-standing flatfoot deformity.

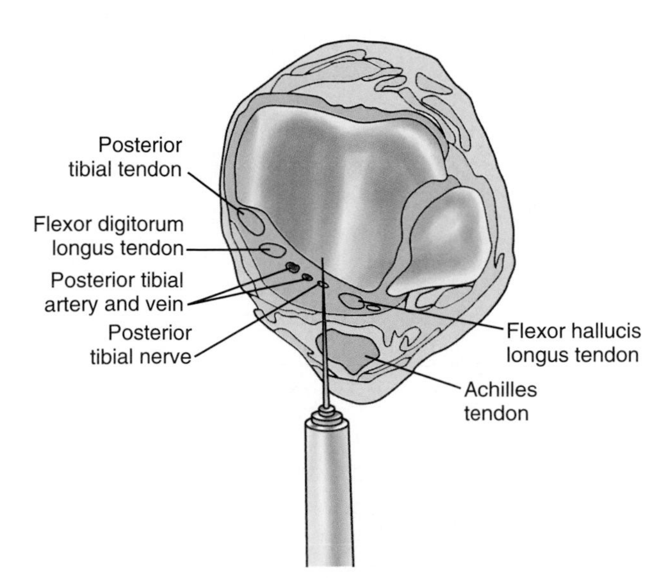

Figure 177-1 Anatomy of the posterior tibial tendon at the medial ankle.

- Poor vascularity of the PTT as it courses posterior to the medial malleolus leads to poor healing potential and degeneration.
- Complete rupture of the tendon is rare, with failure more commonly due to multiple longitudinal split tears, mucoid degeneration, and loss of normal collagen architecture.

History

- Acute tendinitis
  - Can occur with any mechanism of ankle sprain/lower extremity injury
  - Medial and posteromedial ankle pain and swelling
  - Pain worse with walking, especially on stairs
- Chronic tendinitis
  - Insidious onset with no relation to traumatic event
  - Medial and posteromedial ankle pain with or without swelling
  - The patient may report "collapse" of the arch and progressive flatfoot deformity.

Physical Examination

- Observation
  - Gait
  - Heel alignment: Have the patient remove shoes and socks and roll pants to above the knees. Stand behind him/her to observe.
    - Assess varus/valgus of the heel and compare with the contralateral side.
    - Describe the arch as high (cavus) or collapsed (planovalgus or flatfoot).
- Palpation
  - Tenderness along course of the posterior tibial tendon
  - Sinus tarsi tenderness

- Range of motion
  - Ankle, subtalar, and talonavicular range of motion
  - Assess for gastrocnemius contracture by testing ankle dorsiflexion with the knee extended and flexed. Gastrocnemius contracture, if present, will limit ankle dorsiflexion with the knee extended. Limited dorsiflexion with the knee flexed indicates a contracture of the ankle capsule and Achilles tendon.
- Special tests
  - Single heel rise (Fig. 177-2)
    - — Patient stands facing the examiner, holding the examiner's hands for balance.
    - — Alternatively, the patient may place his or her hands on the wall for balance.
    - — The contralateral leg is elevated, and the patient should be able to elevate on the toes on the affected side.

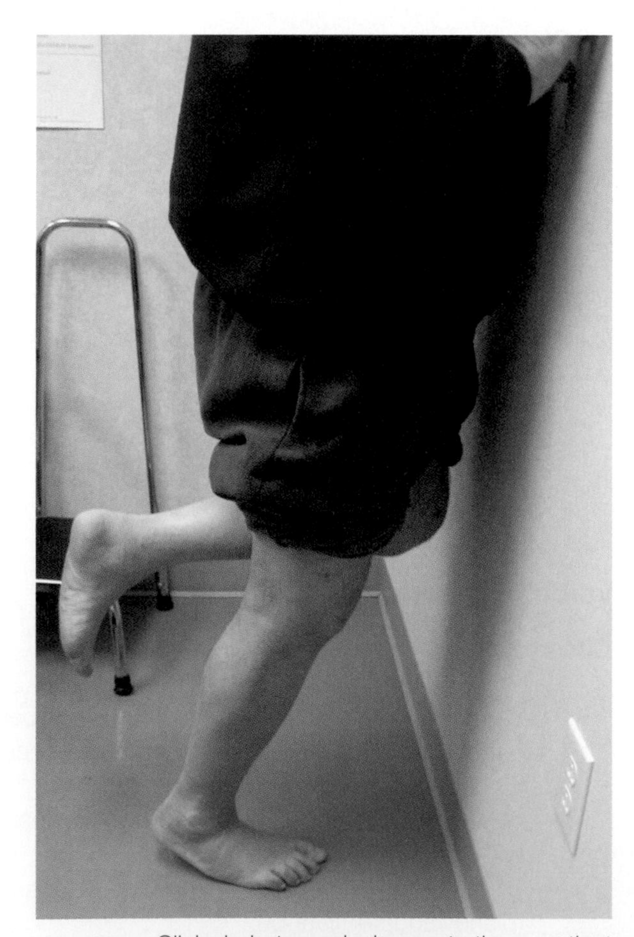

Figure 177-2 Clinical photograph demonstrating a patient with the ability to perform a single heel rise, consistent with an intact and functioning posterior tibial tendon. The contralateral leg should be fully off the ground and the hands lightly on the wall for balance.

    - — Inability to do so reflects PTTI
    - — Watch for the patient who cheats and uses his or her arms to push up to initiate the single heel rise.
  - "Too many toes" sign (Fig. 177-3)
    - — With patient standing, observe heel alignment from behind.
    - — With PTTI, more of the lesser toes will be visible lateral to the heel due to excessive heel valgus.

Imaging

- Radiographs
  - Weight-bearing anteroposterior, lateral, and oblique views of the foot
    - — Check for arthritis of the talonavicular, subtalar, calcaneocuboid, and midfoot joints.
    - — Look for stress fractures.
    - — Check for an accessory navicular.
  - Weight-bearing anteroposterior, lateral, and mortise views of the ankle
    - — Check for valgus tilting of the talus within the mortise, a sign of long-standing PTTI and deltoid ligament insufficiency.
- Magnetic resonance imaging
  - Not required for diagnosis or planning treatment
  - May assist in narrowing the differential diagnosis if the initial diagnosis of PTTI is not clear
  - Frequently demonstrates multiple longitudinal split tears, thickening, synovitis, and fluid surrounding the diseased tendon (Fig. 177-4)

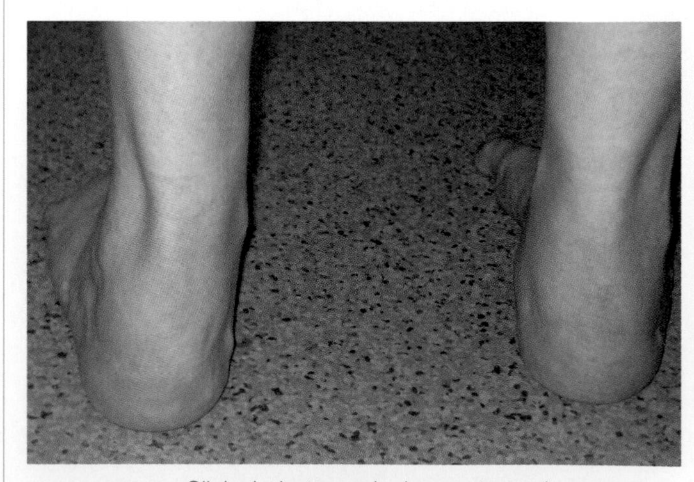

Figure 177-3 Clinical photograph demonstrates increased left heel valgus compared with the normal right side. Also demonstrated is the "too many toes" sign with more of the lesser toes visible in this patient with left posterior tibial tendon insufficiency.

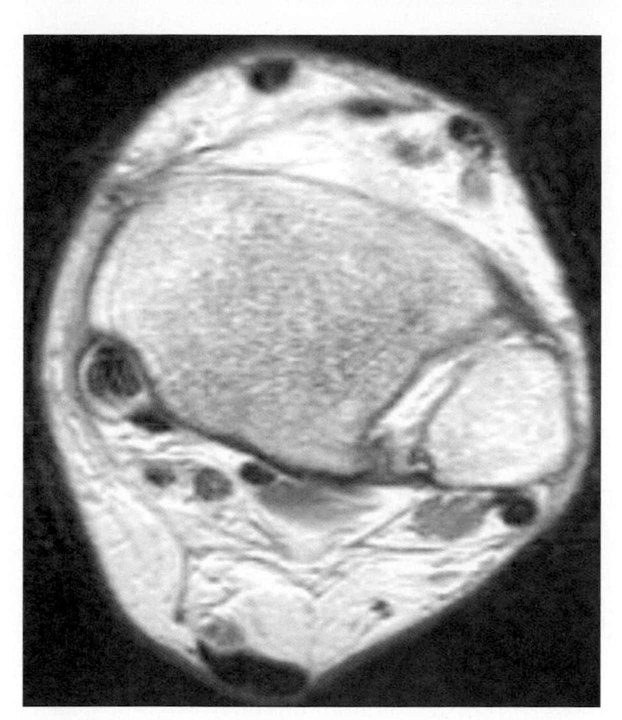

Figure 177-4 T1-weighted axial magnetic resonance imaging at a level just proximal to the ankle joint demonstrates thickening, multiple vertical split tears, and synovitis of a degenerated posterior tibial tendon.

Differential Diagnosis

- Painful congenital flatfoot deformity: ability to perform repetitive single heel rise, long-standing flatfoot deformity with plantar medial pain
- Painful accessory navicular: tenderness over the navicular tuberosity, ability to perform repetitive single heel rise, evident on radiographs
- Rheumatoid arthritis: systemic findings and arthropathy of multiple joints, decreased joint space with arthrosis on weight-bearing radiographs
- Neuropathic arthropathy: warm, erythematous ankle/subtalar/midfoot joints in a patient with long-standing diabetes or peripheral neuropathy, progressive flatfoot or rocker-bottom deformity, decreased plantar foot sensation
- Tarsal coalition: usually long-standing flatfoot deformity, calcaneonavicular or talocalcaneal bony coalition on radiographs
- Osteoarthritis or posttraumatic arthritis of the midfoot/hindfoot: tenderness over the first, second, or third tarsometatarsal or subtalar articulations, flatfoot deformity, joint space narrowing on radiographs

Treatment

- At diagnosis
  - Initial treatment of PTTI focuses on decreasing swelling and synovitis around the PTT.
  - Complete rest of the tendon is accomplished with a tall boot walker or a short leg walking cast to immobilize the ankle and hindfoot. Simple ankle and stirrup braces are insufficient.
  - The patient is encouraged to ice the area of maximum swelling daily and take nonsteroidal anti-inflammatory drugs as needed.
  - The patient can be weight bearing as tolerated in the boot or walking cast.
- Later
  - If the patient has significant resolution of symptoms after 4 to 6 weeks of cast or boot immobilization *and* is able to perform a single heel rise repetitively, a less obtrusive support may be used. The patient may try a custom or over-the-counter orthosis with a 3-degree medial heel wedge to reduce the work required by the PTT or a PTT dysfunction brace, which incorporates an air bladder into the brace to support the PTT and longitudinal arch.
  - Patients who continue to have pain and are unable to perform a single heel rise may be tried on continued boot or cast immobilization. Many will require either a tenosynovectomy or a reconstruction with tendon transfer of the flexor digitorum longus tendon to the navicular to replace the PTT (Fig. 177-5).
  - Patients with a long-standing flatfoot deformity that is rigid through the subtalar and talonavicular joints may require a triple arthrodesis to correct the deformity and restore the longitudinal arch.

When to Refer

- Patients with persistent pain, tenderness, swelling, and an inability to perform a single heel rise at 6 weeks should be referred to an orthopaedic surgeon. Persistent pain and a nonfunctioning PTT can lead to a long-standing rigid, flatfoot deformity that limits reconstructive options. Magnetic resonance imaging is not required for referral.

Prognosis

- Excellent with aggressive early immobilization
- Patients who develop persistent pain and PTTI do quite well with reconstruction and tendon transfer,

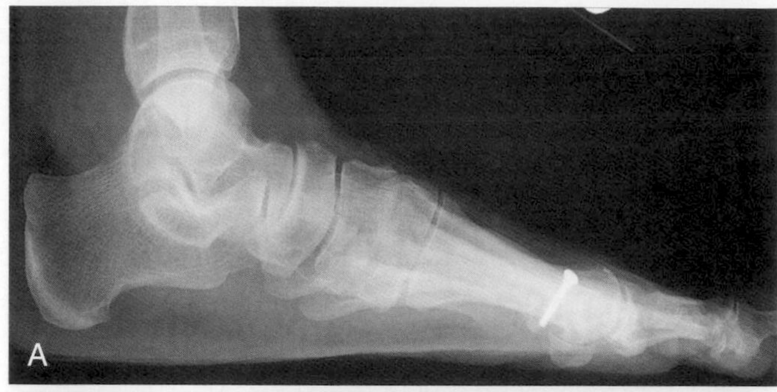

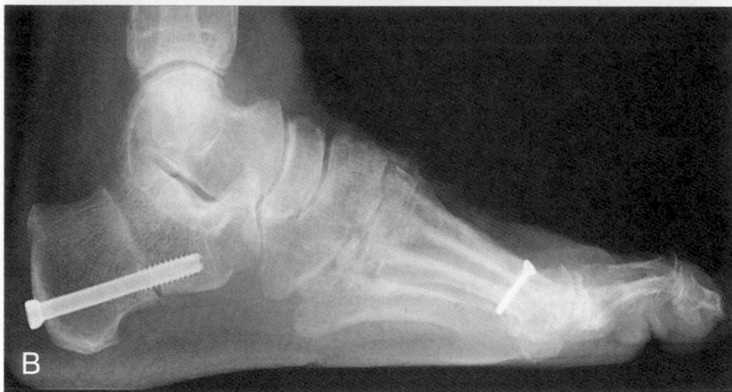

Figure 177-5 Lateral radiographs before (**A**) and after (**B**) calcaneal osteotomy and tendon transfer for reconstruction of flatfoot deformity demonstrate re-creation of the longitudinal arch.

although the transferred tendon is never as strong as the healthy, native PTT.

- Patients with rigid flatfoot deformity who require a triple arthrodesis may experience early ankle arthritis.

Troubleshooting

- The benefits of reconstruction usually outweigh the risks because it leads to pain relief, decreased deformity, and return to an active lifestyle.
- The risks of surgical intervention include neuritis, wound complications, infection, and weakness of inversion due to transfer of a weaker tendon to replace the PTT.
- Injection of the tendon and/or tendon sheath with steroids should be avoided because it can lead to tendon rupture.
- Simple suture repair of the tendon has been shown to fail due to the poor vascularity of the tendon.

Patient Instructions

- Patients should be instructed that insufficiency of the tendon holding up the arch has led to the continued pain.
  - Strict rest of the tendon with boot or cast immobilization can lead to marked improvement in symptoms.
  - Surgery may be required if immobilization is unsuccessful.
- Patients should be reassured that magnetic resonance imaging is not required for diagnosis.

Considerations in Special Populations

- Young (younger than 40 years) and very active individuals may benefit from a tenosynovectomy alone.
- Elderly and sedentary individuals are likely best treated with a triple arthrodesis due to the rehabilitation required after a reconstruction and tendon transfer.

Suggested Reading

- Beals TC, Pomeroy GC, Manoli A: Posterior tendon insufficiency: Diagnosis and treatment. J Am Acad Orthop Surg 1999;7: 112–118.
- Guyton GP, Jeng C, Krieger LE, et al: Flexor digitorum longus transfer and medial displacement calcaneal osteotomy for posterior tibial tendon dysfunction: A middle-term clinical follow-up. Foot Ankle Int 2001;22:627–632.
- Mann RA: Flatfoot in adults. In Mann RA (ed): Surgery of the Foot and Ankle. St. Louis: Mosby, 1999, pp 745–761.
- Myerson MS: Adult acquired flatfoot deformity. J Bone Joint Surg Am 1996;78A:780–792.
- Thordarson DB: Stage II adult acquired flatfoot deformity: Treatment options and indications. In Nunley JA, et al (eds): Advanced Reconstruction: Foot and Ankle. Rosemont, IL: American Academy of Orthopaedic Surgeons, 2004, pp 109–114.

Chapter 178 Peroneal Tendon Disorders

Benjamin J. Jacobs and Anand Vora

ICD-9 CODE
726.79 *Peroneal Tendinitis*

Key Concepts

- The peroneal tendons are the primary evertors/pronators of the foot and are important to maintain proper foot alignment and dynamic ankle stabilization.
- The peroneus longus and brevis run behind the lateral malleolus, with the brevis inserting onto the fifth metatarsal base and the longus inserting on the first and second metatarsals and the medial cuneiform (Fig. 178-1).
- The peroneus brevis tendon is immediately adjacent to the lateral malleolus in the fibular groove and is compressed by the peroneus longus, which is the likely reason that it is more frequently torn.
- The peroneus brevis has a more distal musculotendinous junction, which may help to differentiate it from the peroneus longus.
- The peroneal tendons are held in place behind the lateral malleolus by a fibrous peroneal retinaculum and the normal concave shape of the fibula.
- The os peroneum is an ossicle within the peroneus longus near the base of the fifth metatarsal. It is a normal anatomic variant, but may be painful with injury or fracture.
- Peroneal tendon injuries include subluxation/dislocation, longitudinal split tears (brevis most common), or a painful os peroneum. These can be acute/traumatic (in young athletes) or chronic (in older individuals) injuries.
- Peroneal tendon tears (or neuromuscular weakness) may be associated with a cavus forefoot and varus hindfoot.
- Lateral ankle instability is a common associated finding.

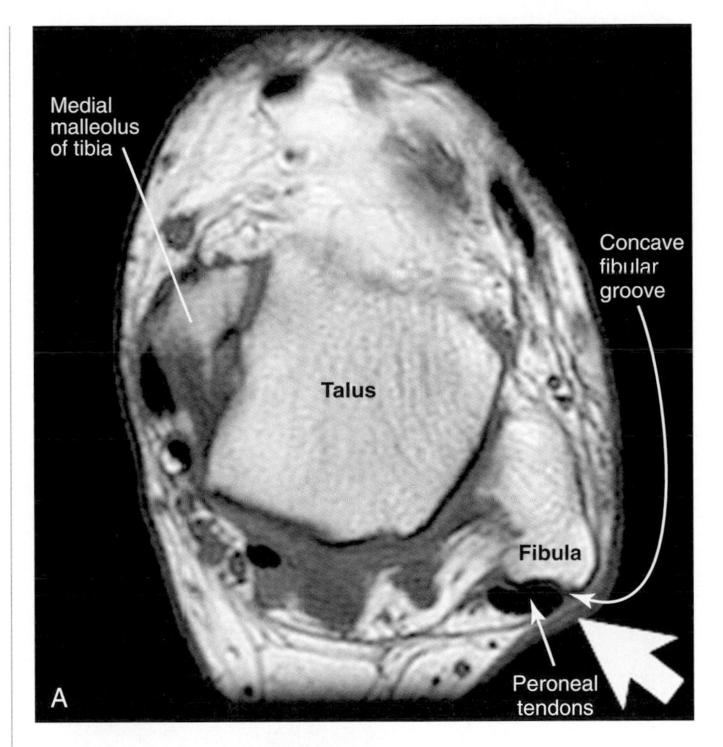

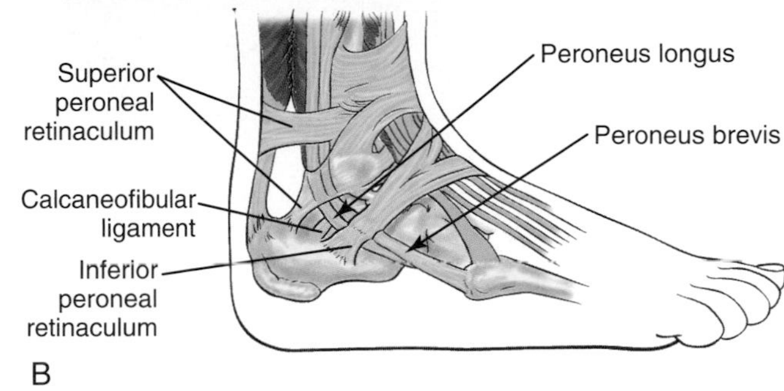

Figure 178-1 **A**, Axial magnetic resonance image at the level of the ankle. **B**, Sagittal drawing of the lateral ankle.

History

- Tendon tear
  - Often confused with ankle sprain
  - Can be chronic lateral ankle pain
  - With or without swelling or ankle instability
  - Young athletes with acute injury or, more commonly, older patients with attritional injury
- Subluxation/dislocation (Fig. 178-2)
  - "Snap" or "pop"
  - Due to forceful contraction of tendons with dorsiflexed foot
  - Often relocate spontaneously, which delays diagnosis
  - Chronic "giving way"

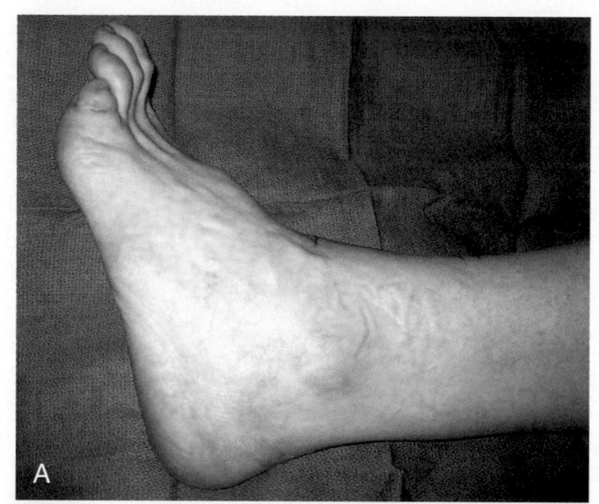

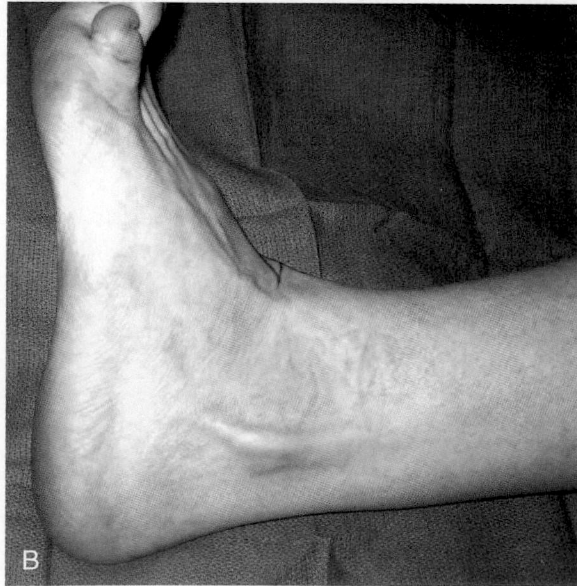

Figure 178-2 Peroneal tendon subluxation. **A**, With plantarflexion and inversion, the tendons are reduced in the fibular groove. **B**, With dorsiflexion and eversion, tendon instability is reproduced. Note the subluxed position of the peroneal tendons.

- Painful os peroneum
  - Acute or chronic
  - May present similar to an ankle sprain

Physical Examination

- Observation
  - Swelling and ecchymosis in acute injuries
  - Watch for tendon "popping."
- Palpation
  - Tenderness over fibular groove or distally over the course of the tendon with tears and instability
  - Feel for tendon subluxation or dislocation.
  - Pain just proximal to the fifth metatarsal base with painful os peroneum
- Range of motion
  - Usually normal, but may be painful/weak with resisted eversion
  - Pain with resisted first ray plantarflexion, toe rise, or supination and inversion of the foot is common in painful os peroneum due to involvement of the peroneus longus.
- Special tests
  - Observe for cavovarus foot deformity by standing behind the patient and judging the overall alignment of the leg relative to the heel.
    - — A varus hindfoot leads to overload at the lateral border of the foot with subsequent ankle instability and peroneal tendinitis. This combination ultimately leads to tendon tear (Fig. 178-3).

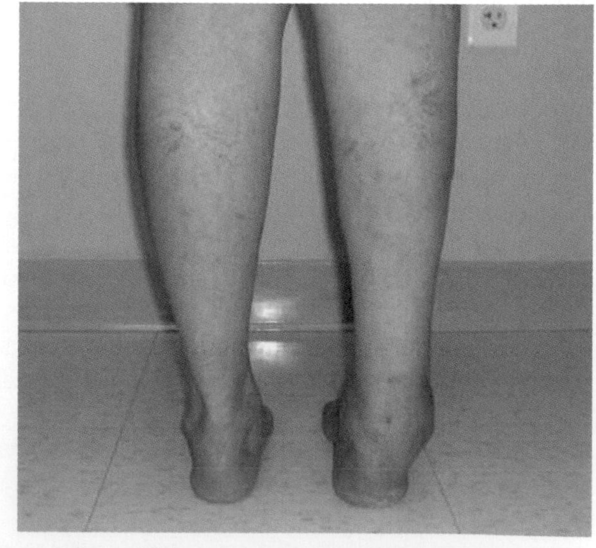

Figure 178-3 Right cavovarus foot deformity. The left side displays normal alignment.

- Provocative maneuver for tendon instability
  — Moving the ankle from plantarflexed, inverted position to dorsiflexed, everted position may reproduce tendon subluxation/dislocation.
- Painful os peroneum
  — Compression of the fibular groove with movement from plantarflexion/inversion to dorsiflexion/eversion reproduces pain.

Imaging

- Radiographs: weight-bearing anteroposterior, mortise, and lateral views of the ankle
  - Often normal; may have fleck sign from avulsion of the superior peroneal retinaculum
  - Evaluate for arthritis or previous fracture.
  - Anteroposterior, lateral, and oblique views of the foot to visualize os peroneum; compare with contralateral foot; fractured os may appear multipartite
- Magnetic resonance imaging
  - Useful in identifying tendon tears and associated bony or ligamentous injuries
  - Tendon subluxation better diagnosed clinically
  - May identify a fractured os peroneum
- Ultrasonography
  - Superior method to evaluate the tendons; can be very useful in identifying peroneal tendon tears and can be done dynamically if subluxation or dislocation is suspected but the diagnosis is uncertain

Differential Diagnosis

- Ankle sprain
- Ankle fracture
- Fifth metatarsal base fracture
- Talus lateral process fracture
- Painful trochlear process
- Arthritis
- Anterior process calcaneus fracture
- Osteochondral injury of the ankle
- Tarsal coalition
- Ankle synovitis
- Neuromuscular disease

Treatment

- At diagnosis
  - There is evidence to suggest that acute peroneal tendon tears and acute traumatic peroneal tendon subluxation/dislocation should be treated surgically and may have improved outcomes if treated acutely.
  - Chronic attritional peroneal tendon tears are treated with rest, nonsteroidal anti-inflammatory drugs, and physical therapy; braces and immobilization may also be considered.
  - Painful os peroneum is treated with casting/cam boot for 1 month
    — Avoid steroid injections.
- Later
  - Tendon tear
    — Surgical treatment involves repair or excision of the torn portion of the tendon.
    — Many surgeons advocate a concurrent valgus calcaneal osteotomy with or without first ray osteotomy, if cavovarus deformity is present, to reduce the risk of recurrence.
  - Subluxation or dislocation
    — Surgical treatment includes repair of the torn or attenuated peroneal retinaculum and any associated tendon tears.
    — Many surgeons include a fibular groove deepening (improved outcomes versus nonoperative management).
  - Painful os peroneum
    — Surgical excision of the offending os peroneum and repair or tenodesis of the peroneus longus tendon

When to Refer

- In the case of acute peroneal tendon tears and subluxation or dislocation, nonemergent but prompt referral to a specialist is appropriate.
- Chronic tendon tears and subluxations should also be referred, but do not require as prompt a referral.
- Referral for painful os peroneum can wait for a trial of conservative management.

Prognosis

- The prognosis varies with the pathology, but, in general, acute injuries repaired surgically have an excellent prognosis.
- Chronic tendon injuries have a more guarded prognosis for high-level function.
- Prognosis is improved when associated pathology (i.e., varus hindfoot/lateral ankle instability) is also addressed.

Patient Instructions

- Patients with chronic tendon tears and a painful os peroneum should be instructed to avoid activities that cause pain and use nonsteroidal anti-inflammatory drugs as tolerated.
- Patients with acute tendon tears and subluxation/dislocation should be instructed to rest, elevate the extremity, and see a specialist.

Suggested Reading

- Chambers HG: Ankle and foot disorders in skeletally immature athletes. Orthop Clin North Am 2003;34:445–459.
- Dombek MF, Lamm BM, Saltrick K, et al: Peroneal tendon tears: A retrospective review. J Foot Ankle Surg 2003;42:250–258.
- MacDonald BD, Wertheimer SJ: Bilateral os peroneum fractures: Comparison of conservative and surgical treatment and outcomes. J Foot Ankle Surg 1997;36:220–225.
- Steel MW, DeOrio JK: Peroneal tendon tears: Return to sports after operative treatment. Foot Ankle Int 2007;28:49–54.
- Vienne P, Schöniger R, Helmy N, et al: Hindfoot instability in cavovarus deformity: Static and dynamic balancing. Foot Ankle Int 2007;28:96–102.

Chapter 179 Haglund's Deformity (Pump Bump)

Scott Van Aman and M. Truitt Cooper

ICD-9 CODES
726.91 *Haglund's Exostosis*
727.06 *Retrocalcaneal Bursitis*

Key Concepts

- Haglund's deformity is a prominence on the superior aspect of the calcaneus.
- Usually developmental in origin, but may be related to chronic apophysitis in childhood
- Termed "pump bump" when overlying irritation is associated with tight, constricting shoes and closely contoured heel counter
- Bony prominence and constrictive shoe wear lead to irritation of overlying bursa, primarily posterolateral prominence and pain
- Retrocalcaneal bursa (between Achilles tendon and calcaneus) normally functions to protect the tendon from posterosuperior calcaneus and provide lubrication
- Inflammation may develop in the retrocalcaneal space, leading to retrocalcaneal bursitis.
- Although the term "pump bump" refers specifically to irritation of the superficial soft tissues, there is significant overlap with retrocalcaneal bursitis in both clinical presentation and treatment.
- Rarely associated with Achilles tendinitis and generally does not involve the tendon proper at all
- Conservative management is successful in most patients.

History

- Frequently occurs in those younger than 30 years of age, although may be seen at any age
- Insidious onset of dull pain in the retrocalcaneal area, localized over the posterosuperior and lateral margins of the calcaneus
- May be aggravated by activity or shoe wear, specifically associated with tight-fitting shoes with constrictive heel counter, leading to skin irritation, erythema, and swelling, thus the term "pump bump"
- Acute onset of pain after trauma is uncommon; may indicate tear of a degenerated Achilles tendon

Physical Examination

- Observation
  - Gait
  - Look for obvious prominence at the heel, specifically the lateral side of the Achilles insertion (Fig. 179-1)
  - Callus or erythema over prominence from shoe wear irritation
- Palpation
  - Prominence and tenderness at superolateral margin of calcaneal tuberosity
  - Swelling may be present in the retrocalcaneal bursa. (Although not part of true Haglund's disease, retrocalcaneal bursitis is often present, with overlap between the two entities.)
  - Note tenderness or nodularity along the course of the Achilles tendon.
- Range of motion
  - Bilateral ankle dorsiflexion: frequently lose at least 5 degrees of dorsiflexion with Achilles disorders

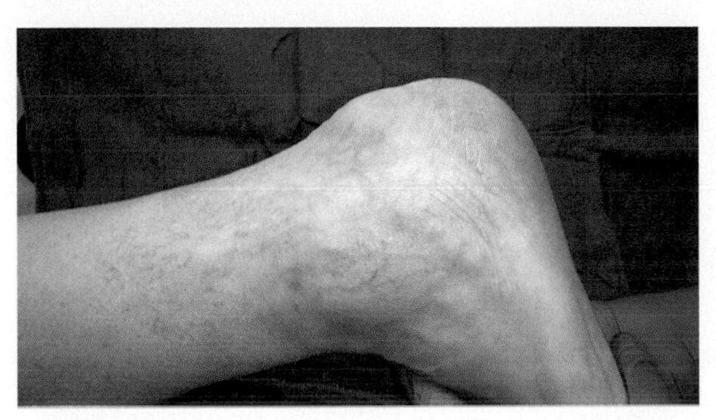

Figure 179-1 Note the prominence located on the superolateral aspect of the heel, just lateral to the insertion of the Achilles tendon.

   - Measure with knee flexed and extended
   - Significant decrease in dorsiflexion with knee extended indicates that the primary origin of tightness is the gastrocnemius muscle.
- Should be able to perform single leg-heel rise

Imaging

- Radiographs: standing anteroposterior, lateral, and oblique views of the foot
   - Haglund's deformity is seen as a prominence or exostosis on the posterosuperior border of the calcaneal tuberosity on a lateral view (Fig. 179-2).
   - May see calcification within substance of Achilles tendon on lateral or oblique views
- Ultrasonography
   - Rarely indicated; may demonstrate increased bursal fluid
- Magnetic resonance imaging
   - Used to evaluate quality of the Achilles tendon and bony changes in refractory cases
   - Increased fluid signal in the retrocalcaneal bursa (Fig. 179-3)

Differential Diagnosis

- Retrocalcaneal bursitis may be present with Haglund's disease, pain with forced dorsiflexion of the foot; ultrasonography/magnetic resonance imaging reveal increased fluid in the retrocalcaneal space.
- Achilles tendinitis/tendinosis: pain over the Achilles tendon or insertion; magnetic resonance imaging reveals edema around the tendon or tendinopathic regions
- Periostitis/calcaneal stress fracture: tenderness over the medial or lateral border of calcaneus
- Sever's disease: usually adolescent males; tenderness directly over the posterior Achilles insertion

Treatment

- At diagnosis
   - Conservative treatment is usually successful and is similar to the treatment for Achilles tendinitis.
   - The goal is to decrease friction between the heel counter and inflamed bursa; this includes shoe wear modifications, including a heel wedge to lift the heel from the shoe and alter the contact pattern.
   - Additionally, nonsteroidal anti-inflammatory drugs and stretching may be beneficial.
   - Corticosteroid injections in and around the Achilles tendon are contraindicated due to an increased risk of rupture.
- Later
   - Surgical interventions typically involve removal of the excess bone on the superior margin of the calcaneal tuberosity, along with débridement of bursal tissue and any diseased areas of the Achilles tendon itself.

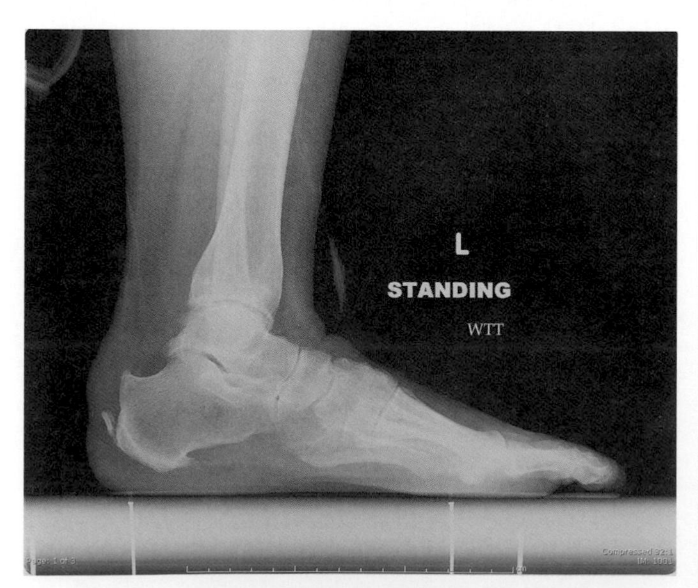

Figure 179-2 Lateral radiograph demonstrating the bony prominence on the superior margin of the calcaneus. This patient also demonstrates calcification at the insertion of the Achilles tendon.

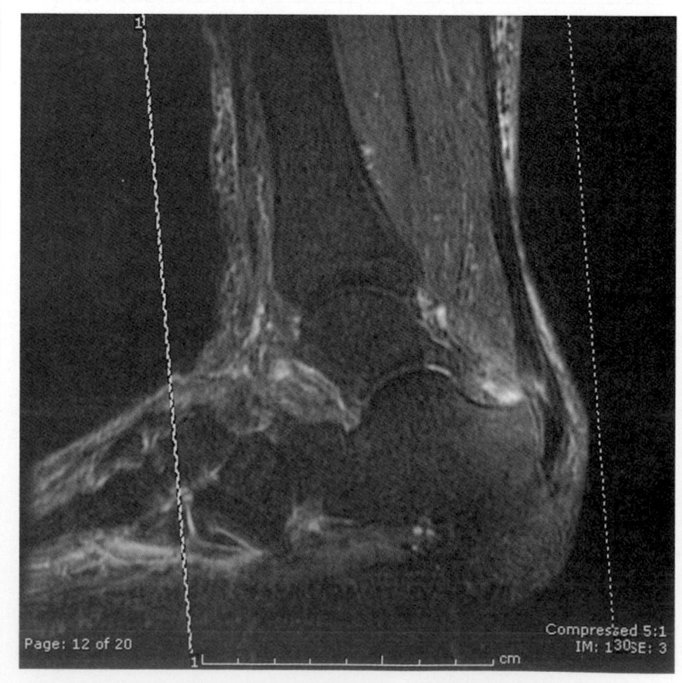

Figure 179-3 T2-weighted sagittal magnetic resonance imaging demonstrating increased fluid in the retrocalcaneal bursa with a small associated bony prominence.

When to Refer

- If nonoperative methods fail, surgical treatment may be required and referral is indicated.

Prognosis

- The prognosis for Haglund's deformity is generally very good, particularly in the absence of retrocalcaneal bursitis and Achilles tendon disorders.
- Approximately 90% of patients are successfully treated with nonoperative management.

Patient Instructions

- Inform patients with true Haglund's disease that the vast majority will improve with nonoperative treatment.
    - Although the bony prominence will remain, the inflamed bursa and irritated skin overlying it can be expected to decrease with several weeks of shoe wear modification.
- Surgery is only considered when strict compliance with nonoperative treatment does not lead to resolution.
- Patients with retrocalcaneal bursitis should be instructed in calf-stretching exercises and perform these multiple times daily.
- Patients should also be advised regarding the safety of nonsteroidal anti-inflammatory drugs.

Suggested Reading

- Haglund P: Beitrage zur klinik der Achillessehne. Z Orthop Chir 1928;49:49–58.
- Heneghan MA, Pavlov H: The Haglund painful heel syndrome. Experimental investigation of cause and therapeutic implications. Clin Orthop Relat Res 1984;187:228–234.
- Myerson MS, McGarvey W: Disorders of the insertion of the Achilles tendon and Achilles tendinitis. Instr Course Lect 1999;48:211–218.
- Reinherz RP, Smith BA, Henning KE: Understanding the pathologic Haglund's deformity. J Foot Surg 1990;29:432–435.
- Stephens MM: Haglund's deformity and retrocalcaneal bursitis. Orthop Clin North Am 1994;25:41–46.

Chapter 180 Plantar Fasciitis

Chin Khoon Tan and Andrew Molloy

ICD-9 CODE
728.71 *Plantar Fasciitis*

Key Concepts

- Plantar fasciitis is the most common cause of inferior heel pain. Ten percent of the population experiences heel pain at some point during their life time.
- Frequently seen in athletes, but also in sedentary individuals, particularly middle-aged women
- Generally a self-limiting condition
- The plantar aponeurosis is a modification of the deep fascia. The central portion is a thick band of tissue superficial to the flexor digitorum brevis. The medial and lateral portions are thinner and lie superficial to the abductor hallucis and abductor digiti minimi, respectively. The three portions (or bands) of the plantar aponeurosis are coextensive (Fig. 180-1).

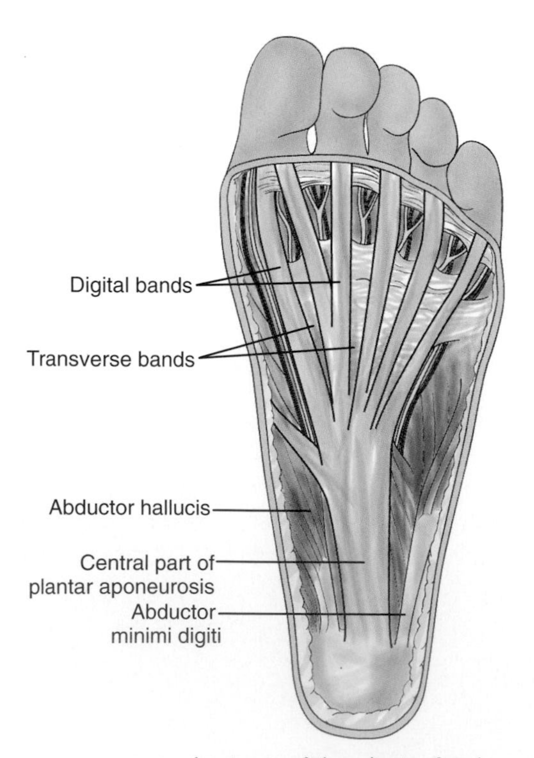

Figure 180-1 Anatomy of the plantar fascia.

- The posterior tibial nerve has one or two superficial branches proximal to the medial malleolus, termed the medial cutaneous nerve. The posterior tibial nerve then divides into medial and lateral plantar branches, which pass deep to the abductor hallucis muscle belly (Fig. 180-2).
- Dorsiflexion of the metatarsophalangeal joint increases tension in the plantar fascia and simultaneously increases arch height while decreasing arch length (windlass mechanism) (Fig. 180-3).
- The cause of plantar fasciitis is poorly understood. Risk factors include reduced ankle dorsiflexion (most important), obesity, mechanical overload, foot biomechanical abnormalities, and unaccustomed walking/running.
- Heel spurs are not a primary cause of heel pain. However, if of significant size, they can be a secondary

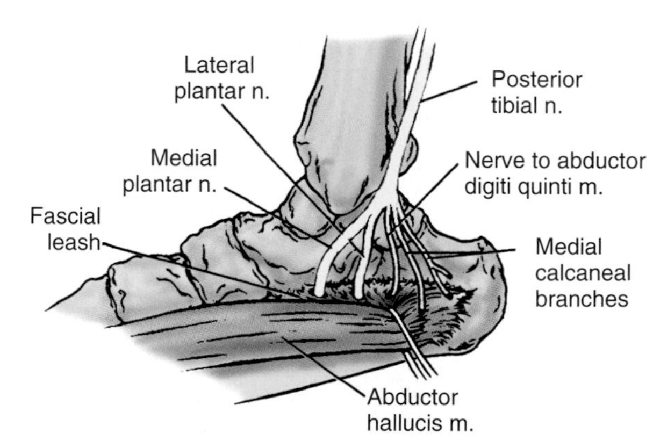

Figure 180-2 Posterior tibial nerve and its branches.

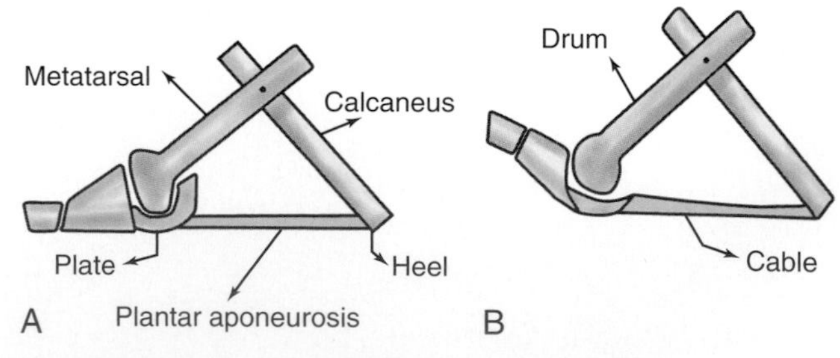

Figure 180-3 **A**, The windlass mechanism. **B**, The plantar aponeurosis functions like a cable in the windlass mechanism, maintaining the plantar arch.

cause of pain by entrapping the nerve to the abductor digiti minimi, a branch of the lateral plantar nerve.

History

- Pain (medial calcaneal tuberosity), swelling, and difficulty walking
- Gradual onset of pain; worse on initial weight bearing in the morning or after a period of inactivity; may lessen with gradual increased activity, but worsen with high-intensity activity (e.g., jogging)
- Nocturnal pain should raise the suspicion of other causes of heel pain, such as tumor, infection, and neuropathic pain.
- Associated paresthesias are uncommon.

Physical Examination

- Observation
  - Weight-bearing evaluation of the arch may reveal a cavus foot or excessive pronation of the heel upon heel strike.
- Palpation
  - Maximal tenderness at the anteromedial calcaneus; exacerbated by passive dorsiflexion of the toes or having the patient stand on the tips of toes
- Range of motion
  - Decreased ankle dorsiflexion due to tightness of the Achilles tendon
- Special tests
  - Neurologic examination is mandatory.
  - Positive Tinel's sign indicates nerve entrapment.

Imaging

- Imaging plays a limited role, although it may be useful to rule out other causes of heel pain if the diagnosis is uncertain.
- Radiographs may rule out calcaneal stress fracture and other bony lesions.
- A bone scan provides objective evidence of an inflammatory process at the enthesis.
- Ultrasonography may be diagnostically useful, although it is not routinely used.
- Magnetic resonance imaging can also be used to visualize the plantar fascia, but is rarely indicated.

Differential Diagnosis

- Achilles tendinopathy: pain with resisted plantarflexion, tenderness over tendon
- Haglund's deformity: noticeable bump on back of heel, possible insertional Achilles tendinopathy
- Tarsal tunnel syndrome: paresthesia/pain over the plantar aspect, exacerbated by exercise; symptoms radiate posterior to medial malleolus
- Other: systemic disorders (seronegative arthropathies, rheumatoid arthritis, fibromyalgia, gout), trauma (fracture, stress fracture), infection (soft tissue or bone), calcaneal apophysitis (Sever's disease), and benign or malignant tumors

Treatment

- At diagnosis
  - Nonsurgical treatment includes activity modification, physical therapy, nonsteroidal anti-inflammatory agents, shoe alterations/inserts/heel pads, night splints, walking cast, and shock wave therapy.
  - Physical therapy: stretching exercises of the Achilles and plantar fascia, plantar fascia massage, ice, taping
  - Cortisone injections: generally limited to two per side; rarely a third may be given; complications include plantar fascia rupture (~10%) and fat pad atrophy
  - Shoe modifications: Shoes with a thicker, well-cushioned mid-portion of the insole decrease the pain associated with walking or standing. A wide variety of custom and prefabricated orthoses, including heel pads/cups, are designed to elevate/cushion the heel and provide medial arch support.
  - Night splints: Individuals usually sleep with the feet plantarflexed, a position that causes the plantar fascia to foreshorten. Night splints are designed to keep the ankle in a neutral position with or without dorsiflexion of the metatarsophalangeal joints.
  - Extracorporeal shock wave therapy: Success rates are mixed.
- Later
  - Surgical intervention should be considered only for intractable pain that has not responded to 12 months of proper conservative management.
  - Surgical procedures include plantar fascia release with or without calcaneal spur excision, excision of abnormal tissue, and nerve decompression.
    - — Open release, endoscopic fasciectomy, and percutaneous or radiofrequency lesioning are various techniques of plantar fascia release.

When to Refer

- If no improvement is noted within 6 to 12 weeks of appropriate conservative care, the patient should be referred for consideration of more intensive conservative therapies or possibly surgery.

Prognosis

- Self-limiting condition
- More than 90% of patients respond to nonsurgical treatment within 6 to 10 months.
- Initiation of conservative treatment within 6 weeks after the onset of symptoms may hasten recovery.

Troubleshooting

- Occasionally, patients present with bilateral heel pain (20% to 30%). This must raise suspicion as to the possibility of an underlying systemic etiology, such as inflammatory arthropathy.
- Patients should receive no more than three corticosteroid injections. Failure of injections may be due to inaccuracy, although obesity and underlying biomechanical abnormality of the foot should also be considered.
- Multiple steroid injections predispose a patient to plantar fascia rupture.
- Potential complications of surgery include transient swelling of the heel pad, calcaneal fracture, injury to the posterior tibial nerve or its branches, and flattening of the longitudinal arch.

Patient Instructions

- There are certain things a patient can do to try to prevent plantar fasciitis, especially if he/she has had it before:
    - Regularly changing shoes used for running or walking
    - Wearing shoes with good cushioning in the heels and good arch support
    - Losing weight, if overweight
    - Avoiding exercise on hard surfaces
- Medical attention should be sought on an elective basis if any of the classic symptoms of plantar fasciitis are present consistently for 2 to 3 weeks:
    - Gradual onset of mild to moderate heel pain (usually aggravated by the commencement of ambulation and also higher-intensity activities)
- The patient should seek medical help urgently if he/she has the following symptoms:
    - Heel pain that occurs at night or resting
    - Swelling or discoloration of the back of the foot
    - Signs of an infection, including fever, redness, warmth
    - Any other unusual symptoms

Suggested Reading

- DiGiovanni BF, Nawoczenski DA, Malay DP, et al: Plantar fascia-specific stretching exercise improves outcomes in patients with chronic plantar fasciitis. A prospective clinical trial with two-year follow-up. J Bone Joint Surg Am 2006;88A:1775–1781.
- Gill LH: Plantar fasciitis: Diagnosis and conservative management. J Am Acad Orthop Surg 1997;5:109–117.
- Pribut SM: Current approaches to the management of plantar heel pain syndrome, including the role of injectable corticosteroids. J Am Podiatr Med Assoc 2007;97:68–74.
- Riddle DL, Schappert SM: Volume of ambulatory care visits and patterns of care for patients diagnosed with plantar fasciitis: A national study of medical doctors. Foot Ankle Int 2004;25:30–33.
- Schepsis AA, Leach RE, Gorzyca J: Plantar fasciitis: Etiology, treatment, surgical results, and review of the literature. Clin Orthop Relat Res 1991;266:185–196.
- Wearing SC, Smeathers JE, Urry SR, et al: The pathomechanics of plantar fasciitis. Sports Med 2006;36:585–611.

Chapter 181 Os Trigonum

Edward V. Wood and Andrew Molloy

ICD-9 CODE

718.97 *Unspecified Derangement of Ankle and Foot Joint*

Key Concepts

- The os trigonum is a discrete accessory ossicle of the posterolateral talus (Fig. 181-1).
- Etiology is either failure of fusion of the secondary ossification center of the talus or fracture of the trigonal/Stieda's process of the talus.
- The secondary ossification center appears between 8 and 11 years of age and normally fuses 1 year after its appearance.
- When pathology of the os trigonum causes symptoms, it is called os trigonum syndrome. It may also be referred to as talar compression syndrome, posterior ankle impingement, and posterior ankle block.

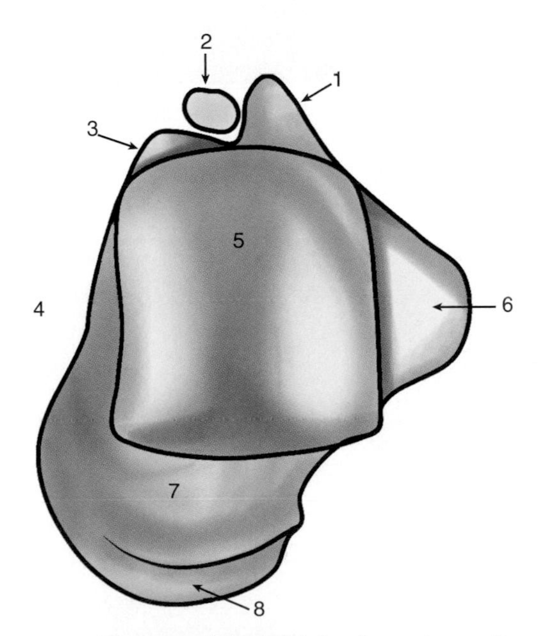

Figure 181-1 Diagram of the left talus from above. Os trigonum/lateral tubercle (1), flexor hallucis longus tendon (2), medial tubercle (3), medial aspect (4), trochlear surface (5), surface for lateral malleolus (6), neck (7), head with articular surface for navicular (8).

- Although the syndrome is uncommon, an os trigonum is not uncommonly discovered as an incidental finding on radiographs, with a prevalence of 2.7% to 7.7%. When present, it is frequently bilateral.

History

- Forced plantarflexion injury of the ankle
- Impingement symptoms may also arise from repetitive ankle plantarflexion.
- Common in ballet dancers and soccer players, but the syndrome is by no means confined to these groups.
- Pain over the posterolateral aspect of the heel on deep plantarflexion of the ankle
- Posteromedial symptoms if the flexor hallucis longus tendon (FHL) is involved

Physical Examination

- Findings are often vague.
- Observation
  - Posterior swelling in acute injury
- Palpation
  - Posterolateral heel tenderness (Fig. 181-2)
- Range of motion
  - Asymmetrical ankle plantarflexion
- Triggering of pain on flexion/extension of the great toe if the FHL is involved
- Special tests
  - Howse test: Forced plantarflexion of the ankle followed by rotation of the calcaneus reproduces impingement pain (Fig. 181-3).
  - Local anesthetic agent: Fluoroscopy-guided injection between the os trigonum and the talus can be diagnostic and correlates with a good outcome after surgical excision.

Imaging (Fig. 181-4)

- Radiographs: lateral weight-bearing view
  - Acute fractures have a rough/irregular edge; ossicles have a smooth edge.

- Ossicles may be a normal finding in 2.7% to 7.7% of people and are often bilateral.
- A lateral view of 25 degrees of external rotation may reveal an os trigonum masked by the medial tubercle.
- Bone scan
  - Useful in excluding os trigonum syndrome when negative
- Computed tomography
  - Useful in identifying fractures of the trigonal process and excluding other differentials
- Magnetic resonance imaging
  - Technique of choice for identifying os trigonum pathology and excluding other differentials

Differential Diagnosis

- Noninsertional Achilles tendinopathy: fusiform swelling, tenderness along tendon
- Insertional Achilles tendinopathy: focal tenderness over posterior/posterolateral heel
- FHL tendinitis: may be associated with os trigonum, young athletes (gymnasts and dancers), posteromedial ankle pain, tenderness, crepitus, and triggering of FHL on movement of the hallux
- Retrocalcaneal bursitis: tenderness and swelling just anterior to the Achilles tendon
- Peroneal tendon subluxation: pain, tenderness, and swelling over the distal fibula; resisted eversion and dorsiflexion of the ankle reproduce subluxation

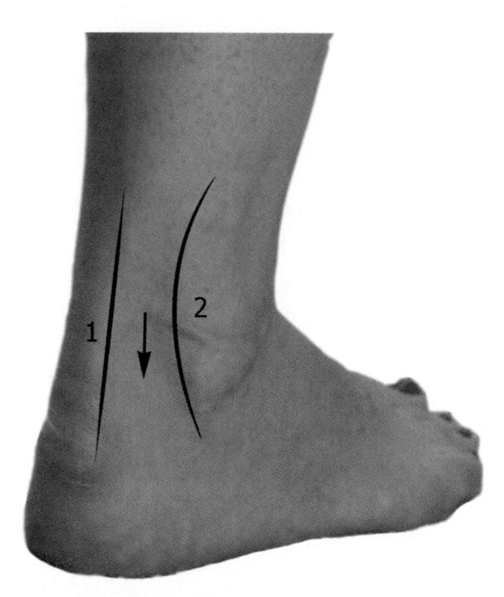

Figure 181-2 Posterolateral view of the right foot. The *arrow* indicates the point where the posterior process of the talus can be palpated between the Achilles tendon (1) and the peroneal tendons (2).

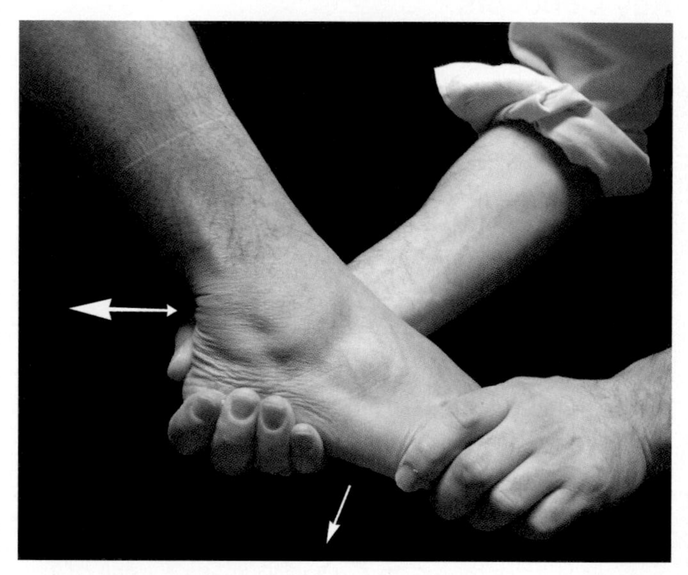

Figure 181-3 Howse test. The foot is forcibly plantarflexed while rotating the calcaneus, causing impingement against the posterior tibial plafond.

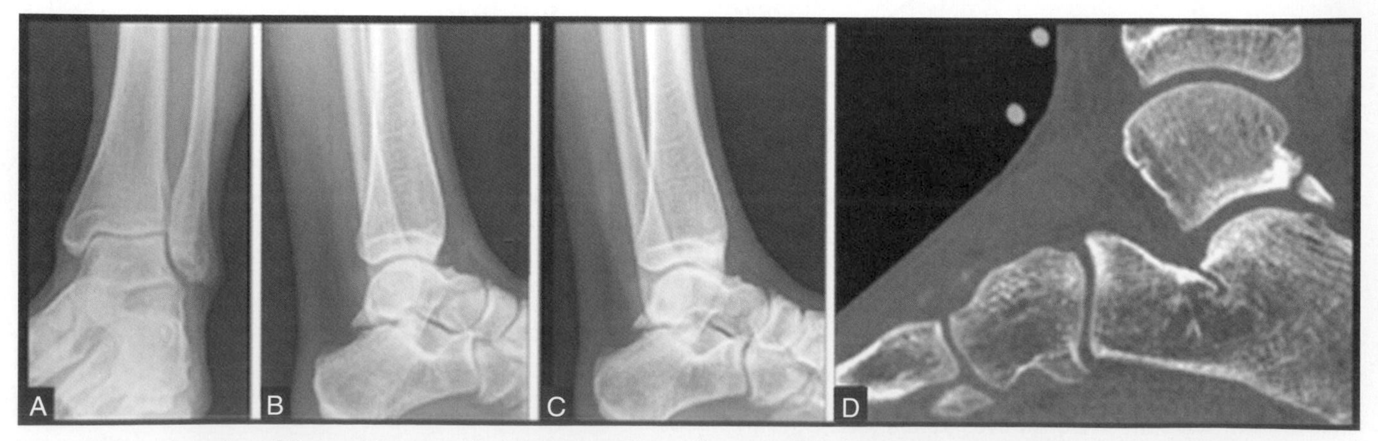

Figure 181-4 Imaging of the os trigonum. **A**, Anteroposterior radiograph. **B**, Lateral radiograph with suspicion of an os trigonum. **C**, Lateral radiograph of 25 degrees of external rotation with a prominent posterior talar process and the os trigonum better visualized. **D**, Sagittal computed tomography scan clearly reveals the os trigonum. (Courtesy of Professor C. Niek van Dijk and Peter de Leeuw.)

- Tarsal tunnel syndrome: vague paresthesia radiating distally along plantar foot; positive Tinel's sign, worse with eversion and dorsiflexion of ankle and metatarsophalangeal joints
- Osteoarthritis of ankle/subtalar joints: anterior/anterolateral pain, stiffness
- Osteonecrosis of the talus: deep aching or sharp ankle pain, mechanical symptoms
- Osteochondral fracture of the talus: chronic ankle swelling, pain, mechanical symptoms after an injury to the lateral ligament complex

Treatment

- At diagnosis
  - The initial treatment is conservative with activity modification, nonsteroidal anti-inflammatory drugs, physiotherapy, and weight-bearing short leg cast immobilization for 4 to 6 weeks.
  - Corticosteroid injections in the region of the os trigonum have been advocated; however, they place the FHL at risk of weakening or rupture.
- Later
  - Surgery is indicated when conservative treatment fails. It involves open or endoscopic excision of the os trigonum.
  - Open surgical excision generally involves a short posterolateral incision and a short period of postoperative immobilization.
  - Alternatively, a posteromedial incision allows concurrent management of associated FHL pathology.
  - FHL decompression is also possible during endoscopic excision. Weight bearing is allowed as soon as it is tolerated.

When to Refer

- Although an os trigonum may be present on radiographs, the syndrome is uncommon. Therefore, other diagnoses should be excluded.
- Refer the patient if there is uncertainty about the diagnosis or if symptoms fail to respond to 3 to 6 months of conservative measures.

Prognosis

- The success rate of conservative treatment is difficult to determine, but may be in the region of 50%.
- Regarding surgical treatment, endoscopic and open techniques offer similar results with patients requiring 3 to 6 months to fully recover. The success rate is approximately 85%.
- Patients with symptoms for more than 2 years fare worse.
- Patients with impingement do better than those with acute fracture.

Troubleshooting

- Patients should be treated conservatively, proceeding to surgery only if symptoms persist.
- The benefits of surgery include improvement of pain and function, including a return to sports in the majority of patients.
- The risks include bleeding, infection, nerve injury (particularly of the sural nerve in the posterolateral approach), stiffness, and recurrence of symptoms.

Patient Instructions

- Os trigonum syndrome is uncommon. Initial treatment is conservative with activity modification, nonsteroidal anti-inflammatory drugs, and physiotherapy.
- If conservative treatment is unsuccessful, a period of immobilization for 4 to 6 weeks may be required.
- If symptoms persist for more than 3 months, referral to a foot and ankle specialist is indicated. The specialist may conduct further investigations before proceeding to either open or endoscopic surgery.

Suggested Reading

- Abramowitz Y, Wollstein R, Barzilay Y, et al: Outcome of resection of a symptomatic os trigonum. J Bone Joint Surg Am 2003;85A:1051–1057.
- Coughlin MJ, Mann RA (eds): Surgery of the Foot and Ankle, 7th ed. St. Louis: Mosby, 1999.
- Howse AJ: Posterior block of the ankle joint in dancers. Foot Ankle 1982;3:81–84.
- Karasick D, Schweitzer ME: The os trigonum syndrome: Imaging features. AJR Am J Roentgenol 1996;166:125–129.
- van Dijk CN: Anterior and posterior ankle impingement. Foot Ankle Clin 2006;11:663–683.

Chapter 182 Tarsal Tunnel Syndrome

Jonathan Smerek

ICD-9 CODES
355.5 *Tarsal Tunnel Syndrome*
355.7 *Other Mononeuritis of the Lower Limb*

Key Concepts

- Tarsal tunnel syndrome (TTS) is an uncommon disorder, and the diagnosis should not be made without a careful history and examination.
- TTS is more common in females, and there is no age predilection.
- A specific etiology is found in only 60% to 80% of individuals and may include a space-occupying lesion, trauma, venous engorgement, or foot deformity (pes planovalgus or severe "flatfoot").
- History is the key to diagnosis.
- Electromyography (EMG) can be extremely unreliable and should not be the basis for diagnosis.
- The posterior tibial nerve supplies the majority of the sensation on the plantar foot.
- The tarsal tunnel is a fibro-osseous structure posterior to the medial malleolus and formed by the flexor retinaculum, which originates from the tibia and inserts onto the posterior process of the calcaneus and talus laterally. The retinaculum blends with the sheaths of the posterior tibial tendon, flexor digitorum longus tendon, posterior tibial nerve/artery, and flexor hallucis longus tendon (Fig. 182-1).

History

- Often vague symptoms
- Burning, sharp, electric pain, tingling, or numbness on the plantar foot
- Rest pain common and symptoms often worse at night, with inability to tolerate socks or sheets on the feet
- Radiation of pain proximally to the posteromedial aspect of the distal tibia (Valleix phenomenon)
- Although pain can be worse with activity, symptoms usually do not correlate with the amount or duration of activity.

Physical Examination

- Observation
  - Gait
  - Heel alignment: Observe patient standing from behind with shoes and socks removed; assess heel varus/valgus and note whether arch is high (cavus) or collapsed (planovalgus or "flatfoot").
- Palpation
  - Tenderness along course of the posterior tibial nerve
  - Positive Tinel's sign: the patient's symptoms reproduced with gentle percussion along the course of the posterior tibial nerve
  - Palpate for tenderness over the plantar fascia.

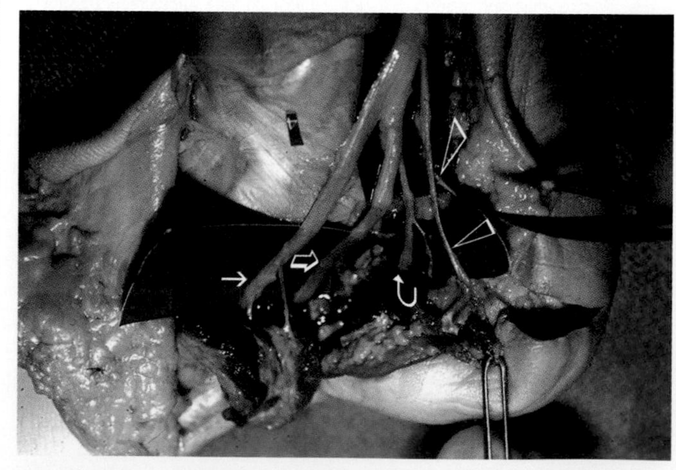

Figure 182-1 Anatomy of the tarsal tunnel demonstrating the boundaries and surrounding structures. *Thin arrow* indicates the medial plantar nerve; *thick arrow* indicates the lateral plantar nerve; *curved arrow* indicates the nerve to the flexor digitorum brevis; *triangles* indicate the medial calcaneal branches.

- Range of motion
  - Ankle, subtalar, and talonavicular range of motion
- Special tests
  - Tarsal tunnel compression test: Reproducing the patient's symptoms by pressure over the nerve (compress against the posteromedial tibia for 30 seconds) is a highly specific finding (Fig. 182-2).

Imaging

- Radiographs: weight-bearing anteroposterior, lateral, and oblique/mortise views of the foot/ankle
  - Look for acute and malunited fractures, arthrosis, accessory ossicles, and tarsal coalitions.
- Magnetic resonance imaging (MRI)
  - Useful if radiographs are normal and index of suspicion for a space-occupying lesion of the tarsal tunnel is high (Fig. 182-3)
  - Lesions are more common in pediatric patients.

Additional Tests

- Electrodiagnostic studies: Decreased mixed motor and sensory conduction velocity is the most specific and sensitive for TTS.
  - There is a false-negative rate of at least 10%, so the diagnosis is not eliminated with a normal EMG.
  - Studies have demonstrated no correlation between EMG results and clinical outcomes.
  - May rule out peripheral neuropathy, proximal compression, or double crush injury

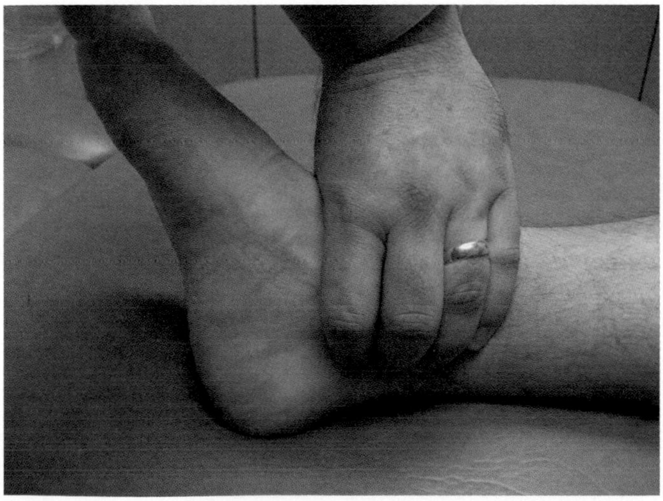

Figure 182-2 Tarsal tunnel compression test demonstrating compression over the posterior tibial nerve in an attempt to recreate the patient's symptoms. The light compression should be held for at least 30 seconds.

Differential Diagnosis

- Herniated nucleus pulposus: radiating leg pain, positive straight leg raise, back pain
- Plantar fasciitis: heel pain, worse with first step in morning
- Peripheral vascular disease: claudication, no palpable pulses
- Peripheral neuropathy: stocking-glove pain and numbness, diabetes, EMG
- Neurolemma/neuroma/ganglion cyst: fullness in the tarsal tunnel, MRI
- Fracture of the ankle/talus/calcaneus: point tenderness; radiographs and computed tomography
- Rheumatoid arthritis: systemic findings; arthrosis on radiographs
- Tenosynovitis: tenderness over posterior tibial tendon, relieved with rest and immobilization
- Venous varicosities: fullness, varicosities on examination
- Tarsal coalition: limited hindfoot motion; radiographs or MRI
- Crush injury/blunt trauma: history of trauma, highly sensitive overlying skin (allodynia)

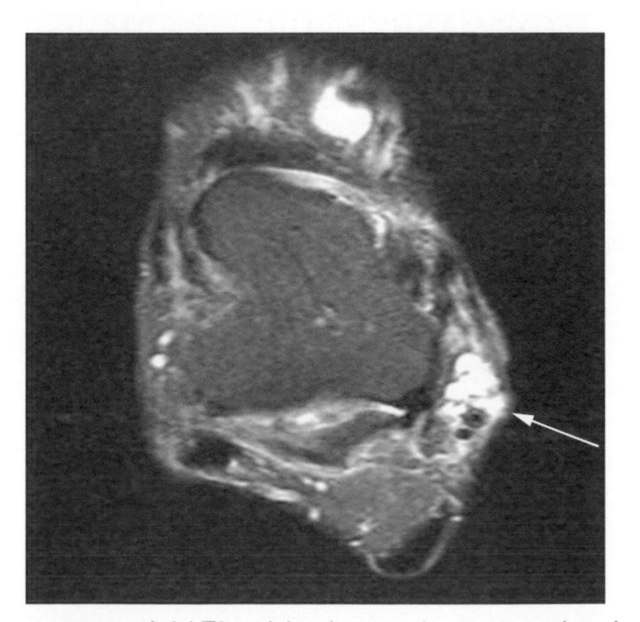

Figure 182-3 Axial T2-weighted magnetic resonance imaging of the ankle demonstrates a multiloculated ganglion cyst (*arrow*) within the tarsal tunnel resulting in compression of the nearby posterior tibial nerve.

Treatment

- At diagnosis
- Unless the patient has a space-occupying lesion compressing the posterior tibial nerve, a prolonged course of conservative management is mandatory.
  - Avoid inciting activities and nonsteroidal anti-inflammatory drugs; physical therapy with adjuvant modalities for desensitization of the posterior tibial nerve may be attempted.
  - In flexible foot deformities, arch supports with a medial heel wedge to decompress the tarsal tunnel can provide significant relief.
  - Neuropathy medications (Neurontin [gabapentin], Lyrica [pregabalin]) may be instituted, but should not be the first line of therapy due to potential side effects.
  - Immobilization with a boot walker or cast is usually not beneficial and may lead to calf atrophy and ankle weakness.
- Later
  - Failure of 6 weeks of conservative therapy with no relief of symptoms warrants a tarsal tunnel injection. This injection can be both therapeutic and diagnostic. Failure of at least 3 months of conservative management, including a tarsal tunnel injection, is sufficient to consider surgical intervention for release of the posterior tibial nerve.

When to Refer

- Diagnosis of TTS requires (1) pain and paresthesias in the foot, (2) positive electrodiagnostic studies, and (3) a positive Tinel's sign or tarsal tunnel compression test. With two of these findings, the patient may have TTS and should be followed closely.

Prognosis

- As many as 75% of patients who undergo release of the posterior tibial nerve can expect nearly complete relief of their symptoms.
- The other 25% do not improve, and in fact, can have worsening of their symptoms after attempted surgical release.
- Repeat surgery has extremely poor outcomes due to scarring around the nerve.
- Patients with a space-occupying lesion have a better prognosis and can expect nearly complete resolution of their symptoms with mass excision and release.

Troubleshooting

- Failure to improve with conservative measures warrants a tarsal tunnel injection, which can be both diagnostic and therapeutic (see Chapter 201).

Patient Instructions

- Patients should be instructed that nerve-related symptoms frequently take many months to resolve and they should expect a slow diminution in symptoms over time.
- Surgery should be only undertaken after at least 3 months of conservative care because surgical outcomes in general are unpredictable. Surgery should not be the first option.

Suggested Reading

- DiGiovanni BF, Gould JS: Tarsal tunnel syndrome and related entities. Foot Ankle Clin 1998;3:405–426.
- Gould JS: Complex nerve problems of the foot and ankle. In Nunley JA (ed): Advanced Reconstruction: Foot and Ankle. Rosemont, IL: American Academy of Orthopaedic Surgeons, 2004, pp 473–479.
- Lau JT, Stavrou P: Posterior tibial nerve—primary. Foot Ankle Clin 2004;9:271–285.
- Mann RA: Diseases of the nerves. In Mann RA (ed): Surgery of the Foot and Ankle. St. Louis: Mosby, 1999, pp 512–516.
- Sammarco GJ, Chang L: Outcome of surgical treatment of tarsal tunnel syndrome. Foot Ankle Int 2003;24:125–131.

Chapter 183 The Diabetic Foot

Alan C. League

ICD-9 CODES
713.5 *Neurogenic Arthropathy*
250.6 *Diabetes with Neurologic Manifestations*

Key Concepts

- Diabetes mellitus is a metabolic disease characterized by high blood glucose levels. More than 20 million Americans have diabetes.
- Common foot problems due to diabetes include pressure ulcers, infection, and Charcot's arthropathy.
- The primary etiology of the diabetic foot is peripheral neuropathy, which results in the following:
  - Loss of protective sensation leads to unperceived trauma and skin breakdown.
  - Autonomic dysfunction results in dry, scaly, cracked skin; at risk of infection
  - Motor dysfunction creates forefoot deformities such as claw toes, which lead to abnormal posturing of the foot and subsequent pressure points.
- Charcot's arthropathy is a progressive degeneration of joints characterized by bony destruction, joint fragmentation, and subsequent deformity. It affects approximately one in 600 patients with diabetes.
  - The etiology of Charcot joints is thought to be repetitive microtrauma or dysregulated resorption of bone.
  - Diabetes is the number one cause of amputation in the United States.

History

- Painless ulcer, typically with an insidious onset
- In later cases, infected ulcer with foul-smelling drainage
- Early stages of Charcot's arthropathy include swelling, erythema, and warmth, which can be difficult to differentiate from infection or gout,
- Progressive deformity of the foot with or without ulceration in later stages of Charcot's arthropathy
- May have neuropathic pain in a stocking-type distribution

Physical Examination

- Observation
  - Ulcers, calluses, erythema, swelling, deformity (Fig. 183-1)
- Palpation
  - Pedal pulses must be documented. Absent pulses require a vascular workup.
  - Warmth may indicate infection, a Charcot joint, or both.
  - Protective sensation is absent if the patient cannot feel the 10-gauge, 5.07-diameter nylon monofilament applied to the plantar foot (Fig. 183-2).

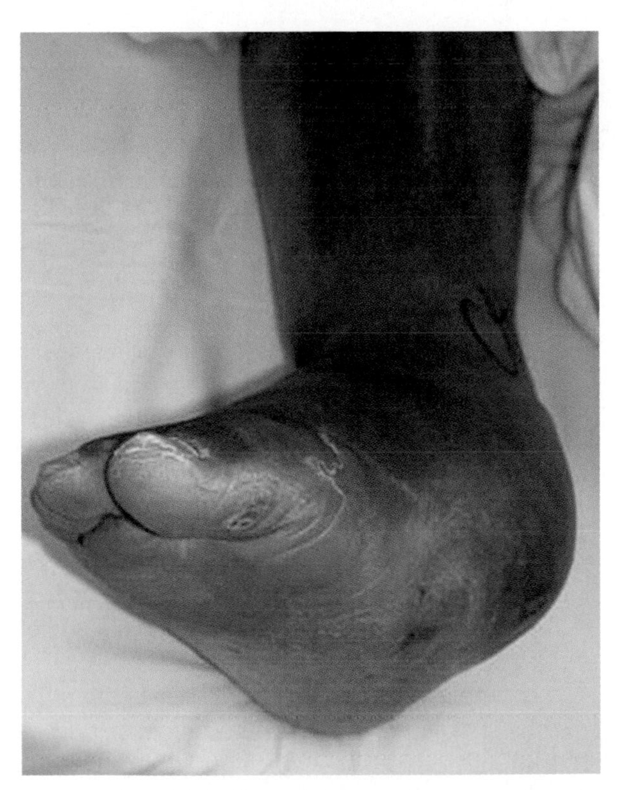

Figure 183-1 Diabetic foot with swelling and deformity.

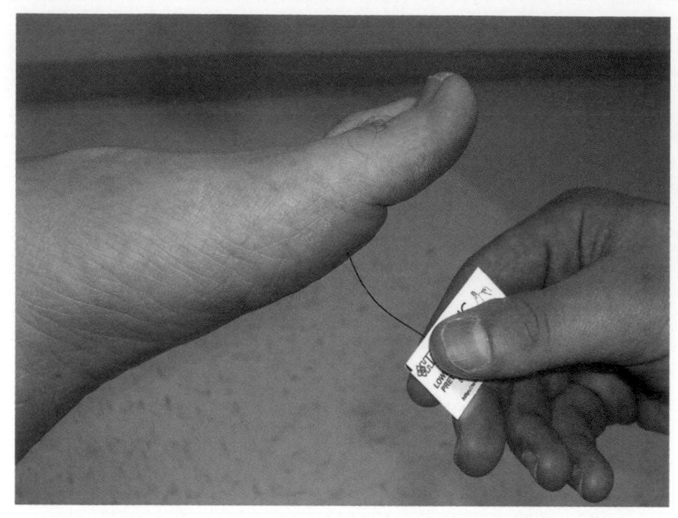

Figure 183-2 Evaluating protective sensation with a 10-gauge, 5.07-diameter nylon monofilament.

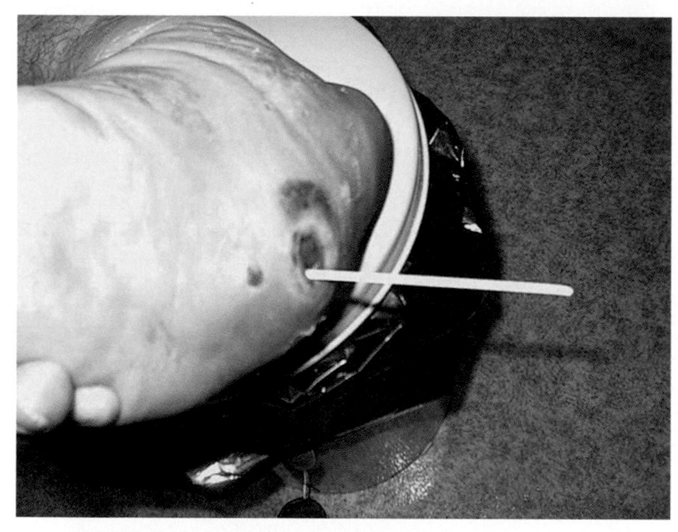

Figure 183-3 Probing to bone in a neuropathic ulcer likely indicates osteomyelitis.

- Range of motion
  - Ankle dorsiflexion is assessed with the knee extended to assess for gastrocnemius contracture, which can result in recurrent forefoot ulcerations.
- Special tests
  - Neuropathic ulcers are insensate and can be easily probed to determine size and depth. If bone is probed, osteomyelitis is likely (Fig. 183-3).
  - One way to differentiate a Charcot joint from infection is to elevate the foot above heart level. After 1 minute of elevation, a foot with Charcot's arthropathy should begin to lose its redness, whereas a foot with cellulitis or osteomyelitis should retain its color.

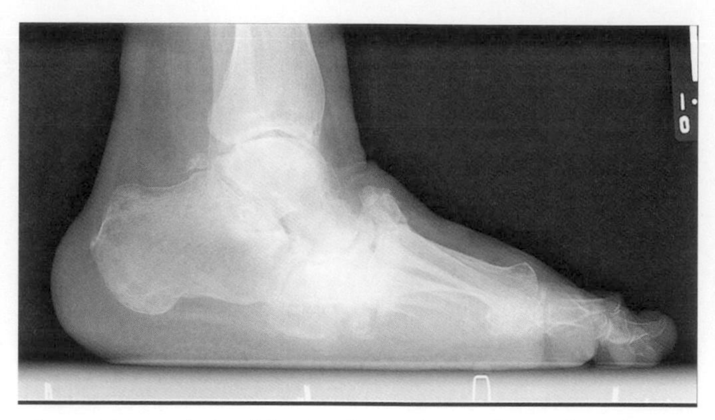

Figure 183-4 Lateral foot radiograph of collapsed midfoot Charcot's arthropathy.

Imaging

- Radiographs: weight-bearing views of the foot and ankle
  - May help identify osteomyelitis, Charcot's arthropathy, and the degree of bone and joint destruction (Fig. 183-4)
  - Triple-phase bone scan
  - Best imaging test to differentiate Charcot's arthropathy from osteomyelitis

Additional Tests

- Vascular studies are appropriate in patients with absent pulses.

Differential Diagnosis

- Cellulitis/abscess: presence of wound drainage; elevation produces no improvement in erythema
- Gout: positive history, improvement with anti-inflammatory drugs
- Osteomyelitis: positive triple-phase bone scan, ulcer probes to bone
- Other neuropathies (Charcot-Marie-Tooth, alcoholic neuropathy, spinal cord neuropathy): positive history, negative diabetes testing

Treatment

- At diagnosis
  - The presence of a callus or ulcer is the result of pressure phenomena. It should be débrided, cleansed, and dressed with a sterile, moist dressing.
  - Orthotic devices such as extra-depth diabetic shoes with accommodative inserts (Fig. 183-5) will help reduce pressure forces.

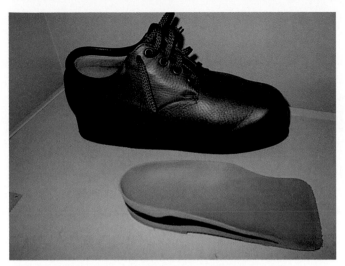

Figure 183-5 Extra-depth diabetic shoes with accommodative insoles may prevent ulcerations.

- Total contact casting is another way to reduce shear forces in the plantar skin and may allow ulcers to heal.
- Treatment of deep ulcers and osteomyelitis requires more aggressive management.
  — Surgical débridement is necessary to allow drainage of an abscess or other deep infection.
  — Bone biopsy is helpful in guiding antibiotic therapy.
- Acute Charcot's arthropathy is best managed by immobilization in a total contact cast or a Charcot restraint orthotic walker (Fig. 183-6).

- Later
  - Chronic Charcot's arthropathy may result in an unstable foot deformity with plantar ulcerations. Many times these can be managed with a Charcot restraint orthotic walker; however, some are unbraceable and require surgical arthrodesis to correct the deformity.

When to Refer

- Any diabetic patient who develops foot ulcers, infection, deformity, or unexplained swelling and pain should be referred to a specialist.

Prognosis

- When managed promptly and aggressively, diabetic foot ulcers will usually heal and their recurrence can be avoided with appropriate diabetic foot gear.

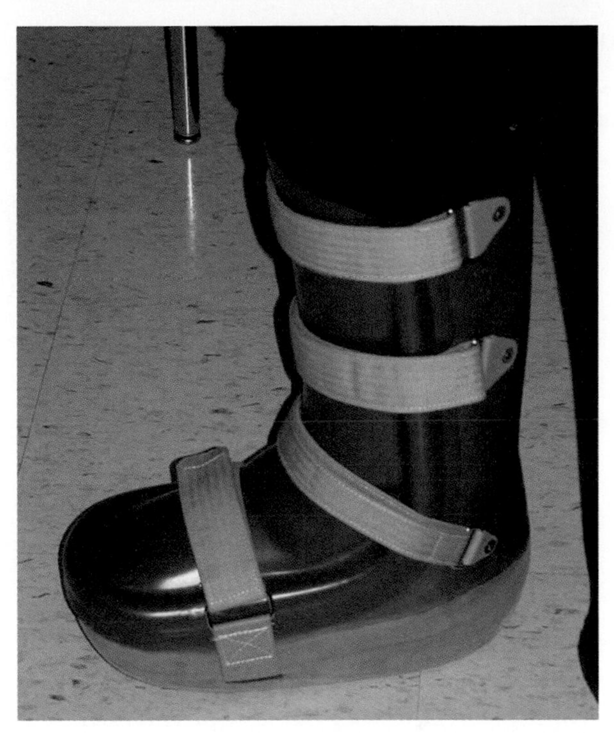

Figure 183-6 The Charcot restraint orthotic walker provides stability and off-loading to a Charcot foot.

- Charcot's arthropathy of the foot results in decreased ability to ambulate, but function can be maximized with appropriate bracing or surgical reconstruction.

Troubleshooting

- Prevention of foot problems through diabetic education is the key to avoiding complications in diabetic patients. Routine diabetic foot care should be taught, and appropriate foot gear should be recommended.
- All diabetic patients should be counseled on the risks of amputation for undertreated foot ulcers.
- The care of diabetic patients with foot problems is often multidisciplinary and may involve primary care physicians, endocrinologists, wound care specialists, podiatrists, infectious disease specialists, orthotists, and others. Efficient communication between these professionals is paramount to achieve the desired results.

Patient Instructions

- An educational brochure on diabetic foot care should be given to all diabetic patients.
- Emphasize the importance of daily foot examinations and appropriate foot gear.

Suggested Reading

- McDermott JE (ed): The Diabetic Foot. Rosemont, IL: American Academy of Orthopaedic Surgeons, 1995.
- Pinzur MS, Slovenkai MP, Trepman E, et al: Guidelines for diabetic foot care: Recommendations endorsed by the Diabetes Committee of the American Orthopaedic Foot and Ankle Society. Foot Ankle Int 2005;26:113–119.
- Strauss MB: The orthopaedic surgeon's role in the treatment and prevention of diabetic foot wounds. Foot Ankle Int 2005;26:5–14.
- Trepman E, Bracilovic A, Lamborn KK, et al: Diabetic foot care: Multilingual translation of a patient education leaflet. Foot Ankle Int 2005;26:64–107.
- Trepman E, Nihal A, Pinzur MS: Current topics review: Charcot neuroarthropathy of the foot and ankle. Foot Ankle Int 2005;26:46–63.

Chapter 184 Morton's Neuroma (Plantar Interdigital Neuroma)

Steven L. Haddad

ICD-9 CODE

355.6 *Lesion of Plantar Nerve; Morton's Metatarsalgia, Neuralgia, or Neuroma*

Key Concepts

- Commonly involves the plantar third web space
- History and physical examination sufficient to make the diagnosis (additional testing unnecessary)
- Conservative care incorporates a pad placed in the shoe to take the pressure off the involved nerve and an injection of cortisone.
- Surgical treatment is reserved for conservative management failure and involves removing the diseased digital nerve.

History

- Insidious onset
- Third intermetatarsal web space most common, followed by the second; rarely, first and/or fourth web space involved
- Burning pain in the affected toes
- Focal paresthesias common, aggravated by specific shoes (i.e., elevated heels, narrow toe box). Patients often remove their shoes and massage their forefoot to eliminate pain.
- Digital numbness may be seen late in the condition.

Physical Examination

- Observation
    - Weight-bearing assessment of the foot specifically looks for a crossover toe or claw toe deformity, conditions that are commonly mistaken for plantar interdigital neuroma due to their presentation with plantar forefoot pain.
- Palpation
    - The hallmark is pain in the plantar web space of the involved digits.
    - Direct pressure between the metatarsal heads or just distal reproduces the pain and paresthesias (Fig. 184-1).
    - Adjacent metatarsal heads are palpated in isolation to differentiate a neuroma from metatarsalgia (seen in isolation or as a component of a claw toe deformity).
    - The volar plate at the plantar metatarsophalangeal (MTP) joint is palpated to differentiate a neuroma from a crossover toe deformity (occurring from a volar plate rupture).

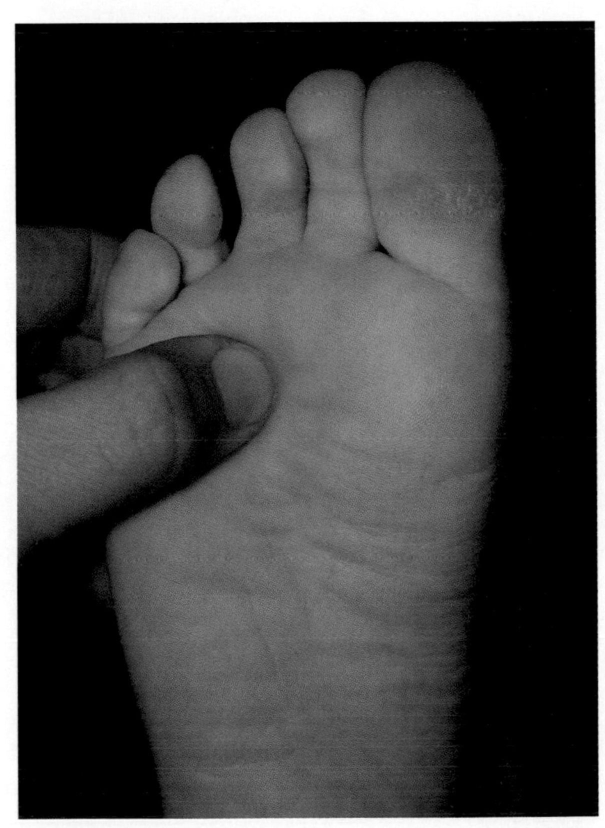

Figure 184-1 Direct palpation of the third web space. It is important not to press on the metatarsal heads or distal to them.

- Special tests
  - Compression test: Firmly squeeze the metatarsal heads together for 30 seconds. Pain is reproduced in the involved web space and digits (Fig. 184-2).
  - Mulder's click: Milk the small mass of nerve/bursal tissue between the involved metatarsal heads by alternating thumb and forefinger pressure while simultaneously compressing the metatarsal heads to reproduce symptoms (Fig. 184-3).
  - Vertical Lachman's test: Grasp the phalanx and firmly place vertical stress on the MTP joint. Reproduction of plantar pain or gross motion/instability is indicative of a crossover toe (and rupture of the volar plate) and not a neuroma.

Imaging

- Radiographs: anteroposterior, lateral, and oblique views of the foot
  - Rule out other conditions such as crossover toe, claw toe, MTP dislocation, Freiberg's infraction (Fig. 184-4), and stress fractures.
- Magnetic resonance imaging
  - May be helpful in equivocal cases and ruling out other forefoot pathology (Fig. 184-5)
- Ultrasonography
  - More economical alternative to assist in diagnosis

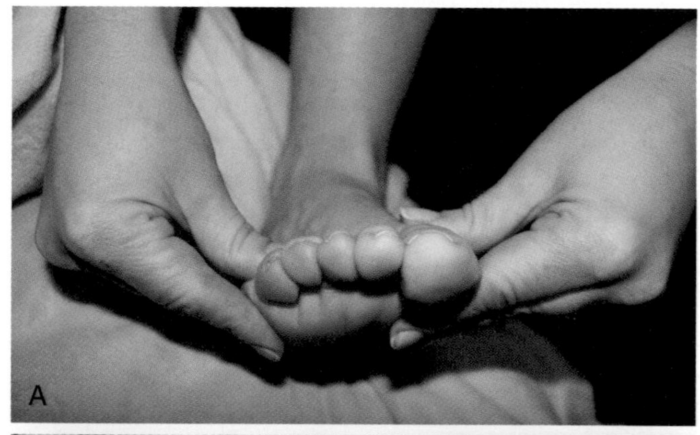

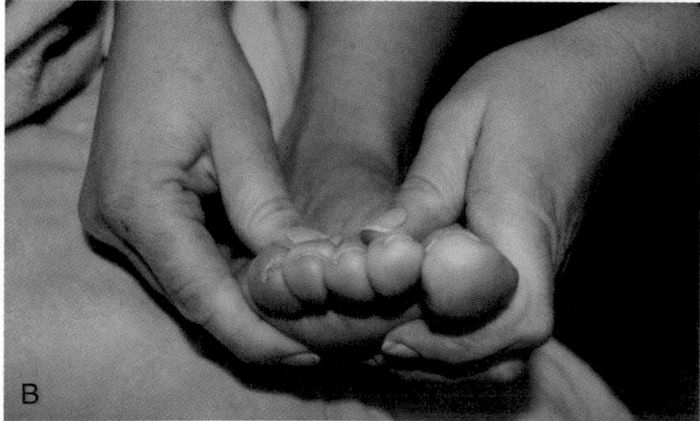

Figure 184-2 The compression test is performed by placing the examiner's hands securely on the metatarsal heads and directing pressure centrally from either side. **A**, Compression of the first and fifth metatarsal heads. **B**, Isolated compression of the third and fourth metatarsal heads.

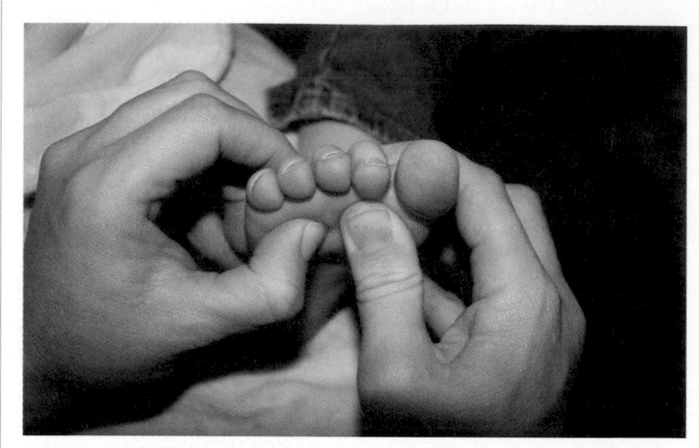

Figure 184-3 The Mulder's click is performed by delivering the dilated nerve into the web space between the metatarsal heads with the examiner's thumb and then performing a compression test to squeeze the third and fourth metatarsal heads, milking the nerve plantarward.

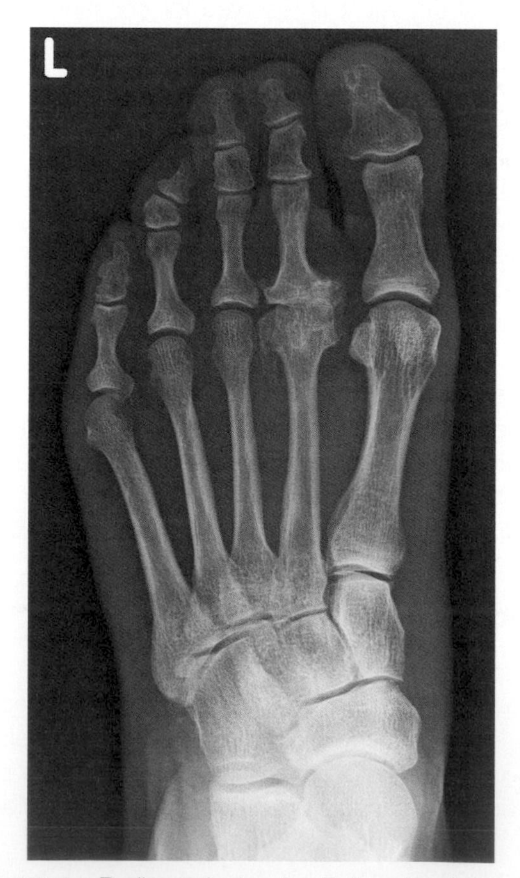

Figure 184-4 Radiograph showing Freiberg's infraction. Note the destruction of the second metatarsophalangeal joint and subsequent arthritic wear.

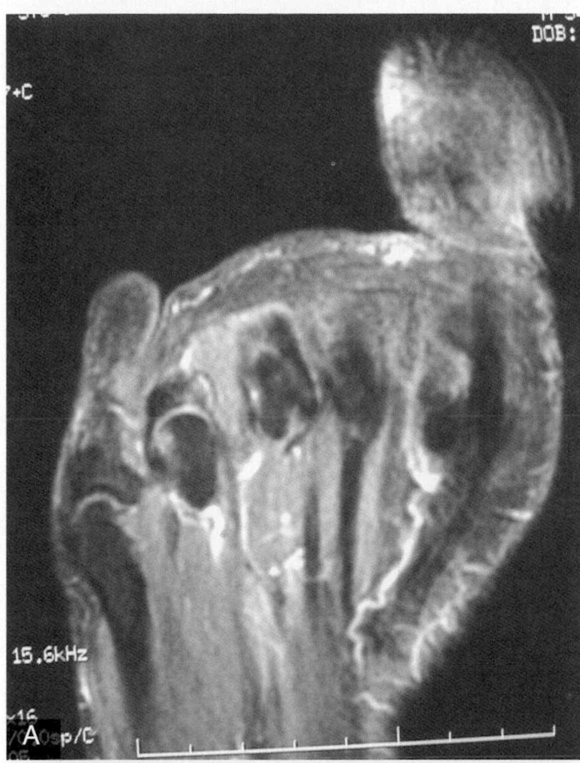

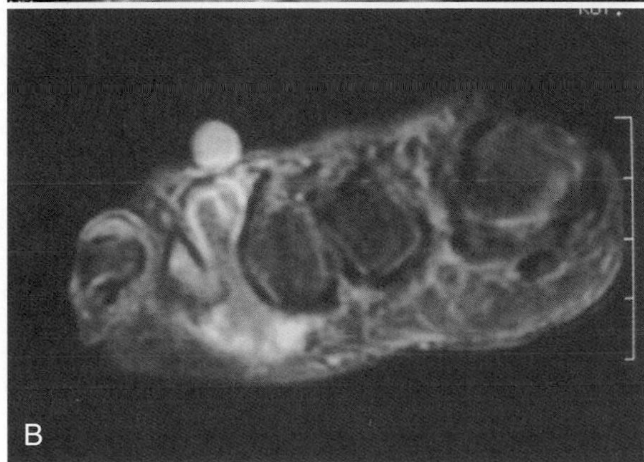

Figure 184-5 Magnetic resonance images of a large Morton's neuroma. **A**, T1-weighted image demonstrates the enlarged digital nerve between the third and fourth metatarsal heads. **B**, T2-weighted image demonstrates the enhanced, inflamed tissue in the same interspace.

- Highly operator dependent; leads to potential misdiagnosis

Additional Tests

- Injection of lidocaine/bupivacaine coupled with cortisone (see Chapter 203)
  - Diagnostic and potentially therapeutic
  - Pain relief may be seen in only 14% of involved patients after a single injection but in 30% after cumulative injections.

Differential Diagnosis

- Volar plate rupture at MTP joint (plantar ligament sprain, early crossover toe)
- Metatarsalgia
- Tarsal tunnel syndrome
- Intractable plantar keratoses (calluses)
- Dislocation of MTP joint after rigid claw toe
- Avascular necrosis of the lesser metatarsal head (Freiberg's infraction)
- Ganglion cyst within a web space

Treatment

- At diagnosis
  - Conservative care consists of shoe wear modifications (wide toe box) to reduce pressure on the involved nerve, and injections for persistent symptoms.
  - Placement of a felt pad just proximal to the metatarsal heads in the involved web space (not at the level of the heads) will help to splay the heads and further reduce pressure on the neuroma.
  - Dilute alcohol injections may be substituted for cortisone. This regimen involves multiple injections (a minimum of five, each separated by 15 days) of this sclerosing agent. Success rates vary from 30% to 94%.
- Later
  - If conservative measures fail, surgical resection of the neuroma is indicated (Fig. 184-6).

When to Refer

- Failure to respond to injections in a patient with intractable pain warrants referral for surgical resection of the Morton's neuroma. Operative intervention is unaffected by the size of the neuroma, and outcomes do not differ after prolonged trials of conservative care. Thus, patients may be reassured that they may wait as long as they like before considering surgery.

Prognosis

- Surgical success rates vary, with the literature suggesting good to excellent results in 50% to 80% of patients.

Troubleshooting

- If injection offers no benefit, it is important to seek other diagnoses to avoid failed surgery.

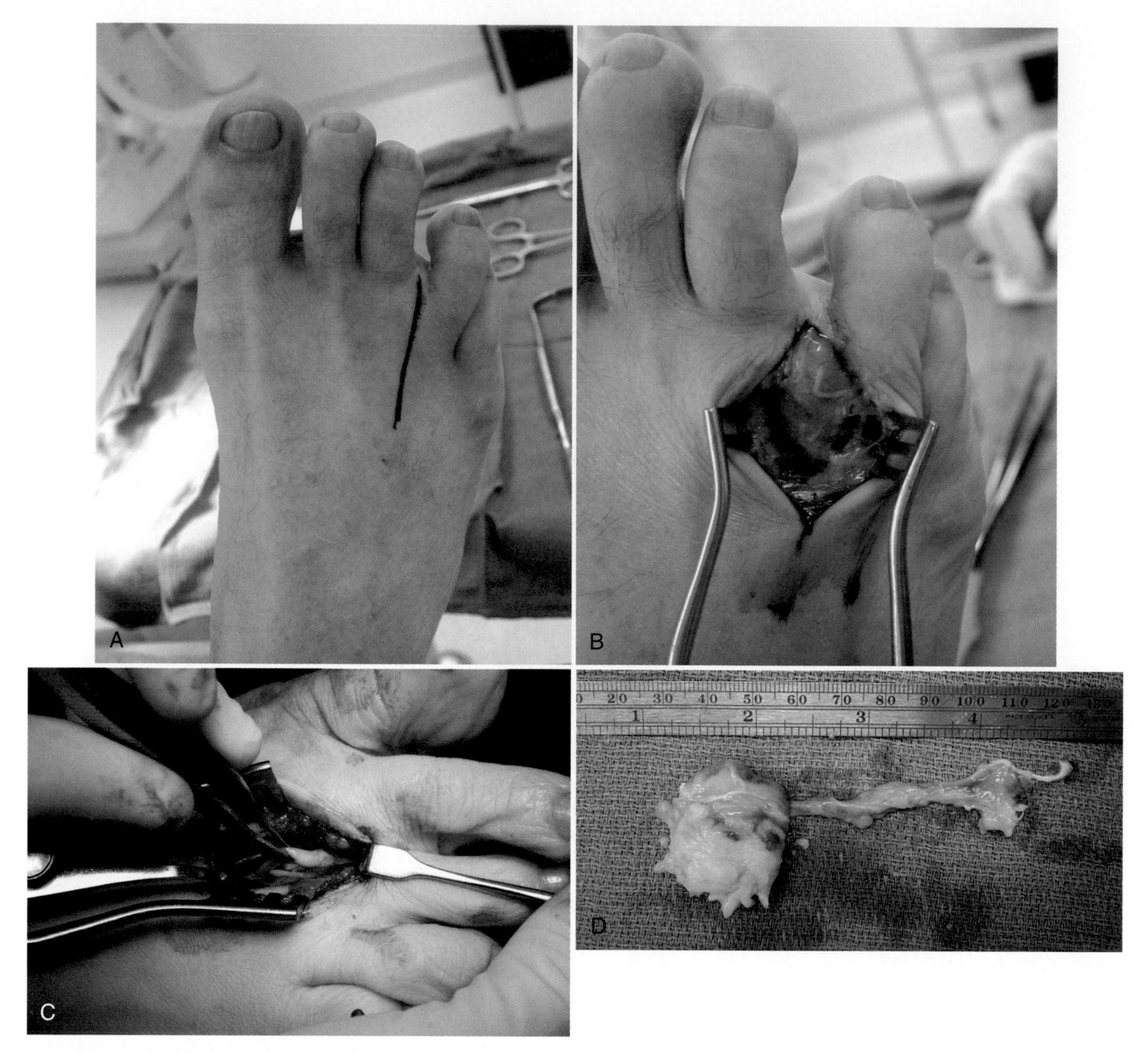

Figure 184-6 Surgical excision of a Morton's neuroma. **A**, Surgical approach. **B**, Example of massive neuroma in the third web space. **C**, Example of a smaller Morton's neuroma in the second web space, completely freed from surrounding soft tissues, with the dilation visible at the level between the metatarsal heads. **D**, Resected Morton's neuroma, with 3 cm of proximal common digital nerve attached to the resected segment.

- Caution patients that pain relief may not be complete after surgical resection.
- Reasons for failure include incorrect diagnosis, stump neuroma (forming at the site of resection), scar tissue entrapment at the resection site, and recurrent neuroma.

Patient Instructions

- Ensure that patients understand the nature of the condition and that they should not rush to surgery.
- Conservative care may eventually result in resolution of pain, although if there is a recurrence, surgery becomes an appropriate option.

Suggested Reading

- Betts LO: Morton's metatarsalgia: Neuritis of the fourth digital nerve. Med J Aust 1940;1:514.
- Bossley CJ, Cairney PC: The intermetatarsophalangeal bursa: Its significance in Morton's metatarsalgia. J Bone Joint Surg Br 1980;62B:184–187.

- Erickson SJ, Canale PB, Carrera GF, et al: Interdigital (Morton) neuroma: High-resolution MR imaging with a solenoid coil. Radiology 1991;181:833–836.
- Greenfield JK, Rea J Jr, Ilfeld FW: Morton's interdigital neuroma: Indications for treatment by local injections versus surgery. Clin Orthop Relat Res 1984;185:142–144.
- Mulder JD: The causative mechanism in Morton's metatarsalgia. J Bone Joint Surg Br 1951;33B:94–95.
- Nissen KI: Plantar digital neuritis: Morton's metatarsalgia. J Bone Joint Surg Br 1948;30B:84–94.
- Redd RA, Peters VJ, Emery SF, et al: Morton neuroma: Sonographic evaluation. Radiology 1989;71:415–417.
- Shapiro PP, Shapiro SL: Sonographic evaluation of interdigital neuromas. Foot Ankle Int 1995;16:604–606.
- Terk MR, Kwong PK, Suthar M, et al: Morton neuroma: Evaluation with MR imaging performed with contrast enhancement and fat suppression. Radiology 1993;189:239–241.
- Womack JW, Richardson DR, Murphy AG, et al: Long-term evaluation of interdigital neuroma treated by surgical excision. Foot Ankle Int 2008;29:574–577.

Chapter 185 Hallux Valgus (Bunion)

Medardo R. Maroto, Daniel K. Park, and Simon Lee

ICD-9 CODES
735.0 *Hallux Valgus (Acquired)*
755.66 *Hallux Valgus (Congenital)*
727.1 *Bunion*

Key Concepts

- Hallux valgus is a deformity of the great toe characterized by adduction (medial deviation) of the metatarsal head and abduction (lateral deviation) of the hallux.
- Hallux valgus is found in at least 2% of children aged 9 to 10 years, and almost half of adults, with a greater prevalence in women.
- Hallux valgus does not directly cause symptoms, but the resulting prominent metatarsal head (bunion) and overlying bursa may become irritated, causing pain.
- The resulting deformity may transfer stress to the second toe, causing more symptoms related to the second toe than the hallux valgus toe (Fig. 185-1).
- Constrictive footwear appears to contribute to creating this deformity.

History

- Etiology
  - Extrinsic causes: constricting footwear (plays a major role)
  - Intrinsic causes: pronated hindfoot, pes planus, metatarsus primus varus, Achilles tendon contracture, generalized joint laxity, hypermobility of the first metatarsocuneiform joint, and neuromuscular disorders
  - Heredity: increased incidence of hallux valgus in families
- Symptomatic patients present with cosmetic concerns, transfer metatarsalgia, second toe deformity, problems with shoe wear, and pain (Fig. 185-2).
- Many patients are minimally symptomatic, but progression of symptoms and deformity can be rapid.
- Patients' occupational and recreational requirements may dictate treatment.
  - Evaluation of shoe wear is crucial.

Physical Examination

- Patients should be examined sitting and standing (accentuates deformity).
- Observation
  - Gait: antalgic or externally rotated
  - Lower extremity alignment: medial longitudinal arch and the relationship between the great toe and lesser toes with patient standing
  - Irritated and inflamed dorsomedial bursa
- Palpation
  - Focal tenderness
  - Synovial thickening, dorsal osteophytes, sesamoid pain, and crepitus
  - Tender, plantar callosities indicate transfer lesions under the lesser metatarsophalangeal (MTP) joints.

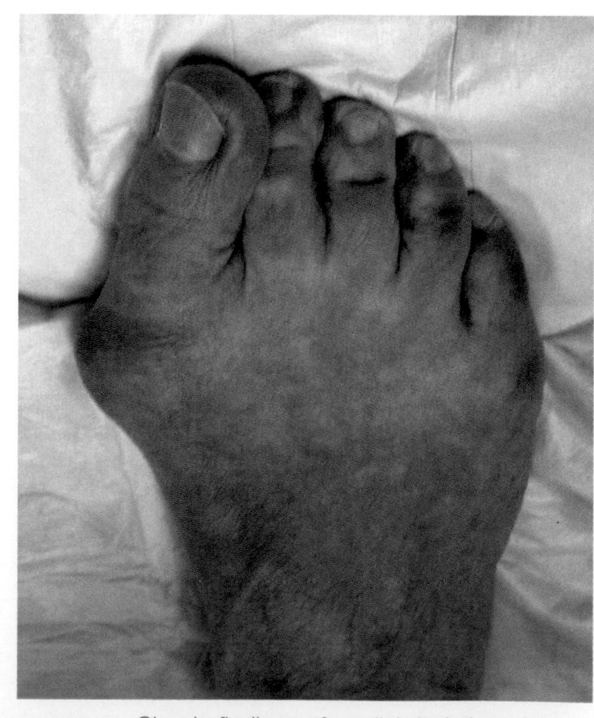

Figure 185-1 Classic findings of medial deviation of the metatarsal and lateral deviation of the phalanx of the hallux. Also note the inflamed bursa over the dorsomedial prominence as well as the overlap deformity developing in the second toe.

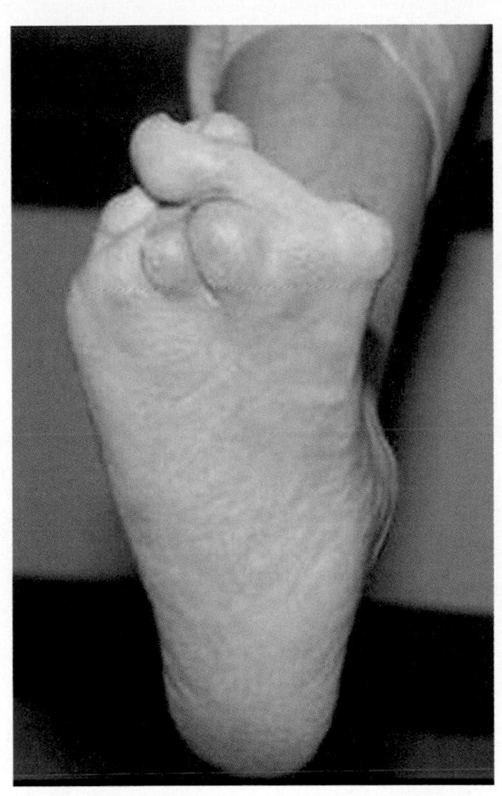

Figure 185-2 Plantar view of the foot showing increased pressure under the second and third metatarsal heads consistent with a transfer metatarsal lesion due to the severe hallux valgus deformity.

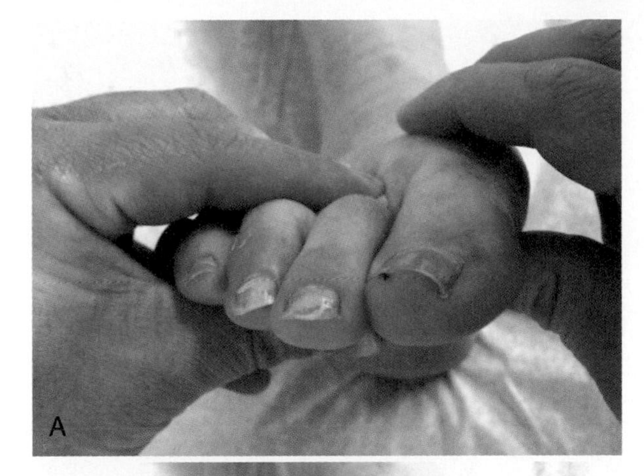

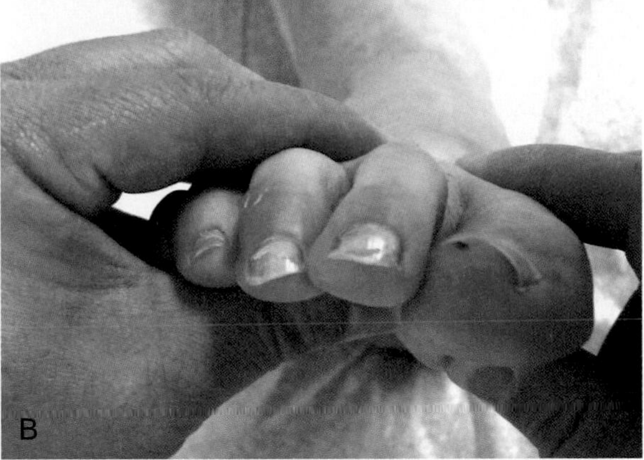

Figure 185-3 Assessment of metatarsocuneiform instability showing maximal dorsiflexion (**A**) and plantarflexion (**B**) stressing in a patient with instability.

   - Occasionally, the dorsal cutaneous nerve overlying the bursa can result in numbness or paresthesia over the dorsomedial distal phalanx.
- Range of motion
   - Ankle, subtalar, and transverse tarsal joints
   - First MTP joint: Dorsiflex and plantarflex while attempting to realign the great toe. Pain or crepitus may indicate degenerative changes.
- Special tests
   - Neurovascular status
   - Stress maneuvers: Increased laxity of the first metatarsocuneiform joint may contribute to deformity.
      — The second metatarsal head is held with one hand while the other hand holds the first metatarsal head and deviates it dorsomedially and then plantar laterally (Fig. 185-3).
      — Deviation greater than the overall width of the metatarsal may indicate contributing instability.
   - The second MTP joint should always be examined.

Imaging

- Radiographs: weight-bearing anteroposterior, lateral, with or without axial (sesamoid) view
   - Hallux valgus angle: Normal is less than 15 degrees (Fig. 185-4).
      — Angle between the long axes of the proximal phalanx and first metatarsal
   - Intermetatarsal angle: Normal is less than 9 degrees (Fig. 185-5).
      — Angle between the first and second metatarsals
   - Distal metatarsal articular angle: Normal is less than 10 degrees.
      — Angle between the distal articular surface and the long axis of the first metatarsal
   - Position of sesamoid in relation to the metatarsal head provides information regarding the severity of the hallux valgus deformity, degree of hallux pronation, and possible pathologic changes in the sesamoid.

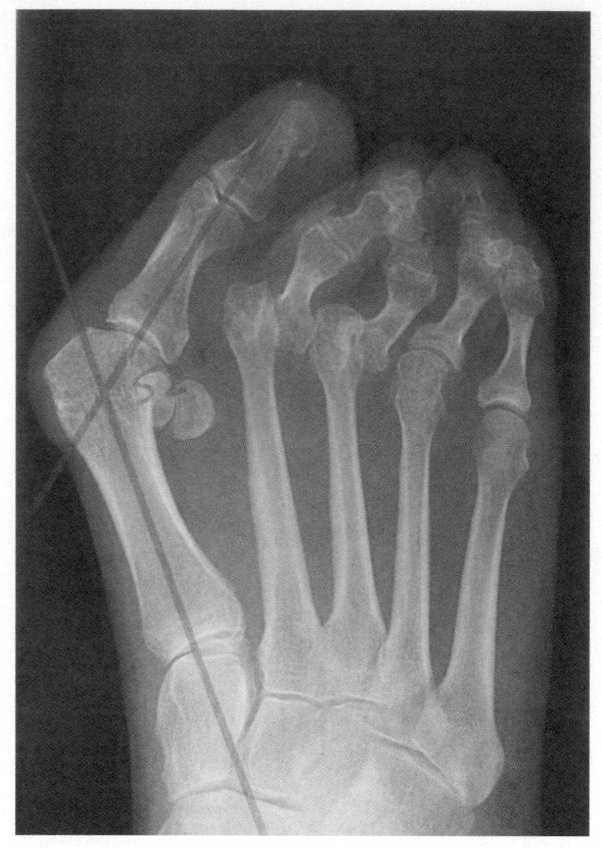

Figure 185-4 Hallux valgus angle.

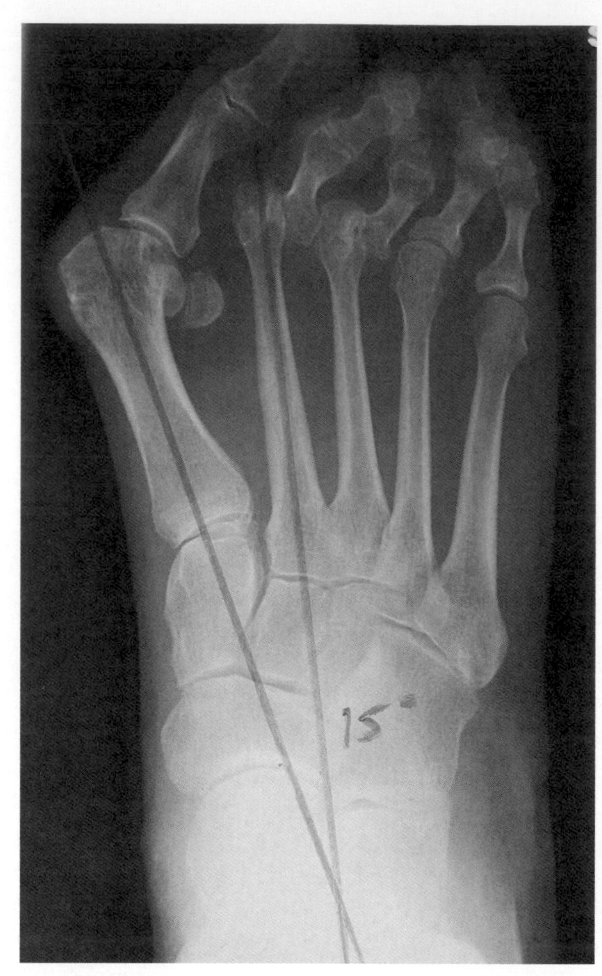

Figure 185-5 Intermetatarsal angle. Note the subluxation and deformity developing in the second and third metatarsophalangeal joints due to transfer metatarsalgia.

- Assess for arthrosis as well as congruence of the proximal phalanx to the metatarsal head.
- Advanced imaging usually not warranted

Additional Tests

- If vascular deficit is suspected, the ankle-brachial index and arterial toe pressures should be performed before surgical intervention.
- The presence of neuropathy should prompt further evaluation, particularly for diabetes.

Differential Diagnosis

- Hallux rigidus
- Interphalangeal hallux valgus
- Hallux varus
- Juvenile hallux valgus
- Inflammatory arthropathy (gout, pseudogout, psoriasis, rheumatoid arthritis)

Treatment

- At diagnosis
  - Conservative treatment is always the first option.
  - Goals include prevention of deformity progression, accommodation of the existing deformity, and redistribution of pressure from transfer lesions.
  - Essentially all hallux valgus deformities can be treated with a wide soft shoe that provides adequate room and sufficient insole padding.
  - Achilles stretching may help if contracture is present.
  - Orthotics provide symptomatic relief in some patients, including those with associated pes planus, and may include medial posting to control pronation, a metatarsal pad/bar for transfer lesions, a bunion flare, and an accommodative extra-depth shoe with an oblique toe box.
- Later
  - Surgical treatment is indicated in patients in whom conservative care has failed and who have realistic expectations of surgery. Surgical intervention must be individualized to each patient.

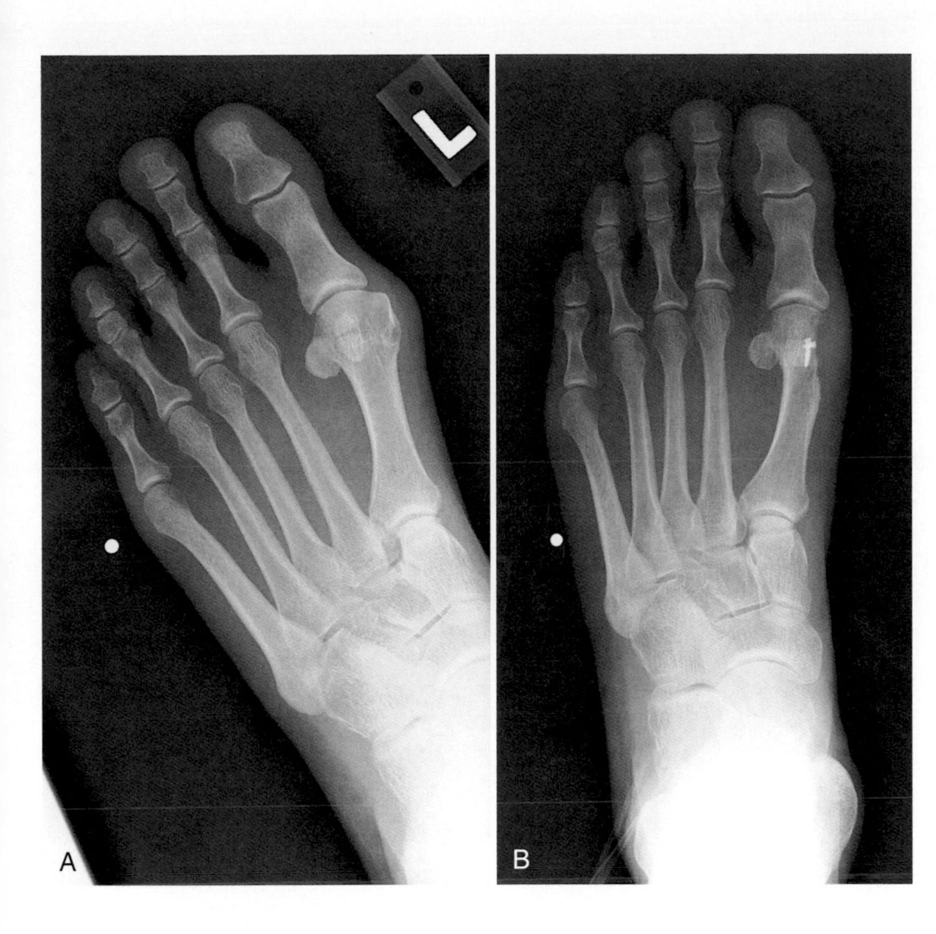

Figure 185-6 Preoperative (**A**) and postoperative (**B**) radiographs showing the most common distal metatarsal osteotomy used to correct mild hallux valgus deformities. Note the decrease in the medial metatarsal border, as well as the correction of the hallux valgus angle.

— Options include MTP soft-tissue reconstruction, distal or proximal first metatarsal osteotomy, cuneiform osteotomy, arthrodesis of the MTP or metatarsocuneiform joint, and excisional arthroplasty (Fig. 185-6).

— Risks of surgery include bleeding, infection, nonunion, recurrence, avascular necrosis, hallux varus, transfer metatarsalgia, neuromas (particularly the dorsomedial nerve), hyperesthesia, degenerative arthritis, and unfulfilled patient expectations.

When to Refer

- When patients fail conservative measures, referral should be made for possible surgical intervention.

Prognosis

- Excellent results have been reported, if the appropriate surgery is selected, to range from 75% to 90%.
  - Relief of pain is the major objective, but ability to wear smaller or narrower shoes is a frequent (often unstated) goal.
  - As many as 41% of patients are not able to return to desired shoe wear choices.
  - If transfer lesions are present before surgery, these should also be addressed. Alternatively, patients may still need cushioned shoes or insoles after surgery.

Patient Instructions

- Educate patients about the progressive nature of hallux valgus as well as treatment options and goals.
- Conservative options often improve symptoms and function.
- Although surgical treatments may have a successful clinical result, unrealistic expectations of future shoe wear and high-impact activity should be tempered.

Considerations in Special Populations

- Symptomatic hallux valgus is uncommon in pediatric patients.
- Surgical correction is associated with high rates of recurrence and variable clinical outcomes. Injury to the epiphysis may occur during surgery, resulting in growth disturbance.
- Most advocate delaying surgery until bony maturity unless an unusual degree of pain and deformity interferes with daily living.

Suggested Reading

- Canale PB, Aronsson DD, Lamont RL, et al: The Mitchell procedure for the treatment of adolescent hallux valgus: A long-term study. J Bone Joint Surg Am 1993;75A:1610–1618.
- Coughlin MJ: Juvenile bunions. In Mann RA, Coughlin MJ (eds): Surgery of the Foot and Ankle. St. Louis: Mosby, 1993, pp 297–339.
- Kato T, Watanabe S: The etiology of hallux valgus in Japan. Clin Orthop Relat Res 1981;157:78–81.
- Kilmartin TE, Barrington RL, Wallace WA: A controlled prospective trial of a foot orthosis for juvenile hallux valgus. J Bone Joint Surg Br 1994;76B:210–214.
- Klaue K, Hansen ST, Masquelet AC: Clinical, quantitative assessment of first tarsometatarsal mobility in the sagittal plane and its relation to hallux valgus deformity. Foot Ankle Int 1994;15:9–13.
- Mann RA, Rudicel S, Graves SC: Repair of hallux valgus with a distal soft-tissue procedure and proximal metatarsal osteotomy: A long-term follow-up. J Bone Joint Surg Am 1992;74A:124–129.
- Robinson AHN, Limbers JP: Modern concepts in the treatment of hallux valgus. J Bone Joint Surg Br 2005;87B:1038–1045.
- Sammarco V, Nichols R: Orthotic management for disorders of the hallux. Foot Ankle Clin 2005;10:191–209.
- Stephens MM: Pathogenesis of hallux valgus. Eur J Foot Ankle Surg 1994;1:7–10.

Chapter 186 Bunionette

Andrew Molloy and Edward V. Wood

ICD-9 CODE
727.1 *Bunionette*

Key Concepts

- A bunionette is a bony prominence of the fifth metatarsal, frequently associated with overlying bursitis and a corn.
- Common etiologies include
  - Idiopathic
  - Rheumatoid arthritis
  - Sporting activities (e.g., long-distance running, skiing)
  - Congenitally short, plantarflexed or dorsiflexed fifth metatarsal
  - Failure or incomplete development of the intermetatarsal ligament
  - Accessory ossicles on lateral side of fourth metatarsal
  - Potentially worse outcome in the presence of peripheral neuropathy (e.g., diabetes, Charcot-Marie-Tooth disease, spinal dysraphism)
- There are a variety of treatments including footwear and orthoses, chiropody, and surgery.
- The prognosis is good, with 90% or more success rates.

History

- Bunionettes are a common abnormality, but the majority are asymptomatic.
- Symptoms are most commonly present from adolescence to middle age.
- Pain around the fifth metatarsal head is most commonly lateral but may be dorsolateral or plantar; symptoms are exacerbated by constrictive footwear.
- May have difficulty purchasing footwear, especially if associated with hallux valgus or splaying of the foot
- Patients almost invariably report a history of a corn over the affected area.
- May be history of predisposing features: increased activity, other foot deformities, inflammatory arthropathy, altered sensation
- There may be a history of swelling, skin color changes, or even ulceration and infection. If either of the latter two is present, careful attention should be paid to the possibility of diabetes or an inflammatory arthropathy.

Physical Examination

- Observation
  - Gait
  - Obvious bony prominence of the fifth metatarsal head, often with an overlying hyperkeratotic area and possible surrounding erythema due to pressure from constrictive footwear (Fig. 186-1)
  - The size of the osseous protuberance may be exacerbated by the presence of an inflamed, hypertrophic bursa.
  - Observe for predisposing foot deformities: hallux valgus, intermetatarsal ligament laxity (splay foot), pes planovalgus, varus hindfoot, hallux rigidus
- Palpation
  - The plantar metatarsal head fat pads may be atrophied in diabetes, neuropathy, or inflammatory arthropathies (especially rheumatoid arthritis).
- Range of motion
  - Fifth metatarsophalangeal joint: emphasis on whether the joint is subluxed or dislocated
- Special tests
  - Careful examination for active or healed ulcers and signs of chronic infection
  - Careful neurovascular examination

Imaging

- Radiographs: weight-bearing anteroposterior (with 15-degree cephalic tilt), lateral, and oblique views (Figs. 186-2 and 186-3)

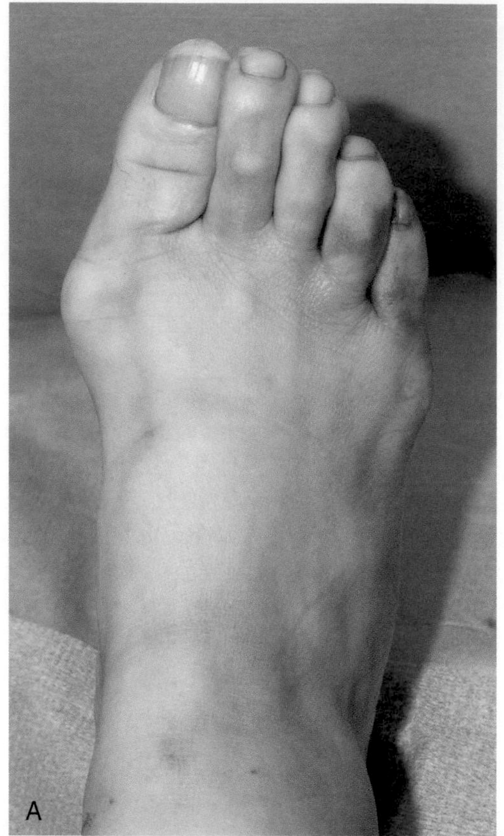

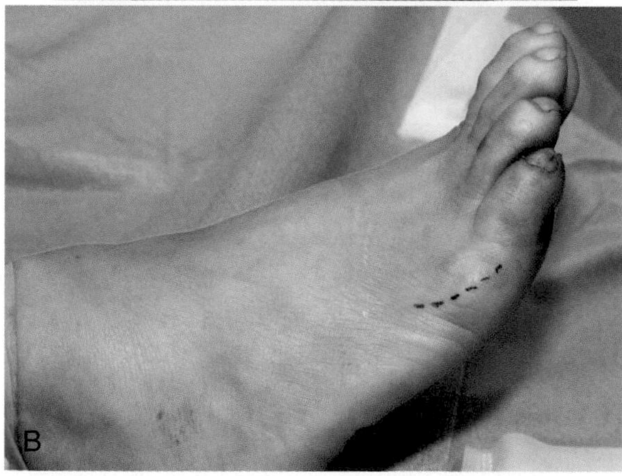

Figure 186-1 Clinical photographs of patient with hallux valgus with splaying of the foot (**A**) and symptomatic bunionette (**B**).

- The intermetatarsal angle between the fourth and fifth metatarsals averages more than 10 degrees in symptomatic patients (normal, <8 degrees).
- The fifth metatarsophalangeal angle averages more than 16 degrees in symptomatic patients (normal, <10 degrees).
- Lateral bowing of the fifth metatarsal averages 8 degrees in symptomatic patients (normal, <3 degrees).
- Bunionettes are classified into four types (Fig. 186-4).

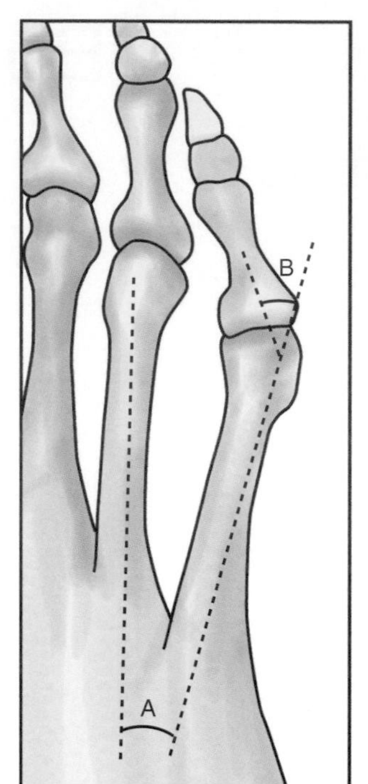

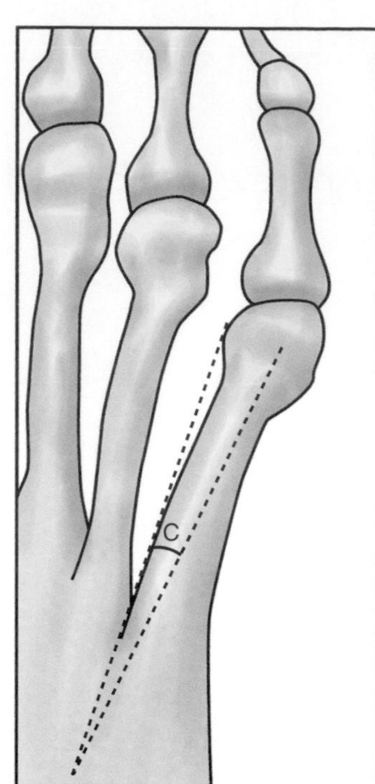

Figure 186-2 Schematic diagram depicting radiographic angular measurements in the assessment of a bunionette. A, Fourth-fifth intermetatarsal angle. B, Fifth metatarsophalangeal angle. C, Angle of lateral bowing of the fifth metatarsal.

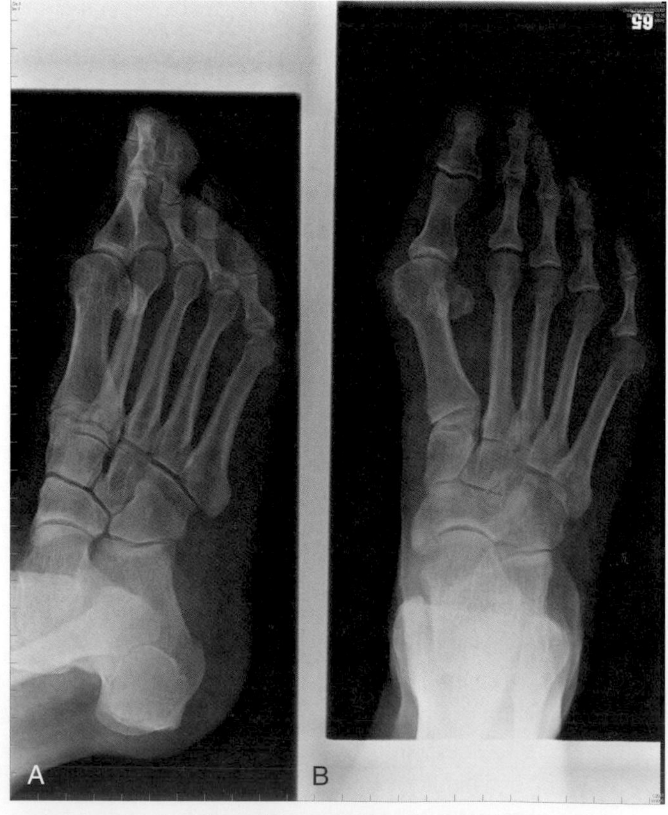

Figure 186-3 Oblique (**A**) and anteroposterior (**B**) radiographs of patient with bunionette and hallux valgus deformities with splaying of the foot.

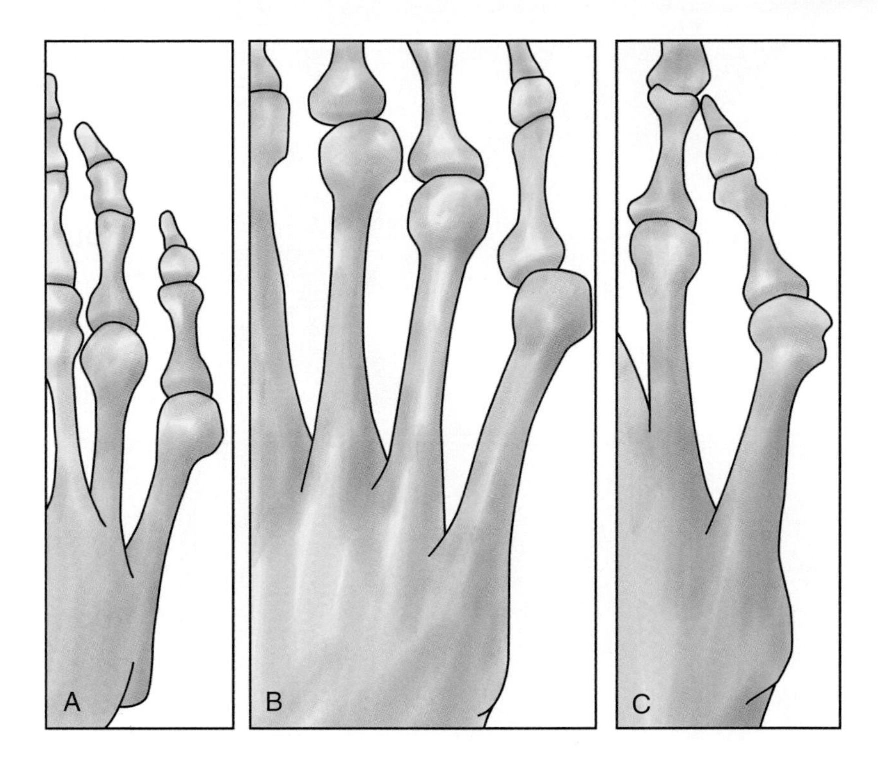

Figure 186-4 Bunionette classification. **A**, Type 1: enlargement of the lateral aspect of the fifth metatarsal head. **B**, Type 2: lateral bowing of the fifth metatarsal. **C**, Type 3: widened fourth-fifth intermetatarsal angle. Type 4 is a combination deformity.

- Magnetic resonance imaging
  - May be useful with gadolinium enhancement if chronic infection is suspected in the setting of previous ulceration (especially in diabetics)
- Bone scan
  - Only of use in rare cases of Charcot-Marie-Tooth disease to confirm presence of infection

Differential Diagnosis

- Malunited fracture of the fifth metatarsal shaft: history of trauma, sudden onset deformity, greater angular deformity
- Bone tumor: extremely rare, rapidly expanding lesion, nocturnal pain, systemic illness, history of other tumors

Treatment

- At diagnosis
  - Conservative management consists of footwear modifications and orthoses, chiropody, and anti-inflammatory drugs.
  - Footwear: wide, deep toe box, semirigid shoes without heels and accommodating insole designs (especially in rheumatoid arthritis, diabetes, peripheral neuropathy); padding of the bunionette may also be used as an adjunct
  - Orthoses: may include hindfoot corrective orthoses if the bunionette is a secondary pathology; midfoot and forefoot orthoses, such as metatarsal pads/bars, have limited success
  - Chiropody: Paring down of any hyperkeratotic lesions can provide symptomatic relief, and should be carried out with caution by experienced practitioners in diabetic patients with neurovascular compromise
  - Medications: Simple analgesics are first-line treatment in the majority of cases. Nonsteroidal anti-inflammatory drugs may lessen the duration of an exacerbation of an inflamed bursa. Disease-modifying agents are of benefit in rheumatoid arthritis patients.
- Later
  - Patients in whom conservative measures fail may benefit from surgical procedures. Options include exostectomy, head resection, and a variety of metatarsal osteotomies, including chevron osteotomy (Fig. 186-5). Patients may fully weight bear in a stiff-soled postoperative shoe immediately. They continue to wear the shoe for 6 weeks.

When to Refer

- Athletic patients in whom the deformity and symptoms are unacceptable to their activity level, patients at risk of skin breakdown and possible infection (e.g., those with neuropathic or rheumatoid conditions), and patients in whom conservative measures failed are appropriate for referral.

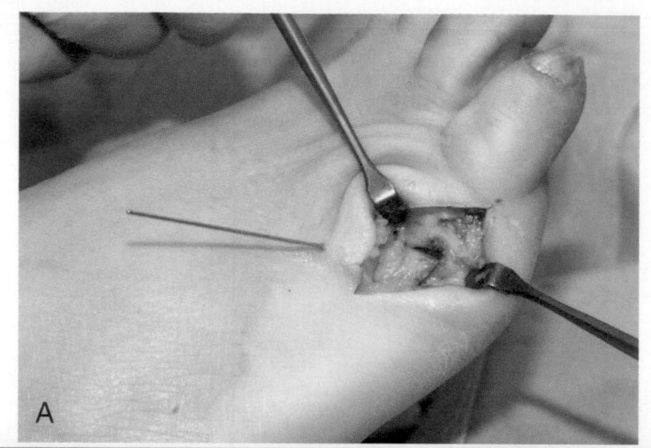

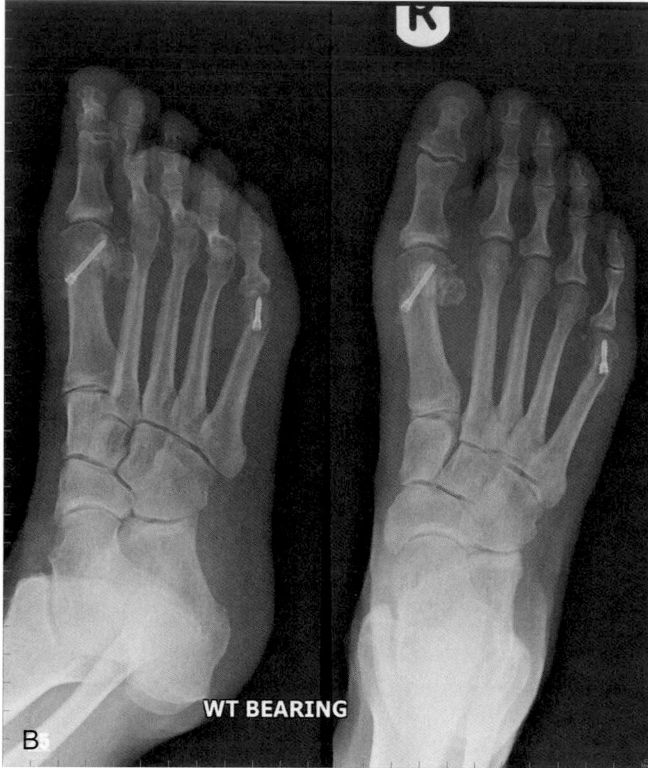

Figure 186-5 Chevron osteotomy. **A**, Intraoperative photograph showing displacement of the osteotomy held with guidewire. **B**, Radiographs 4 weeks postoperatively of a patient who underwent chevron osteotomies of her bunionette and hallux valgus deformities.

Prognosis

- Success rates of conservative treatment are difficult to quantify due to the large variety of patients who are affected by this condition. However, there is a good chance of success in the nonathletic patient with a bunionette of idiopathic origin.
- Surgical success rates vary from 63% to 90% or more depending on the technique. Complication rates depend on the patient cohort and vary from 0% to 15%.

Troubleshooting

- Initial treatment should include the wide range of conservative measures.
- Close attention should be paid to the state of the soft tissues in patients with rheumatoid arthritis, diabetes, and neuropathy of any cause.
- Patients should be referred for a surgical consult if conservative measures have failed or are unacceptable to the patient with continued symptoms.

Information for Patients

- A bunionette is a relatively common deformity that is most often idiopathic, but may be associated with other foot pathology or generalized systemic disease.
- There are many successful conservative therapies including footwear, in-shoe orthoses, chiropody, and medications.
- Modern surgeries have a high chance of excellent results. The complication rate depends on the general health of the patient.

Suggested Reading

- Baumhauer JF, DiGiovanni BF: Osteotomies of the fifth metatarsal. Foot Ankle Clin 2001;6:491–498.
- Coughlin MJ: Treatment of bunionette deformity with longitudinal diaphyseal osteotomy with distal soft tissue repair. Foot Ankle 1991;11:195–203.
- Diebold P: Basal osteotomy of the fifth metatarsal for the bunionette. Foot Ankle 1991;12:74–79.
- Karasick D: Preoperative assessment of symptomatic bunionette deformity: Radiologic findings. AJR Am J Roentgenol 1995; 164:147–149.
- Kitaoka HB, Holiday AD Jr, Campbell DC II: Distal chevron metatarsal osteotomy for bunionette. Foot Ankle 1991;12:80–85.
- Koti M, Maffulli N: Bunionette. J Bone Joint Surg Am 2001; 83A:1076–1082.
- Seide HW, Peterson W: Tailor's bunion: Results of scarf osteotomy for the correction of increased intermetatarsal IV/V angle. Arch Orthop Trauma Surg 2001;121:166–169.

Chapter 187 Hallux Rigidus

Ivan J. Antosh and Eric M. Bluman

ICD-9 CODE
735.2 *Hallux Rigidus*

Key Concepts

- Second most common pathology affecting the first metatarsophalangeal (MTP) joint
- Usually insidious in onset, but may also be posttraumatic
- The progression of arthrosis leads to proliferation of bone over the dorsal aspect of the metatarsal head and alteration of normal joint kinematics (Fig. 187-1).
- Marginal osteophytes restrict motion and lead to pain.
- Conservative interventions aim to provide space for the hypertrophied joint and restrict painful motion of the first MTP joint.
- Surgical interventions include débridement of the first MTP joint, cheilectomy (excision of osteophytes), interposition arthroplasty, prosthetic replacement, and arthrodesis.

History

- Localized pain over dorsum of first MTP joint
- Occasionally, more diffuse lateral forefoot pain secondary to offloading the affected first MTP joint
- Pain with forced dorsiflexion of the great toe, including the toe-off phase of gait
- Possible aggravating factors (e.g., shoe wear, repetitive activities) should be identified.
- Occurs in two populations: adolescents and adults aged 30 to 60 years of age
- The etiology is unknown, but there are multiple proposed mechanisms.
  - Acute: posttraumatic (turf toe, osteochondritis dissecans)
  - Chronic: repetitive microtrauma (running)
  - Congenital: length of first metatarsal, shape of metatarsal head and proximal phalanx, positive family history

Physical Examination

- Observation
  - Skin color: Localized erythema may indicate pressure points from shoe wear irritation over dorsal osteophytes.
  - Increased bulk of joint (Fig. 187-2): compare with the contralateral foot
  - Shoe wear: High-heeled shoes force the first MTP joint into hyperextension and exacerbate pain.
  - Gait: symptoms commonly reproduced during toe-off

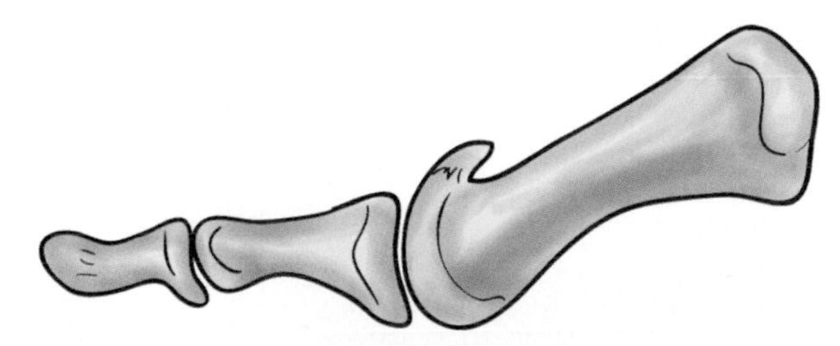

Figure 187-1 Drawing showing lateral view of the first metatarsophalangeal joint with dorsal osteophytes characteristic of hallux rigidus.

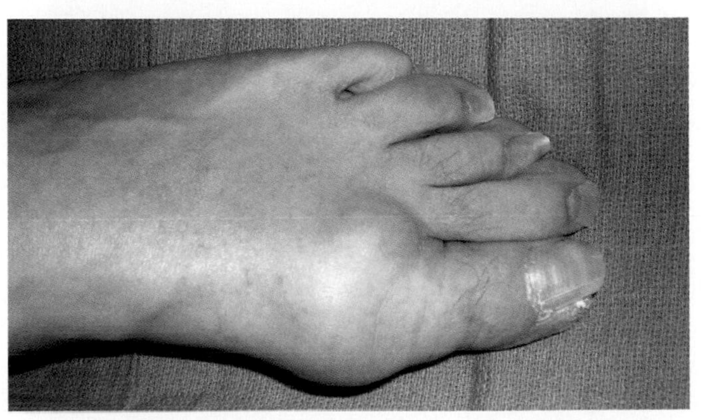

Figure 187-2 Thickening of tissues around the first metatarsophalangeal joint in a patient with severe hallux rigidus.

- Palpation
  - Bony prominence: dorsal with or without lateral osteophytes
  - Neuritic symptoms: dorsal medial cutaneous nerve sensitivity common
- Range of motion
  - Loss of dorsiflexion
  - Lateral deviation may elicit pain if lateral osteophyte is present.
  - Forced plantarflexion may irritate joint capsule and extensor hallucis longus as it passes over dorsal osteophytes.
  - Crepitus may be present in late stages with degenerative arthritis.
  - Interphalangeal joint motion should also be evaluated.
- Special tests
  - Compression of the dorsal cutaneous nerves over the dorsal aspect of the hallux may result in neuritic symptoms distally in the toe.

Imaging

- Radiographs: Ensure that images are centered on the MTP joint itself and not the foot.
  - Weight-bearing anteroposterior view: to evaluate for the presence of lateral osteophytes (Fig. 187-3)
  - Weight-bearing lateral view: to evaluate for dorsal osteophytes (Fig. 187-4)
  - Oblique view: to quantify amount of joint space narrowing

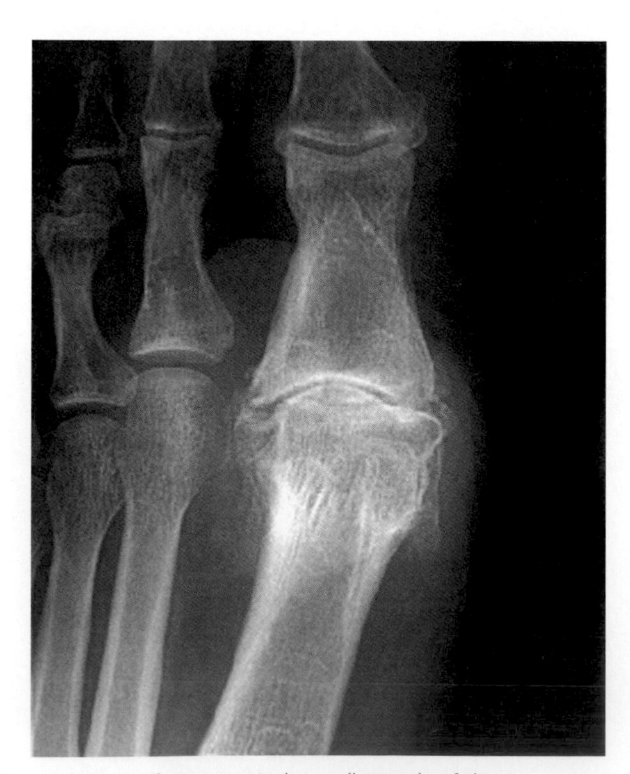

Figure 187-3 Anteroposterior radiograph of the metatarsophalangeal joint with severe hallux rigidus.

Differential Diagnosis

- First MTP joint infection
- Rheumatoid arthritis
- Seronegative spondyloarthropathies
- Gout: uric acid crystals in joint aspirate
- Pseudogout: calcium pyrophosphate crystals in joint aspirate
- Sesamoiditis
- Turf toe: acute injury
- Hallux valgus

Treatment

- At diagnosis
  - Conservative management is appropriate on initial evaluation.
  - Goals include providing adequate space to accommodate the increased joint size, minimizing painful joint motion, and decreasing inflammation in and around the joint.
  - Avoid aggravating shoe wear (high heels) and activities.
  - Convert to shoe wear with a wide toe box and sufficient depth to accommodate the increased joint size.
  - Rigid rocker sole or rigid orthotic with Morton's extension to decrease motion at the first MTP joint (Fig. 187-5)
  - Nonsteroidal anti-inflammatory drugs
  - Corticosteroid injection: diagnostic and therapeutic

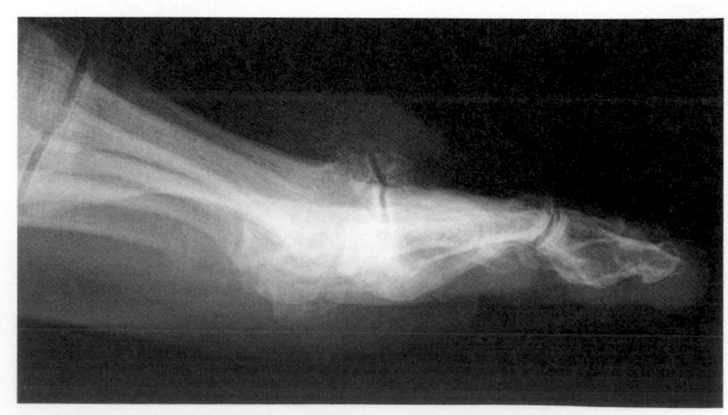

Figure 187-4 Lateral radiograph of the metatarsophalangeal joint with severe hallux rigidus.

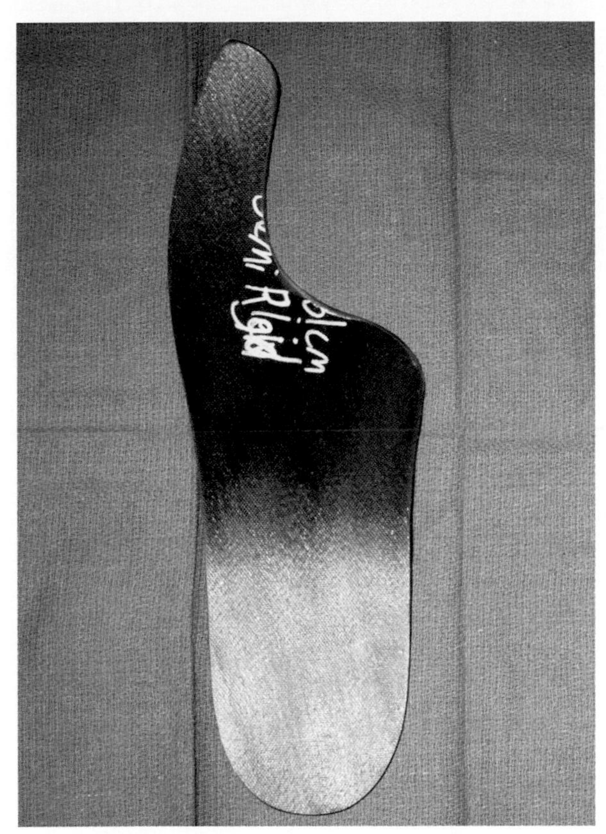

Figure 187-5 Carbon fiber insert with Morton's extension limits the amount of flexion at the first metatarsophalangeal joint.

- Later
  - A number of surgical interventions are available for patients in whom conservative measures fail, depending on the extent of the disease, age, activity level, and expectations of the patient.
    - — Cheilectomy: mild to moderate symptoms and restricted motion or persistent ulcers overlying the dorsal osteophytes; involves surgical resection of the dorsal osteophytes to decrease pain and improve motion
    - — First MTP joint arthrodesis: more severe degenerative joint disease, large osteophytes, and a desire to remain active (Fig. 187-6); although typically very effective for pain relief, arthrodesis is still considered a salvage procedure as it will eliminate motion at the joint and preclude the use of other treatment modalities
    - — Other surgical interventions include interposition arthroplasty, silicone arthroplasty, nonsilicone prosthetic replacement, and osteotomies of both the metatarsal and proximal phalanges.

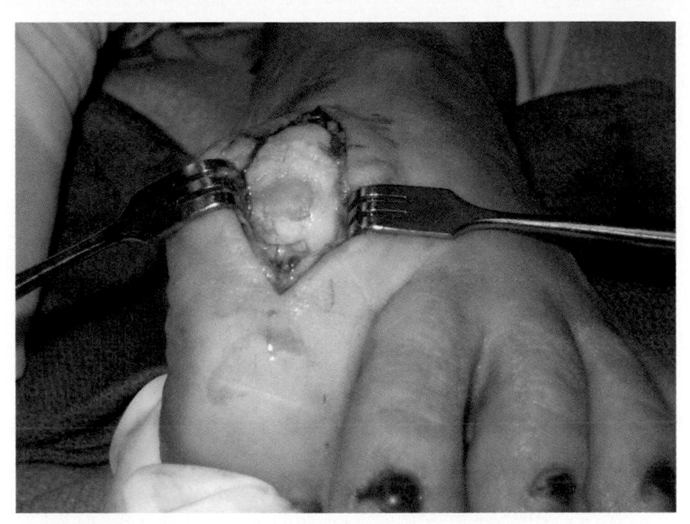

Figure 187-6 Intraoperative image showing loss of metatarsal articular cartilage in advanced hallux rigidus.

When to Refer

- All patients should undergo an initial trial of conservative therapy as many will improve with this intervention alone.
- Patients who have persistent symptoms after 6 months of conservative treatment are candidates for referral for surgical intervention.

Prognosis

- Hallux rigidus is a progressive degenerative disease.
  - Nonoperative therapies are aimed at slowing progression and relieving pain.
  - Once conservative therapies are exhausted, operative therapy is considered.
  - Good to excellent results can be expected in patients with mild to moderate pain and restricted motion who undergo cheilectomy.
  - Patients with advanced degenerative joint disease and more severe symptoms do not have such predictably favorable outcomes. Arthrodesis will generally provide reliable pain relief and allow a return to most activities in these patients.

Troubleshooting

- Patients treated conservatively should be educated regarding the progressive nature of the disease and the goal of slowing disease progression rather than halting it. Surgery should only be discussed after an adequate trial of conservative treatment.
- Patients should be extensively counseled on the benefits and risks of surgery.

- Benefits include elimination of pain, improved range of motion (except arthrodesis), and return to activities.
- Operative risks include bleeding, infection, persistent pain, postoperative neuritis, scarring of the extensor hallucis longus tendon, and hypertrophic dorsal scar. Risks specific to cheilectomy include recurrence of osteophytes and theoretical risk of accelerated joint degeneration. Risks specific to arthrodesis include failure of fusion and painful hardware.

Patient Instructions

- Nonoperative treatment of hallux rigidus may include activity modification, ice, shoe modifications, orthotics, medications, and injections in the joint. Multiple treatment methods may need to be combined.

Suggested Reading

- Coughlin M: Arthritides. In Coughlin M, Mann R (eds): Surgery of the Foot and Ankle, 7th ed. St. Louis: Mosby, 1999, pp 605–650.
- Coughlin M, Shurnas P: Hallux rigidus: Demographics, etiology, and radiographic assessment. Foot Ankle Int 2003;24:731–743.
- Coughlin M, Shurnas P: Hallux rigidus: Grading and long-term results of operative treatment. J Bone Joint Surg Am 2003; 85A:2072–2088.
- Coughlin M, Shurnas P: Hallux rigidus: Surgical techniques (cheilectomy and arthrodesis). J Bone Joint Surg Am 2004; 86A:119–130.
- Jack E: The aetiology of hallux rigidus. Br J Surg 1940; 27:492–497.
- Mann R: Disorders of the first metatarsophalangeal joint. J Am Acad Orthop Surg 1995;3:34–43.
- Mann R, Coughlin M, DuVries H: Hallux rigidus: A review of the literature and a method of treatment. Clin Orthop Relat Res 1979;142:57–63.
- McMaster M: The pathogenesis of hallux rigidus. J Bone Joint Surg Br 1978;60B:82–87.

Chapter 188 Turf Toe

Medardo R. Maroto, Daniel K. Park, and Simon Lee

ICD-9 CODES
845.12 *Sprain, Metatarsal Phalangeal Joint*
838.05 *Dislocation, Metatarsal Phalangeal Joint*

Key Concepts

- The great toe metatarsophalangeal (MTP) joint is important in gait, push-off, forward drive, running, jumping, and crouching.
- MTP stability is created by the surrounding capsuloligamentous (CL) complex, including the joint capsule, plantar plate, flexor hallucis brevis and sesamoids, and collateral ligaments (Fig. 188-1).

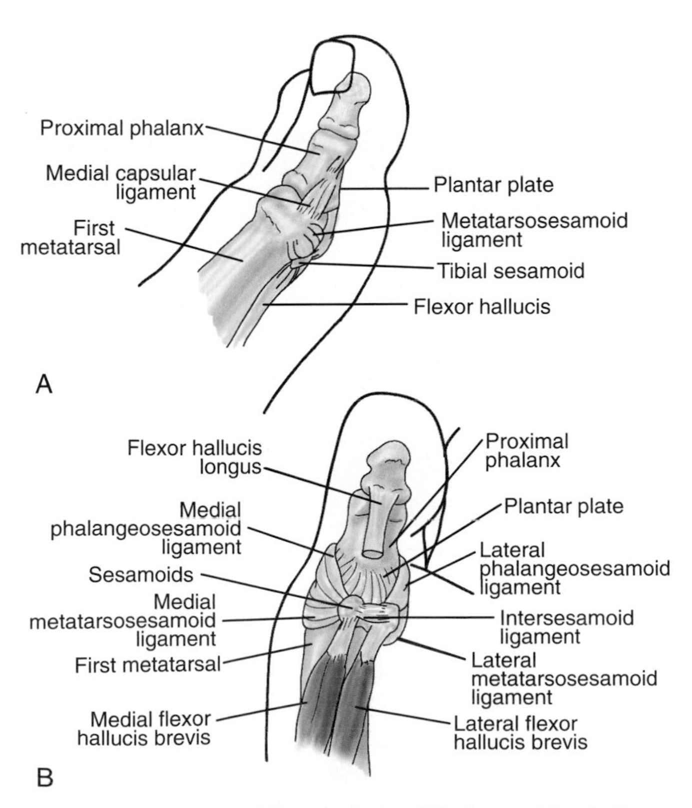

Figure 188-1 Lateral (**A**) and plantar (**B**) views of the hallux metatarsophalangeal joint showing the capsuloligamentous complex.

- Turf toe, in its strictest definition, is a hyperextension injury to the hallux MTP joint. However, the term has been used for any injury to the hallux MTP joint and represents a spectrum of injuries from mild to severe.
- Turf toe primarily occurs in athletes, particularly football players, and is associated with the increased use of flexible shoe wear and increased traction on artificial turf.
- The injury can be debilitating in athletes who need to perform rapid acceleration and cutting maneuvers.
- Most cases are treated nonoperatively; surgery is rarely required.

History

- Acute injury
  - Hyperextension injury of the great toe MTP joint with axial loading of the heel and plantarflexed forefoot (Fig. 188-2)
  - Limp or inability to bear weight
  - Pain and swelling around the MTP joint, primarily on the plantar surface
  - May also result in flexor hallucis brevis tendon rupture, tibial sesamoid fracture, or metatarsal dorsal articular injury (Fig. 188-3)
- Chronic injury
  - Difficulty with push-off activities: accelerating, jumping, and running

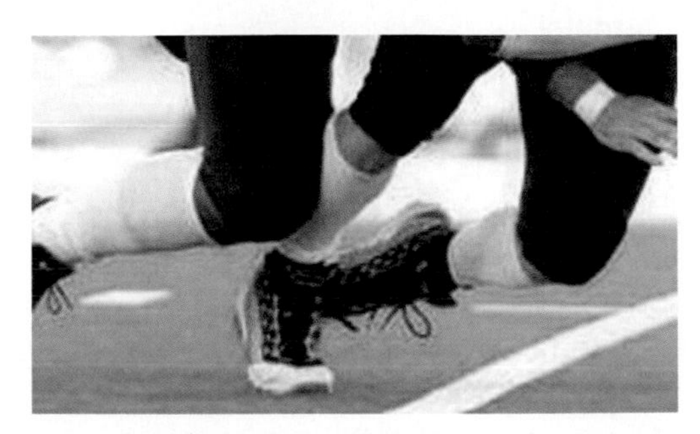

Figure 188-2 Typical turf toe injury mechanism: hyperextension and axial loading.

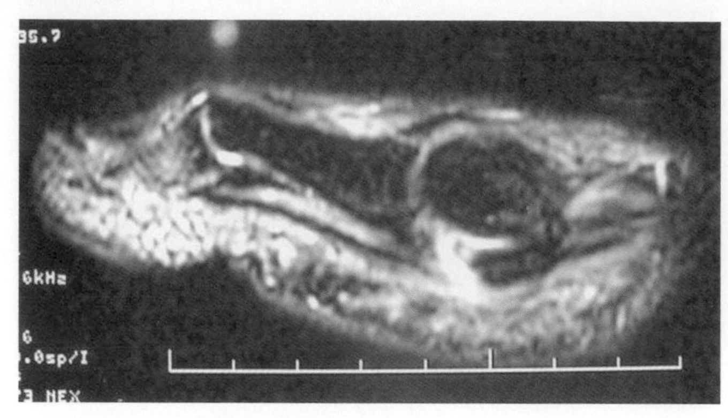

Figure 188-3 Magnetic resonance imaging showing rupture of the plantar complex, edema in the flexor hallucis longus tendon, and proximal migration of the tibial sesamoid.

Physical Examination

- Observation
  - Erythema, ecchymosis, and swelling of the MTP joint
- Palpation
  - Dorsal and plantar tenderness
- Range of motion
  - Stiff MTP joint (normal is 30 degrees of flexion, 80 degrees of extension)
  - Pain on MTP extension
- Special tests
  - Lachman's test of the hallux MTP joint (Fig. 188-4)
  - Injury grading scale
    - — Grade 1: stretching or minor tearing of CL complex; minimal pain, swelling, and restricted motion; able to bear weight and return to play
    - — Grade 2: partial tear of CL complex; moderate pain, swelling, and restricted motion; can bear weight, but with a limp
    - — Grade 3: complete tear of CL complex with plantar plate avulsion from the metatarsal neck; severe injuries may show a tibial sesamoid fracture or a dorsal impaction injury of the metatarsal articular surface; severe pain, swelling, and loss of motion; usually unable to bear weight

Imaging

- Radiographs: anteroposterior, lateral, and oblique views of the foot
  - Usually only show soft-tissue swelling
  - May see proximal/distal migration or fracture of the sesamoids (Fig. 188-5)

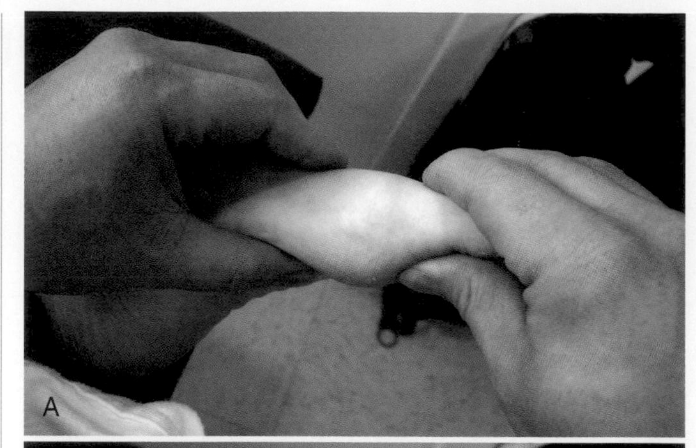

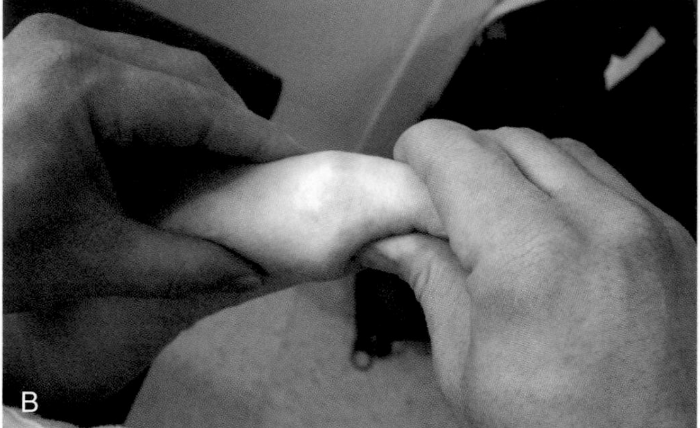

Figure 188-4 **A**, Lachman's test of the hallux metatarsophalangeal joint held in a neutral position. **B**, Lachman's test showing plantar instability with superior stressing of the phalanx while stabilizing the metatarsal with the opposite hand.

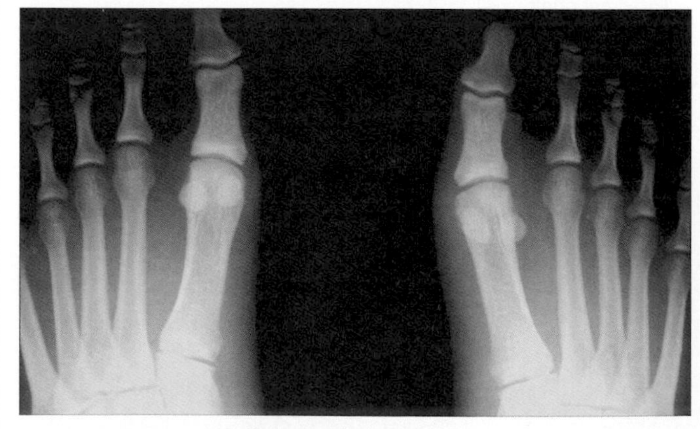

Figure 188-5 Radiograph demonstrating proximal migration of the sesamoids on the right foot.

  - Bilateral forced (stress) dorsiflexion lateral views may assist in determining migration of the sesamoids, indicating plantar plate rupture or sesamoid diastasis (Fig. 188-6).
- Magnetic resonance imaging
  - Recommended for grade 2 and 3 injuries
  - Evaluates degree of soft-tissue injury and possible articular damage

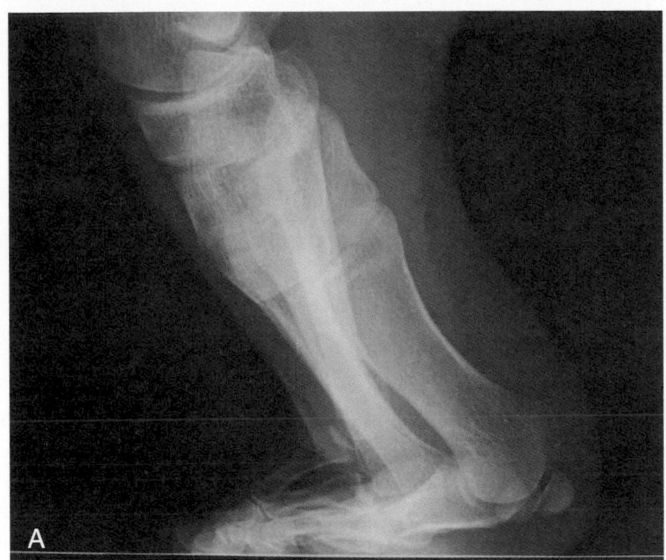

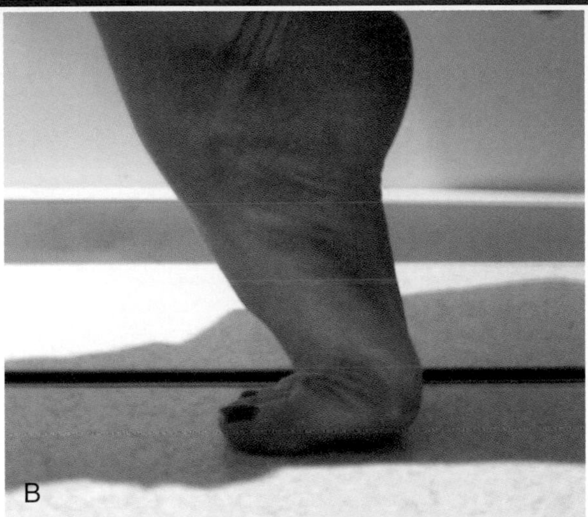

Figure 188-6 **A**, Forced dorsiflexion lateral radiograph showing distal migration of the sesamoids. **B**, Clinical photograph demonstrating this position.

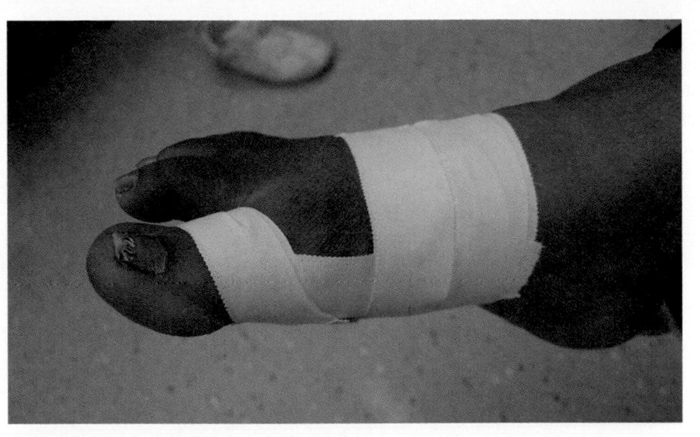

Figure 188-7 Taping procedure for turf toe injury to allow hallux interphalangeal motion but limit metatarsophalangeal dorsiflexion.

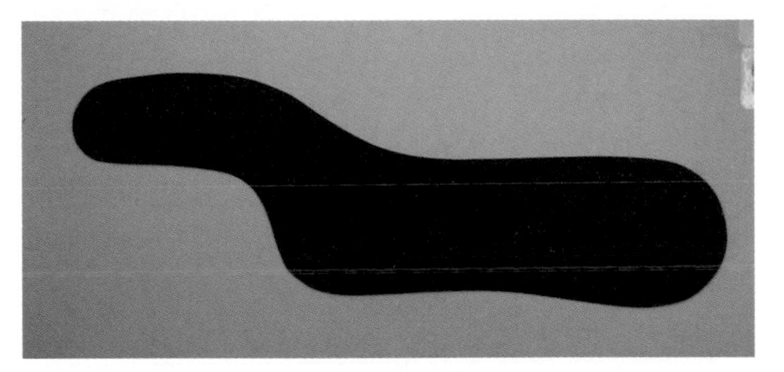

Figure 188-8 Rigid insole to prevent metatarsophalangeal hyperextension.

Differential Diagnosis

- Fracture of the great toe metatarsal or phalanges
- Hallux rigidus

Treatment

- At diagnosis
  - Conservative management includes rest, ice, compression, and elevation (RICE); anti-inflammatory drugs; and possibly a boot or cast. Turf toe taping provides compression and restricts MTP extension (Fig. 188-7). Taping should not cross the interphalangeal joint. Cortisone and lidocaine injections are contraindicated and may exacerbate chronic turf toe.
    - — Grade 1: RICE, taping, stiff-sole shoe, return to play per pain level
    - — Grade 2: as for grade 1 plus 2 weeks of rest (weight bearing as tolerated)
    - — Grade 3: as for grade 1 plus 4 weeks of rest (nonweight bearing)
- Later
  - Return to play is indicated when swelling subsides and painless extension of the MTP joint to 60 degrees (or symmetrical with the opposite side) is achieved. A rigid insole will allow earlier return by limiting motion (Fig. 188-8). Operative indications include a large capsular tear, unstable MTP joint, loose body, traumatic bunion, and sesamoid fracture or proximal migration.

When to Refer

- Referral is indicated if the clinical course does not proceed as expected or there is evidence of significant injury with instability on initial presentation.

Prognosis

- The prognosis is good. Most turf toe injuries are minor and heal with appropriate care without any functional limitations.

Patient Instructions

- Follow-up in a timely manner from the initial injury will allow more rapid diagnosis and initiation of treatment, allowing earlier return to athletic activity.

Suggested Reading

- Clanton TO, Ford JJ: Turf toe injury. Clin Sports Med 1994;13:731–741.
- Mullen JE, O'Malley MJ: Sprains—residual instability of subtalar, Lisfranc, and turf toe. Clin Sports Med 2004;23:97–121.
- Sammarco GJ: Turf toe. Instr Course Lect 1993;42:207–212.

Chapter 189 Sesamoid Disorders of the Hallux

Josef K. Eichinger and Eric M. Bluman

ICD-9 CODES

715.7 *Localized Osteoarthropathy, Idiopathic, Ankle and Foot*

905.4 *Late Effect of Fracture of Lower Extremities*

Key Concepts

- Hallucal sesamoids are an important part of normal static and dynamic foot mechanics.
- The sesamoid complex transmits 50% body weight with stationary weight bearing and as much as 300% during active push-off. These high stresses result in injury and difficulties in healing.
- Stress fractures are the most common injury, occurring frequently in individuals who experience repetitive loading, such as runners and dancers.
- Ten percent of individuals have a bipartite medial sesamoid, which is a normal anatomic variant. In 25% of these individuals, the condition is bilateral. Bipartite lateral sesamoids are rare.
- Treatment involves accurate diagnosis, initial conservative treatment, and surgical intervention in those with refractory symptoms.
- *Sesamoiditis* is a term sometimes used as a diagnosis of exclusion. This condition does not have a clear pathology associated with it and may actually represent chondromalacia or an osteochondral lesion.

History

- Insidious onset of generalized pain about the metatarsophalangeal (MTP) joint with weight bearing, usually concentrated on the plantar aspect
- Acute injury less common
- Increased pain with MTP dorsiflexion
- May walk on lateral border of the foot
- Neuritic symptoms may be described on the plantar aspect of the hallux if swelling results in compression of the plantar nerves.
- Inquire about previous foot surgery.

Physical Examination

- Observation
  - Erythema and swelling
  - Callus formation
  - Standing foot position: The patient may walk on the lateral column of the foot to avoid pressure on the sesamoids. Cavus foot is associated with first ray plantarflexion and resultant increased pressure on the sesamoids.
  - Hallux alignment: Valgus or varus may gradually develop if the medial or lateral sesamoid is fractured or resected, respectively.
- Palpation
  - Focal tenderness: challenging due to close proximity of the sesamoids to each other and other structures that may generate pain (Fig. 189-1).
  - Tinel's sign may be elicited if there is plantar digital nerve compression.
  - Subhallucal sesamoids are located at the plantar interphalangeal joint and may be associated with plantar keratosis (Fig. 189-2).

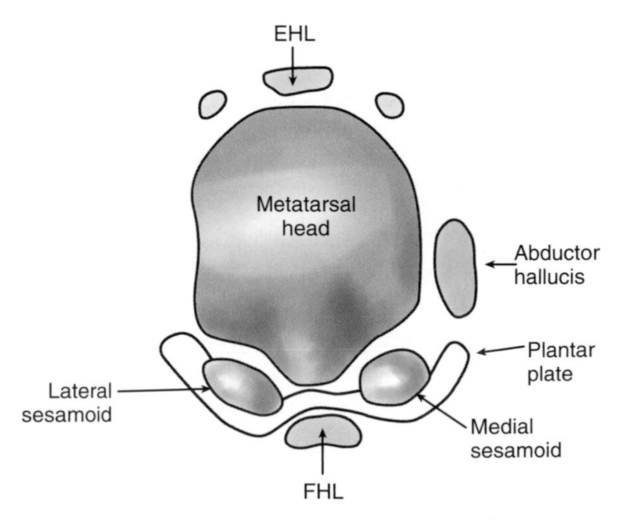

Figure 189-1 Cross section at the level of the first metatarsophalangeal (MTP) joint indicating structures that may be involved in first MTP joint pain. EHL, extensor hallucis longus; FHL, flexor hallucis longus.

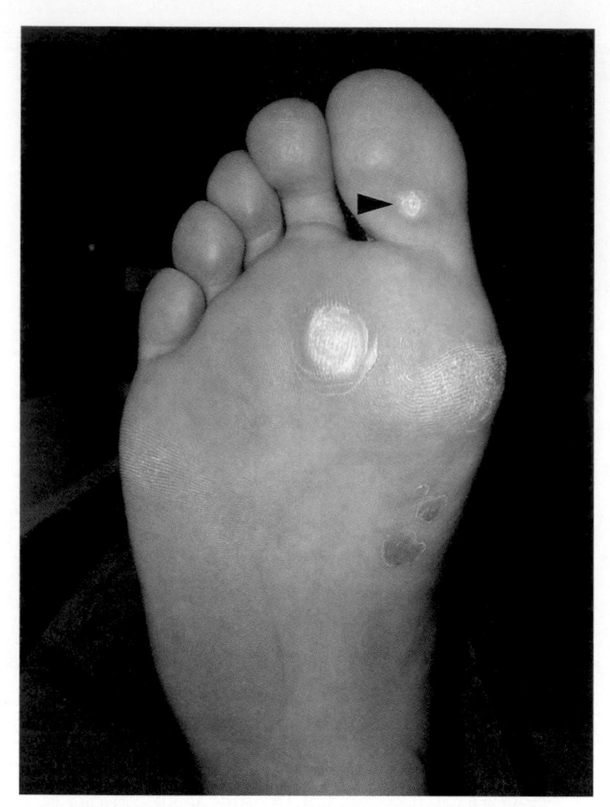

Figure 189-2 Plantar keratosis caused by subhallucal sesamoid (*arrowhead*).

- Range of motion
  - Increased pain with dorsiflexion, relieved with plantarflexion
  - Effusion may restrict MTP joint motion.
  - Pain on resisted hallux interphalangeal joint flexion suggests flexor hallucis longus paratenonitis.

Imaging

- Radiographs: anteroposterior, lateral, and oblique views of the foot (centered on the MTP joint) and axial view of the sesamoids
  - Evaluate for bony deformity of the first metatarsal.
  - Evaluate for arthrosis of the first MTP joint.
  - An axial view aids in evaluation of osteonecrosis, degenerative joint disease of the sesamoids, and plantar exostoses (Fig. 189-3).
  - Evaluate for fractures and bipartite sesamoids (Fig. 189-4).
  - Proximal retraction of the sesamoids may be seen with a severe turf toe injury.
- Bone scan
  - To distinguish between acute fracture and bipartite sesamoid (Fig. 189-5)
  - May aid in distinguishing between osteonecrosis and sesamoiditis

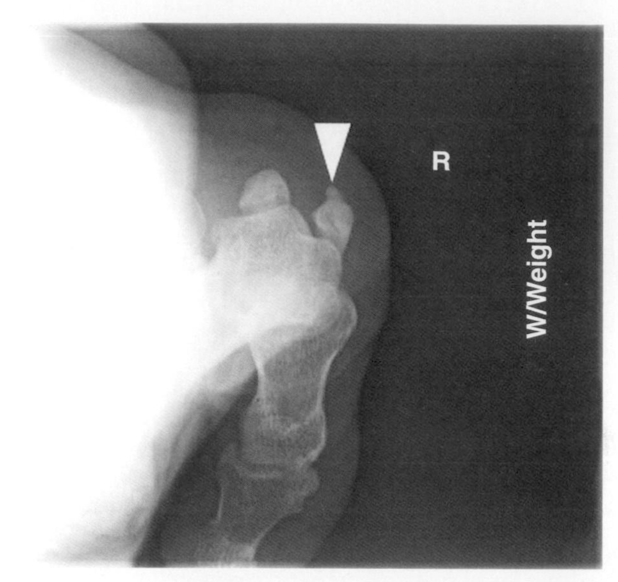

Figure 189-3 Axial radiograph with plantar exostosis of medial sesamoid (*arrowhead*).

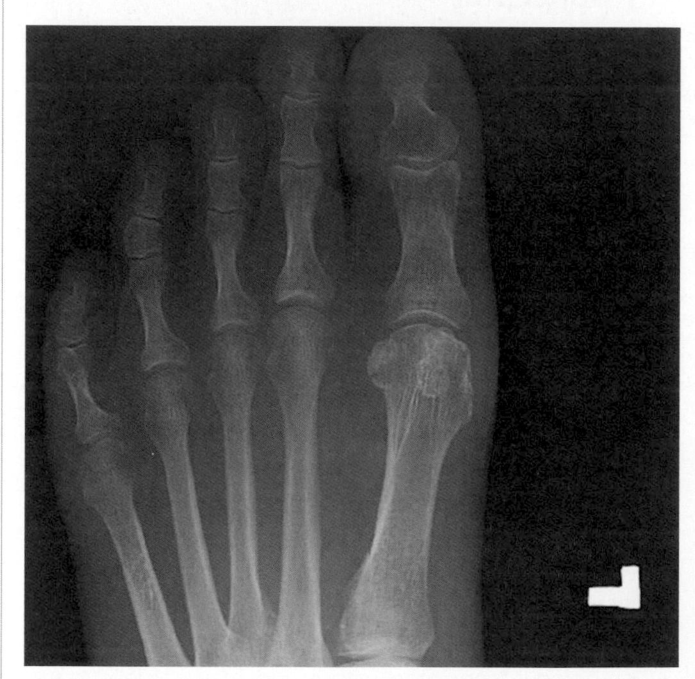

Figure 189-4 Fracture of lateral sesamoid with bipartite medial sesamoid.

- Magnetic resonance imaging
  - Valuable in evaluation of soft-tissue structures such as plantar plate, cartilage, nerves, and flexor tendons
  - May be a useful adjunct in the workup of osteomyelitis, fracture, and tendinitis

Differential Diagnosis

- Acute fracture or stress fracture
- Turf toe
- Osteonecrosis

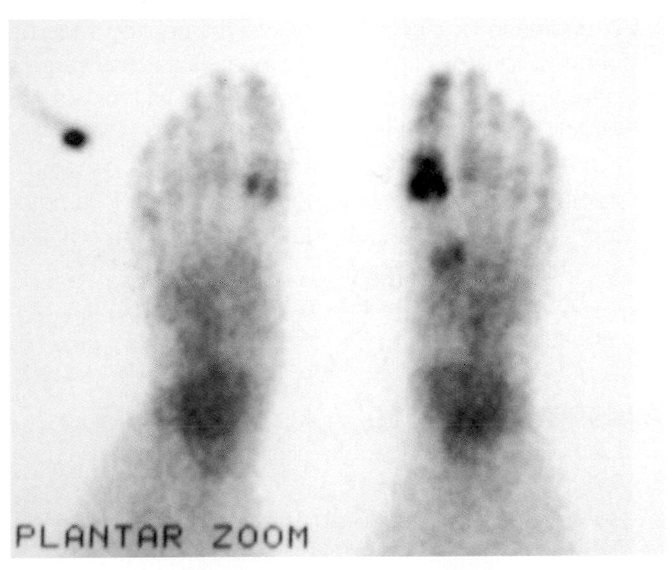

Figure 189-5 Bone scan indicating medial and lateral sesamoid fractures on the right. Compare with normal sesamoids on the left.

- Digital nerve compression/neuroma
- Arthrosis of the first MTP joint or sesamoid-metatarsal joint
- Subluxation of hallucal sesamoids
- Plantar keratosis
- Osteomyelitis
- Flexor hallucis longus paratenonitis

Treatment

- At diagnosis
  - Conservative treatment should be attempted initially for all sesamoid disorders except fractures displaced more than 2 mm. Conservative treatment aims to reduce pressure and stress on the sesamoid complex to allow bony healing and/or resolution of inflammation.
    - — Activity modification
    - — Shoe wear modifications and orthotics: shoe insert with cutout below sesamoids, rocker bottom, metatarsal bar/pad, avoid high heels
    - — Shaving of plantar keratoses
    - — Taping to block dorsiflexion of MTP joint
    - — Nonsteroidal anti-inflammatory drugs for non-fracture pathology
- Later
  - More intensive conservative treatments can be used if initial attempts are unsuccessful and include corticosteroid injections (except in osteonecrosis and fractures) and casting/non-weight bearing for 6 to 8 weeks. Extend cast out past the great toe to prevent unintended motion at the MTP joint.

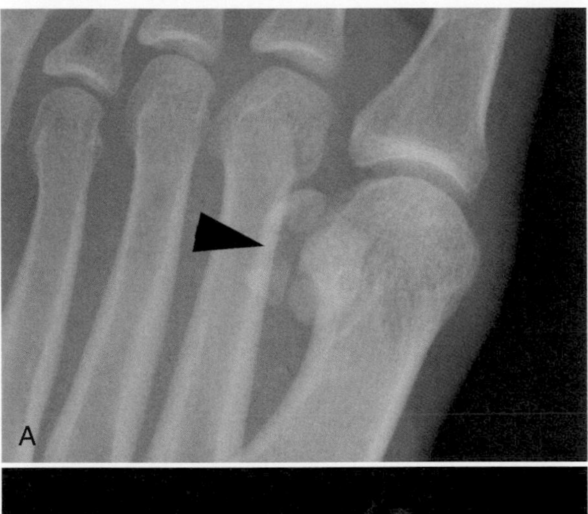

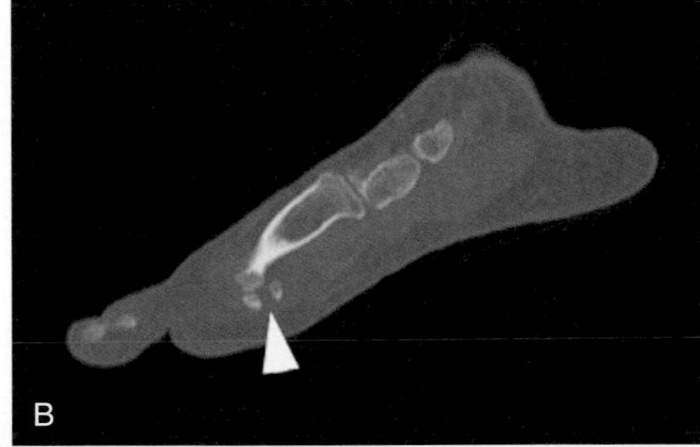

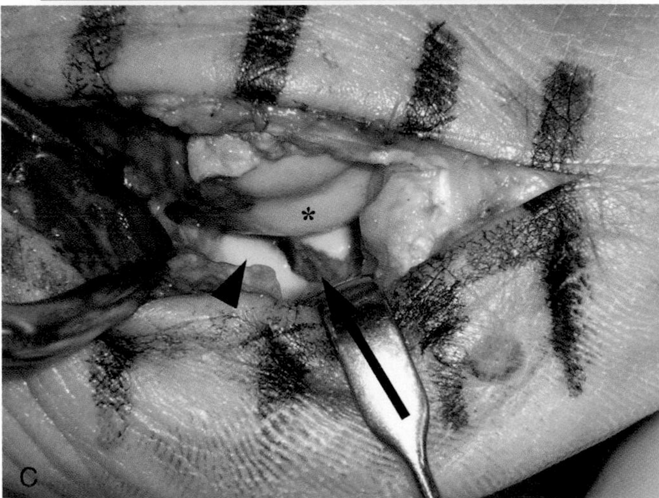

Figure 189-6 **A**, Oblique radiograph demonstrating fractured lateral sesamoid with significant displacement. **B**, Sagittal computed tomography reconstruction image. **C**, Intraoperative photograph. Plantar surface of metatarsal head (*asterisk*), distal fragment of fractured lateral sesamoid (*arrow*), articular surface of proximal fragment (*arrowhead*).

When to Refer

- Immediate consultation for potential surgical treatment is recommended for fractures displaced more than 2 mm (Fig. 189-6).

- Chronic conditions treated unsuccessfully for more than 3 to 6 months with appropriate conservative measures should also be referred.
  - Surgical options include bone grafting, shaving of prominences, and excision.
  - Patients with associated hallux varus/valgus or arthrosis of the first MTP joint may benefit from realignment or fusion surgery.

Prognosis

- Prognosis for the majority of sesamoid disorders is excellent with appropriate conservative measures.

Troubleshooting

- Fractures with more than 2 mm displacement will not heal with conservative means.
- These patients should be referred to an orthopaedic surgeon on initial presentation.
- Treatment usually consists of excision of the fractured sesamoid as results are comparable to those of open reduction and internal fixation.

Patient Instructions

- Conservative treatments aim to provide pain relief and immobilization of the hallucal sesamoid complex.
- A decrease or elimination of weight bearing may be needed to allow the injury to heal. This may require orthotics, taping, or cast immobilization with or without crutch weight bearing.
- If the patient has been diagnosed with a sesamoid fracture or osteonecrosis, nonsteroidal anti-inflammatory medications should not be taken without first consulting the physician.
- If conservative measures fail, surgery may be required.

Suggested Reading

- Axe MJ, Ray RL: Orthotic treatment of sesamoid pain. Am J Sports Med 1998;16:411–416.
- Biedert R, Hintermann B: Stress fractures of the medial great toe sesamoids in athletes. Foot Ankle Int 2003;24:137–141.
- Coughlin MJ: Sesamoid pain: Causes and surgical treatment. Instr Course Lect 1990;39:23–35.
- Dedmond BT, Cory JW, McBryde A: The hallucal sesamoid complex. J Am Acad Orthop Surg 2006;14:745–753.
- Richardson EG: Hallucal sesamoid pain: Causes and surgical treatment. J Am Acad Orthop Surg 1999;7:270–278.
- Richardson EG: Injuries to the hallucal sesamoids in the athlete. Foot Ankle 1987;7:229–244.

Chapter 190 Corns and Calluses

Norman Espinosa and Gerardo Juan Maquieira

ICD-9 CODE
700.0 *Corns and Callosities*

Key Concepts

- Corns and calluses are an accumulation of keratotic layers of epidermis as a response to excessive pressure exerted over a bony prominence.
- Loss of the normal fat pad, improper shoe wear, toe deformities, and systemic diseases (rheumatoid arthritis) may contribute to the development of corns and calluses.
- Callus refers to a large lesion with vague boundaries and no central core.
- Corn refers to a smaller focal lesion with well-defined boundaries and a central core. Corns are divided into hard and soft corns.
- A cleavage plane may develop in larger corns making them prone to secondary infection.
- Surgery is rarely indicated.
- Nonoperative treatment consists of modifying shoe wear and trimming the calluses and corns. Patient education is also important.
- Corns and calluses have a tendency to recur unless the underlying pathology is properly addressed.

History

- Discomfort in normal shoe wear or when walking barefoot (advanced corn)
- Inquire about a history of Charcot-Marie-Tooth disease, previous compartment syndrome, or systemic disease (rheumatoid arthritis) as these can be causes for the toe deformities associated with corns and calluses.

Physical Examination

- Observation (Fig. 190-1)
  - Calluses are typically located on the plantar aspect of foot.
  - Hard corns are typically found on the fibular aspect of the fifth toe or dorsal aspect of the proximal interphalangeal or the distal interphalangeal joints.
    - — Sometimes associated with hammer toe, mallet toe, or claw toe deformity
    - — Hyperkeratotic area with a lighter conical center (without vessels)

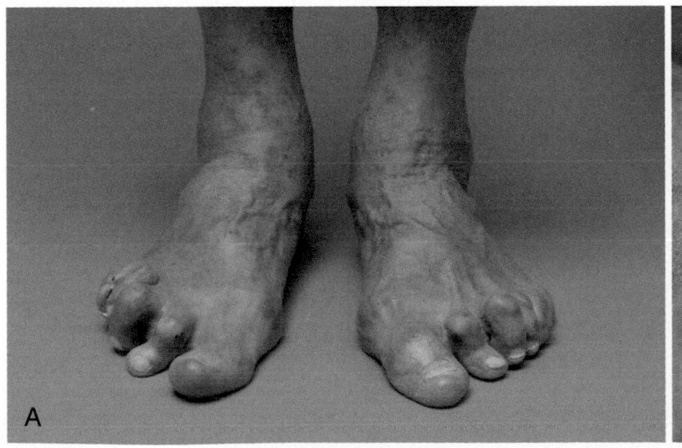

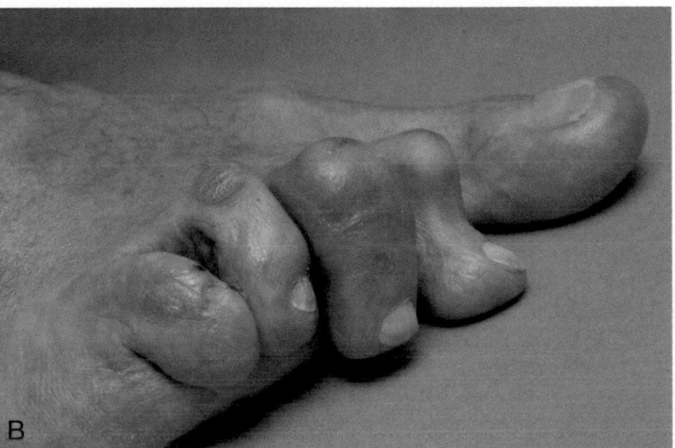

Figure 190-1 **A**, Clinical photograph of the feet of a patient with multiple calluses over his toes. **B**, Close-up view of the toe deformities that are a cause of corn and callus formation.

- Soft corns present as a maceration between the lesser toes.
  - — Manifest as medial lesion overlying the condyle of the proximal phalanx
  - — Sometimes reddish appearance
- Palpation
  - Hard and soft corns eventually tender

Imaging

- Usually not necessary; clinical diagnosis
- Radiographs: weight-bearing anteroposterior and lateral views of the foot
  - Sometimes helpful in identifying osteomyelitis in the case of an ulcerated lesion
  - Osseous changes are rarely found as the cause of corns and calluses.

Differential Diagnosis

- Plantar warts: fine capillaries perpendicular to the surface, exhibit punctuate bleeding after trimming
- Skin ulceration: skin layer is destroyed and exposes underlying soft tissues or bone
- Mycotic infection

Treatment

- At diagnosis
  - Conservative management is appropriate.
    - — Reduction of hyperkeratotic area by trimming with a scalpel
    - — Shoe wear adaptations (soft-soled shoes with large toe box)
    - — Padding of the symptomatic area
    - — Toe sleeves or toe crests for dorsal corns
    - — Instruct patient how to shave the callus/corn with pumice stone
    - — In cases with maceration, lamb's wool, soft gauze, or a pad can be applied to desiccate the area, which promotes healing.
    - — Carbofuchsin or alcohol may also accelerate healing of soft corns.
- Later
  - In rare cases, the corn or callus cannot be controlled by conservative measures and surgical intervention may be warranted.

When to Refer

- Failure of conservative measures warrants referral to an orthopaedic surgeon.
- Surgical options include correction of the toe deformity and isolated condylectomy.
- Deformity correction is performed by resection of the head of the proximal phalanx and temporary Kirschner wire fixation (3 weeks).
- If the examiner is not confident in excluding a true mycotic infection, referral to a dermatologist can be considered.

Prognosis

- Generally good when there is no infection associated with osteomyelitis

Troubleshooting

- Complications include bleeding after trimming the corn or callus, mycotic infection when maceration is not managed adequately, and, in rare cases, deeper infection with osteomyelitis of the phalanx.
- Infection with swelling, redness, and warmth of the toe combined with pain is an absolute indication for immediate referral. Under such circumstances, intravenous antibiotic therapy should be considered.

Patient Instructions

- Patients should be educated about the causes of corns and calluses and counseled to wear appropriate shoe wear.
- Patients must be instructed in the use of a pumice stone to trim calluses without injuring the skin.

Suggested Reading

- Brahms MA: Common foot problems. J Bone Joint Surg Am 1967;49A:1653–1664.
- Coughlin MJ: Common causes of pain in the forefoot in adults. J Bone Joint Surg Br 2000;82B:781–790.
- Coughlin MJ: Mallet toes, hammer toes, claw toes, and corns. Causes and treatment of lesser-toe deformities. Postgrad Med 1984;75:191–198.
- Gillet HG: Interdigital clavus: Predisposition is the key factor of soft corns. Clin Orthop Relat Res 1979;142:103–109.

Chapter 191 Lesser Toe Deformities

Aaron Hoblet and Eric M. Bluman

ICD-9 CODES
735.4 *Hammertoe*
735.5 *Claw Toe*
735.8 *Other Acquired Deformities of Toe*

Key Concepts

- Lesser toe deformities include mallet toe, hammertoe, and claw toes; crossover and curly toe deformities; and instability of the metatarsophalangeal (MTP) joints.
- Lesser toe deformities may cause disabling pain.
- Conventionally, deformities with neurologic etiologies are termed claw toes. Those caused by improper shoe wear are hammertoes.
- The etiology may be an anatomic abnormality of the affected toe, adjacent toe, metatarsal, or forefoot. Neurologic conditions, repetitive injury, inflammatory arthropathies, and ill-fitting/high-fashion shoes may also contribute.
- Diagnosis and elimination of causative factors aid in treatment and prognosis.
- Treatment is initially nonoperative with the goal of alleviating symptoms. The aim is to passively diminish or correct supple deformities and cushion or relieve pressure in rigid deformities.

History

- Painful callosities are common in all deformities due to abnormal pressure points.
- Mallet toe, hammertoe, and claw toes: difficulty with shoe wear; pain on tips of toes, dorsal interphalangeal joints, plantar callosities, and soft tissues around toenail
- MTP joint instability: ill-defined forefoot pain with walking; initially plantar (plantar plate rupture); generalized synovitis over time; pain precedes deformity
- Crossover toe deformity: progressive worsening of second toe alignment in conjunction with hallux valgus
- Curly toe deformity: passively correctable, asymptomatic, overlapping toe in young children; usually bilateral and familial; third and fourth toes most common

Physical Examination

- Observation
  - Examine patient sitting and standing. When standing, flexible deformities may correct.
  - Forefoot/hindfoot malalignment may contribute to toe abnormalities.
  - Thick, painful plantar callosities are common (Fig. 191-1).
  - Hammertoes (Fig. 191-2): proximal interphalangeal (PIP) joint flexion; frequent MTP joint hyperextension; distal interphalangeal (DIP) joint variable position
  - Claw toes (Fig. 191-3): The primary deformity is MTP hyperextension and PIP and DIP flexion. Plantar position of the metatarsal head results in painful plantar callosities or ulcers.

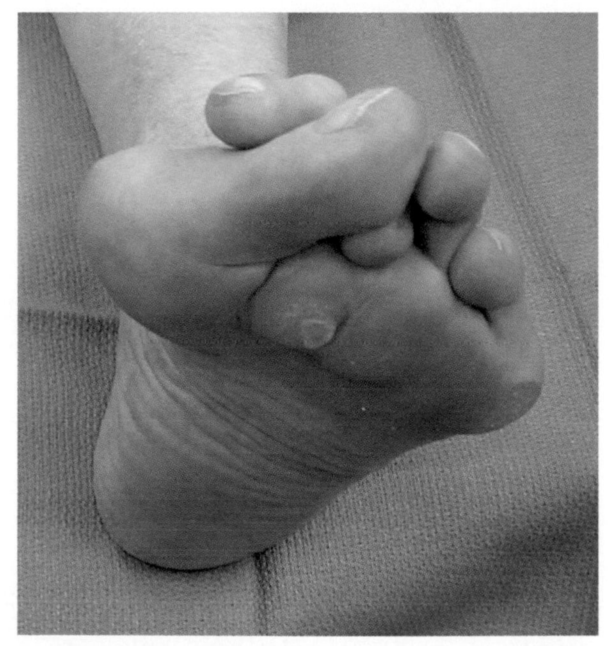

Figure 191-1 Plantar callosities in a patient with multiple severe lesser toe deformities.

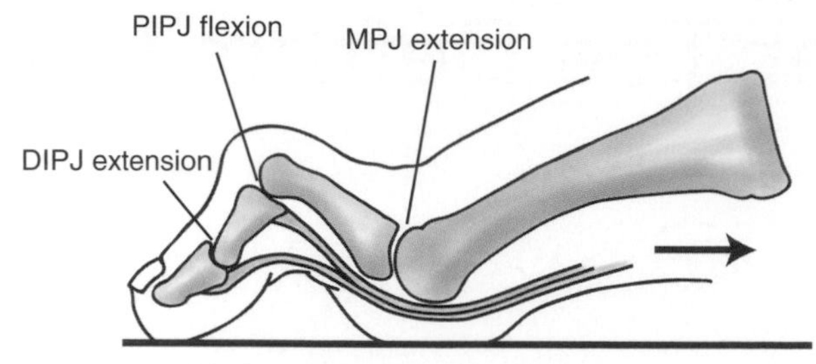

Figure 191-2 Hammertoe deformity. DIPJ, distal interphalangeal joint; MPJ, metatarsophalangeal joint; PIPJ, proximal interphalangeal joint.

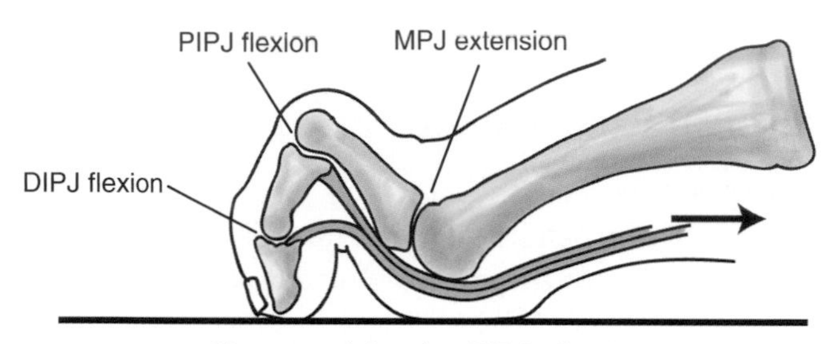

Figure 191-3 Claw toe deformity. DIPJ, distal interphalangeal joint; MPJ, metatarsophalangeal joint; PIPJ, proximal interphalangeal joint.

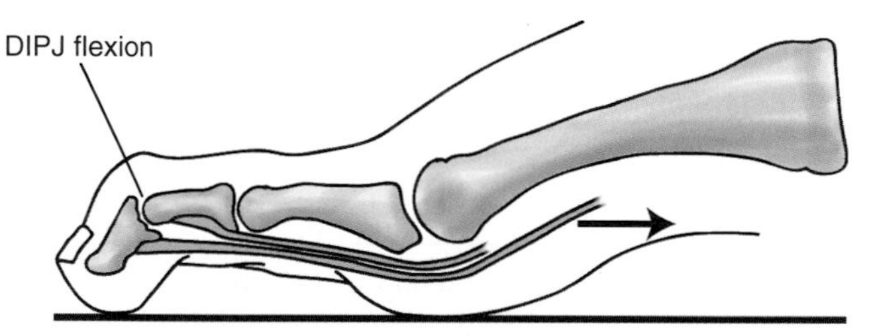

Figure 191-4 Mallet toe deformity. DIPJ, distal interphalangeal joint.

- Mallet toes (Fig. 191-4): isolated DIP flexion (attenuation of the terminal extensor tendon leads to unopposed pull of the flexor digitorum longus); callosities at tip of toe or dorsal DIP joint
- Crossover toes (Fig. 191-5): varus, dorsiflexion deformity of the second toe allowing it to lie over the top of the hallux (capsular instability of the second MTP joint); commonly associated with hallux valgus
- MTP joint instability (Fig. 191-6): medial toe deviation, occasional MTP joint hyperextension or lateral deviation
- Curly toes (Fig. 191-7): toe flexion, medial deviation (lies under the adjacent toe), and external rotation (nail faces laterally); caused by tight toe flexor tendon

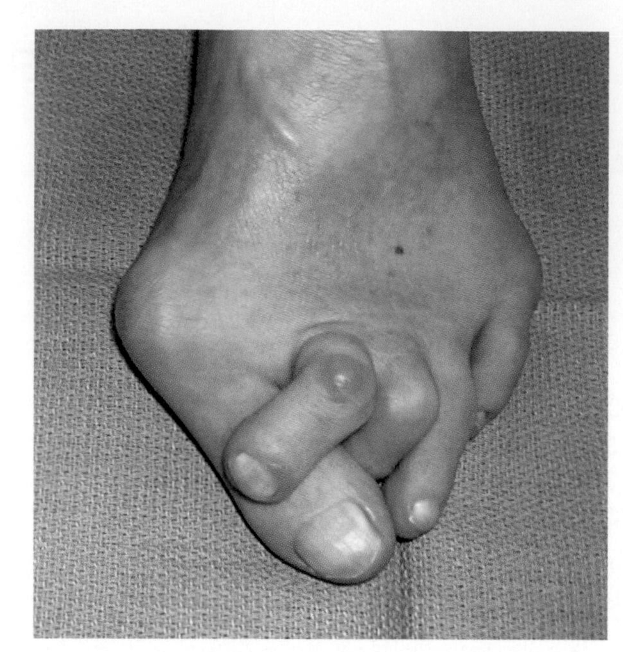

Figure 191-5 Crossover toe deformity in a patient with hallux valgus.

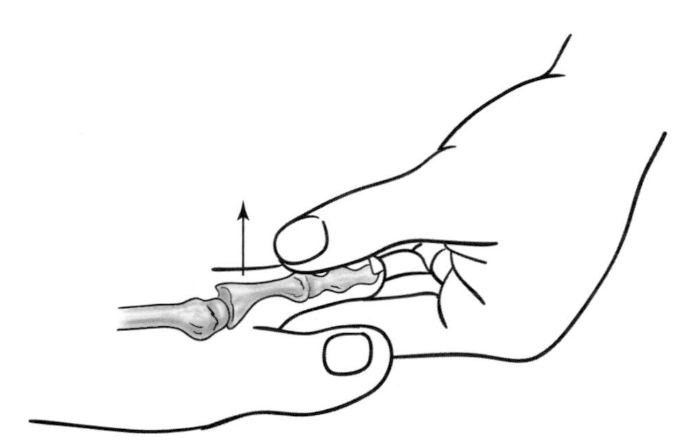

Figure 191-6 Metatarsophalangeal drawer test for the diagnosis of joint instability.

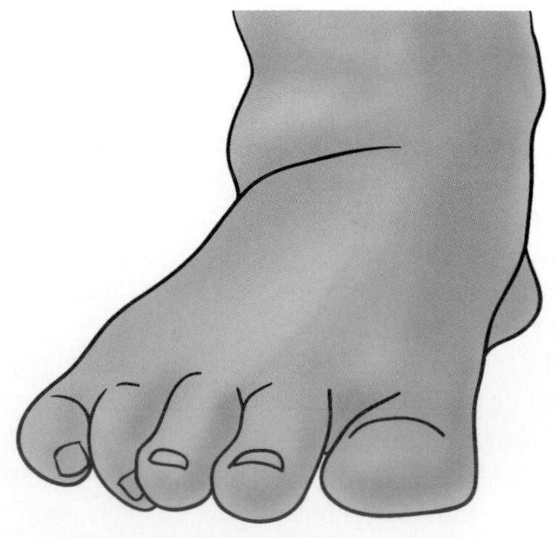

Figure 191-7 Curly toe deformity of the fourth digit.

- Palpation
  - Palpate for tenderness at the metatarsal heads.
- Range of motion
  - Determine whether deformities are flexible or rigid.
- Special tests
  - Drawer test for MTP joint instability: Grasp the proximal phalanx of the involved toe between the thumb and index finger and pull the toe dorsally; when performed on an unstable MTP joint, this produces dorsal translation and pain (see Fig. 191-6).
  - Assess for associated neurologic or inflammatory conditions (e.g., Charcot-Marie-Tooth disease, rheumatoid arthritis).

Imaging

- Radiographs: weight-bearing anteroposterior, lateral, and oblique views of the foot (Fig. 191-8)
  - Check for concomitant pathology and alternate sources of pain such as arthritis, Freiberg's infraction, and fractures.
- Magnetic resonance imaging
  - Not usually required, but can show stress fractures and Freiberg's infraction

Additional Tests

- Diagnostic injection: Local anesthetic and steroid solution can be injected into the MTP joint or around the digital nerve to distinguish between the causes of pain.

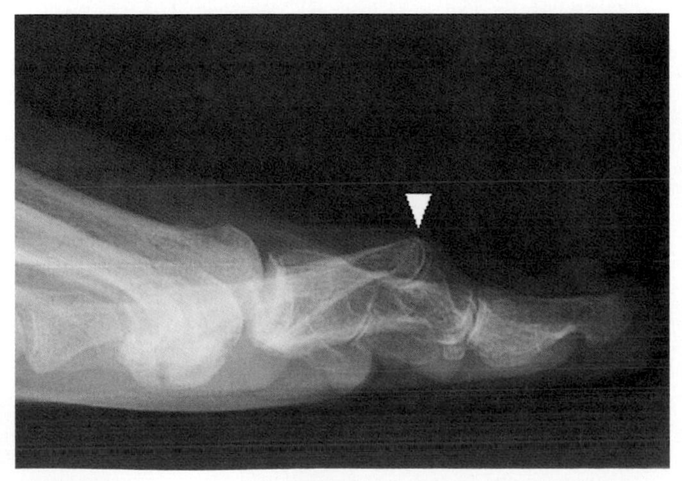

Figure 191-8 Lateral radiograph of patient with second hammertoe deformity (*arrowhead*).

Differential Diagnosis

- Metatarsal fracture
- Corn
- Interdigital neuroma
- Freiberg's infraction
- Stress fracture

Treatment

- At diagnosis
  - Conservative management includes activity modification to reduce synovitis, shoe wear modifications and orthotics to relieve pressure and accommodate deformities, passive stretching exercises to keep joints supple, and careful trimming of calluses. Nonsteroidal anti-inflammatory drugs may decrease pain and inflammation.
    - Shoe wear modifications: Extra-depth shoes with a wide toe box and flat heel prevent crowding of the toes. Patients unwilling to change shoes may have their current leather shoes modified with stretching or cutouts.
    - A firm-soled shoe, with or without a rocker bottom, decreases flexion at the MTP joints.
    - Buddy taping of the toes for 10 to 12 weeks in those with MTP joint instability may also aid in resolution of associated synovitis.
    - Orthotics: A toe crest, pad, or cap may be used to decrease pressure (Fig. 191-9). Soft insoles with metatarsal pads may decrease the pressure on the affected metatarsal heads. Options depend on the stiffness of the deformity.
- Later
  - If nonsurgical measures fail, surgical realignment may be required.

When to Refer

- Patients with deformities and pain unresponsive to conservative therapy should be referred to an orthopaedic surgeon.

Prognosis

- Conservative management often is all that is required for alleviation of pain and callosities. Curly toe deformities frequently correct spontaneously; stretching and taping have no proven efficacy.

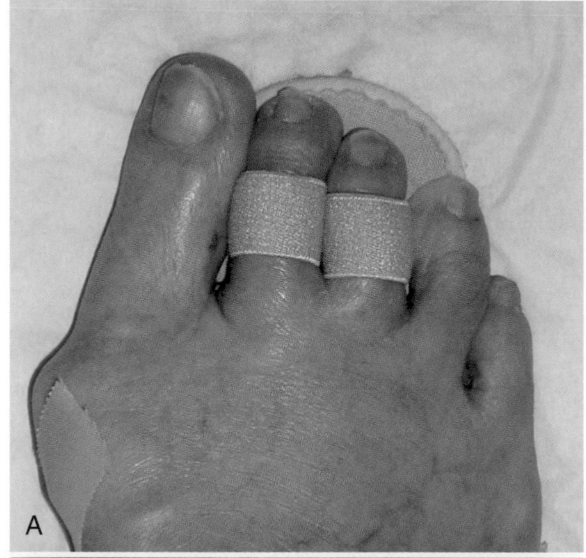

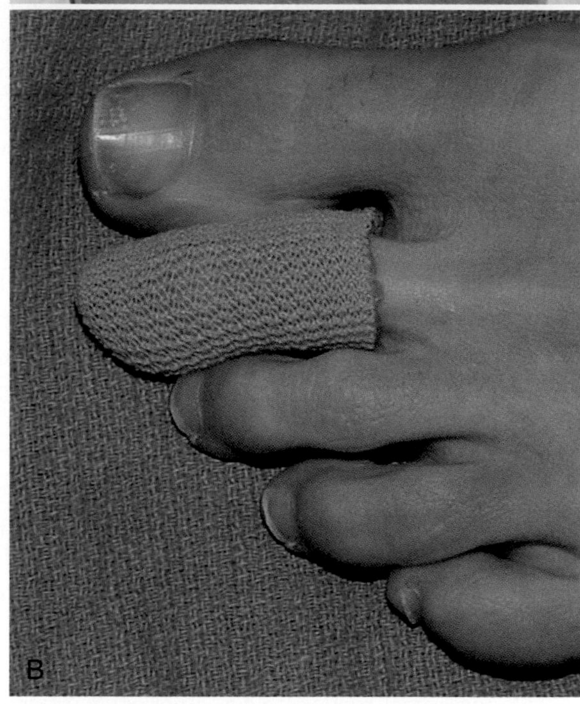

Figure 191-9 Commercially available orthotics for hammertoe deformity. **A**, Splint for reduction of deformity. **B**, Silicone toe sleeve for padding of deformity.

Troubleshooting

- In patients who do not improve, ensure that they have instituted the therapies prescribed. If improper use is noted or decreased compliance is suspected, further education may lead to greater success with nonoperative measures.

Patient Instructions

- Patients should be instructed on the importance of appropriate shoe wear and the use of recommended orthotics.
- Educate patients on the need for daily foot inspections to check for redness, ulcers, and blisters.

Consideration in Special Populations

- Neuropathic patients may develop unrecognized ulcerations due to insensate feet. These patients need to be further educated about soft-tissue breakdown and the need to inspect their feet daily. Toe strapping and bracing devices may cause pressure sores and should be avoided. Management problems should be referred to an orthopaedic surgeon immediately.
- Vasculopathic patients: Even small amounts of pressure or constriction applied by orthotic devices may lead to digit-threatening ischemia. Use of these devices should be done with extreme care or avoided altogether.
- Rheumatoid arthritics: Because of progressive soft-tissue inflammation and destruction that is a hallmark of the disease, conservative management may not be possible. If optimally managed with pharmacotherapy and shoe wear/orthotics fail to give relief, referral should be made for surgical options.

Suggested Reading

- Coughlin MJ: Lesser-toe abnormalities. J Bone Joint Surg Am 2002;84A:1446–1469.
- Easley ME, Aydogan U: Lesser toe deformities and bunionettes. In Thordarson DB (ed): Orthopedic Surgery Essentials: Foot and Ankle. Philadelphia: Lippincott Williams & Wilkins, 2004, pp 131–152.
- Kasser JR: The foot. In Morrissy RT, Weinstein SL (eds): Lovell and Winter's Pediatric Orthopaedics, 6th ed. Philadelphia: Lippincott Williams & Wilkins, 2006, pp 1302–1303.
- Myerson MS: Arthroplasty of the second toe. Semin Arthroplasty 1992;3:31–38.
- Myerson MS, Shereff MJ: The pathological anatomy of claw and hammer toes. J Bone Joint Surg Am 1989;71A:45–49.
- Shurnas PS, Sanders A: Second MTP joint capsular instability with clawing deformity: Metatarsal osteotomy, flexor transfer with biotenodesis, hammer toe repair, and MTP arthroplasty without the need for plantar incisions. Tech Foot Ankle Surg 2005;4:196–201.
- Thompson GH: Bunions and deformities of the toes in children and adolescents. J Bone Joint Surg Am 1995;77A:1924–1936.

Chapter 192 Nail Disorders

Nicholas R. Seibert and Robert E. Meehan

ICD-9 CODES
703.0 *Ingrowing Nail (Onychocryptosis)*
110.1 *Dermatophytosis of Nail (Onychomycosis)*

Key Concepts

- Diseases and deformities of the toenail are common foot ailments.
- Onychocryptosis is the most common toenail abnormality.
- Most toenail disorders are caused by intrinsic factors related to fungal or bacterial infections.
- The remaining deformities are caused by mechanical problems from shoe wear or adjacent toes.
- The nail plate and bed can also be damaged by direct trauma.

ONYCHOCRYPTOSIS (INGROWN NAIL)

History

- Virtually limited to the great toe
- Report of pain along nail edge, worse with closed-toe shoes
- Occasional drainage from the nail undersurface
- Causes include narrow toe box or tight-fitting footwear, improper nail trimming, and trauma

Physical Examination

- Observation
  - Edge of the nail plate penetrates adjacent nail fold (Fig. 192-1)
  - Hyperplasia of nail groove
  - Nail plate deformity is relatively uncommon.
  - Stages
    - — Stage 1: swelling, erythema, irritated nail fold
    - — Stage 2: increased pain, drainage, active infection
    - — Stage 3: granulation tissue, hypertrophy, chronic infection
- Palpation
  - Tenderness along the affected nail fold
  - Purulence expressed underneath the nail

Imaging

- Radiographs: anteroposterior, lateral, and oblique views of the phalanx
  - Useful in stages 2 and 3 to rule out subungual exostosis or osteomyelitis

Differential Diagnosis

- Onychomycosis: fungal infection of the nail
- Paronychia: superficial infection of nail fold
- Subungual exostosis: underlying bony growth
- Onychophosis: accumulation of callus in nail groove
- Trauma

Treatment

- At diagnosis
  - Stage 1 onychocryptosis treated with warm soaks, accommodative footwear, and proper nail trimming

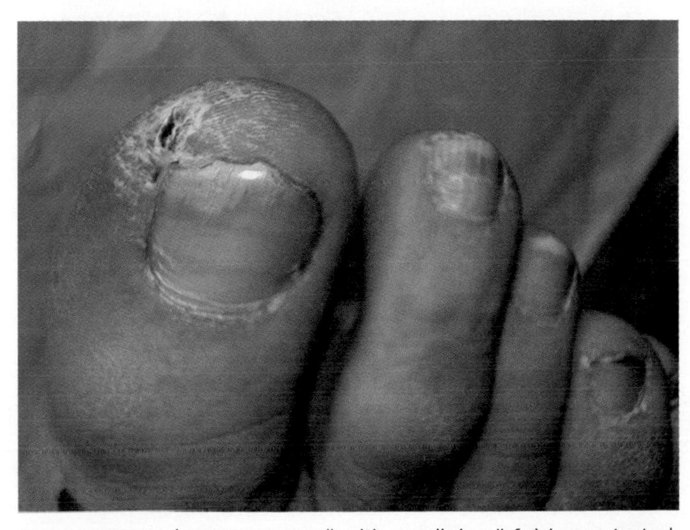

Figure 192-1 Ingrown toenail with medial nail fold penetrated.

- Later
  - Stage 2 ingrown nails are treated as previously described, with or without oral antibiotics, and partial nail excision under digital block (see Chapter 207). Stage 3 may also involve partial versus complete nail excision and ablation of the nail matrix for recurrent problems.

When to Refer

- Failure of nonoperative treatment or recurrent stage 3 disease

Prognosis

- Recurrence is common.

Patient Instructions

- Proper footwear and nail care are essential to prevent recurrence.

Considerations in Special Populations

- Diabetic patients (Fig. 192-2) and patients with total joint replacements have a lower threshold for treatment to prevent recurrent infections and sepsis. Surgery should be performed sooner.
- Excessive forefoot pronation may benefit from an orthotic to unload the medial border of the great toe, if affected.

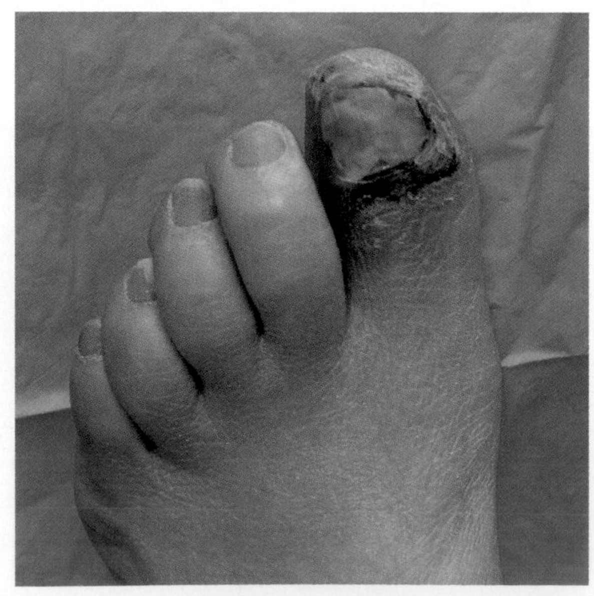

Figure 192-2 Ingrown toenail in a diabetic patient with superinfection.

ONYCHOMYCOSIS (NAIL FUNGAL INFECTION)

History

- Four times more common in the toes than fingers
- Common: 20% incidence in the general population
- Elderly: 75% incidence in adults older than 60 years of age
- *Trichophyton rubrum* and *Trichophyton mentagrophytes* most common

Physical Examination

- Observation
  - Thickened, discolored, deformed, brittle nail plate (Fig. 192-3)
  - Interference with shoe wear due to thickened, raised nail plate
- Palpation
  - Thickened, rough nail
  - With or without tenderness
- Special tests
  - Nail scrapings examined under light microscopy prepared with potassium hydroxide may exhibit hyphae.
  - Nail debris may be sent for fungal culture.

Differential Diagnosis

- Onychocryptosis: ingrown toenail
- Onychogryphosis: severe thickening and curling of the nail plate (Fig. 192-4)
- Psoriasis
- Trauma

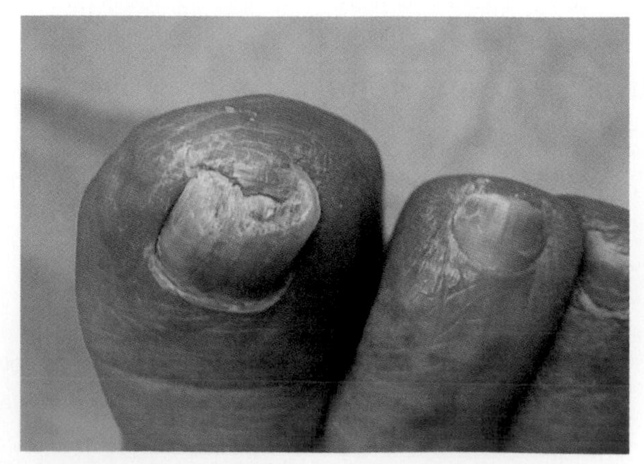

Figure 192-3 Fungal infection of the great toenail. Note the lateral border is also ingrown.

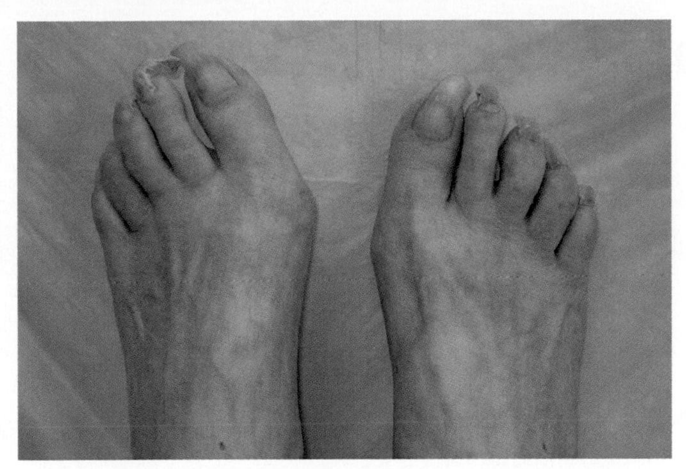

Figure 192-4 Onychogryphosis with nail plate thickening and curling.

Treatment

- At diagnosis
  - Simple trimming and débridement of the hypertrophic nail plate may relieve the pain and discomfort associated with shoe wear, but will not result in a cure.
- Later
  - Topical medications are less effective than systemic ones due to their inability to penetrate the thickened nail plate. Systemic antifungal medications result in mycologic cure in 60% to 100% of patients with extended treatment (3–12 months).

When to Refer

- Refractory cases necessitating nail matrix ablation

Prognosis

- Good in small lesions that respond to local treatment including débridement and medications
- Poor in larger lesions, which do better in the long term with permanent nail removal

Patient Instructions

- General foot hygiene

Considerations in Special Populations

- Avoid systemic antifungals in pregnant women and patients with hepatic disease.

Suggested Reading

- Alavi A, Woo K, Sibbald RG: Common nail disorders and fungal infections. Adv Skin Wound Care 2007;20:346–357.
- Coughlin MJ, Mann RA (eds): Surgery of the Foot and Ankle, 8th ed. St. Louis: Mosby, 2006.
- Griffin LY (ed): Essentials of Musculoskeletal Care, 3rd ed. Rosemont, IL: American Academy of Orthopaedic Surgeons, 2005.
- Mayeaux EJ Jr: Nail disorders. Prim Care 2000;27:333–351.

Chapter 193 Subtalar Dislocation

Jeremy Kinder and Anand Vora

ICD-9 CODE
838.01 *Subtalar Dislocation*

Key Concepts

- Subtalar dislocations typically occur from high-energy mechanisms (motor vehicle collision, fall from height), but can also occur from low-energy mechanisms (athletic injuries).
- Relatively infrequent injury, accounting for 1% of all dislocations
- Approximately 20% to 45% of subtalar dislocations are open injuries.
- The subtalar joint consists of the articulations between the calcaneus and talus. The talonavicular and calcaneocuboid joints are also considered part of the subtalar complex (Fig. 193-1).
- Subtalar dislocations can cause avascular necrosis of the talus due to disruption of the blood supply.
- Subtalar dislocations are described by the direction that the foot takes in relation to the talus, which usually remains in its anatomic place. Medial dislocations are most common and account for more than 75% of these injuries.
- Occult fractures are common.

History

- History of major trauma (motor vehicle collision, fall from height); less commonly result from "rolling" or "twisting" the ankle
- Medial dislocations occur from forced inversion of the foot with the ankle in plantarflexion, whereas lateral dislocations occur from forced eversion of the foot with the ankle in plantarflexion.
- May give history of gross deformity that "snapped" back into place
- Unable to bear weight

Physical Examination

- Observation
  - Skin: Assess for tenting, which can cause soft-tissue compromise or necrosis. Lacerations may indicate an open injury (Fig. 193-2).
  - Gross deformity: forefoot and heel significantly everted or inverted depending on the type of dislocation (Fig. 193-3)
  - Swelling
- Palpation
  - Tenderness

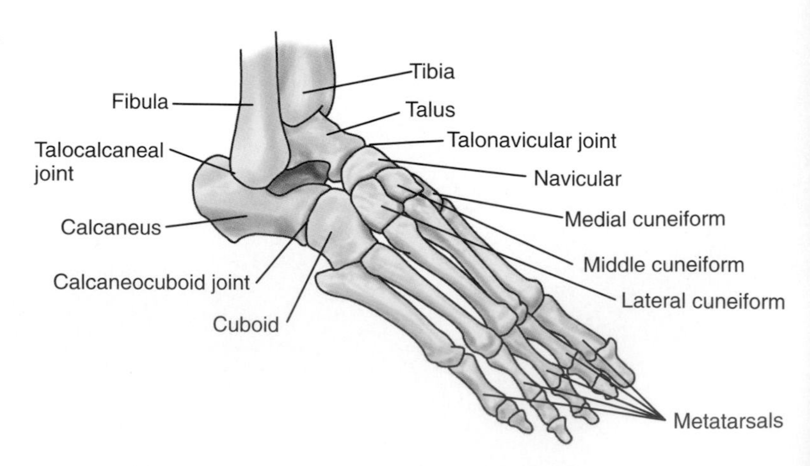

Figure 193-1 Basic anatomy of the subtalar complex.

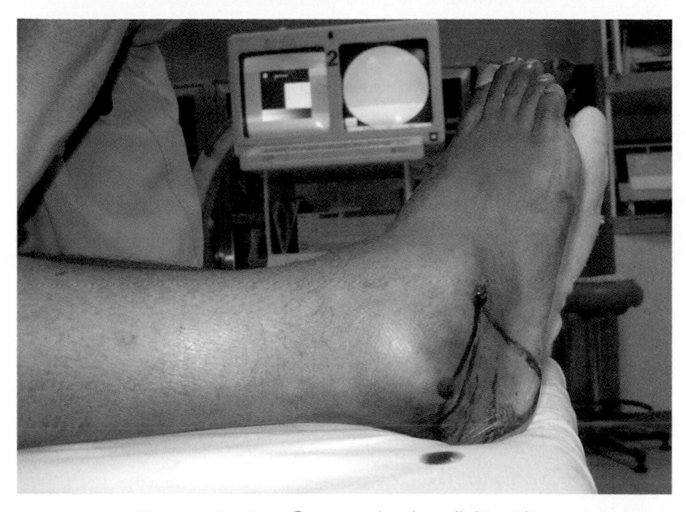

Figure 193-2 Open subtalar dislocation.

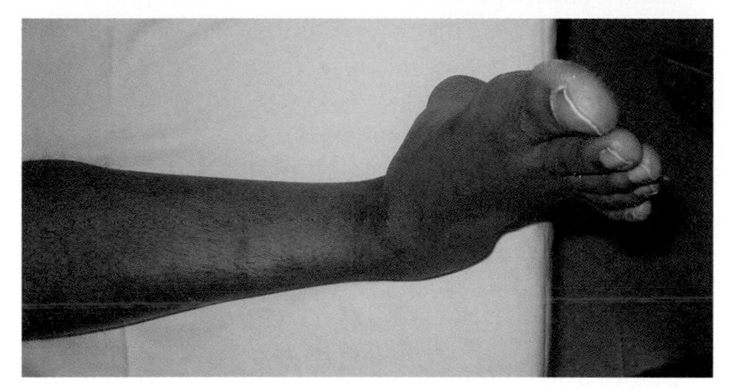

Figure 193-3 Obvious deformity associated with a medial subtalar dislocation.

- Special tests
  - Neurovascular examination: Evaluate for injury to the tibial nerve and/or posterior tibial artery, particularly with open injuries.

Imaging

- Radiographs: anteroposterior and lateral radiographs of the ankle (Fig. 193-4)
  - Typically normal relationship between the talus, tibia, and fibula
  - The anteroposterior view best demonstrates talonavicular dislocation.
  - Lateral view: Note the absence of the talar head within the "cup" of the navicular. The head of the talus usually lies superior to the navicular and cuboid in medial dislocations and appears inferior in lateral dislocations.
- Computed tomography
  - Should be ordered after reduction to assess reduction and identify associated articular fractures, osteochondral defects, and nondisplaced fractures

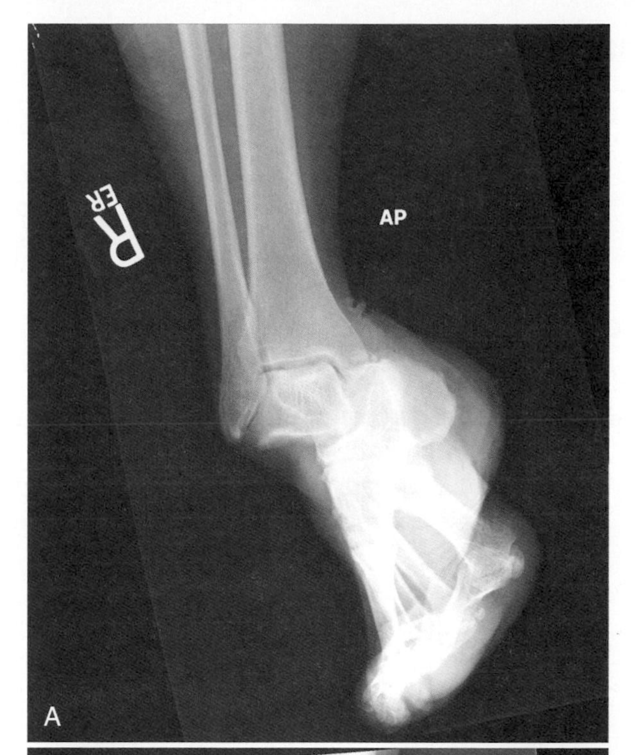

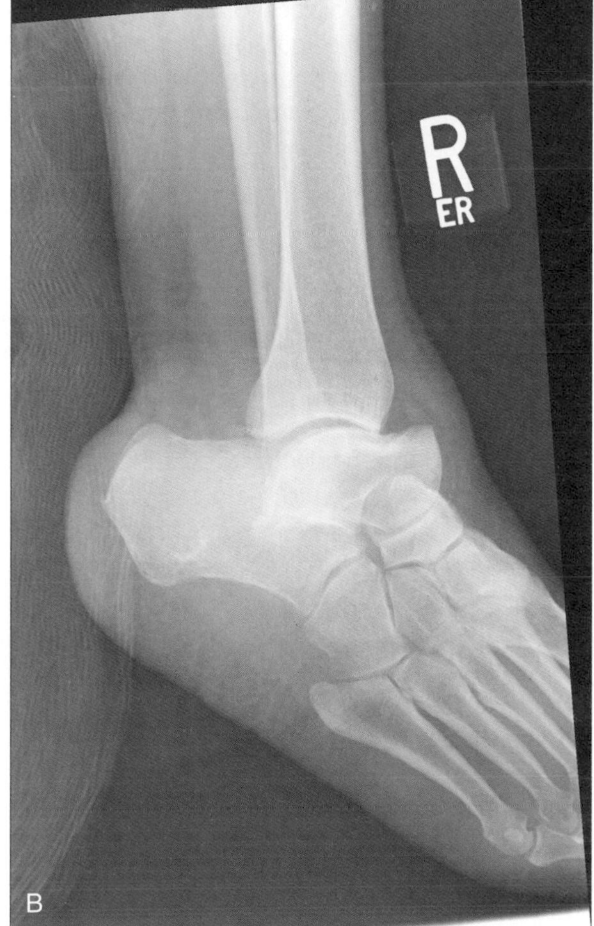

Figure 193-4 Anteroposterior (**A**) and lateral (**B**) radiographs of a medial subtalar dislocation.

Differential Diagnosis

- Displaced ankle fracture-dislocation: talonavicular and talocalcaneal joints intact on radiographs
- Total talar dislocation: talus completely disrupted (including tibiotalar articulation) and may be extruded in open injuries

Treatment

- At diagnosis
  - All subtalar dislocations require a gentle and timely reduction; most can be performed closed in the emergency department setting with intravenous sedation or in the operating room with general anesthesia.
  - Reductions are performed by knee flexion to relieve deforming forces of the gastrocnemius muscle, longitudinal traction through the heel with the foot plantarflexed, accentuation of the deformity to unlock the calcaneus from the talus, and eversion (medial dislocations) or inversion (lateral dislocations) of the foot to complete reduction. A satisfying clunk accompanies reduction. Normal alignment of the foot and normal range of motion of the subtalar and midtarsal joints should be achieved.
  - After reduction, a bulky splint is applied with the foot in neutral position.
  - Postreduction radiographs are mandatory to confirm reduction. Computed tomography is highly recommended to further assess reduction and look for associated fractures.
- Later
  - After swelling and edema are controlled, the patient should be switched to a short leg cast for 3 to 6 weeks if there is no associated fracture. Approximately 50% of subtalar dislocations do have associated fractures (medial or lateral malleolus, fourth or fifth metatarsal, osteochondral fractures of the subtalar or talonavicular joints) that may require surgical open reduction and internal fixation, prolonged immobilization, or excision of intra-articular fragments. A vigorous exercise and range of motion program should be instituted after the cast has been removed and all associated fractures are stable to minimize stiffness.

When to Refer

- Immediate orthopaedic consultation is indicated for all subtalar dislocations for urgent closed reduction of the joint. Open injuries additionally require immediate irrigation and débridement of the open wound.
- If closed reduction is unsuccessful, open reduction and stabilization are necessary. With medial dislocations, the talar head can become trapped by the talonavicular joint capsule, extensor tendons, or extensor digitorum brevis muscle. With lateral dislocations, articular surface impaction of the talar head or the posterior tibial tendon may impede reduction.

Prognosis

- Most patients with subtalar dislocations can be managed with a short leg walking cast and have satisfactory outcomes. Poorer results are associated with lateral dislocations due to the high-energy cause of the injury and resultant associated injuries. Most patients with subtalar dislocation will experience some loss of subtalar motion, and the majority will have posttraumatic subtalar arthritis at long-term follow-up. Some patients may benefit significantly from subtalar arthrodesis or triple arthrodesis for pain relief.

Troubleshooting

- Associated fractures, loose bodies, or other injuries should be addressed after reduction to maximize outcome.
- If pain and instability are severe and worsen over time, subtalar fusion may be necessary.

Patient Instructions

- After successful reduction, patients can weight bear in a short leg cast.
- Patients will require frequent follow-up to assess stability and reduction.
- The length of immobilization will be 3 to 6 weeks depending on other associated injuries.
- Most patients will have a decrease in subtalar motion and are prone to subtalar arthritis.

Suggested Reading

- Bibbo C, Lin SS, et al: Missed and associated injuries after subtalar dislocation: The role of CT. Foot Ankle Int 2001; 22:324–328.
- Bohay DR, Manoli A: Subtalar joint dislocations. Foot Ankle Int 1995;16:803–807.
- DeLee JC, Curtis R: Subtalar dislocation of the foot. J Bone Joint Surg Am 1982;64A:433–437.

- Goldner JL, Poletti SC, et al: Severe open subtalar dislocations: Long-term results. J Bone Joint Surg Am 1995;77A:1075–1079.
- Heck BE, Ebraheim NA, Jackson WT: Anatomic considerations of irreducible medial subtalar dislocation. Foot Ankle Int 1996;17:103–106.
- Malenkovic S, Radenkovic M, Mitkovic M: Open subtalar dislocation treated by distractional external fixation. J Orthop Trauma 2004;18:638–640.
- MerChan EC: Subtalar dislocations: Long-term follow-up of 39 cases. Injury 1992;23:97–100.

Chapter 194 Lisfranc Injuries

Hany El-Rashidy and Anand Vora

ICD-9 CODE
838.03 *Lisfranc (Tarsometatarsal) Fracture-Dislocation*

Key Concepts

- The Lisfranc joint represents the junction between the midfoot and forefoot.
- Three metatarsal-cuneiform articulations (first, second, and third tarsometatarsal joints) and two metatarsal-cuboid articulations (fourth and fifth tarsometatarsal joints) (Fig. 194-1)
- Proper alignment and stability of these joints are essential for normal foot function.
- The Lisfranc joint is very stable because of its bony anatomy and strong ligamentous attachments. The base of the second metatarsal ("keystone") is recessed and locks between the medial and lateral cuneiforms. Plantar ligaments are stronger than dorsal ligaments.

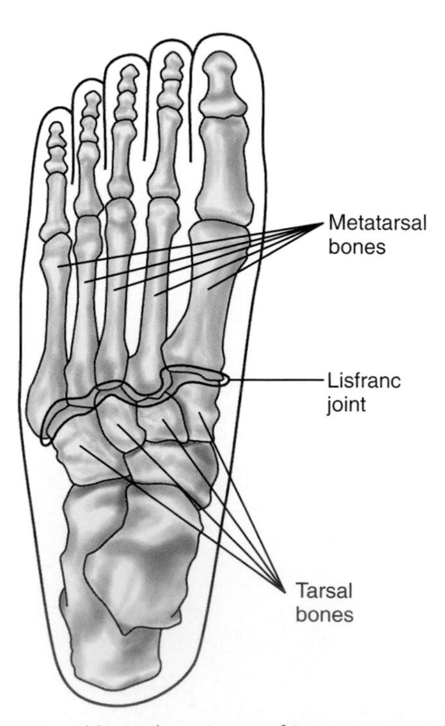

Figure 194-1 Normal anatomy of tarsometatarsal joints.

- The Lisfranc ligament is the strongest ligament and runs from the base of the second metatarsal to the medial cuneiform.
- Injuries to this joint range from mild sprains to widely displaced, unstable, debilitating injuries.
  - Injuries can be bony, ligamentous, or a combination of the two.
- As many as 20% of Lisfranc injuries initially go unrecognized. When suspected, weight-bearing and/or stress radiographs are critical.
- Injuries to the tarsometatarsal joints require early accurate diagnosis with prompt anatomic reduction and internal fixation for optimal results. Severe long-term morbidity may occur if injuries are not properly treated at initial presentation.

History

- Mild to severe pain in the midfoot at rest and with weight bearing; may be unable to bear weight
- Acute injury; may be direct or indirect (Fig. 194-2)
  - Direct: crush injury
  - Indirect (more common): axial load in fixed planted foot (football, missed step off curb, landing dance jump) or twisting injury with forceful abduction of forefoot on midfoot (motor-vehicle collision)
- Any traumatic mechanism with significant midfoot pain should raise suspicion of a possible Lisfranc injury.

Physical Examination

- Observation
  - Abrasions, lacerations
  - Bruising (especially medial plantar surface of the foot)
  - Swelling around dorsal midfoot
  - Loss of normal arch or midfoot contour with weight bearing
- Palpation
  - Pain with palpation or manipulation of the tarsometatarsal joints

- Range of motion
  - Passive dorsiflexion and plantarflexion of the metatarsals elicits pain.
- Special tests
  - Pain at the midfoot with attempted single leg heel rise suggests a Lisfranc injury.

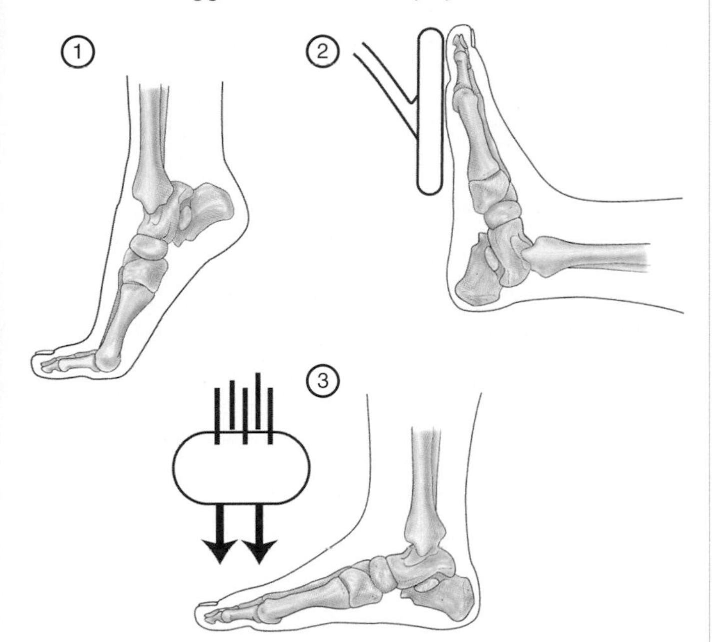

Figure 194-2 Common mechanisms of injury. Axial load in a planted foot (1), motor-vehicle collision trauma (2), direct crush injury (3).

- Careful neurovascular examination emphasizing sensation and perfusion is essential. Lisfranc dislocation can be associated with impingement or laceration of a branch of the dorsalis pedis artery or the deep peroneal nerve, both of which cross dorsally between the base of the first and second metatarsals.
- Severe swelling, especially in high-energy mechanisms, should alert the physician to possible compartment syndrome of the foot.

Imaging

- Radiographs: anteroposterior, lateral, and oblique views of the foot (Fig. 194-3)
  - Should be weight bearing if possible to load the ligaments and test their integrity; if not possible, obtain stress views
  - Anteroposterior view: The medial border of the second metatarsal should align with the medial border of the middle cuneiform.
  - Oblique view: The medial border of the fourth metatarsal should align with the medial border of the cuboid.
  - Lateral view: The superior border of the metatarsal base should align with the superior border of the medial cuneiform.

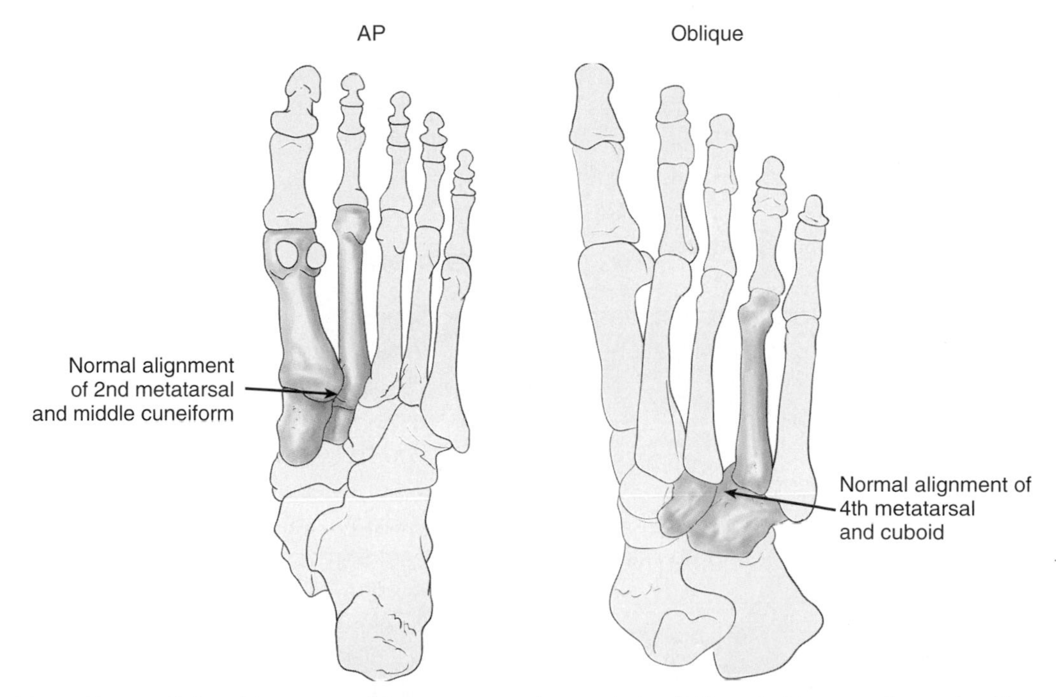

Figure 194-3 Normal bony relationships as would appear on anteroposterior (AP) and oblique radiographs. The second metatarsal should align with the medial border of the middle cuneiform on the AP view, and the medial border of the fourth metatarsal should align with the cuboid on the oblique view.

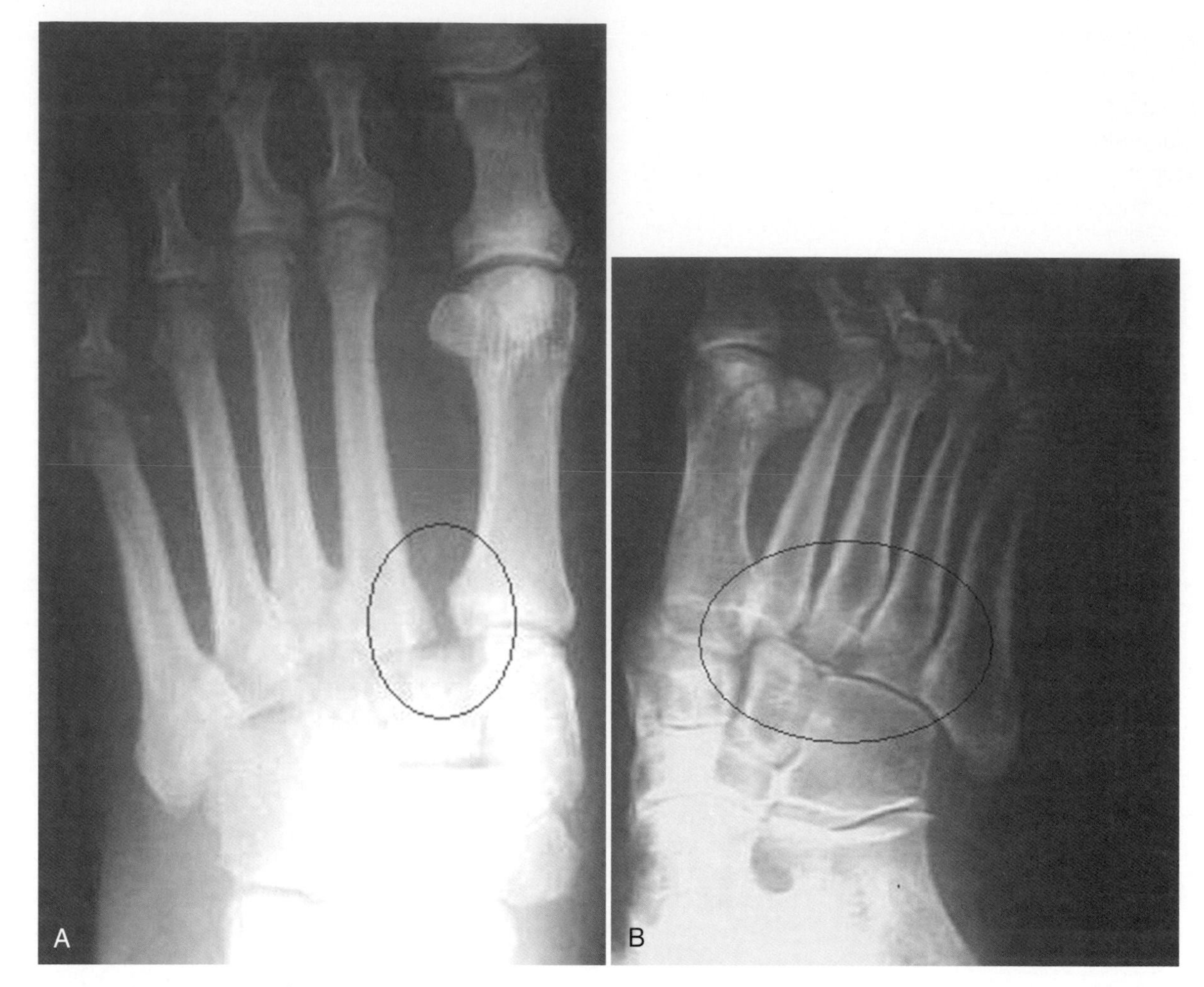

Figure 194-4 Lisfranc injury. **A**, On the anteroposterior view, note the abnormal alignment between the medial borders of the second metatarsal and middle cuneiform (*circle*). **B**, On the oblique view, note the abnormal alignment between the medial borders of the fourth metatarsal and cuboid (*circle*).

  - Disruption of any these defined relationships is indicative of a Lisfranc injury (Fig. 194-4).
  - Stress views help reveal displacement in subtle cases with spontaneous reduction (Fig. 194-5). Ankle block or sedation may be required.
- Computed tomography
  - Better for discerning minor displacement, associated fractures, comminution, and dislocations
- Magnetic resonance imaging
  - To assess soft-tissue damage

Additional Tests

- Compartment pressure monitoring in selected cases

Differential Diagnosis

- Tarsal, metatarsal, or phalangeal fractures of the foot
- Ligamentous injury outside the Lisfranc joint
- Soft-tissue damage around foot without fracture or ligament injury

Treatment

- At diagnosis
  - Initial treatment of a Lisfranc injury focuses on soft-tissue evaluation and diagnosing instability and associated fractures/dislocations.
  - For truly nondisplaced, stable injuries (negative weight-bearing and stress radiographs) with a normal soft-tissue/neurovascular examination, cast immobilization can be used.
  - A non–weight-bearing short leg cast for 6 weeks is followed by a walking cast for an additional 6 weeks until pain and tenderness have resolved.
  - All other injuries should be referred acutely (see the following).

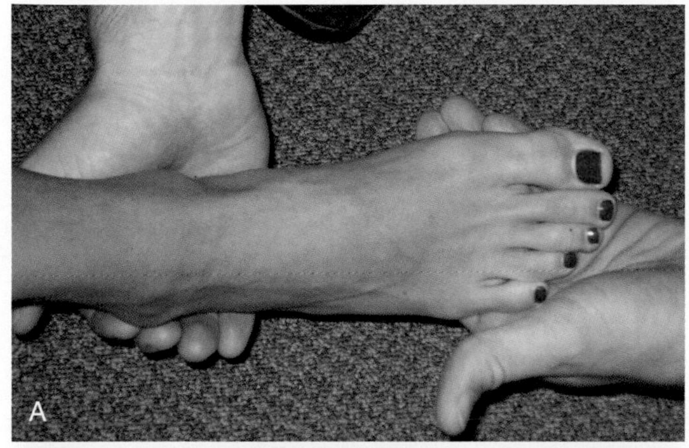

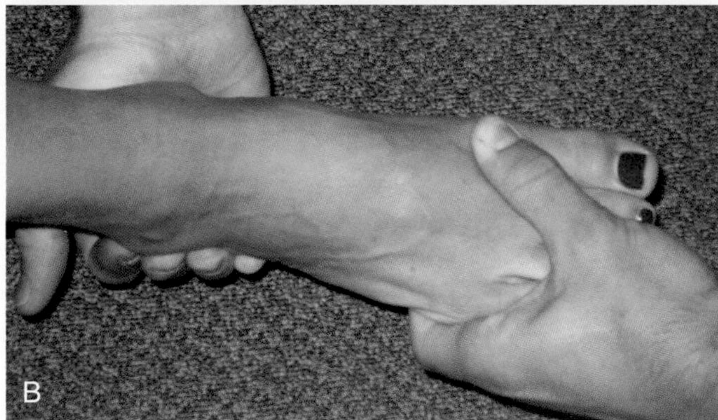

Figure 194-5 **A**, To obtain a stress view radiograph, stabilize the hindfoot with one hand and grasp the forefoot with the opposite hand. **B**, With the heel stabilized, place abduction/pronation stress on the forefoot. Widening of more than 2 mm or severe pain indicates a Lisfranc injury.

- Later
  - For stable injuries, follow-up weight-bearing radiographs should be repeated at 10 to 14 days. If the injury remains stable (<2 mm displacement) and pain is decreasing, continued cast management with serial repeat radiographs in 2 weeks is recommended.
  - Any evidence of displacement or instability on follow-up examination warrants immediate orthopaedic referral for operative planning.

When to Refer

- Any Lisfranc injury with displacement or instability requires operative intervention and anatomic reduction for optimal results.
- Urgent/emergent referral is essential for any question of compartment syndrome (severe swelling and pain), dislocation, open fracture, or abnormal neurovascular examination.

Prognosis

- As many as 20% of Lisfranc injuries are overlooked, especially in polytrauma patients, with severe long-term morbidity.
- The severity of even subtle Lisfranc injuries is often underestimated, and healing may be prolonged.
- Patients should be provided with an accurate prognosis at the time of diagnosis.
- The best results (95% good to excellent functional recovery) are seen in those patients who undergo open reduction and internal fixation.
- Inadequate reduction or initial damage to the joint surface directly correlates with the development of posttraumatic arthritis.
- Symptoms after Lisfranc injury may persist, but continue to subside for several years.

Troubleshooting

- Compartment syndrome usually occurs only with a high-energy Lisfranc fracture-dislocation and should be considered in any injury with severe swelling and a painful, tense foot. Any suspicion warrants immediate orthopaedic evaluation.
- Counsel patients that posttraumatic arthritis is common and related to both the initial injury and the adequacy of reduction.
- Be very wary of diagnosing a simple midfoot sprain. If a patient with a foot injury is unable to bear weight or has severe midfoot pain, he or she should be referred for orthopaedic evaluation.
- Standard radiographs may only show slight incongruity of the joint; gross instability may only be seen on stress or weight-bearing views. In any patient with a midfoot sprain, it is essential to obtain such studies to avoid missing an unstable injury.

Patient Instructions

- Instruct patients on the importance of elevation to decrease swelling, weight-bearing restrictions, and orthopaedic follow-up.
- Accurately outlining the prognosis associated with Lisfranc injuries, including a likely prolonged recovery time (immobilization up to 3 to 4 months), is an important component of the treatment plan.

Considerations in Special Populations

- Athletes with traumatic foot injury and resultant midfoot pain should be referred to an orthopaedic specialist for appropriate evaluation.

- Diabetic patients may have an underlying neuropathic (Charcot's) arthropathy contributing to the Lisfranc pathology, especially with a history of minimal trauma.

Suggested Reading

- Arntz CT, Veith RG, Hansen ST: Fractures and fracture-dislocations of the tarsometatarsal joint. J Bone Joint Surg Am 1988;70A:173–181.
- Coetzee JC, Ly TV: Treatment of primarily ligamentous Lisfranc joint injuries: Primary arthrodesis compared with open reduction and internal fixation. J Bone Joint Surg Am 2007;89A:122–127.
- Davis E: Lisfranc joint injuries. Trauma 2006;8:225–231.
- Desmond EA, Chou LB: Current concepts review: Lisfranc injuries. Foot Ankle Int 2006;27:653–660.
- Kuo RS, Tejwani NC, DiGiovanni CW, et al: Outcome after open reduction and internal fixation of Lisfranc joint injuries. J Bone Joint Surg Am 2000;82A:1609–1617.
- Mulier T, Reynders P, Dereymaeker G: Severe Lisfranc injuries: Primary arthrodesis or ORIF. Foot Ankle Int 2002;23:902–905.
- Richter M, Wipperman B, Krettek C: Fractures and fracture dislocations of the midfoot: Occurrence, causes, and long-term results. Foot Ankle Int 2001;22:392–398.
- Sands AK, Grose A: Lisfranc injuries. Injury 2004;35:71–76.

Chapter 195 Stress Fractures of the Foot

Scott Van Aman and M. Truitt Cooper

ICD-9 CODES
733.94 *Stress Fracture of Metatarsal*
733.95 *Stress Fracture of Other Bone*

Key Concepts

- Stress fractures can affect any bone in the foot.
- Caused by failure of bone to adequately respond and remodel to repetitive stress (cumulative effects of uncompensated loading)
- May result from abnormal loading patterns or stresses applied to normal bone
- May also be due to abnormal bone or healing response (chronic disease states) that is unable to meet the demands of physiologically normal stresses
- Females are at higher risk, especially those with the female athlete triad of amenorrhea, anorexia, and osteoporosis.
- Many stress fractures of the foot can be treated conservatively with activity modification and rest.
- Underlying causative factors (systemic or mechanical abnormalities) must be addressed.
- High-risk stress fractures, such as navicular, talus, and proximal fifth metatarsal fractures, have a propensity to develop into nonunions and require more aggressive treatment.

History

- Insidious onset of pain, frequently worsened with activity
- Recent increase or alteration of physical activity, such as beginning a running program or enlisting in boot camp
- A history of stress fractures is common.
- Important to note predisposing medical conditions
  - Hormonal abnormalities
  - Osteoporosis/osteopenia
  - Anorexia
  - Medications (corticosteroids)
  - Chronic disease (diabetes or rheumatoid arthritis)
- Certain stress fractures are classically associated with specific activities.
  - March fractures: second or third metatarsal shaft fracture seen in military recruits
  - Second metatarsal base fractures are seen in ballerinas who dance *en pointe*.

Physical Examination

- Observation
  - Minimal swelling, ecchymosis, or erythema
  - Gait: most will be able to bear weight
  - Deformity or leg length discrepancy
  - Foot morphology
  - High arch with varus heel may predispose to fifth metatarsal stress fracture (increased lateral column load)
  - Flatfoot deformity with hypermobile first ray may predispose to second metatarsal stress fracture (load transfer)
- Palpation
  - Point tenderness
  - Palpate each metatarsal individually to elicit pain.
  - Squeeze medial/lateral heel to elicit pain and differentiate from pain over the Achilles insertion (Achilles tendinitis) or plantar heel (plantar fasciitis)
- Range of motion
  - Tight gastrocsoleus complex may predispose to forefoot stress fractures
  - Increased first ray motion may lead to second or third metatarsal stress fractures.
  - Dorsiflexion of the great toe elicits pain with stress fractures of the sesamoids.

Imaging

- Radiographs: standing anteroposterior, lateral, and oblique views of the foot
  - Frequently normal; findings lag behind clinical symptoms by at least 2 to 3 weeks (Fig. 195-1)

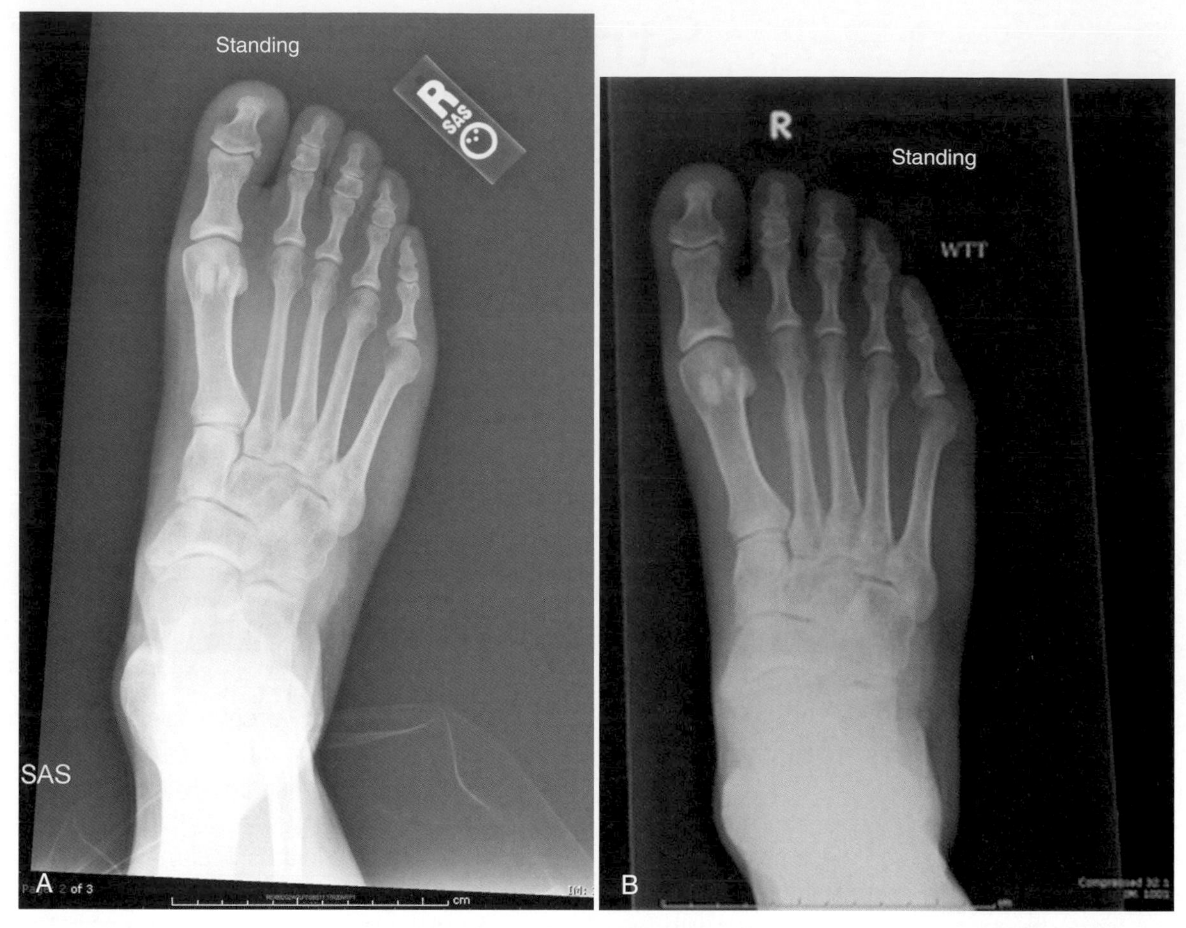

Figure 195-1 **A**, Normal-appearing anteroposterior radiograph of the foot in a patient with forefoot pain. **B**, Repeat radiograph 3 weeks later shows callus formation around the second metatarsal shaft, indicating a healing response of the stress fracture.

- If stress fracture has been present for an extended period, may see early callus or distinct fracture line
- If there is a high level of suspicion for stress fracture, particularly in high-risk area such as the navicular, talar neck, or proximal fifth metatarsal, proceed with advanced imaging.

- Nuclear imaging
  - Increased uptake in region of fracture
  - Highly sensitive, but not specific
- Computed tomography
  - Best modality to demonstrate bony anatomy
  - Particularly useful for navicular
- Magnetic resonance imaging
  - It is very sensitive for bone marrow edema; an increase in a T2-weighted signal indicates edema (Fig. 195-2) as does a decrease in intensity of marrow on T1-weighted images. T1-weighted images will also demonstrate a fracture as a dark line across the bone.

Differential Diagnosis

- Synovitis: pain isolated to specific joint with range of motion; may have instability at affected joint
- Arthritis: pain located at joint; radiographs reveal loss of joint space and subchondral sclerosis
- Infection: erythema usually present, frequently in patients with systemic illness (diabetes)
- Tendinitis: pain located over a major tendon, worsened when tendon stressed
- Acute fracture: acute pain with traumatic incident

Treatment

- At diagnosis
  - Except for high-risk stress fractures, most can be treated initially with conservative management. Any offending activities (such as distance running) should be discontinued.

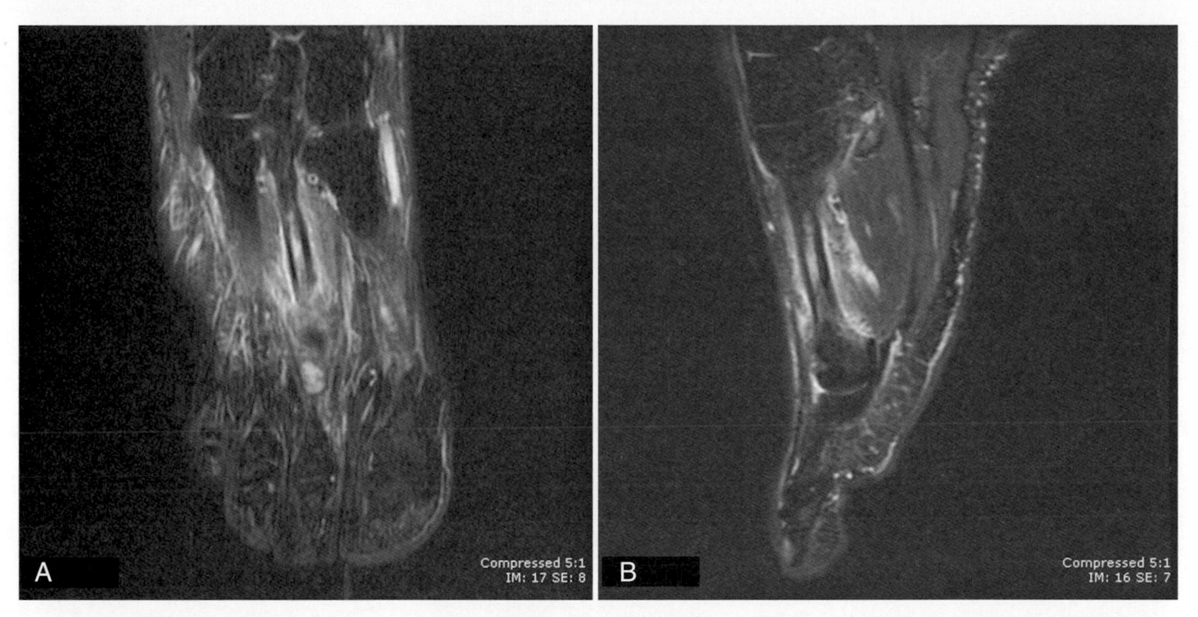

Figure 195-2 Coronal (**A**) and sagittal (**B**) T2-weighted magnetic resonance images demonstrate edema in the shaft of the second metatarsal consistent with a stress reaction or early stress fracture.

- — Middle metatarsal shaft stress fractures: hard-soled shoe with gradual return to activity when symptomatically improved (usually approximately 6 weeks)
- — Calcaneal stress fractures: activity avoidance, heel wedges, and stretching of the calf musculature
- — Sesamoids, navicular, and fifth metatarsal base; short leg non–weight-bearing cast for 6 to 8 weeks

- Later
  - If any deformity (varus foot) or mechanical abnormality is present, appropriate orthotics should be used to prevent recurrence.

When to Refer

- Stress fractures that remain symptomatic despite appropriate nonoperative management should be referred.
- Consider immediate referral of high risk fractures such as the proximal fifth metatarsal (Fig. 195-3), talus, and navicular as these have a high propensity for nonunion. Additionally, stress fractures in high-level athletes may benefit from early operative fixation and should be referred.

Prognosis

- Generally good for most healthy patients, with healing in 6 to 8 weeks with nonoperative treatment
- High-risk fractures also have a good prognosis when they are diagnosed early and treated appropriately. Nonunion may develop and often requires open reduction and internal fixation with bone grafting.

Troubleshooting

- In patients with stress fractures resistant to conservative treatment, it is imperative to ascertain whether compliance is an issue. Many patients with stress fractures are highly driven athletes who may continue to participate in athletics despite pain.
- In patients with a history of multiple stress fractures, causative factors must be delineated including an appropriate laboratory workup to rule out metabolic abnormalities.
- Despite operative treatment, there is a risk of completion of fracture or refracture if activity is resumed too quickly.

Patient Instructions

- Patients should be instructed to discontinue offending activities. For athletes for whom continued conditioning is crucial, they may participate in alternative low-impact training, such as water running or cycling. For the high-risk stress fractures, including those of the navicular and proximal fifth metatarsal, patients must be informed that there is a significant risk of nonunion.

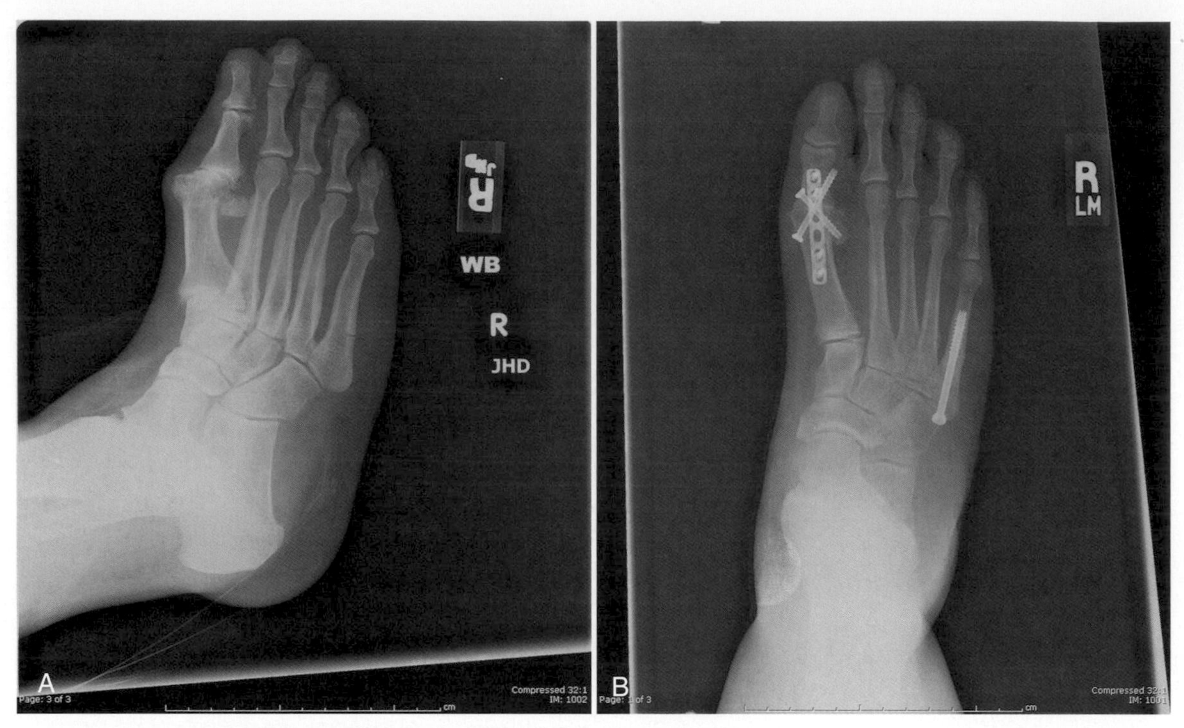

Figure 195-3 **A**, Oblique radiograph of the foot in a patient with severe first metatarsophalangeal joint arthritis and recent onset of atraumatic lateral foot pain demonstrates a fracture line of the proximal fifth metatarsal. The patient had been walking with an altered gait to unload the great toe, thus transferring force to the lateral side of the foot. **B**, Anteroposterior radiograph after operative fixation of the fifth metatarsal stress fracture and first metatarsophalangeal arthrodesis.

Considerations in Special Populations

- High-level athletes may require more aggressive treatment to allow for a faster return to activity and continued conditioning.
- Patients with suspected endocrinopathy should be referred for appropriate diagnostic testing and treatment.
- Diabetic patients will frequently require longer periods of treatment due to a slowed healing response.

Suggested Reading

- Boden BP, Osbahr DC: High-risk stress fractures: Evaluation and treatment. J Am Acad Orthop Surg 2000;8:344–353.
- Gehrmann RM, Renard RL: Current concepts review: Stress fractures of the foot. Foot Ankle Int 2006;27:750–757.
- Khan KM, Fuller PJ, Brukner PD, et al: Outcome of conservative and surgical management of navicular stress fracture in athletes. Eighty-six cases proven with computerized tomography. Am J Sports Med 1992;20:657–666.
- Konkel KF, Menger AG, Retzlaff SA: Nonoperative treatment of fifth metatarsal fractures in an orthopaedic suburban private multispecialty practice. Foot Ankle Int 2005;26:704–707.
- Korpelainen R, Orava S, Karpakka J, et al: Risk factors for recurrent stress fractures in athletes. Am J Sports Med 2001;29:304–310.
- Wall J, Feller JF: Imaging of stress fractures in runners. Clin Sports Med 2006;25:781–802.

Chapter 196 Ankle Fractures

Robert E. Meehan

ICD-9 CODES

824 *Ankle Fracture*
845.01 *Deltoid Ligament Rupture*
845.03 *Syndesmotic Ligament Rupture*

Key Concepts

- Ankle fractures are generally the result of a rotational or angular force on the foot relative to the leg.
- The ankle joint is highly conforming and must transmit large forces over a small surface area. Any abnormal shift of the talus relative to the tibia alters joint pressures and will result in arthrosis.
- It is important to differentiate between stable and unstable ankle fractures. Treatments, surgical or nonsurgical, are based on ankle stability.

History

- Twisting, noncontact injury; less commonly, direct trauma
- Stable fracture: often able to bear weight on the extremity with some discomfort
- Unstable fracture: unable to bear weight on the injured limb; may have an obvious deformity that requires immediate attention, such as reduction

Physical Examination

- Observation
  - Ecchymosis and swelling
  - Fracture blisters may develop later and are a sign of significant soft-tissue trauma. Serum-filled blisters are a sign of superficial skin damage, whereas blood-filled blisters are typically a sign of deeper, more severe soft-tissue injury (Fig. 196-1).
  - Open wounds indicative of an open or compound fracture
  - Deformity or gross malalignment may indicate the presence of fracture-dislocation.
- Palpation
  - Tenderness over the fractured medial and/or lateral malleoli. The medial ankle gutter may be tender if the deltoid ligament has been injured.
- Range of motion
  - Gentle manipulation of the ankle may reveal gross instability and thus an unstable injury.
- Special tests
  - Associated neurovascular injuries are rare but should be ruled out with a careful examination.
  - Compartment syndrome is occasionally associated with high-energy fractures, and if it is suspected on the clinical examination, pressures should be measured (see Chapter 15).

Imaging

- Radiographs: anteroposterior, lateral, and mortise views of the ankle
  - Look for fracture lines and displacement.
  - Mortise view (true anteroposterior view of the ankle) obtained with the foot in 15 to 20 degrees

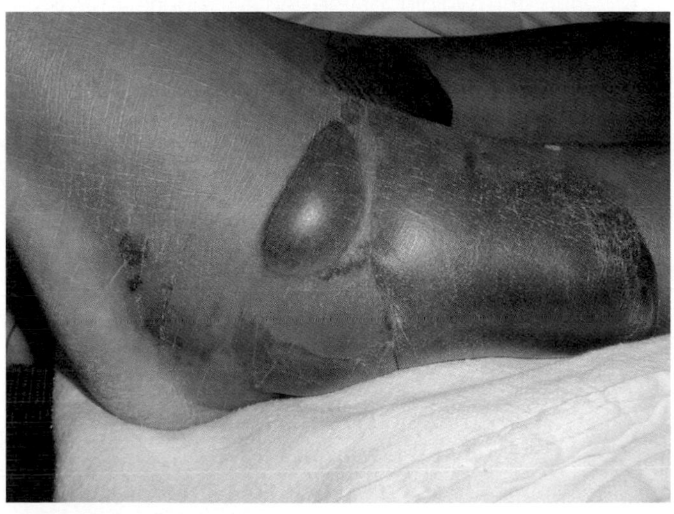

Figure 196-1 Blood-filled fracture blisters are indicative of a deep, dermal soft-tissue injury.

of internal rotation; asymmetry of the clear space, such as medial widening, indicative of injury

- Stress radiographs: mortise view with foot externally rotated
  - Obtained when it is unclear whether the deltoid ligament has been disrupted; medial clear space greater than 3 mm typically an indication of deltoid ligament incompetence
- Computed tomography
  - Quantifies the size of a posterior malleolar fragment in relation to the distal tibial articular surface; helpful for surgical planning (Fig. 196-2)
  - Identifies osteochondral fractures of the talus
- Magnetic resonance imaging
  - Typically not helpful

Differential Diagnosis

- Ankle sprain
- Syndesmotic injury
- Maisonneuve fracture
- Osteochondral fracture of the talus
- Tarsal bone fracture/dislocation

Treatment

- At diagnosis
  - The ankle is placed in a well-padded, posterior molded splint and elevated to heart level.
  - Subluxations or frank dislocations are reduced by pulling in-line traction with the deformity. Quigley's traction involves hanging the great and second toes from a weighted IV pole and allowing the position of the ankle (plantarflexion and inversion) and the weight of the leg to reduce the ankle. The ankle is splinted in situ to hold the reduction (Fig. 196-3).
  - Open wounds are dressed with povidone-iodine–soaked gauze. The tetanus immunization is updated, and intravenous antibiotics appropriate for the grade of wound are given (Table 196-1).
- Later
  - Definitive management is by surgical or closed methods (Table 196-2).
    - — The primary indications for surgery are unstable bi- or trimalleolar injuries and isolated displaced fractures of the medial malleolus (Fig. 196-4).
    - — Surgery is rarely indicated for an isolated fibula fracture without ligamentous injuries (deltoid or syndesmotic) (Fig. 196-5).

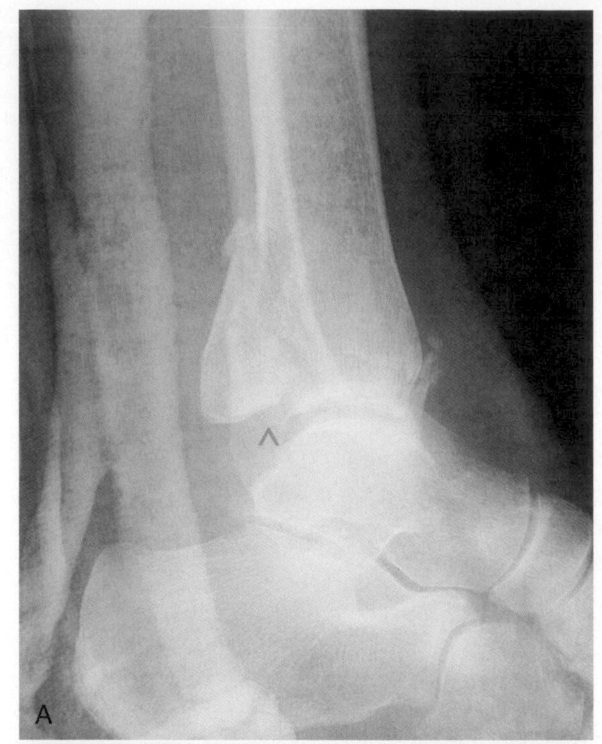

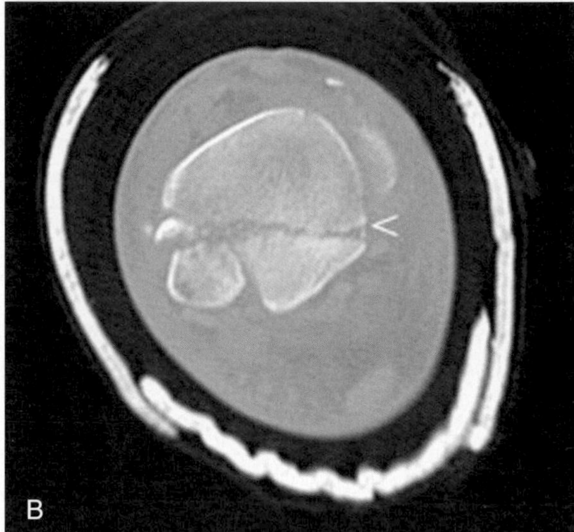

Figure 196-2 **A**, Lateral radiograph of a large, displaced posterior malleolar fracture, part of a trimalleolar injury. **B**, Computed tomography demonstrates the large posterior malleolar fragment (*arrowhead*) involving more than 25% of the articular surface.

- Nondisplaced/stable fractures can be treated safely with a short leg walking cast for 4 to 6 weeks and then conversion to a removable cast or brace for the next 4 to 6 weeks.
  - — Monthly radiographs are used to monitor healing.

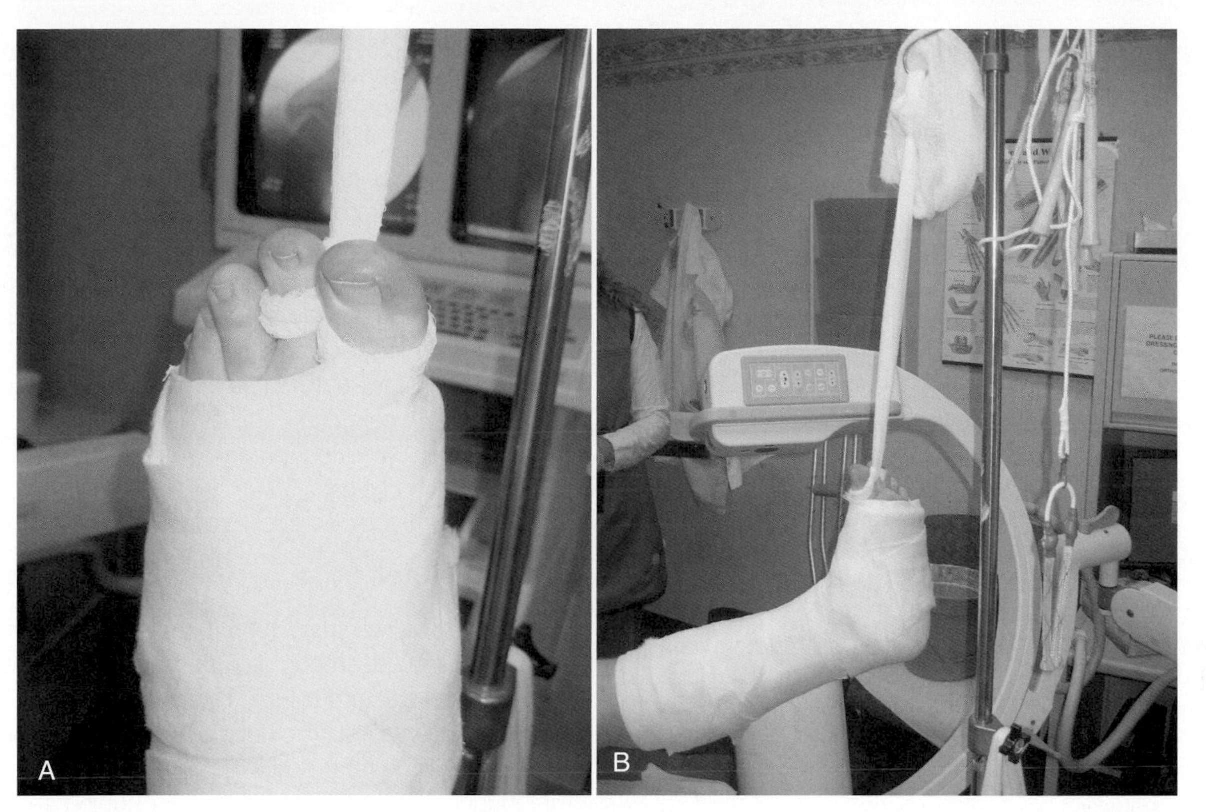

Figure 196-3 **A**, Quigley's traction involves hanging the toes with Kerlix gauze. **B**, The toes are hung from a weighted IV pole, allowing the weight of the leg to reduce the fracture. The ankle is splinted in situ (plantarflexion and inversion) to hold the reduction.

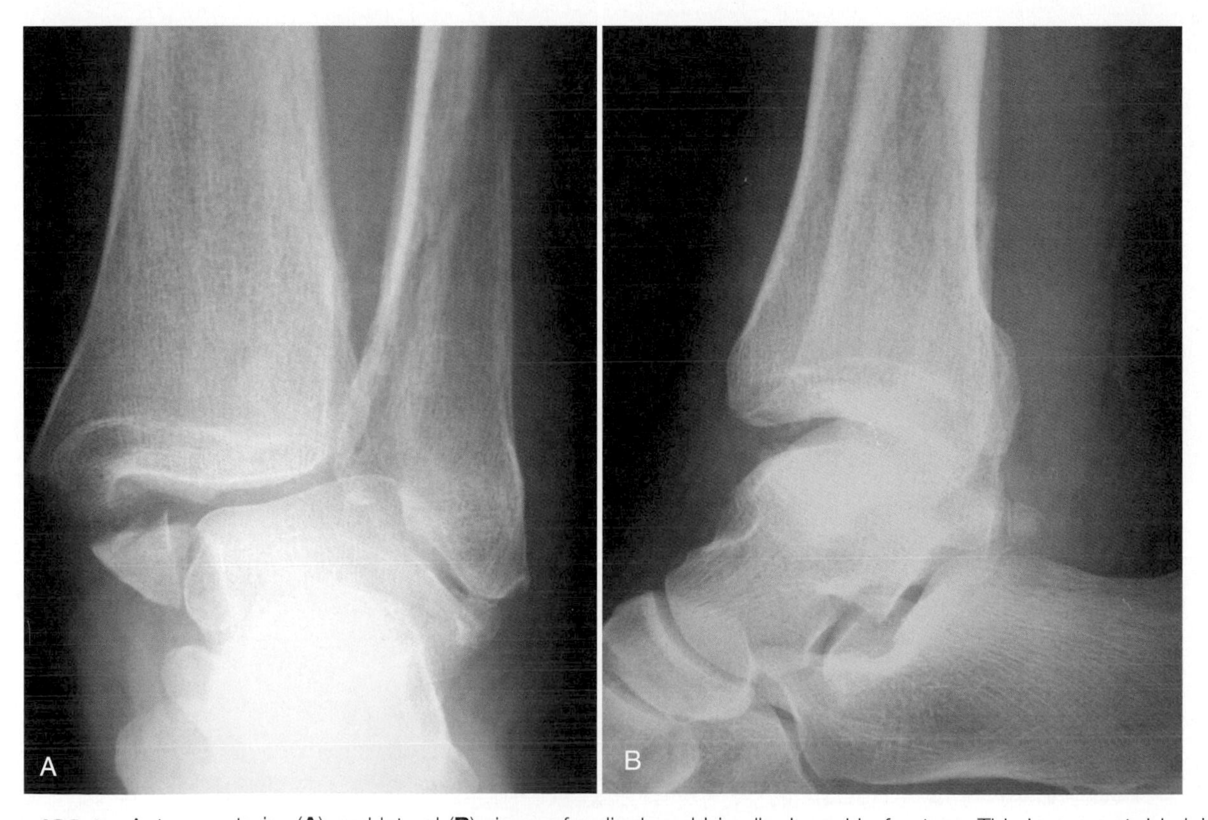

Figure 196-4 Anteroposterior (**A**) and lateral (**B**) views of a displaced bimalleolar ankle fracture. This is an unstable injury.

TABLE 196-1 *Open Fracture Antibiotic Treatment Algorithm*

Type	Wound Size	Antibiotic
I	<1 cm	Cephalosporin first-generation
II	1–10 cm	Cephalosporin first-generation
III	>10 cm	Cephalosporin first-generation and gentamicin
Anaerobic contaminant		Add penicillin, clindamycin, or metronidazole (Flagyl)

TABLE 196-2 *Examples of Stable and Unstable Ankle Fractures*

Stable	Unstable
Isolated lateral malleolus without deltoid or syndesmotic disruption	Lateral malleolus with deltoid and/or syndesmotic disruption
Isolated nondisplaced medial or posterior malleolus	Isolated displaced (>2 mm) medial or posterior malleolus
	Bi- or trimalleolar fracture
	Deltoid and syndesmotic disruption (i.e., Maisonneuve injury with a high fibular fracture)

- Displaced/unstable fractures should be internally fixed. Even when anatomically reduced, these tend to re-displace and therefore should be treated surgically.
  - Surgical fixation can be performed immediately, as in the case of an open or irreducible fracture.
  - More often, closed fractures can be reduced, splinted, and referred to an orthopaedic surgeon for operative treatment.
  - Surgical treatment is often delayed (as long as 1–2 weeks) until soft-tissue swelling is reduced (skin wrinkles present) and fracture blisters have healed.

When to Refer

- Unstable ankle fractures (bimalleolar, trimalleolar, deltoid, or syndesmotic disruption) should be referred for surgical treatment (Fig. 196-6).
- Isolated displaced fractures of the medial malleolus should also be referred for surgical fixation due to the high incidence of delayed union/nonunion secondary to periosteum interposed in the fracture site with closed treatment.

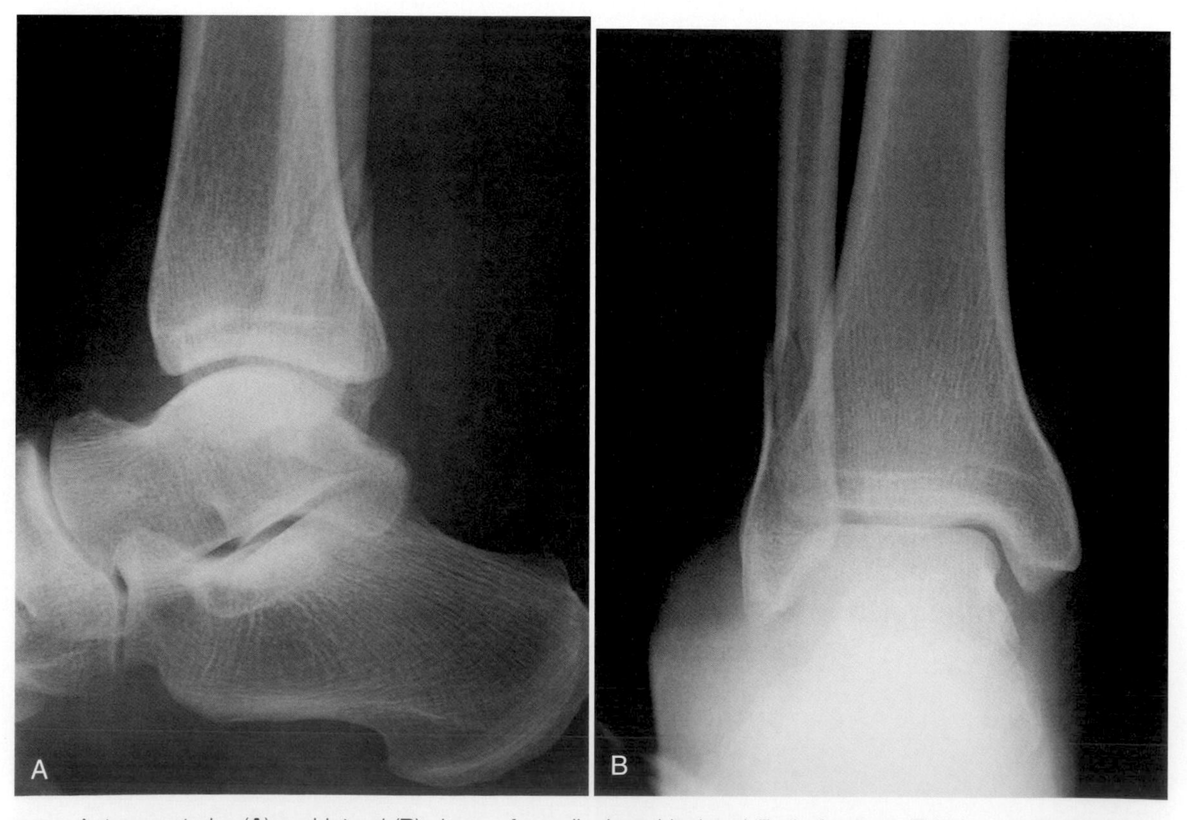

Figure 196-5 Anteroposterior (**A**) and lateral (**B**) views of nondisplaced isolated fibula fracture. This is a stable injury and does not require operative intervention.

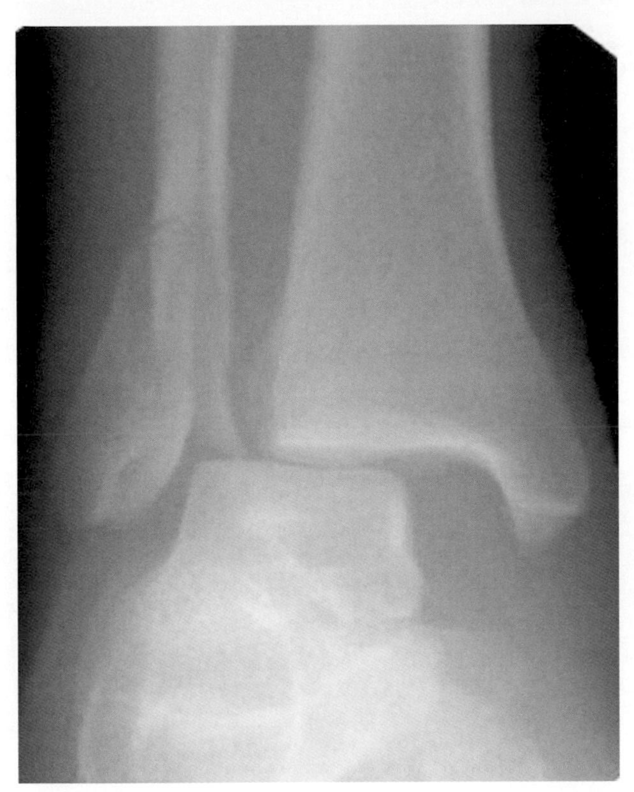

Figure 196-6 Mortise radiograph of a bimalleolar equivalent fracture. The deltoid and syndesmotic ligaments are ruptured. This is an unstable ankle injury and will require operative intervention.

Prognosis

- Good to excellent results can be expected for 80% to 90% of all ankle fractures.
- Stable, nonoperative fractures fair better overall, mainly because the injury sustained was less severe.
- Some unstable fractures, ankle fractures-dislocations in particular, treated operatively have unrecognized or untreatable injuries to the articular cartilage and result in early posttraumatic arthritis.

Troubleshooting

- Unstable ankle fractures treated without surgery have a high risk of malunion, nonunion, stiffness, chronic pain, and early posttraumatic arthritis.
- The inherent risks of any fracture surgery include wound infection or dehiscence; damage to nerves, blood vessels, or tendons; nonunion; malunion; failure of hardware; the need for hardware removal; chronic pain; stiffness; posttraumatic arthritis; and the general risks of anesthesia.
- The benefits of surgery for an unstable fracture far outweigh these risks, and surgery is highly recommended to restore stability, expedite fracture healing, and improve functional outcome.

Patient Instructions

- Elevation of the injured extremity at heart level is recommended to help control swelling.
- Weight-bearing restrictions must be strictly obeyed.
  - Unstable injuries require non–weight-bearing limitations, whereas stable fractures are allowed to bear weight as tolerated and not risk further damage.

Considerations in Special Populations

- Patients with diabetes mellitus, neuropathy, and medical comorbidities such as peripheral vascular disease present a challenge to the treating orthopaedist, with higher rates of wound complications and mechanical failure.
- The elderly and patients with osteoporosis present difficulties with surgical fixation and skin closure secondary to poor bone and soft-tissue quality.
- Care of these special populations is best handled by an orthopaedic surgeon for stable or unstable injuries.

Suggested Reading

- Belcher GL, Radomisli TE, Abate JA, et al: Functional outcome analysis of operatively treated malleolar fractures. J Orthop Trauma 1997;11:106–109.
- Egol KA, Amirtharajah M, Tejwani NC, et al: Ankle stress test for predicting the need for surgical fixation of isolated fibular fractures. J Bone Joint Surg Br 2004;86B:2393–2398.
- Giordano CP, Koval KJ. Treatment of fracture blisters: A prospective study of 53 cases. J Orthop Trauma 1995;9:171–176.
- Jones KB, Maiers-Yelden KA, Marsh JL, et al: Ankle fractures in patients with diabetes mellitus. J Bone Joint Surg Br 2005;87B:489–495.
- Lantz BA, McAndrew M, Scioli M, et al: The effect of concomitant chondral injuries accompanying operatively reduced malleolar fractures. J Orthop Trauma 1991;5:125–128.
- Pankovich AM: Fractures and dislocations of the ankle. In Perry CR, Elstrom JA, Pankovich AM (eds): The Handbook of Fractures. New York: McGraw-Hill, 1995, pp 290–303.
- Raasch WG, Larkin JJ, Draganich LF: Assessment of the posterior malleolus as a restraint to posterior subluxation of the ankle. J Bone Joint Surg Am 1992;74A:1201–1206.
- Ramsey PL, Hamilton W: Changes in tibiotalar area of contact caused by lateral talar shift. J Bone Joint Surg Am 1976;58A:356–357.

Chapter 197 Tarsal Fractures

Robert E. Meehan

ICD-9 CODES
825.21 *Talus (Astragalus) Fracture*
825.0 *Calcaneus Fracture*
825.22 *Navicular Fracture*
825.23 *Cuboid Fracture*

Key Concepts

- The tarsal bones play a key role in transmitting forces from the ankle to the foot.
- Functionally, the tarsal joints account for the extremes of sagittal motion at the ankle (dorsiflexion/plantarflexion) and are the major location for side-to-side (inversion/eversion) motion.
- The four bones that make up the tarsus (the talus, calcaneus, navicular, and cuboid) are unique in the types of fractures that they sustain and their mechanism of injury.
- Dislocations associated with tarsal fractures must be promptly reduced to prevent pressure necrosis on areas of tented skin.
- Overall, surgical management of displaced tarsal fractures is successful in restoring anatomy and healing the fracture. However, some loss of hindfoot motion should be expected, and heavy labor jobs may not be advised.

History

- Typically fall from height or motor vehicle accident
- Talus fractures: forced dorsiflexion of the foot against the tibia
  - Talar neck fractures most common (50%) (Fig. 197-1)
  - Excessive dorsiflexion ruptures the posterior ankle capsule and may result in subluxation/dislocation of the talar body from the ankle or subtalar joint.
- Calcaneal fractures: axial loading injury with direct impact to the plantar heel (Fig. 197-2)
- Navicular fractures: twisting injury (Fig. 197-3)
- Cuboid fractures: violent abduction of the forefoot on the hindfoot
  - Often termed nutcracker fractures with compression of the lateral wall of the cuboid (Fig. 197-4)
  - Uncommon

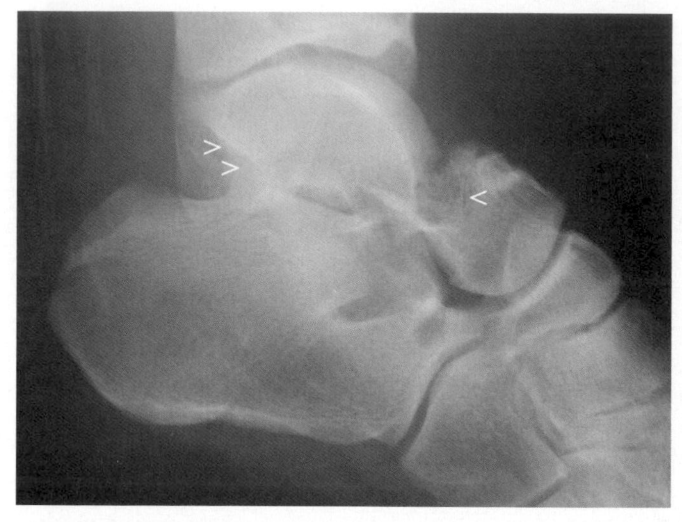

Figure 197-1 Displaced talar neck fracture (*single arrowhead*) with subluxation of the subtalar joint (*double arrowhead*).

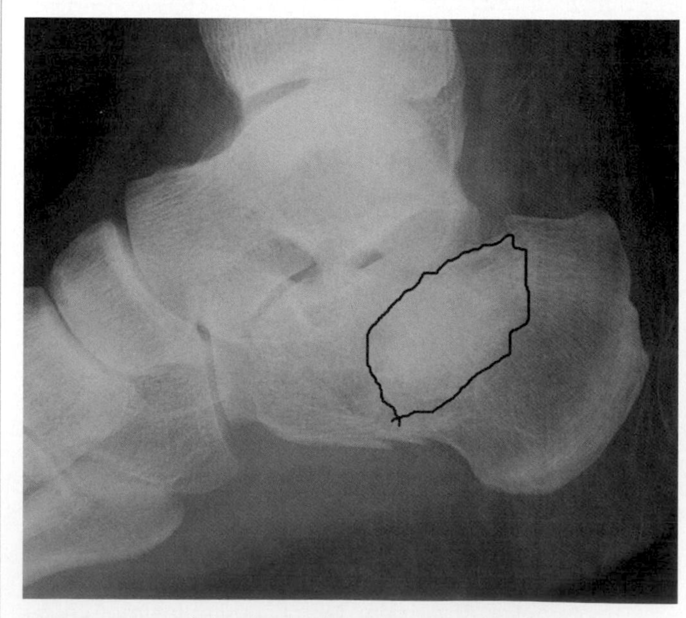

Figure 197-2 Joint depression–type calcaneus fracture. The posterior facet (*outlined in black*) has been depressed and rotated into the calcaneal body.

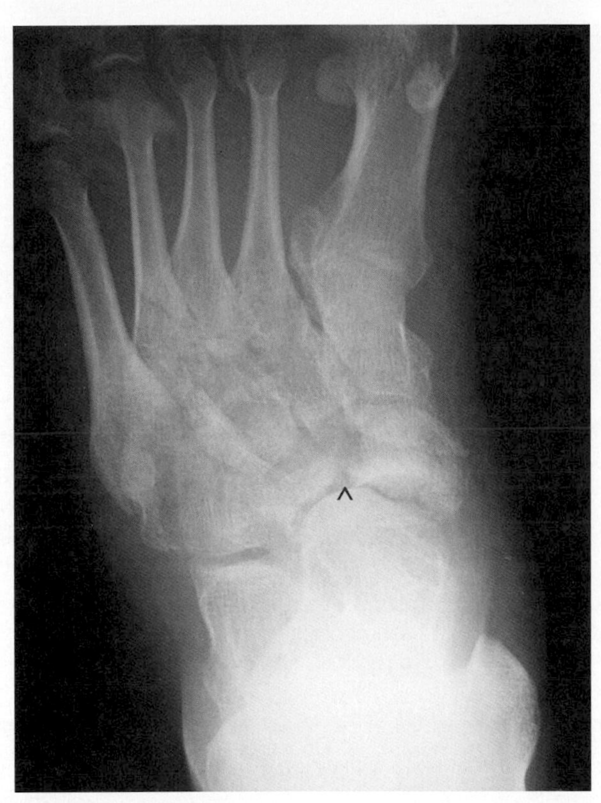

Figure 197-3 Navicular fracture (*arrowhead*) involving the lateral half of the navicular body.

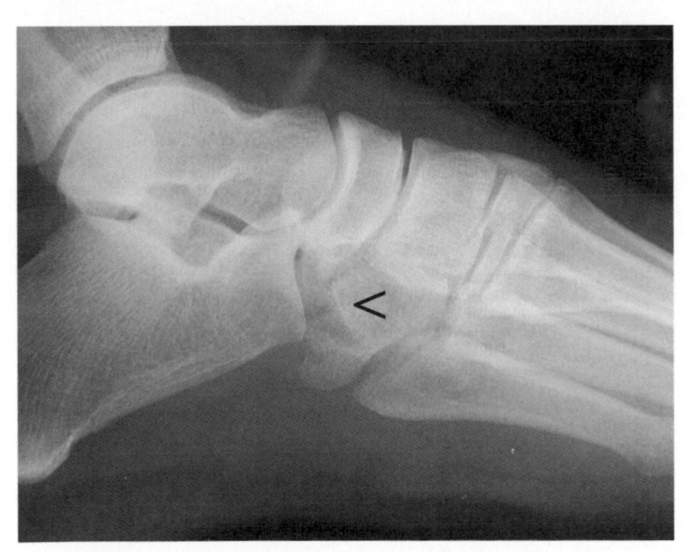

Figure 197-4 Depressed joint surface (*arrowhead*) in an isolated cuboid fracture.

Physical Examination

- Observation
  - Swelling, fracture blisters, ecchymosis (hindfoot and plantar)
  - Open wounds, indicative of open fracture
  - Deformity or gross malalignment of the hindfoot may indicate a fracture/dislocation.
- Palpation
  - Tenderness in the hindfoot or over the specific tarsal bone fractured
  - Squeeze test identifies occult or stress fracture of the calcaneus; compression of the medial and lateral sides of the calcaneus elicits pain if a fracture is present.
- Special tests
  - Associated neurovascular injuries are rare but should be ruled out with careful examination.
  - Compartment syndrome of the foot is occasionally associated with high-energy crush injuries. If suspected on clinical examination, pressures should be measured.
  - Occult injuries of the thoracolumbar spine need to be ruled out because they have been associated with tarsal bone fractures.

Imaging

- Radiographs: anteroposterior, lateral, and oblique views of the foot and ankle
  - To identify fracture lines and displacement
  - Canale/Kelly view (talus): modified anteroposterior view of the foot; allows visualization of the talar neck and evaluates for displacement
  - Harris/axial view (calcaneus): useful in evaluating the calcaneal tuberosity for angulation and shortening
  - Broden's view (calcaneus): lateral radiograph with the foot internally rotated and the beam focused on the sinus tarsi; evaluates for displacement of the posterior and middle facet joints
- Computed tomography
  - Necessary for all tarsal fractures; axial, sagittal, and semicoronal images give useful information about fracture pattern and extent of comminution (Fig. 197-5)

Differential Diagnosis

- Ankle sprain or fracture
- Osteochondral lesion of the talus
- Subtalar or Chopart's joint dislocation
- Lisfranc joint injury

Treatment

- At diagnosis
  - Subluxations or frank dislocations are reduced by flexing the knee (relaxes the Achilles tendon) and pulling in-line traction with the deformity.

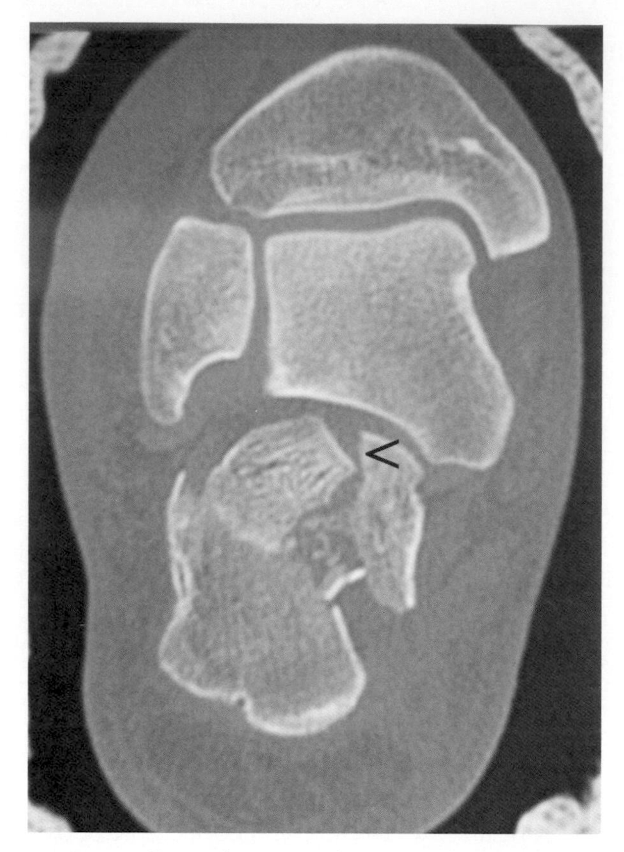

Figure 197-5 Coronal computed tomography image of a joint depression calcaneus fracture. The lateral half of the posterior facet (*arrowhead*) is displaced and rotated.

- After closed reduction, the foot is placed in a well-padded posterior molded splint and elevated to heart level.
- If the fracture is irreducible, immediate open reduction is indicated to prevent pressure necrosis on compromised skin and further damage to the articular cartilage.
- Open wounds are dressed with povidone-iodine–soaked gauze. The tetanus immunization is updated, and IV antibiotics are given appropriate for the grade of wound.

- Later
  - Definitive management is dependent on the fracture type. In general, nondisplaced fractures are treated with non–weight-bearing immobilization for 6 weeks, followed by a removable walking cast for an additional 4 weeks.
    — Early range of motion may prevent excessive ankle/subtalar stiffness.
    — Radiographs should be monitored to ensure absence of displacement.
    — Displaced fractures are typically treated with open reduction and internal fixation.
  - Talar neck fracture may require as much as 10 weeks of non-weight bearing.

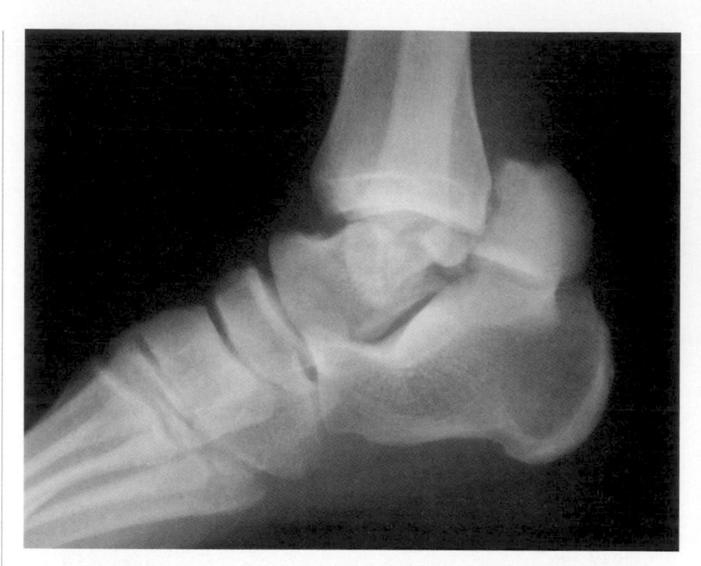

Figure 197-6 Talar neck fracture with a dislocation of the talar body. Emergent surgical reduction is recommended to prevent further soft-tissue compromise.

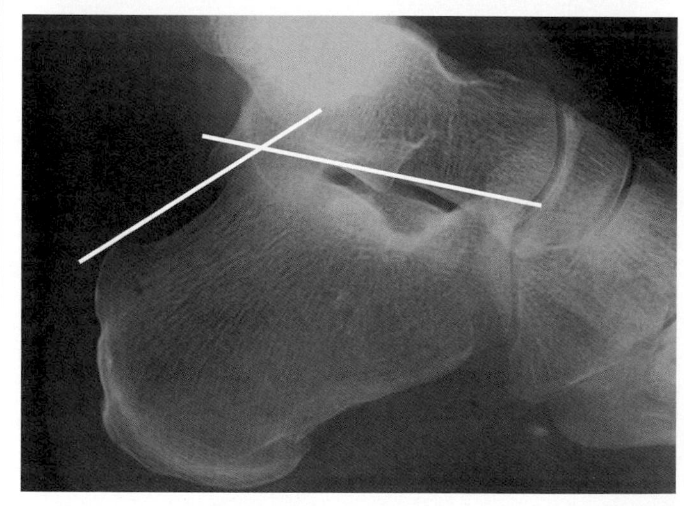

Figure 197-7 Lateral view of a normal calcaneus. A normal Bohler's angle (20–40 degrees) is drawn where the white lines intersect.

    — Talar neck fractures with dislocation of the talar body are an emergency and require immediate surgical reduction (Fig. 197-6).
  - Calcaneus fracture: Fractures with a Bohler's angle greater than 20 degrees are treated nonoperatively (Fig. 197-7).
    — Surgical treatment of displaced fractures has a high wound complication rate (10% to 40%).
    — Patients with drug/alcohol addiction, mental illness, or neurologic disorders may be unable to cooperate with postoperative protocols and are probably better treated nonoperatively.

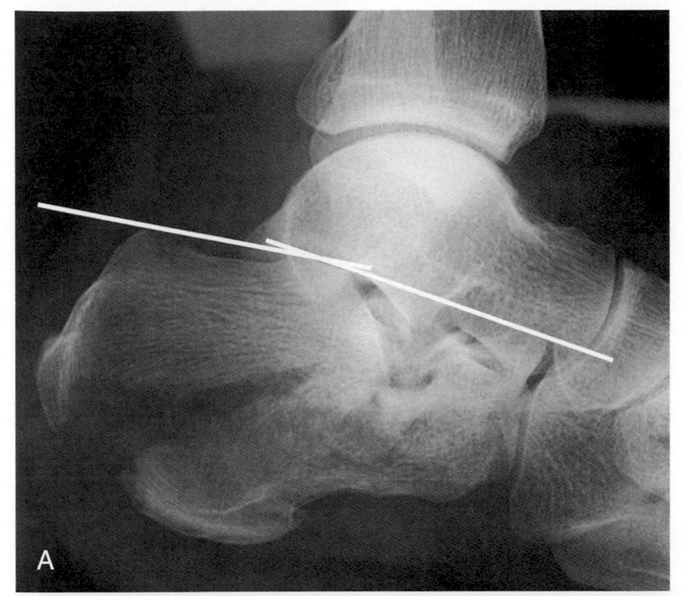

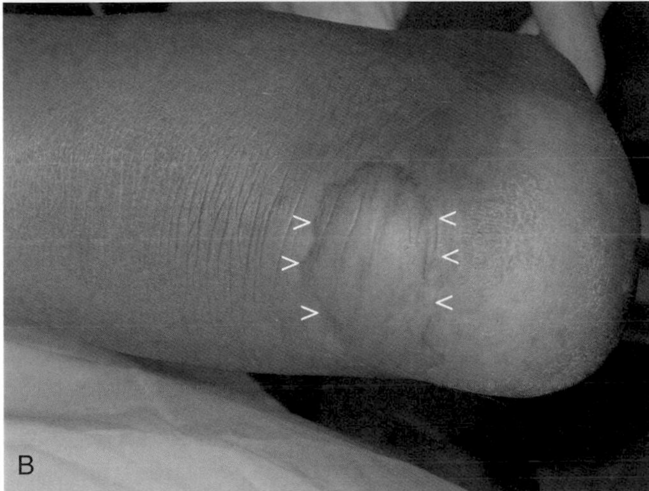

Figure 197-8 **A**, Displaced tongue-type calcaneus fracture with flattening of Bohler's angle (indicated by crossed *white lines*). **B**, Posterior heel blister (*arrowheads*) developed immediately after an unreduced tongue-type fracture.

- — Nicotine use, diabetes, and peripheral vascular disease are also relative contraindications to surgery.
  — Severely displaced tongue-type fractures require immediate surgical attention to prevent devastating skin problems (skin necrosis/ulceration) on the posterior heel (Fig. 197-8).
- Navicular fracture: Dorsal chip fractures (capsular avulsion most common) and minimally displaced tuberosity fractures (avulsion of the posterior tibial tendon) are treated nonoperatively. Body fractures (least common) or displaced tuberosity fractures require open reduction and internal fixation (Fig. 197-9).

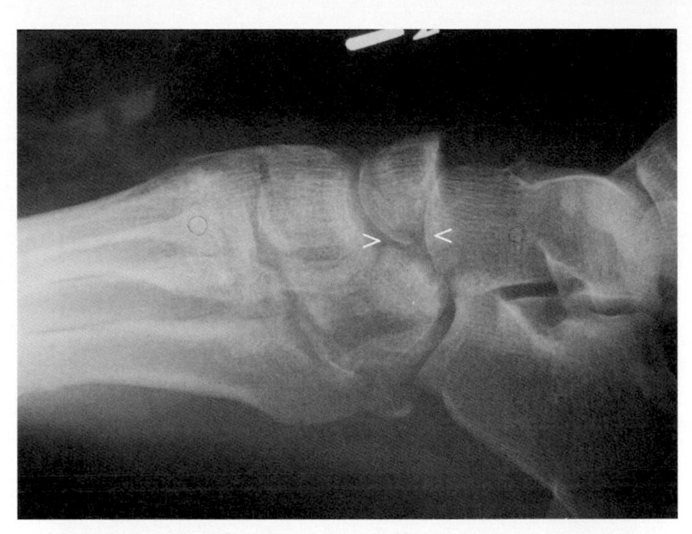

Figure 197-9 Fracture of the navicular body (*arrowheads*) with dorsal subluxation at the talonavicular joint.

- Cuboid fracture: Failure to surgically treat displaced fractures can result in lateral column shortening (pes planus deformity) and painful arthritis (Fig. 197-10).

When to Refer

- All injuries to the tarsal bones can be referred to an orthopaedist. However, some nondisplaced fractures of the tarsal bones, such as the navicular chip fracture, can be safely treated by a general practitioner using the management guidelines outlined previously.

Prognosis

- The outcomes for nondisplaced tarsal fractures are good. Patients may have occasional stiffness but are able to return to preinjury activities.
- The prognosis for displaced tarsal fractures is guarded, even with anatomic reduction.
  - Many patients develop chronic stiffness with restricted inversion/eversion. Posttraumatic arthritis may develop, resulting in the need for long-term treatment with bracing, nonsteroidal anti-inflammatory drugs, cortisone injections, and even surgical arthrodesis.
  - Many tarsal fractures occur in young male laborers, many of whom will never return to their previous line of work because they will no longer be able to "trust" their foot and navigate job sites that require climbing ladders or working at heights.

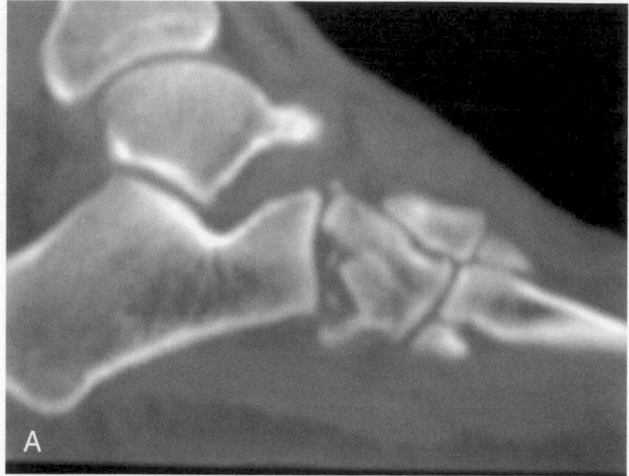

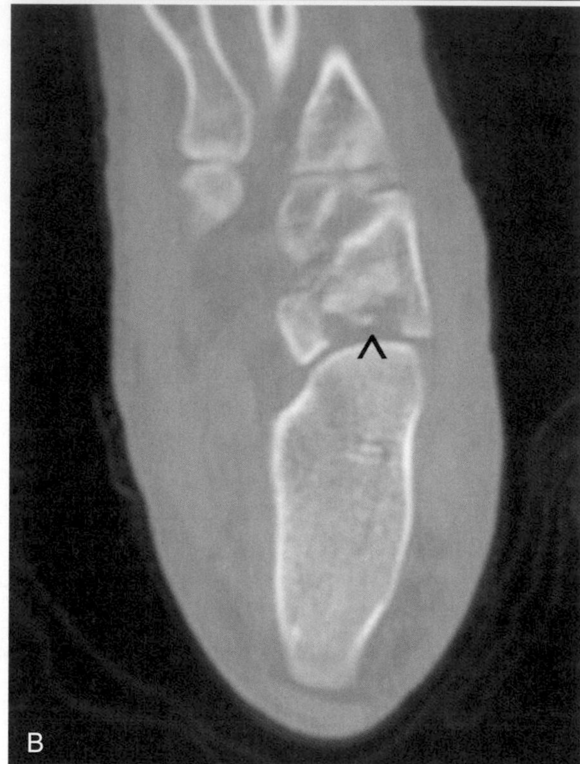

Figure 197-10 Sagittal (**A**) and axial (**B**) computed tomography images of a cuboid fracture with depression of the joint surface (*arrowhead*).

Troubleshooting

- Swelling of the foot/ankle and distortion of the anatomic prominences will make it difficult at times to clinically identify the specific injury. Imaging studies are crucial to the diagnosis.
- Displaced tarsal fractures treated without surgery have a high risk of malunion, nonunion, stiffness, chronic pain, and early posttraumatic arthritis.
- Although the risks of surgery remain high for certain populations, such as open reduction and internal fixation for a calcaneal fracture in high-risk patients, secondary reconstruction at a later date is easier and safer with a well-aligned foot.

Patient Instructions

- Elevation of the injured foot at heart level is recommended to help control swelling.
- Weight-bearing restrictions must be strictly obeyed. Weight bearing on a displaced fracture may risk further damage to an already injured articular surface.

Considerations in Special Populations

- Patients with diabetes mellitus, neuropathy, and medical comorbidities, such as peripheral vascular disease, present a challenge to the treating orthopaedist with higher rates of wound complications and mechanical failure.
- In the diabetic patient, a tarsal bone fracture or dislocation may be the first sign of an evolving neuropathic (Charcot's arthropathy) joint. These patients often present with a painless, yet severely swollen ankle/foot and deny any trauma. These patients should be referred to an orthopaedist for definitive management.

Suggested Reading

- Buckley RE, Tough S: Displaced intra-articular calcaneal fractures. J Am Acad Orthop Surg 2004;12:172–178.
- Buckley R, Tough S, McCormack R, et al: Operative compared with nonoperative treatment of displaced intra-articular calcaneus fractures: A prospective, randomized, controlled multicenter trial. J Bone Joint Surg Am 2002;84A:1733–1744.
- DiGiovanni CW: Fractures of the navicular. Foot Ankle Clin 2004;9:25–63.
- Fortin PT, Balazsy JE: Talus fractures: Evaluation and treatment. J Am Acad Orthop Surg 2001;9:114–127.
- Kanlic E, Clayton PR: Foot injuries. In Perry CR, Elstrom JA, Pankovich AM (eds): The Handbook of Fractures. New York: McGraw-Hill, 1995, pp 310–333.
- Mihalich RM, Early JS: Management of cuboid crush injuries. Foot Ankle Clin 2006;11:121–126.
- Sangeorzan BJ, Benirschke SK, Mosca V, et al: Displaced intra-articular fractures of the tarsal navicular. J Bone Joint Surg Am 1989;71A:1504–1510.
- Vallier HA, Nork SE, Barei DP, et al: Talar neck fractures: Results and outcomes. J Bone Joint Surg Am 2004;86A:1616–1624.

Chapter 198 Metatarsal Fractures

Scott Van Aman and M. Truitt Cooper

ICD-9 CODE
825.25 *Metatarsal Fracture*

Key Concepts

- Most metatarsal fractures may be treated nonoperatively with excellent results.
- The fifth metatarsal is most commonly fractured, usually by an avulsion of the base as the result of a twisting injury.
- The goal of treatment is to maintain alignment of all five metatarsals to preserve longitudinal and transverse arches of the foot and normal weight-bearing distribution under the metatarsal heads.
- The first and fifth metatarsals are most important for weight bearing, and malalignment is poorly tolerated.
- The history is important to rule out a previous stress fracture.
- High-risk fractures include the proximal fifth metatarsal, first metatarsal shaft, proximal second metatarsal (Lisfranc joint injury), and multiple fractures of the middle metatarsals.

History

- Multiple injury mechanisms include falls, direct crush injuries, and indirect twisting injuries of the leg with the forefoot fixed. Avulsion fractures of the base of the fifth metatarsal may result from the supination mechanism.
- Severe trauma may lead to multiple fractures.
- Swelling, pain, and ecchymosis
- Usually able to bear some weight, except in cases of severe trauma

Physical Examination

- Observation
  - Gait
  - Swelling, ecchymosis
  - Deformity, including rotation and angulation of toes
  - Check for open wounds.
- Palpation
  - Determine the area of maximum tenderness.
  - Careful sensory and vascular examinations
  - Palpate the hindfoot and ankle to rule out additional injuries.
- Range of motion
  - Must range toes; pain out of proportion to what would be expected on passive extension of toes, in conjunction with massive swelling, may indicate compartment syndrome
  - Ankle range of motion

Imaging

- Radiographs: weight-bearing (if possible) anteroposterior, lateral, and 45-degree oblique views
  - Usually sufficient to diagnose fracture
  - Check alignment of second metatarsal base with middle cuneiform to rule out Lisfranc joint injury.
  - Occasionally, a nondisplaced fracture will not appear for more than 2 weeks on plain radiographs.
- Advanced imaging
  - Computed tomography scan only indicated for complex intra-articular fractures
  - Magnetic resonance imaging and bone scan rarely indicated for acute injuries; more commonly used with stress fractures

Differential Diagnosis

- Lisfranc joint injury: pain located at tarsometatarsal joint, exacerbated by pronating/supinating forefoot; may see fracture at base of second metatarsal
- Tendon rupture/avulsion: pain located over tendon insertion or tendon proper; weakness to resistance testing
- Stress fracture: prodromal pain present
- Charcot's arthropathy: patients with neuropathy (any type); erythema of foot that decreases with elevation

Treatment

- At diagnosis
  - Dependent on the metatarsal involved, location (head, neck, shaft, base), and displacement

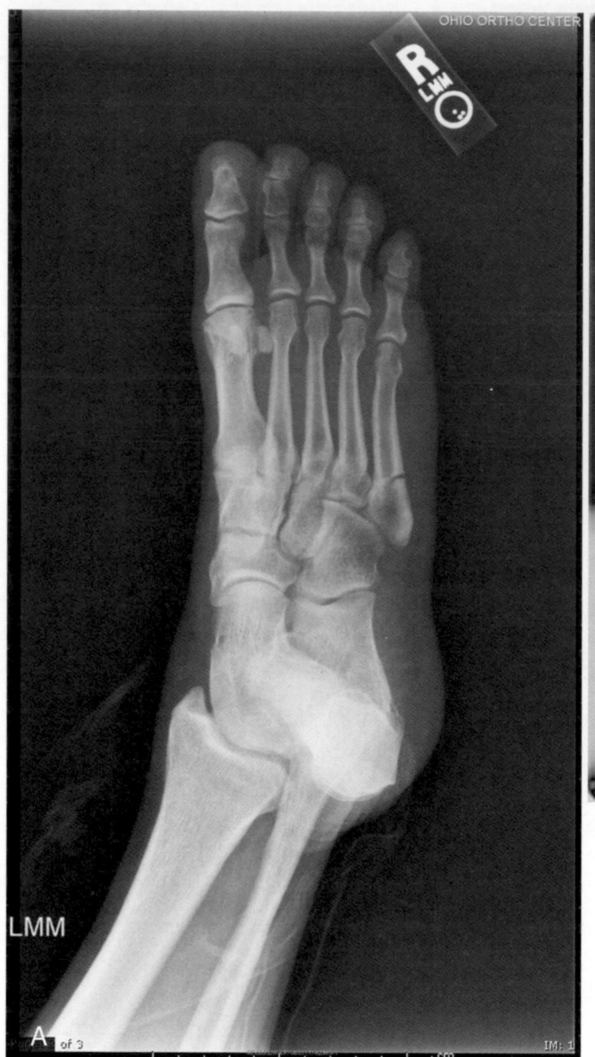

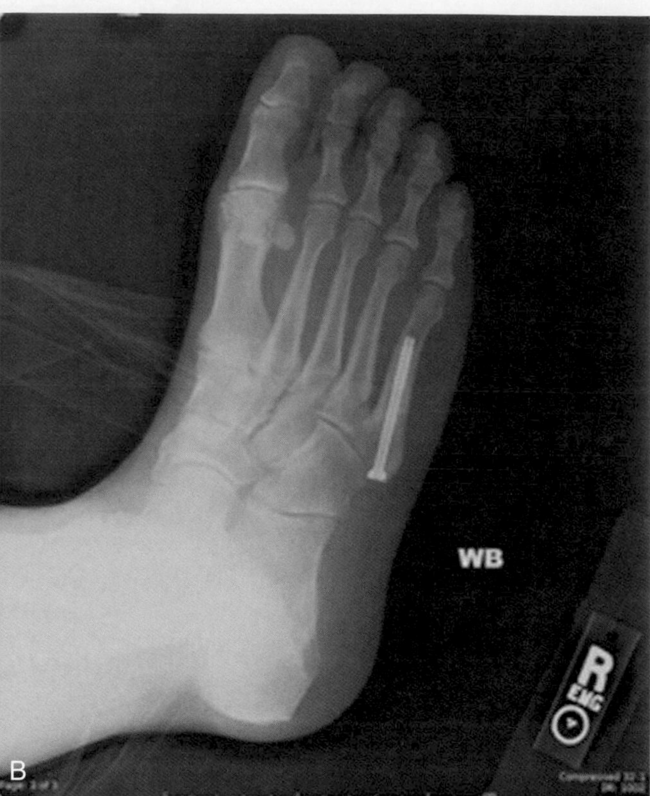

Figure 198-1 **A**, Anteroposterior radiograph of the foot displays a fracture of the fifth metatarsal at the junction of the diaphysis and metaphysis. **B**, Postoperative radiograph shows a healed fracture treated with an intramedullary screw.

- Treatment is primarily symptomatic and includes compressive wrapping with a hard-soled shoe and weight bearing as tolerated for 5 to 6 weeks.
- If necessary, a fracture boot may be applied to further immobilize the foot.
- Close follow-up is recommended with early repeat radiographs to check for changes in alignment.
- Avulsions of the fifth metatarsal base should be treated with a walking cast or fracture boot with restricted weight bearing until the foot is completely pain free.

- Later
  - Rarely, metatarsal fractures go on to symptomatic malunion or nonunion, and surgical osteotomy, bone grafting, and internal fixation may be beneficial.

When to Refer

- Several fracture patterns require referral for surgical consideration.
  - Displaced fractures of the first or fifth metatarsal; may lead to abnormal loading patterns
  - Fractures of the proximal fifth metatarsal (with the exception of small avulsions); high risk of nonunion; frequently treated with intramedullary screw fixation (Fig. 198-1)
  - Multiple metatarsal shaft or neck fractures: treated with percutaneous wires or plate and screw constructs
  - Possible Lisfranc joint injury: fixed with screws or fusion of the tarsometatarsal joints depending on the extent of injury

- Intra-articular fractures of the proximal or distal first metatarsal; may lead to posttraumatic arthritis; fixation frequently includes plate and screw constructs

Prognosis

- Generally good, especially for isolated mid–metatarsal shaft fractures
- Appropriate management of neck fractures, as well as first and fifth metatarsal fractures, should also lead to a good outcome.
- Although good outcomes can be anticipated for fifth metatarsal base avulsion fractures, it may be several months before a return to preinjury activity level
- Intra-articular fractures may lead to posttraumatic arthritis.
- Missed Lisfranc joint injuries may lead to devastating arthritic collapse of the arch of the foot.

Troubleshooting

- Patients should be counseled on the risks associated with certain fractures as discussed previously.
- Surgical risks include bleeding, infection, superficial nerve injury, and hardware irritation.

Patient Instructions

- Patients should be counseled on the nature of their injury.
- They should be instructed in the importance of ice and elevation in the acute period in an effort to reduce swelling.
- For most fractures other than isolated mid-metatarsal shaft fractures, patients should be instructed in appropriate crutch use and the importance of non-weight bearing on the affected limb to allow for proper healing.

Considerations in Special Populations

- Diabetic patients require longer periods of treatment due to delayed healing, even in young patients.
  - Fractures may precipitate Charcot's arthropathy.
  - Malalignment is poorly tolerated as altered weight bearing predisposes the patient to the development of skin ulceration.
- High-level athletes/dancers may benefit from surgical fixation.
- Patients with previous or recurrent stress fractures may also benefit from surgical fixation.

Suggested Reading

- Egol K, Walsh M, Rosenblatt K, et al: Avulsion fractures of the fifth metatarsal base: A prospective outcome study. Foot Ankle Int 2007;28:581–583.
- Fetzer GB, Wright RW: Metatarsal shaft fractures and fractures of the proximal fifth metatarsal. Clin Sports Med 2006;25:139–150.
- Jones R: Fracture of the base of the fifth metatarsal bone by indirect violence. Ann Surg 1902;35:697–700.
- Kell IP, Glisson RR, Fink C, et al: Intramedullary screw fixation of Jones fractures. Foot Ankle Int 2001;22:585–589.
- Petrisor BA, Ekrol I, Court-Brown C: The epidemiology of metatarsal fractures. Foot Ankle Int 2006;27:172–174.
- Reese K, Litsky A, Kaeding C, et al: Cannulated screw fixation of Jones fractures. A clinical and biomechanical study. Am J Sports Med 2004;32:1736–1742.
- Sanders RW, Papp S: Fractures of the midfoot and forefoot. In Coughlin MJ, Mann RA, Saltzman CL (eds): Surgery of the Foot and Ankle, 8th ed. Mosby: Philadelphia, 2007, p 2199.
- Schenck RC, Heckman JD: Fractures and dislocations of the forefoot: Operative and non-operative treatment. J Am Acad Orthop Surg 1995;3:70–78.

Chapter 199 Phalangeal Fractures of the Foot

Alan C. League

ICD-9 CODES

826.0 *Fracture of One or More Phalanges of Foot, Closed*

826.1 *Fracture of One or More Phalanges of Foot, Open*

Key Concepts

- Phalangeal fractures are caused by the toe striking an object or being crushed by a falling object.
- Low-energy closed injuries are the most common.
- More severe injuries can occur as a result of being run over by a vehicle or lawnmower.
- The fifth digit is most commonly injured.
- Nonoperative treatment is the rule for most toe phalanx fractures.
- The hallux is most likely to cause long-term impairment; operative treatment may be necessary in some fractures.

History

- Pain and swelling after direct trauma to toe

Physical Examination

- Observation
  - Inspect the nail for signs of injury.
  - Degree of swelling
  - Ecchymosis is often found distant to the zone of injury as blood migrates along tissue planes.
  - Skin integrity
  - Angular deformity
- Palpation
  - Sites of tenderness
  - Palpate the entire foot and ankle to rule out additional fractures or dislocations.
- Range of motion
  - Check for pain and stiffness at all metatarsophalangeal (MTP) joints and interphalangeal joints to help isolate the zone of injury.

Imaging

- Radiographs: anteroposterior, lateral, and oblique views of the toes (Fig. 199-1)
  - To prevent superimposing toes on lateral radiographs, the affected toe may be manually elevated above the remaining toes.

Differential Diagnosis

- Freiberg's infraction: osteonecrosis of the second metatarsal head seen on an anteroposterior radiograph
- Nail bed injury: hematoma under the nail, normal radiographs (unless associated with distal phalanx fracture)
- Ingrown toenail, paronychia: erythema, drainage at nail folds; normal radiographs
- Metatarsalgia: pain located in the ball of the foot; normal radiographs
- MTP joint synovitis: subacute history; joint deviation on radiographs with no fracture

Treatment

- At diagnosis
  - Immobilize in a stiff, open, postoperative shoe and buddy tape to adjacent toe (Fig. 199-2)

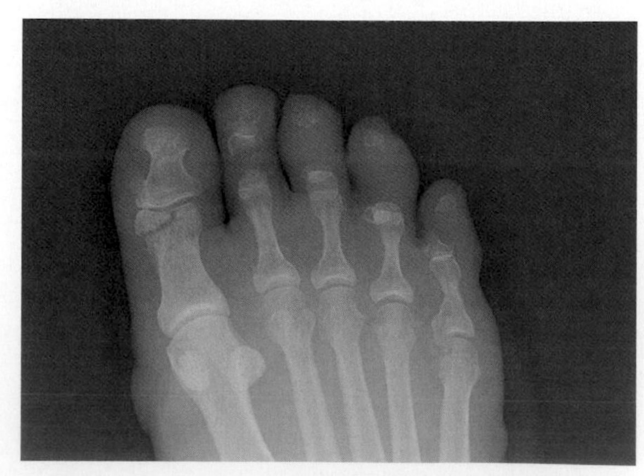

Figure 199-1 Hallux intra-articular phalangeal fracture with lesser toe middle phalanx dissociations after a forklift crush injury.

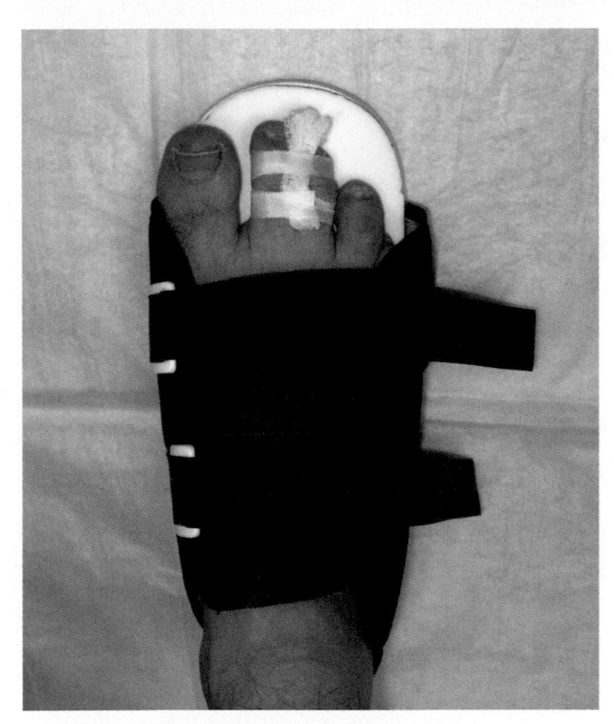

Figure 199-2 Buddy taping of second and third toes with foot in a stiff-soled postoperative shoe.

- Later
  - Transition to athletic shoes when tenderness and swelling allow, usually 2 to 4 weeks

When to Refer

- Fractures with obvious angular deformity (such as an overlapping toe), open fractures, intra-articular fractures of the MTP joint, displaced fractures of the hallux, and other associated injuries to the foot and ankle should be referred.

Prognosis

- Return to full function is expected in the majority of these injuries; however, patients should be warned that some degree of long-term swelling and stiffness is common.

Patient Instructions

- Patients may bear weight as tolerated, but should decrease the level of activity.
- Crutches may be helpful for several days if pain is severe.
- Elevate the foot several times daily to limit swelling.
- Use buddy taping and a postoperative shoe to maintain immobilization.
- Expect swelling to persist for several months, even after full function is regained.

Considerations in Special Populations

- Diabetics must be very cautious with the use of buddy tape to avoid ulceration.
  - To avoid maceration, a layer of gauze should be placed between the tape and skin and between the toes.
  - The tape should not be tight and should be changed daily to allow inspection of the skin.
  - Buddy taping should not be used in insensate diabetics.

Suggested Reading

- Bucholz RW, Heckman JD (eds): Rockwood and Green's Fractures in Adults: Rockwood, Green, and Wilkins' Fractures, 5th ed. Philadelphia: Lippincott Williams & Wilkins, 2001.
- Coughlin MJ, Mann RA, Saltzman CL (eds): Surgery of the Foot and Ankle, 8th ed. St. Louis: Mosby, 2006.

Chapter 200 Ankle Aspiration and/or Injection Technique

Nicholas R. Seibert and Anish R. Kadakia

CPT CODE

20605 *Arthrocentesis, Aspiration and/or Injection; Intermediate Joint or Bursa*

Procedure Name

- Ankle aspiration (arthrocentesis) and injection

Equipment

- 25-gauge needle if local anesthesia planned
- Injection needle (21 gauge)
- Large-bore aspiration needle (16–18 gauge)
- Stopcock, optional for combined aspiration and injection
- Injection syringe (5–10 mL)
- Aspiration syringe (10–20 mL)
- Local anesthetic agent
- Sterile cup and/or appropriate laboratory tubes for aspiration
- Sterile tray
- Sterile gloves
- Sterile prep solution (i.e., povidone-iodine)
- Ethyl chloride, optional
- Injectable agent (e.g., steroid, local anesthetic agent)
- Sterile gauze and bandage

Indications

- Aspiration
  - Suspected joint infection
  - Gouty arthritis
  - Large painful effusion
  - Loss of motion secondary to effusion
- Injection
  - Osteoarthritis
  - Rheumatoid arthritis
  - Crystalloid deposition disease

Contraindications

- Aspiration
  - Generalized sepsis without evidence of infected joint
- Injection
  - Active or recent joint infection
  - Overlying skin disease
  - Impending surgical procedure

Technique

- Verbal consent is obtained from the patient, and the correct limb is identified.
- The medication is prepared on a sterile tray with a stopcock and extra syringe available if aspiration is indicated.
- Ethyl chloride, if used, should be administered topically before sterile skin preparation.
- With sterile gloves in place, the skin is prepared with a sterile prep solution (Fig. 200-1).

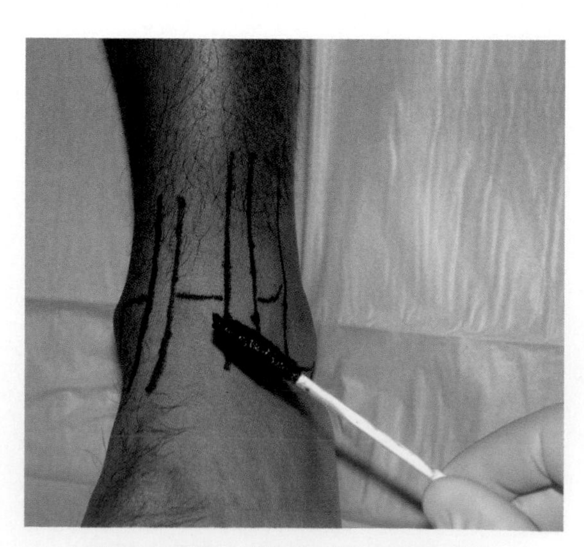

Figure 200-1 Sterile skin preparation.

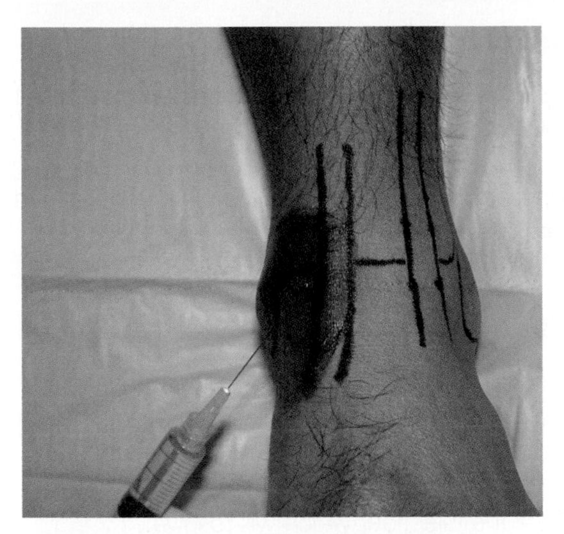

Figure 200-2 Local anesthetic is administered subcutaneously.

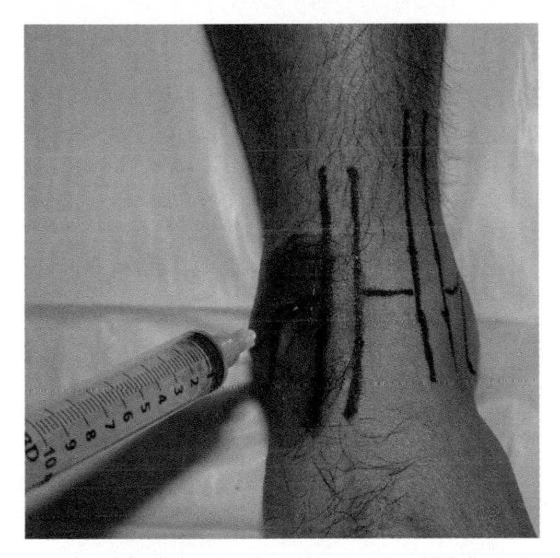

Figure 200-3 Medial entry is between the tibialis anterior tendon and the medial malleolus.

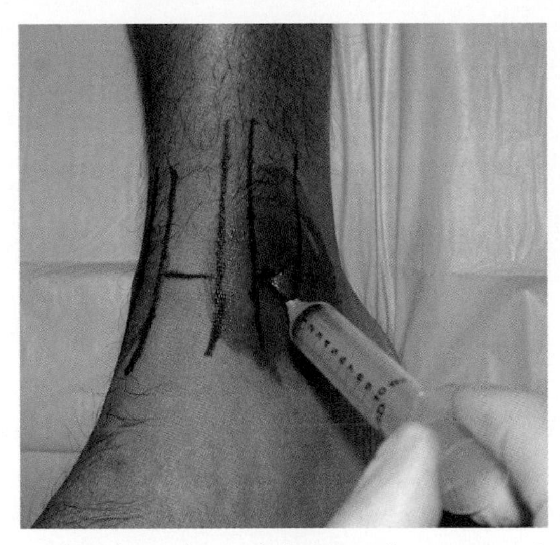

Figure 200-4 Lateral entry is between the peroneus tertius tendon and the lateral malleolus.

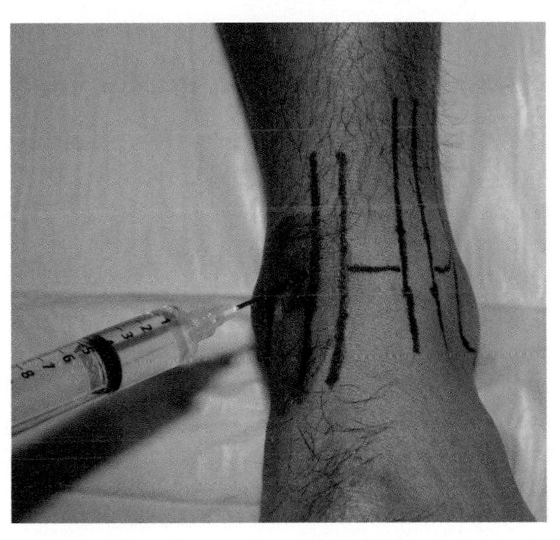

Figure 200-5 The plunger is gently withdrawn to aspirate the joint space.

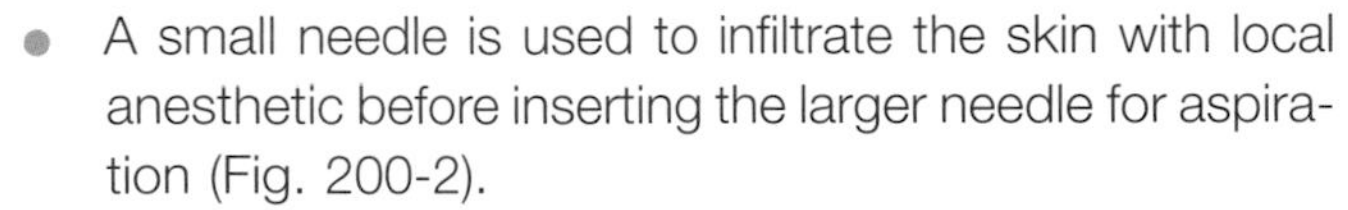

- A small needle is used to infiltrate the skin with local anesthetic before inserting the larger needle for aspiration (Fig. 200-2).
- A large-bore aspiration needle is passed into the ankle between the anterior border of the medial malleolus and the tibialis anterior tendon at the level of the joint line (Fig. 200-3).
  - Alternatively, the ankle may be entered laterally between the anterior border of the lateral malleolus and the peroneus tertius and extensor digitorum longus tendons at the level of the joint line (Fig. 200-4).
- After feeling the needle pass into the joint capsule, aim across the joint to facilitate the procedure. Attempting to place the needle posteriorly between the tibia and talus is difficult and can damage the articular surface.
  - Gentle pressure is applied to the plunger of the syringe to aspirate the fluid (Fig. 200-5).
- Using a stopcock will allow the same needle to be used for the injection after the aspiration is complete.
- After ensuring that the needle tip is unobstructed and in place inside the joint capsule, turn the stopcock and inject the steroid or local anesthetic preparation.
  - Alternatively, the injection can be done without the use of a stopcock by using a second needle and syringe (Fig. 200-6).
- Apply dressing per routine

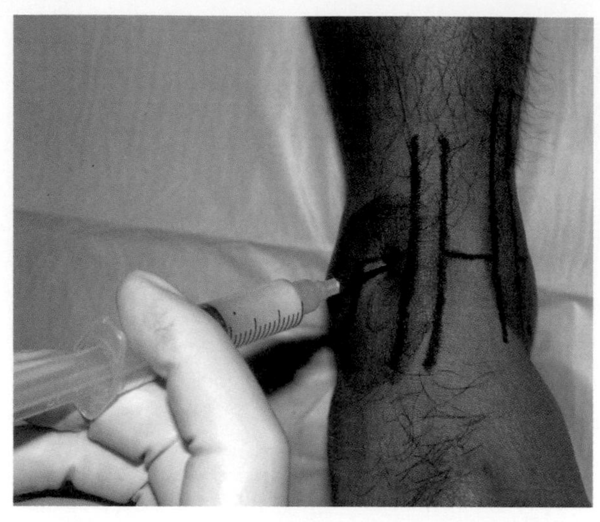

Figure 200-6 Injection of corticosteroid.

Considerations in Special Populations

- Injury to the terminal branches of either the saphenous nerve or the superficial peroneal nerve is possible.
- Atrophy can occur with subcutaneous injection of the corticosteroid.
- Skin discoloration can occur in darker-skinned individuals.
- If joint infection is suspected, synovial fluid obtained during aspiration should be sent for cell count with differential, crystal analysis, Gram stain, and aerobic/anaerobic cultures, and steroid injection is avoided.

Troubleshooting

- "Bumping" bone: Gently redirect the needle into the joint space.
- No fluid on aspiration: Make sure that you are in the synovial capsule and push the plunger back in to clear any obstructions in the needle tip.

Patient Instructions

- The dressing can be removed the following day.
- Use ice to treat any local soreness at the injection site.
- Some patients have worsening pain for 3 to 5 days after the injection, which will resolve.
- The physician's office should be contacted immediately if any redness, warmth, increased swelling, severe increase in pain, fever, or chills develop.
- Diabetic patients may notice a slight transient elevation in the blood glucose level.

Suggested Reading

- Coughlin MJ, Mann RA (eds): Surgery of the Foot and Ankle, 8th ed. St. Louis: Mosby, 2006.
- Myerson MS (ed): Foot and Ankle Disorders. Philadelphia: WB Saunders, 2000.
- Tallia AF, Cardone DA: Diagnostic and therapeutic injection of the ankle and foot. Am Fam Physician 2003;68:1356–1362.
- Tehranzadeh J, Mossop EP, Golshan-Momeni M: Therapeutic arthrography and bursography. Orthop Clin North Am 2006;37:393–408.

Chapter 201 Tarsal Tunnel Injection

Jonathan Smerek

CPT CODE

90772 *Tarsal Tunnel Injection (Add -25 Modifier if Billing in Addition to EM Visit Code)*

Procedure Names

- Tarsal tunnel injection
- Posterior tibial nerve block

Equipment

- 25-gauge, 1.5-inch needle for injection
- 18-gauge needle for drawing up steroid and local anesthetic agent
- 5-mL injection syringe
- Short-acting local anesthetic agent without epinephrine
- Injectable steroid
- Sterile tray
- Povidone-iodine swabs and alcohol swabs for sterile prep solution
- Sterile gloves
- Ethyl chloride, optional
- Sterile gauze
- Sterile dressing

Indications

- Compliant patient with documented tarsal tunnel syndrome (see Chapter 182)
- Failure to improve with noninvasive conservative modalities, such as medially posted orthotics, shoe wear modifications, lifestyle modifications, and medications such as gabapentin (Neurontin) and pregabalin (Lyrica)

Contraindications

- Magnetic resonance imaging demonstrating a significant mass within the tarsal tunnel or significant fullness within the tunnel
- Active infection, sepsis, cellulitis, or open sores near the injection site
- Impending surgical procedure

Technique

- Verbal patient consent is obtained, and the correct ankle is identified.
- The patient is placed supine on the examination table with the affected extremity externally rotated to easily visualize and access the medial malleolus and posterior neurovascular structures.
- The medication is prepared on a sterile tray. In general, 2 mL of steroid and 3 mL of an injectable, short-acting anesthetic agent (without epinephrine) are used.
- The tip of the medial malleolus is palpated and marked. A horizontal line is drawn two fingerbreadths proximal to the medial malleolus to mark the site of injection on the medial border of the Achilles tendon (Fig. 201-1).
- Ethyl chloride, if used, should be administered topically before sterile skin preparation (Fig. 201-2).
- In general, the overlying skin is not anesthetized with an injection because this would require two injections that combined are as painful as one injection.

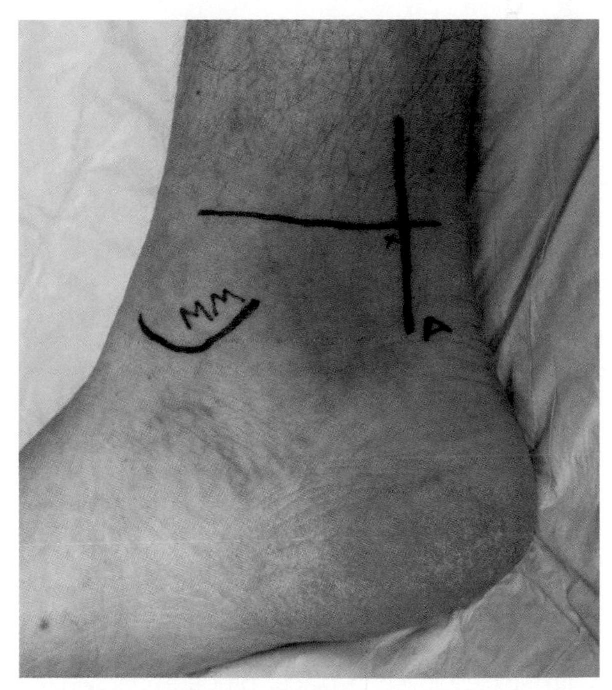

Figure 201-1 Landmarks, including the medial malleolus (MM), Achilles tendon (A), and *horizontal line* two fingerbreadths above the medial malleolus, are marked on the skin. The intersection of this line and the medial border of the Achilles tendon is the site of injection, marked with an *X*.

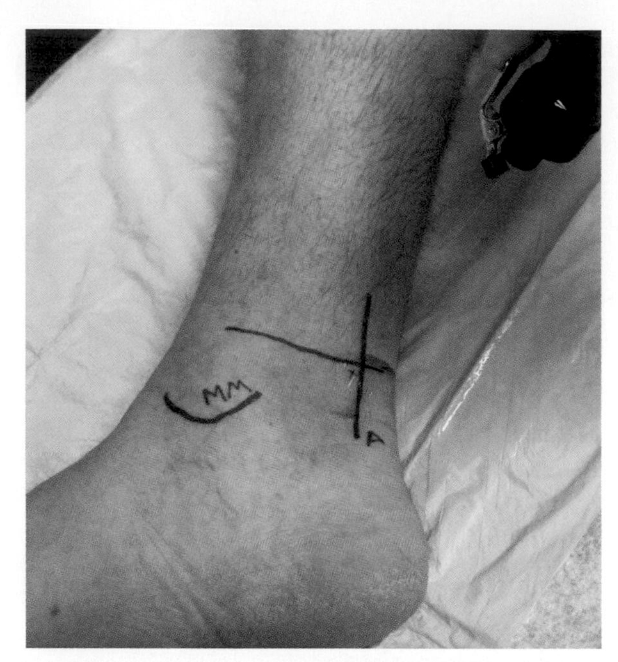

Figure 201-2 Application of ethyl chloride to topically anesthetize the skin before injection.

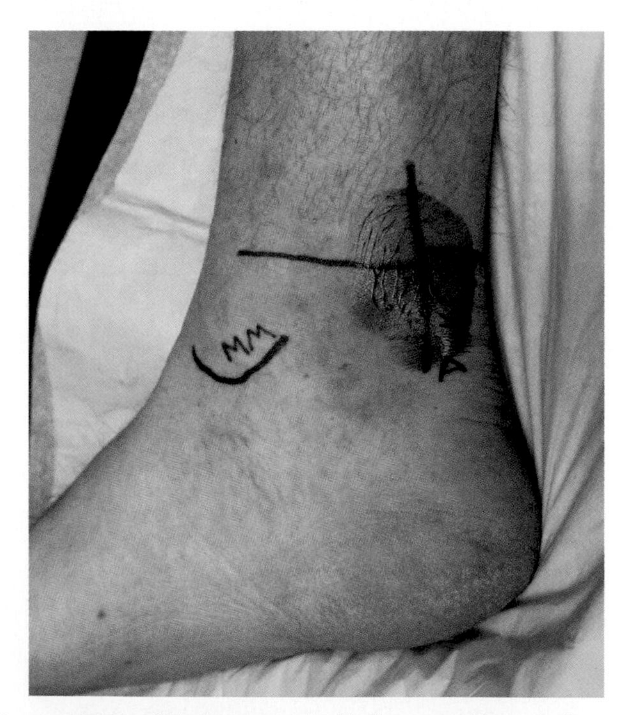

Figure 201-3 Skin is prepped with three povidone-iodine swabs, starting at the site of injection and moving circumferentially outward.

- With sterile gloves in place, prepare the skin with a sterile prep solution (Fig. 201-3).
- Insert the needle at the medial border of the Achilles tendon and advance the needle until the posterior cortex of the distal tibia is palpated (Fig. 201-4).

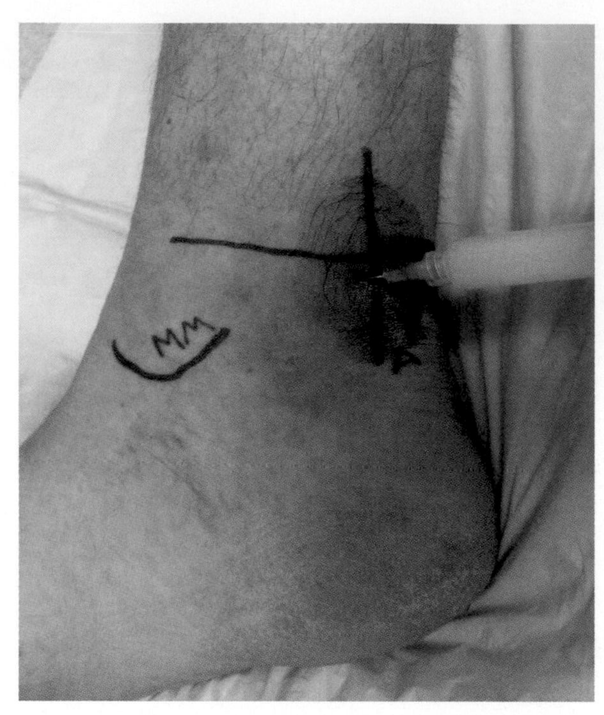

Figure 201-4 The needle is advanced until the posterior cortex of the tibia is encountered, and then the needle is withdrawn 2 to 3 mm and aspirated. If no blood is returned, the steroid mixture is injected.

- Withdraw the needle 2 or 3 mm and attempt to aspirate. If no blood is returned, inject the 5 mL of fluid around the posterior tibial nerve.
- If blood is aspirated or paresthesia is elicited, repeat the previous step.
- Withdraw the needle when finished and apply a sterile bandage.

Considerations in Special Populations

- In extremely obese individuals, a longer needle may be required.
- Pediatric patients should not undergo the injection due to pain and the extreme sensitivity of the ankle region.

Troubleshooting

- Make sure to aspirate before injection. A large amount of blood may indicate positioning in the posterior tibial artery or vein due to their close proximity (Fig. 201-5). Advance or withdraw a few millimeters and re-aspirate to avoid injecting a vascular structure.
- If, during injection, the patient experiences a shooting, electric shock sensation to the plantar aspect of the

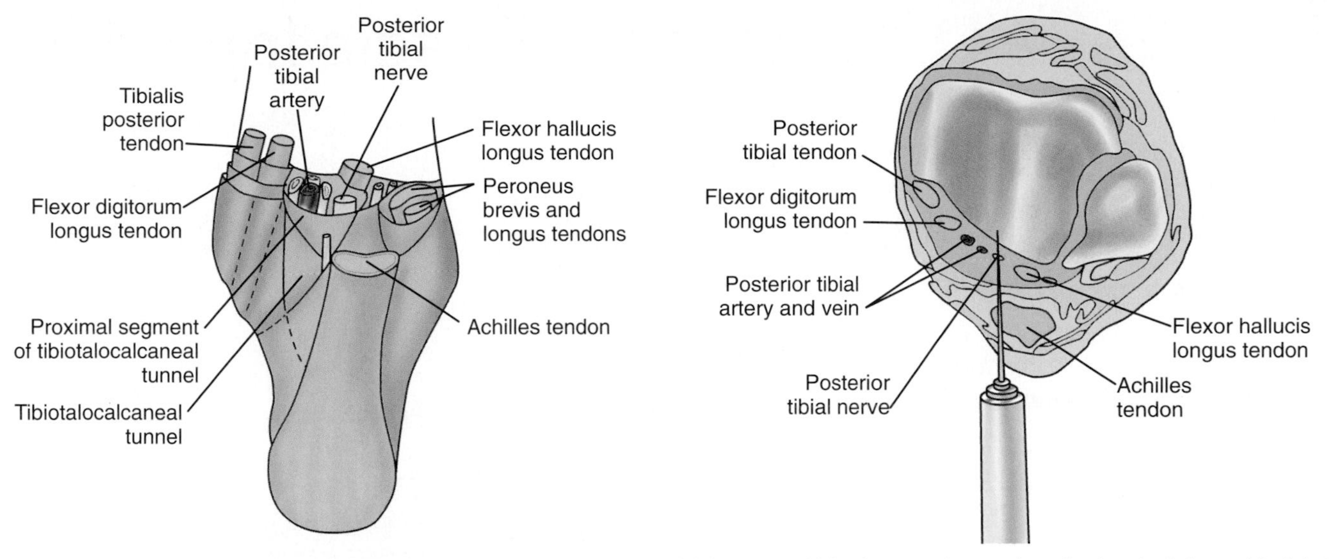

Figure 201-5 Illustration of injection around the posterior tibial nerve within the tarsal tunnel at the level of the ankle joint.

foot, stop injection immediately. The needle may be positioned intraneurally and needs to be redirected.

- The injection should proceed fairly easily with minimal resistance.
- Always redirect the needle small distances (2–3 mm) and avoid withdrawing the needle completely from the skin and repuncturing the skin.

Patient Instructions

- The bandage can be removed the night of the injection.
- Soreness secondary to the injection may be present for 2 to 3 days and is typically most severe on the first postinjection day.
- Apply ice to the injection site for 20 minutes every other hour until resolution of the soreness.
- The physician's office should be called immediately if any redness, warmth, increased swelling, fever, or chills develops or there is a sudden increase in pain.
- Diabetic patients may notice a small increase in the usual blood glucose levels.

Suggested Reading

- Coughlin MJ: Peripheral anesthesia. In Coughlin MJ, Mann RA (eds): Surgery of the Foot and Ankle, 7th ed. St. Louis: Mosby, 1999, pp 139–142.
- Lau J I, Stavrou P: Posterior tibial nerve—primary. Foot Ankle Clin 2004;9:271–285.
- Mann RA: Diseases of the nerves. In Coughlin MJ, Mann RA (eds): Surgery of the Foot and Ankle, 7th ed. St. Louis: Mosby, 1999, pp 512–516.

Chapter 202 Plantar Fascia Injection

Chin Khoon Tan and Andrew Molloy

CPT CODE

20550 *Injection(s); Single Tendon Sheath, or Ligament, Aponeurosis (e.g., Plantar "Fascia")*

Procedure Name

- Plantar fascia injection

Equipment

- Injection syringe (5 mL)
- Injection needle (25 gauge)
- Local anesthetic agent: lidocaine (1%) or bupivacaine (0.25% or 0.5%)
- Corticosteroid (40 mg): triamcinolone acetonide (Kenalog) or methylprednisolone (Depo-Medrol)
- Sterile tray
- Sterile gloves
- Sterile prep solution (povidone-iodine)
- Sterile gauze and bandage

Indications

- Symptoms persist after more than 8 weeks of conservative management

Contraindications

- Infection

Technique

- Obtain verbal consent and identify the correct foot.
- Palpate and locate the most tender spot, usually the anterior aspect of the medial plantar calcaneus (Figs. 202-1 and 202-2).
- Prepare the injection equipment: Aspirate a mixture of 2 mL of local anesthetic agent and 1 mL of steroid (Figs. 202-3 to 202-5).
- Aseptic technique: The injection site is cleansed with appropriate topical antiseptic (e.g., povidone-iodine).
- The needle may be introduced from either the plantar aspect or the medial side of the calcaneus.

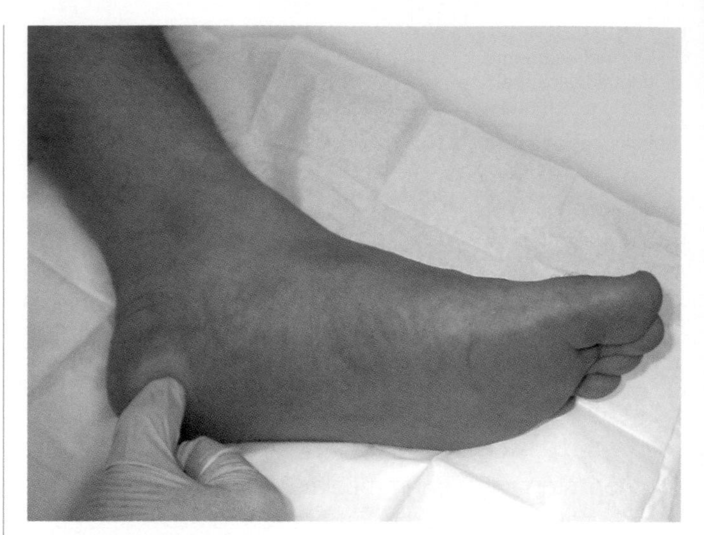

Figure 202-1 Locate the tender spot.

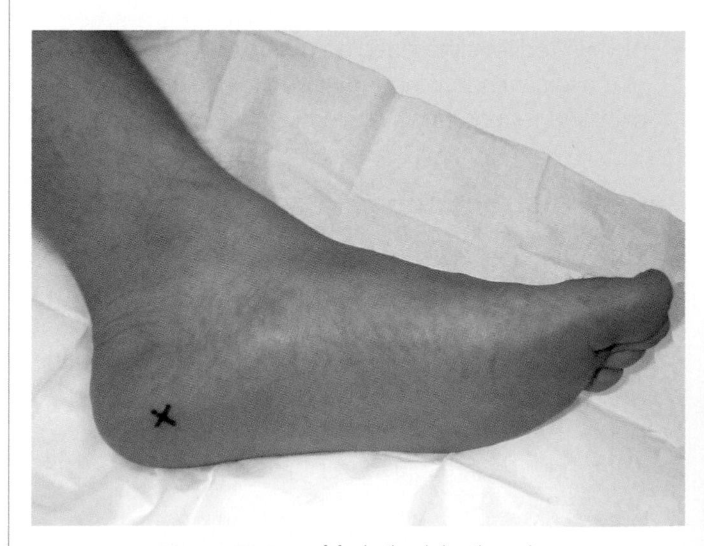

Figure 202-2 Mark the injection site.

- The needle is advanced until it reaches the medial plantar calcaneal tuberosity (Fig. 202-6).
- Avoid injecting within subcutaneous tissue, which may result in fat pad atrophy and necrosis, resulting in loss of shock absorption of the plantar heel.

Considerations in Special Populations

- Patients with coagulation disorders: see Troubleshooting section

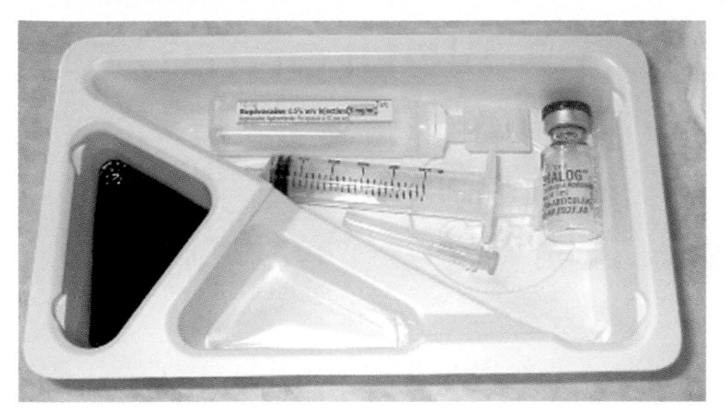

Figure 202-3 Injection equipment.

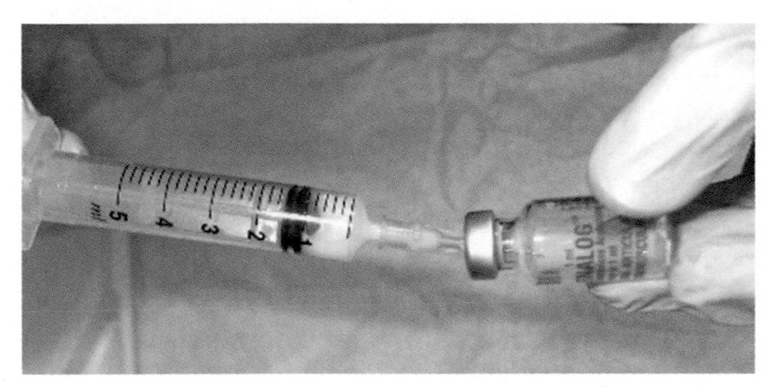

Figure 202-4 Aspirate 1 mL (40 mg) triamcinolone acetonide (Kenalog).

- Diabetic patients: A transient elevation of blood glucose levels may occur.
- Generally limited to two injections per side; rarely, a third may be given. If three injections have not been successful, it seems fruitless to continue this form of treatment. This may be secondary to inaccuracy of injection or obesity. Underlying biomechanical abnormality of the foot should also be considered.

Troubleshooting

- Bleeding or bruising can occur in patients who have a bleeding disorder or are on anticoagulants. Remember to check the international normalized ratio in patients who have a history of a clotting disorder or liver failure or are taking anticoagulant drugs.

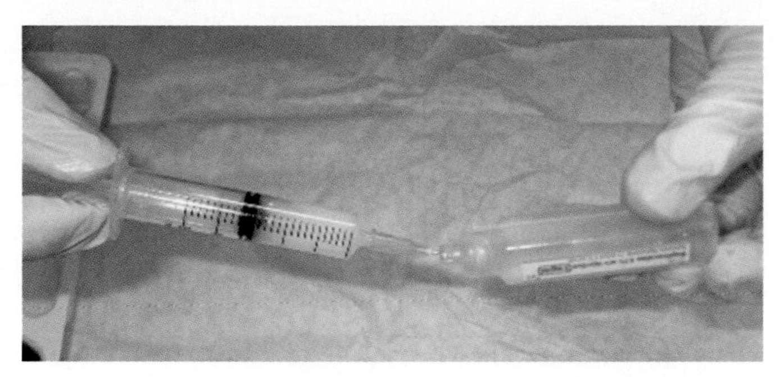

Figure 202-5 Aspirate 2 mL 0.5% bupivacaine.

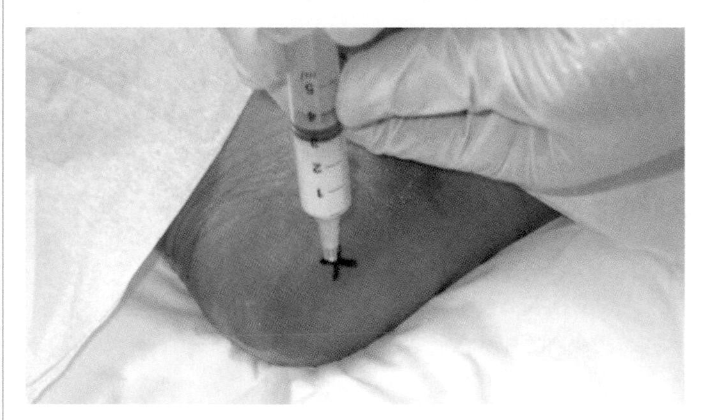

Figure 202-6 Inject the plantar fascia under sterile technique.

- Rupture of the plantar fascia has been found in 10% of patients after injection. The symptoms of most of these patients resolve with rest and rehabilitation.
- Lateral plantar nerve injury is a potential complication if the local anesthetic is injected either close to or within the nerve.
- Ultrasonography has also been used to precisely localize the inflamed area and guide needle placement.

Patient Instructions

- Appropriate medical attention should be sought if redness, discharge, or increasing pain develops at the injection site or generally unwell.
- Diabetic patients may notice a slight increase in the blood sugar level, which is a transient phenomenon.

Chapter 203 Morton's Neuroma Injection

Medardo R. Maroto, Daniel K. Park, and Simon Lee

CPT CODE
20600 *Arthrocentesis, Aspiration and/or Injection; Small Joint or Bursa*

Procedure Name

- Morton's neuroma injection

Equipment

- 25-gauge injection needle; 1.5-cm length
- Syringe (3–5 mL)
- Local anesthetic (1% lidocaine without epinephrine and 0.25% bupivacaine)
- Steroid solution (methylprednisolone [Depo-Medrol], triamcinolone acetonide [Kenalog], betamethasone [Celestone])
- Sterile tray
- Sterile gloves
- Sterile prep solution
- Ethyl chloride (topical anesthetic)
- Sterile gauze and bandage

Indications

- Painful interdigital neuroma (Morton's neuroma); most commonly, the second or third common digital branch of the medial plantar nerve and corresponding second or third web space
- Diagnostic tool to confirm interdigital neuroma as the cause of forefoot pain
- Therapeutic tool for painful interdigital neuromas resistant to other nonoperative modalities (nonsteroidal anti-inflammatory drugs, metatarsal pads, orthoses, proper footwear) and patients in whom surgical intervention is contraindicated.

Contraindications

- Overlying infection in the area
- Overlying skin disease

Technique

- Verbal consent is obtained, and the correct extremity is identified.
- The patient is positioned supine with the knee supported underneath with a pillow. The ankle is in neutral position.
- The medication mixture of a local anesthetic agent and corticosteroid is prepared on a sterile tray, typically, 2 mL of anesthetic agent (1 mL lidocaine and 1 mL bupivacaine) to 1 mL of steroid.
- The area of maximal tenderness to palpation is identified dorsally, just proximal to and between the affected metatarsal heads (Fig. 203-1).
- Ethyl chloride should be administered topically before sterile skin preparation.
- The skin is prepared in the usual sterile fashion.
- In a distal to proximal direction, the needle is advanced through the dorsal skin at a 45-degree angle between the metatarsal heads (Fig. 203-2).
- The needle can typically be inserted 0.75 to 1 inch to adequately approach the nerve, which is slightly plantar to the metatarsal heads.
- Care should be taken to avoid overshooting the neuroma and inadvertently injecting the plantar fat pad, which can result in fat pad atrophy.

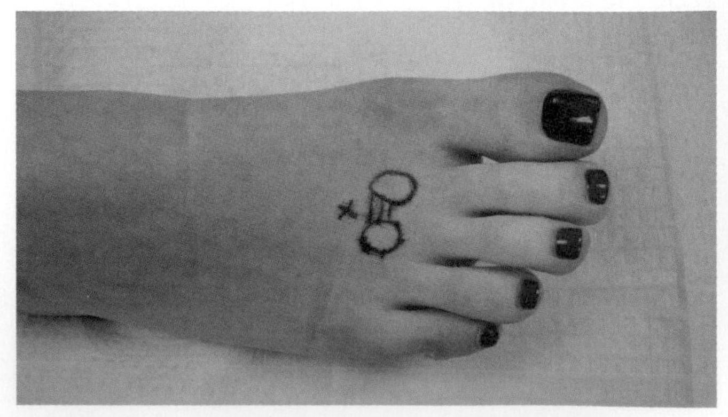

Figure 203-1 The area of maximal tenderness on the dorsum of the forefoot between the metatarsal heads (marked with an X).

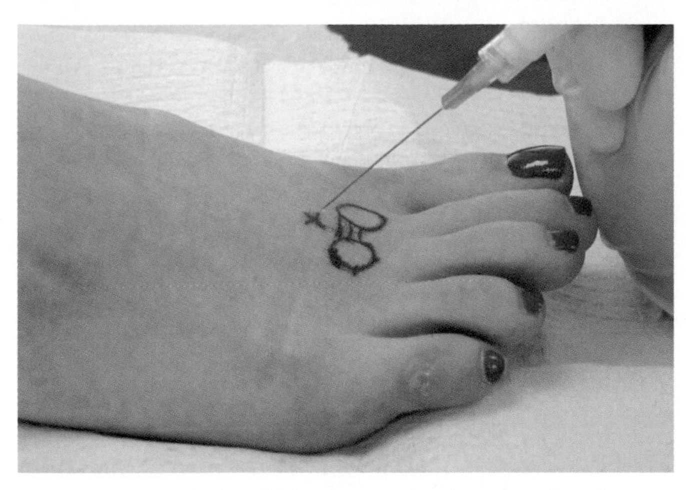

Figure 203-2 Angle of injection on the dorsal surface is shown.

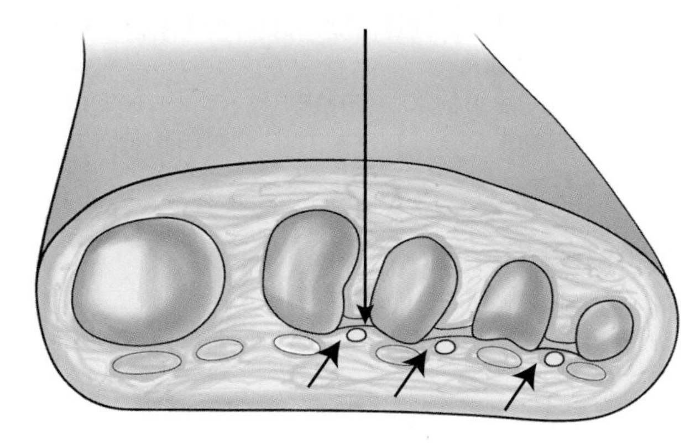

Figure 203-3 Diagram of the relative location of the metatarsal heads (*long arrow*), the deep transverse ligament (*arrows*), and the location of the nerve (*short arrows*).

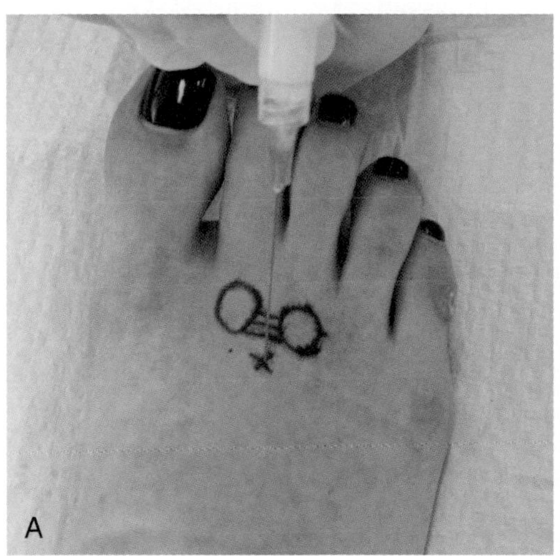

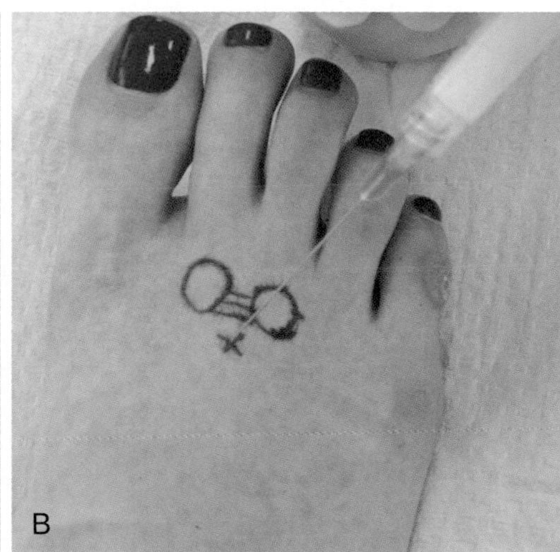

Figure 203-4 The relative angle of approach for a pes planus foot (**A**) versus that for a high arch foot (**B**).

- The mixture is injected proximally and distally after the needle tip passes the deep transverse metatarsal ligament (Fig. 203-3).
- Apply a dressing per routine

Special Considerations

- Complete or partial pain relief is variable, with reported success rates of as high as 80%.
- Repeat injections can be successful in alleviating pain, but at the risk of increased complications.
  - Plantar fat pad atrophy
  - Tendon or ligament rupture
  - Dermal thinning
  - Hyperpigmentation of skin
  - Infection
- If the injection fails to alleviate the pain, consider other causes of forefoot pain.

Troubleshooting

- "Bumping" bone: gentle redirection of the needle medial or lateral to find the intermetatarsal region
- Patients with pes planus typically can be approached with a more perpendicular approach to the axis of the foot, whereas those with high arches will require a more lateral to medial approach to account for the angulation of the metatarsals (Fig. 203-4).

Patient Instructions

- The bandage can be removed later in the day.
- Use ice to treat any local soreness at the site.
- Diabetic patients may notice a slight transient increase in the blood glucose level.
- The physician's office should be called immediately if any purulent drainage, redness, warmth, increased

swelling, or fevers/chills develops or there is a severe increase in pain.
- There may be painful symptoms for several days at the injection site before the desired effects are obtained.

Suggested Reading

- Miller SD: Technique tip: Forefoot pain: Diagnosing metatarsophalangeal joint synovitis from interdigital neuroma. Foot Ankle Int 2001;22:914–915.
- Rasmussen MR, Kitaoka HB, Patzer GL: Nonoperative treatment of plantar interdigital neuroma with a single corticosteroid injection. Clin Orthop Relat Res 1996;326:188–193.
- Weinfeld SB, Myerson MS: Interdigital neuritis: Diagnosis and treatment. J Am Acad Orthop Surg 1996;4:328–335.

Chapter 204 First Metatarsophalangeal Joint Aspiration and/or Injection Technique

Eric M. Bluman

CPT CODE
20600 *Arthrocentesis, Aspiration and/or Injection; Small Joint or Bursa*

Procedure Name

- First metatarsophalangeal joint aspiration and injection

Equipment

- 23- or 25-gauge needle
- 5-mL injection syringe
- Three-way stopcock
- Ethyl chloride (optional)
- Local anesthetic agent (2% lidocaine)
- Appropriate laboratory collection tubes for aspiration
- Sterile gloves
- Povidone-iodine or other skin prep agent
- Injectable agent (e.g., steroid)
- Small adhesive bandage

Indications

- Aspiration
  - Suspected joint infection
  - Gouty arthritis
  - Large painful effusion
  - Painful hemarthrosis
- Injection
  - Hallux rigidus
  - Rheumatoid arthritis
  - Osteochondral lesion of joint
  - Sesamoiditis
  - Pseudogout

Contraindications

- Aspiration
  - Generalized sepsis without evidence of infected joint
  - No joint space visualized on radiographs
- Injection
  - No joint space visualized on radiographs
  - Active or recent joint infection
  - Overlying skin disease

Technique

- Verbal patient consent is obtained, and the site and side are confirmed.
- The medication is prepared on a sterile tray with an extra syringe if aspiration is indicated.
- Visual examination and palpation are used to locate the joint line and site for needle insertion. Needle insertion is most easily done at the dorsomedial aspect of the joint, just medial and inferior to the dorsomedial sensory nerve. Any marking of the insertion site should be done before antiseptic skin preparation (Fig. 204-1).
- Ethyl chloride, if used, should be applied topically to the area into which the needle will be inserted (Fig. 204-2).
- While wearing sterile gloves, the skin is prepared with a sterile prep solution (Fig. 204-3).
- A small-bore needle (23- or 25-gauge) is inserted in the joint (Fig. 204-4). The metatarsal head is convex, whereas the proximal articular surface of the proximal phalanx is concave. To successfully access the joint without penetrating cartilage or bone, the needle should be directed distally and laterally from a

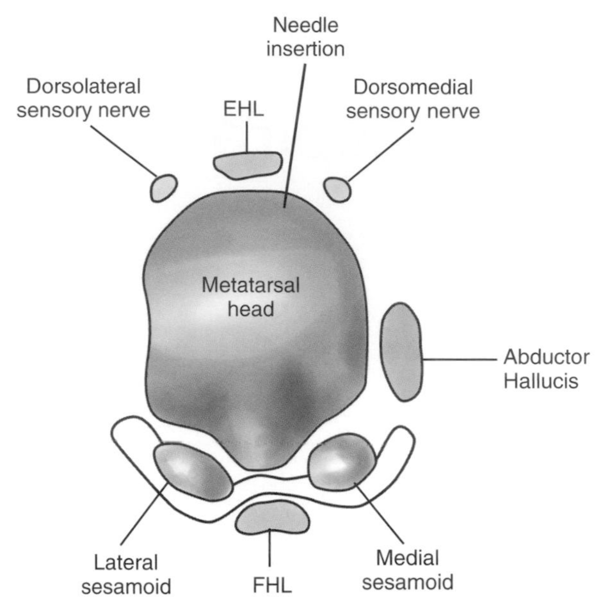

Figure 204-1 Drawing depicts the location of needle placement to obtain safe access to metatarsophalangeal joint. EHL, extensor hallucis longus; FHL, flexor hallucis longus.

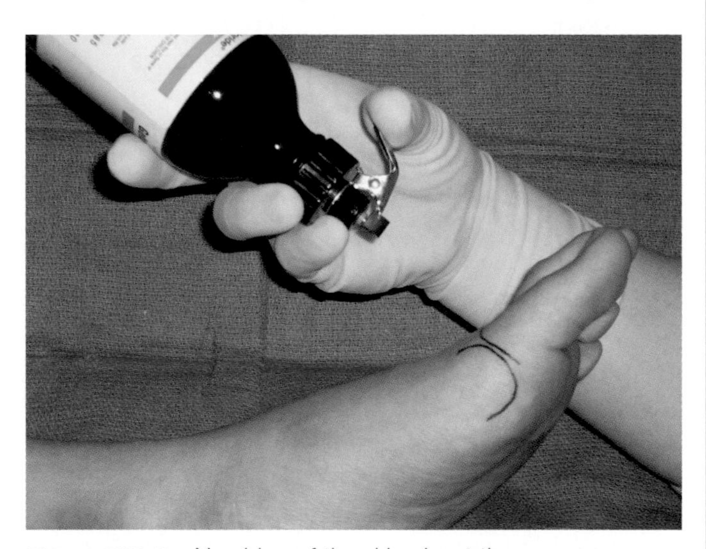

Figure 204-2 Numbing of the skin about the metatarsophalangeal joint with ethyl chloride spray solution.

dorsomedial point of entrance. Aspiration is easier with a larger-bore needle.

- After feeling the needle pass through the joint capsule, the plunger of the syringe is withdrawn to aspirate joint fluid/hemarthrosis.
- If no joint fluid can be obtained, the stopcock setting is switched to the syringe containing sterile saline, and a small amount (approximately 1 mL) is injected into the joint (see Special Considerations section).
- The lavage fluid is then withdrawn into the aspiration syringe after the stopcock has been switched back to its initial position.
- The syringe is withdrawn, and the site is dressed with a small adhesive bandage.

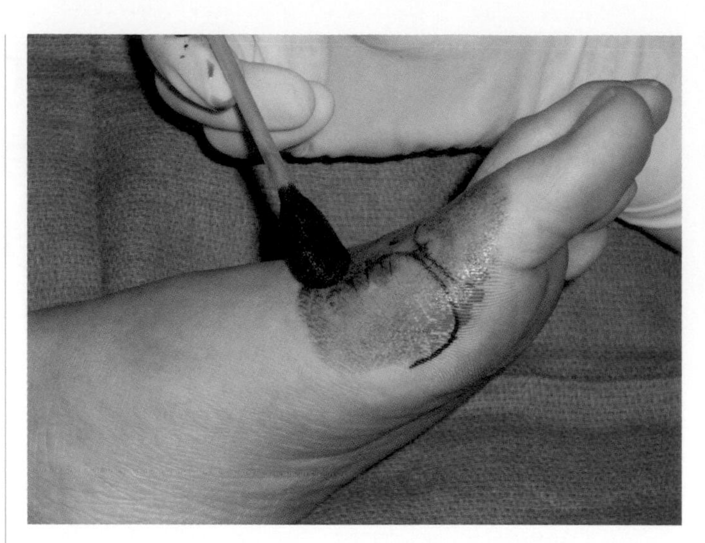

Figure 204-3 Preparation of the skin at the injection site with a povidone-iodine solution.

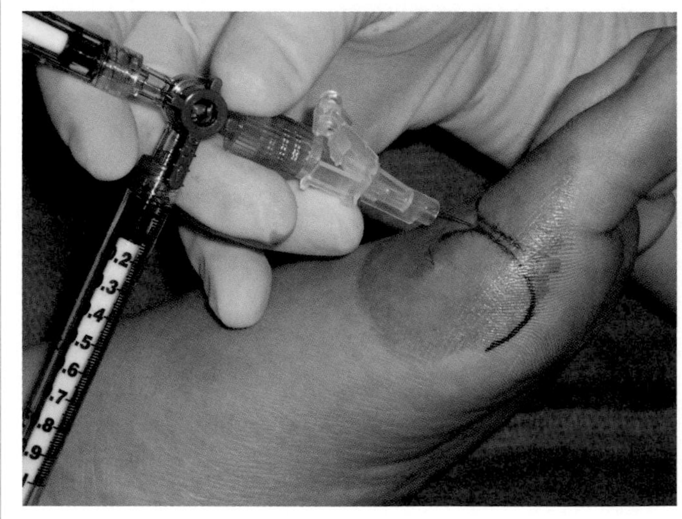

Figure 204-4 Insertion of the needle to access the metatarsophalangeal joint.

Special Considerations

- The dorsomedial aspect of the joint is chosen because it avoids all neurovascular structures, ligaments, and tendons. An insertion point just medial to the extensor hallucis longus tendon, which runs over the dorsal aspect of the joint, is safe (see Fig. 204-1).
- Laboratories differ on how they prefer to receive specimens. Before sending joint fluid aspirates for analysis, the clinician should check to determine his or her laboratory's preferences.
- Unless the clinician is absolutely certain that the pathology within the joint is not infectious in nature, cultures should be sent off with other fluid analyses to be done.

The clinician may have to be selective about the number of analyses to be performed because the volume of aspirate obtained may be limiting.

- The first metatarsophalangeal joint usually contains very little synovial fluid. Although pathologic processes may increase this amount and make aspiration easier, there may be times when fluid must be added to the joint (lavage) before fluid can be aspirated for analysis. The clinician must be cautious in doing this as it may affect the results obtained.
- Uric acid (gout) and calcium pyrophosphate (pseudogout) crystals are soluble in dilute aqueous solutions. Addition of saline to joint fluid containing these crystals may cause their dissolution. Injection of saline into the joint should not be done if crystal analysis is planned.
- Some sodium chloride solutions contain a bacteriostatic substance. Saline with a bacteriostatic additive should not be used for joint lavage if cultures are to be performed. The label will indicate whether such an additive is present.
- Injection of fluid into a joint capsule distends it and causes pain. The patient should be educated about this pain before the procedure is performed. A toe block may be done before aspiration (see Chapter 207). This will significantly decrease the pain experienced by the patient.

Troubleshooting

- In some individuals who have a limited amount of joint space, distraction of the joint may aid in placing the needle within the metatarsophalangeal joint. With the hand not being used to inject, longitudinal traction is applied to the distal toe. A sulcus sign may be seen, which indicates distraction of the joint surfaces (Fig. 204-5). Insertion of the needle should be at this location. The angle of insertion of the needle should proceed so that the tip avoids the articular cartilage of the metatarsal head (see Fig. 204-4).
- "Bumping" bone: At no point during the injection or aspiration should a rigid surface be felt. This indicates that the needle has been placed in cartilage or bone. If this occurs, gently redirect the needle into the joint.
- If examination, manual palpation, or gentle traction does not allow easy identification of the joint line, fluoroscopy may help to insert hypodermic needles into the joint.

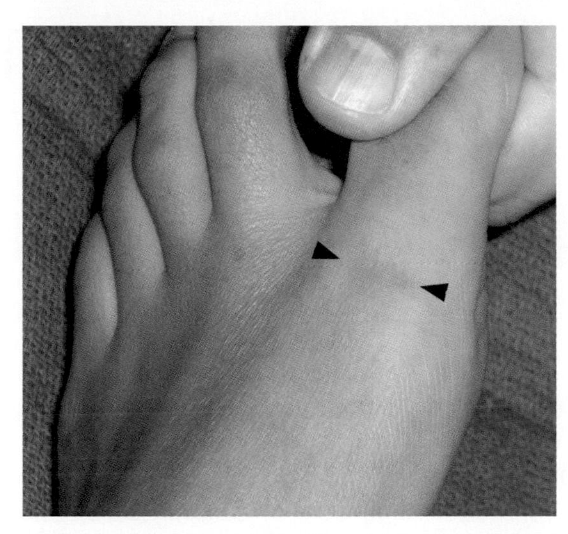

Figure 204-5 Sulcus created with axial traction on the great toe is shown between *arrowheads*.

Patient Instructions

- The patient can remove the bandage the day after the injection.
- Use ice to treat any local soreness at the injection site.
- If the patient received an injection of steroid mixed with a local anesthetic agent, there will likely be pain relief before leaving the doctor's office. This pain relief is due to placement of local anesthetic in the joint. The pain relief obtained from the local anesthetic will last only a few hours. Pain relief from the steroid will not begin for a day or so after the injection. In the time between the local anesthetic wearing off and the onset of pain relief from the steroid, the patient may feel a heightened sense of pain. This has been termed the flare reaction. This is normal and may be treated with oral medications prescribed by the physician.
- The physician's office should be contacted immediately if there is persistent redness, swelling, or increase in pain after the flare reaction occurs. Fever or chills any time after the injection/aspiration should be brought to the attention of the physician.

Chapter 205 Trimming of Corns and Calluses

Norman Espinosa

CPT CODES

11055 *Paring or Cutting of Benign Hyperkeratotic Lesion (e.g., Corn or Callus); Single Lesion*
11056 *Two to Four Lesions*
11057 *More Than Four Lesions*

Procedure Name

- Trimming of corns and calluses

Equipment

- No. 17 or 20 blade scalpel
- Sterile cup
- Sterile tray
- Gloves (sterile ones preferred, but not ultimately necessary)
- Sterile prep solution (e.g., alcohol, povidone-iodine)
- Sterile gauze and adhesive bandage

Indications

- Symptomatic corns and calluses

Contraindications

- Localized, acute infection (e.g., cellulitis) surrounding the callus

Technique

- Verbal patient consent is obtained and the symptomatic corn identified.
- Prepare the sterile prep solution for disinfection of the area (Fig. 205-1).
- Use a sufficient light source to identify the lesion (Fig. 205-2).
- With gloves in place, the skin is prepared with the sterile prep solution.
- Hold the scalpel blade tangentially to the surface of the skin (Fig. 205-3).
- Start removing the superficial layers of the hyperkeratotic epidermis tangentially to the surface of the skin (see Fig. 205-3).
- Intermittently palpating how much keratosis has been removed is important to define the correct depth of keratotic resection (Fig. 205-4).
- After the corn is completely removed, apply an adhesive bandage or dressing as needed (Fig. 205-5).

Special Considerations

- Be sure not to cut too deeply because of possible injury to the skin and risk of infection. This is especially important when treating patients with an insensate foot.

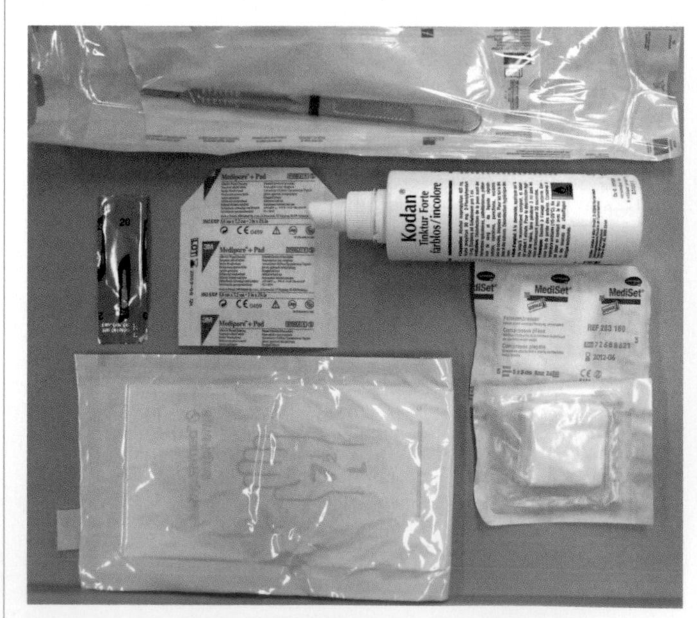

Figure 205-1 Setup includes the sterile prep solution (alcohol), a no. 20 blade scalpel, sterile gloves, sterile gauze, and a simple dressing.

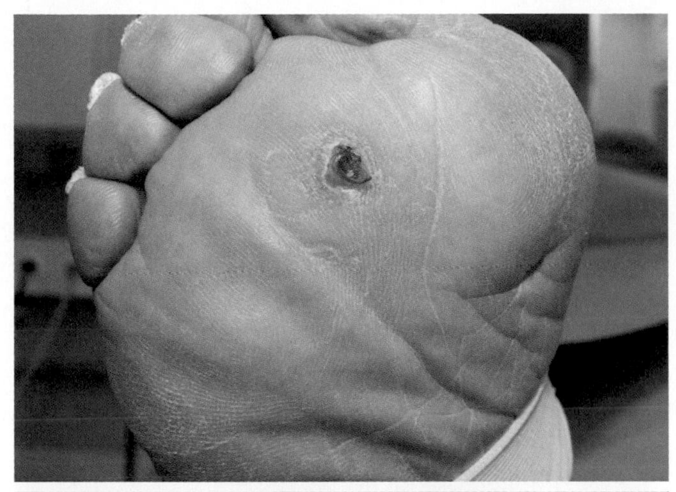

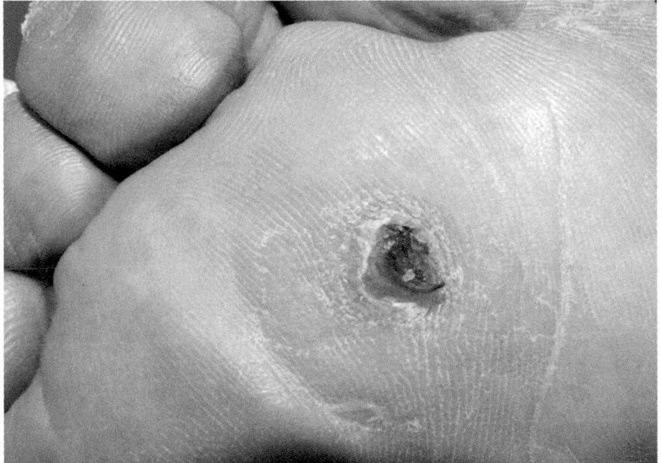

Figure 205-2 Use a powerful light source to identify the lesion and its margins.

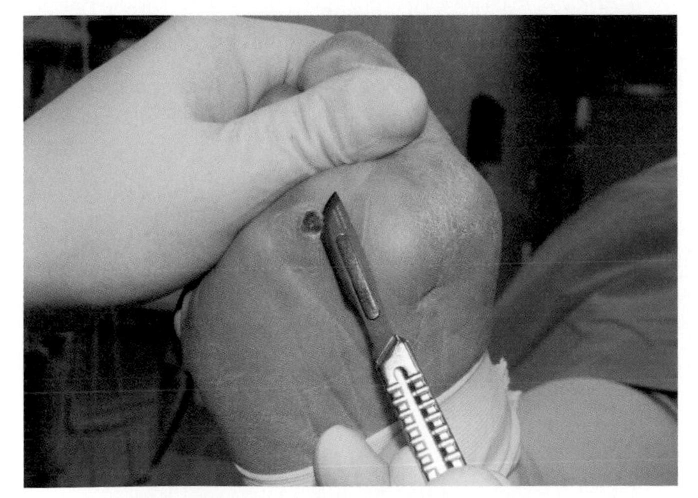

Figure 205-3 Hold the blade tangentially to the surface of the skin to begin trimming the edges of the callus or corn.

Troubleshooting

- In the case of too much removal, associated with a skin lesion (bleeding spot), the patient should be seen the next day to make sure that the wound has healed.

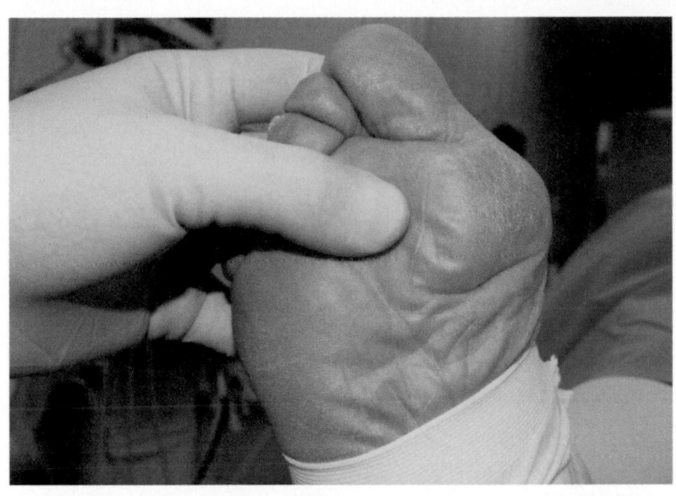

Figure 205-4 Intermittent palpation of the trimmed lesion allows estimation of depth. Do not go too deeply because this can result in subcutaneous lesions, which may be the source of possible infection.

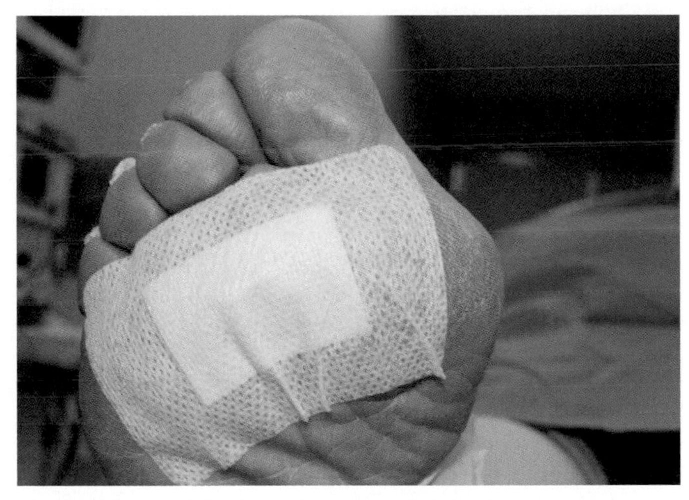

Figure 205-5 After trimming of the lesion, the wound is disinfected and covered with an adhesive bandage.

This is particularly important in patients with an insensate foot.
- Skin care is essential.

Patient Instructions

- The dressing can be removed 3 to 5 hours after the procedure.
- The patient should continue to wear modified footwear.
- The physician's office should be contacted if any redness, warmth, swelling and severe pain, fever, or chills develops.

Chapter 206 Ulcer Débridement

Alan C. League

CPT CODES
11042 *Débridement; Skin and Subcutaneous Tissue*
97597 *Removal Devitalized Tissue from Wound*

Procedure Name

- Ulcer débridement
- Diabetic foot débridement

Equipment

- No. 15 blade scalpel, curet, rongeur
- Protective pad or towel
- Sterile gloves
- Alcohol prep pads and povidone-iodine solution
- Suture removal kit with scissors and forceps
- Sterile gauze and bandage supplies

Indications

- Diabetic skin ulceration with hypertrophic callus formation and fibrinous debris

Contraindications

- Large, infected, or ischemic ulcers require a full evaluation, and routine outpatient débridement is not advised for these lesions.

Technique

- An ulcer débridement in the office setting should be performed with optimal lighting and sterile technique.
- The patient should be seated or supine on the examination table with feet at the edge of the table (Fig. 206-1).
- A pad or towel should be placed on the floor under the foot to catch debris.
- The clinician should be seated comfortably on a rolling stool to maximize ergonomic positioning.
- The ulcer should be cleansed with povidone-iodine solution and alcohol pads to create a clean environment.
- The edges of the ulcer are typically hyperkeratotic and should be sharply débrided so that they become flush with the surrounding skin (Fig. 206-2). This reduces shear forces on the ulcer.
- The ulcer itself should be débrided of all nonviable material, including any white or yellow material. Once the ulcer bed has achieved a beefy-red appearance, a sterile moist dressing should be applied.
- Appropriate pads, orthotics, and casting should be used to unload any pressure points.

Special Considerations

- This outpatient technique is practical only for débridement of noninfected, nonischemic neuropathic diabetic foot ulcers.
- Bedside cultures of infected ulcers are rarely helpful because multiple organisms are typically found.
- Document the size and depth of the ulcer after each débridement.

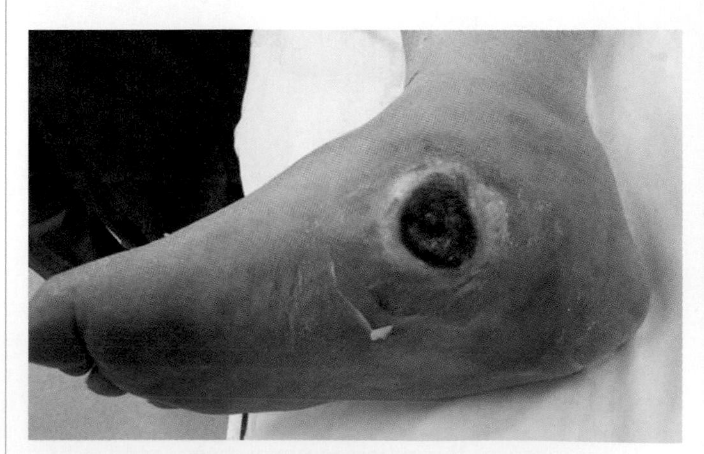

Figure 206-1 Example of diabetic pressure ulcer before débridement. Note the hyperkeratotic rim and beefy-red granulation tissue.

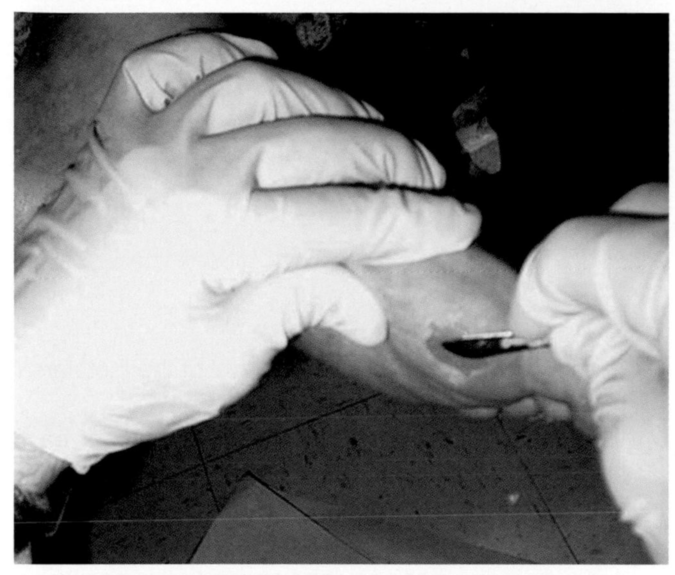

Figure 206-2 Ulcer edges are sharply débrided to the level of the surrounding skin.

Troubleshooting

- This procedure is a means to convert a chronic wound to an acute one and, when systematically performed, may aid in the healing of an ulcer. Often, serial débridements may be necessary to keep the ulcer clean and prevent chronic fibrinous overgrowth.
- The underlying etiology of the pressure ulcer (e.g., claw toe, gastrocnemius contracture, Charcot's arthropathy) should be addressed with appropriate pads, braces, or surgery.

Patient Instructions

- Any dressing changes should be performed as instructed by the physician.
- The feet should be examined daily and immediate medical attention sought at any sign of infection such as redness, swelling, drainage, fever, and chills.

Suggested Reading

- Pinzur MS, Slovenkai MP, Trepman E, Shields NN: Guidelines for diabetic foot care: Recommendations endorsed by the diabetes committee of the American Orthopaedic Foot and Ankle Society. Foot Ankle Int 2005;26:113–119.
- Strauss MB: The orthopaedic surgeon's role in the treatment and prevention of diabetic foot wounds. Foot Ankle Int 2005;26:5–14.

Chapter 207 Digital Block

Alan C. League

CPT CODE

64450 *Injection Anesthetic Agent; Other Peripheral Nerve or Branch*

Procedure Names

- Digital anesthetic block (foot)
- Toe block

Equipment

- Sterile gloves
- Alcohol swab
- Iodine-based swab
- Ethyl chloride spray
- 10-mL syringe
- 18-gauge needle
- 25-gauge, 1.5-inch needle
- 2% lidocaine *without* epinephrine
- 0.5% bupivacaine *without* epinephrine
- 2 × 2-inch sterile gauze
- Small adhesive bandage

Indications

- Closed reduction of digit
- Nail procedures
- Paronychia drainage

Contraindications

- Infection
- Allergy to any items used

Technique

- Mark the digit with your initials, obtain consent, and have an assistant perform a time out confirming the planned procedure.
- Instruct the patient to lay supine with his or her foot at the edge of the examination table (Fig. 207-1). Place a mark on the dorsal skin at the level of the metatarsal head on either side of the affected digit.
- Using the 18-gauge needle, aspirate 5 mL of each anesthetic solution into the 10-mL syringe. Aseptically exchange for the 25-gauge, 1.5-inch needle.
- Prepare the dorsal skin over both marks with three separate iodine-based swabs and then use an alcohol wipe to remove excess iodine solution.
- Don sterile gloves and grasp the affected foot with the left hand (for a right-handed clinician).
- Grasp the syringe in the right hand while an assistant freezes the dorsal skin with ethyl chloride spray.
- Introduce the needle perpendicularly to the skin at one of the marked spots and advance until the needle tip begins to tent the plantar skin (Fig. 207-2). Remember that the digital nerves are located more plantar than dorsal, so be sure that the needle is adequately advanced.
- Withdraw the needle approximately 5 mm so that the tip of the needle is near the plantar edge of the metatarsal head.
- Aspirate to prevent intravascular injection.
- Inject 3 mL of solution at this location and an additional 2 mL while slowly withdrawing the needle, including some subcutaneous infiltration.

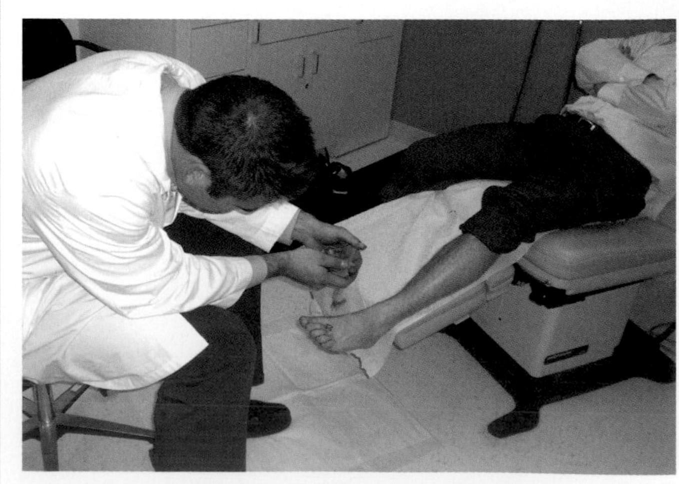

Figure 207-1 Patient and clinician are comfortably positioned for the injections.

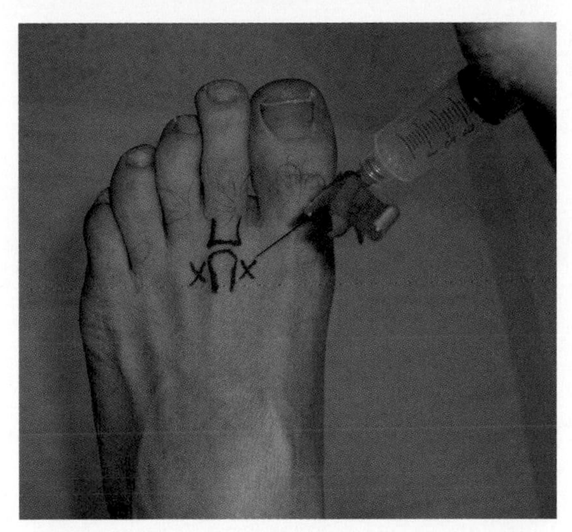

Figure 207-2 The needle should be directed perpendicular to the skin at the level of the metatarsal head.

- Repeat the previous four steps for the other side of the metatarsal head.
- Hold pressure with sterile gauze until bleeding stops and apply a small adhesive bandage to each injection site. Because of the two different anesthetics used, expect anesthesia to occur within 5 to 10 minutes and to last as long as several hours.

Special Considerations

- Use anesthetic agents without epinephrine. Injection of epinephrine near the digits may result in necrosis.
- When applying a dressing to an anesthetized toe, be sure that the dressing is not tight and that toe color is normal.

Patient Instructions

- Sensation may return to the digit as early as an hour or as late as a day.
- Pain medicine should be taken as soon as sensation begins to return. This allows pain relief to begin before the block wears off entirely.

Chapter 208 Nail Removal

Andrew Moore and Robert E. Meehan

CPT CODE
11730 *Removal of Nail Plate, Partial or Complete*

Procedure Name

- Removal of nail plate

Equipment

- Ethyl chloride (optional)
- 25-gauge needle
- 10-mL injection syringe
- Local anesthetic agent
- Sterile gloves
- Iodine solution
- Sterile fenestrated drape
- Small Penrose drain or wide rubber band
- Two small hemostats
- Periosteal elevator
- Nail splitter
- Iris scissors or equivalent
- Antibiotic ointment
- Sterile dressing
- Matricectomy supplies: electrosurgical unit, sharp instrument or sterile cotton-tip applicators, and phenol solution (88%)

Indications

- Partial removal
  - Onychocryptosis (ingrown toenail)
- Complete removal
  - Onychogryposis (deformed, curved toenail)
  - Onychomycosis
  - Chronic or recurrent paronychia
  - Nail bed biopsy

Contraindications

- Bleeding disorders: prolonged bleeding time
- Active infection, cellulitis: All active infections should be eradicated before matricectomy to prevent seeding of deeper tissues or bone.
- Dysvascular toe: gangrenous toe

Technique

- Verbal patient consent is obtained, and the correct toe is identified (Fig. 208-1).
- Medication and supplies are prepared on a sterile tray or Mayo stand.
- The toe is washed and prepped with povidone-iodine solution, prepping proximally to the level of the metatarsal head, and a fenestrated drape is applied.
  - Optional: Have an assistant anesthetize the skin with ethyl chloride at the injection site for a digital block.

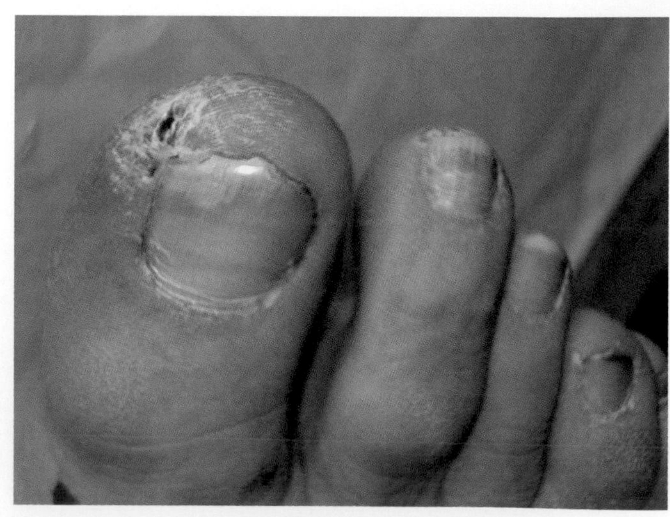

Figure 208-1 Example of an ingrown nail on the medial margin.

- A digital block is performed (see Chapter 207).
  - Optional: Use a sterile rubber band, Penrose drain, or a cut piece of glove clasped tightly with a hemostat as a tourniquet.
- Grasp the toe in your nondominant hand and use a periosteal elevator to separate the eponychial fold from the dorsal aspect of the nail plate (Fig. 208-2).
- Slide the periosteal elevator or small curved hemostat under the nail plate with gentle dorsal pressure, separating the nail matrix from the nail plate (Fig. 208-3).
- If removing only the lateral or medial fourth of the nail (as for onychocryptosis), incise the nail longitudinally with a nail splitter or strong scissors, taking care to avoid lacerating the underlying nail bed (Fig. 208-4).

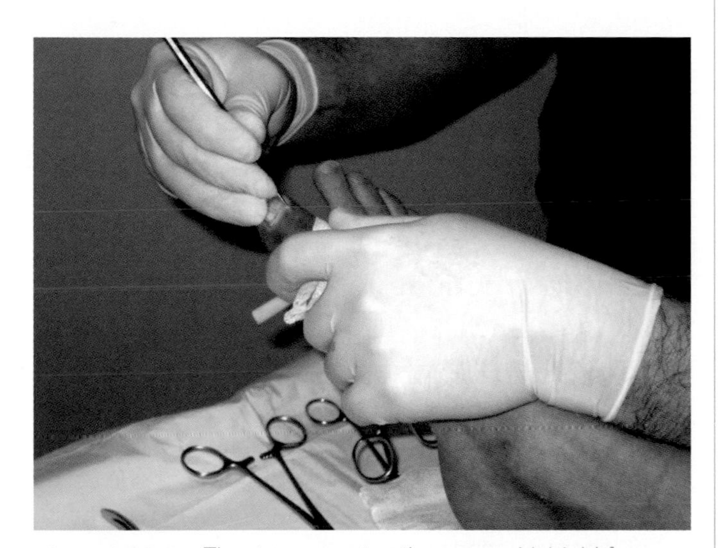

Figure 208-2 Elevator separates the eponychial fold from the nail plate.

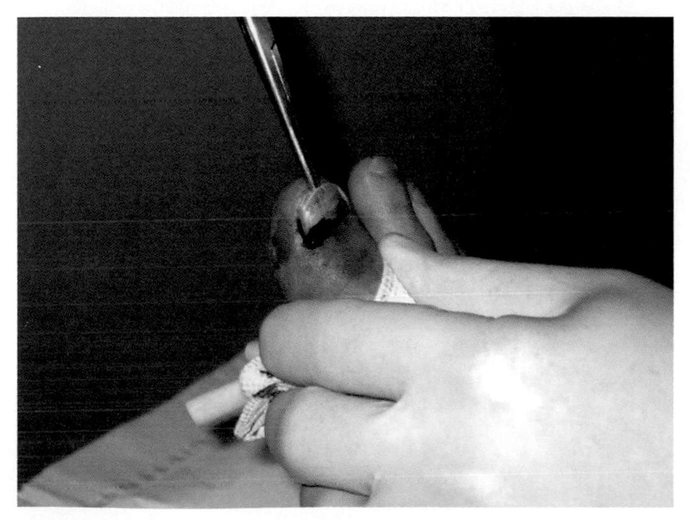

Figure 208-3 Hemostat used to bluntly elevate the nail from the nail bed.

- Grasp the nail with a hemostat; remove the nail plate using gentle traction and elevation (Fig. 208-5).
- Perform matricectomy (ablation of germinal matrix) with electrocautery, a sharp instrument (no. 15 scalpel or Beaver blade), or topical phenol (88% solution applied to germinal matrix with cotton-tipped applicator for 1–2 minutes) (Fig. 208-6).
- Remove the tourniquet. Apply antibiotic ointment and a sterile dressing (Figs. 208-7 and 208-8).

Special Considerations

- Matricectomy decreases the recurrence rate of onychocryptosis, but slightly increases the infection rate. Patients should be counseled that after matricectomy, the nail will be narrower than before.
- If present, granulation tissue should be débrided back to normal tissue. This will leave a concavity that will gradually fill in over time.

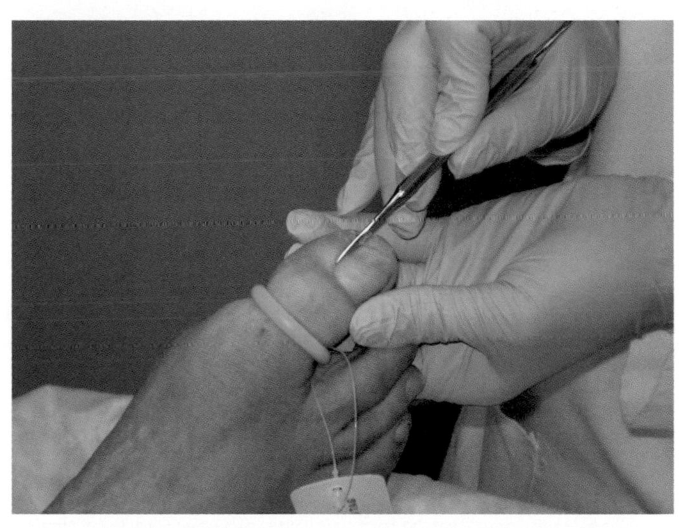

Figure 208-4 Nail splitter used to cut nail longitudinally.

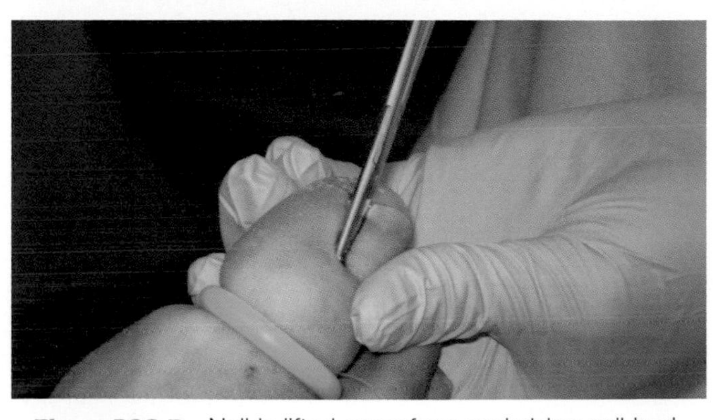

Figure 208-5 Nail is lifted away from underlying nail bed.

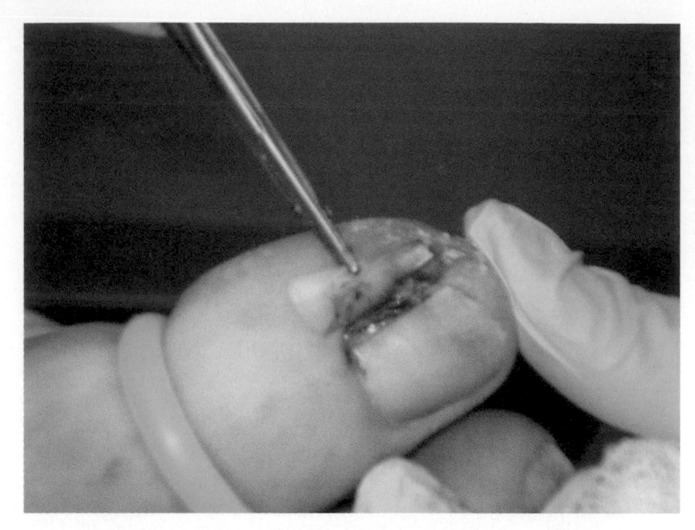

Figure 208-6 Avulsion of the nail is complete.

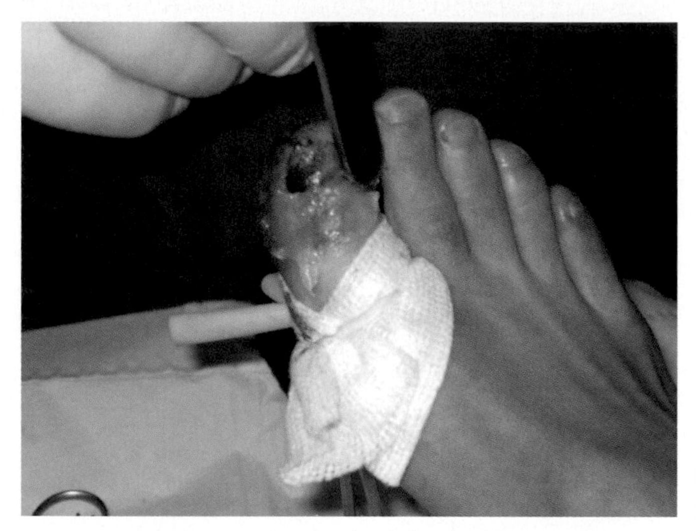

Figure 208-7 Apply bacitracin.

- The development of increasing pain, swelling, or drainage suggests postprocedural infection, which usually responds to oral antibiotics. Consider plain radiographs to assess for underlying osteomyelitis if drainage and erythema are persistent. If present, surgical referral should be considered.
- After performing complete nail plate removal, adhesions may form between the nail fold and matrix, impairing the growth of a new nail plate. Interposing a part of the old nail (or a piece of packaging foil) in this space for 3 weeks is recommended to prevent this complication. This material should be securely affixed to the underlying matrix with absorbable suture.

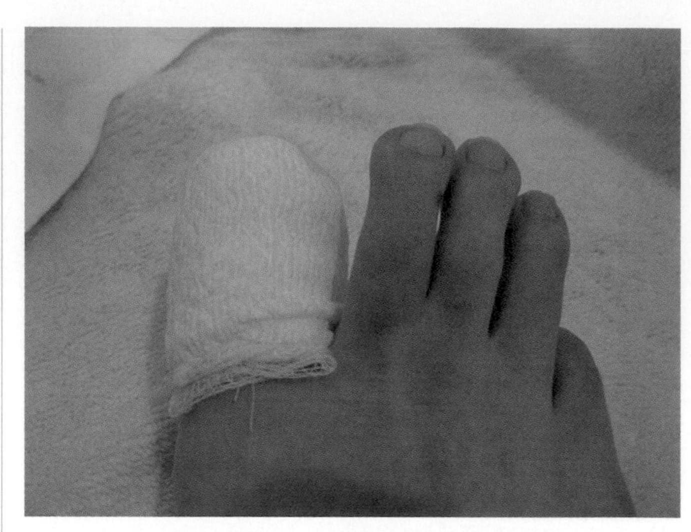

Figure 208-8 Compression dressing.

Patient Instructions

- The dressing can be removed in 48 to 72 hours; antibiotic ointment is applied daily for 2 weeks.
- For postprocedural pain, over-the-counter ibuprofen and acetaminophen are generally sufficient. A piece of dental floss under the advancing nail edge should be applied for the next few months to prevent recurrence of ingrown toenail.

Suggested Reading

- Benjamin RB: Excision of ingrown toenail. In Benjamin RB (ed): Atlas of Outpatient and Office Surgery, 2nd ed. Philadelphia: Lea & Febiger, 1994, pp 357–359.
- Quill G, Myerson M: A guide to office treatment of ingrown toenails. Hosp Med 1994;30:51–54.
- Sanders M: Marginal toenail ablation. In Kitaoka HB, Ravin D (eds): Masters Techniques in Orthopaedic Surgery: The Foot and Ankle, 2nd ed. Philadelphia: Lippincott Williams & Wilkins, 2002, pp 3–10.
- Zuber TJ: Ingrown toenail removal. Am Fam Physician 2002;65:2547–2552, 2554.

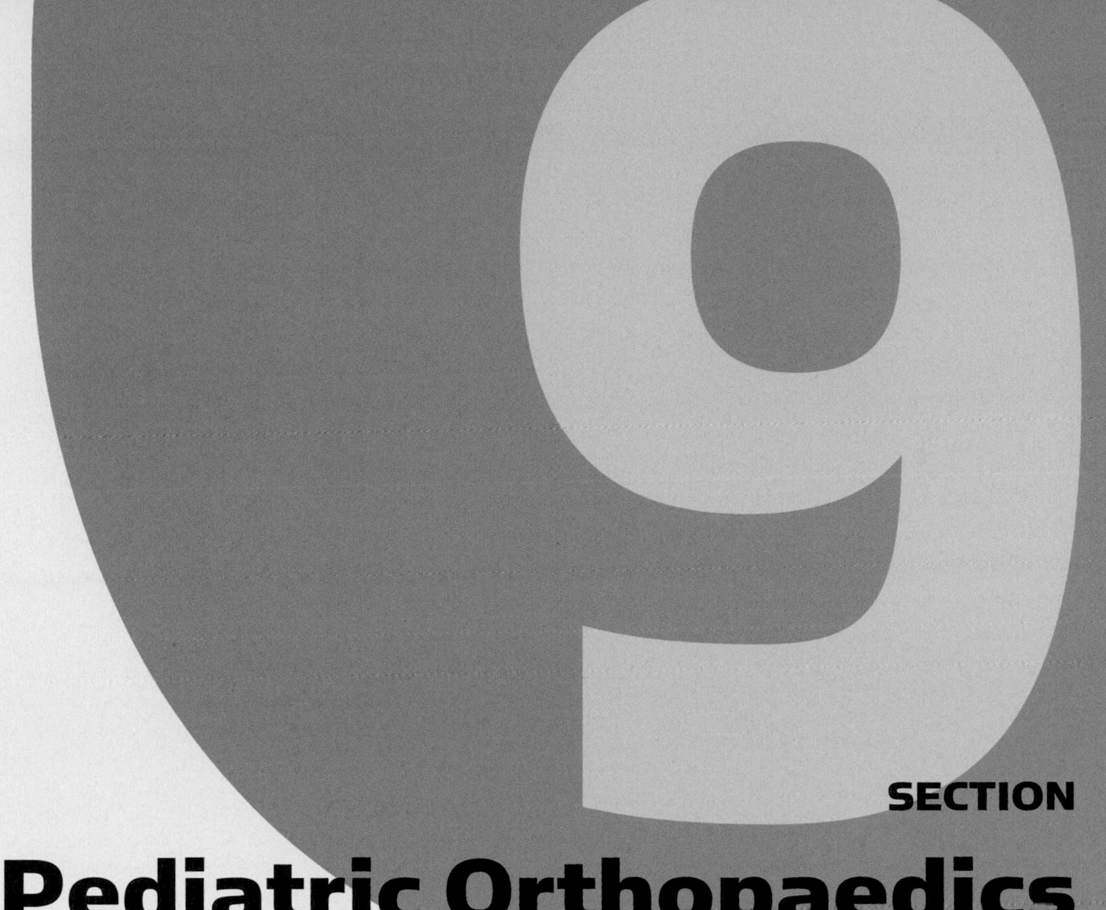

SECTION 9

Pediatric Orthopaedics

Chapter 209 Overview of Pediatric Orthopaedics

Jennifer A. Hart

Approach to the Pediatric Patient

- Pediatric patients provide a very different interaction during an orthopaedic examination than is typical of adult patients. For this reason, we present a unique section to discuss these differences both in general terms and with regard to the conditions that are particular to this patient population.

Infants

- Because infants are unable to communicate their symptoms directly, one is forced to use visual cues and history points provided by the parents to make a diagnosis.
- Crying is nonspecific and may be the result of pain or fear during the examination but can be useful in localizing the problem.
- History and observation of the interaction between the parent(s) and child become even more important in this age group.

Toddlers

- Toddlers can be slightly more descriptive than infants but still do not have the full vocabulary to provide the information needed.
- Toddlers respond well to games (Fig. 209-1), so be firm but creative to make the experience fun and less frightening for them. A simple game of "Simon says" can go a long way to getting a full examination from a cooperative toddler (Fig. 209-2).

Young Children

- Young children can be a difficult group to examine because they have developed the memory necessary to be afraid of health care providers.
- Explain what you are going to do before you do it for every step of the examination. The child will be less frightened if he or she does not feel that he or she is being tricked into something painful.

Adolescents

- For some health care professionals, adolescents prove to be the hardest group to work with because they are often reluctant to communicate personal feelings, including pain and experiences, to someone with whom they are unfamiliar.
- Be open and up front about the examination and the potential diagnoses.
- Be aware of the fact that an adolescent patient is not an adult with the level of maturity necessary to understand everything that you might have to say, but be respectful of the fact that he or she is likely old enough to want to be an active participant in his or her care.

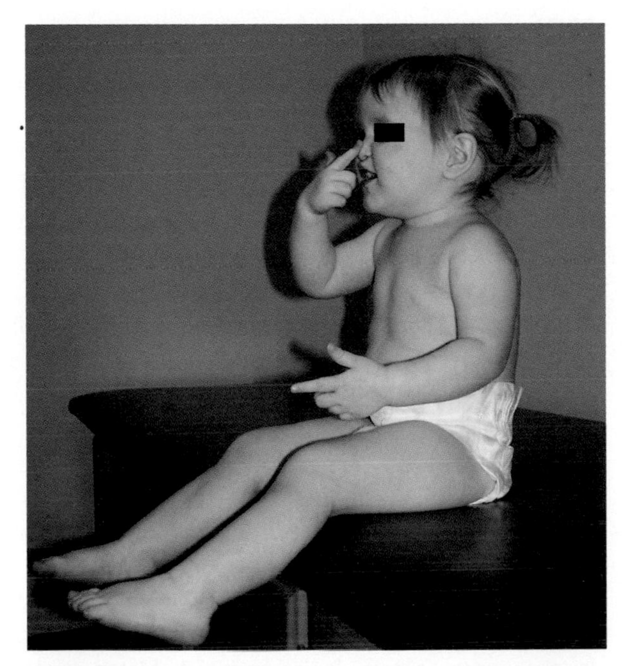

Figure 209-1 Toddlers and young children respond very well to games that can distract them from their natural fear and anxiety.

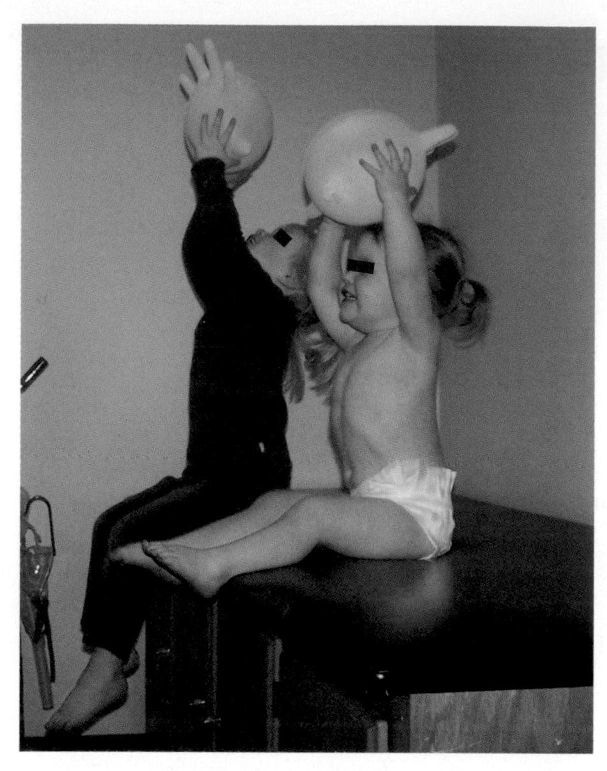

Figure 209-2 "Simon says" can be a useful method to obtain a cooperative toddler examination. Involving a sibling can also ease patient anxiety.

History

- For most young children, the history will come from the parents.
  - For cases of trauma, try to find someone who witnessed the injury to collect detailed information regarding when the accident happened, the mechanism of injury, and the forces involved.
  - For nontraumatic conditions, ask questions about the timing, apparent location, and frequency of pain. Ask about any patterns the parents have noticed and any history of similar difficulty.
- For many conditions, especially congenital deformities, a detailed pregnancy and birth history will be helpful as well as information on family members with similar disorders.
- Finally, do not make the mistake of discounting the child's own contributions to the history. Although usually unable to provide the complete history that you need, a child's ability to communicate is often underestimated.

Physical Examination

- Inspection and palpation
  - Inspection should begin the first time that you see the patient, even if that is in the parking lot, waiting room, or the hallway of the office.
  - Useful information regarding gait abnormalities, movement disorders, and parental interaction can be obtained simply by observing the child walking and playing in the examination room (Fig. 209-3).
  - There are a variety of congenital and acquired deformities for which patients seek orthopaedic care. Each deformity should be carefully evaluated and compared with the other side. The use of digital photography or measurement may prove useful for later comparison.
- Range of motion and strength
  - Passive range of motion is much easier to test than active motion in the young child. Be creative and create a game by having the child mimic your own motions to try to get an accurate idea of active joint motion and spasticity with movement.
  - Strength can be tested in a similar manner. It may be useful to have one of the parents or caregivers help to demonstrate (Fig. 209-4).
- Special tests
  - Barlow test (Fig. 209-5)
    - — Purpose: evaluation for congenital hip instability
    - — How to perform: Flex the hips to 90 degrees with the examiner's thumbs along the medial thighs and the index finger along the lateral femur. Apply gentle pressure in the posterior direction at the knee.
    - — Positive: indicated by a palpable "clunk" as the hip dislocates
  - Ortolani maneuver (Fig. 209-6)
    - — Purpose: evaluation for congenital hip instability
    - — How to perform: Gently abduct the hip while pushing anteriorly with the index finger over the greater trochanter.
    - — Positive: indicated by a palpable "clunk" as the hip relocates
  - Galeazzi's sign (Fig. 209-7)
    - — Purpose: evaluation for congenital hip instability after 3 months of age
    - — How to perform: Flex the hip to 90 degrees and observe the location of the knees.
    - — Positive: indicated by the knee on the affected side being lower

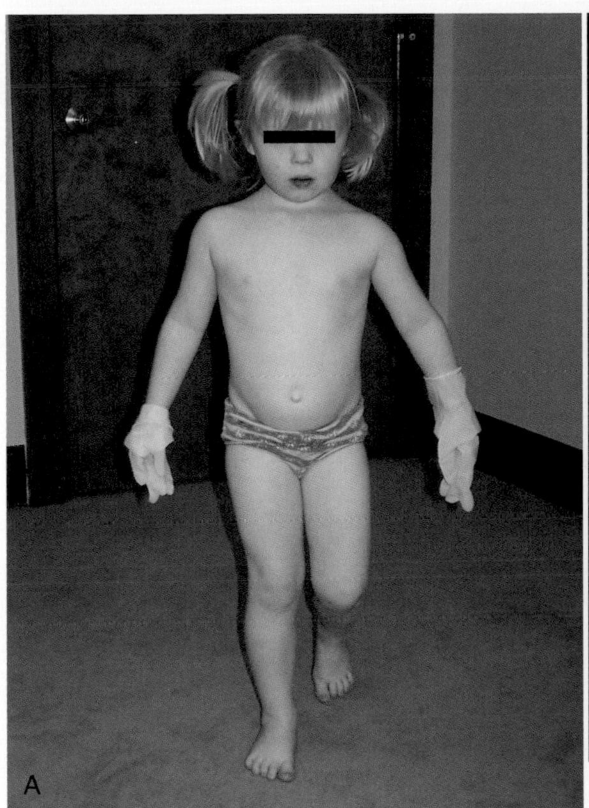

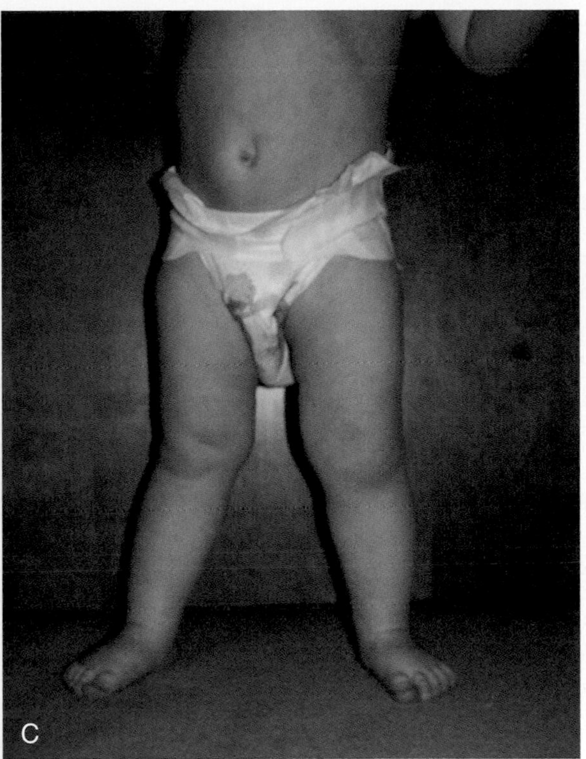

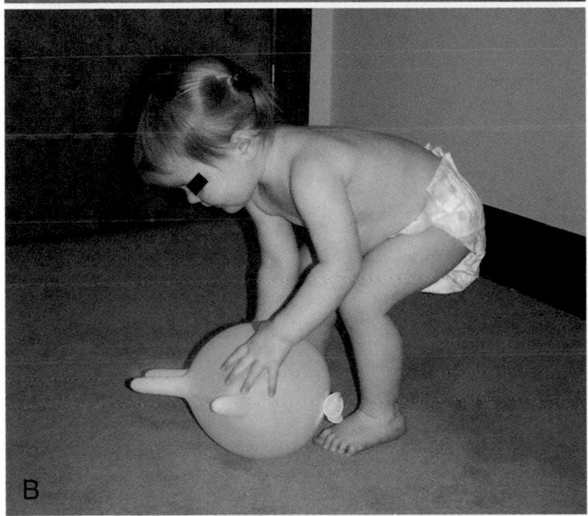

Figure 209-3 Observe the child walking (**A**), playing (**B**), and standing normally (**C**) for clues as to pain and movement abnormalities.

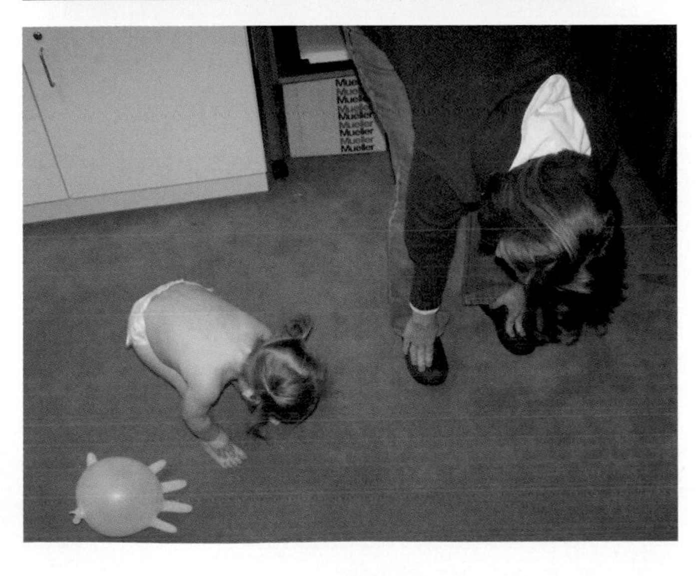

Figure 209-4 Having a parent demonstrate the activity can help with evaluation of range of motion and spasticity with movement.

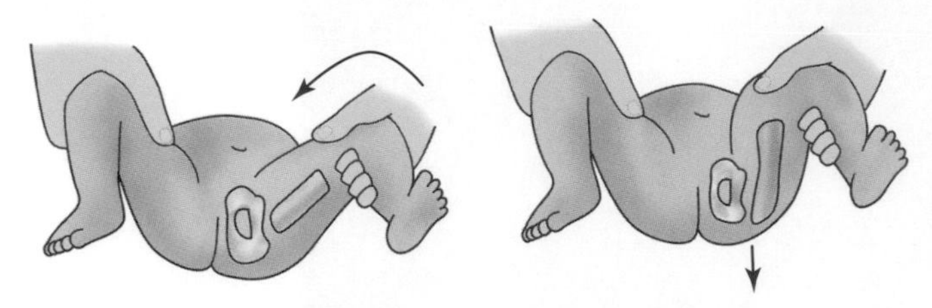

Figure 209-5 Barlow test.

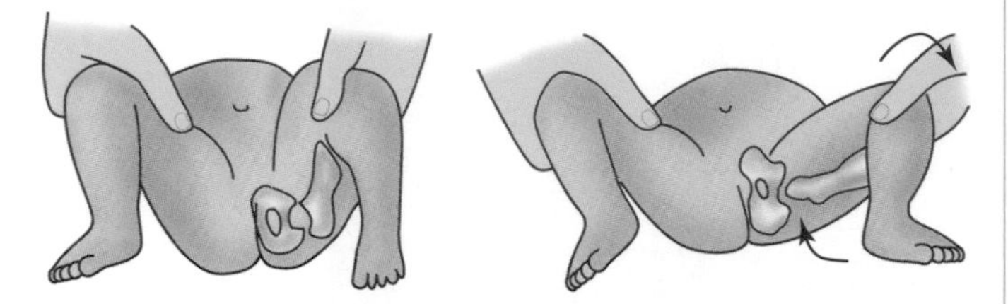

Figure 209-6 Ortolani test.

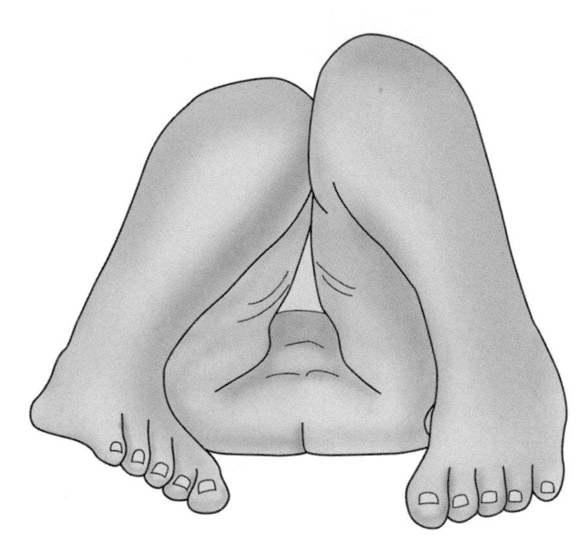

Figure 209-7 Galeazzi's sign.

- Thomas test (Fig. 209-8)
  - — Purpose: evaluation for a flexion contracture of the hip
  - — How to perform: With the patient lying supine, flex the opposite hip and knee up toward the chest to flatten the lumbar spine and correct anterior pelvic tilt.
  - — Positive: indicated by the opposite hip remaining flexed as the patient will be unable to keep it extended on the table
- Scoliosis (Adams) forward bend test (Fig. 209-9)
  - — Purpose: evaluation for spinal scoliosis
  - — How to perform: Ask the patient to face away from you and, with his or her arms hanging in front of the body, bend forward as if trying to touch the toes until the spine is parallel with the floor.

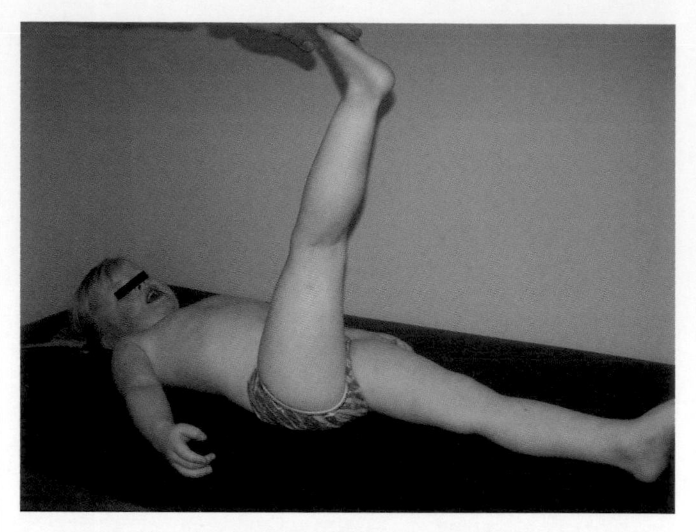

Figure 209-8 Thomas test.

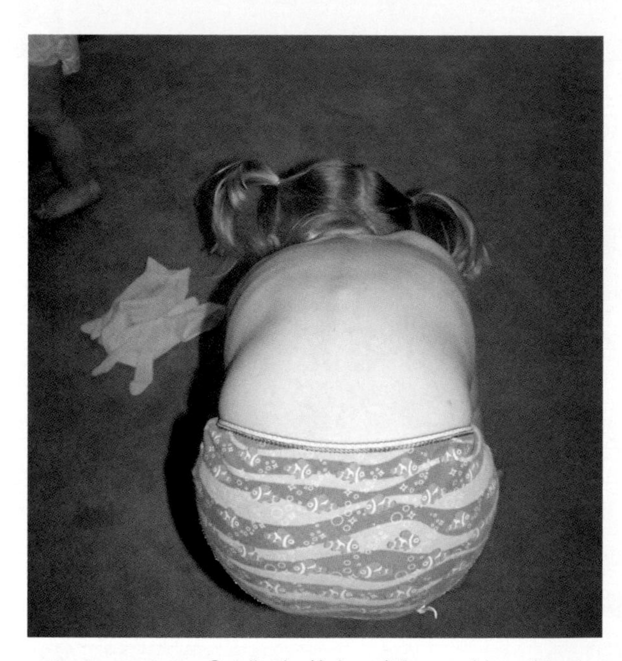

Figure 209-9 Scoliosis (Adams) forward bend test.

  - — Positive: indicated by an asymmetry of the rib cage, the degree of which can be measured using a scoliometer

Imaging

- Radiography
  - Evaluating radiographs in pediatric patients involves unique challenges due to the multiple physes in the growing skeleton.
  - Plain radiographs remain the mainstay of initial bony evaluation and as always should be ordered in at least two planes.

- Stress radiographs may be necessary to evaluate for physeal injury as a result of local trauma.
- Plain radiography is also useful in evaluating bone age when skeletal maturity is in question.
- Typically a single view of the wrist, hand, and fingers is used and compared with age-related "normals" in an atlas such as that by Greulich and Pyle.

- Magnetic resonance imaging
  - Magnetic resonance imaging has been used with increased frequency to evaluate a variety of pediatric disorders because it can provide information about soft-tissue anatomy that is not as easily assessed with other available studies.
  - It is especially useful in evaluating joint pathology such as cartilage disorders (osteochondritis dissecans), osteomyelitis, tumors, physeal injury, and soft-tissue spinal abnormalities.
- Computed tomography
  - Computed tomography has a much higher contrast resolution than traditional radiography and is most useful when evaluating traumatic bony lesions (fractures).
  - It also can be useful in conditions of the physis such as slipped capital femoral epiphysis because physeal irregularity and femoral head displacement can be more clearly seen.
  - Other common uses are to evaluate and measure anatomic bony orientation (i.e., glenoid version, femoral anteversion, or tibial torsion).
- Ultrasonography
  - Ultrasonography is employed in pediatric patients because it is safe, easy to perform, and very inexpensive compared with many other available tests.
  - It is primarily useful for evaluating such things as developmental dysplasia of the hip, the presence of joint effusion and hemarthrosis, and vascularity.
- Bone scan
  - Scintigraphy is a useful examination with a high sensitivity for bony abnormalities but a low specificity.
  - It is especially useful for evaluating tumors, bony metastasis, avascular necrosis, and trauma.
  - It can be especially useful in cases of suspected child abuse.

Suggested Reading

- Darmonov AV, Zagora S: Clinical screening for congenital dislocation of the hip. J Bone Joint Surg Am 1996;78A:383–388.
- Greulich WW, Pyle SI: Radiographic Atlas of Skeletal Development of the Hand and Wrist, 2nd ed. Stanford, CA: Stanford University Press, 1959.
- Hoppenfeld S: Physical examination of the spine and extremities. Norwalk, CT: Appleton & Lange, 1976.
- Morrissey RT, Weinstein SL: Lovell and Winter's Pediatric Orthopaedics. Philadelphia: Lippincott Williams & Wilkins, 2001.
- Storer SK, Skaggs DL: Pearls and pitfalls in the evaluation of pediatric congenital and developmental disorders. Instr Course Lect 2006;55:615–623.

Chapter 210 Little Leaguer's Shoulder

Mininder S. Kocher, Olabode Ogunwole, and Modern Weng

ICD-9 CODE
733.9 *Epiphysitis*

Key Concepts

- Little leaguer's shoulder is a clinical term used to describe proximal humeral pain associated with throwing and radiographic evidence of a widened proximal humeral physis. Chronic changes such as demineralization, sclerosis, or fragmentation of the proximal humeral metaphysis can also be seen.
- It is not known whether little leaguer's shoulder is caused by inflammation secondary to overuse or a stress fracture at the proximal humeral physis.
- Little leaguer's shoulder has also been described as proximal humeral epiphysitis, proximal humeral epiphysiolysis, and rotational stress fracture of the proximal humeral epiphyseal plate.
- Little leaguer's shoulder typically occurs in patients between the ages of 11 and 16. Although classically this clinical syndrome occurs in baseball pitchers, it can also arise in a baseball player of any position, racquet sport athletes (i.e., tennis, badminton), swimmers, and even gymnasts.
- If properly diagnosed and treated, little leaguer's shoulder is a benign and self-limiting condition.
- However, if proper time off from throwing is not given, little leaguer's shoulder may manifest into premature closure of the proximal humeral physis and thus growth retardation of the humerus.

History

- Progressive pain at the proximal humerus with throwing, especially with high-velocity pitches and at higher pitch counts, over several months. The symptom of pain usually worsens to the point where the child develops pain even with light throwing and at low pitch counts. Furthermore, pitch control and command are lost as symptoms advance.
- The symptoms of pain and discomfort can occur at any point of the pitching motion.
- Initially, the symptoms of pain resolve over the course of 24 hours. However, increased recovery time is evident as a child continues to throw with this condition. An athlete who has rested a few days may not present with pain in the clinic.
- It is common to receive a history of a child that is on multiple baseball teams during the season and plays a throwing sport year around.

Physical Examination

- Tenderness to palpation of the proximal humerus, specifically at the lateral aspect
- Discomfort can also be elicited with shoulder abduction at 90 degrees with external or internal rotation against resistance.
- Moreover, it may be uncomfortable for the patient when testing the supraspinatus muscle with the thumb down and the shoulder in 90 degrees of abduction and 30 degrees of horizontal flexion.
- Simple abduction of the shoulder at 90 degrees against resistance may also be distressing (Fig. 210-1).
- There is typically no effusion, muscle atrophy, or loss of active or passive range of motion.

Imaging

- When little leaguer's shoulder is suspected, plain anteroposterior radiographs of both shoulders in internal and external rotation should be taken for comparison (Fig. 210-2).
- Classically, a widening of the proximal humeral physis will be seen, although symptoms may precede radiographic changes. On occasion, chronic changes such

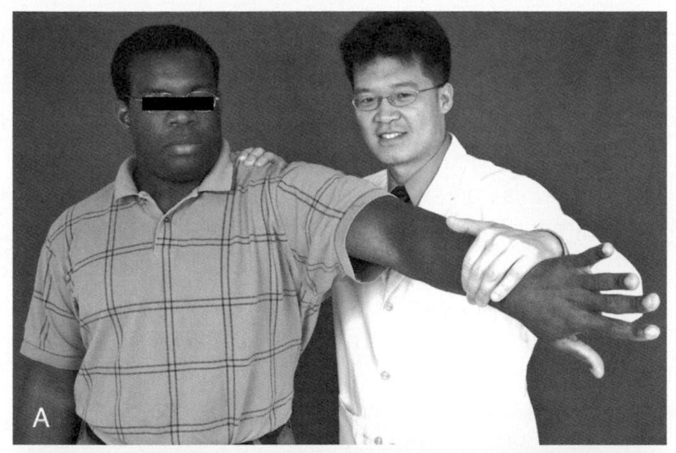

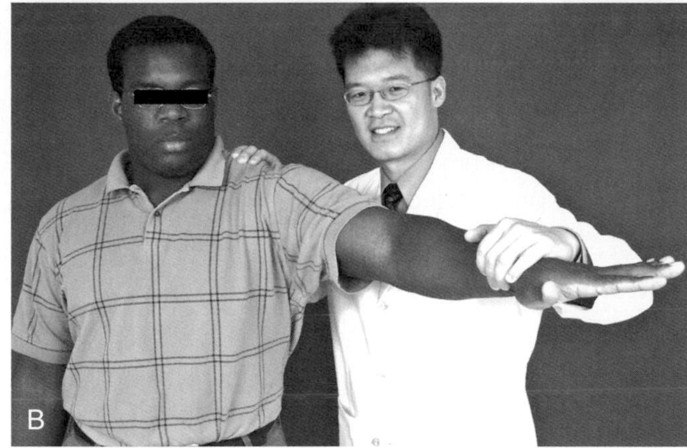

Figure 210-1 **A**, To evaluate the supraspinatus muscle, the thumb should be pointed down and the shoulder needs to be at 90 degrees of abduction and 30 degrees of horizontal flexion. **B**, Simple resistance of the shoulder at 90 degrees of abduction may elicit discomfort at the proximal humerus in a patient with little leaguer's shoulder.

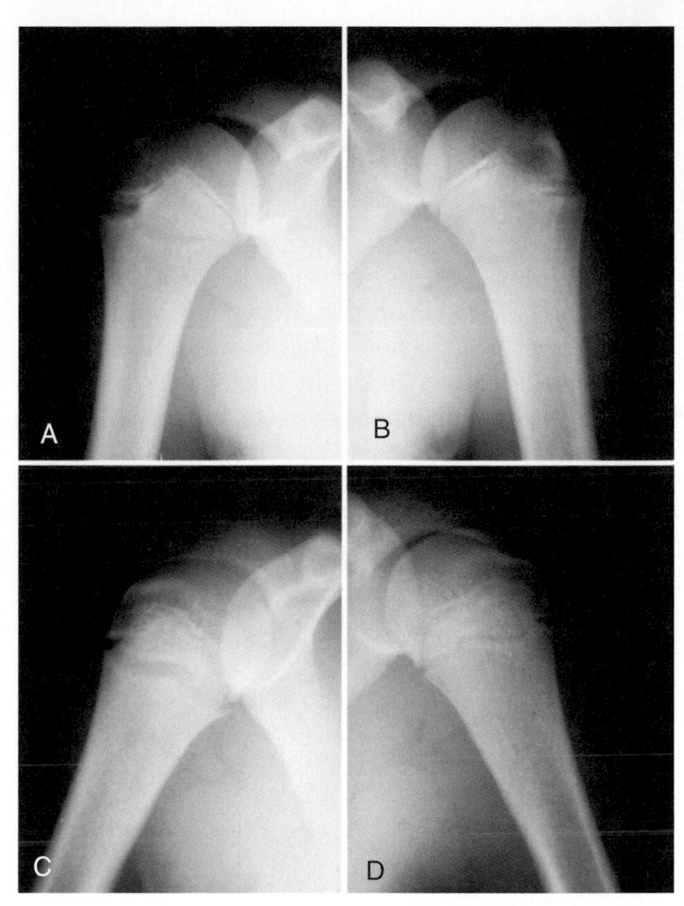

Figure 210-2 External (**A**, right shoulder and **B**, left shoulder) and internal (**C**, right shoulder and **D**, left shoulder) rotation anteroposterior comparison radiographs of the proximal humerus show widening of the physis (*arrow*) compared with the opposite side.

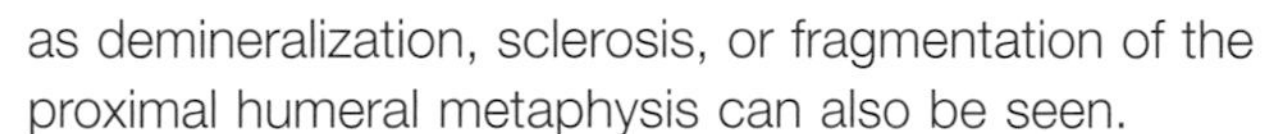

as demineralization, sclerosis, or fragmentation of the proximal humeral metaphysis can also be seen.

- Magnetic resonance imaging, computed tomography, and single-photon emission computed tomography bone scans are not needed to make the diagnosis of little leaguer's shoulder and should not be ordered.

Differential Diagnosis

- Please see Table 210-1.

Treatment

- Little leaguer's shoulder is a benign and self-limited condition if properly diagnosed and treated. Treatment is almost always nonsurgical.
- At diagnosis
    - Nonsteroidal anti-inflammatory drugs can be started for acute pain relief. The athlete should be

TABLE 210-1 *Differential Diagnosis*

Differential Diagnosis	Differentiating Feature
Shoulder impingement syndrome	Pain with impingement test
Subacromial bursitis	Pain with impingement test
Rotator cuff tear	Weakness
Labral tear	Positive Speed's test, positive O'Brien's test
Shoulder instability	Instability on examination
Acromioclavicular joint inflammation	Pain and tenderness over acromioclavicular joint
Biceps tendinitis	Pain and tenderness over biceps tendon

taken out of sports that require any kind of throwing or swinging of the symptomatic shoulder. It is recommended that these activities should be avoided for a total of at least 3 months.

- Later
  - Physical therapy can be started when the patient is clinically asymptomatic. Rotator cuff strength, scapular stability, and general shoulder flexibility should be emphasized during physical therapy. However, if the patient has any symptoms of discomfort at the proximal humeral physis during therapy, then shoulder rehabilitation should be temporarily stopped.
  - Before gradual progressive throwing can be reinstituted, the patient needs to be completely asymptomatic on physical examination. This includes testing for apprehension, range of motion limitations, and weakness or discomfort in the rotator cuff muscles.
  - Gradual progressive throwing is defined as subtle increases in the number of pitches, the types of pitches, throwing distance, and pitching velocity over a 1- to 2-month period. Any return of symptoms during this planned pitching progression indicates that the athlete needs to rest and decrease his or her throwing regimen.
  - The decision to allow an athlete to resume throwing should not be based on radiographic evidence of healing, which may take several months. In fact, proximal humeral physeal widening is possibly an adaptive change in throwing athletes and thus would signify a normal finding if not associated with any symptoms.

When to Refer

- If the patient continues to have symptoms despite an adequate rest period, then the clinician may need to reconsider the diagnosis. Conditions that are not relieved with rest in the differential diagnosis include shoulder instability, labral tear, and rotator cuff tear. A referral to an orthopaedic surgeon may be considered at this time.

Prognosis

- If properly diagnosed and treated, little leaguer's shoulder is a benign and self-limited condition.
- More than 90% of athletes who develop little leaguer's shoulder are asymptomatic on return to sports.
- The most prominent long-term sequelae of little leaguer's shoulder is premature closure of the affected proximal humeral physis.
- Although not many long-term studies have been done on this condition, it appears that premature physeal closure is an extremely rare complication after treatment.

Troubleshooting

- Physical therapy exercises may exacerbate symptoms of little leaguer's shoulder and therefore should be delayed until the patient is completely asymptomatic on physical examination.
- The patient should be counseled on the expected time frame to recovery. Compliance to therapy is essential to a full recovery. Often adolescents will become more active and resume throwing or swinging when symptoms of pain have decreased.

Patient Instructions

- Pitch count limitations, rest days between pitching outings, and a gradual increase in the types of pitches thrown are the keys to preventing upper extremity pathology in a young athlete. Listed in Tables 210-2 to 210-4 are the USA Baseball Medical and Safety Advisory Committee's pitching recommendations for injury prevention.

TABLE 210-2 *Recommended Maximum Number of Pitches by Age of Athlete*

Age (yr)	Maximum Pitches/Game	Pitchers Ages 7–16 Must Adhere to the Following Rest Requirements
<10	75	If a player pitches 61 or more pitches in a day, 3 calendar days of rest must be observed.
11–12	85	If a player pitches 41–60 pitches in a day, 2 calendar days of rest must be observed.
13–16	95	If a player pitches 21–40 pitches in a day, 1 calendar day of rest must be observed.
17–18	105	If a player pitches 1–20 pitches in a day, no calendar day of rest is required before pitching again.

TABLE 210-3 *Recommended Minimum Number of Rest Days after Throwing a Certain Number of Pitches*

Age (yr)	1 Day of Rest after Throwing (Pitches)	2 Days of Rest after Throwing (Pitches)	3 Days of Rest after Throwing (Pitches)	4 Days of Rest after Throwing (Pitches)
8–10	20	35	45	50
11–12	25	35	55	60
13–14	30	35	55	70
15–16	30	40	60	80
17–18	30	40	60	90

TABLE 210-4 *Proper Age to Learn Certain Types of Pitches*

Pitch Type	Age (yr)
Fastball	8
Change-up	10
Curveball	14
Knuckleball	15
Slider	16
Forkball	16
Split-finger fastball	17
Screwball	17

Suggested Reading

- Alber MJ, Drvaric DM: Little League shoulder: Case report. Orthopedics 1990;13:779–781.
- Cahill BR, Tullos HS, Fain RH: Little League shoulder: Lesions of the proximal humeral epiphyseal plate. J Sports Med 1974;2:150–151.
- Carson WG, Gasser SI: Little Leaguer's shoulder: A report of 23 cases. Am J Sports Med 1998;26:575–580.
- Chen FS, Diaz VA, Loebenberg M, Rosen JE: Shoulder and elbow injuries in the skeletally immature athlete. J Am Acad Orthop Surg 2005;13:172–185.
- Ireland ML, Andrews JR: Shoulder and elbow injuries in the young athlete. Clin Sports Med 1988;7:473–494.
- Kocher MS, Waters PM, Micheli LJ: Upper extremity injuries in the paediatric athlete. Sports Med 2000;30:117–135.
- Petty DH, Andrews JR, Fleisig GS, Cain EL: Ulnar collateral ligament reconstruction in high school baseball players: Clinical results and injury risk factors. Am J Sports Med 2004;32:1158–1164.

Chapter 211 Little Leaguer's Elbow

Mininder S. Kocher, James MacDonald, and Olabode Ogunwole

ICD-9 CODE

718.82 *Little Leaguer's Elbow (Variously Termed "Little League" or "Little Leaguer" Elbow)*

Key Concepts

- This condition is an eminently preventable and classic overuse syndrome that represents a valgus overload to the skeletally immature elbow typically seen in throwing athletes.
- A comprehensive definition of the condition includes several specific injuries seen most frequently over the medial elbow, but also over the lateral and posterior aspects of the joint.
- Classic little leaguer's elbow refers specifically to an apophysitis of the medial epicondylar growth plate, an overuse injury similar to Osgood-Schlatter's lesion of the knee or Sever's disease of the calcaneus.
- Other medial-side injuries are age dependent and can include epicondylar avulsion fractures and, in the more mature athlete, ligamentous injuries.
- Lateral-side injuries can be seen as well and include Panner's disease and osteochondritis dissecans (OCD) of the capitellum and radial head.
- Posterior injury patterns include olecranon apophysitis, posteromedial impingement, and flexion/capsular contractures.
- In the throwing motion, tensile forces affect the medial elbow, compressive forces affect the lateral elbow, and shear forces affect the posterior elbow.
- It is helpful for the clinician to have an understanding of the throwing phases of pitching (windup, early cocking, late cocking, early acceleration, late acceleration, deceleration, and follow-through) because stress forces through the elbow vary depending on the phase.
    - Distracting forces affecting the medial elbow tend to be seen in early and late cocking phases.
    - Compressive forces affecting the lateral elbow tend to be seen in late cocking and early acceleration phases.
    - Shear forces affecting the posterior elbow tend to be seen in follow-through.
- Prevention and treatment require strict attention to the following.
    - Keeping track of pitch counts
    - Avoidance of year-round training and participation in multiple leagues
    - Learning specific pitch types (e.g., breaking balls) only at the appropriate age
    - Pitching mechanics and core stability
- Examination and possibly imaging of the unaffected, contralateral, nonthrowing arm can be helpful in resolving questions of pathology versus physiology.
- The diagnosis of little leaguer's elbow should be entertained in all throwing athletes with even minor complaints of elbow pain. Such pain should never be considered "normal."
- Elbow pain is a frequently seen condition; the annual incidence of elbow pain in the 9- to 12-year-old age range in baseball is 20% to 40%.
- Classic little leaguer's elbow is a condition that all primary care practitioners should feel comfortable managing. It is also important to know which pathologies seen in the spectrum of other childhood/adolescent elbow injuries should be referred to a specialist.

History

- Several key features of the history are important for the evaluating physician to remember.
    - The patient's age, both skeletal and chronologic, is crucial because many of the injury patterns are age dependent.
        - For instance, medial-side pain in an 8 year old is more likely to be a classic apophysitis. In a 13 year old, such pain may indicate an avulsion fracture of the medial epicondyle, or in the even older adolescent, this pain may represent a medial collateral ligament injury.
    - Regarding pain, two "where" questions are of vital importance in history taking: Where in the elbow (e.g., medial, lateral, or posterior aspect) does the

patient experience pain (Fig. 211-1)? Where in the throwing motion (e.g., late cocking, deceleration) does the patient feel pain (Fig. 211-2)?
- Likewise, assessing the chronicity or duration of the pain is crucial. An acute onset of symptoms is more suggestive of an avulsion-type injury, whereas long-standing pain is more typical of a chronic overuse phenomenon.
- It is incumbent on the practitioner likewise to elicit a thorough history of the patient's participation in baseball: what positions are played, how many months of the year does the patient play, in how many different leagues, does he or she play other sports or cross-train, what different types of pitches does the youngster throw?

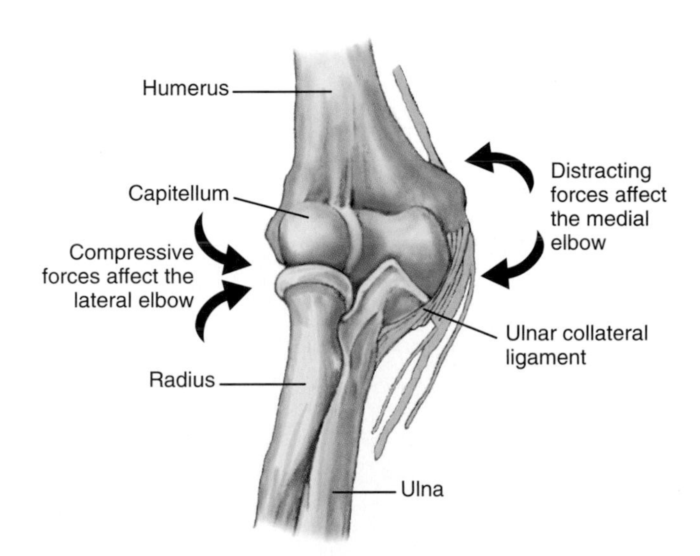

Figure 211-1 Functional anatomy of the elbow.

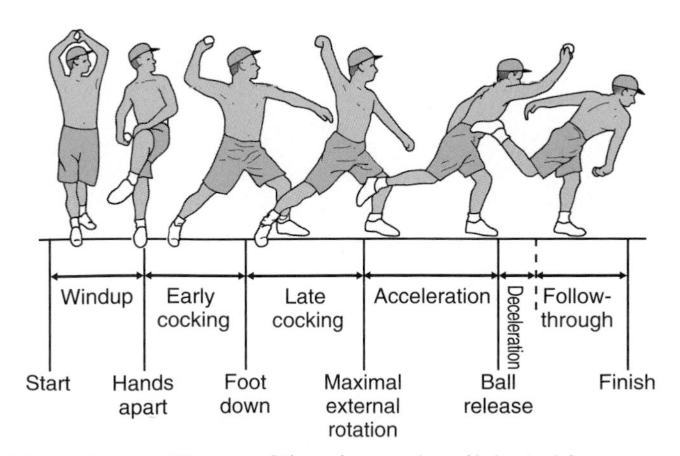

Figure 211-2 Phases of throwing motion. (Adapted from Limpisvasti O, ElAttrache NS, Jobe FW: Understanding shoulder and elbow injuries in baseball. J Am Acad Orthop Surg 2007;15:139–146, Fig. 1.)

- Family history is important to elicit because a positive history of osteochondrosis increases the likelihood of it being found in another family member (i.e., puts the throwing patient at a higher risk of Panner's disease).
- A review of systems is always important: Does the patient have locking, recurrent effusions, or decreased active range of motion in the elbow? Asking more comprehensive questions about fevers, weight loss, nocturnal pain, or the presence of rashes can rule out more insidious causes of the patient's pain.

Physical Examination

- The physical examination begins with an inspection of both elbows, assessing for overall alignment, carrying angle, and any obvious asymmetry such as atrophy, hypertrophy, and contractures.
  - The range of motion should be tested and documented, comparing flexion, extension, pronation, and supination with the contralateral nonthrowing arm.
  - Palpation of all bony protuberances, including the medial epicondyle, laterally the radiocapitellar joint, and posteriorly the olecranon apophysis, is mandatory.
  - Stress testing (applying varus/valgus stresses) to the elbow through an arc of motion is important to assess for "gapping" of the joint. Valgus stressing at 30 degrees of flexion is especially important to evaluate the degree of ulnar collateral ligament stability.
- When assessing the youth with elbow pain, it is important to keep in mind a broad differential diagnosis initially, including, for example, cervical radiculopathies and referred pain. Therefore, a general examination of the neck, shoulder, and wrist is warranted, as well as a thorough neurovascular examination of the upper extremity. The ulnar nerve specifically should be examined for subluxation or the presence of Tinel's sign in the cubital tunnel.
- More broadly, height and weight should be obtained and an assessment of general ligamentous laxity should be done.

Imaging

- Although the diagnosis of little leaguer's elbow is primarily a clinical one, imaging should be considered, recognizing that as many as 85% of patients will have normal radiographs.

- A series of plain radiographs, including anteroposterior, lateral, and oblique views of the affected elbow, is typically obtained. Occasionally, stress views can play a role. Obtaining a series of plain radiographs of the contralateral, nonaffected arm is often helpful in resolving questions of pathology versus physiology (Fig. 211-3).
- During evaluation of radiographs, it is important to keep in mind the chronologic order of ossification centers (apophyses) in the elbow; the mnemonic CRITOE can be helpful (*c*apitellum, *r*adius, "*i*nternal" or medial epicondyle, *t*rochlea, *o*lecranon, "external" or lateral epicondyle).
- The first ossification center appears approximately at age 1 to 2 years, with each of the remaining five centers subsequently appearing approximately every 2 years.
- The apophyses close by ossification as the elbow matures, with all apophyses completely closed by the mid-teen years in most cases.

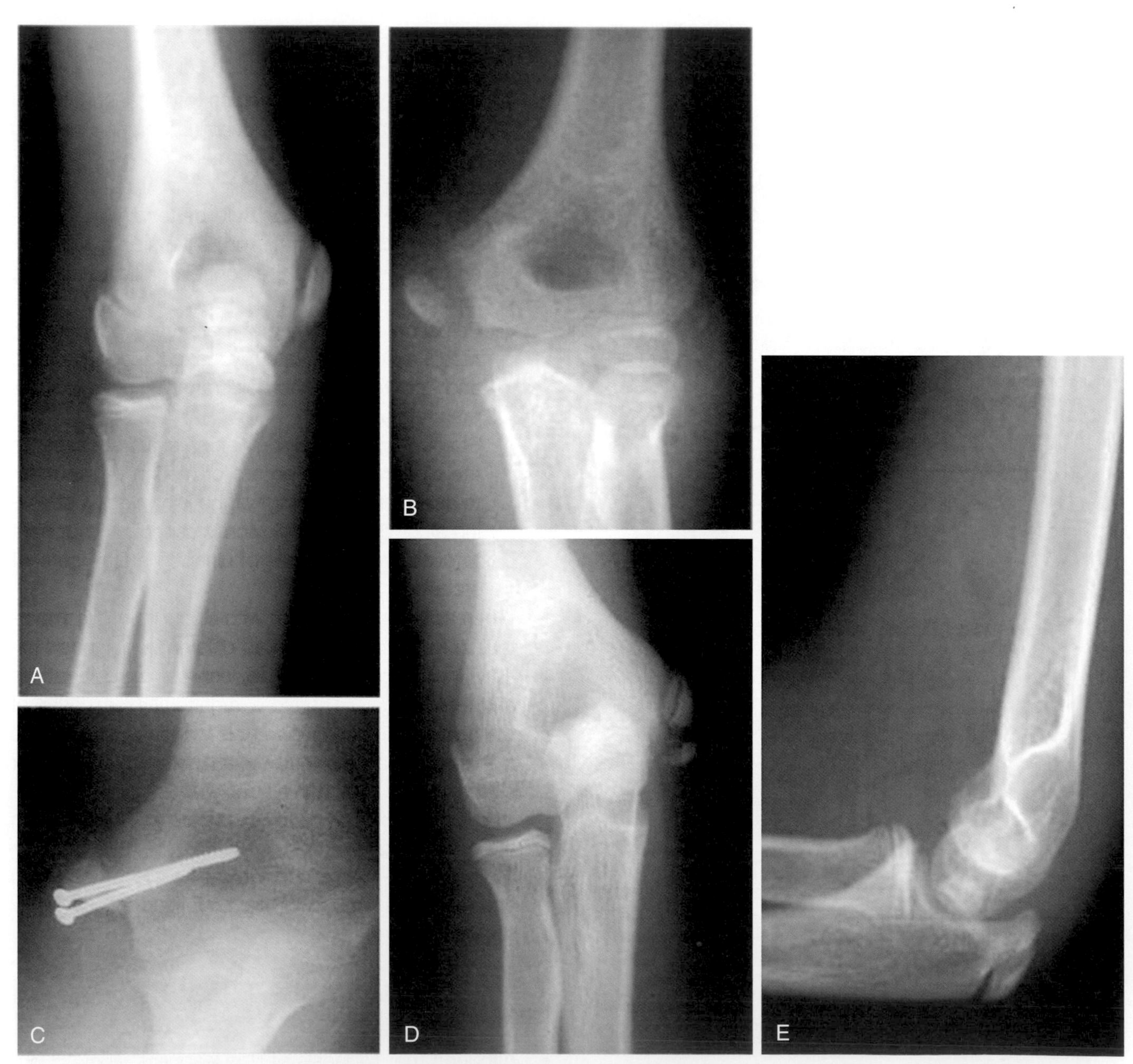

Figure 211-3 Injury patterns of the medial epicondyle. **A,** Medial epicondyle apophysitis with widening. **B,** Displaced medial epicondyle fracture requiring open reduction internal fixation (**C**). **D,** Chronic medial epicondyle apophysitis with fragmentation. **E,** Entrapment of a displaced medial epicondyle fracture within the elbow joint requiring emergent open reduction internal fixation. (From Klingele K, Kocher M: Little league elbow: Valgus overload injury in the paediatric athlete. Sports Med 2002;32:1005–1015.)

- An understanding of this pattern is crucial in making a proper reading of plain radiographs (Fig. 211-4).
- When lateral pain is present, the plain radiographs should be scrutinized for evidence of Panner's disease or OCD. When posterior pain is present and olecranon apophysitis or avulsion fractures are being considered, there is typically a widening of the olecranon apophysis in the former and frank fracture in the latter.
- Magnetic resonance imaging plays a role in some cases, especially when there is suspicion of pathologies in addition to classic apophysitis. For instance, magnetic resonance imaging can assess the degree of displacement in an avulsion fracture, delineate the extent of OCD, rule out the presence of loose bodies, and assess the integrity of associated ligaments.

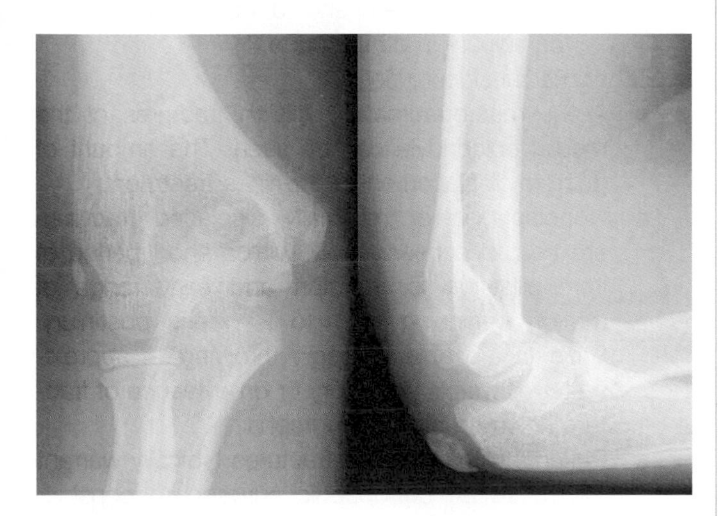

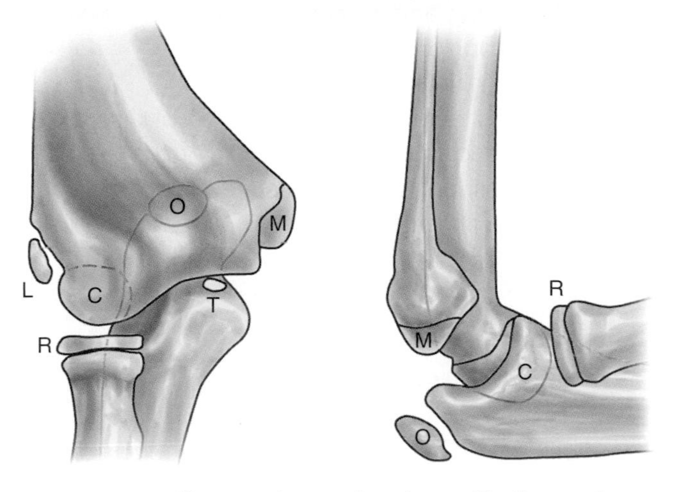

Figure 211-4 The apophyses close by ossification as the elbow matures, with all apophyses completely closed by the mid-teen years in most cases. An understanding of this pattern is crucial in doing a proper reading of plain radiographs. C, capitellum; L, lateral epicondyle; M, medial epicondyle; O, olecranon; R, radius; T, trochlea. (From [part A] and adapted from [part B] Benjamin H, Briner W: Little league elbow. Clin J Sports Med 2005;15:37–40.)

Differential Diagnosis

- The term *little leaguer's elbow* frequently is broadly defined. A comprehensive listing of the various elbow injuries seen in young throwers follows.
  - Medial
    - — Medial epicondyle
      - — Apophysitis
      - — Avulsion fracture
      - — Fragmentation
      - — Growth disturbance
    - — Ulnar collateral ligament injury
    - — Common flexor origin stress
    - — Ulnar nerve neuritis
  - Lateral
    - — Capitellum injuries
      - — Osteochondrosis (Panner's disease)
      - — OCD
      - — Traumatic osteochondral fracture
    - — Radial head injuries
      - — OCD
      - — Deformation
    - — Lateral extension overload
    - — Extensor origin stress
  - Posterior
    - — Olecranon
      - — Apophysitis/osteochondrosis
      - — Avulsion fracture/lack of apophyseal fusion
      - — Posteromedial impingement/osteophytes
- In addition, there are other etiologies of elbow pain that should be considered in the differential diagnosis.
  - Stress fractures
  - C8 radiculopathy

Treatment

- The treatment of classic little leaguer's elbow is addressed first and most comprehensively because many of the principles of treatment discussed are generally applicable to the treatment of other elbow injuries in young pitchers. Then, some attention is given to other specific injuries seen in the medial, lateral, and posterior elbow of young throwers. The details of the treatment of these less common, often more complicated injuries is beyond the scope of this chapter.

- Medial epicondylar apophysitis
  - At diagnosis
    - — The most important initial step should be complete rest from pitching for a minimum of 4 to 6 weeks. If even nonpitch throwing causes pain, a period of enforced rest with no throwing at all should be entertained.
    - — Adjunctive treatment with ice massage and nonsteroidal anti-inflammatory drugs is helpful. In a patient with a flexion contracture or loss of range of motion, an elbow extension brace may be used.
    - — During this period, physical therapy can begin. The initial focus is on general endurance activities and work on core strength.
      - — A thrower's physical therapy program includes attention to the entire kinetic chain from the lower extremity through the core up to the arm/elbow/shoulder.
      - — Interestingly, although it stands to reason that a focus on pitch mechanics would be part of a sound rehabilitation program, some recent studies have not correlated "poor" pitching mechanics with elbow pain. The authors of this chapter do routinely recommend a review of pitch mechanics to our patients.
  - Later
    - — Once an athlete is injured, relative rest from pitching followed by a slow progressive symptom-free return to competition is essential for complete recovery. Any return of clinical symptoms during this period should mandate immediate cessation of throwing activities for a minimum of 2 to 3 days.
    - — Overall, the patient, parents, and coaches are educated about the need to keep a strict account of pitch counts. The patient should be encouraged to incorporate regular rest into his or her training and to avoid incorporating certain pitch types into his or her routine until the patient is suitably mature. All involved parties should be aware of the crucially important information in Table 211-1.
  - Prognosis
    - — The prognosis for classic little leaguer's elbow is very good if the patient can completely rest from pitching as described previously. The average time to return to competitive pitching is 12 weeks.
  - When to refer
    - — It is rare that uncomplicated little leaguer's elbow requires referral.
  - Patient instructions
    - — Finally, the practitioner should emphasize the importance of cross-training and avoiding participation in multiple leagues or year-round play. The patient should be encouraged to participate in other sports.
- Other medial-side injuries
  - Acute macrotraumatic avulsion fractures of the medial epicondyle can be seen. The amount of fracture displacement determines treatment.
  - Nondisplaced or minimally displaced fractures are treated conservatively, with a short period of immobilization for comfort and early range of motion beginning at 1 to 2 weeks postinjury. Patients are able to begin throwing at approximately 6 weeks postinjury or on evidence of fracture union on plain radiographs.
  - Patients with displaced fractures typically warrant referral to an orthopaedic surgeon to consider either a long-arm cast or open reduction and internal fixation.
- Lateral-side injuries
  - OCD of the capitellum especially but also of the radial head is seen as a result of the repetitive compressive forces on the lateral side of the elbow and the shear forces across the radiocapitellar joint. OCD of the capitellum is the leading cause of permanent elbow disability in adolescent athletes.

TABLE 211-1 *Recommended Pitch Counts and Types by Age*

Age (yr)	OK to Throw	Pitches/Game	Pitches/Week	Pitches/Season	Pitches/Year
8–10	Fastball	50	75	1000	2000
11–12	Change-up	75	100	1000	3000
13–14	Curve	75	125	1000	3000
15–16	Slider, splitter	90	N/A	N/A	3000
17–18	Screwball	105	N/A	N/A	N/A

Data from USA Baseball Medical and Safety Advisory Committee Guidelines; May 2006. Available at www.asmi.org/asmiweb/usabaseball.htm. Accessed Jan. 11, 2009.

- Staging of capitellar OCD can be done with magnetic resonance imaging as well as arthroscopically and can help determine appropriate treatment plans (Fig. 211-5). It is also important to determine radiographically the patient's bone age because the prognosis for juvenile OCD can be good, whereas the prognosis for adult OCD (when the elbow bone physeal plates have closed) tends to be poor.
- It is typical to obtain consultation with an orthopaedist familiar with OCD of the elbow once the diagnosis has been made. Treatment can range from conservative to drilling and/or the fixation of the osteochondral lesion.
- Osteochondrosis of the capitellum or Panner's disease is the most common cause of chronic lateral elbow pain seen in the athlete younger than 10 years of age. It is of vital importance to distinguish this condition from OCD because Panner's disease is self-limited, has no long-term sequelae, and responds favorably to a period of decreased activity, similar to classic little leaguer's elbow (medial apophysitis).
- Radial head deformation can also be seen with chronic, repetitive microtrauma to the lateral side of the elbow. Treatment entails referral to an orthopaedist for the removal of loose bodies, the burring down of osteophytes, or, for severe disease, excision of the radial head.

- Posterior injuries
  - Olecranon apophysitis is the most common injury seen in the posterior elbow of the young pitcher and results from shear forces seen in both the acceleration and deceleration phases of throwing. In slightly older adolescents, olecranon avulsion fractures can result from the same forces.
  - Olecranon apophysitis and medial epicondylar apophysitis are treated similarly, with several weeks of rest and immobilization if needed, proceeding to a physical therapy program and a gradual return to throwing. Most athletes are able to return to throwing after 6 weeks.
  - Acute, nondisplaced avulsion fractures of the apophysis are treated with casting, whereas displacement of more than 2 mm requires open reduction and internal fixation. In these circumstances, orthopaedic consultation/referral is indicated.

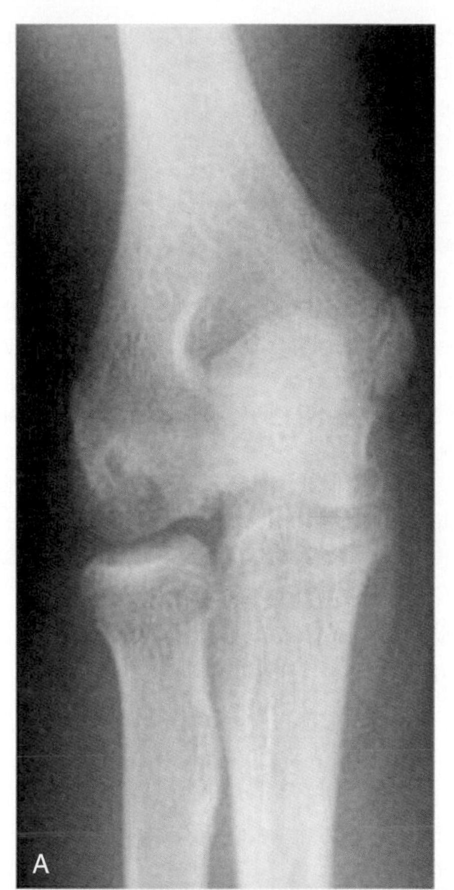

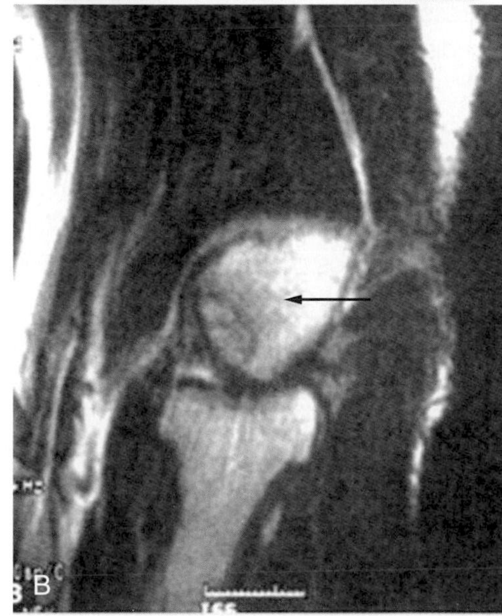

Figure 211-5 Osteochondritis dissecans of the capitellum. **A**, Anteroposterior radiograph of the elbow reveals a well-demarcated subchondral lesion of the capitellum. **B**, Magnetic resonance imaging demonstrates a stage I lesion (*arrow*) with an intact articular surface. (From Klingele K, Kocher M: Little league elbow: Valgus overload injury in the paediatric athlete. Sports Med 2002;32:1005–1015.)

Troubleshooting

- Pitch counts have superseded innings pitched as the measure by which overuse is determined in young baseball players. There has been some confusion over the term *pitch count,* so educating parents, coaches, and young patients pays off.

- Pitch counts describe pitches in a game situation with throws at maximal effort. Other throws do not need to be counted rigorously but should nevertheless be considered, for instance, if a clinician is mandating a period of complete rest from throwing.
  - Emphasizing to parents and coaches the importance of keeping a strict count (using count meters) of true pitches is important, and getting the patient to "buy in" and understand is also important. The young patient should know that, for instance, if he or she is playing backyard ball with friends and attempting to throw at maximal effort, these throws should be counted as pitches and should be reported to the appropriate adult(s).
  - Reminders should be given to patients who pitch in more than one league that pitch counts refer to total pitches and are not independently evaluated for each league.
  - As with most overuse injuries in youngsters, it is also important to get the patient to buy in to the idea of reporting early on symptoms of pain. The earlier an incipient little leaguer's elbow can be addressed, the more likely it is that it will heal expeditiously and without long-term sequelae.

Patient Instructions

- The American Academy of Orthopaedic Surgeons has an excellent patient information guide. Available at http://orthoinfo.aaos.org/topic.cfm?topic=A00328.
- The Little League organization has published online statements regarding pitch counts and rest days at www.littleleague.org/asp.

Suggested Reading

- American Academy of Pediatrics Committee on Sports Medicine: Risk of injury from baseball and softball in children 5 to 14 years of age. Pediatrics 1994;93:690–692.
- Benjamin H, Briner W: Little league elbow. Clin J Sports Med 2005;15:37–40.
- Cain EL Jr, Dugas JR, Wolf RS, Andrews JR: Elbow injuries in throwing athletes: A current concepts review. Am J Sports Med 2003;31:621–635.
- Chen F, Diaz VA, Loebenberg M, Rosen JE: Shoulder and elbow injuries in the skeletally immature athlete. J Am Acad Orthop Surg 2005;13:172–185.
- Hang DW, Chao CM, Hang YS: A clinical and roentgenographic study of little league elbow. Am J Sports Med 2004;32:79–84.
- Klingele K, Kocher M: Little league elbow: Valgus overload injury in the paediatric athlete. Sports Med 2002;32:1005–1015.
- Limpisvasti O, ElAttrache NS, Jobe FW: Understanding shoulder and elbow injuries in baseball. J Am Acad Orthop Surg 2007;15:139–146.
- Lyman S, Fleisig GS, Andrews JR, Osinski ED: Effect of pitch type, pitch count, and pitching mechanics on risk of elbow and shoulder pain in youth baseball pitchers. Am J Sports Med 2002;30:463–468.
- Olsen S, Fleisig GS, Dun S, et al: Risk factors for shoulder and elbow injuries in adolescent baseball pitchers. Am J Sports Med 2006;34:905–912.
- USA Baseball Medical and Safety Advisory Committee. Guidelines: May 2006. Available at www.asmi.org/asmiweb/usabaseball.htm. Accessed Jan. 11, 2009.

Chapter 212 Nursemaid's Elbow

Justin Kunes and Todd Milbrandt

ICD-9 CODE
832.00 *Closed Dislocation of the Elbow*

CPT CODE
24640 *Closed Reduction of the Elbow*

Key Concepts

- The radiocapitellar joint is the key to rotational movement in the forearm and hand.
- It is a secondary restraint to elbow stability.
- Radial head subluxation is a common injury in young children and most common at 5 years of age.
  - Until this point, the radial head has a spherical shape, and thus the joint is less constrained than the adult's cup-shaped head.

History

- The usual mechanism is a sudden jerking of the upper limb, as when an adult attempts to prevent a child from falling.
  - Elbow extended, forearm pronated position
  - Injury occurs to the annular ligament (restraint for the radial head) and remains interposed in the radiocapitellar joint.
- Most likely to occur in children younger than 4 years of age and rarely in those older than 5 years.
  - May occur in children younger than 6 months of age
- Pain in the elbow

Physical Examination

- Observation
  - Presenting position: forearm pronated, elbow flexed and held at patient's side
  - Skin condition: Look for lacerations, abrasions, and ecchymosis to rule out other conditions (these are usually not present in this condition).
- Palpation
  - Tenderness to palpation over the radial head (lateral structure)
  - Feel the medial epicondyle, lateral condyle, and olecranon process for other injuries.
- Range of motion
  - Attempts can be made to passively range the child's elbow if it is tolerated (usually not well tolerated).
- Special tests
  - Neurovascular examination
    - — Check the median nerve. The OK sign must show a true O shape, tip to tip, and show an intact anterior interosseous nerve (by demonstrating that the flexor pollicis longus and flexor digitorum profundus tendons are intact) as opposed to the volar pads pinching.
    - — Check the ulnar nerve (crossing the patient's fingers and spreading the fingers apart demonstrates intact interosseous innervations).
    - — Check the radial nerve (check thumb extension to show that the extensor pollicis longus tendon is intact).
    - — Check the radial and ulnar pulses.

Imaging

- Radiographs
  - Obtain two views of the humerus (anteroposterior and lateral), three views of the elbow (anteroposterior, lateral, and oblique), and two views of the forearm (anteroposterior and lateral) (this confirms that there are no other injuries).
  - The center of the radial head and the capitellum should line up normally.

TABLE 212-1 *Differential Diagnosis*

Differential Diagnosis	Differentiating Feature
Congenital radial head dislocation	Look for bilateral involvement; no pain, no trauma
Monteggia's fracture (ulna fracture with associated radial head dislocation)	Look for subtle plastic deformation (slight bend without obvious fracture line) of the ulnar shaft or even the olecranon
Supracondylar humerus fracture	Associated with trauma, ecchymosis, and swelling

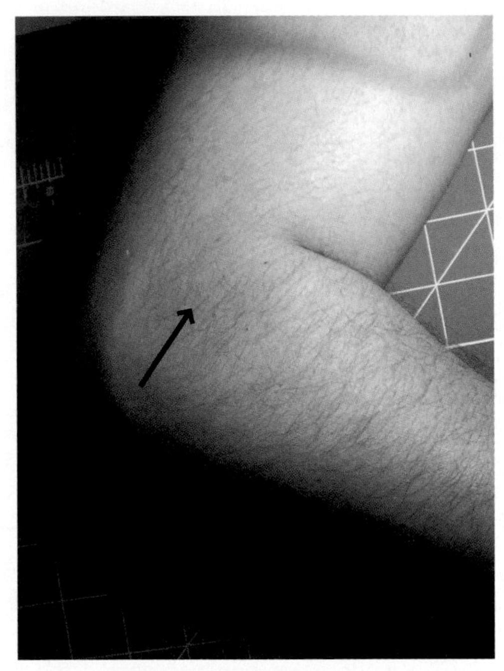

Figure 212-1 Lateral aspect of the elbow with *arrow* indicating location of the radial head.

Differential Diagnosis

- Please see Table 212-1.
- Congenital radial head dislocation
  - Look for bilateral involvement, no pain, and no trauma.
- Monteggia's fracture (fracture of the ulna with associated radial head dislocation)
  - Look for subtle plastic deformation (slight bend without obvious fracture line) of the ulnar shaft or even of the olecranon.
  - Usually associated with severe trauma
- Supracondylar humerus fracture, associated with trauma, ecchymosis, and swelling

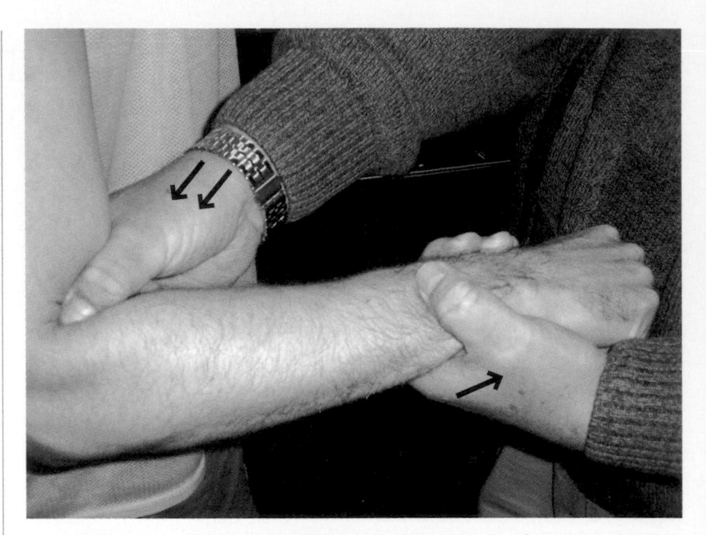

Figure 212-2 Clinical picture showing hand 1 (*single arrow*) and hand 2 (*double arrow*) placement for reduction.

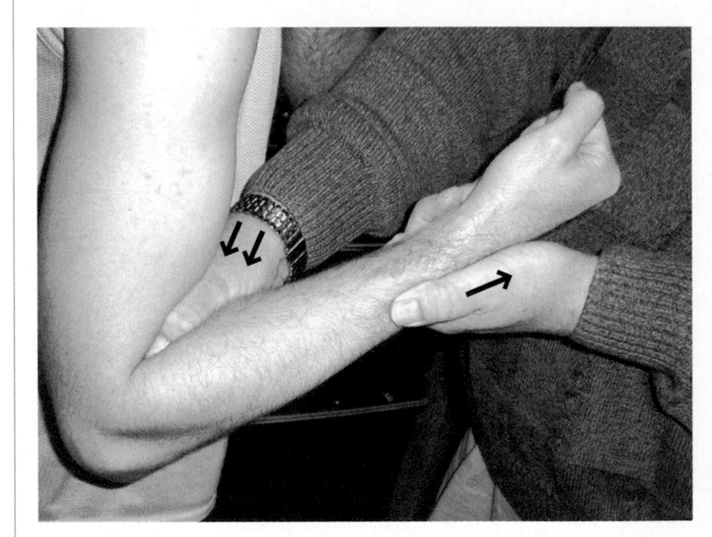

Figure 212-3 Hand 1 (*single arrow*) has now supinated the forearm, whereas hand 2 (*double arrow*) places posterior force on the radial head.

Treatment

- At diagnosis
  - Reduction of nursemaid's elbow (Figs. 212-1 to 212-4)
    - — Where to hold the arm and wrist (see Fig. 212-2)
      - — One hand at distal forearm (hand 1)
      - — Other hand at distal humerus with thumb on radial head (hand 2)
    - — Manipulation (see Figs. 212-3 and 212-4)
      - — Hand 1 flexes and supinates the forearm and gently extends the elbow from 90 to 0 degrees.

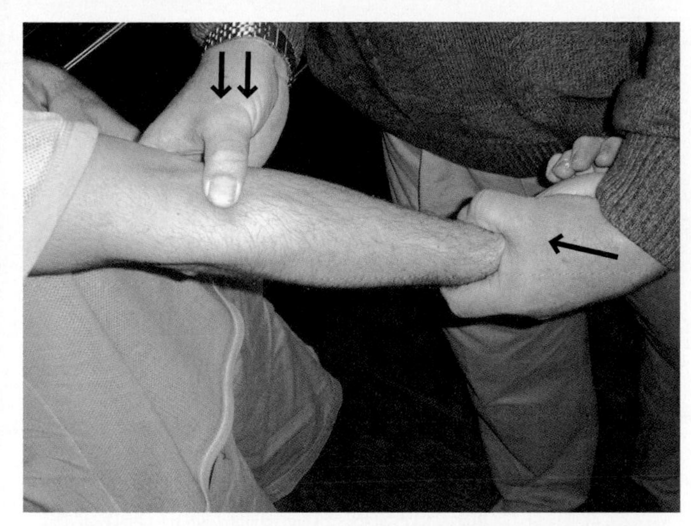

Figure 212-4 Hand 1 (*single arrow*) has extended the elbow, whereas hand 2 (*double arrow*) continues to apply posterior force on the radial head. This completes the reduction maneuver.

  - — Hand 2 applies posteriorly directed force on the radial head and feels for reduction of the radial head.
  - — Allowing the parent to attempt this reduction while described by the physician over the telephone has been reported; subsequent follow-up is recommended.
- — Immobilization
- — The first episode requires no immobilization unless reduction is delayed more than 12 hours.
- — Delayed for more than 12 hours: 10 days in a posterior long arm splint, 90 degrees of flexion and full supination
  - — Recurrent episodes: After three recurrences, the patient should wear a cast for 3 weeks in the same position as a long arm splint.

When to Refer

- Children who develop recurrent subluxation after 3 weeks of cast immobilization should be referred to an orthopaedist comfortable with dealing with pediatric upper extremity injuries.
- Occasionally such children will require surgical intervention to reconstruct the annular ligament to prevent further instability.

Troubleshooting

- Many patients will have reduced on the way to the office.

Patient Instructions

- Have the family watch for the expected recovery after relocation, which is increasing use of the elbow by the child. If this does not occur, then a re-evaluation must be performed.

Suggested Reading

- Choung W, Heinrich SD: Acute annular ligament interposition into the radiocapitellar joint in children (nursemaid's elbow). J Pediatr Orthop 1995;15:454–456.
- Kaplan RE, Lillis KA: Recurrent nursemaid's elbow (annular ligament displacement) treatment via telephone. Pediatrics 2002;110:171–174.
- Newman J: "Nursemaid's elbow" in infants six months and under. J Emerg Med 1985;2:403–404.

Chapter 213 Common Congenital Hand Conditions

Scott A. Riley

ICD CODES

755.11 *Syndactyly*
762.8 *Constriction Ring Syndrome*
755.01 *Polydactyly (Duplication)*
755.5 *Common Digital Deformities*
755.59 *Hypoplasia*
727.03 *Congenital Trigger Thumb*
754.89 *Radial Club Hand*

Key Concepts

- Congenital hand deformities affect approximately 1 in 500 newborns.
- The child's parents are usually quite anxious and have concerns regarding appearance and functional abilities.
- These children need comprehensive physical evaluations because many upper extremity anomalies are associated with other organ system disorders.
- Unless extremity vascular problems are found in the neonatal period, most children can be referred to a specialist by 3 months of age.

Specific Conditions

Syndactyly (Fig. 213-1)
Key Concepts
- Failure of digital separation
- Frequency is 1 in 2000 births
- More common in males; both hands involved 50% of the time

History
- Apparent in neonatal period
- May have history of other affected family members (autosomal dominant pattern)

Examination
- Fingers may be joined simply by a skin bridge, or conjoined digits may share nail and bone elements.
- The middle and ring fingers are the most common sites.

Studies
- Radiographs help to define the shared bony elements between the digits.

Associated Conditions
- Polydactyly
- Chest wall deformities (Poland's syndrome)
- Spinal deformities
- Constriction ring syndrome

Treatment
- Border digits (thumb and small finger) are released sooner to prevent finger deformity (6–9 months of age).
- Central digits can be treated at 12 months of age.

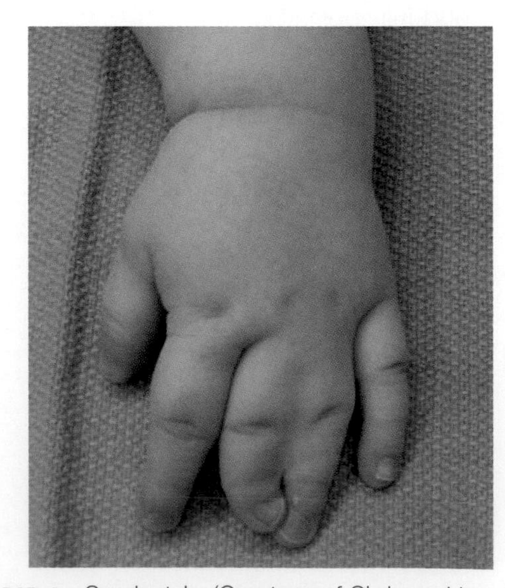

Figure 213-1 Syndactyly. (Courtesy of Shriners Hospital of Lexington, Lexington, KY.)

Constriction Ring Syndrome

Key Concepts

- Occurs in 1 in 15,000 births

History

- Deficiencies are not hereditary.

Examination

- A deep crease that encircles a digit or body part
- May cause vascular or lymphatic drainage compromise

Treatment

- If the vascular supply of the body part is compromised, urgent surgical release of the crease is necessary.

Polydactyly (Duplication) (Figs. 213-2 and 213-3)

Key Concepts

- Three types: radial side of hand (preaxial), central, and ulnar side of hand (postaxial)

History

- Incidence in black population is 1 in 300 births (usually postaxial type)
- Incidence in white population is 1 in 3000 births (often involves the thumb and can be associated with other congenital anomalies)

Treatment

- The central duplication type requires surgical reconstruction.
- Ulnar-side polydactyly may present with a small nubbin or skin tag that can be ligated at the base soon after birth.
- Thumb duplication requires reconstruction because neither thumb is normal in size.

Common Digital Deformities

- Camptodactyly
  - Flexion deformity of the proximal interphalangeal joint; usually treated by splinting and stretching, unless deformity is severe
- Clinodactyly
  - Angular digital deformity thought to be due to an abnormally shaped middle phalanx
  - Treatment is surgical osteotomy if the deformity is severe.
  - Can be seen in as many as 79% of patients with Down syndrome
- Kirner's deformity
  - Flexion deformity of the distal phalanx
  - Often bilateral
  - Usually no treatment needed

Common Thumb Conditions

- Hypoplasia
  - "Short thumb," which is staged from type I (small with all anatomic elements present) to type V (total absence)
  - Surgery may be needed for the more severe types (Fig. 213-4).
- Congenital trigger thumb
  - One of the most common pediatric hand conditions seen
  - Presents as a flexion posture of the interphalangeal joint

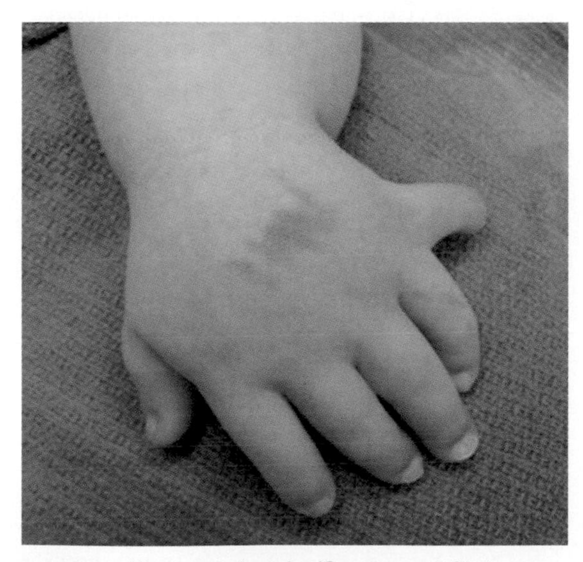

Figure 213-2 Ulnar polydactyly. (Courtesy of Shriners Hospital of Lexington, Lexington, KY.)

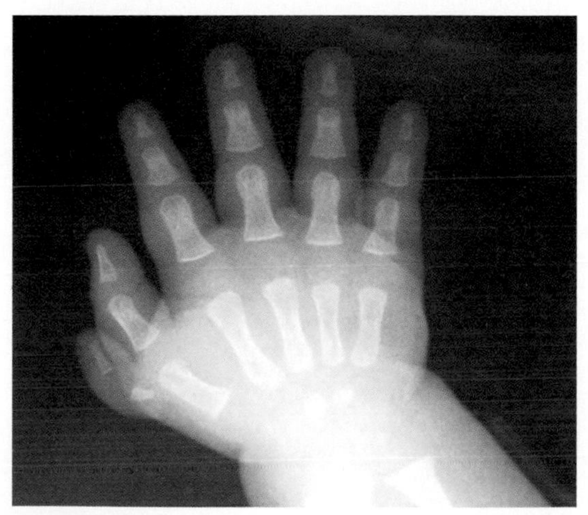

Figure 213-3 Radial polydactyly. (Courtesy of Shriners Hospital of Lexington, Lexington, KY.)

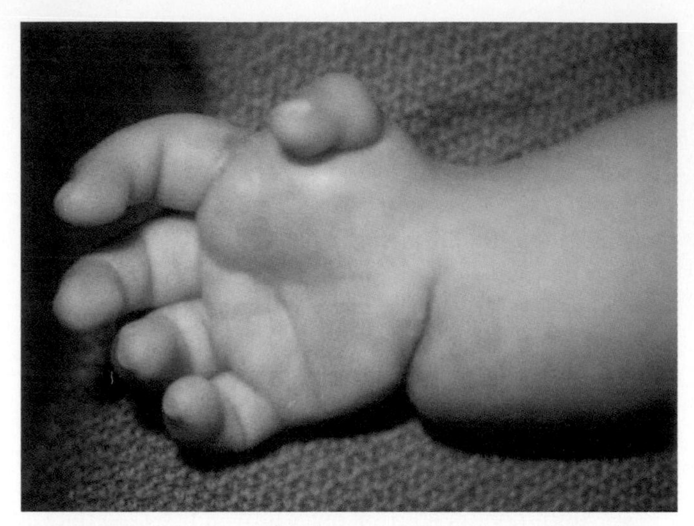

Figure 213-4 Hypoplasia. (Courtesy of Shriners Hospital of Lexington, Lexington, KY.)

- Many cases resolve by 1 year of age; if not, surgical release gives good functional results.

Radial Clubhand (Fig. 213-5)

Key Concepts

- Four clinical types that vary from a short radial bone to the complete absence of the radius
- Occurs in 1 in 100,000 live births

History

- Fifty percent of cases are bilateral; most cases occur sporadically.

Examination

- The classic finding is a hand that deviates to the radial side of the forearm.
- The remaining ulna is short and bowed; the thumb may be absent.

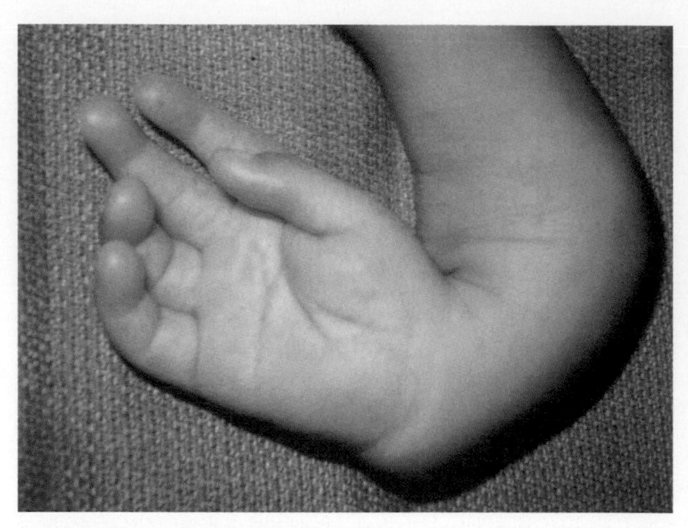

Figure 213-5 Radial clubhand. (Courtesy of Shriners Hospital of Lexington, Lexington, KY.)

Associated Conditions

- Aplastic anemia, thrombocytopenia, and cardiac anomalies

Treatment

- Depends on the severity of deformity
    - Mild cases respond to stretching and splinting.
    - More severe cases may benefit from surgical repositioning of the hand on the forearm.

Suggested Reading

- Dobyns JH, Wood VE, Bayne LG: Congenital hand deformities. In Green DP (ed): Operative Hand Surgery, 3rd ed. New York: Churchill Livingstone, 1993, pp 251–548.
- Flatt AE: The Care of Congenital Hand Anomalies, 2nd ed. St. Louis: Quality Medical Publishing, 1994.
- Gallant GG, Bora FW Jr: Congenital deformities of the upper extremity. J Am Acad Orthop Surg 1996;4:162–171.

Chapter 214 Scoliosis

Joseph A. Janicki

ICD-9 CODES
737.30 *Idiopathic Scoliosis*
754.2 *Congenital Scoliosis*

Key Concepts

- Scoliosis is a lateral deviation of the normal vertical line of the spine consisting of a lateral curvature with rotation of the vertebrae within the curve.
- Classified broadly as congenital, neuromuscular, syndrome related, idiopathic, and spinal curvature due to secondary reasons
- Adolescent idiopathic scoliosis is the most common and is the focus of this chapter.
- Idiopathic scoliosis is a spinal curve without an identifiable cause.
  - A prevalence of 1 to 3 per 100 (curves >10 degrees) in an equal proportion of boys and girls
  - The prevalence of curves greater than 30 degrees is 1 to 3 per 1000 with a 1:8 ratio of boys to girls.
  - Multifactorial etiology: genetic component and also related to multiple syndromes
  - Idiopathic scoliosis classification is based on age at presentation:
    - — Infantile, 0 to 3 years (0.5% of idiopathic scoliosis)
    - — Juvenile, 4 to 10 years (10.5%)
    - — Adolescent, after age 10 (89%)
- After skeletal maturity, scoliosis curves less than 30 degrees do not progress, whereas most curves greater than 50 degrees tend to progress (~1 degree per year).
- The risk of curve progression in idiopathic scoliosis and hence its treatment and prognosis are based on gender, remaining spinal growth, curve type, and magnitude.

History

- Age at onset
- Evidence of maturation
  - Age at menarche, adolescent growth spurt, breast development, signs of puberty
- Presence of back pain
  - Where located, intensity, and whether worsening
- Neurologic symptoms
  - Gait abnormalities, weakness, or sensory changes
  - Bowel and bladder difficulties
- Feelings about overall appearance and back shape
  - Posterior chest wall prominence
  - Shoulder asymmetry, postural balance
- Genetic component to this condition, with siblings (seven times more frequently) and children (three times) of patients with scoliosis having a higher incidence

Physical Examination

- Observation
  - Overall body shape (marfanoid, joint hyperlaxity)
  - Skin inspection (café au lait spots, hairy patch on back)
  - Pubertal development (Tanner staging)
  - Foot shape (high-arched feet associated with Charcot-Marie-Tooth disease)
  - Height measurement, at multiple ages if possible
- Neurologic examination
  - Motor and sensory
  - Reflexes: patellar, Achilles, umbilical, Babinski's sign
  - Gait check
  - Symmetry of shoulders and iliac crests
- Back examination (Fig. 214-1)
  - Scapular prominence
  - Flexibility with forward, backward, and side bending
  - Adams forward bending test (scoliometer helpful)

Imaging

- Radiographs
  - Standing posteroanterior 3-foot spine (preferably on one radiograph)
    - — Comparison with previous radiographs important, if possible

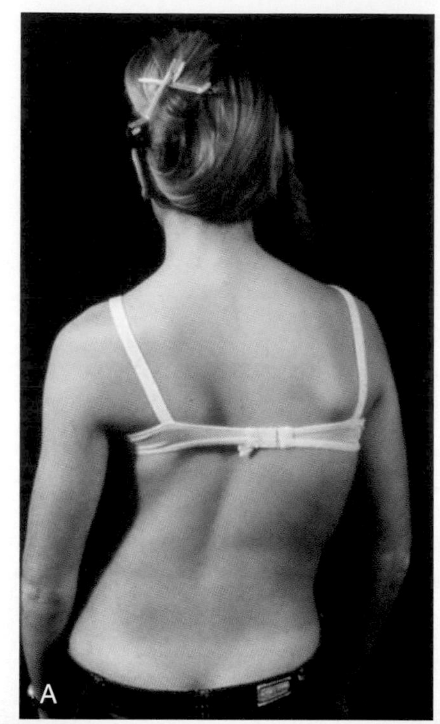

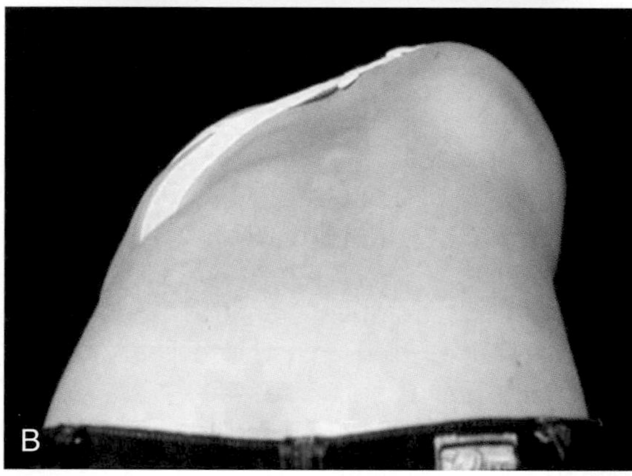

Figure 214-1 Patient with idiopathic scoliosis upright (**A**) and forward bending (**B**) test. Note the rotational asymmetry of the back.

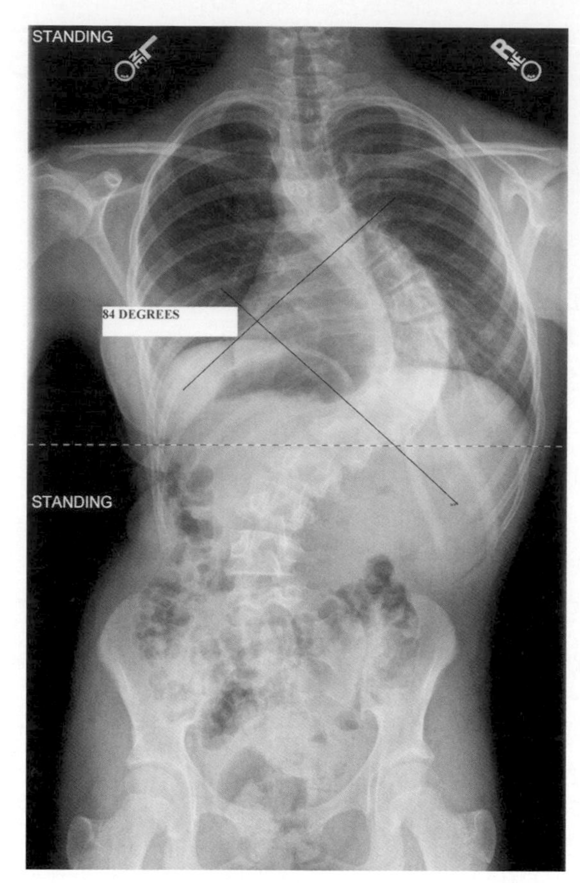

Figure 214-2 Severe adolescent idiopathic scoliosis. Cobb angles of the main curve are drawn. Each curve in the spine would also have a Cobb angle measurement.

- Examine vertebral bodies
  - Two pedicles at every level
  - Vertebral rotation: maximum at apex of curve
- Cobb angles for curve magnitude
  - A Cobb angle is measured by selecting the most tilted vertebrae of each curve (end vertebrae).
  - Lines are drawn along the superior endplate of the cephalad vertebrae and the inferior endplate of the caudal vertebrae.
  - The measurement of these intersecting lines is the Cobb angle (Fig. 214-2).
- Limb length discrepancy (pelvic obliquity while standing)
- Growth remaining
  - Risser sign and triradiate cartilage
- Shape of curvature
  - Sharp versus gradual
  - Left versus right thoracic
  - Primarily thoracic, lumbar, or both
- Position of left shoulder: if elevated, denotes proximal thoracic curve

- Lateral view
  - Sagittal alignment
  - Examine for vertebral body abnormalities, spondylolysis, and spondylolisthesis

- Magnetic resonance imaging
  - Controversial, but generally not necessary with standard idiopathic scoliosis
  - Recommended for patients younger than 10 years of age at presentation (juvenile and infantile scoliosis), with left thoracic curves, with an abnormality on the neurologic examination and with quickly progressing curves
  - If concern exists for infection or bony tumors (e.g., osteoid osteoma), intraspinal pathology (syringomyelia and masses), and nerve root irritation

- Bone scan
  - Evaluate for spondylolysis if suspected in an adolescent with significant low back pain

Additional Tests

- Ultrasonography of the kidneys and an echocardiogram should be obtained in cases of congenital scoliosis.

Differential Diagnosis

- Leg length discrepancy
  - Unequal pelvic height causes oblique take-off of spine and apparent scoliosis
- Scoliosis due to secondary causes (minimal or no vertebral rotation) (Fig. 214-3)
- Tumor: osteoid osteoma, intradural mass
  - Vertebral destruction, neurologic abnormalities
- Syringomyelia
  - Neurologic abnormalities, magnetic resonance imaging abnormalities
- Discitis or osteomyelitis
  - Fevers, vertebral changes, significant pain
- Muscle spasm
  - Intermittent back pain, usually precipitating event
- Mechanical back pain
  - Long-standing back pain with no other abnormality on radiograph or examination
- Disc herniation
  - Back pain with radicular symptoms
- Congenital scoliosis
  - Abnormalities noted on radiographic examination
- Neuromuscular scoliosis or other syndrome (cerebral palsy)

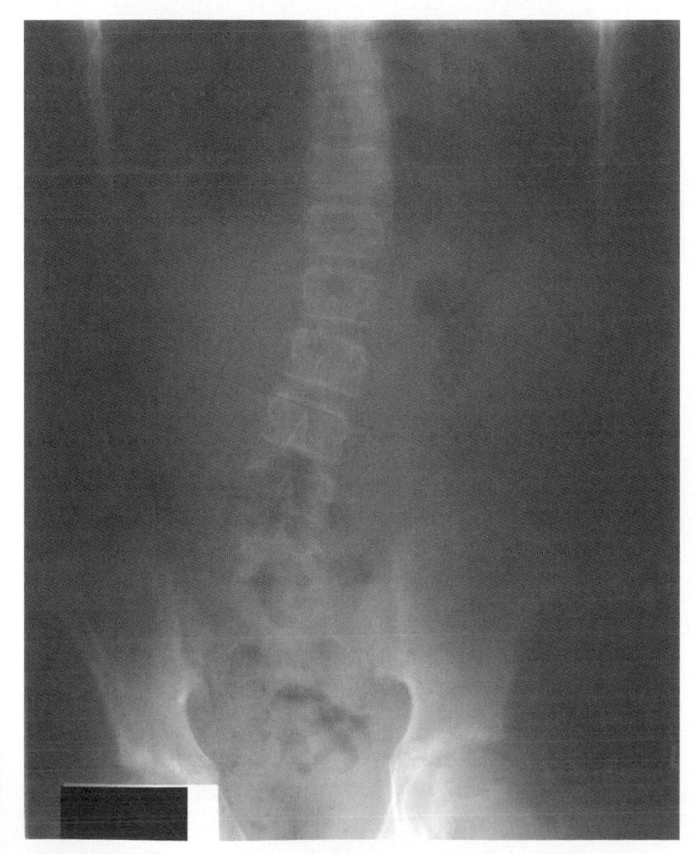

Figure 214-3 Spinal curvature without rotation. Other diagnoses apart from idiopathic scoliosis must be considered.

Treatment

- At diagnosis and later
  - The treatment of scoliosis is based on the type of scoliosis, the magnitude of the curve, the number of years of growth remaining, and the patient's opinion about the shape of his or her back. Although many other factors must be considered, the general goal is to keep curves less than 50 degrees at maturity
  - Observation is recommended for immature patients with curves less than 25 degrees; no treatment necessary for mature patients with curves less than 25 degrees
  - Orthotic management is recommended for immature patients with progressing curves between 25 and 45 degrees.
  - Surgical correction of idiopathic scoliosis is considered for curves greater than 45 degrees in immature patients and in curves greater than 50 degrees in mature patients.
  - The treatment of patients with congenital, neuromuscular, and syndrome-associated scoliosis and those with idiopathic curves who are younger than 10 years of age presents a number of controversies. These patients should be treated at specialized facilities.
  - The goals of surgical treatment are to prevent progression and to improve spinal alignment and balance. The hips and shoulders should be level and the head over the sacrum while maintaining sagittal alignment. The spine is corrected with some combination of rods, hooks, screws, and wires while being fused by bone graft. Strategies include fusion with and without instrumentation anteriorly, posteriorly, or both depending on the curve type, patient's age, and surgeon preference (Figs. 214-4 and 214-5).

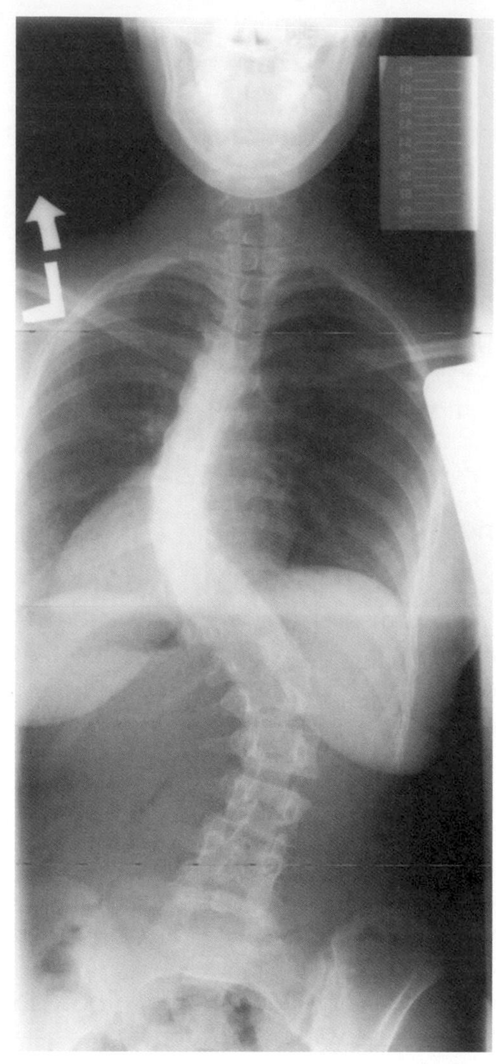

Figure 214-4 Typical adolescent idiopathic scoliosis requiring correction and fusion.

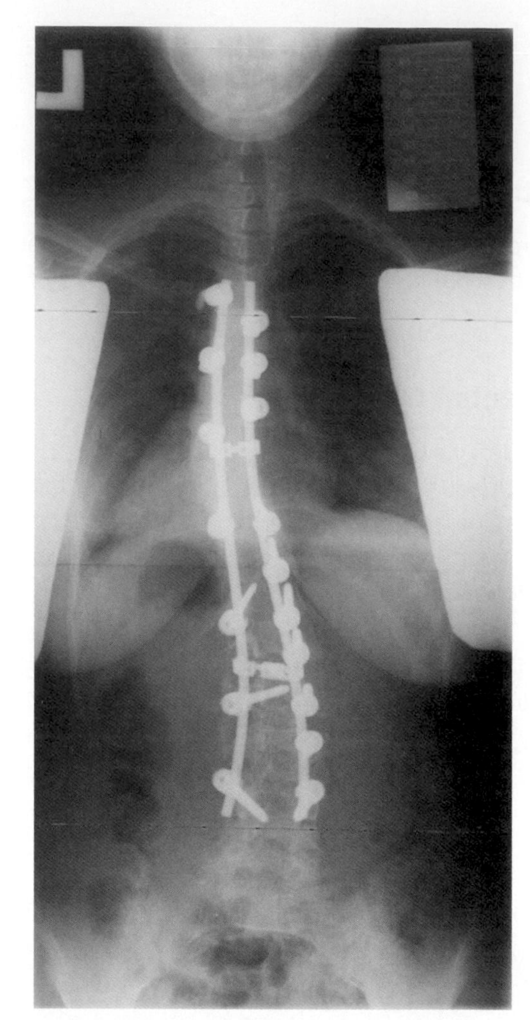

Figure 214-5 Fused spine with hook and screw construct.

When to Refer

- Any child with an atypical curve greater than 10 degrees including patients younger than 10 years of age, with left thoracic curves, neurologic abnormalities, or significant pain
- A child older than the age of 10 and less than skeletal maturity can be referred at any time but definitely once the curve reaches 20 to 25 degrees.
- A referral is usually indicated within 3 months for typical scoliosis and within 1 month for atypical scoliosis.

Prognosis

- In untreated scoliosis after skeletal maturity, curves less than 30 degrees do not progress, whereas most curves greater than 50 degrees continue to progress. The progression is approximately 1 degree per year.
- In patients with severe thoracic curves (>90–100 degrees), there is an increased risk of cardiac and pulmonary complications.
  - However, an increased mortality rate has not been found in long-term studies of patients with adolescent idiopathic scoliosis.
  - Back pain is common in the normal population, making studies evaluating back pain in scoliosis difficult.
  - Some studies show a slightly higher rate of back pain in patients with adolescent idiopathic scoliosis.
- Scoliosis has also been found to be a risk factor for psychosocial issues and health-compromising behavior. However, there have been no studies comparing treated and untreated patients with scoliosis and their rates of back pain and self-image.
- The techniques for correction and fusion change quickly, and long-term results have not been obtained

for the newest techniques. However, with older technology, good results have been found at 20-year follow-up.

Troubleshooting

- The patient should be counseled on the benefits and risks of treatment and nontreatment.
- Bracing is controversial. It is the current standard of care and the only proven nonoperative treatment to prevent curve progression.
  - Currently, it can be difficult to convince image-conscious teenagers that bracing can be beneficial.
  - A prospective, randomized trial examining the efficacy of bracing in the treatment and prevention of curve progression with idiopathic scoliosis is under way.
- Curves will not cause cardiovascular changes until they reach 90 degrees. Patients with curves that begin during adolescence do not reach this magnitude, whereas curves that begin before age 10 often will reach this magnitude unless they are treated.
- Surgical correction with fusion is the only proven method of improving the shape of the back and halting scoliotic curve progression.
- Risks of surgery include bleeding, nonunion, infection, and nerve injury. Significant nerve complications occur in less than 1% of cases.
- Scoliosis is associated with multiple other conditions including Marfan syndrome, neurofibromatosis, muscular dystrophy, and various tumors. The practitioner must be watchful for these other diagnoses, which often need treatment.

Information for Patients

- Scoliosis is a curvature of the spine with rotation of the vertebrae.
- Scoliotic curves more than 50 degrees after maturity tend to continue to progress, so the goal is to prevent curves from reaching 50 degrees.
- Bracing is the only proven nonoperative treatment that may prevent curve progression. Bracing will not correct the scoliosis.
- Surgical correction and fusion with instrumentation is the only proven treatment that corrects scoliosis and prevents progression.
- Despite the fact that a curve is less than 50 degrees, a patient may still be unhappy with his or her appearance and request surgical correction.
- Patients with scoliosis should be aware that their siblings and eventual children have an increased risk of scoliosis and should be examined in early adolescence.

Considerations in Special Populations

- Scoliosis can be related to neurologic conditions, muscular abnormalities, and global syndromes. This long list of diagnoses would typically have other signs, symptoms, and physical manifestations as well as scoliosis. Usually these varying diagnoses are treated at tertiary care facilities with special expertise in the management of patients with complex multisystem problems. The caregiver who treats these patients should be familiar with the nonspinal manifestations of these conditions.
- Congenital scoliosis is due to skeletal abnormalities of the spine that are present at birth. These anomalies are the result of and broadly classified as a failure of formation or of segmentation (or both) during vertebral development.
  - It is important to identify associated anomalies with a thorough evaluation of the neurologic, cardiovascular, and genitourinary system including a good neurologic and cardiac physical examination and an abdominal ultrasound scan and echocardiogram.
  - Treatment is based on age of the patient, progression of the curve, and location and type of the anomaly.
  - The options for surgical treatment include in situ fusion and resection with correction of the deformity.
- Infantile idiopathic scoliosis may be associated with neuroaxial abnormalities, plagiocephaly, hip dysplasia, congenital heart disease, and mental retardation. It usually (90% of cases) resolves spontaneously.
- Juvenile scoliosis is often progressive and has the potential for severe trunk deformity and eventual cardiac or pulmonary compromise.
  - Curves that reach 30 degrees are usually progressive if left untreated.

Suggested Reading

- Basu PS, Elsebaie H, Noordeen MH: Congenital spinal deformity: A comprehensive assessment at presentation. Spine 2002;27:2255–2259.
- Dickson JH, Mirkovic S, Noble PC, et al: Results of operative treatment of idiopathic scoliosis in adults. J Bone Joint Surg Am 1995;77A:513–523.

- Lenke LG, Betz RR, Harms J, et al: Adolescent idiopathic scoliosis: A new classification to determine extent of spinal arthrodesis. J Bone Joint Surg Am 2001;83A:1169–1181.
- Little DG, Song KM, Katz D, et al: Relationship of peak height velocity to other maturity indicators in idiopathic scoliosis in girls. J Bone Joint Surg Am 2000;82A:685–693.
- Montgomery F, Willner S: The natural history of idiopathic scoliosis: Incidence of treatment in 15 cohorts of children born between 1963 and 1977. Spine 1997;22:772–774.
- Nachemson AL, Peterson LE: Effectiveness of treatment with a brace in girls who have adolescent idiopathic scoliosis. A prospective, controlled study based on data from the Brace Study of the Scoliosis Research Society. J Bone Joint Surg Am 1995;77A:815–822.
- Peterson LE, Nachemson AL: Prediction of progression of the curve in girls who have adolescent idiopathic scoliosis of moderate severity. Logistic regression analysis based on data from the Brace Study of the Scoliosis Research Society. J Bone Joint Surg Am 1995;77A:823–827.
- Schwend RM, Hennrikus W, Hall JE, et al: Childhood scoliosis: Clinical indications for magnetic resonance imaging. J Bone Joint Surg Am 1995;77A:46–53.
- Weinstein SL, Ponseti IV: Curve progression in idiopathic scoliosis. J Bone Joint Surg Am 1983;65A:447–455.

Chapter 215 Spondylolysis and Spondylolisthesis

Henry J. Iwinski, Jr., Vishwas Talwalkar, and Todd Milbrandt

ICD-9 CODES
756.12 *Spondylolysis*
738.4 *Spondylolisthesis*

Key Concepts

- Spondylolysis and spondylolisthesis are common conditions in the child or adolescent presenting with low back pain.
  - Rarely seen before the age of 5 years
  - Adult prevalence of 4% to 6%
  - More common in males (6:1 male-to-female ratio)
  - More common in those participating in sports that require hyperextension and loading of the spine
    — Gymnastics, football, weight lifting, soccer, wrestling
- Spondylolysis is an acquired condition caused by repetitive hyperextension of the lumbar spine resulting in a stress reaction or fracture of the pars interarticularis, most commonly at L5.
- Spondylolisthesis is the forward translation of one vertebra on the adjacent caudal vertebra, most frequently seen between L5 and S1.
- Classified by type (Wiltse-Newman) and amount of displacement (Myerding)

History

- Activity-related low back pain
  - Insidious in nature
  - Occasional radiation to buttock or posterior thigh
  - Night pain unusual
- Radicular symptoms or sacral anesthesia with bowel and bladder dysfunction seen in high-grade slips
- Inquire about type of sporting activity
  - Gymnastics, football, wrestling

Physical Examination

- Paraspinal tenderness and spasm
- Limited lumbar mobility
- Loss of normal lumbar lordosis
- Tight hamstrings
- Pain with hyperextension
- Late findings
  - Waddling gait
  - Increased hip and knee flexion
  - Reduced stride length
- High-grade slip
  - Lumbosacral kyphosis
  - Palpable step-off between L4 and L5 spinous process
- Scoliosis can be seen secondary to muscle spasm or in a patient with spondyloptosis.
- Rare neurologic findings
  - Positive straight leg raise
  - Weakness, particularly of extensor hallucis longus muscle (L5)
  - Cauda equina with bladder dysfunction and sacral anesthesia in case of severe or dysplastic slip

Imaging

- Radiographs
  - Anteroposterior and lateral standing views of the spine on a scoliosis cassette
  - Supine right and left oblique views
    — Look for Scotty dog sign (fracture of the pars interarticularis) (Fig. 215-1),
  - Lateral view of lumbosacral junction
    — Most sensitive view
    — Quantify amount of forward displacement (Myerding classification) (Fig. 215-2)
    — Quantify amount of lumbosacral kyphosis (slip angle) (Fig. 215-3)

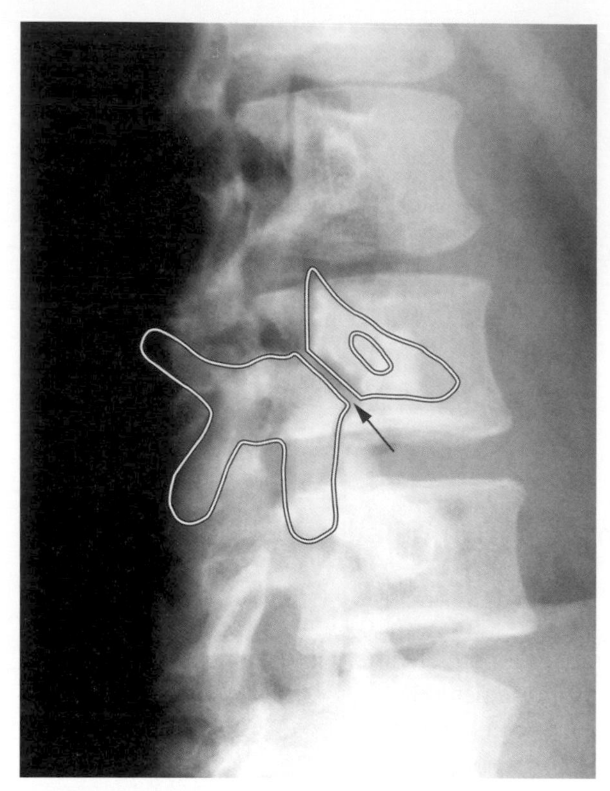

Figure 215-1 "Scotty dog" sign showing fracture (*arrow*) through the pars interarticularis at L4-L5.

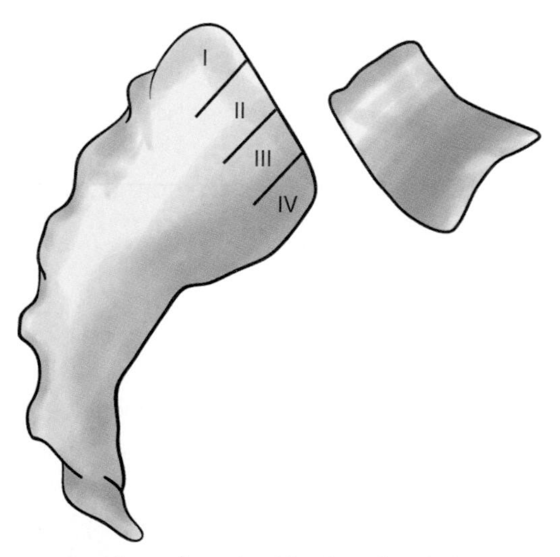

Figure 215-2 Meyerding classification. Grade I, 0–25%; grade II, 26–50%; grade III, 51–75%; grade IV, 76–100%.

- Bone scan
  - Helpful early in the disease course
    — Increased activity at the pars interarticularis
    — Single-photon emission computed tomography (SPECT) is the best means for identifying spondylolysis when radiographs are normal and assists in identifying increased bone turnover at the site of impending stress fracture.
  - Contraindicated in an asymptomatic patient with a long-standing defect

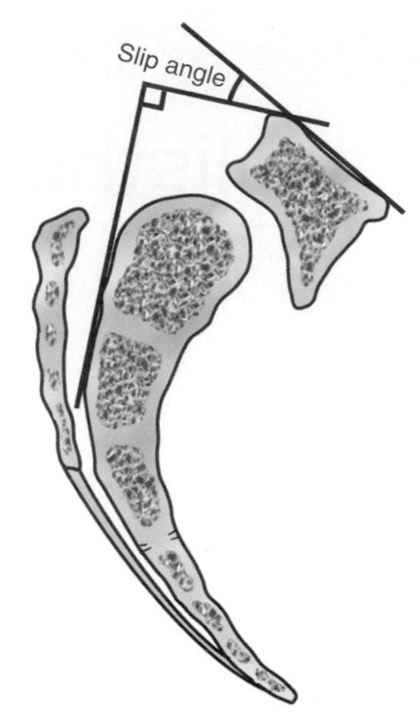

Figure 215-3 Slip angle.

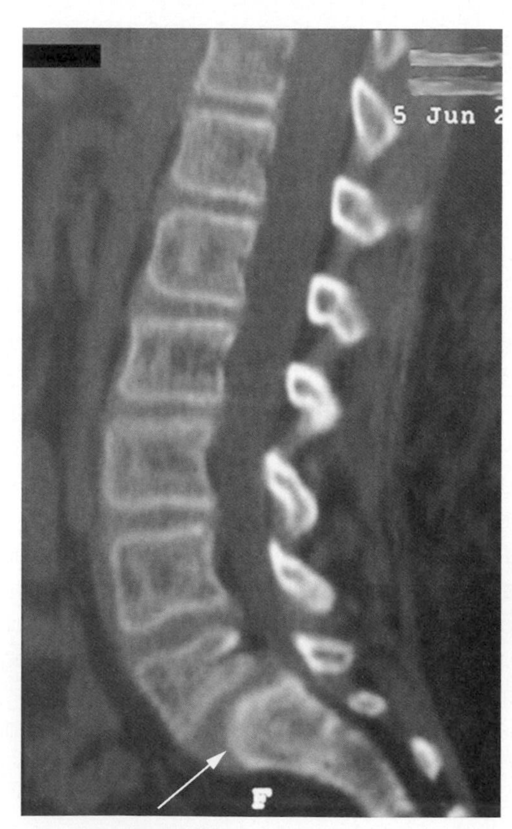

Figure 215-4 Sagittal reconstruction computed tomography of dysplastic spondylolisthesis (note rounded sacrum, *arrow*) and stenosis.

- Computed tomography (CT)
  - Thin-cut CT more sensitive than plane radiographs
    — Helpful in delineating anatomy (Fig. 215-4)
  - Can be used to monitor healing of stress reactions

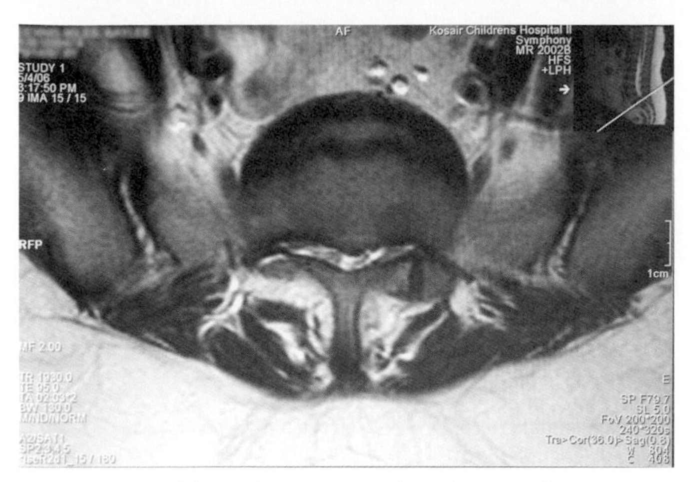

Figure 215-5 Magnetic resonance imaging revealing severe stenosis at S1 in a dysplastic slip,

- Magnetic resonance imaging
  - Not as useful in imaging a pars defect
  - Useful in evaluating nerve root compression, disc abnormalities, or stenosis or to rule out other sources of back pain such as tumor and infection (Fig. 215-5)

Classification

- Wiltse-Newman classification
  - Grade I: dysplastic (congenital), 14% to 21% of the cases, abnormality of the lumbosacral articulation, poorly formed pars interarticularis, abnormal facets, and dome-shaped sacral promontory (see Fig. 215-4)
  - Grade II: isthmic, results from defect in the par interarticularis (Figs. 215-1 and 215-6)
    - — Grade IIA: disruption of the pars as a result of stress fracture, most common subtype
    - — Grade IIB: elongation of the pars without disruption (repeated healed microfractures)
    - — Grade IIC: acute fracture through the pars (rare)
  - Grade III: degenerative
  - Grade IV: traumatic
  - Grade V: pathologic
- Meyerding classification (see Fig. 215-2)
  - Radiographic system for measuring the amount of translation of the cranial vertebra on the caudal vertebra
  - The superior endplate of the caudal vertebra is divided into quadrants, and the amount of translation is noted based on the quadrant where the posterior aspect of the cranial body is located.

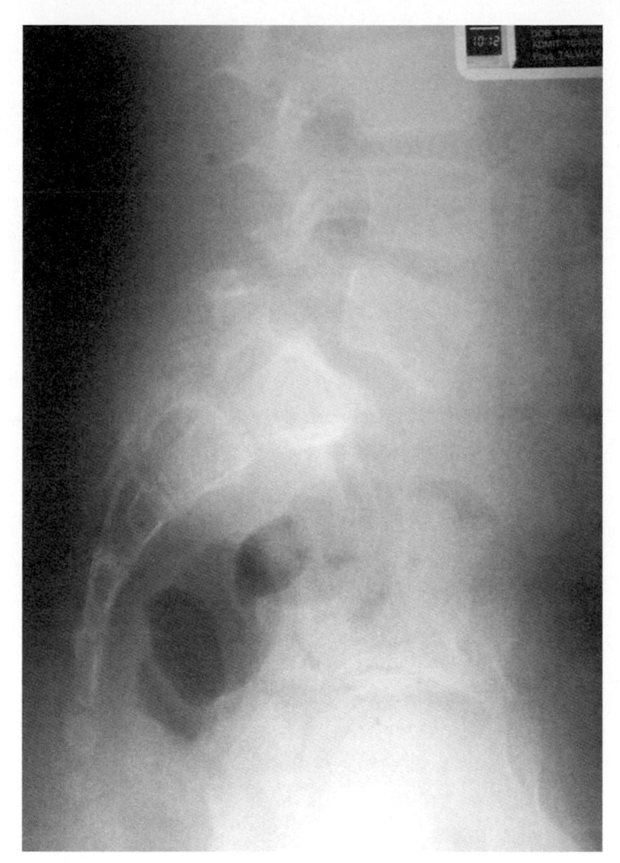

Figure 215-6 Lateral view of L5-S1 showing Meyerding grade I spondylolisthesis.

    - — Grade I translation, as much as 25%; grade II, 26% to 50%; grade III, 51% to 75%; and grade IV, 76% to 100%
    - — Spondyloptosis describes the complete anterior displacement of the vertebral body on the adjacent caudal segment.

Treatment

- Conservative treatment
  - Observation
    - — Asymptomatic patients with spondylolysis or spondylolisthesis grade I or II
    - — Majority of children
    - — Many cases are found incidentally on radiographs.
  - Physical therapy
    - — For symptomatic patients with established nonunion (spondylolysis) or grade I or II spondylolisthesis
    - — Focus on pain reduction and return to function
    - — Abdominal and core back strengthening, stretching of lumbodorsal and hamstring muscles

- Bracing
  - — Stress reaction by SPECT or CT
    - — Try to prevent progression to fracture and fibrous union
    - — Full-time bracing with thoracolumbosacral orthosis with physiologic lordosis for 6 to 12 weeks
    - — Follow until resolution of symptoms and repeat SPECT showing diminution of uptake
  - — Patient who fails to improve with physical therapy alone (rare)
    - — Four to 6 weeks of rest and bracing followed by a reconditioning program with gradual resumption of sporting activities
- Monitoring of patient
  - — The rate of slip progression is low for patients with symptomatic spondylolysis.
  - — Dysplastic slips need to be monitored with radiographs every 6 months due to a greater risk of slip progression.

- Surgical treatment
  - Indications
    - — A patient with mild slips (grade I or II) and uncontrolled pain after at least 6 months of conservative measures
    - — Slippage of greater than 50% on initial evaluation
    - — Young patient with progressive dysplastic spondylolisthesis, slip angle greater than 30 degrees, or significant nerve root irritation or cauda equina
  - Direct repair of the pars defect
    - — Symptomatic spondylolysis without listhesis
    - — Preserve motion segment
  - Noninstrumented posterolateral fusion
    - — Gold standard
    - — L5-S1 for low-grade slip, L4-S1 for higher-grade slip (>50%)
    - — Excision of posterior elements of L5 (Gill procedure) not recommended in patients without neurologic deficits and can lead to slip progression
    - — Postoperative casting or bracing to reduce slip angle and until fusion is solid
  - Instrumented spinal fusion
    - — With reduction of slip
      - — Reduction carries risk of neurologic injury
      - — Controversial
      - — With wide decompression
    - — With partial or no reduction
      - — Better environment for fusion by limiting motion and restoring spinal balance
  - Anterior spinal fusion
    - — May be indicated in high-grade slips to improve fusion rate

When to Refer

- Symptomatic patients with failure of conservative measures
- Young patients with dysplastic slips
- Any patient with neurologic findings

Patient Instructions

- Most cases respond to physical therapy.
- Young patients need to be monitored for progression of the slip with radiographs every 6 months.
- Surgery is recommended for severe slips, unrelenting pain, or neurologic symptoms.

Suggested Reading

- Bellah RD, Summerville DA, Treves ST, Micheli LJ: Low-back pain in adolescent athletes: Detection of stress injury to the pars interarticularis with SPECT. Radiology 1991;180:509–512.
- Blanda J, Bethem D, Moats W, Lew M: Defects of pars interarticularis in athletes: A protocol for nonoperative treatment. J Spinal Disord 1993;6:406–411.
- Boxall D, Bradford DS, Winter RB, Moe JH: Management of severe spondylolisthesis in children and adolescents. J Bone Joint Surg Am 1979;61A:479–495.
- Fredrickson BE, Baker D, McHolick WJ, et al: The natural history of spondylolysis and spondylolisthesis. J Bone Joint Surg Am 1984;66A:699–707.
- Harris IE, Weinstein SL: Long-term follow-up of patients with grade III and IV spondylolisthesis. Treatment with and without posterior fusion. J Bone Joint Surg Am 1987;69A:960–969.
- Lamberg T, Remes V, Helenius I, et al: Uninstrumented in situ fusion for high-grade childhood and adolescent isthmic spondylolisthesis: Long-term outcome. J Bone Joint Surg Am 2007;89A:512–518.
- Meyerding HW: Spondylolisthesis. Surg Gynecol Obstet 1932;54:371–377.
- Poussa M, Schlenzka D, Seitsalo S, et al: Surgical treatment of severe isthmic spondylolisthesis in adolescents. Reduction or fusion in situ. Spine 1993;18:894–901.
- Sys J, Michielsen J, Bracke P, et al: Nonoperative treatment of active spondylolysis in elite athletes with normal X-ray findings: Literature review and results of conservative treatment. Eur Spine J 2001;10:498–504.
- Wiltse LL, Newman PH, Macnab I: Classification of spondylolysis and spondylolisthesis. Clin Orthop Relat Res 1976;117:23–29.

Chapter 216 Pediatric Discitis

Michael P. Horan, Todd Milbrandt, Henry J. Iwinski, Jr., and Vishwas Talwalkar

ICD-9 CODES

722 *Intervertebral Disc Disorders*
722.9 *Other and Unspecified Disc Disorder*
Calcification of Intervertebral Cartilage or Disc
Discitis
722.90 *Unspecified Region*
722.91 *Cervical Region*
722.92 *Thoracic Region*
722.93 *Lumbar Region*

Key Concepts

- Discitis is an inflammatory condition of the intervertebral disc. It is also referred to as spondylodiscitis when adjacent vertebral bodies are involved.
- The cause is usually infection, but no organism is identified in more than 25% of cases.
- Much less common than adult discitis; incidence is one to two cases per year in a large tertiary referral center
- Trimodal distribution of patients: neonates/infants, toddlers, and young teenagers
- The most common organism in developed countries is *Staphylococcus aureus,* followed by *Kingella kingae* and *Streptococcus*. There are isolated reports of other rare bacteria.
    - *Escherichia coli*, *Proteus*, and *Pseudomonas* are more common after invasive procedures.
    - *Salmonella* may be present in the setting of a sickle cell patient.
    - A fungus or tuberculosis cause may be present in immunocompromised patients.
    - No viral isolates have been reported in the literature.
- The classic cause is tuberculosis, especially in underdeveloped countries.
- Commonly affects lumbar and thoracic spine but can occur at any spine level
- Disease process more destructive in infants

History

- Variable presentation
- The most common presentation is back pain (50%) or change in gait (limp).
- Symptoms may have a gradual onset and last for weeks.
- May or may not present with a history of fever (<30% with a fever of >100.3°F reported)
- Presentation is related to age and verbal skills
- Patients younger than 2 years old will most commonly have a refusal to bear weight (refusal to sit, crawl, or walk depending on ambulatory status) or a gait disturbance.
- Those aged 2 years to young adult will commonly report back, pelvis, or abdominal pain; some may report extremity pain arising from irritated nerve roots.
- Rare presentation of neurologic changes such as muscle weakness, sensory changes, and incontinence
- Rare presentation of a septic patient
- Delays in diagnosis for as long as 4 to 6 months have been reported because of the benign appearance of the patient.

Physical Examination

- Variable presentation of fever
- Children younger than 3 years may refuse to bear weight on either leg, refuse to walk, or refuse to crawl, depending on their ambulatory status.
- Patients may find relief of symptoms when they are lying supine.
- Patients usually will avoid flexing/extending the spine to perform simple activities such as picking up an object and bending the neck to look down at the ground/extending to look up at the ceiling.
- Important to test range of motion of hip, knee, and spine

- Pain to palpation may be appreciated along symptomatic regions of the axial spine.
- Rarely, neurologic changes, such as lower extremity weakness, may be seen.
- Must assess for intra-abdominal or retroperitoneal process

Imaging

- Plain radiographs
  - Initial films at onset of symptoms are often benign.
  - These should be standing posteroanterior and lateral views of the entire spine if possible.
  - If the patient is unable to stand, the radiographs may be done as supine anteroposterior and lateral views of the spine.
  - The first changes may be noted at 3 to 4 weeks after the onset of symptoms, and decreased disc space may be the only positive finding (Fig. 216-1).
  - Certain infections and osteomyelitis may show destructive lesions on plain films (cavitary tuberculosis).
- Bone scan
  - Can localize lesions to the spine; advanced studies are needed to differentiate infection versus other process (Fig. 216-2)
- Magnetic resonance imaging (MRI)
  - Early MRI reduces a delay in diagnosis.
  - More than 95% of patients with discitis show abnormal findings.
  - Edema and suppuration are illustrated by a high-intensity signal on T2-weighted MRIs and a low-intensity signal on T1-weighted MRIs.
  - The disadvantage is the need for sedation in young patients (Fig. 216-3).

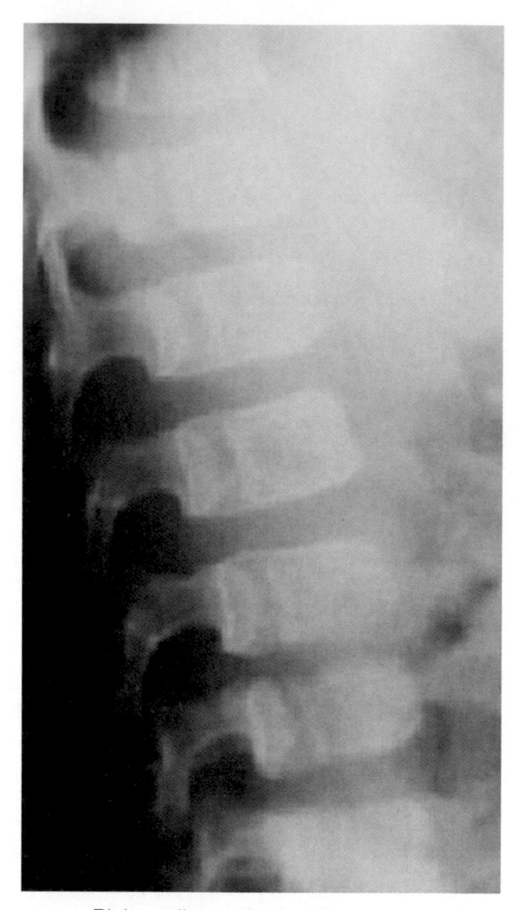

Figure 216-1 Plain radiograph showing narrowed disc space.

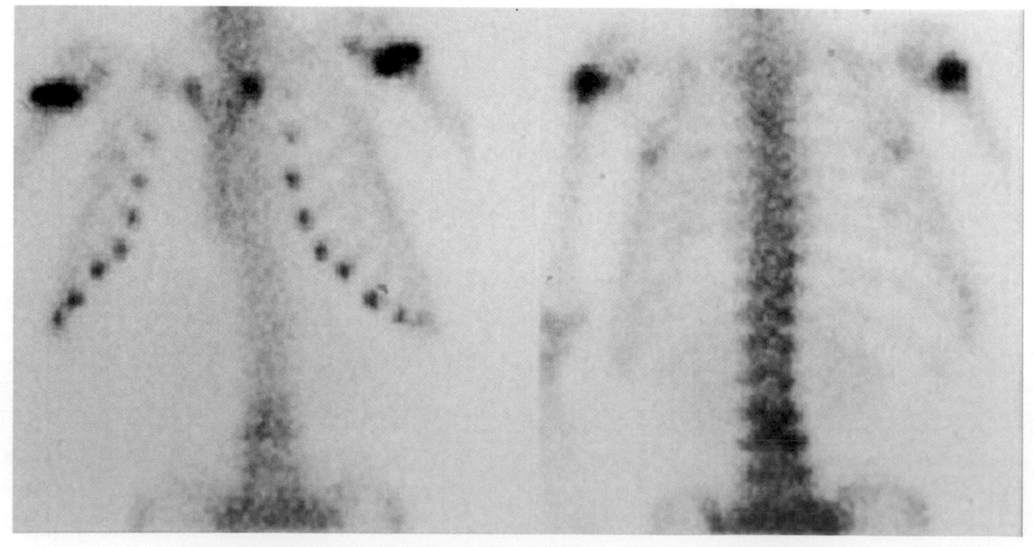

Figure 216-2 Increased lumbar tracer uptake on bone scan.

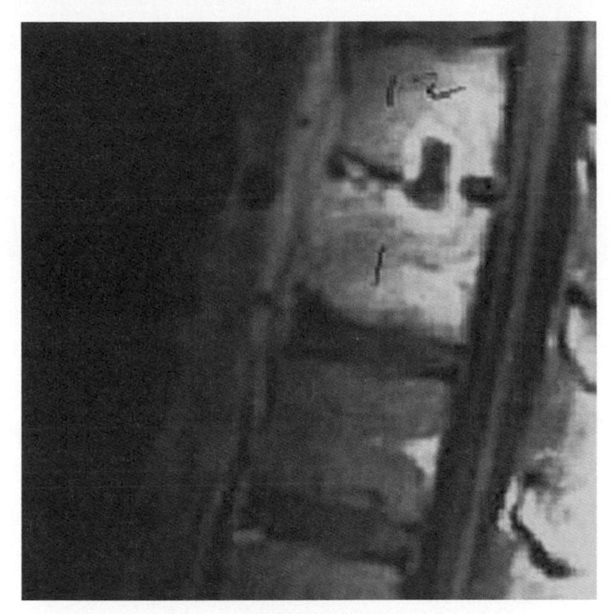

Figure 216-3 Magnetic resonance imaging showing involvement of vertebral bodies.

- Computed tomography scan
  - Useful for bony analysis and can show fluid collection, but limited soft-tissue examination

Additional Tests

- Laboratory tests are mandatory, but often normal or only slightly elevated.
  - Complete blood count, erythrocyte sedimentation rate, C-reactive protein
  - Erythrocyte sedimentation rate and C-reactive protein are useful for tracking the progress of the condition, with C-reactive protein being the most specific for improvement during treatment.
  - Blood cultures should be sent, but are most often negative.
  - Urinalysis may also help to distinguish between gastrointestinal and genitourinary processes.
- Aspiration: only in cases of an unusual clinical course or failure to respond to initial empiric therapy
  - As many as 60% of aspirations isolate no bacteria.
  - Performed under fluoroscopic or computed tomography guidance
  - If fluid collection is identified, fine-needle aspiration can be performed with guidance.

Differential Diagnosis

- Please see Table 216-1.

TABLE 216-1 *Differential Diagnosis*

Condition	Feature
Discitis	Back pain, refusal to walk, gait disturbance
Tumor	Neurologic involvement, localized unrelenting night pain
Hip pathology: septic arthritis/ toxic synovitis	Vague hip or knee pain; refusal to walk or gait disturbance; unable to bear weight; fever; elevated C-reactive protein, erythrocyte sedimentation rate, complete blood count
Stress fracture, spondylolysis	Classic: teenager with repetitive activities, pain relieved with rest

Treatment

- At diagnosis
  - Initial treatment includes bed rest, empiric antistaphylococcal IV antibiotics for 5 to 7 days plus oral antibiotics for 2 to 4 weeks and nonsteroidal anti-inflammatory drugs
  - Bracing often necessary
  - Expect clinical response within 2 to 3 days; otherwise consider aspiration or further imaging
- Later
  - Continued clinical surveillance until erythrocyte sedimentation rate normalizes
  - Disc height may remain diminished or even proceed to fusion, but patients are asymptomatic.

Prognosis

- Generally good unless there is significant bony destruction

When to Refer

- Referral to a pediatric orthopaedist should be made as soon as the diagnosis is made or suspected. A physician with access to an infectious disease specialist would be preferred.

Troubleshooting

- Beware the child with new-onset neurologic symptoms or lack of response to therapy. Both of these could signal that the organism is not being adequately treated or the process is something other than discitis.
- Bracing is sometimes necessary for 3 to 6 weeks for comfort.

Suggested Reading

- Dormans JP, Moroz L: Infection and tumors of the spine in children. J Bone Joint Surg Am 2007;89A(Suppl 1):79–97.
- Early SD, Kay RM, Tolo VT: Childhood discitis. J Am Acad Orthop Surg 2003;11:413–420.
- Eismont FJ, Bohlman HH, Soni PL, et al: Vertebral osteomyelitis in infants. J Bone Joint Surg Br 1982;64B:32–35.
- Fernandez M, Carrol CL, Baker CJ: Discitis and vertebral osteomyelitis in children: An 18-year review. Pediatrics 2000;105:1299–1304.
- Karabouta Z, Bisbinas I, Davidson A, Goldsworthy L: Discitis in toddlers: A case series and review. Acta Paediatr 2005;94:1516–1518.
- Ring D, Johnston CE, Wenger D: Pyogenic infectious spondylitis in children: The convergence of discitis and vertebral osteomyelitis. J Pediatr Orthop 1995;15:652–660.
- Tay BK, Deckey J, Hu SS: Spinal infections. J Am Acad Orthop Surg 2002;10:188–197.

Chapter 217 The Limping Child

Todd Milbrandt

Key Concepts

- Discovering that a child is limping is a scary situation for parents. The causes of a childhood limp can vary from the very benign to the malignant, from growing pains to septic hip.
- It is crucial that the evaluating practitioner should approach these children in a systematic fashion to not miss or delay the diagnosis to prevent lifelong consequences.
- Examination of the involved limb includes inspection for redness, palpation for swelling, and range of motion testing of the major joints.
- In addition to a physical examination, an observation of the child's gait pattern can give the practitioner insights as to which diagnosis is correct.
- The tests to order are directed by the findings on physical examination and include blood work for inflammation markers, radiography, ultrasonography for effusions, bone scintigraphy, and magnetic resonance imaging.
- Treatment is based on the diagnosis and ranges from simple observation to emergent surgical drainage of infection.
- Overall, the prognosis is good if the diagnosis is made in a timely manner.

History

- Acute onset
  - May be related to minor trauma
  - May have fever and malaise
  - Refusal to bear weight or move extremity (pseudoparalysis)
  - Can also be painless
- Chronic onset
  - Can be associated with premature birth
  - Not usually associated with trauma
  - Pain may be transient throughout the day.

Physical Examination

- Observation
  - Normal gait
    - — Normal gait in children can vary by age and neuromuscular development. At the beginnings of a child's gait pattern, typically between 12 to 16 months, the child will have a shorter stride length and a fast cadence.
    - — By the age of 7, a child has obtained a mature gait pattern of a smooth and rhythmic cadence with a minimal expenditure of energy.
  - Antalgic gait
    - — Antalgic gait is an avoidance pattern with less time in the stance phase of gait. By decreasing the time in single limb stance, the child limits the overall pressure during gait on that limb. This is also described as "short stepping."
    - — Children may simply refuse to walk as another strategy to prevent pain in the limb, especially if the pain is severe enough and the child's verbal skills are not well developed.
  - Short-limbed gait
    - — Children will present with toe walking on the shortened limb and a flexed knee and hip in the stance phase of the longer limb.
  - Trendelenburg gait
    - — Children will shift their body weight over the affected hip, thus lateralizing the center of gravity. This gait pattern does not hurt the patient.
  - Spastic gait
    - — Weakened quadriceps muscles in combination with hamstring tightness can lead to a crouched knee gait in which the knee does not come out to full extension. This leads to a shortened stride length.
    - — If the quadriceps muscles are strong or very spastic, the opposite deformity may be created.

This is known as the stiff knee gait pattern in which the child walks with the knees in extension.
    - Other spastic patterns also exist such as the scissoring gait in which the hip adductors are hypertonic, thus making it difficult during the swing phase of gait. Isolated toe walking may also indicate a spastic process.
- Palpation
  - Tenderness along the affected extremity may indicate minor trauma or infection.
- Range of motion
  - All the affected joints in the leg in question must go through a passive range of motion evaluation (including the hip, knee, and ankle) and compared with joints on the contralateral side.

Imaging

- Plain radiographs
  - The entire limb in two views, an anterior to posterior view and a lateral view, including the hip
- Bone scan
  - Can reveal pathology across a large segment of the body; it will be positive in areas of high bone turnover (fracture, tumor, infection)
  - Most helpful when evaluating a nonverbal child
- Ultrasound scan of the hip
  - Will determine whether there is effusion and does not require sedation of the patient
- Magnetic resonance imaging
  - Magnetic resonance imaging of the limb provides the best detail possible for the extremity.
  - The physical examination should limit the study to a small area.
  - This study will delineate tumor, infection, and fracture.
  - Most pediatric patients will require sedation.

Additional Tests

- Laboratory tests
  - Screening complete blood count with differential, erythrocyte sedimentation rate, and C-reactive protein will indicate infection but can also screen for leukemia
  - Joint or bone aspiration
    - Joint aspiration is required if infection of the joint is suspected.
    - Aspiration of the bone is required if purulence is seen in or around the bone on magnetic resonance imaging.

Differential Diagnosis

- The differential diagnosis is very long. An algorithm is presented as a suggested way to work through the many possible diagnoses (Fig. 217-1).
- Juvenile myalgias ("growing pains")
  - Diagnosis of exclusion
- Osteomyelitis
  - Bone infection, most commonly *Staphylococcus aureus*
- Discitis
  - Infection of the intervertebral disc, most commonly *S. aureus*
- Transient synovitis
  - Inflammation of the joint without infection
- Septic arthritis
  - Inflammation of joint with infection; surgical emergency
- Toddler fracture
  - Spiral fracture of the tibia
- Cerebral palsy
  - Static encephalopathy
  - Usually associated with an abnormal birth history
- Developmental dysplasia of the hip
  - May see apparent leg length discrepancy and Trendelenburg gait
- Inflammatory arthritis
  - Will present with effusion and stiffness in the morning
- Neoplasia
  - Leukemia, lymphoma much more common than primary bone tumors
- Legg-Calvé-Perthes disease
  - Idiopathic avascular necrosis of the femoral head
- Discoid lateral meniscus
  - May cause locking and catching symptoms
- Leg length discrepancy
  - May be congenital or from previous infection/trauma
- Slipped capital femoral epiphysis
  - Rotation through the growth plate of the proximal femur
  - Must get hip radiographs (anteroposterior pelvis and frog pelvis views)
- Overuse syndromes
- Osteochondritis dissecans
  - Area of cartilage delamination within a joint
- Tarsal coalition
  - Congenital fusion of bones of the feet

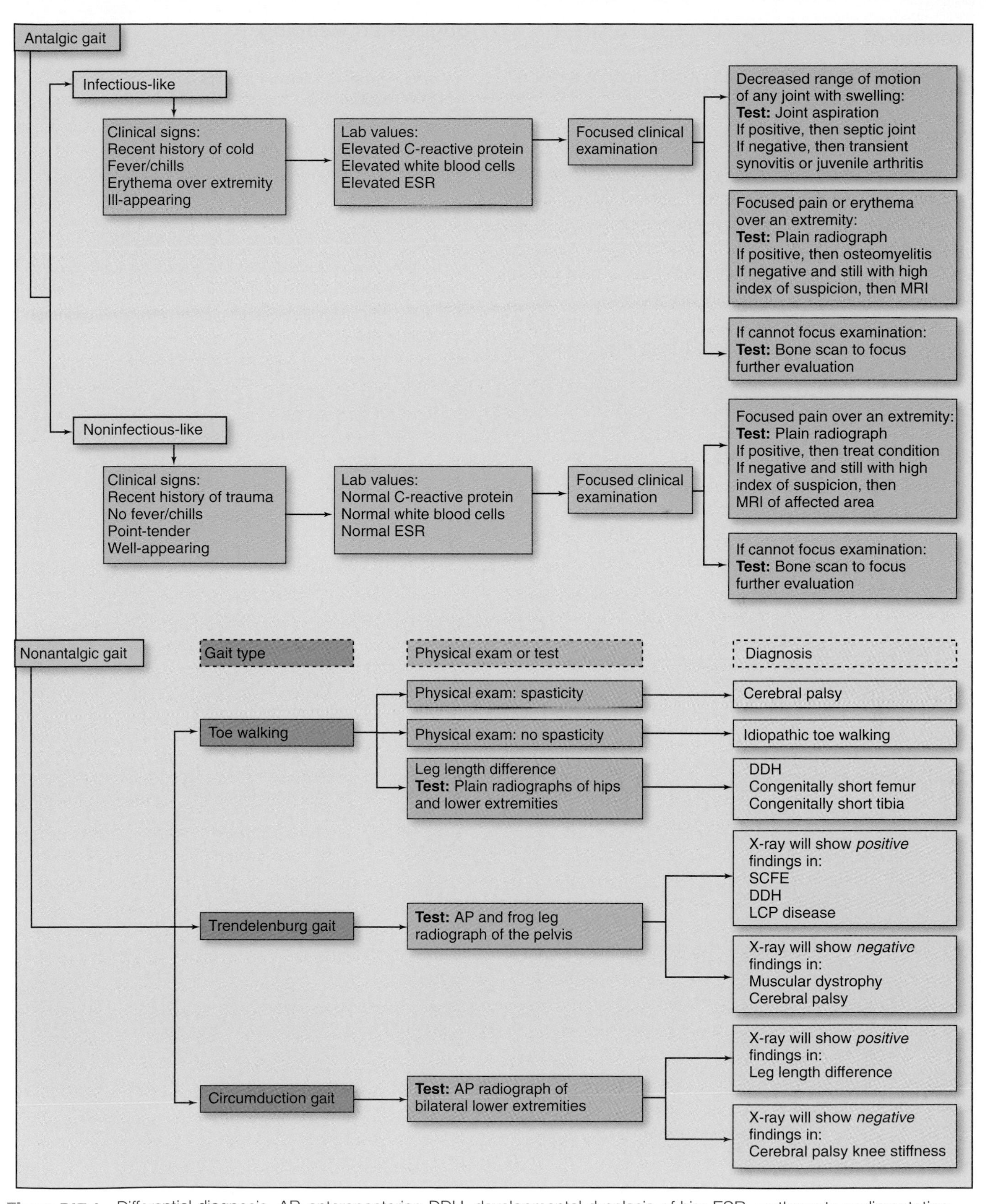

Figure 217-1 Differential diagnosis. AP, anteroposterior; DDH, developmental dysplasia of hip; ESR, erythrocyte sedimentation rate; LCP, Legg-Calvé-Perthes; SCFE, slipped capital femoral epiphysis.

Treatment

- Treatment depends on the specific diagnosis made.

When to Refer

- If a diagnosis cannot be made or is in question, it must be evaluated by a specialist urgently. Many of the listed conditions will worsen within months if they are not addressed.
- Once the diagnosis is confirmed, then urgent referral to an orthopaedic surgeon is appropriate.
- If a septic joint is suspected, then an emergent transfer to a facility to confirm and treat the condition is appropriate.

Suggested Reading

- Aronsson DD, Loder RT, Breur GJ, Weinstein SL: Slipped capital femoral epiphysis: Current concepts. J Am Acad Orthop Surg 2006;14:666–679.
- Barkin RM, Barkin SZ, Barkin AZ: The limping child. J Emerg Med 2000;18:331–339.
- De Boeck H, Vorlat P: Limping in childhood. Acta Orthop Belg 2003;69:301–310.
- Flynn JM, Widmann RF: The limping child: Evaluation and diagnosis. J Am Acad Orthop Surg 2001;9:89–98.
- Leet AI, Skaggs DL: Evaluation of the acutely limping child. Am Fam Physician 2000;61:1011–1018.
- Leung AK, Lemay JF: The limping child. J Pediatr Health Care 2004;18:219–223.

Chapter 218 Normal Lower Extremity Anatomic Variants

Jasmin McGinty

ICD-9 CODES
736.41 *Genu Valgum, Acquired*
736.42 *Genu Varum, Acquired*
736.89 *Acquired Deformity of the Lower Limb*
781.2 *Abnormality of Gait*

Key Concepts

- Knowledge of the natural history of lower limb growth is important for any practitioner who evaluates children.
- Deformity of the lower limb is a very common reason for parents to seek orthopaedic advice.
- The angular and rotational alignment of the growing child's lower extremity goes through several predictable stages as the child matures to adult stature.
- Recognition of normal variations seen in the pediatric lower extremity is key in the accurate assessment of the patient and allows for sound counsel for parents or referring practitioners.

Angular Alignment

- The normal alignment of the knees at birth is approximately 10% to 15% of varus at birth.
- As the child grows, the femoral-tibial alignment becomes neutral at approximately 14 months of age.
- The limb then begins to develop a valgus knee position at 2 years.
- Maximum physiologic genu valgum peaks between 3 and 4 years of age and is typically symmetrical and may also be associated with asymptomatic flatfeet.
- Genu valgum then gradually decreases to the normal adult femoral-tibial angulation of 5 to 7 degrees by age 6 to 7 years.
- It is important to note that there can be a wide variation among children, and normal femoral-tibial angulation generally falls within two standard deviations of the mean.
- Anterior or posterior bowing of the femur or tibia is almost never normal and should be an indication for radiographic evaluation.

Rotational Alignment

- The range of normal rotation of the pediatric lower extremity can be vast, especially before the age of 5 years.
- The rotation of the limb is not limited to the bony architecture, but is affected by soft-tissue constraints and muscular control.
- Most rotational variations of normal are symmetrical, and the gait cycle is generally normal.
- Neonatal femoral anteversion is approximately 40 degrees.
- The version slowly decreases to the average adult femoral anteversion of 15 degrees by age 8 or 9 years.
- It is within the normal spectrum of development for a disproportionate amount of femoral anteversion to persist until the age of 4 or 5 years, causing in-toeing, which usually normalizes by the age of 8 years.
- Persistent increased femoral anteversion has not been associated with degenerative joint disease, but has been associated with knee pain, especially when tibial torsion is also present.
- More commonly in-toeing is caused by excessive internal tibial torsion, especially in the 1- to 2-year-old age group; it can be unilateral or bilateral.
- Internal tibial torsion generally spontaneously resolves by age 4 years and is not affected by shoe wear, bracing, or physical therapy.
- Persistent isolated unilateral or bilateral internal tibial torsion past the age of 4 years, in general, does not increase with age and is not associated with degenerative joint disease.

- Excessive external tibial torsion, which is associated with out-toeing, usually presents in adolescence as parents better tolerate its cosmesis; it is more commonly unilateral and can progress until the child stops growing.
- Excessive external tibial torsion is strongly associated with patellofemoral pain and patellar instability.

Limb Length

- Leg length discrepancies of 2.5 cm or less are generally well tolerated and do not increase the mechanical work required for ambulation.

History

- Any child presenting with a questionable lower limb deformity should have a thorough history taken, which should include the birth history, dates and age development milestone achievement, and family history of illness/congenital abnormalities.

Physical Examination

- The physical evaluation should include both static and dynamic examination of the lower limbs.
- The clinical assessment of gait, joint mobility, and muscle tone is as important as the clinical appearance of the limb.
- The inspection should consist of an unobstructed view of the child's lower limbs.
  - The child should be dressed in comfortable attire.
  - Infants should be undressed, leaving the diaper in place.
  - It is preferable for older children to wear shorts.
  - Children who can stand or walk should be observed both lying down and standing.
  - Look for any asymmetry in the limb length, knee and ankle angulation, and muscle bulk and tone.
  - The pelvis should also be inspected for any sign of tilt because this can be a sign of significant limb length discrepancy.
  - The child who walks should also be observed walking and running over a distance that allows the practitioner to view the patient through a full gait cycle.
- Palpate the entire length of the leg and the hip, knee, and ankle joints to evaluate for tenderness or soft-tissue abnormalities such as masses or crepitus.
- The lower limb length can be assessed with a measuring tape, starting at the anterior superior iliac spine to the medial malleolus.
  - Alternatively, the measurement can start at the umbilicus.
  - Blocks of different known sizes may also be placed under the shorter limb, stopping when the pelvis is level, to assess limb length discrepancies.
- Hip rotation should be evaluated with the child lying on his or her abdomen in the prone position on an examination table with the knees flexed to 90 degrees.
  - To assess internal rotation of the hip, rotate the legs outward.
  - To assess external rotation of the hip, rotate the legs inward.
  - Hip rotation is equal to the maximal angular difference between vertical and the axis of the tibia.
  - Hip internal rotation of more than 80 degrees is associated with excessive femoral anteversion.
  - Also compare hip rotation side to side because rotation is typically symmetrical.

Imaging

- Radiographic evaluation is indicated in any child who presents with clinical limb asymmetry, short stature, or clinically excessive rotational or angulated limbs (>15–20 degrees) outside of the typical age range of the normal physiologic growth pattern. Full-length, weight-bearing plain radiographs, centered on the knees, should be the first radiographic imaging obtained.

Differential Diagnosis

- Blount's disease: asymmetrical, older children, obesity, radiograph of bilateral tibia/fibula
- Infantile tibia vara: early ambulation, radiograph of bilateral lower extremities
- Hip dysplasia: family history, more prevalent in girls than boys, first-born child, ultrasound scan of hips, physical examination, radiograph of bilateral hips
- Femoral anteversion: physical examination, radiographs of hip in two views
- Tibial torsion: physical examination, radiograph
- Foot deformity: physical examination, radiograph
- Neurologic pathology (e.g., cerebral palsy, myelodysplasia, diastematomyelia, Charcot-Marie-Tooth disease, muscular dystrophy): birth/family history, genetic testing

- Tumor: radiograph, clinical examination, magnetic resonance imaging/computed tomography, bone scan
- Metabolic bone disease: serum calcium, serum phosphate, kidney function
- Congenital deformity: family history, genetic testing
- Fracture: radiograph to confirm
- Infection: elevated erythrocyte sedimentation rate, C-reactive protein, +/– radiographic changes consistent with osteomyelitis

Considerations in Special Populations

- Obesity is a risk factor for Blount's disease.
- Early ambulation (walking before the age of 1 year) is associated with infantile tibia vara and is more common in African Americans.

Chapter 219 Pelvic Avulsion Fractures

Michael Kwon

ICD-9 CODES

808.41 *Fracture of the Pelvis, Closed; Ilium*
808.42 *Fracture of the Pelvis, Closed; Ischium*

Key Concepts

- Pelvic avulsion fractures are uncommon injuries that typically occur in adolescents and young adults participating in athletics.
- Injury occurs during a violent muscle contracture or eccentric contracture as in floor exercises in gymnastics or kicking in soccer.
- Fractures occur at secondary ossification centers because these points are weaker than the musculotendinous attachments.
- The most common sites of injury are the adductor muscle attachments to the ischial tuberosity (IT), the sartorius muscle attachment to the anterior superior iliac spine (ASIS), and the attachment of the direct head of the rectus femoris muscle to the anterior inferior iliac spine (AIIS) (Fig. 219-1)
- Other less common sites include the lesser trochanter (LT) and iliac crest (IC).
- Treatment generally entails rest with a gradual return to activities and rarely requires surgical intervention.

History

- Acute injury
  - Athletic activities with a severe muscle strain (e.g., groin pull); the patient may report hearing a "pop"
  - IT injuries associated with a hamstring stretch as in gymnastic floor exercises, ASIS and AIIS associated with swinging a baseball bat and high kicking as in soccer, IC associated with abrupt changes in direction as in power serves in tennis
  - Immediate shooting pain, focal tenderness, swelling around the site of injury
  - Inability or difficulty bearing weight
- Chronic injury
  - Repetitive activities without a clear history of a traumatic event
  - Pain with limited joint motion that progresses over time

Physical Examination

- Observation
  - Focal swelling and ecchymosis
  - Inability to bear weight
- Palpation
  - Focal tenderness at fracture site
- Range of motion and motor strength
  - May be limited secondary to pain

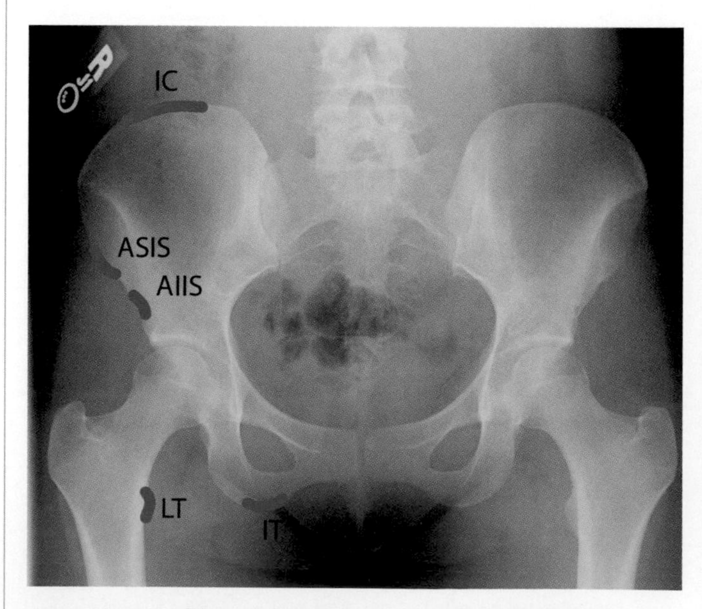

Figure 219-1 Plain radiograph of an adolescent patient demonstrating the common sites associated with pelvic avulsion fractures. AIIS, anterior inferior iliac spine; ASIS, anterior superior iliac spine; IC, iliac crest; IT, ischial tuberosity; LT, lesser trochanter.

- Special examinations
  - IT avulsion
    - Increased pain with hip flexed, knee extended, and leg abducted
    - Pain may also occur with sitting or scooting on the involved side.
  - ASIS avulsion
    - Painful hip flexion and external rotation
  - AIIS avulsion
    - Painful hip flexion with knee in extension

Imaging

- Radiographs
  - Anteroposterior (AP) view of the pelvis
    - Check for symmetry on the contralateral hemipelvis.
    - Look for subtle signs of soft-tissue swelling and evidence of nondisplaced or minimally displaced fractures.
    - Common sites of injury are the IT, ASIS, and AIIS. Less common sites are the IC and LT.
  - AP/frog leg lateral view of the hip
    - Rule out other possible diagnoses (e.g., slipped capital femoral epiphysis)
    - May give better dedicated resolution of the hip
  - Judet, inlet, outlet pelvis views
    - May add little to the diagnosis unless there is a history of significant direct trauma indicating an acetabular or pelvic ring injury
  - AP/lateral view of the knee
    - Consider evaluating the knee as another potential source of pain.
- Magnetic resonance imaging
  - In the case of a nondisplaced fracture, bone marrow edema may be evident as well as a fracture line not seen on plain radiographs, but magnetic resonance imaging is rarely indicated to make this diagnosis.

Additional Tests

- In a chronic and sometimes an acute setting in which an athletic injury may be in doubt, other tests to rule out infection, rheumatologic conditions, and neoplasm may be indicated
  - Temperature, complete blood count with differential, erythrocyte sedimentation rate, C-reactive protein, rheumatoid factor, antinuclear antibody, Lyme titers

Differential Diagnosis

- Muscle strain (see Chapters 127 and 134)
  - Similar history and presentation without evidence of fracture
  - Recovery is typically faster than with an avulsion fracture
- Slipped capital femoral epiphysis (see Chapter 221)
  - More prevalent in younger teens and preteens
  - May or may not be able to bear weight
  - Can also be activity related
- Septic arthritis/osteomyelitis (see Chapters 18 and 19)
  - Fever, elevated white blood cell count, erythrocyte sedimentation rate, C-reactive protein; inability to bear weight
  - Usually younger age group
  - Recent history of upper respiratory infection
- Lyme disease (see Chapter 19)
  - History of tick exposure and bull's-eye rash
  - Insidious onset
  - Knee involvement more common
- Rheumatologic disease (see Chapter 18)
  - Hip pain may be the initial presenting symptom.
  - History of other joint pain and other systemic symptoms
  - No trauma- or activity-related pain
- Neoplastic disease (see Chapter 24)
  - Radiographs may reveal significant findings.
  - Evaluate complete blood count and differential
  - Other constitutional signs

Treatment

- At diagnosis
  - Initial treatment focuses on rest with the hip in a relaxed position of least tension on the muscle groups involved.
  - Crutches are recommended for at least 2 weeks with a gradual return to weight bearing and sports-related activity.
  - Rehabilitation should be guided by clinical as well as radiographic recovery.
  - A premature return to activity may cause re-injury and prolong the overall recovery time of 6 weeks to several months.
- Later
  - Surgical intervention is rarely indicated.
  - A steady course of rehabilitation will likely lead to a full recovery.

When to Refer

- Pelvic avulsion fractures typically can be managed with conservative measures. If displacement is greater than 2 cm on radiographs, consider early referral for possible surgical intervention.
- If follow-up shows evidence of a fracture nonunion (e.g., persistent pain and serial radiographs demonstrating a lack of fracture healing), refer the patient for surgical evaluation.
- If long-term follow-up shows radiographs with exuberant callus and the patient has symptoms of painful myositis ossificans, consider referral for surgical excision.

Prognosis

- Good with conservative measures
- Surgery is rarely indicated except for significant displacement.
- Most athletes are able to return to full activities, with disability mostly occurring in patients with IT avulsions.

Troubleshooting

- Patients and families should be counseled on the time to recovery with conservative measures. Full recovery and return to full activity may take several months.
- It should be stressed that surgery is rarely indicated, even in displaced fractures. It may only be advocated in cases of fracture nonunion, which would be defined as a failure to heal by conservative measures.

Patient Instructions

- The patient should rest the hip in a position of comfort to decrease strain on the muscle groups involved in the avulsion fracture.
- Strict non-weight bearing for 2 weeks with crutches
- Weight bearing can begin after 2 weeks.
    - Guidance of a physical therapist may be helpful.
- Sports-directed therapy should be gradually introduced.
- Any significant pain during rehabilitation should delay the advancement of therapy to prevent reaggravation of injury.
- Repeat clinical examinations and radiographs are necessary to monitor the progress of healing.

Considerations In Special Populations

- High-level athletes need to understand that although a quick return to play may be desired, careful and cautious rehabilitation is necessary to obtain full healing.

Suggested Reading

- Busch MT: Sports medicine in children and adolescents. In Morrissy RT, Weinstein SL (eds): Lovell and Winter's Pediatric Orthopaedics. Philadelphia: Lippincott Williams & Wilkins, 2001.
- Canale ST: Fractures and dislocations in children. In Canale ST (ed): Campbell's Operative Orthopaedics. Philadelphia: Mosby, 2003.
- Canale ST, Beaty JH: Fractures of the pelvis. In Beaty JH, Kasser JR (eds): Rockwood and Wilkin's Fractures in Children. Philadelphia: Lippincott Williams & Wilkins, 2001.
- Ferbach SK, Wilkinson RH: Avulsion injuries to the pelvis and proximal femur. Am J Radiol 1981;137:581–584.
- Kaneyama S, Yoshida K, Matsushima S, et al: A surgical approach for an avulsion fracture of the ischial tuberosity: A case report. J Orthop Trauma 2006;20:363–365.
- Metzmaker JN, Pappas AM: Avulsion fracture of the pelvis. Am J Sports Med 1985;13:349–358.
- Rosenberg N, Noiman M, Edelson G: Avulsion fractures of the anterior superior iliac spine in adolescents. J Orthop Trauma 1996;10:440–443.
- Rossi F, Dragoni S: Acute avulsion fractures of the pelvis in adolescent competitive athletes: Prevalence, location and sports distribution of 203 cases collected. Skeletal Radiol 2001;30:127–131.
- Sundar M, Carty H: Avulsion fractures of the pelvis in children: A report of 32 fractures and their outcome. Skeletal Radiol 1994;23:85–90.
- Vandervliet EJ, Vanhoenacker FM, Snoeckx A, et al: Sports-related acute and chronic avulsion injuries in children and adolescents with special emphasis on tennis. Br J Sports Med 2007;41:827–831.
- White KK, Williams SK, Mubarak SJ: Definition of two types of anterior superior iliac spine avulsion fractures. J Pediatr Orthop 2002;22:578–582.

Chapter 220 Legg-Calvé-Perthes Disease

Vishwas Talwalkar, Henry J. Iwinski, Jr., and Todd Milbrandt

ICD-9 CODES
732.1 *Osteochondrosis of Hip*
729.5 *Limb Pain*

Key Concepts

- Idiopathic osteonecrosis of the capital femoral epiphysis causing varying degrees of pain, deformity, gait disturbance, and ultimately risk of premature arthrosis of the hip
- Simultaneously described in 1909 by Legg, Calvé, and Perthes
- Onset of symptoms at ages 2 to 12 years
- Male-to-female ratio of 5 : 1
- 1 in 4000 incidence
- Ethnic variation exists (rare in African Americans)
- Ten percent to 12% bilateral
- Most patients with skeletal age less than chronologic age
- Proposed etiologies include coagulation disorder, trauma, bone dysplasia, venous hypertension, collagen abnormality, environmental

Disease Course

- Disease progresses through stages described by Waldenström
- The initial stage includes the inciting event and inflammation of the hip.
- The fragmentation stage starts with subchondral fracture and progresses to significant radiographic irregularity and shape distortion of the femoral epiphysis. It is usually the most symptomatic phase.
- The reossification stage is characterized by increasing new bone formation in the epiphysis with decreasing pain.
- The remodeling stage is the final phase that progresses from the completion of reossification to skeletal maturity.

History

- Insidious onset of limp and pain, often a remote traumatic history
- Pain may be localized to the hip, groin, thigh, knee, or entire limb.
- Symptoms exacerbated by activity, partially relieved by rest
- Usually several months of symptoms before diagnosis
- Rarely any family history; if present, consider other etiology

Physical Examination

- Examination of the hip usually reveals limited abduction and internal rotation.
- Motion is limited by pain early in the disease process and by deformity later.
- Trendelenburg gait evident
- Muscle atrophy may also be evident.
- Late in the course, fixed adduction deformity and leg length discrepancy may also be seen.

Imaging

- Radiographs are most widely used to diagnose, classify, treat, and monitor the disease process.
    - The initial radiographic finding is a relatively smaller femoral epiphysis with an apparently widened joint space.
    - Subsequent findings during the fragmentation phase include subchondral fracture (crescent sign), increased radiodensity, fragmentation of the ossific nucleus, flattening of the ossific nucleus, physeal irregularity, broadening and shortening of the femoral neck, and flattening and widening of the acetabular roof (Figs. 220-1 to 220-4).
- Technetium-99 bone scan has been described as an additional imaging modality to track reperfusion of the epiphysis.

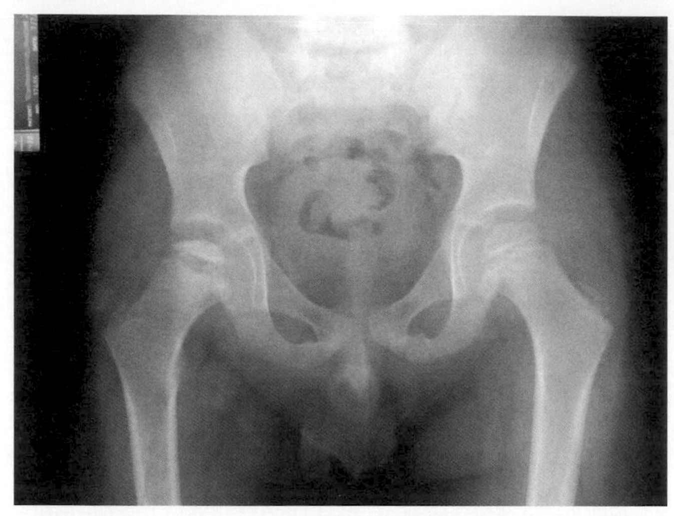

Figure 220-1 Anteroposterior view of the pelvis of a 6-year-old child with lateral pillar C Legg-Calvé-Perthes disease.

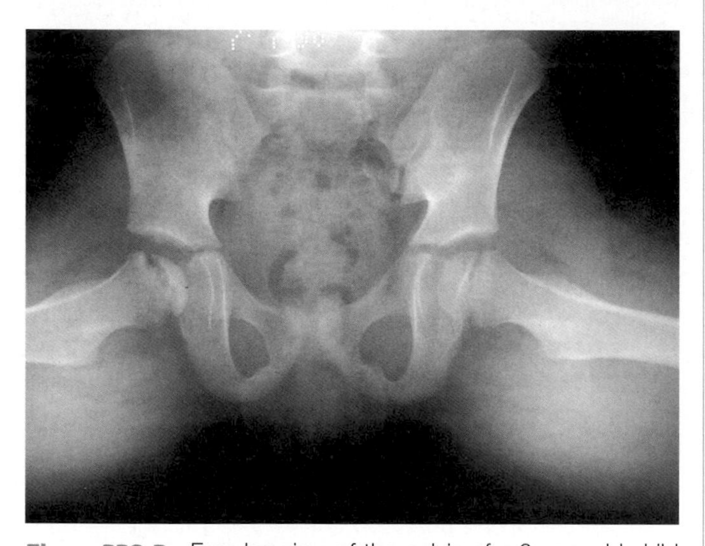

Figure 220-2 Frog leg view of the pelvis of a 6-year-old child with lateral pillar C Legg-Calvé-Perthes disease.

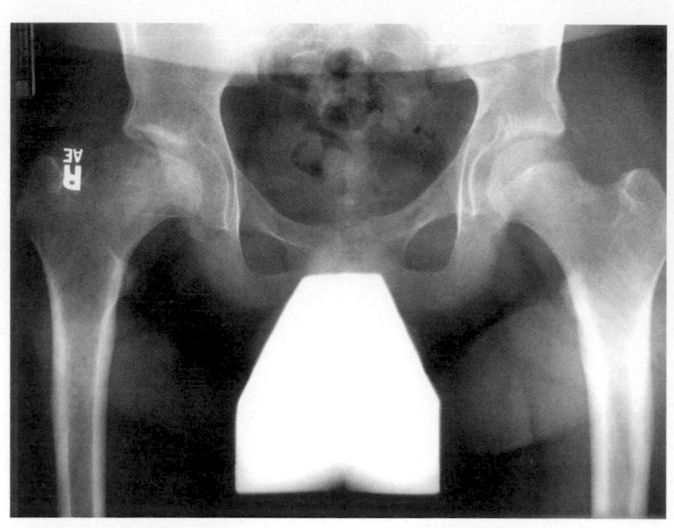

Figure 220-3 Anteroposterior view of the pelvis of the same child shown in Figures 220-1 and 220-2 at age 15 displaying a Stulberg class IV result.

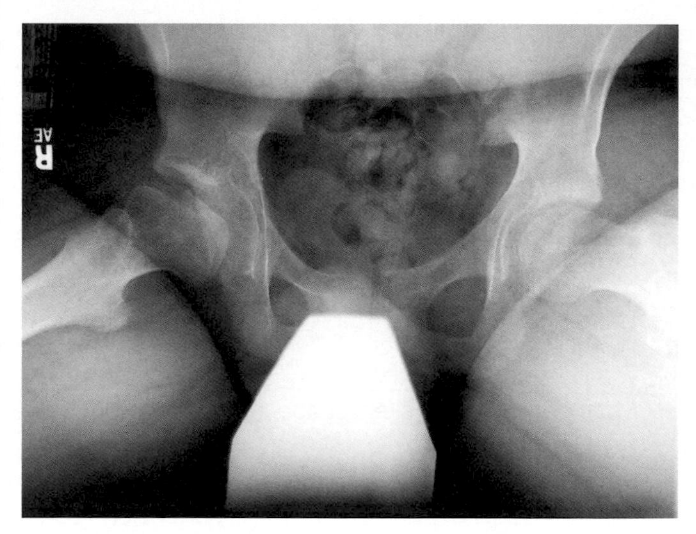

Figure 220-4 Frog leg view of the pelvis of the same child shown in Figures 220-1 and 220-2 at age 15 displaying a Stulberg class IV result.

- Magnetic resonance imaging occasionally useful for diagnosis in the initial stage of disease or to identify intra-articular and cartilage pathology (i.e., labral tears, osteochondritic lesions, articular cartilage injuries)
- Computed tomography, particularly with three-dimensional reconstruction, is useful for assessing shape deformity and for possible osteotomy planning in young adult patients.

Differential Diagnosis (Table 220-1)

- Steroid-induced osteonecrosis
- Postinfectious osteonecrosis
- Multiple epiphyseal dysplasia
- Spondyloepiphyseal dysplasia
- Gaucher's disease
- Sickle cell disease

Classification

- Severity
  - Catterall: stages I through IV with increasing volume of head deformity
  - Salter-Thompson: A, less than 50% head involvement as determined by the width of the crescent sign; B, more than 50% involvement

TABLE 220-1 *Differential Diagnosis*

Differential Diagnosis	Differentiating Feature
Steroid-induced osteonecrosis	Bilateral, shoulders and knees involved
Postinfectious osteonecrosis	History of infection
Multiple epiphyseal dysplasia	Bilateral, symmetrical, multiple sites
Spondyloepiphyseal dysplasia	Bilateral symmetrical with spine abnormality
Gaucher's disease	Signs of systemic disease
Sickle cell disease	Signs of systemic disease

- Lateral pillar: currently the most popular and widely applied; measured during the fragmentation phase
  - A: no loss of height of the lateral one third of the epiphysis (lateral pillar)
  - B: loss of as much as 50% of the height of the lateral pillar
  - B/C border: preservation of 50% of the lateral pillar height, but abnormal bone quality in the lateral pillar
  - C: more than 50% loss of height of the lateral pillar
- Deformity: measures of sphericity and congruity, measured at skeletal maturity
  - Mose: femoral head sphericity compared with circular overlay
  - Stulberg: measure of femoral head flattening and congruity related to risk of developing arthritis
    - I: spherical
    - II: minimal deformity, spherical head
    - III: ovoid head, congruent hip
    - IV: flat head, congruent hip
    - V: flat head with incongruent hip

Natural History

- In general, outcomes related to the age at onset and amount of femoral head involvement
- Most patients do well clinically into the fifth decade of life, but approximately half have hip arthritis at age 50 years.
- Patients with incongruous hips and hinged abduction are at highest risk of premature arthritis developing in the third or fourth decade.
- Patients with age at onset younger than 8 years have the best prognosis, those with age at onset of 8 to 10 years have an intermediate prognosis, depending on severity of disease, and those older than 10 years have a poor prognosis.
- Patients with lateral pillar C hips have a poor prognosis across all ages.

Treatment

- The goal of all methods of treatment is a congruent, spherical, mobile, pain-free hip. Most hips fall short of this goal.
- Due to the great variability of this disease process, it is very difficult to compare treatment methods and their ability to reliably alter the natural history of the disease.
- The concept of containment is still the primary idea behind treatment.
  - Containment is the idea that maintaining the mechanically softer femoral epiphysis within the spherical acetabulum during the critical phase of the disease can prevent flattening and preserve sphericity while the damaged femoral head regains mechanical integrity.
- Various methods of containment have been described including abduction casting and bracing, varus proximal femoral osteotomy, redirectional pelvic osteotomy, or combinations of these methods.
- Noncontainment treatment is also performed to reposition the leg without changing the hip relationship (proximal femoral valgus osteotomy) or to accommodate the enlarged femoral head (shelf acetabuloplasty).
- More recently, methods of treatment to address late intra-articular pathology including hip arthroscopy and surgical dislocation have been applied, but the long-term efficacy of these procedures is still under review.
- The use of pharmaceutical agents to prevent deformity and femoral head collapse is a promising area of ongoing research and future intervention.

When to Refer

- Immediate but not emergent referral to an orthopaedic surgeon is indicated for any child with any radiographic abnormality of the hip, persistent complaints of hip pain, abnormal physical examination, or a limp that lasts more than a few days.

Suggested Reading

- Herring JA, Kim HT, Browne R: Legg-Calve-Perthes disease. Part I: Classification of radiographs with use of the modified lateral pillar and Stulberg classifications. J Bone Joint Surg Am 2004;86A:2103–2120.
- Herring JA, Kim HT, Browne R: Legg-Calve-Perthes disease. Part II: Prospective multicenter study of the effect of treatment on outcome. J Bone Joint Surg Am 2004;86A:2121–2134.
- McAndrew MP, Weinstein SL: A long-term follow-up of Legg-Calve-Perthes disease. J Bone Joint Surg Am 1984; 66A:860–869.
- Salter RB: Experimental and clinical aspects of Perthes' disease. In Proceedings of a Joint Meeting of the American Physicians' Fellowship and the Israeli Orthopaedic Society. J Bone Joint Surg Br 1966;48B:393–394.
- Stulberg SD, Cooperman DR, Wallensten R: The natural history of Legg-Calve-Perthes disease. J Bone Joint Surg Am 1981; 63A:1095–1108.

Chapter 221 Slipped Capital Femoral Epiphysis

Henry J. Iwinski, Jr.

ICD-9 CODE
732.2 *Slipped Capital Femoral Epiphysis*

Key Concepts

- Slipped capital femoral epiphysis (SCFE) is a common cause of adolescent hip, groin, thigh, or knee pain.
- Disorder of the proximal femoral physis with displacement of the head/neck relationship
- Associated with increased body mass index
- Classified by the patient's ability or inability to walk (stable versus unstable) on presentation and degree of displacement (Southwick angle)
- Diagnosis of a stable slip is frequently delayed due to a lack of recognition.
- Treatment is surgical with in situ fixation with a percutaneously placed cannulated screw.

Epidemiology

- Onset during adolescent growth spurt (boys, 13–15 years; girls, 11–13 years)
- Incidence 10.8 in 100,000 children between ages of 9 and 16 years
- More common in boys and black and Hispanic children

Etiology

- Mechanical forces
  - Femoral neck retroversion
  - Increased acetabular depth
  - Weakness of growth plate during rapid growth
  - Thinning of perichondral ring during adolescence
  - Change in orientation of proximal femoral growth plate
  - Obesity creating increased mechanical forces
    - — Associated with a body mass index higher than the 95th percentile
- Endocrine factors
  - Hypothyroidism
  - Renal failure
  - Growth hormone

Classification

- Temporal
  - Acute slip: a symptomatic period of 2 to 3 weeks or less frequently with a sudden onset of severe hip pain from a minor traumatic event
  - Chronic slip: the majority of patients (85%) with a few months' history of vague hip, groin, thigh, or knee pain
  - Acute on chronic slip: sudden onset of severe pain after a prodromal period consistent with a chronic slip
- Ability to bear weight
  - Stable: able to walk even with assistive devices; avascular necrosis rate of 0%
  - Unstable: unable to bear weight; avascular necrosis rate of 15% to 50%
- Magnitude of displacement (Southwick): head-shaft angle on frog leg lateral views compared with opposite side
  - Mild: less than a 30-degree difference
  - Moderate: 30- to 60-degree difference
  - Severe: more than a 60-degree difference

Clinical Presentation

- Chronic, stable SCFE
  - Obese adolescent with brief history of hip, groin, thigh, or knee pain
  - Mild to moderate limp
  - Progressive out-toeing
  - Decreased internal rotation or obligatory external rotation with hip flexion
  - Pain with motion is variable.
    - — Need to be astute and aware of physical examination findings to prevent delay

  - Knee and/or thigh pain can be the only symptom
  - Delay in diagnosis is frequent; misdiagnoses as hip strain or groin pull
- Unstable SCFE
  - Sudden onset of severe hip pain
  - Unable to walk, even on crutches
  - The patient seeks prompt medical attention.
  - Lies with leg externally rotated and resists any motion of hip
- Atypical SCFE
  - Frequently present outside the narrow age range (younger than 10 or older than 16 years of age)
  - Less than the 50th percentile for weight or less than the 10th percentile for height
  - Endocrine disorders (hypothyroidism), renal failure, radiation therapy

Imaging

- Always obtain anteroposterior (AP) (Fig. 221-1) and frog leg lateral view radiographs in any adolescent presenting with hip, thigh, groin, or knee pain.
  - Look for a widening of the growth plate and any displacement of the epiphysis on the metaphysis.
  - Klein's line (Fig. 221-2)
- There is little role for magnetic resonance imaging, computed tomography, or bone scan. Additional studies will only further delay the diagnosis.
- The key is prompt recognition of the typical patient with his or her presenting signs and symptoms.

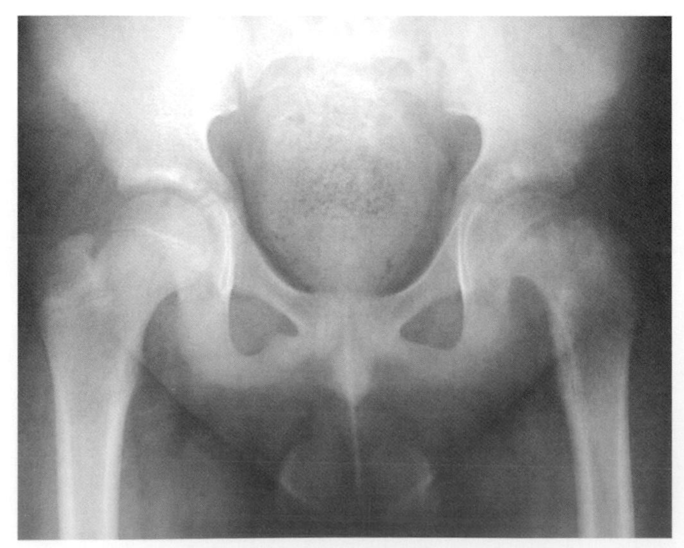

Figure 221-1 Radiographic representation of a slipped capital femoral epiphysis on the left hip.

Treatment

- Stable SCFE
  - Prompt in situ fixation with a single stainless steel cannulated screw (Fig. 221-3)
  - Place the screw perpendicular to the orientation of the displaced femoral neck in both AP and lateral planes
  - Screw threads should bridge the physis.
  - The starting point is anterior on the femoral neck
  - Need to ensure placement of the screw tip in the center of the femoral head on both views (center-center)
  - Before leaving the operating room, the surgeon must ensure that the screw tip does not violate the joint.
    - Persistent joint penetration can cause iatrogenic chondrolysis.
  - Allowed to weight bear as tolerated or with crutches for 4 to 6 weeks
  - Need to follow closely for a slip on the opposite side

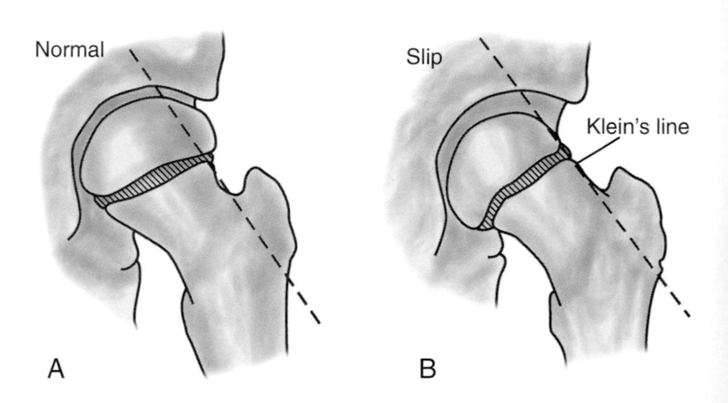

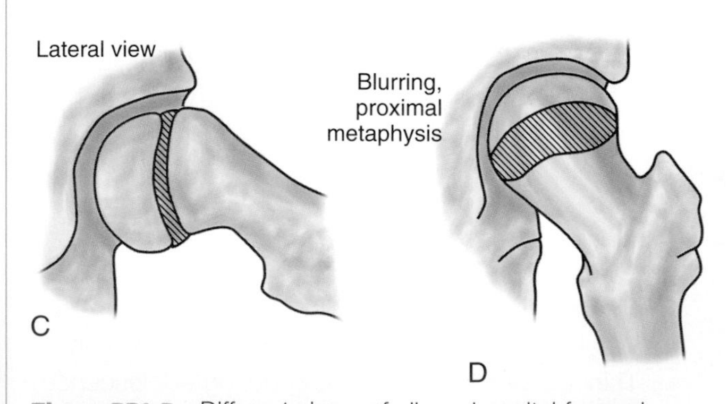

Figure 221-2 Different views of slipped capital femoral epiphysis (SCFE). **A**, Normal. Note that Klein's line intersects the epiphysis. **B**, In an SCFE, Klein's line does not intersect the epiphysis. **C**, In an SCFE, the epiphysis is posteriorly displaced compared with the metaphysis. **D**, In a valgus SCFE, blurring of the proximal metaphysis is seen.

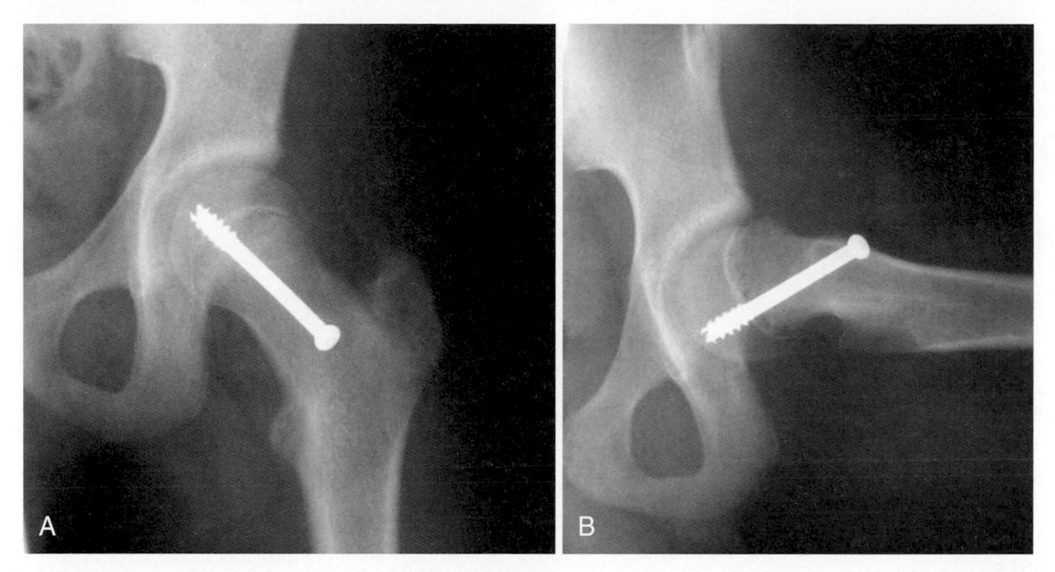

Figure 221-3 Anteroposterior (**A**) and frog leg lateral (**B**) radiographs of a single in situ pinning of a left slipped capital femoral epiphysis (SCFE). Note that in the image on the left, the relationship between the epiphysis and metaphysis would be considered normal. However, on the lateral view, a large posterior displacement of the epiphysis is seen, thus confirming the SCFE. This emphasizes the necessity of lateral radiographs in making this diagnosis.

- Unstable SCFE
  - High rate of avascular necrosis
  - Urgent treatment with gentle repositioning of the slip
  - Consider two-screw fixation.
  - Consider a mini-arthrotomy or aspiration for joint decompression.
- Atypical SCFE
  - High risk of bilateral slips
  - Pin the opposite side in young patients (younger than 10 years of age) or those with underlying endocrine or metabolic disorders.

When to Refer

- Immediate referral to an orthopaedic surgeon of any patient with an SCFE
- Patients with a stable SCFE should be made non-weight bearing due to the risk of progression to an unstable slip.

Troubleshooting

- Have a high index of suspicion in any obese adolescent with hip, thigh, groin, or knee pain.
- Check for limited hip internal rotation or obligatory external rotation with hip flexion.
- Always obtain AP and frog leg views of the pelvis.

Patient Instructions

- Parents, coaches, and trainers need to be aware of the typical patients and initial symptoms to prevent a delay in presentation.

Considerations in Special Populations

- An SCFE can occur in patients with Down syndrome, patients on growth hormone replacement, and patients with hypothyroidism.

Suggested Reading

- Carney BT, Weinstein SL, Noble J: Long-term follow-up of slipped capital femoral epiphysis. J Bone Joint Surg Am 1991;73A:667–674.
- Katz DA: Slipped capital femoral epiphysis: The importance of early diagnosis. Pediatr Ann 2006;35:102–111.
- Lehmann CL, Arons RR, Loder RT, et al: The epidemiology of slipped capital femoral epiphysis: An update. J Pediatr Orthop 2006;26:286–290.
- Loder RT: Controversies in slipped capital femoral epiphysis. Orthop Clin North Am 2006;37:211–221, vii.
- Loder RT, Richards BS, Shapiro PS et al: Acute slipped capital femoral epiphysis: The importance of physeal stability. J Bone Joint Surg Am 1993;75A:1134–1140.
- Manoff EM, Banffy MB, Winell JJ: Relationship between body mass index and slipped capital femoral epiphysis. J Pediatr Orthop 2005;25:744–746.
- Rahme D, Comley A, Foster B, et al: Consequences of diagnostic delays in slipped capital femoral epiphysis. J Pediatr Orthop B 2006;15:93–97.

Chapter 222 Developmental Dysplasia of the Hip

Mark J. Romness

ICD-9 CODES
754.3 *Congenital Dislocation of Hip*
755.63 *Other Congenital Deformity of Hip*

Key Concepts

- The term developmental dysplasia of the hip (DDH) encompasses *all* forms of hip dysplasia including acetabular dysplasia, instability, subluxation, and dislocation.
- The term congenital dysplasia of the hip implies that the deformity was present at birth, which is not always true.
- Teratologic dislocations occur before birth, have more severe deformity, and are often associated with other disorders.
- Instability is present in 0.5% to 1% of babies at birth.
  - Sixty percent recover by 1 week old
  - Eighty-eight percent recover by 2 months old
  - Underdevelopment or dysplasia may persist.
- Classic DDH persists in 1 in 1000 births.
  - Persistent instability
  - Persistent dislocation
- Diagnosis as early as possible is key to the best outcome.

History

- Perinatal risk factors
  - First-born child
  - Female
    - Eighty percent of DDH patients are female.
    - Female babies twice as likely as males to be breech
  - Breech position in utero
    - Seventeen percent to 23% of breech babies have DDH.
    - Two percent to 4% of births are breech.
  - Family history
    - Present in 10% to 30% of DDH patients
  - Any condition with intrauterine crowding including oligohydramnios and twin or multiple birth
- Conditions that may also have DDH associated
  - Torticollis: 8%
  - Metatarsus adductus: 1.5%
  - Clubfoot or other foot deformities
  - Oligohydramnios
  - Other syndromes or anomalies

Physical Examination

- Asymmetrical inguinal folds
- Klisic line from the greater trochanter to the anterosuperior iliac spine directed below the umbilicus
- The greater trochanter palpable above Nelaton's line connecting the anterosuperior iliac spine and ischial tuberosity
- Decreased hip abduction
- Galeazzi's sign of apparent femoral shortening
- Barlow's test to subluxate the hip
- Ortolani test to reduce a dislocated hip (Fig. 222-1)
- A simple hip click is not associated with DDH.
- Be aware of bilateral dislocations.
  - Decreased abduction bilaterally
  - Klisic line below the umbilicus bilaterally
  - Both greater trochanters above Nelaton's line

Imaging

- Ultrasonography: up to 4 months of age
- Anteroposterior radiograph of pelvis if older than 4 months or ossific nucleus present on the ultrasound scan
- Computed tomography or magnetic resonance imaging if additional information is needed, but usually requires sedation
- Additional study: arthrography

Differential Diagnosis

- Please see Table 222-1.
- A congenital short femur will have femoral shortening on Galeazzi's test.

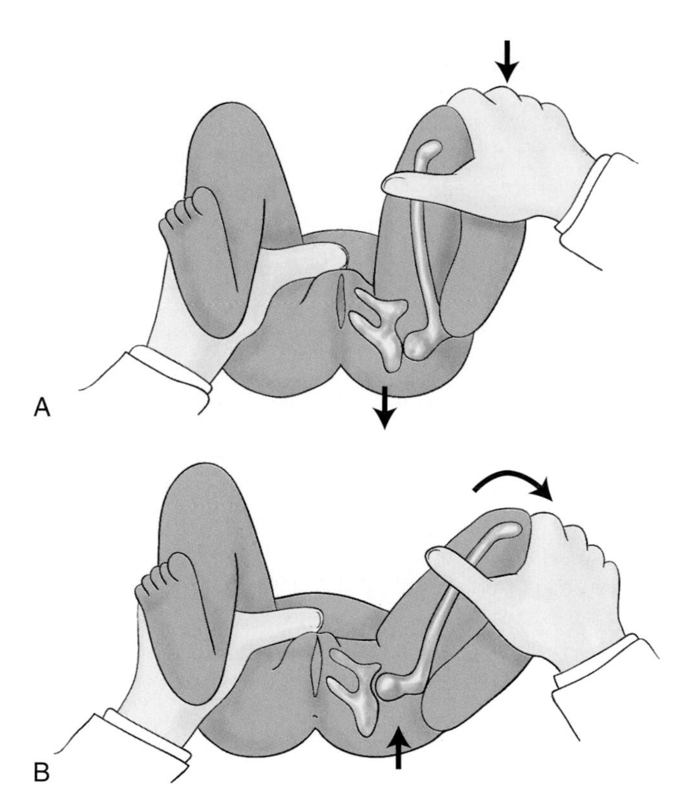

Figure 222-1 **A**, Barlow's test with posteriorly directed loading of the hip from the flexed and adducted position to try to dislocate or subluxate a reduced hip. **B**, The Ortolani test with medially directed force at the greater trochanter while the hip is actively abducted to try to reduce a dislocated hip. (Adapted from Hüftdysplasie. Available at www.ebenhoeh-dr.com/Schulerseite/Huftdysplasie/huftdysplasie.html. Accessed Jan. 11, 2009.)

TABLE 222-1 *Differential Diagnosis*

Differential Diagnosis	Differentiating Features	Chapter Reference
Congenital short femur	Femoral shortening on Galeazzi's test	223
Congenital coxa vara (with shepherd's crook deformity of the proximal femur)	May have decreased abduction	223

- Congenital coxa vara (with a shepherd's crook deformity of the proximal femur) may have decreased abduction.

Treatment

- Close observation of the newborn for spontaneous improvement
- Positioning devices such as a Pavlik harness

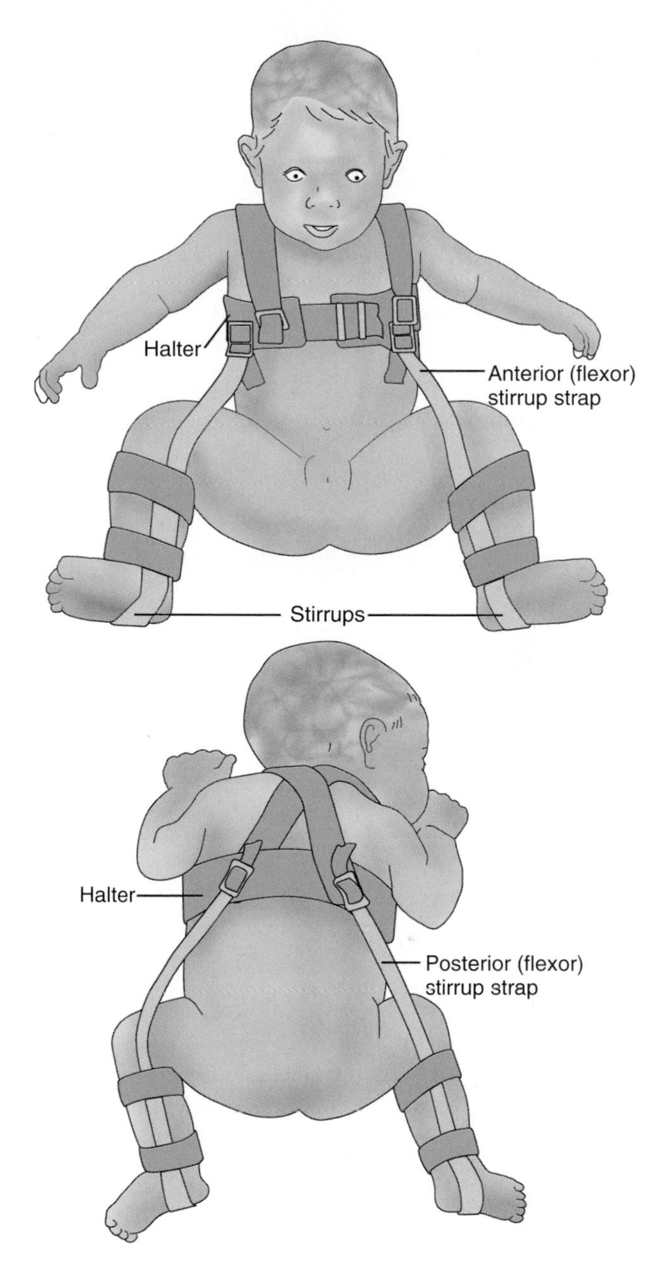

Figure 222-2 Standard strap position of the Pavlik harness to prevent certain hip positions but allow some active motion. The anterior strap prevents hip extension and is set with the hip flexed at 90 to 100 degrees. Overtightening of the anterior strap increases the risk of femoral nerve or artery impingement. The posterior strap prevents adduction and is set to allow hip adduction to 0 degrees or neutral. The posterior strap should not be overtightened in an attempt to pull the hip into a reduced position or the risk of avascular necrosis is increased.

- Closed reduction and casting
- Open reduction (Fig. 222-2)

Contraindications to Reduction

- Bilateral dislocation more than 8 years old
- Unilateral with medical contraindications

When to Refer

- Any dislocated hip
- Any unstable hip more than a week old
- Persistent acetabular dysplasia

Troubleshooting

- Worse prognosis with delayed diagnosis and treatment
- Hips that are dislocated at rest are more likely to require treatment.

Patient Instructions

- Avoid positioning hips tightly adducted or swaddled.

Prognosis

- When detected early, treatment is very successful.

Considerations in Special Populations

- Patients with other conditions of joint laxity such as Down syndrome or Ehlers-Danlos syndrome may require more aggressive treatments.

Suggested Reading

- Banta JV, Scrutton D (eds): Hip Disorders in Childhood. London: Mac Keith Press, 2004.
- Pavlik A: The functional method of treatment using a harness with stirrups as the primary method of conservative therapy for infants with congenital dislocation of the hip. Original 1957. [Translated and abridged by Leonard F. Peltier, MD, PhD.] Clin Orthop Relat Res 1992;281:4–10.
- Weinstein SL, Mubarek SJ, Wenger DR: Developmental hip dysplasia and dislocation: Part I. Instr Course Lect 2004; 53:523–530.
- Weinstein SL, Mubarek SJ, Wenger DR: Developmental hip dysplasia and dislocation: Part II. Instr Course Lect 2004; 53:531–542.

Chapter 223 Congenital Lower Extremity Disorders

Mark J. Romness

ICD-9 CODES
755.3 *Reduction Deformities of the Lower Limb*
755.69 *Congenital Angulation of the Tibia*

Key Concepts

- The history and physical examination continue to be the most important tools for assessment.
- Deficiencies of the long bones can range from mild shortening or bowing to complete absence.
- Proper diagnosis of the congenital deformity is important for genetic counseling, management, and prediction of progression.
- Hemihypertrophy is associated with Wilms' tumor in 20% of the cases and requires abdominal ultrasound scans biannually until age 4 to screen for Wilms' tumor.
- Tibial deficiencies (previously known as tibial hemimelia) are important to distinguish from fibular deficiencies (previously known as fibular hemimelia) in that tibial deficiencies have an autosomal dominant inheritance pattern.

History

- Major deficiencies are often identified at birth.
- Milder cases may not present until further growth and development uncover the deformity.
- The family often reports some difference noted since birth.

Physical Examination

- Accurate assessment of extremity deformity is critical to both diagnosis and treatment.
- All components of the deformity need to be considered including structural or static deformity and functional or dynamic deformity.
- Structural deformity includes length, rotation, and angular deformity in the frontal, transverse, and sagittal planes.
- Functional impairments include motion, strength, and motor control problems that result in abnormal posturing and an effective deformity.

Imaging

- Standard radiographs remain the primary method of assessment.
- Full-length standing radiographs (teloroentgenograms) in both the frontal and sagittal planes provide a full evaluation including bone and joint structure, alignment, and length assessment (Fig. 223-1).

Additional Tests

- Computed tomography and magnetic resonance imaging have specific indications, depending on the condition.
- Computed tomography remains the best instrument to assess bone structure.
- Magnetic resonance imaging provides better definition of cartilage and soft-tissue structures.
- Genetic evaluation and testing are beneficial for diagnosis and family counseling.

Differential Diagnosis

- Hemihypertrophy
  - Be aware of Wilms' tumor.
- Congenital short femur: proximal femoral focal deficiency
- Tibial deficiencies (hemimelia)
- Fibular deficiencies
- Terminal deficiencies (congenital amputations)
- Posteromedial apex tibial bowing
  - Associated with calcaneovalgus foot deformity
  - Small tibial length discrepancies with growth

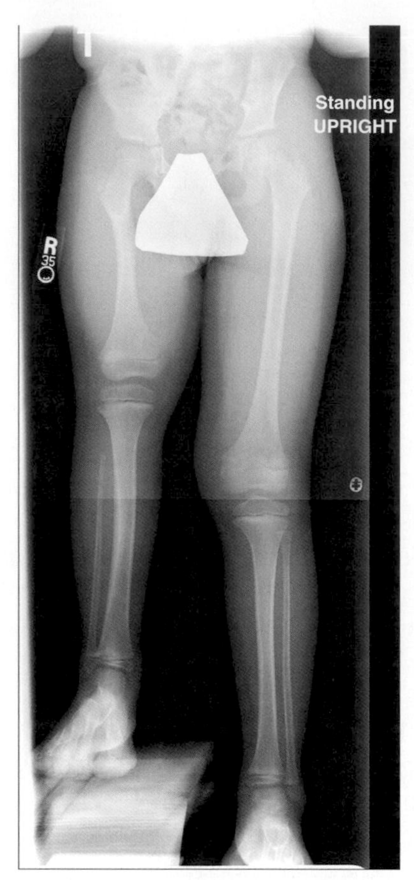

Figure 223-1 Full-length standing radiograph. Radiograph taken from hip to ankle gives assessment of bone structure and development including alignment, length, and formation. This radiograph shows multiple changes associated with a congenital short femur.

- Anterolateral apex tibial bowing
  - Strong association with congenital pseudarthrosis of the tibia and neurofibromatosis (Fig. 223-2)

Treatment

- At diagnosis
  - Proper diagnosis
  - Modifications to accommodate the deformity
  - Family counseling
- Later
  - Monitor change with growth

When to Refer

- If any significant visual deformity

Prognosis

- Depends on the diagnosis
- Influence on the adjacent joints portends outcome

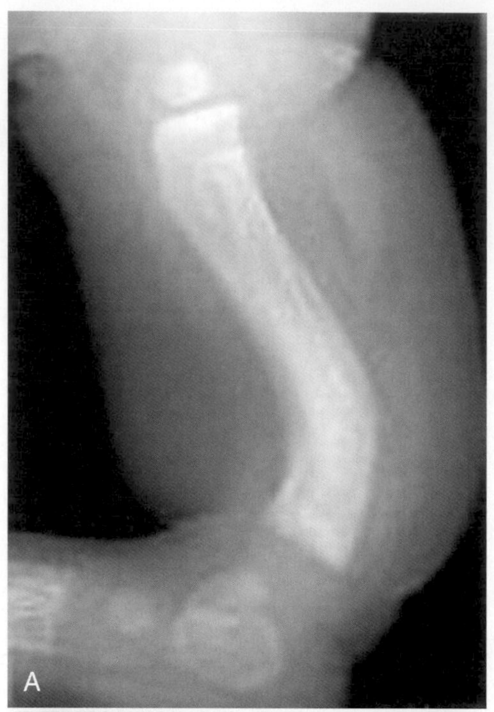

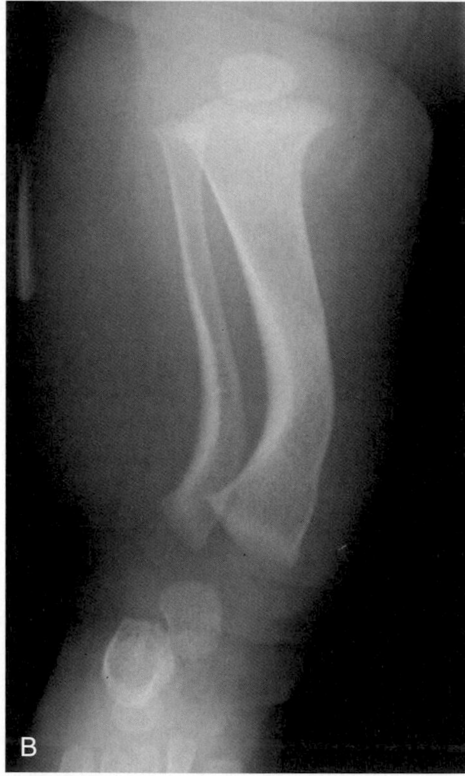

Figure 223-2 Posterior medial tibial bowing. The apex of the deformity is directed in the posterior direction on the lateral view (**A**) and in the medial direction on the anteroposterior view (**B**), which is not associated with neurofibromatosis and congenital pseudarthrosis. The amount of deformity in this child will likely be associated with a leg length discrepancy.

Troubleshooting

- The small size of infant extremities makes it difficult to determine subtle differences between the limb development and positional influences. If there is sufficient concern, monitor with serial examinations and radiographs.

Patient Instructions

- Tibial deficiencies have an autosomal dominant genetic inheritance pattern.
- Congenital deficiencies are usually not genetic, but genetic counseling may be helpful to confirm this.

Suggested Reading

- Finch GD, Dawe CJ: Hemiatrophy. J Pediatr Orthop 2003; 23:99–101.
- Koman LA, Meyer LC, Warren FH: Proximal femoral focal deficiency: Natural history and treatment. Clin Orthop Relat Res 1982;162:135–143.
- Schoenecker PL, Capelli AM, Millar EA, et al: Congenital longitudinal deficiency of the tibia. J Bone Joint Surg Am 1989;71A:278–287.

Chapter 224 Osteochondritis Dissecans

Mininder S. Kocher, Olabode Ogunwole, and Modern Weng

ICD-9 CODE
732.7 *Osteochondritis Dissecans*

Key Concepts

- The etiology of osteochondritis dissecans (OCD) is idiopathic; nonetheless, there appears to be a growing consensus that OCD may be the result of repetitive microtrauma.
- OCD is a condition affecting the subchondral bone characterized by separation of an osteochondral fragment with or without articular cartilage involvement.
- The separation of the osteochondral fragment may be present in situ, incomplete detachment, or complete detachment. Classification of OCD is based on imaging studies (i.e., plain radiographs, single-photon emission computed tomography bone scan, or magnetic resonance imaging [MRI]), surgical findings, and anatomic location of the lesion.
- OCD can also be divided into juvenile and adult forms depending on the physeal maturity. The majority of adult OCD cases are secondary to the persistence of an unresolved juvenile OCD lesion, although de novo cases of adult OCD have been described.
- OCD can be present on any joint surface; however, it most commonly involves the knees, elbows, ankles, and hips, in that order. It is extremely rare to have OCD develop in the shoulder or wrist joints.
- Bilateral involvement is reported in as many as 25% of cases.
- If untreated, the long-term sequela is premature degenerative joint disease.

History

- Presentation depends on the stage of the lesion. Early, stable lesions with an intact articular surface may present as vague episodic knee pain that can be confused with patellofemoral pain. Later, unstable lesions with disrupted articular surfaces present with more pain, swelling, catching, and locking that can be confused with meniscal tears.
- Clinical presentation of adult OCD is typically insidious, progressive, and unremitting joint discomfort that does not resolve over time and with rest.
- Symptoms of juvenile OCD are classically gradual in onset but fairly nonspecific. Patients may exhibit joint effusion, locking, or simply poorly localized joint pain that is exacerbated by activity and improves with rest.
- The patient may also report an antalgic gait if OCD of the knee or ankle is suspected.

Physical Examination

- Observation
  - Joint effusion is often present.
  - An antalgic gait is seen if OCD involves the lower extremity.
- Palpation
  - With OCD of the knee, maximal tenderness to palpation is noted over the medial femoral condyle. This can be best felt with the knee in 90 degrees of flexion with pressure directed just medial to the inferior pole of the patella. More than 70% of OCD lesions are found in the posterolateral aspect of the medial femoral condyle.
  - With OCD of the elbow, the anterolateral aspect of the capitellum is the most common site of the lesion. This area of the elbow is best palpated with the elbow flexed to 90 degrees.
- Range of motion
  - Loss of range of motion may occur secondary to an effusion or a completely detached osteochondral lesion causing locking of the joint.

- Special tests
  - Wilson's sign for OCD of the knee
    - — Pain or discomfort with internal rotation of the tibia with the knee in 90 and 30 degrees of flexion
    - — Relief of pain with external rotation of the tibia
    - — Wilson's sign lacks the sensitivity to detect OCD of the knee; however, it is useful as a clinical monitor during treatment.

Imaging

- Radiographs
  - For OCD of the knee: anteroposterior, lateral, notch, and sunrise views
    - — The notch view will allow for better visualization of the posterior femoral condyle in comparison with the anteroposterior view (Fig. 224-1).
    - — More than 70% of OCD lesions are found in the posterolateral aspect of the medial femoral condyle.
- MRI
  - If an OCD lesion is found on plain radiographs, then MRI needs to be done because it provides vital information about prognosis and management.
  - It will help determine the size of the OCD lesion, the status of the articular cartilage and subchondral bone, the extent of bony edema, and the presence of any possible loose bodies, as well as other knee injuries.

Classification of Osteochondritis Dissecans

- Juvenile OCD is first differentiated from the adult form based on the closure of the physes. In juvenile OCD, the physes remain open, whereas in the adult form, the physes are closed.
- There are different classification schemes based on anatomic location or imaging modalities (Figs. 224-2 and 224-3).

Differential Diagnosis of Osteochondritis Dissecans of the Knee

- Please see Table 224-1.

Treatment

- The treatment goal of OCD is to have complete healing of the lesion.

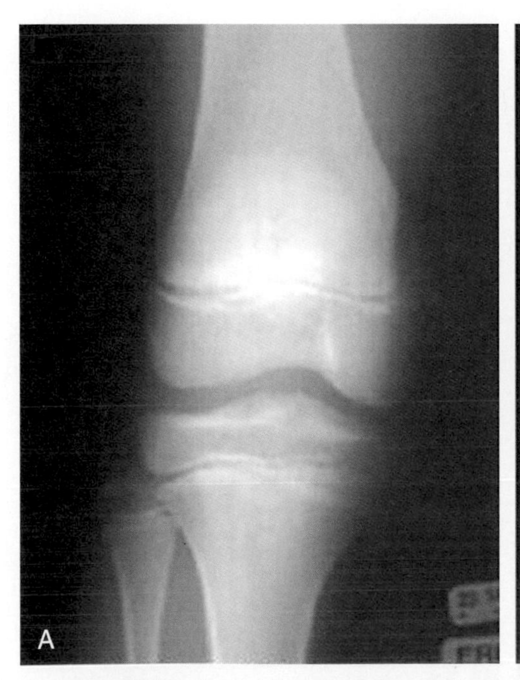

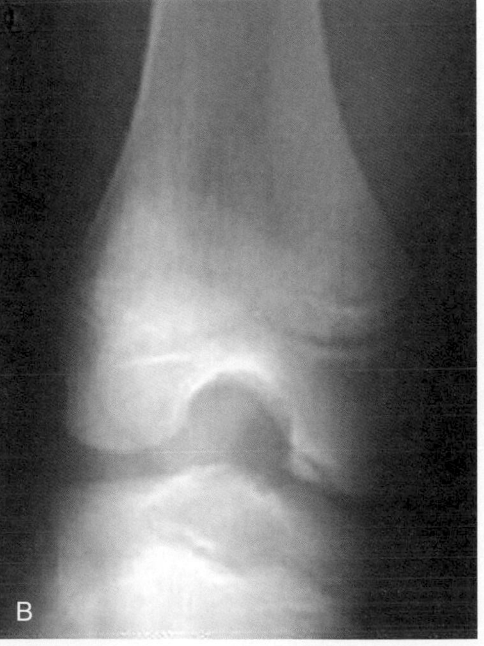

Figure 224-1 **A**, Anteroposterior view of the knee does not reveal an osteochondritis dissecans (OCD) lesion in the posterolateral aspect of the medial femoral condyle. However, once a notch view is obtained (**B**), it is clearly evident that an OCD lesion is present.

- At diagnosis
  - The initial treatment of OCD depends on the classification of the lesion.
  - Nonoperative management is the treatment of choice for stable juvenile OCD lesions, which are defined based on the MRI classification as either stage I or II.
  - The first 4 to 6 weeks of treatment involve immobilization of the knee with a knee immobilizer and partial weight bearing with crutches. A plain radiograph should be repeated at the end of this phase to see whether there is any healing of the OCD lesion.
  - During the second 4 to 6 weeks, the knee immobilizer is discontinued as the patient is weaned off crutches and advanced to weight bearing as tolerated. Physical therapy is initiated emphasizing knee range of motion and low-impact quadriceps and hamstring muscles strengthening exercises.
- Later
  - MRI should be repeated to evaluate for healing after a total of 12 weeks of treatment. If there is

TABLE 224-1 *Differential Diagnosis*

Differential Diagnosis	Differentiating Features
Meniscal tear (see Chapter 148)	Joint line tenderness, positive McMurray's test, pain with provocation maneuvers of hyperflexion and hyperextension
Chondromalacia patella (see Chapter 153)	Crepitus and pain with compression of the patella during flexion and extension, apprehension with manipulation of patella, patellar facet tenderness, positive grind test (pain with compression of the superior pole of the patella as the patient contracts the quadriceps muscle)
Osteoarthritis (see Chapter 151)	Knee effusion, crepitus with flexion and extension

Figure 224-2 Anatomic classification of osteochondritis dissecans of the knee.

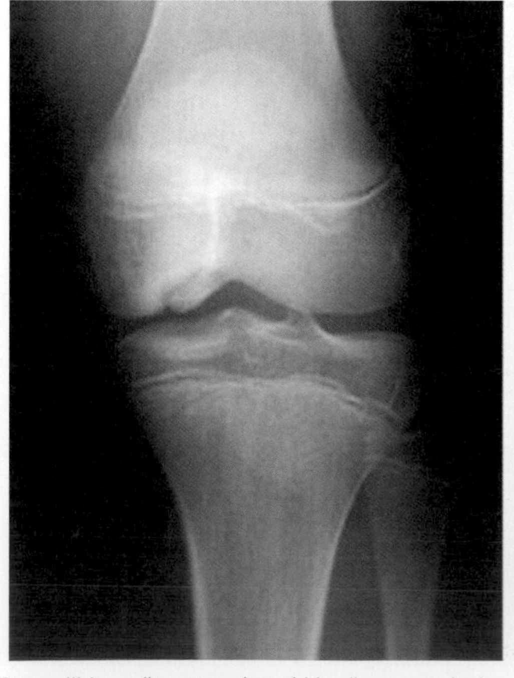

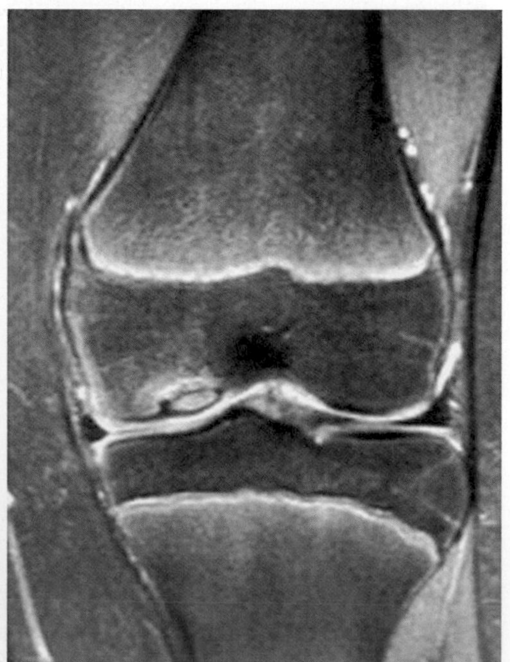

Figure 224-3 Stage III juvenile osteochondritis dissecans lesion of the medial femoral condyle. The lesion is clearly demarcated with fluid between the lesion and the subchondral bone.

radiographic and clinical evidence of healing, then the patient is ready to begin the third phase of therapy, which includes sport-specific physical therapy with supervised running, cutting, and jumping. The patient is then permitted to gradually return to sports as symptoms allow.

When to Refer

- OCD lesions that are MRI classification stage III or higher require a referral to an orthopaedic surgeon. This includes any detached or unstable lesions. Referral is also recommended for any adolescents approaching physeal closure as well as any adult with OCD. Adult OCD lesions present typically with insidious, progressive, and unremitting joint discomfort that does not respond to nonsurgical management.
- Patients with stable lesions that have not healed with 6 to 9 months of nonsurgical treatment should also be referred to an orthopaedic surgeon.

Prognosis

- Fifty percent of juvenile OCD lesions will heal within 10 to 18 months provided the physes remain open and the patient complies with treatment.
- Nonoperatively managed juvenile OCD lesions of MRI classification stage III or higher typically do not heal.
- Surgical drilling results in significant pain reduction and radiographic healing in 83% of adolescents with open physes and 75% with closed physes.
- Surgical fixation is indicated for unstable lesions. Healing rates are approximately 85% for juvenile OCD lesions.
- Excision of large fragments should be avoided as this leads to degenerative joint disease. If excision has been performed, chondral resurfacing procedures may be indicated.

Troubleshooting

- Radiographs can be taken at the 6-week mark and MRI performed at the 12-week mark to evaluate for healing of the OCD lesion. A notch view is helpful to identify the lesion.
- Persistent pain symptoms and no radiographic improvement often result from poor compliance with treatment in an adolescent patient.
- Nonweight-bearing with slow but gradual advancement to partial and then full weight bearing is the key to nonoperative therapy.
- If symptoms return after treatment or follow-up radiographs show lesion recurrence, repeated nonoperative treatment can be considered.
- Bilateral involvement is reported in as many as 25% of cases.

Patient Instructions

- Counsel the patient as to the importance of compliance with therapy. Often, adolescents will become more active when symptoms of pain have decreased. However, decreased pain symptoms are not the equivalent of a healed OCD lesion.
- Counsel the patient that complete resolution of the OCD lesion either nonoperatively or surgically requires 3 to 6 months.
- Unsuccessful treatment of OCD may lead to progressive degenerative joint disease and worsening of pain symptoms.

Considerations in Special Populations

- Adult OCD lesions present typically with insidious, progressive, and unremitting joint discomfort that does not respond to nonsurgical management. Early orthopaedic referral is recommended.
- Nonoperative initial management of stable juvenile OCD lesions is advised. Surgical treatment is indicated for any detached or unstable lesions in which physeal closure is imminent or nonoperative management has failed.

Suggested Reading

- Anderson AF, Richards DB, Pagnani MJ, Hovis WD: Antegrade drilling for osteochondritis dissecans of the knee. Arthroscopy 1997;13:319–324.
- Cahill BR: Osteochondritis dissecans of the knee: Treatment of juvenile and adult forms. J Am Acad Orthop Surg 1995; 3:237–247.
- Cahill BR, Phillips MR, Navarro R: The results of conservative management of juvenile osteochondritis dissecans using joint scintigraphy: A prospective study. Am J Sports Med 1989; 17:601–606.
- Conrad JM, Stanitski CL: Osteochondritis dissecans: Wilson's sign revisited. Am J Sports Med 2003;31:777–778.
- Ganley TJF, Amro RR, Gregg JR, et al: Antegrade drilling for osteochondritis dissecans of the knee. Paper presented at the Pediatric Orthopaedic Society of North America 2002 Annual Meeting, May 3–5, 2002, Salt Lake City, Utah.
- Garrett JC: Osteochondritis dissecans. Clin Sports Med 1991;10:569–593.
- Glancy GL: Juvenile osteochondritis dissecans. Am J Knee Surg 1999;12:120–124.

- Hefti F, Beguiristain J, Krauspe R, et al: Osteochondritis dissecans: A multicenter study of the European Pediatric Orthopedic Society. J Pediatr Orthop B 1999;8:231–245.
- Kocher MS, Micheli LJ: The pediatric knee: Evaluation and treatment. In Insall JN, Scott WN (eds): Surgery of the Knee, 3rd ed. New York: Churchill Livingstone, 2001, pp 1356–1397.
- Kocher MS, Micheli LJ, Czarnecki JJ, Andersen JS: Internal fixation of juvenile osteochondritis dissecans lesions of the knee. Am J Sports Med 2007;35:712–718.
- Kocher MS, Tucker R, Ganley TJ, Flynn JM: Management of osteochondritis dissecans of the knee. Am J Sports Med 2006;34:1181–1191.
- Twyman R, Kailish D, Aichroth P: Osteochondritis of the knee: A long-term study. J Bone Joint Surg Br 1991;73B:461–464.

Chapter 225 Discoid Meniscus

Mininder S. Kocher, Olabode Ogunwole, and Modern Weng

ICD-9 CODE
717.5 *Congenital Discoid Meniscus*

Key Concepts

- A discoid meniscus is a congenital variant in which there are thickening and widening of the normal crescentic, semilunar-shaped meniscus.
- There are three types of discoid meniscus (Fig. 225-1): complete, incomplete, and Wrisberg types.
  - The difference between the complete and incomplete types of discoid meniscus is the amount of meniscus tissue covering the tibial plateau (see Fig. 225-1A and B). The incomplete discoid meniscus is more of a crescentic semilunar shape that covers less of the tibial plateau than the complete meniscus.
  - The Wrisberg type has only one attachment posteriorly, the meniscofemoral ligament (which is also called the ligament of Wrisberg). This type lacks a ligamentous attachment at the posterior horn to the tibial plateau.
- The overall incidence of discoid meniscus syndrome has been reported from between 1.4% and 15.5%. However, only a small percentage of cases are symptomatic. There appears to be a higher incidence of discoid meniscus in the Asian population (16.6%).
- The lateral meniscus is most likely to be involved. A discoid meniscus appears bilaterally in approximately 15% to 20% of cases.

History

- The most common symptoms are knee snapping, lateral knee pain, and lack of full extension without knee effusion. A child younger than 10 years old who has this set of symptoms has a discoid lateral meniscus until proven otherwise.
- These symptoms may be associated with a discoid meniscal tear.
- The snapping knee sound is typically associated with the unstable Wrisberg type of discoid meniscus. However, the snapping sound by itself is not deleterious unless it is accompanied by pain or effusion of the knee.
- There may also be a history of the knee becoming stuck in flexion (knee locking) requiring the patient to manipulate the knee range of motion to unlock the joint. This typically occurs when there is an extensive meniscal tear associated with a discoid meniscus.

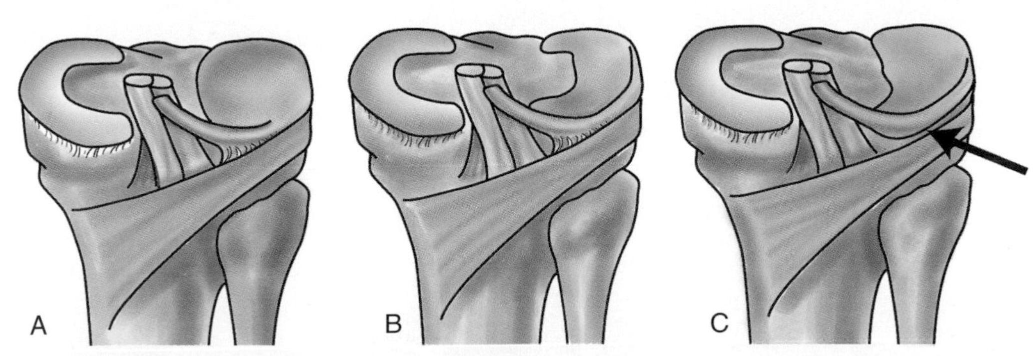

Figure 225-1 Posterior view of the three types of discoid meniscus. Complete (**A**), incomplete (**B**), and Wrisberg (**C**) types. Note that the Wrisberg type of discoid meniscus lacks a posterior horn ligamentous attachment to the tibial plateau (*arrow*), whereas the complete and incomplete types of discoid meniscus have a firm attachment at the posterior horn to the tibial plateau.

Physical Examination

- There is often a lack of full extension with lateral joint line tenderness if a patient has a symptomatic discoid meniscus.
- A snapping sound can be heard when the knee goes from flexion to extension. Hence, a snapping sound may be heard with walking or running and may be more salient with going up stairs.
- A positive McMurray's test will be evident when a complete or incomplete type of discoid meniscus is associated with a meniscal tear. In this case, knee effusion may be evident and locking of the knee joint may occur.

Imaging

- Plain radiographs are the first imaging modality that should be used when evaluating any knee pain. Ideally, standing anteroposterior, lateral, notch, and sunrise views should be obtained.
  - Radiographic findings that are suggestive of a discoid lateral meniscus include lateral joint space widening (Fig. 225-2), squared-off lateral femoral condyle, and cupping of the lateral aspect of the tibial plateau. The tibial plateau is normally flat or convex, but with a lateral discoid meniscus, it becomes more concave in shape.
- Magnetic resonance imaging is the modality of choice when surgery is being considered for a discoid meniscus. A discoid meniscus is likely when meniscal tissue can be seen on three or more contiguous sagittal cuts (Fig. 225-3).
- However, magnetic resonance imaging has a low sensitivity (57%) but a high specificity (92%) for the detection of a discoid meniscus. There can be a classic false-negative finding with a Wrisberg type of discoid meniscus.

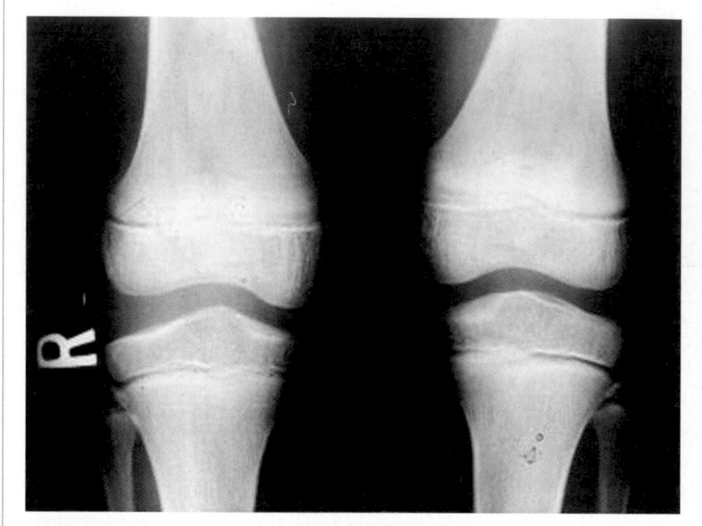

Figure 225-2 Standing anteroposterior view of both knees reveals a widening of the joint space of the right knee compared with the left, which is suggestive of a lateral discoid meniscus. Mild cupping of the lateral aspect of the tibial plateau is also noted.

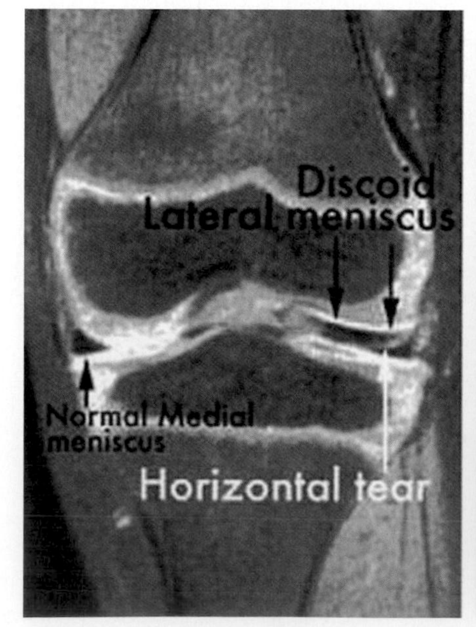

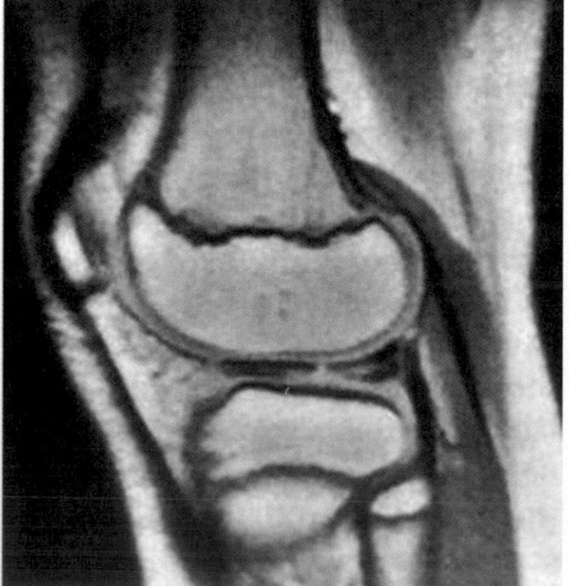

Figure 225-3 Coronal and sagittal views of the knee reveal a lateral discoid meniscus with a horizontal tear.

Differential Diagnosis

- Please see Table 225-1.

Treatment

- At diagnosis
  - Asymptomatic discoid meniscus found incidentally does not require treatment, and the prognosis is generally good. However, symptomatic discoid meniscus typically will require surgical intervention. The initial management involves quadriceps and hamstring muscle physical therapy as well as pain control with nonsteroidal anti-inflammatory drugs.
- Later
  - Symptomatic discoid meniscus will generally require arthroscopic surgical intervention. Surgical options differ depending on the type of discoid meniscus and whether there is an additional meniscal tear.

When to Refer

- A history of knee locking or the knee joint stuck in flexion on presentation requires immediate referral to an orthopaedic surgeon.
- Discoid meniscus syndrome is a diagnosis based on a solid history, physical examination, and proper imaging studies. If magnetic resonance imaging confirms the diagnosis or if the patient does not show symptomatic relief with nonoperative management, then an orthopaedic referral is recommended.

TABLE 225-1 *Differential Diagnosis*

Differential Diagnosis	Differentiating Features
Meniscal tear (see Chapter 148)	Joint line tenderness, positive McMurray's test, pain with provocation maneuvers of hyperflexion and hyperextension
Osteochondritis dissecans (see Chapter 224)	Antalgic gait, maximal tenderness to palpation over the medial femoral condyle, positive Wilson's sign (pain with internal rotation of the tibia with the knee in 90 and 30 degrees of flexion)
Chondromalacia patella (see Chapter 153)	Crepitus and pain with compression of the patella during flexion and extension, apprehension with manipulation of the patella, patellar facet tenderness, positive grind test (pain with compression of the superior pole of the patella as the patient contracts the quadriceps muscle)
Osteoarthritis (see Chapter 151)	Knee effusion, crepitus with flexion and extension

Prognosis

- Surgical treatment typically involves arthroscopic saucerization, which is reshaping the meniscus to a more normal shape with a 6- to 8-mm rim. After saucerization, the meniscus should be probed to assess stability. Meniscal instability may require meniscal repair. Total meniscectomy should be avoided as it leads to early degenerative joint disease.
- Although not many long-term studies have been done, it is believed that in a small percentage of patients who have had a total meniscectomy, there may be a risk of degenerative joint disease or osteochondritis dissecans decades after the procedure.

Troubleshooting

- Plain radiographs may be obtained in a patient who has had a total meniscectomy for a discoid meniscus to evaluate for degenerative joint changes. If there are degenerative changes, one should observe for joint space narrowing, bony ridge formation along the margin of the lateral femoral condyle, and spurring and sclerosis of the tibial plateau.
- The benefits of a total or subtotal meniscectomy for a discoid meniscus would be the elimination of pain, knee locking, decreased range of motion, and knee effusion.
- There is a less than 1% risk of bleeding, infection, and nerve injury with this arthroscopic procedure.

Patient Instructions

- Physical therapy before and after the procedure is essential for a seamless recovery and return to sports.
- The patient will be partially weight bearing and then weaned off crutches during the first week after surgery. Full recovery is expected typically 4 weeks after the operation.

Considerations in Special Populations

- In a child younger than 10 years of age, symptoms of knee snapping, lateral knee pain, and lack of full extension without knee effusion signify a lateral discoid meniscus until proven otherwise.

Suggested Reading

- Cosgarea AJ, Ryan A: Repair of a bucket-handle tear of a complete discoid lateral meniscal incarcerated in the posterolateral compartment. Am J Sports Med 2000;28:737–740.
- Dickhaut SC, DeLee JC: The discoid lateral-meniscus syndrome. J Bone Joint Surg Am 1982;64A:1068–1073.
- Fujikawa K, Iseki F, Mikura Y: Partial resection of the discoid meniscus in the child's knee. J Bone Joint Surg Br 1981; 63B:391–395.
- Hayashi LK, Yamaga H, Ida K, Miura T: Arthroscopic meniscectomy for discoid lateral meniscus in children. J Bone Joint Surg Am 1988;70A:1495–1500.
- Kaplan E: Discoid lateral meniscus of the knee joint. J Bone Joint Surg Am 1957;39A:77–87.
- Kocher MS, Micheli LJ, DiCanzio J, Zurakowski D: Diagnostic performance of clinical examination and selective magnetic resonance imaging in the evaluation of intra-articular knee disorders in children and adolescents. Am J Sports Med 2001;29:292–296.
- Kocher MS, Micheli LJ, Klingele KE, et al: Discoid lateral meniscus: Prevalence of peripheral rim instability. J Pediatr Orthop 2004;24:79–82.
- Monllau JC, Leon A, Cugat R, Ballester J: Ring-shaped lateral meniscus. Arthroscopy 1998;14:502–504.
- Räber DA, Friederich NF, Hefti F: Discoid lateral meniscus in children: Long-term follow-up after total meniscectomy. J Bone Joint Surg Am 1998;80A:1579–1586.
- Smillie IS: The congenital discoid meniscus. J Bone Joint Surg Br 1948;30B:671–682.
- Woods GW, Whelan JM: Discoid meniscus. Clin Sports Med 1990;9:695–706.

Chapter 226 Osgood-Schlatter/ Sinding-Larsen-Johansson Lesions

Mininder S. Kocher and James MacDonald

ICD-9 CODES
732.4 *Osgood-Schlatter Disorder*
732.4 *Sinding-Larsen-Johansson Disorder*

Key Concepts

- Osgood-Schlatter lesion (OSL) and Sinding-Larsen-Johansson lesion (SLJL) are both disorders of the extensor mechanism of the knee seen typically in active youngsters during the time of ossification of characteristic anatomic sites in the knee.
- OSL is a disorder of the formation and growth of the proximal tibial apophysis.
  - OSL typically presents with pain and tenderness at the tibial tuberosity with or without a history of local trauma.
  - OSL is a common cause of disability in active adolescents. Some studies have found more than 20% of active 13-year-olds have signs and symptoms of OSL.
- SLJL is a disorder of the normal ossification process involving the inferior pole of the patella.
  - SLJL typically presents with pain and tenderness at the inferior pole of the patella with or without a history of local trauma.
  - SLJL is seen exclusively in youngsters with open physes; it is similar to the condition of patellar tendinitis (jumper's knee) seen in more mature athletes.
- SLJL is seen less commonly than OSL. Both disorders are typically reviewed concurrently and considered in the spectrum of extensor mechanism problems of the adolescent knee.
- The diagnosis of both OSL and SLJL is typically made clinically; imaging can occasionally be helpful but often is not necessary initially.
- Treatment of OSL and SLJL is conservative in the majority of cases.
- Symptoms of both disorders are typically self-limited. Late sequelae of OSL and SLJL tend to be mild and insignificant, such as a prominent tibial tuberosity.
- Surgery including excision of painful ossicles is rarely indicated in refractory cases. Surgery is indicated in OSL for complete tibial tubercle avulsion fractures, but this is a rare complication.

History

- OSL and SLJL commonly present as anterior knee pain in children 10 to 15 years of age who participate in running, cutting, and jumping sports such as basketball and soccer.
- OSL and SLJL disorders have been associated with the adolescent growth spurt. Girls typically present at a younger age (mean age of about 11.5 years compared with 13 years for boys).
- The onset of pain is typically insidious, but can commonly be associated with trauma. If there has been recent acute trauma, there should be heightened suspicion of a tibial tubercle apophyseal fracture (in the case of OSL) or a sleeve fracture of the patella (in the case of SLJL).
- Knee pain caused by OSL or SLJL is typically well localized and is not associated with mechanical symptoms such as recurring effusions, locking, and instability.
- Twenty percent to 30% of patients with OSL will report bilateral knee symptoms. If a patient presents with unilateral symptoms, some attention should be paid to the contralateral knee in the history and physical examination.
- A careful review of systems should be done to rule out more insidious etiologies of pain, particularly when the patient presents with unilateral symptoms. A review of systems should include (not exclusively) queries about weight loss, fevers or night sweats, nocturnal pain or pain that awakens a patient, and hip/groin pain.

Physical Examination

- Both knees should be examined, even if the patient is reporting pain exclusively in one knee.
- Inspection
  - Patients may walk with an antalgic gait.
  - There can be swelling over the corresponding anatomic locations (OSL, tibial tubercle; SLJL, inferior patella).
  - There should be no effusion.
  - There may be associated quadriceps muscle atrophy if the condition has been long-standing before presentation.
- Palpation
  - There will be tenderness to palpation and palpable swelling over the tibial tubercle in OSL and the inferior pole of the patella in SLJL.
  - There should be no tenderness over the joint line.
- Range of motion
  - There should be full range of motion in the knee.
  - The patient should be able do a straight leg raise and perform active terminal knee extension; if the patient cannot do that, especially if seen in the setting of acute trauma, there may be an associated fracture.
- Flexibility assessment
  - Patients with OSL and SLJL will typically have a marked degree of inflexibility.
  - The popliteal angle (to assess hamstring muscle flexibility) and the Thomas test (to assess hip flexor flexibility) should be done.
  - The popliteal angle is measured to assess the tightness of the patient's hamstring muscle.
    - — This assessment is done by the practitioner initially flexing the patient's hip to 90 degrees and then passively extending the leg.
    - — The angle formed between a perpendicular line to the femoral shaft and the tibial shaft is the hamstring-popliteal angle.
    - — In an ideal situation (i.e., excellent flexibility), the angle approaches 0 degrees.
  - The Thomas test is done to assess hip flexor flexibility.
    - — The patient is assessed supine.
    - — The examiner asks the patient to flex both hips into the chest; this movement should abolish the normal lumbar lordosis (this can be confirmed by the practitioner attempting to place a hand under the back with the patient in this position).
    - — Asking the patient to continue to hold one hip into the chest, the other leg is held by the practitioner, extended passively, and then lowered to the table.
    - — The practitioner should ensure that the pelvis does not tip to the side during this maneuver.
    - — Any flexion deformity (hip extension should be to 180 degrees or flat on the bed) should be measured.
    - — The procedure should be repeated on the other leg.
- Examination of the hip
  - An examination of the hip should be done to rule out causes of referred pain to the knee.
  - Specifically, the patient should have full and pain-free internal and external range of motion of the hips.

Imaging

- Often imaging is not indicated when OSL or SLJL are the working diagnoses. With cost and radiation exposure potential considerations, clinicians may elect to proceed with treatment and careful follow-up in the majority of cases.
- That being said, plain radiographs can be invaluable in ruling out more insidious etiologies of knee pain (e.g., fractures, osteosarcomas, osteochondritis dissecans).
- Plain radiographs in OSL may include a four-view series of the affected knee(s), including anteroposterior, lateral, skyline, and notch/tunnel views.
    - — The lateral view is especially revealing of the tibial apophysis.
    - — The notch view can rule out osteochondritis dissecans if that is included in the working differential diagnosis.
    - — Comparison views of the contralateral unaffected knee are sometimes helpful, especially if there is significant tibial tubercle fragmentation seen radiographically and the clinician wants to rule out associated fracture (Fig. 226-1).
  - Plain radiographs in SLJL likewise may include a four-view series of the affected knee(s).
    - — Again, comparison views of the unaffected knee can be helpful in resolving potential questions that may arise from initial radiography.
  - Often a radiograph will show a small bone fragment adjacent to the inferior patella; this should be correlated clinically.

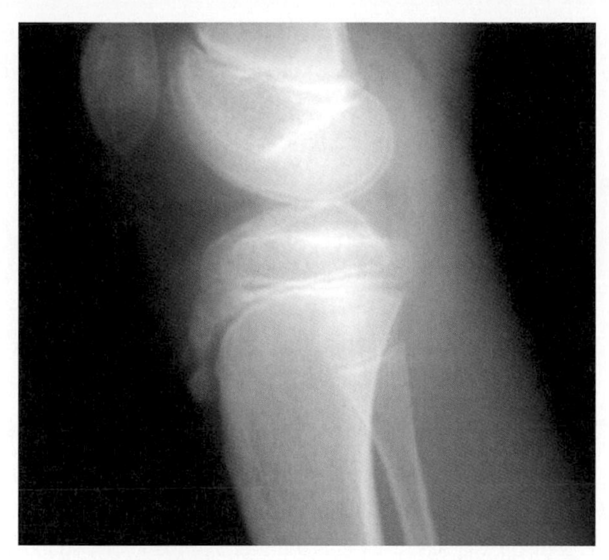

Figure 226-1 Osgood-Schlatter lesion.

 — One can see this finding in either SLJL or a patellar sleeve fracture. In the latter, there should be strong clinical evidence such as a significant hemarthrosis and significant disability (e.g., inability to extend the knee) (Fig. 226-2).
- Advanced imaging (e.g., magnetic resonance imaging, bone scans, computed tomography) is rarely indicated unless other diagnoses (e.g., stress fractures) are being seriously considered.

Differential Diagnosis

- Please see Table 226-1.

Treatment

- Treatment is typically conservative and usually begins with a period of rest to decrease a patient's symptoms followed by rehabilitation to address deficits in flexibility and strength.
- Activity limitation should include not only the patient's sport, but consideration should also be given to provocative activities such as participation in physical education classes or kneeling in church or when gardening.
- The duration of initial rest typically is 2 to 3 weeks. When the patients are symptom free with activities of daily living, they can return gradually to their sport.
- In moderately severe cases, consideration may be given to casting or bracing for 2 to 3 weeks to "cool off" the severely inflamed lesion.
- Ice therapy should be used liberally. Nonsteroidal anti-inflammatory drugs can be considered but should be

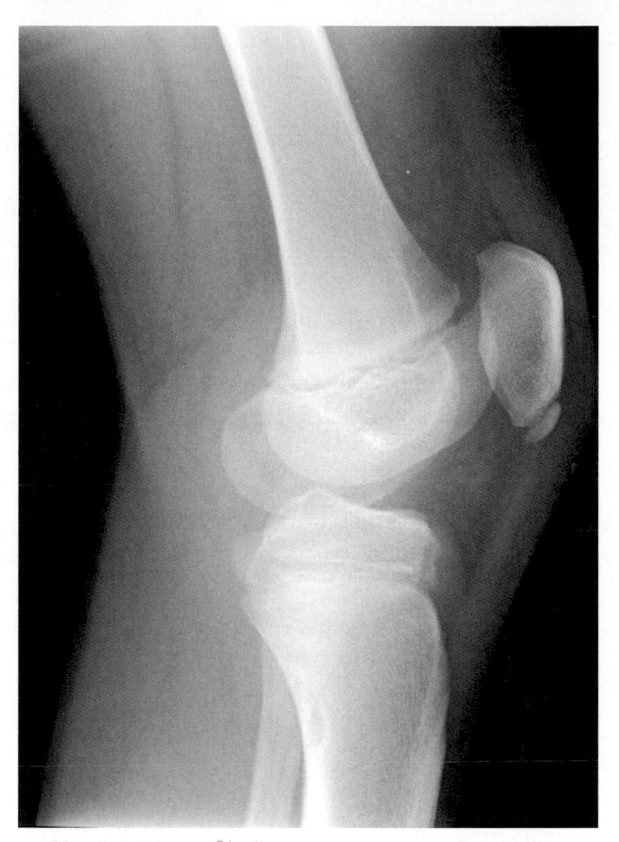

Figure 226-2 Sinding-Larsen-Johansson lesion.

TABLE 226-1 *Differential Diagnosis*

Condition	Differentiating Features
Fracture (e.g., tibial tubercle to patella) (see Chapters 165, 230, and 231)	Inability to do terminal extension of leg and significant radiographic abnormalities
Osteogenic sarcoma/ osteomyelitis (see Chapter 19)	Red flags in history, review of systems, and significant radiographic abnormalities
Hoffa's disease (see Chapter 153)	Tenderness at different anatomic site
Patellofemoral pain syndrome (see Chapter 153)	More diffuse discomfort
Osteochondritis dissecans (see Chapter 224)	Mechanical symptoms; abnormal notch view typically seen on radiograph
Patellar/quadriceps tendinitis (see Chapter 156)	Skeletally mature individual
Patellar stress fracture (see Chapter 165)	Significant disability; abnormal plain radiographs with or without abnormal bone scan/ magnetic resonance imaging
Pre- or infrapatellar bursitis (see Chapter 168)	Significant fluctuance typically seen
Painful multipartite patella (see Chapter 165)	Radiographic abnormality
Referred pain (e.g., slipped capital femoral epiphysis) (see Chapter 221)	Abnormal hip examination; hip radiography abnormal

used sparingly. They should never be taken as premedication so that the patient can engage in activities that have been forbidden or limited.
- Equipment such as protective padding and patellar tendon straps (for SLJL especially) may be useful.
- Quadriceps/hamstring/gastrocnemius muscle strengthening and stretching should be done, in formal physical therapy, with a school athletic trainer, or at home.
- Above all, time is necessary. The natural history of OSL and SLJL is that, in the vast majority of cases, the patient will outgrow the condition without any residual sequelae.
- Avoid cortisone injections.
- Consider referral when concerned about
  - Possible fracture, especially in the setting of recent acute trauma
  - Refractory cases; excision of ossicles and tibial tubercle plasty are done in the case of OSL

Troubleshooting

- Expectations should be managed. Patients and parents can typically expect a waxing and waning course of symptoms corresponding to activity levels during rapid phases of growth in adolescence. Patience is a virtue: The patient will almost inevitably outgrow the disorder.
- Imaging should be performed at times, as in acute trauma, when physical examination findings are atypical, and in prolonged/refractory cases.

Patient Instructions

- Both the American Academy of Orthopaedic Surgeons (http://orthoinfo.aaos.org/topic.cfm?topic=A00411&return_link=0) and the American Academy of Family Practice (http://familydoctor.org/online/famdocen/home/children/parents/special/bone/135.html) have excellent Web resources for patients.

Suggested Reading

- Bloom OJ, Mackler L: What is the best treatment for Osgood-Schlatter disease? J Fam Pract 2004;53:153–156.
- Cassas K, Cassettari-Wayhs A: Childhood and adolescent sports-related overuse injuries. Am Fam Physician 2006;73:1014–1022.
- Krause BL, Williams PR, Catterall A: Natural history of Osgood-Schlatter disease. J Pediatr Orthop 1990;10:65–68.
- Smith A: Osgood-Schlatter disorder and related extensor mechanism problems. In Kocher M, Micheli L (eds): The Pediatric and Adolescent Knee. Philadelphia: Saunders, 2006.
- Wall EJ: Osgood-Schlatter disease: Practical treatment for a self-limited condition. Physician Sports Med 1998;26:29–34.
- Weiss JM, Jordan SS, Andersen JS, et al. Surgical treatment of unresolved Osgood-Schlatter disease: Ossicle resection with tibial tubercleplasty. J Pediatr Orthop 2007;27:844–847.

Chapter 227 Tarsal Coalition

Mark J. Romness

ICD-9 CODE
755.67 *Anomalies of Foot, Not Elsewhere Classified*

Key Concepts

- Tarsal coalition is due to the failure of the bones in the foot to separate completely during formation.
- Depending on the position of the coalition, there may be stiffness, deformity, or pain.
- Asymptomatic coalitions may not need treatment.
- Symptomatic coalitions often need surgery.
- The most common are calcaneonavicular and talocalcaneal coalitions (Fig. 227-1).

History

- Clinical signs rarely manifest before preadolescent age.
- The initial symptom is a limp or pain.

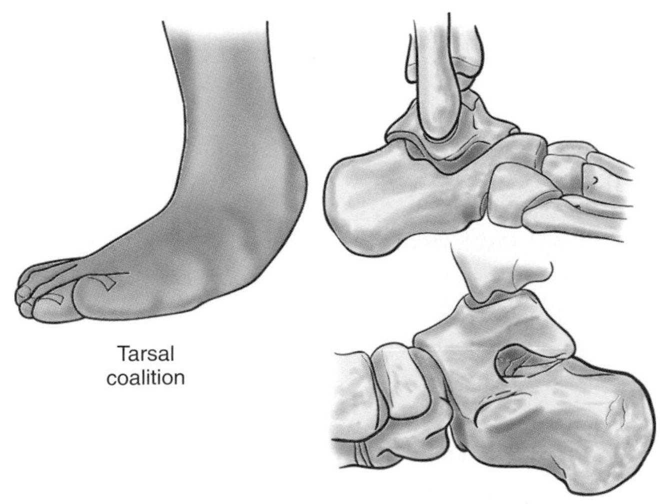

Figure 227-1 Coalitions. A more severe foot position is shown on the *left.* Calcaneonavicular coalition is demonstrated at *top right.* Talocalcaneal coalition is demonstrated at *bottom right.*

- Pain is usually medial or dorsolateral.
- Recurrent ankle sprains may be secondary to a coalition.

Physical Examination

- Asymmetrical position of the foot in standing position
- Usually more valgus or pronation of the foot with a coalition
- Decreased motion actively and passively
- Lack of arch accentuation and heel varus on tip-toe position (Fig. 227-2)
- Tenderness at the area of the coalition
  - Sinus tarsi for a calcaneonavicular coalition
  - Medial for a talocalcaneal coalition

Imaging

- Plain radiographs may be diagnostic, but special views must be ordered.
  - An oblique radiograph of the foot shows most calcaneonavicular coalitions (Fig. 227-3).
  - The axial view of the calcaneus may show a talocalcaneal coalition, but usually computed tomography or magnetic resonance imaging is necessary.
- Computed tomography is more accurate than magnetic resonance imaging in the diagnosis.
- A bone scan is rarely necessary, but may be helpful in equivocal cases.

Additional Tests

- Serology studies and nerve conduction studies should be considered if there is no definitive coalition radiographically and there is a suggestion of muscle disease or a neuropathy.

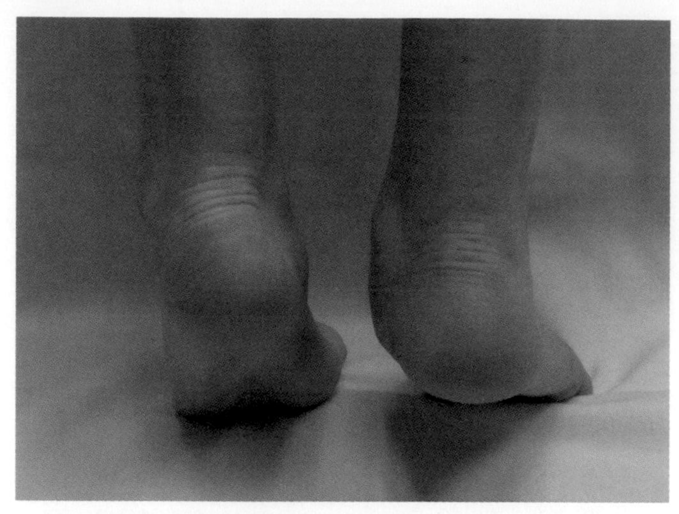

Figure 227-2 Feet in tip-toe position. The right foot with a coalition does not correct out of pronation, but the left does with restoration of the arch and hindfoot varus in tip-toe position.

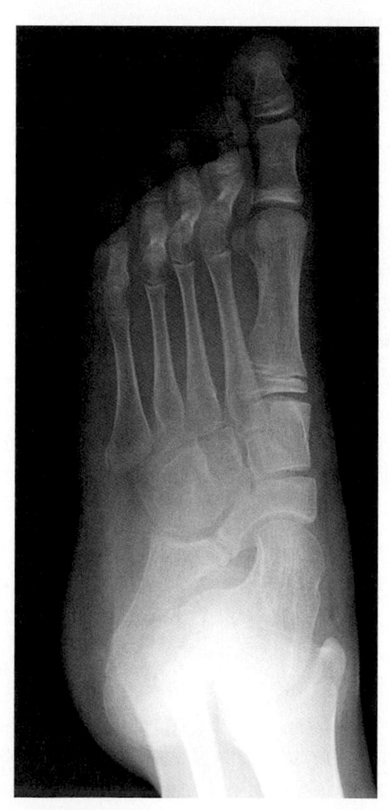

Figure 227-3 Oblique radiograph of the foot with a well-defined calcaneonavicular coalition.

Differential Diagnosis

- The historical term of peroneal spastic flatfoot for coalition is thought to describe the secondary contracture of the peroneal tendons, but primary contracture of the peroneals may occur and mimic a coalition.
- Conditions such as juvenile rheumatoid arthritis that can affect the subtalar joint may have similar complaints and presentation.
- Muscle disease or a neuropathy should be considered, but it usually is associated with an opposite position (cavovarus) of the foot.

Treatment

- At diagnosis
  - Proper diagnosis
  - Symptomatic treatment with limited activity, inserts or orthoses, anti-inflammatory medication, and immobilization in a boot or cast
- Later
  - Monitor the foot position with growth.
  - Consider surgery for significant deformity or pain.

When to Refer

- Persistent pain despite symptomatic treatment
- Significant deformity or stiffness

Prognosis

- Depends on the location and extent of the coalition
- Calcaneonavicular coalitions have better prognosis than talocalcaneal coalitions
- More initial deformity has worse prognosis

Troubleshooting

- Magnetic resonance imaging may not detect the coalition.
- Secondary changes in the adjacent joints, such as beaking of the talar head, may be misinterpreted as the primary condition if appropriate radiographic views are not obtained.

Patient Instructions

- Bilateral involvement is present in 50% to 60% of cases, and studies of the opposite foot are indicated if clinical evidence is present.
- Asymptomatic feet with only mild deformity do not require treatment.

Considerations in Special Populations

- Tarsal coalitions are present in some genetic conditions, such as fibular deficiencies (hemimelia; see Chapter 223), clubfoot, Apert's syndrome, and Nievergelt-Pearlman syndrome.

Suggested Reading

- Drennan JC: Tarsal coalitions. Instr Course Lect 1996; 45:323–329.
- Gonzalez P, Kumar SJ: Calcaneonavicular coalition treated by resection and interposition of the extensor digitorum brevis muscle. J Bone Joint Surg Am 1990;72A:71–77.
- McCormack TJ, Olney B, Asher M: Talocalcaneal coalition resection: A 10-year follow-up. J Pediatr Orthop 1997;17:13–15.
- Mosier KM, Asher M: Tarsal coalitions and peroneal spastic flat foot: A review. J Bone Joint Surg Am 1984;66A:976–984.
- Takakura Y, Sugimoto K, Tanaka Y, Tamai S: Symptomatic talocalcaneal coalition: Its clinical significance and treatment. Clin Orthop Relat Res 1991;269:249–256.

Chapter 228 Congenital Clubfeet

Mark J. Romness

ICD-9 CODE
754.51 *Talipes Equinovarus*

Key Concepts

- Spectrum of equinovarus deformity from mild to severe
- Rarely associated with other anomalies
- Incidence averages 1.24 per 1000 births
- Boys have twice the incidence of girls.
- 50% bilateral
- Multifactorial cause
- Less operative treatment than previously when principles developed by Ponseti are followed

History

- Family history of clubfeet
- Clubfeet may be seen in the following neuromuscular conditions:
  - Myelomeningocele (spina bifida)
  - Arthrogryposis
  - Muscular dystrophy
  - Spinal muscular atrophy

Physical Examination (Fig. 228-1)

- Check the spine and hips.
- Rare leg length discrepancy with shortening on the clubfoot side
- Common calf atrophy
- Foot postured in equinus, varus, and adductus
- Limited flexibility to passive range of motion
- Incomplete passive correction to neutral
- Active motor function limited by contractures

Imaging

- Imaging is not required for diagnosis.
- Plain radiographs helpful for atypical foot positions or in complex cases

Differential Diagnosis (Tables 228-1 and 228-2)

- Many foot deformities are called clubfeet erroneously.
- The key distinguishing component of the clubfoot is limited dorsiflexion of the hindfoot (Fig. 228-2).

Treatment

- At diagnosis
  - Weekly casting for five to six casts
  - Percutaneous tenotomy of Achilles tendon in 80% to 90%
  - Three-week cast after tenotomy
  - Brace (foot abduction orthosis full time for 3 months) (Fig. 228-3)
- Later
  - Foot abduction orthosis at night for 3 years
  - Possible extensive release if casting not successful
  - Transfer of the tibialis anterior for persistent forefoot supination at 3 to 5 years of age in 10% to 20%

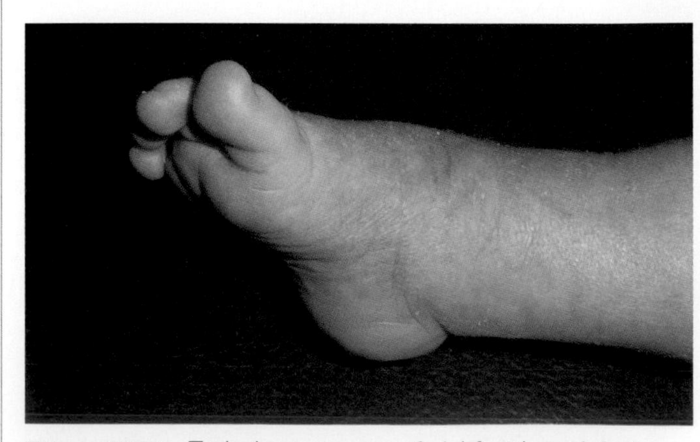

Figure 228-1 Typical appearance of clubfeet in an infant. Note the high arch for an infant and the varus plus plantar-flexed (equinus) position of the heel. The heel pad is less well defined than normal.

TABLE 228-1 *Differential Diagnosis*

Differential Diagnosis	Differentiating Features
Calcaneovalgus feet	Common at birth with the foot dorsiflexed all the way into the tibia
Metatarsus adductus	Similar forefoot adductus but a mobile hindfoot
Skewfoot	Atypical and more severe form of metatarsus adductus

TABLE 228-2 *Foot Positions at Birth*

Condition	Forefoot	Midfoot	Hindfoot
Calcaneovalgus	Neutral	Neutral or lateral	Hyperdorsiflexed
Metatarsus adductus	Adduction	Normal	Normal
Skewfoot	Adduction	Lateral	Valgus
Clubfoot	Adduction	Medial	Varus/equinus

When to Refer

- Immediately if rigid for weekly casting
- If not tolerating cast or brace
- Persistent deformity despite casting and bracing

Troubleshooting

- Inability to maintain the cast on the leg, usually due to casting technique
- Inability to keep the foot in the foot abduction orthosis, usually due to a lack of family persistence in maintaining the brace wear schedule or inadequate motion of the foot to tolerate the foot abduction orthosis

Patient Instructions

- Casting is successful in 80% or more of feet if the family adheres to brace wearing.
- Children are expected to walk, run, and play sports at age-appropriate stages.
- Risk for subsequent children
  - Baby boy with clubfoot
    - 1:40 chance for brother
    - Minimal for sister
  - Baby girl with clubfeet
    - 1:16 for brother
    - 1:40 for sister
  - Parent and child with clubfoot
    - 1:4 for siblings

Figure 228-2 A calcaneovalgus foot is hyperdorsiflexed and can often be positioned flush with the anterior shin. A more severe calcaneovalgus deformity may be associated with posterior medial apex bowing of the tibia and limb shortening.

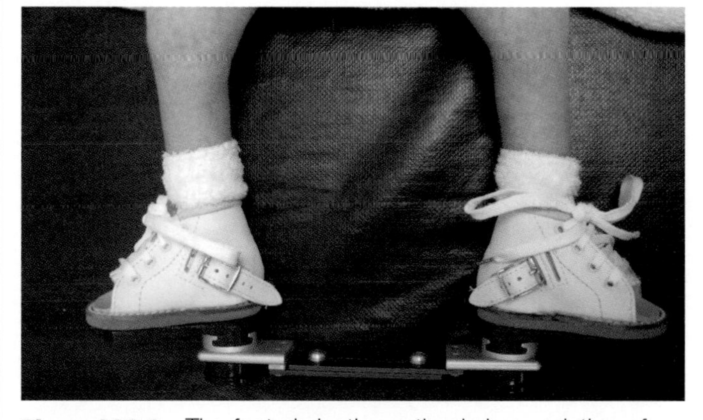

Figure 228-3 The foot abduction orthosis is a variation of the Dennis-Brown bar used frequently in the past and less often now for internal tibial torsion. The clubfoot is externally rotated 70 degrees. The foot abduction orthosis is worn full time for 3 months and then during sleep for as long as 3 years.

Considerations in Special Populations

- Clubfeet associated with neuromuscular conditions may be more resistant to casting and nonoperative treatment, but casting is still attempted.
- An atypical clubfoot has been described in which the foot is smaller, more deformed, and more rigid than the standard foot and requires special attention for casting and bracing.

Suggested Reading

- Morcuende JA, Dolan LA, Dietz FR, Ponseti IV: Radical reduction in the rate of extensive corrective surgery for clubfoot using the Ponseti method. Pediatrics 2004;113:376–380.
- Ponseti IV: Congenital Clubfoot. Fundamentals for Treatment. Oxford: Oxford University Press, 1996.
- Siapkara A, Duncan R: Congenital talipes equinovarus: A review of current management. J Bone Joint Surg Br 2007;89B:995–1000.
- Staheli L, Ponseti IV, Morcuende JA, et al: Clubfoot: Ponseti Management, 3rd ed. Available at www.global-help.org/publications/books/help_cfponseti.pdf. Accessed February 23, 2009.

Chapter 229 Cavus Foot

Mark J. Romness

ICD-9 CODES
736.73 *Cavus Deformity of Foot, Acquired*
736.75 *Cavovarus Deformity of the Foot, Acquired*

Key Concepts

- Progressive cavus foot deformity may be the first sign of other pathologic conditions that must be identified.
- Treatment for the foot is generally symptomatic.

History

- A family history of any neurologic condition should be defined.
- Clinical signs rarely manifest before age 3 years.
- A visual deformity or a limp is the common symptom in the young child.
- Pain or shoe wear problems occur later.
- Neurologic problems such as bowel or bladder incontinence and subtle weakness signs such as problems with stairs must be asked about specifically.

Physical Examination

- The foot shows a progression of deformity.
  - Toe dorsiflexion and clawing
  - Plantar fascia contraction and increased arch height
  - First metatarsal plantarflexion
  - Asymmetrical muscle weakening, especially of the peroneals
  - Hindfoot varus as the first metatarsal plantarflexion increases
  - Rigidity of the foot with maturity (Fig. 229-1)
- Comprehensive neurologic examination, including tone assessment, reflexes, strength, and motor control
- Spine examination for scoliosis or other deformity
- Lower extremity examination to assess length, alignment, and development

Imaging

- Plain radiographs define the degree and location of the deformity.
  - Standing radiographs are recommended.
  - The position of the calcaneus is usually dorsiflexed relative to the tibia, indicating that the Achilles tendon is not shortened.
- Magnetic resonance imaging of the spinal axis, including the entire spinal cord if upper motor neuron findings are present
  - Magnetic resonance imaging of the brain if indicated by symptoms and findings

Additional Tests

- Nerve conduction studies may help classify the condition.
- Serology studies
  - Hereditary sensorimotor neuropathy type IA is caused by duplication of the gene for peripheral myelin protein 22 (*PMP-22*) in chromosome region 17p11.2.

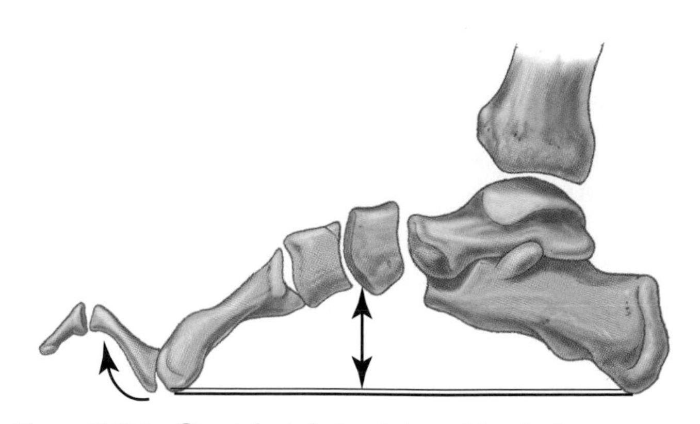

Figure 229-1 Cavus foot. Lateral view of the foot demonstrating the clawing of the toes, plantar fascia contraction, and increased arch height leading to first metatarsal plantarflexion. (Adapted from Schwend RM, Drennan JC: Cavus foot deformity in children. J Am Acad Orthop Surg 2003;11:201–211.)

- Eighteen genes and 11 additional loci harboring candidate genes have been associated with hereditary sensorimotor neuropathy and related peripheral neuropathies.

Differential Diagnosis

- Many conditions have been associated with cavus foot deformity and are grouped by cause in Box 229-1.
- Hereditary sensorimotor neuropathy type I is the most prevalent neuromuscular cause and is commonly known as Charcot-Marie-Tooth disease type I.

Treatment

- At diagnosis
  - Determination of the cause if there is one
  - Maintain flexibility with stretching as possible
  - Shoe modifications or foot orthosis if symptomatic
- Later
  - Flexibility of the deformity determines treatment options.
  - Surgical reconstruction if severely symptomatic

When to Refer

- If unable to determine the etiology
- If foot is rigid or symptomatic

Prognosis

- Depends on the etiology
- Most forms are treatable and do not prevent light-duty daily activities.

Troubleshooting

- Many of the conditions that cause cavus foot deformity also cause scoliosis and hip dysplasia.

Patient Instructions

- There is no effective medical treatment to prevent progression of hereditary sensorimotor neuropathy (Charcot-Marie-Tooth disease).
- Hereditary sensorimotor neuropathy types Ia and II are autosomal dominant and type Ix is X-linked dominant.

BOX 229-1 Conditions Associated with Cavus Foot Deformity Grouped by Cause

Central Nervous System
Spastic hemiplegia
Friedreich's ataxia
Brain tumors

Spinal Abnormalities
Diastematomyelia
Myelodysplasia
Syringomyelia
Poliomyelitis
Spinal cord tumors
Intrathecal lipoma
Tethered cord syndrome
Guillain-Barré syndrome

Peripheral Nerves
Hereditary sensorimotor neuropathy
Polyneuritis
Small muscular atrophy
Atypical polyneuritis
Neuromuscular choristoma

Other Causes
Isolated injuries to selected nerves, muscles, and tendons
Clubfoot or residual clubfoot deformity
Idiopathic

Adapted from Schwend RM, Drennan JC: Cavus foot deformity in children. J Am Acad Orthop Surg 2003;11:201–211.

Considerations in Special Populations

- Before skeletal maturity of the foot there is usually more flexibility.
- A rigid foot with skeletal maturity is less likely to respond to nonoperative treatment for severe symptoms.

Suggested Reading

- Aktas S, Sussman MD: The radiological analysis of pes cavus deformity in Charcot Marie Tooth disease. J Pediatr Orthop B 2000;9:137–140.
- Mosca VS: The cavus foot. J Pediatr Orthop 2001;21:423–424.
- Olney B: Treatment of the cavus foot. Deformity in the pediatric patient with Charcot-Marie-Tooth. Foot Ankle Clin 2000; 5:305–315.
- Saifi GM, Szigeti K, Snipes GJ, et al: Molecular mechanisms, diagnosis, and rational approaches to management of and therapy for Charcot-Marie-Tooth disease and related peripheral neuropathies. J Investig Med 2003;51:261–283.
- Schwend RH, Drennan JC: Cavus foot deformity in children. J Am Acad Orthop Surg 2003;11:201–211.

Chapter 230 Salter-Harris Fractures

Joseph A. Janicki

Key Concepts

- Approximately 15% to 30% of childhood fractures involve the physis.
- The risk of growth arrest depends on the site of injury with growth disturbance of fractures in the distal tibia (25%), distal femur (25%), distal ulna (60%), and distal radius (4%).
- Injury classically occurs through the zone of provisional classification of the physis, although multiple layers can be involved.
- Salter-Harris classification (Fig. 230-1)
    - Type I: transverse fracture through the physis
    - Type II: fracture line through the physis exiting into the metaphysis
    - Type III: transverse fracture line through the physis and exiting into the epiphysis (intra-articular fracture)
    - Type IV: fracture line passes through the metaphysis, physis, and epiphysis
    - Type V: crush injury to the physis, which is usually not apparent initially
    - Type VI (added by Rang): localized injury to the perichondrium
- Fractures heal quickly, so avoid manipulation and reduction more than 5 days postinjury.
- Follow patients for 6 to 12 months after healing to watch for growth arrest (partial or complete).
- Treatment of physeal growth arrest relies on the location, extent of involvement, and remaining growth.
- Growth arrests are more common in Salter-Harris III, IV, and V fractures because the reserve cell layer is involved.

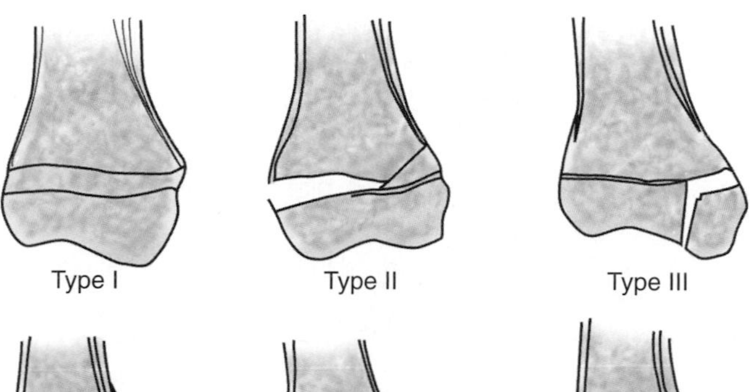

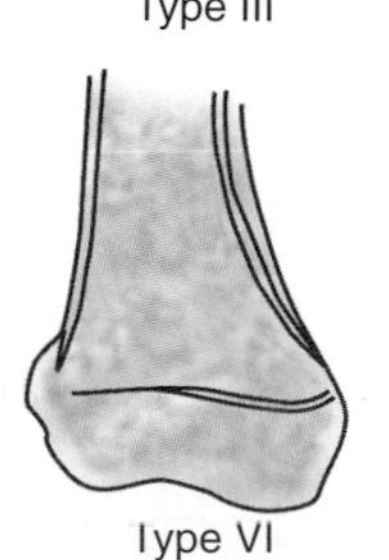

Figure 230-1 Salter-Harris classification of growth plate injuries.

History

- Acute
    - Basic trauma history including mechanism of injury, areas of pain or deformity, and other associated injuries or previous injuries to extremity
- Chronic or at follow-up
    - Whether pain exists
    - What type of deformity
    - Evidence of maturation and amount of growth remaining
        - — Age at menarche, adolescent growth spurt, Tanner staging
    - Feeling of limb length discrepancy

Physical Examination

- Examination specific to extremity involved
- Acute
    - Observation: deformity and bruising/swelling
    - Palpation: tenderness or crepitus
    - Neurovascular examination
- Chronic or at follow-up
    - Examine for limb length discrepancy
    - Angular deformity

Imaging

- Acute
  - Radiographs
    - — Anteroposterior and lateral views of the affected joint
    - — Stress radiographs of the knee can be performed for a distal femoral or proximal tibial injury with normal initial radiographs (not recommended with magnetic resonance imaging availability)
  - Magnetic resonance imaging
    - — Examining for physeal edema and separation
  - Computed tomography
    - — Aids in assessment of reduction and joint congruence
- Follow-up
  - Radiographs
    - — Anteroposterior and lateral views of affected bone and joint
      - — Look for Harris growth arrest lines to aid with assessment.
    - — Three-foot standing hips to ankles on one cassette with patellas pointing forward to assess mechanical axis alignment and limb length
    - — Left-hand anteroposterior view to assess bone age
  - Computed tomography or magnetic resonance imaging to assess physeal closure and determine the percentage of involvement

Differential Diagnosis

- Depends on extremity involved
- All extremities could have fractures of the metaphysis without physeal injury (e.g., distal radius), dislocation of the joint (e.g., shoulder, elbow, hip), ligamentous injury (e.g., knee medial collateral ligament injury), osteochondral injury (e.g., knee), labral or meniscal injury (e.g., hip, shoulder, or knee).

Treatment

- At diagnosis
  - Depends on fracture and age
  - In general, avoid multiple reduction attempts and fixation through the physis and, if necessary, use smooth pins.
  - Distal radius and ulna: closed reduction and casting
  - Proximal radius (rare, usually fractures through the metaphysis)
    - — Attempt closed reduction; often needs percutaneous or open reduction with or without pinning
- Distal humerus
  - — Supracondylar humerus fracture: arthrogram often helpful to aid in diagnosis and to judge joint congruence; pin fixation necessary
  - — Lateral condyle fracture (see Chapter 231)
- Proximal humerus
  - — Observation: This injury rarely needs manipulation despite significant deformity due to the shoulder's great remodeling potential and range of motion.
- Proximal femur
  - — Often difficult to distinguish from unstable or acute slipped capital femoral epiphysis
  - — Anatomic reduction and fixation; this injury has a very high rate of avascular necrosis (>80% in some series) and should be managed at specialized facilities
- Distal femur
  - — Neurovascular examination important because popliteal vessel injuries can occur
  - — Closed reduction alone usually not sufficient to maintain reduction so fixation usually necessary
  - — With Salter-Harris I, crossed pins through physis are necessary if displaced (Fig. 230-2)
  - — With Salter-Harris II, reduce and place screws in the metaphyseal fragment (Thurston-Holland fragment) for fixation, avoiding crossing the physis, if possible (Fig. 230-3).
  - — Salter-Harris III and IV: screw fixation; articular surface should be congruent
- Proximal tibia
  - — Injuries through the physis are equivalent to knee dislocations due to tethering of vessels.
    - — Careful neurovascular examination is a necessity.
  - — Injuries also have a high rate of compartment syndrome.
  - — Reduction and pin fixation are usually necessary.
  - — Tibial tubercle avulsions (see Chapter 231)
- Distal fibula
  - — Physeal tenderness after "ankle sprain" mechanism common
    - — Treat as a physeal injury with 4 to 6 weeks of immobilization.
- Distal tibia
  - — Salter Harris I and II fractures: typically closed reduction and casting adequate

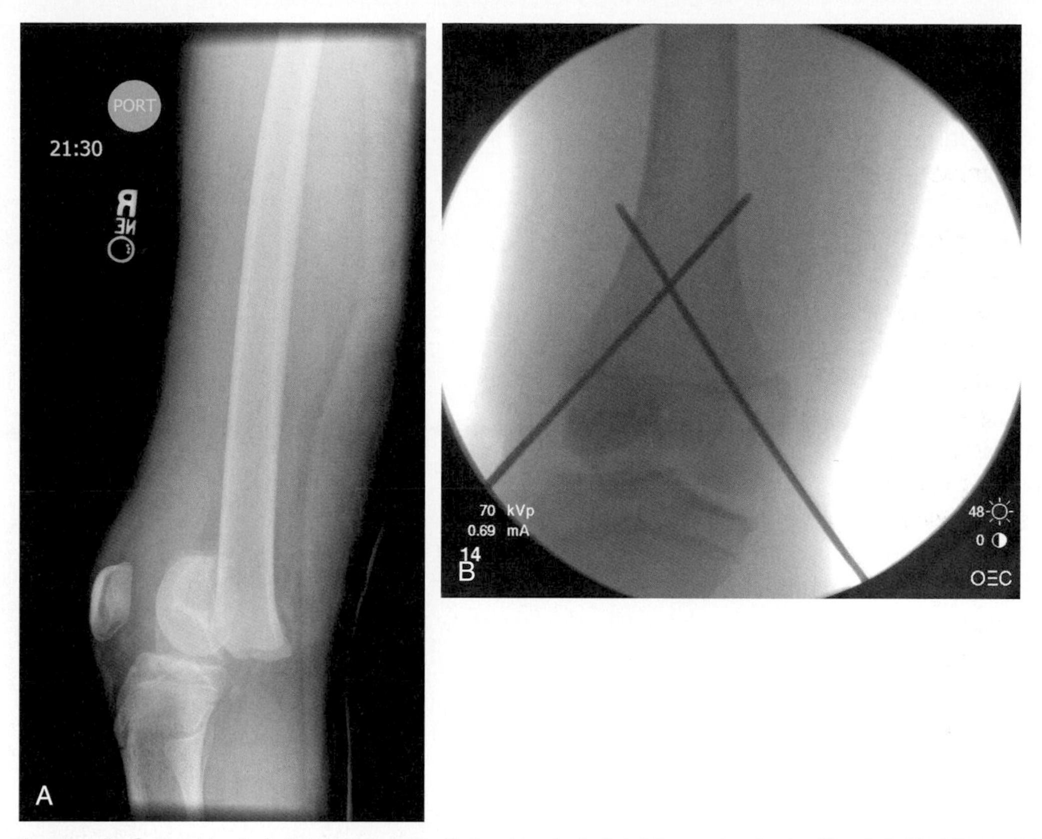

Figure 230-2 **A**, Salter-Harris I distal femur. **B**, Salter-Harris I distal femur treated with smooth Kirschner wires.

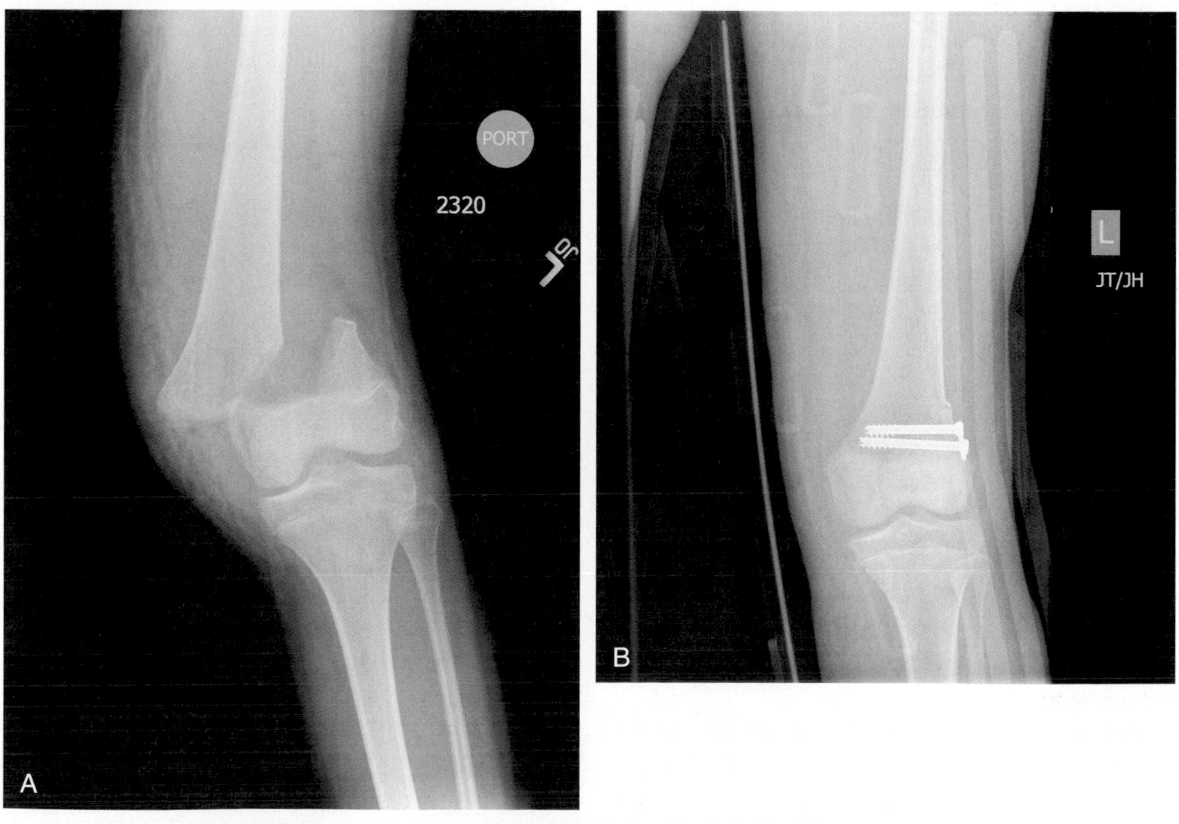

Figure 230-3 **A**, Salter-Harris II distal femur. **B**, Salter-Harris II distal femur treated with screws.

- Medial malleolus fracture: usually Salter-Harris IV due to small metaphyseal flag
  - Requires open reduction and screw placement (articular congruence); usually possible to keep screw epiphyseal
- Triplane and Tillaux (see Chapter 231)

- Later
  - Must monitor for 6 to 12 months postinjury for partial or complete growth arrest
  - Site of injury and mechanism affect likelihood of growth arrest (e.g., growth disturbance rare in the distal radius but common in the distal femur and proximal tibia)
  - If complete growth arrest in the lower extremity, must calculate the remaining growth and treat according to anticipated leg length discrepancy
    - Observation if anticipated leg length discrepancy less than 2 cm
    - Epiphysiodesis of contralateral side at appropriate time if leg length discrepancy 2 to 5 cm
    - Lengthening or shortening procedures if anticipated leg length discrepancy more than 5 cm
  - If incomplete growth arrest or physeal bar, treatment is based on the remaining growth, percentage of physis involved, and location
    - Central bars often halt growth, whereas peripheral bars can result in more problematic angular deformity (Fig. 230-4).
    - In general, epiphyseolysis (physeal bar removal) is attempted when less than 50% of the physis is involved (Fig. 230-5).
    - With a potential for angular deformity, the decision must be made whether to complete the partial epiphysiodesis or attempt a bar resection.

When to Refer

- In the management of acute fractures, referrals are based on the comfort level of the treating physician in managing the fracture.
- In general, distal radius fractures should be able to be treated by most orthopaedic surgeons, whereas fractures of the lower extremities and elbow are usually referred to pediatric trauma centers.
- Monitoring for growth arrest can be completed by community surgeons, whereas addressing leg length discrepancies and angular deformities associated with growth arrest often requires more expertise.

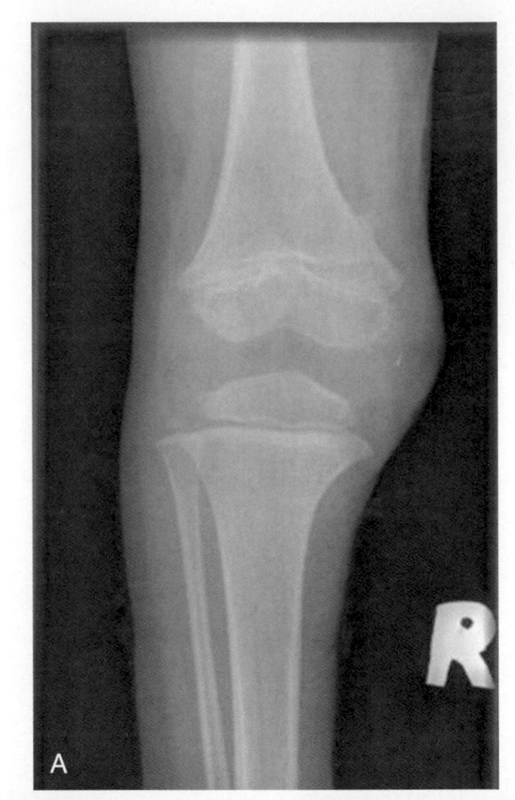

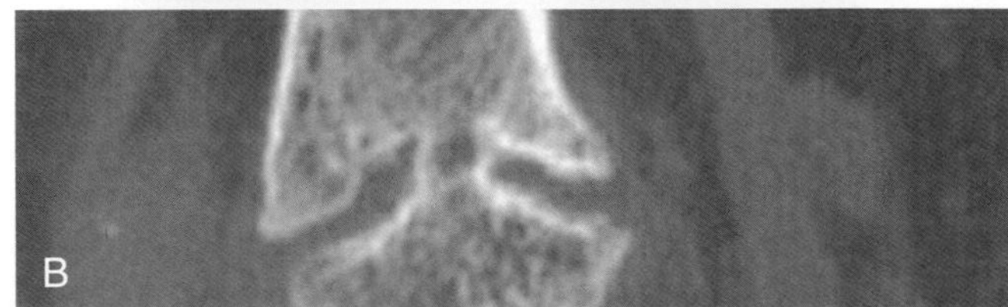

Figure 230-4 **A**, Growth arrest in the distal femur, anteroposterior view: central bar. Note growth lines. **B**, Growth arrest in the distal femur: computed tomography scan.

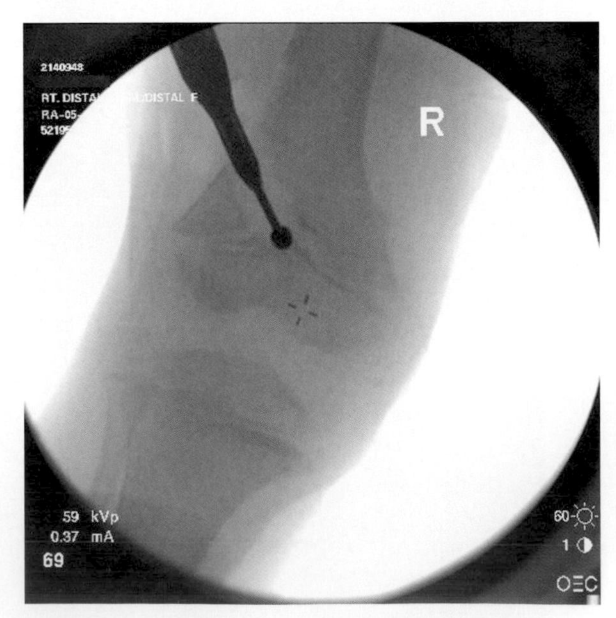

Figure 230-5 Growth arrest treated with physeal bar resection.

Prognosis

- Depends on the site of fracture, age of the patient, and energy of the mechanism
- Generally, fractures involving the growth plate heal more rapidly (often <4 weeks) and almost never have problems with union.

Troubleshooting

- Attempt only one closed reduction in the emergency department under block or conscious sedation. If this fails, the patient should be paralyzed in the operating room setting.
- Multiple reduction attempts have been associated with growth arrest.
- Use advanced imaging to help with the diagnosis.

Patient Instructions

- Patients and their parents should be aware that any physeal injury has the potential for growth disturbance. The frequency and implications depend on the site of injury, age of the patient (and remaining growth), and the energy of the injury mechanism.
- Fortunately, most physeal injuries do not result in a clinically significant problem.

Suggested Reading

- Birch JG: Surgical treatment of physeal bar resection. In Eilert RE (ed): Instructional Course Lectures. Rosemont, IL: American Academy of Orthopaedic Surgeons, 1992, pp 445–450.
- Hynes D, O'Brien T: Growth disturbance lines after injury of the distal tibial physis. Their significance in prognosis. J Bone Joint Surg Br 1988;70B:231–233.
- Khoshhal KI, Kiefer GN: Physeal bar resection. J Am Acad Orthop Surg 2005;13:47–58.
- Peterson HA: Physeal fractures: Part 3. Classification. J Pediatr Orthop 1994;14:439–448.
- Salter R, Harris WR: Injuries involving the epiphyseal plate. J Bone Joint Surg Am 1963;45A:587–622.

Chapter 231 Special Fractures in Pediatrics

Joseph A. Janicki

ICD-9 CODES

812.41 *Supracondylar Fracture*
812.42 *Lateral Condyle Fracture*
823.00 *Tibial Tubercle and Spine Fracture*
824.8 *Distal Tibial Intra-articular Fracture (Triplane and Tillaux)*

COMMON FRACTURES: ELBOW (SUPRACONDYLAR AND LATERAL CONDYLE FRACTURES)

Key Concepts

- Elbow fractures common in pediatrics
- Supracondylar humerus fractures
  - Neurovascular injury common, with 15% of cases involving nerve injury and as many as 20% without pulse (although often the hand remains perfused)
  - Avoid cubitus varus deformity with supracondylar fractures.
  - Compartment syndrome higher when treated with closed reduction, hyperflexion, and without pinning
- Lateral condyle fractures
  - Intra-articular fractures need anatomic reduction of the articular surface.
  - Risk of nonunion that is decreased by fixation
  - Prolonged casting may be necessary, often for 6 weeks.

History

- Acute: basic trauma history including mechanism of injury, areas of pain or deformity, and other associated injuries or previous injuries to extremity

Physical Examination

- Observation: deformity, bruising/swelling, skin condition
- Palpation: tenderness or crepitus at fracture site as well as in the forearm and shoulder
- Neurovascular examination critical

Imaging

- Radiographs
  - Anteroposterior and lateral views of elbow
    - — The anterior humeral line should intersect the capitellum in a true lateral view.
    - — The radial shaft should point to the capitellum in all views; if not, the elbow is dislocated.
    - — Baumann's angle (humeral capitellar angle) should be in valgus and typically greater than 9 degrees.
    - — A posterior fat pad seen on a lateral view denotes an occult fracture.
  - Oblique elbow radiographs helpful if high index of suspicion of lateral condyle fracture
- Arthrography or magnetic resonance imaging helpful if suspect transphyseal fractures or with fractures involving the articular surface

Differential Diagnosis

- Please see Table 231-1.

Treatment

Supracondylar Humerus Fracture

- At diagnosis
  - If hand nonperfused, flexion alone often adequate to restore capillary refill
    - — If remains nonperfused, emergent operative treatment necessary
  - Splint in 30 to 50 degrees of flexion
  - If pinning necessary, treat within 20 hours for displaced fractures and within 2 to 3 days for angulated fractures with minimal swelling.

TABLE 231-1 *Differential Diagnosis: Common Injuries of the Elbow*

Differential Diagnosis	Differentiation Features
Other fractures Supracondylar Lateral condyle Radial neck Medial condyle Olecranon	Location of pain and tenderness, radiographic differences
Elbow dislocation	Radiographic differences: radial head not aligned with the capitellum
Osteochondral injury	Persistent discomfort (often after elbow dislocation), radiographic diagnosis difficult; joint incongruity noted on magnetic resonance imaging

- Later
  - Closed treatment and casting in 90 degrees in nondisplaced fractures and those in which the anterior humeral line touches the capitellum and have a normal valgus Baumann's angle
  - Closed reduction and percutaneous pinning for displaced fractures and fractures in extension (anterior humeral line does not touch the capitellum) and in varus (Fig. 231-1)
    — Crossed pins (increased risk of iatrogenic ulnar nerve injury) versus lateral-only pins (potentially not as stable) both acceptable
  - Open reduction reserved for open fractures, fractures unable to be reduced due to interposed tissue, and those without a pulse

When to Refer

- Cold, nonperfused extremity and if any question with treatment
- Transfer to treating facility with displaced fractures
- Refer within 24 hours for nondisplaced or minimally displaced fractures.

Prognosis

- Generally excellent
- Healing problems are very rare, and as long as the elbow is not in varus, patients will do well.
- Stiffness after immobilization can improve for as long as 2 years after casting or pinning.

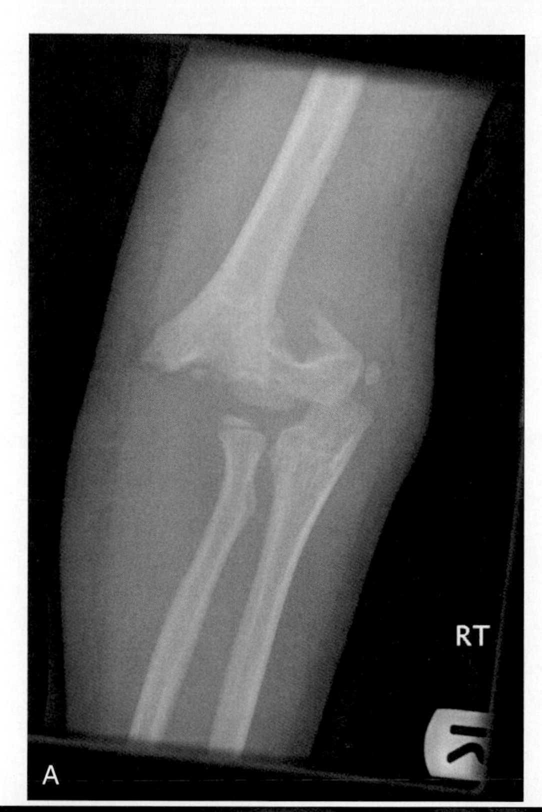

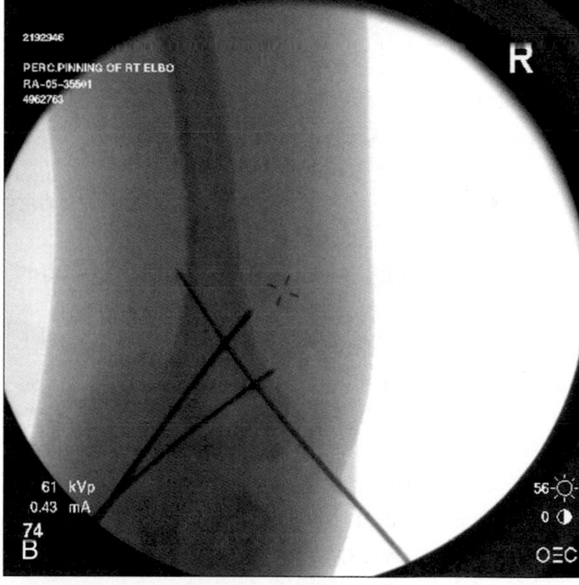

Figure 231-1 **A**, Displaced supracondylar humerus fracture requiring reduction and pinning. **B**, Closed reduced and pinned supracondylar humerus fracture; three pins were used, including a medial pin, because of persistent instability.

Lateral Condyle Fracture

- At diagnosis
  - Splint
  - Nondisplaced (≤2 mm) fractures with an intact articular surface can be treated nonoperatively with casting. It is sometimes necessary to take the cast off weekly to make sure displacement has not occurred.

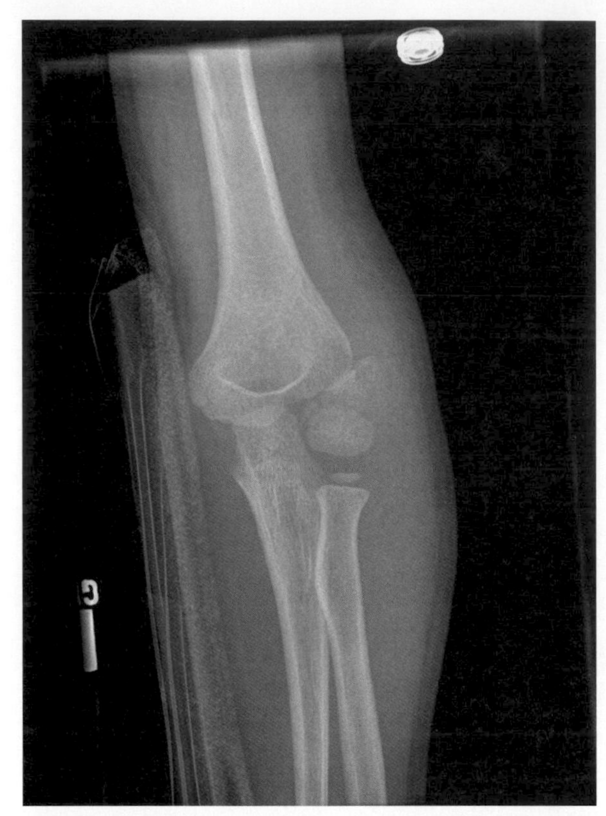

Figure 231-2 Displaced lateral condyle fracture requiring open reduction.

- Later
  - With more than 2 mm of displacement, operative treatment is indicated.
  - If the articular surface is intact, percutaneous pinning is adequate.
  - With significant displacement, open reduction, anatomic reduction of the articular surface, and pinning are needed (Fig. 231-2).
    - — Do not dissect posteriorly; lateral trochlea blood supply comes from the posterior nonarticular portion (disruption may result in avascular necrosis of the fragment).
  - May take 4 to 6 weeks to heal

When to Refer
- Late presenting lateral condyle fractures are often difficult to treat and have a high risk of nonunion and cubitus varus.

Prognosis
- Usually heal well but increased risk of complications including nonunion, late fracture displacement, and cubitus valgus
- Also, there will usually be a prominence laterally after an open reduction.
- The fracture involves the physis, but is of little consequence with good reduction and healing.
- Stiffness is occasionally a problem after open reduction and prolonged casting.

Troubleshooting

- Vascular compromise not uncommon.
  - With perfused hand, acceptable to watch even without a pulse
  - With cold, pulseless hand, emergent reduction needed (and sometimes vascular surgery)
- Nerve injuries are not uncommon with supracondylar fractures (either caused by the injury or iatrogenic).
  - Nerve palsies usually improve with time.

Patient Instructions

- Warn patients about the risks of nonunion and stiffness with lateral condyle fractures as well as a likely prominence laterally on the elbow.

SPECIAL FRACTURES: KNEE (TIBIAL SPINE AND TIBIAL TUBERCLE FRACTURES)

Key Concepts

- The tibial spine fracture mechanism of injury similar to the anterior cruciate ligament or posterior cruciate ligament in skeletally mature patients
- If more than 2 mm of displacement, the meniscus may be interposed, and surgical reduction and fixation may be necessary.
- Tibial tubercle fractures are actually Salter-Harris fractures of the anterior proximal tibial physis.
- Typically occurs in teenage boys (near skeletal maturity), usually during a jumping sport
- Fixation is typically necessary due to the pull of the extensor mechanism.
- Associated with compartment syndrome despite being a low-energy injury

History

- See anterior/posterior cruciate ligament injury and extensor mechanism injuries.
- Acute: age of patient, basic trauma history including the mechanism of injury, areas of pain or deformity, and other associated injuries or previous injuries to extremity

Physical Examination

- See anterior/posterior cruciate ligament injury and extensor mechanism injuries.
- Observation: deformity, bruising/swelling, effusion
- Palpation: tenderness, crepitus, effusion
- Range of motion, if able
- Whether extensor mechanism is intact

Imaging

- Radiographs: anteroposterior and lateral views of the knee
- Computed tomography or magnetic resonance imaging confirms the diagnosis or the amount of displacement of the tibial spine fracture.

Differential Diagnosis

- Please see Table 231-2.

Treatment

Tibial Spine Fracture (Fig. 231-3)

- At diagnosis
  - Extension with knee immobilization or cast often reduces fracture
    — If any question, obtain advanced imaging
- Later
  - Treatment of 4 weeks if minimal displacement with extension followed by range of motion
  - If displaced (>2 mm with knee extended), the tibial spine should be repaired to origin
    — Can be performed arthroscopically or open depending on surgeon's preference
    — Fixation options include suture, cannulated screws, and pins.

When to Refer

- If the examiner has any concern about management, the patient should be placed in a knee immobilizer and evaluated within 3 to 5 days.

Prognosis

- Generally good
- The spine typically heals well.
- Due to stretching of the anterior cruciate ligament, there may be some laxity to the knee after treatment. This does not appear to be clinically significant and may even improve with growth.
- Arthrofibrosis can be a problem with prolonged knee immobilization and open treatment.

TABLE 231-2 *Differential Diagnosis: Special Injuries of the Knee*

Differential Diagnosis	Differentiating Features
Anterior/posterior cruciate ligament tear	Positive Lachman's test, knee instability, radiographs negative for fracture, magnetic resonance imaging diagnostic
Patellar sleeve fracture	Extensor mechanism disrupted, patellar tenderness, patellar fracture noted on radiograph
Meniscal tear	Joint line tenderness, mechanical symptoms, magnetic resonance imaging diagnostic
Patellar dislocation	History of kneecap "popping out," medial patellar tenderness, apprehension with lateral patellar translation
Proximal tibial fracture	Proximal tibial pain and tenderness, swelling, radiographs diagnostic
Osgood-Schlatter disease	Chronic knee pain localized over tibial tubercle, intact extensor mechanism

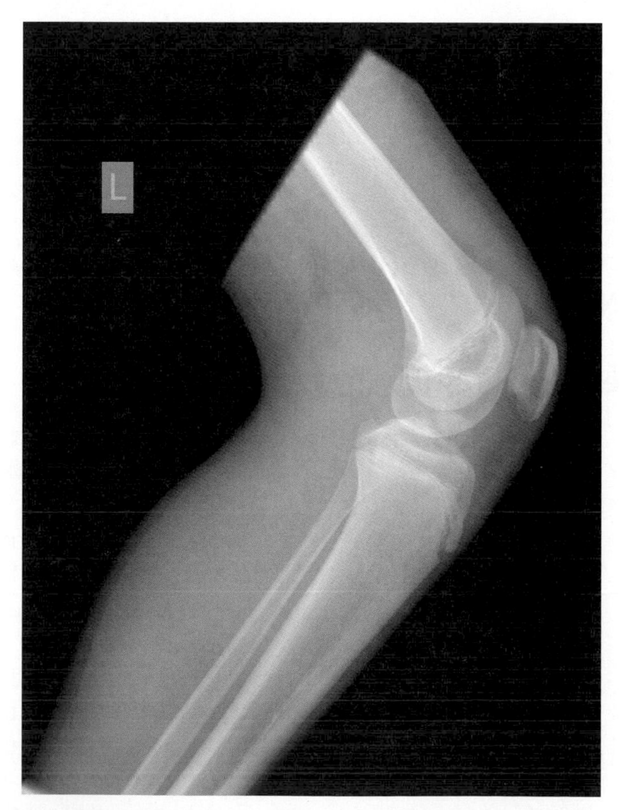

Figure 231-3 Tibial spine fracture requiring reduction, either arthroscopic or open.

Tibial Tubercle Fracture (Fig. 231-4)

- At diagnosis
  - Knee immobilizer
  - Watch for compartment syndrome.
- Later
  - Typically operative fixation needed; bicortical screws usually adequate
  - If extends to the joint, may have associated meniscal or ligamentous injury and needs anatomic reduction of the articular surface

When to Refer

- If the examiner has any concern about management, the patient should be placed in a knee immobilizer and evaluated within 3 to 5 days.

Prognosis

- Bone healing is typically good.
- Despite the fact that this is a physeal injury, clinically significant growth arrest is unusual due to the lack of remaining growth.
- However, in children with 1 year or more of growth remaining, watch for partial physeal arrest.

Troubleshooting

- Use advanced imaging to determine tibial spine displacement after closed reduction.
- In a younger child with tibial tubercle fractures (usual), clinically relevant growth disturbance is possible and results in difficult-to-treat recurvatum deformity.
- Complete physeal closure electively if any growth deformity is noted.

SPECIAL FRACTURES: ANKLE (TRIPLANE AND TILLAUX FRACTURES)

Key Concepts

- Transitional fractures (Tillaux and triplane) occur due to the asymmetrical closure of the distal tibial physis during early adolescence.
- A triplane fracture has a sagittal fracture line through the epiphysis, a transverse fracture line through the physis, and a coronal fracture line through the metaphysis (Fig. 231-5).
- A Tillaux fracture occurs when the anterolateral portion of the distal tibial epiphysis (the last portion of the physis to close) is avulsed anteriorly by a pull from the anterior inferior tibiofibular ligament.
- Both fractures require anatomic reduction of the articular surface.

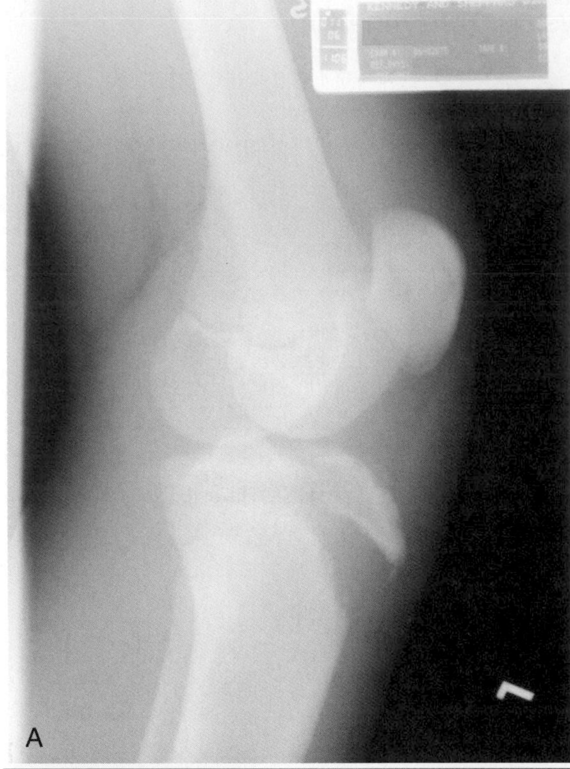

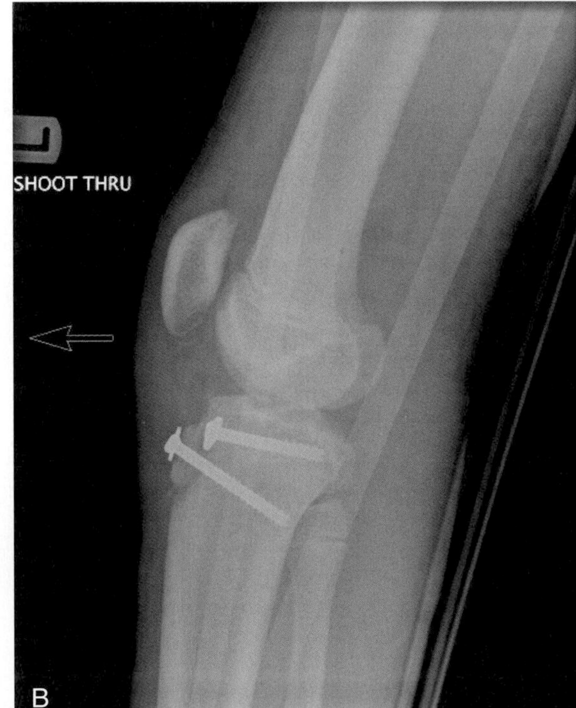

Figure 231-4 **A**, Displaced tibial tubercle fracture. **B**, Tibial tubercle fracture treated with open reduction and internal fixation.

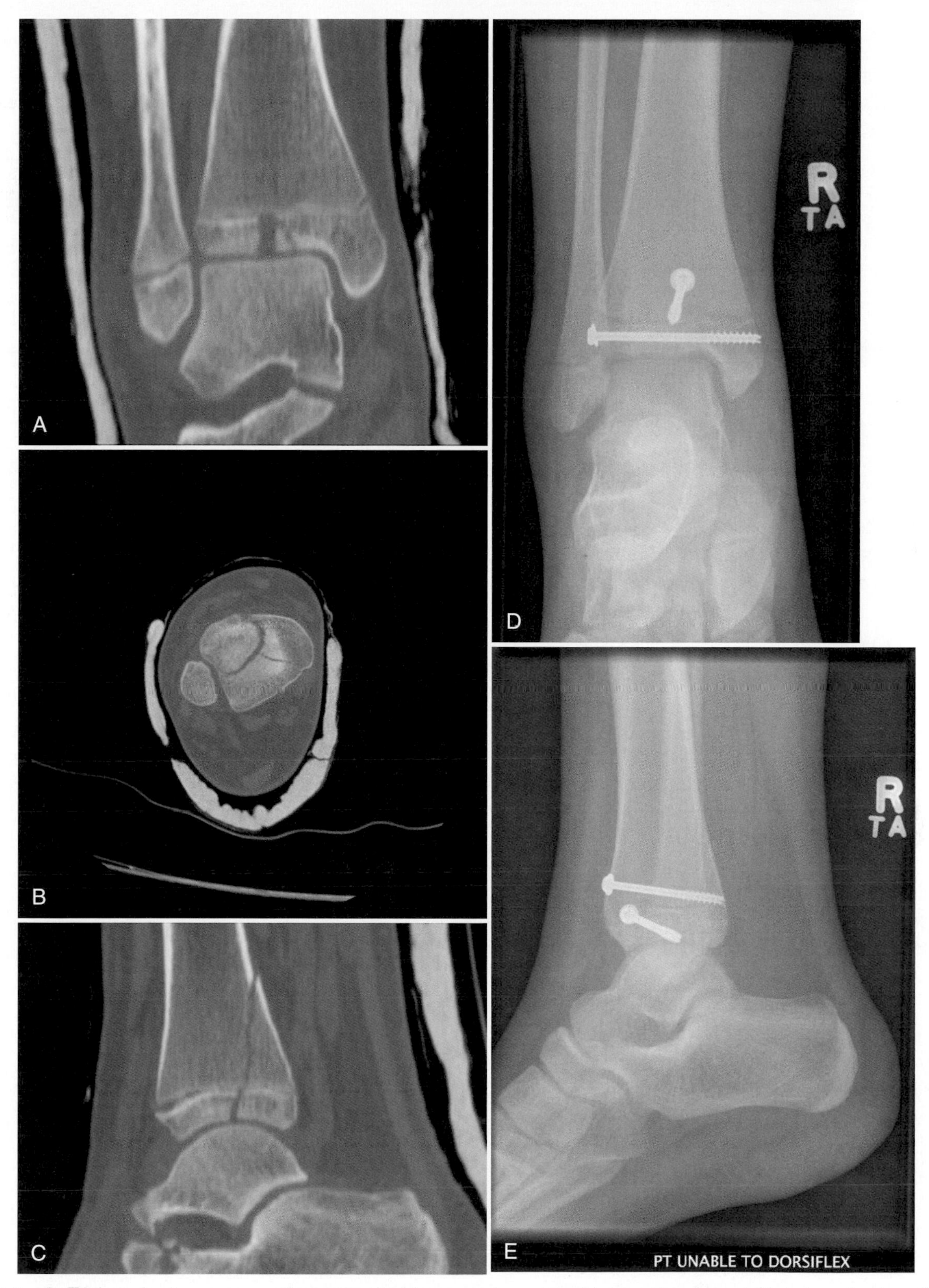

Figure 231-5 **A**, Triplane fracture preoperative computed tomography: coronal image showing sagittal plane fracture through the epiphysis. **B**, Triplane fracture preoperative computed tomography: axial image showing transverse plane fracture through the physis. **C**, Triplane fracture preoperative computed tomography: sagittal image showing coronal plane fracture through the metaphysis. **D**, Triplane fracture treated with open reduction and internal fixation, anteroposterior radiograph. **E**, Triplane fracture treated with open reduction and internal fixation, lateral radiograph.

History

- Acute: age of the patient, basic trauma history including mechanism of injury, areas of pain or deformity, and other associated injuries or previous injuries to extremity

Physical Examination

- Observation: deformity, bruising/swelling, skin condition
- Palpation: tenderness or crepitus at the fracture
- Neurovascular examination

Imaging

- Radiographs: anteroposterior, lateral, and mortise views of the ankle
  - Fibula often fractured with triplane fractures
- Computed tomography critical in determining joint congruence and need for open reduction

Differential Diagnosis

- Please see Table 231-3.

Treatment

Triplane and Tillaux fractures

- At diagnosis
  - Can attempt closed reduction in casting; usual maneuver is anterior translation of the ankle with internal rotation; long leg cast is necessary
  - Perform computed tomography to determine joint congruity.
- Later
  - With more than 2 mm of displacement and any articular step-off, open reduction is necessary; some displacement of the metaphysis is acceptable.
  - Usually need screw fixation from the lateral to medial epiphysis to close down the articular surface in a triplane fracture (see Fig. 231-5D and E)
  - Screw fixation for Tillaux fractures also recommended

When to Refer

- If any question of reduction or decision making

TABLE 231-3 *Differential Diagnosis: Special Injuries of the Ankle*

Differential Diagnosis	Differentiating Features
Ankle sprain	Tenderness isolated on soft tissue, no fracture on radiographs
Medial or lateral malleolar fracture	Tenderness at bone, fracture noted on radiographs
Osteochondritis dissecans lesion of the ankle	Often more chronic history of pain, radiographic abnormality, magnetic resonance imaging diagnostic
Nonarticular fractures of the distal tibia	Deformity and radiographic findings

Prognosis

- Heals well generally
- Increased risk of arthritis but decreased with good anatomic joint reduction
- Growth plate injury not usually a problem because of the fact that fractures occur due to growth plate closure

Troubleshooting

- Articular congruence key to a good long-term result
- Screws in the epiphysis may change the articular cartilage joint mechanics so it is advised to remove the screws after healing.

Suggested Reading

- Finnbogason T, Karlsson G, Lindberg L, Mortensson W: Nondisplaced and minimally displaced fractures of the lateral humeral condyle in children: A prospective radiographic investigation of fracture stability. J Pediatr Orthop 1995;15:422–425.
- Mosier SM, Stanitski CL: Acute tibial tubercle avulsion fractures. J Pediatr Orthop 2004;24:181–184.
- Rapariz JM, Ocete G, González-Herranz P, et al: Distal tibial triplane fractures: Long-term follow-up. J Pediatr Orthop 1996;16:113–118.
- Skaggs DL: Elbow fractures in children: Diagnosis and management. J Am Acad Orthop Surg 1997;5:303–312.
- Skaggs DL, Hale JM, Bassett J, et al: Operative treatment of supracondylar fractures of the humerus in children: The consequences of pin placement. J Bone Joint Surg Am 2001;83A:735–740.
- Wiley JJ, Baxter MP: Tibial spine fractures in children. Clin Orthop Relat Res 1990;255:54–60.

Index

Note: Page numbers followed by f indicate figures; those followed by t indicate tables; and those followed by b indicate boxed material.

B

D

E

F

G

Q

R

T